MW01077199

TEMPESTS, POXES, PREDATORS, AND PEOPLE

OXFORD SERIES IN BEHAVIORAL NEUROENDOCRINOLOGY

Series Editors

Gregory F. Ball, Jacques Balthazart, and Randy J. Nelson

Hormones and Brain Plasticity
Luis Miguel Garcia-Segura

Biology of Homosexuality
Jacques Balthazart

Brain Aromatase, Estrogens, and Behavior
Edited by Jacques Balthazart and Gregory F. Ball

Losing Our Minds: How Environmental Pollution Impairs Human Intelligence and Mental Health
Barbara Demeneix

Tempests, Poxes, Predators, and People: Stress in Wild Animals and How They Cope
L. Michael Romero and John C. Wingfield

TEMPESTS, POXES, PREDATORS, AND PEOPLE

Stress in Wild Animals and How They Cope

L. MICHAEL ROMERO

JOHN C. WINGFIELD

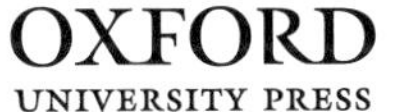

OXFORD
UNIVERSITY PRESS

Oxford University Press is a department of the University of Oxford. It furthers the University's objective of excellence in research, scholarship, and education by publishing worldwide.

Oxford New York
Auckland Cape Town Dar es Salaam Hong Kong Karachi
Kuala Lumpur Madrid Melbourne Mexico City Nairobi
New Delhi Shanghai Taipei Toronto

With offices in
Argentina Austria Brazil Chile Czech Republic France Greece
Guatemala Hungary Italy Japan Poland Portugal Singapore
South Korea Switzerland Thailand Turkey Ukraine Vietnam

Oxford is a registered trademark of Oxford University Press in the UK and certain other countries.

Published in the United States of America by
Oxford University Press
198 Madison Avenue, New York, NY 10016

Library of Congress Cataloging-in-Publication Data

Romero, L. Michael.
Tempests, predators, poxes, and people : stress in wild animals and how they cope / L. Michael Romero and John C. Wingfield.
pages cm.—(Oxford series in behavioral neuroendocrinology)
Includes bibliographical references and index.
ISBN 978-0-19-536669-3
1. Stress (Physiology) 2. Veterinary physiology. 3. Animal welfare.
4. Animals—Effect of human beings on. I. Wingfield, John C., 1948- II. Title.
QP82.2.S8R66 2015
591.5′3—dc23
2014030406

1 3 5 7 9 8 6 4 2
Printed in the United States of America
on acid-free paper

CONTENTS

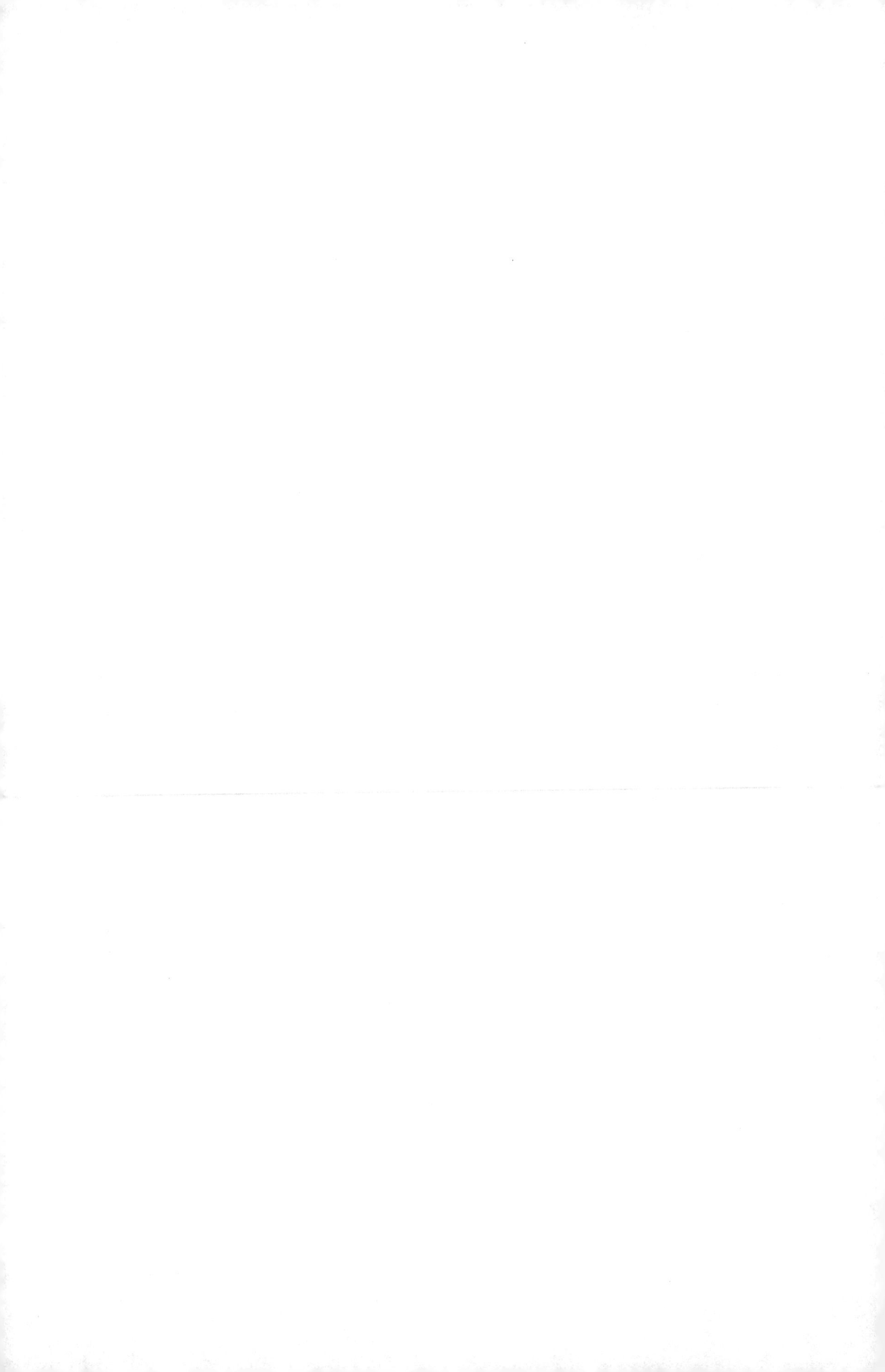

ACKNOWLEDGMENTS

As with any large work, this book is a culmination of the efforts of many people, all of whom we should thank. First and foremost are our families, who sacrificed considerably to allow us time to think and to write. Gauri Bhide and Marilyn Ramenofsky have been incredibly patient throughout the process, and our children, Vikas and Vishal Romero and Emma and Anna Wingfield, have been very supportive. This book is as much for them as it is for us.

This book also owes a huge debt to all our collaborators throughout the years. We have both been incredibly fortunate to have had so many amazing people work with us. To name them all here would court the unforgivable sin of omitting someone. Consequently, we will simply issue a blanket and heartfelt "thank you" to all of you. We feel privileged to share with the readers the work of talented undergraduates, graduate students, postdoctoral fellows, and senior colleagues. The quality of the science is a testament to their skills, but if there are any misrepresentations of their work, that is entirely our fault.

We need to provide a special thanks to Randy Nelson, Jacques Balthazart, and Greg Ball, the senior editors of this series. They originally approached us about writing this book, and then showed the infinite patience to overlook an almost 6-year extension of the original deadline for providing a complete manuscript. Randy, Jacques, and Greg then passed our manuscript into the capable hands of the staff at Oxford University Press. Their expert guidance, and especially the help of Louis Gulino, successfully midwifed the final product.

Finally, none of our work would have been possible without generous financial support over the years. Grants from the US National Institutes of Health, US Department of Defense, US Environmental Protection Agency, and The Guggenheim Foundation have all contributed to our studies. However, the generous support from the US National Science Foundation (NSF) provided the bedrock funding for both of us. Without NSF support, this book would be significantly shorter and more limited in scope.

L. Michael Romero
John C. Wingfield

PART I

Biology of Stress

1

Environment and the Earth

A Stressful Planet

In Nature there are unexpected storms and in life unpredicted vicissitudes.

WU CHENG-EN, *"Journey to the West" (circa sixteenth-century China)*

I. INTRODUCTION: WHAT IS STRESS?

We live on a small but changeable planet whose environment is always challenging us. Every day we hear about natural and human-made disasters somewhere on earth, and the media references stress constantly. But what is stress? Say this word and everyone knows what you mean. Stress has become an extraordinarily important concept to our society today. A recent search on Google on the word "stress" brought up over 600 million hits. Compare this to Google searches on diabetes (305 million hits), heart disease (279 million hits), obesity (99 million hits), alcohol (512 million hits), depression (271 million hits), aging (205 million hits), and mental health (275 million hits). Only cancer (621 million hits) brought up more hits. One conclusion to draw from this is that we, as a society, are more concerned with stress than with getting old or getting too fat—not bad for a concept that was introduced only about 100 years ago by Walter Cannon (reviewed by Cannon 1932) and popularized by Hans Selye in the 1940s (Selye 1946).

Say the word "stress" and everyone knows what you mean. Actually, that is not true. "Stress" may get over 600 million hits on Google, but "stress" is a very slippery word to define. Stress is a bit like pornography in that it fits the famous description by a jurist of the United States, Potter Stewart: "I shall not today attempt further to define [pornography] . . . but I know it when I see it." Say the word "stress" and everyone brings his or her own experience and preconceptions to bear on what you mean. What is stressful for one person, extreme sports for example, might be a pleasant diversion for another. Perhaps this is the reason for the great success of the term—"stress" can mean virtually whatever you want it to mean, constrained only by a vague shared consensus.

The consensus usually involves some psychosocial pressure (feeling) to do something you don't desire to do. Typical things that most people will cite as causing stress include interacting with coworkers or family, public speaking, school exams, and so on. When we tell laypeople that we study stress, the typical response is: "You should study me!" In fact, neither of us has ever encountered someone who did not think that they were under stress. But what exactly do they want us to study? The strength of the psychosocial pressure, that is, feelings that they have? The depth of their antipathy to do something? Both of us have done extensive fieldwork in the Arctic and especially near the Inupiaq Eskimos at Barrow, Alaska. We are told that the Inupiaq word for scientist, when translated literally, means "one who measures things." Although we don't know if there is, in fact, such a word (it is not in the Inupiaq online dictionary), the essence is correct. If we cannot measure it, we cannot use science to study it.

So, how do you measure feeling or desire? Quantifying these emotions usually has been in the realm of the poet, not the scientist, and perhaps only free-market economics has found a way to measure someone's desire. Science, especially those branches that study animals, has failed miserably at this task. In fact, every few years there is a movement to jettison the word "stress" from the entire scientific enterprise. Inevitably these movements fail, primarily because the concept of stress is so useful and the proposed substitute suffers from the syndrome of "... that which we call a rose / By any other name would smell as sweet" (*Romeo and Juliet*, Act II, Scene 2). After a while, most researchers simply return to using the word "stress" (Levine and Ursin 1991).

Human perspectives of stress notwithstanding, if we take a look at how other organisms deal with perturbations of the environment, all of which have the potential for stress, there are many things we can measure. Although all of us experience a changing environment every day of our lives, some changes are expected, such as dawn and dusk, with related activity; others are not expected, such as infection, a car accident, or loss of a loved one. We respond to these changes in the best way possible and adjust our lives accordingly. These basic concepts of coping apply to all free-living organisms because none lives in a truly constant environment. Fluctuations in environmental conditions can sometimes be extreme. For example, in arctic habitats, temperature, food availability, and snow cover vary dramatically in a yearly seasonal cycle, and in the tropics dry and rainy periods occur at specific times of year. However, the amount and duration of snow, cold temperatures, rain, or drought vary dramatically from year to year. Even in localities that are frequently regarded as unchanging, if data are collected over long periods then perturbations do occur. For example, in caves yearly temperature fluctuations may only be on the order of 2°C—pretty constant. Nonetheless, seasonal flooding, which provides essential nutrient input from non-cave sources, occurs in varying intensity and sometimes can be so enormous that some cave-dwelling organisms are expelled from their recluse and all probably die (Poulson 1964). The deep oceanic abyss has been regarded as being a dark, cold, and relatively constant environment, but even here "benthic storms" caused by surface winds such as hurricanes and typhoons can change currents, even at great depths, for weeks at a time (Gage and Tyler 1991). How organisms that live in benthic regions of oceans respond to these perturbations is entirely unknown.

Superimposed on these weather and climate events (tempests) are other environmental changes such as disease (poxes), changes in predator numbers, and in recent times exploding human populations that change ecosystems dramatically, introducing toxic chemicals and generally disturbing other organisms. Human disturbances include, unfortunately, some of our favorite recreational activities. Every organism, including ourselves, is exposed to a barrage of environmental changes every day. Some are benign, some are dangerous, but many can be tolerated if exposure is of short duration or infrequent. However, all environmental changes can become detrimental if the duration and frequency of these events increase. Just about every environmental change we can think of has been called "stressful" at some point, and indeed the "stress of life" is a global concept shared by many.

In this book we explore this nebulous concept that has captured our constant attention, try to dissect it apart, and examine underlying concepts of coping with the environment in general. It is important to remember that the physiological responses to stress are often vital for successful coping and thus serve a useful purpose. It is only when those systems are activated for too long that problems arise, as we shall explore in future chapters. Natural systems offer vast examples of organism-environment interactions that we can investigate and measure, looking for underlying and unifying concepts. All these natural systems are vulnerable to climate and other types of global change because environmental conditions may exceed the organism's capacity to respond (reaction norm). Others with greater flexibility may thrive (IPCC 2001). Although the debate on global climate change rages back and forth, one clear concept that is emerging is that shifts in expected weather and increases in unpredictable weather, such as the frequency, duration, and intensity of floods, droughts, and severe storms, are occurring. Combine this with human disturbance, pollution, habitat degradation, and invasive species, and we see a much greater phenomenon—global change (Travis 2003). Significant and irreversible damage may result. Clearly research on "stress" has reached a new level of urgency. Biomedical and agricultural studies have been ongoing for many decades and are critical for our welfare, but environmental stress exaggerated by human impacts has the potential for catastrophic loss of biodiversity, introduction of invasive species, and emerging diseases that has only recently been a focus of research. Determining the mechanisms by which organisms cope with a capricious world will be critical for understanding why some organisms thrive in the face of change and others do not. Ultimately we will also understand our own abilities to cope with this same world.

II. PALEONTOLOGY DATA: THE HISTORY OF ENVIRONMENTAL CHANGE ON EARTH

Daily to seasonal cycles, tempests, poxes, and predators on Earth are not recent phenomena. Evidence gleaned from geological strata and fossils indicates that seasonality is ancient and that unpredictable events, perturbations of environment, were common. Furthermore, evidence from deep time (i.e., Precambrian, more than a billion years ago) to the present suggests that climates can change quickly (Soreghan 2004). Evidence from the early Cambrian indicates minor local and short-lived perturbations in sediment movements of organisms, which enhanced fossilization, but also probably affected the life cycles of local living organisms (Babcock et al. 2001).

At the Eocene-Oligocene boundary (33 million years ago), there is evidence for marked changes in seasonality. Summer temperatures remained the same but winters became colder, resulting in ice age effects (Ivany et al. 2000). In another example, two mass extinction events occurred at the end of the Permian (250 million years ago) eliminating 70%–80% of marine invertebrate species, possibly due to global cooling and other causes (Fraiser and Bottjer 2004). A number of glaciations accompanying cold periods, intermingled with warmer periods, occurred at this time (DiMichele et al. 2001). Although these shifts were short in terms of geological time, they occurred over hundreds of thousands or even millions of years, probably allowing the evolution of coping mechanisms in those species that survived. Climate change at present is occurring on a scale of decades, and the question of whether organisms will be able to adapt to new environmental challenges remains to be answered.

Fossil specimens and other material from South African formations showed a plant and animal community living in a climate with cool winters but without significant frost and seasonal precipitation (Glasspool 2003; Soreghan 2004). Summer vegetation was coniferous as well as broad-leaved deciduous. This suggested considerable seasonality, leading to winter scarcity of food, at least for herbivores, so much so that many of the larger dinosaurs may have migrated (Tokaryk and Bryant 2004). The paleo-environment of the Maastrichian period (65.5–65 million years ago) in southwestern Saskatchewan was meso-thermal (mild), with no frost but a seasonal drought. The deciduous nature of the vegetation at this time was probably related to short days of winter at this high latitude. This contrasts strongly with vegetation a few degrees farther south. These data again raise questions about how dinosaurs coped with this seasonality (McIver 2002; see Figure 1.1), how and when they migrated, and to what extent facultative movements may also have occurred (Paul 1997).

In other areas, studies of isotope changes in bivalve shells from the late Cretaceous (90 million years ago) of Greece, Turkey, Somalia, and the Arabian Peninsula indicate distinct cyclic variations in temperature and salinity, consistent with seasonality (Steuber 1999). Other evidence for seasonality, especially flooding in a wetland in the lower Cretaceous, provided evidence for seasonal fires as well as floods. Variation from

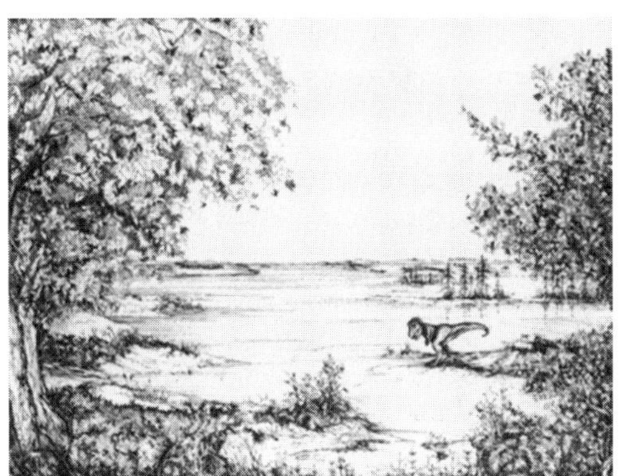

FIGURE 1.1: Artistic reconstruction of a river system that might have included *Tyrannosaurus rex* (from southwestern Saskatchewan, drawn by A. Tait). Plant taxa include *Vitis stantonii* (large tree on left); cycads, horsetails, cattails, *Trochodendron flabella* seedlings (center and small tree, lower right), ferns, *Parataxodium*, *Ginkgo* (tree on right). Such environments were highly seasonal, with the degree of seasonality varying from year to year, punctuated by further perturbations such as floods, fires, and so on. The animals living in these habitats were susceptible to diseases and parasites that may have had a profound effect on how they responded to seasons and other perturbations (Poiner and Poiner 2008).

From McIver (2002) with permission.

year to year suggests that the degree of flooding is variable on top of seasonality (Wright et al. 2000). Growing evidence indicates that there were many sources of unpredictable perturbations over hundreds of millions of years of life on earth. Evidence from the distribution of gastropod fauna in the early Triassic (245 million years ago) suggests long-term severe environmental perturbations, including storms that may have had a major impact on organisms (Fraiser and Bottjer 2004). Profiles of Mg/Ca across bivalve shells in a Jurassic (200 million years ago) deposit of northern Scotland reveal inundations of a brackish-water lagoon with cooler seawater, leading to a temporary increase in metabolic activity in the bivalves (Hendry et al. 2001). Fossil charcoal deposits in the Late Cretaceous (90–94 million years ago) indicate that all the plant communities were fire prone. The environment was warm and humid with a short dry season, when fires occurred (Falcon-Lang et al. 2001). Early Permian coal seams in South Africa show evidence for distinct seasonality, including cool seasons with drying. However, this led to widespread fires of varying intensity (Glasspool 2003). Some ancient organisms such as Silurian brachiopods may have been opportunists, taking advantage of rapid sediment accumulation created after intermittent storms in a "high-stress" environment (Harper and Doyle 2003).

Evidence from inoceramid bivalves in the late Mesozoic indicates that evolution of predators may have led to the extinction of many groups, especially locally. Changes in predator numbers therefore could have had significant effects on coping styles in these animals. There is also evidence for the spread of disease with similar effects (Ozanne and Harries 2002). Poinar and Poinar (2008) present convincing evidence that dinosaurs were continually attacked by insects and other parasites, probably resulting in open sores from infected bites. This in turn could have led to other infections and illnesses, making dinosaurs more vulnerable to additional perturbations of the environment (Poiner and Poiner 2008), much as we see in many vertebrate species today.

The evidence for environmental change, seasonality, and perturbations of many kinds, going back to the beginnings of life on earth, is vast and only a few examples are given here. An important take-home message is that there has been over a billion years of selection for coping mechanisms by which organisms of all kinds respond to a changing planet.

III. THE NATURAL HISTORY OF STRESS

From this point, we focus on vertebrates, but with the full realization that invertebrates, plants, and other organisms also must cope. Although many cellular mechanisms, such as responses of heat-shock proteins, DNA repair, and amelioration of oxidative damage, probably have common themes throughout the spectrum of life, hormonal signals, our emphasis here, appear to be less well conserved except, perhaps, within the vertebrates.

A. Predictable versus Unpredictable Environmental Changes

All vertebrates must adjust to changing environmental conditions at some point in their life cycle. All of the bewildering host of changes that can occur can, however, be classified into two major types that have implications for control mechanisms (Figure 1.2). Most organisms live in fluctuating environments in which conditions change in a *predictable* manner, such as daily/circadian cycles (night, day, high tide, low tide) or seasons (spring, summer, autumn, winter, wet and dry seasons). Organisms also must cope with *unpredictable* events in their environment, such as bad weather, social stress, predators, infection and, in recent years, pollution, human disturbance, and so on (Figure 1.2). Humans have been aware of this division through much of our history, as described by Wu Cheng-En in his epic "Journey to the West" (circa sixteenth-century China): "In Nature there are unexpected storms and in life unpredicted vicissitudes." It is only very recently that we have realized that such a division of environmental changes also indicates fundamentally different control mechanisms.

Thus an individual must respond to environmental change in two fundamentally different ways. Typically, vertebrates show changes in morphology, physiology, and behavior in *anticipation* of the predictable changes so that they can respond appropriately to the changing seasons and so on (Figure 1.2). An example is the development of the reproductive system before the breeding season so that individuals are able to begin reproducing as soon as environmental conditions are favorable. On the other hand, when responding to unpredictable changes in the environment, the facultative physiological and behavioral changes that occur take place *during* or *after* a perturbation (Figure 1.2). In some cases it is possible that an individual could predict the onset

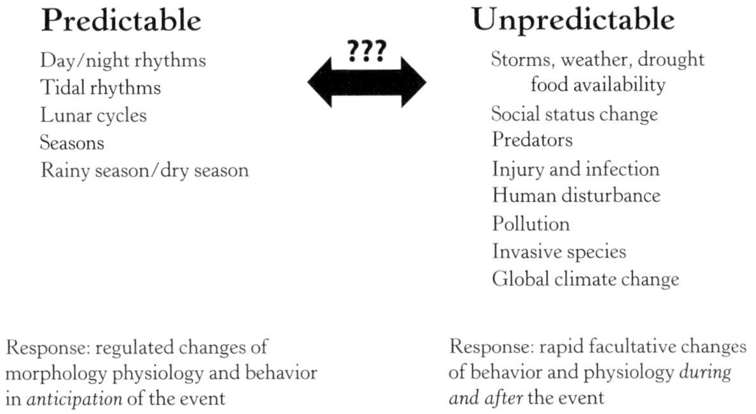

Predictable

Day/night rhythms
Tidal rhythms
Lunar cycles
Seasons
Rainy season/dry season

Unpredictable

Storms, weather, drought food availability
Social status change
Predators
Injury and infection
Human disturbance
Pollution
Invasive species
Global climate change

Response: regulated changes of morphology physiology and behavior in *anticipation* of the event

Response: rapid facultative changes of behavior and physiology *during and after* the event

FIGURE 1.2: Responses of organisms to environmental change can be divided into two major components. Predictable changes as part of daily or annual routines (e.g., circadian rhythms, seasonal changes), and unpredictable events that may lead to stress. Neuroendocrinological implications are that responses in physiology, morphology, and behavior occur in anticipation of predicable events, and thus environmental signals must contain information about those future events. In contrast, responses to unpredictable events require rapid physiological and behavioral changes that occur during and after perception of the change. These two types of environmental change indicate fundamentally different neuroendocrine and endocrine pathways from perception, transduction, and response. There is growing evidence for interactions of predictable and unpredictable environmental changes (e.g., global climate change), but how this may affect neuroendocrine control systems remains obscure (Wingfield 2005a; Wingfield and Sapolsky 2003).

From Wingfield (2006), courtesy of Elsevier Press.

of a perturbation (such as an approaching storm), but this would be a brief period of minutes, or at most a few hours. Anticipatory changes before predictable changes in the environment are initiated days or weeks ahead. This concept of two major types of response to environmental change—anticipatory and facultative—is probably applicable to many organisms, including plants, invertebrates, and vertebrates. All animals use these environmental changes to signal morphological, physiological, and behavioral adjustments that make up an appropriate response. An important series of events must occur that will be central to understanding mechanisms. First, the individual must perceive the environmental change through some sensory modality, or cells may be able to respond directly (e.g., de Wilde 1978; Wingfield 2006). The information is then transduced by the brain or within a cell and the response is mediated directly, either neurally or through neuroendocrine and endocrine mechanisms. This chain of events, perception-transduction-response, pertains to all responses to environmental change and in all organisms. In vertebrates, this will involve sensory ecology and the central processing of information.

B. Types of Perturbations

First, it is important to put the multitude of environmental changes, predictable and unpredictable, into further context. These environmental signals, predictable and unpredictable, can be further classified according to their actions on the life cycles of individuals (Figure 1.3). Predictive cues come in two groups: initial predictive and local predictive information. Initial predictive information provides long-term information about future events and their timing. A classic example is the response to the annual cycle of photoperiod (day length) that initiates reproductive development so that the gonads are fully mature when it is time for breeding to begin (Figure 1.3). Photoperiod has been shown to regulate many aspects of the life cycle including molt, migration, growth, and so on. Then there are many examples of local predictive cues that speed up (accelerators) or slow down (inhibitors) the development of life-history stages according to local conditions that vary from year to year (Figure 1.3). Local environmental temperature can speed up or slow down photoperiodically induced gonadal growth in many species. Other local predictive cues include the availability of food, the presence of predators, and rainfall.

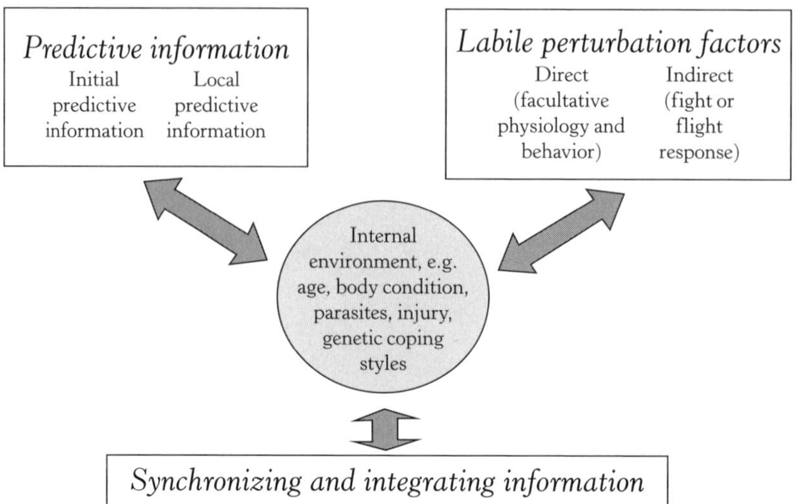

FIGURE 1.3: There are three major types of environmental factors that can regulate changes in the morphology, physiology, and behavior of organisms. Predictive information allows individuals to anticipate changes in the environment (such as seasons) so that an appropriate life-history stage (such as breeding, molting, migrating, etc.) can be developed and expressed at the appropriate time. There are two subtypes of predictive information—initial predictive (long-term) and local predictive (short-term) cues. Labile perturbation factors are the result of unpredictable events in the environment that trigger the emergency life-history stage that allows an individual to cope with the potential stress of the perturbation. There are also two subtypes of this class of environmental information. The first are direct perturbation factors (such as storms) that trigger facultative physiology and behavior. The second are indirect perturbation factors (such as attacks by predators) that trigger rapid coping mechanisms such as the "fight-or-flight" response. The third major type of environmental factor includes all the social interactions among individuals that synchronize and integrate many aspects of the predictable life cycle *and* responses to perturbation factors. All three types of environmental information can thus influence how an organism responds accordingly, through responses of the internal environment (central circle) and subsequent behavior.

Modified after Wingfield (2006), courtesy of Elsevier Press.

The social environment is also critical for many species, and even solitary animals must interact with others to reproduce. Social interactions over mates, territories, and access to food and other resources have been termed "synchronizing and integrating factors" and can influence the responses of an individual to predictive cues and to unpredictable cues (Figure 1.3; see also Wingfield 2006). Social "stress" is widespread in humans and animals, and as yet it has not been classified satisfactorily as part of synchronizing and integrating information, or as potential perturbation factors, described next. This topic will be the subject of considerable discussion later in this volume.

The third major group of environmental factors encompasses the unpredictable events known as labile perturbation factors (Figure 1.3). They are called "labile" because they will pass but on different time scales (Jacobs 1996). Some are brief and are over in minutes to hours, whereas others may persist for days or even months. Such time scales can determine how an individual responds. Indirect labile perturbation factors include brief but disruptive events that do not affect the individual directly in terms of condition, infection, or ability to defend resources; however, these factors do require the individual to make rapid and major behavioral and physiological adjustments, such as a fight-or-flight response to survive the perturbation (Figure 1.3). Examples are the loss of a mate or offspring to a predator, sudden but brief severe storms such as a tornado, or temporary withdrawal of food by freezing rain (Figure 1.4). Large groups of animals can temporarily displace smaller ones, resulting in a brief perturbation. Within a few minutes or hours, the individual can then return to the routines of that life-history stage and resume the life cycle.

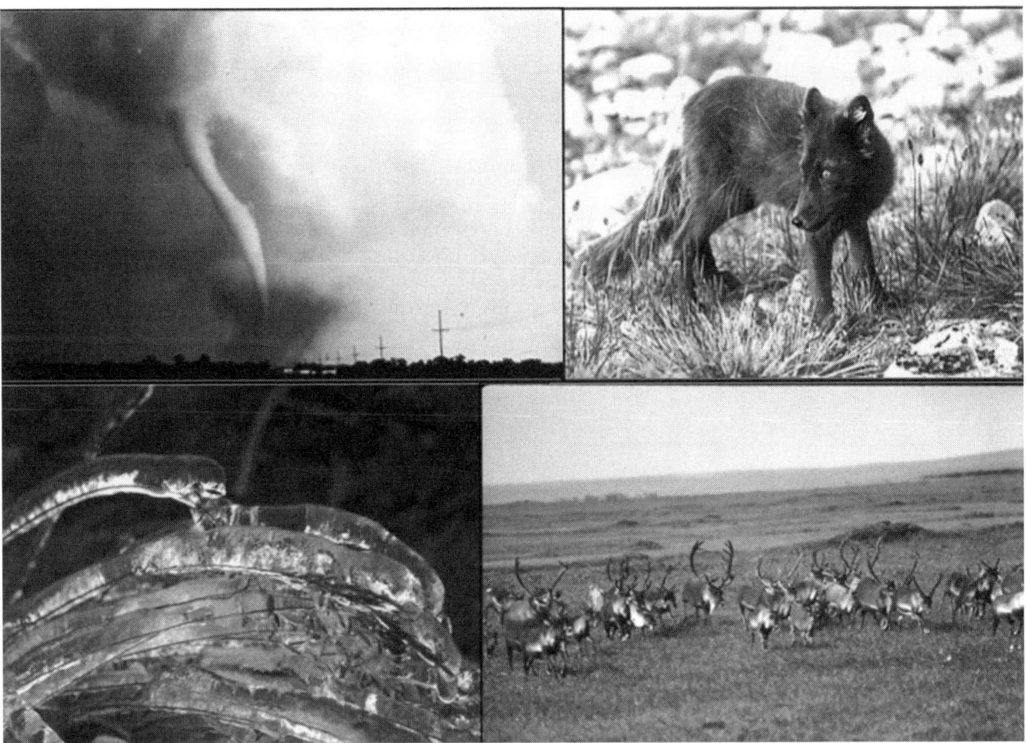

FIGURE 1.4: Examples of indirect perturbation factors that temporarily disrupt the life cycle, but may demand strong behavioral and physiological responses. Brief but severe storms such as tornadoes (top left) temporarily force animals to shelter or leave the immediate area. But within minutes the storm is over and the individual can return to the daily routines of its life-history stage. A predator (e.g., Arctic fox, top right) can take offspring or a mate, or an individual may have to undergo energetically demanding escape maneuvers, following which it will return to daily routines. Freezing rain (bottom left) can cover food resources, triggering local movements. But this kind of event rarely persists more than a few hours. Bottom right shows a migrating heard of caribou on the North Slope of Alaska. Herds of large animals may force small resident animals to temporarily move aside while the herd moves by. Again, the individual can then return to daily routines within a few minutes to hours. Indirect perturbation factors are short-lived (minutes to hours) and do not result in major changes in body condition, resource-holding ability, or social status.

Photo credits: top left courtesy of NOAA. All other photos by J. C. Wingfield.

Direct labile perturbation factors (Figure 1.3) tend to be longer term—many hours, days, or even weeks—resulting in loss of condition, for example body weight, as the individual attempts to maintain daily routines. If the perturbation persists, then the individual is eventually forced to abandon its current life-history stage and initiate changes in behavior and physiology that allow it to survive the perturbation in the best condition possible. After the perturbation passes, there may be a recovery period before the individual can return to the normal life-history stage and daily routines. Examples of direct labile perturbation factors include persistent storms such as rain, resulting in floods or high winds that change habitat (Figure 1.5). In these cases, nesting songbirds were forced off their territories for several days and had to survive in the best condition possible before the storm passed and they could return to resume normal daily routines (e.g., Wingfield 1984). In some cases, direct perturbation factors may persist for months, for example El Niño Southern Oscillation events.

Finally, another important subdivision of the unpredictable environmental changes is a group of unpredictable events that are permanent. These are particularly severe because permanent and deleterious changes in the environment mean

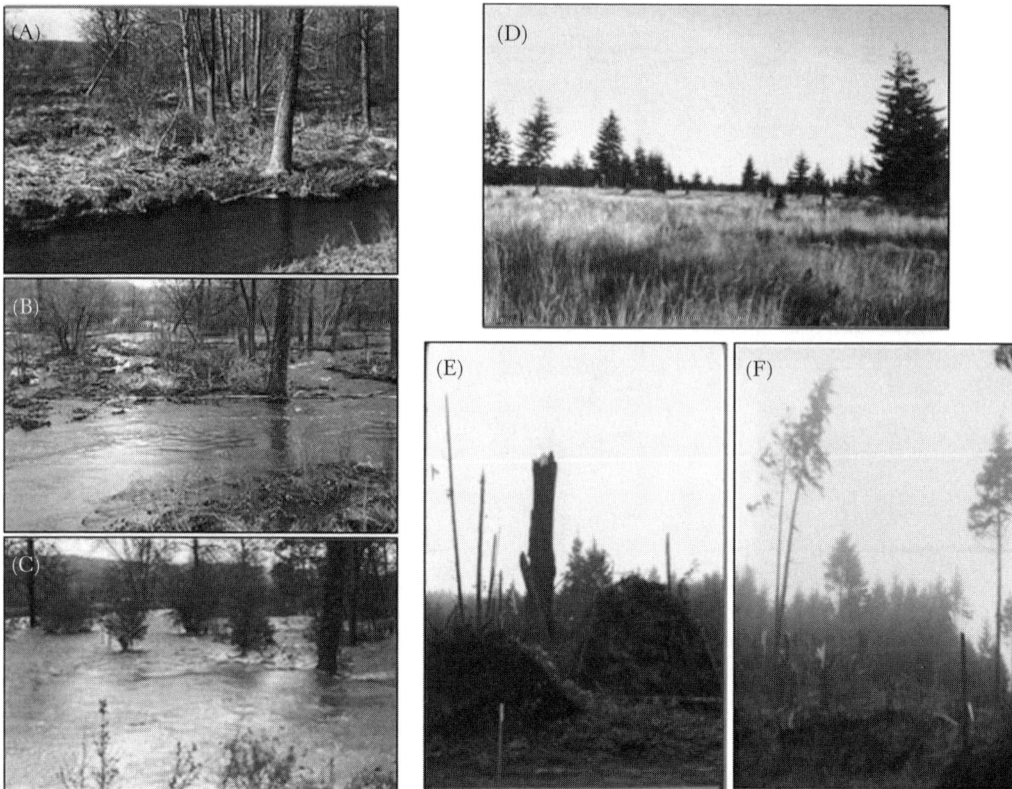

FIGURE 1.5: Examples of direct labile perturbation factors. Left panels show Ham Creek, a tributary of the Hudson River in the mid-Hudson Valley of New York State. (A) Normal flow. (B) In May 1982 a 3-day rain storm resulted in flooding. Many organisms (especially vertebrates) were forced to abandon territories and move to higher ground. After the flood receded, these organisms returned. (C) In June 1982, more than 5 days of heavy rain resulted in an even greater flood. Once again, organisms were forced to move to higher ground. The right set of panels shows the effects of a major wind storm in May 1980 on Camano Island and western Washington State. (D) A typical forest clearing in a non-storm year. (E and F) Effects of the severe wind storm with large trees uprooted. During this storm many organisms abandoned breeding until conditions improved. For hormonal responses of birds to these storms see Wingfield (1985a, 1985b) and Wingfield et al. (1983).

From Wingfield (2005b). Photographs by J. C. Wingfield

that organisms probably must leave and find alternate habitat, or the density of that species in the affected habitat must decrease. Some individuals may find alternate habitat, others may not and probably die. If the entire habitat is lost, then all of the population may die out, or selection may favor a few individuals that can survive in a different habitat and found a new population. Examples of permanent perturbation factors include many anthropogenic activities such as urbanization, in which natural habitat is lost forever, and the exploitation of resources, such as clear cuts of forest that may never recover fully, or may regenerate as different species of trees (Figure 1.6). Some permanent perturbation factors such as fire occur naturally (Figure 1.6), but it may take many years for the habitat to regenerate (although populations may be able to move to a similar habitat nearby). Moreover, in recent years global climate change has resulted in greater frequency and intensity of fires; many are started by humans and quickly get out of control, resulting in habitat devastation over huge areas. Populations of animals forced to leave such areas also interact with resident populations, providing further competition, social stress, and so on. Thus, a perturbation in one area can have a domino effect, resulting in further perturbation of populations in areas not

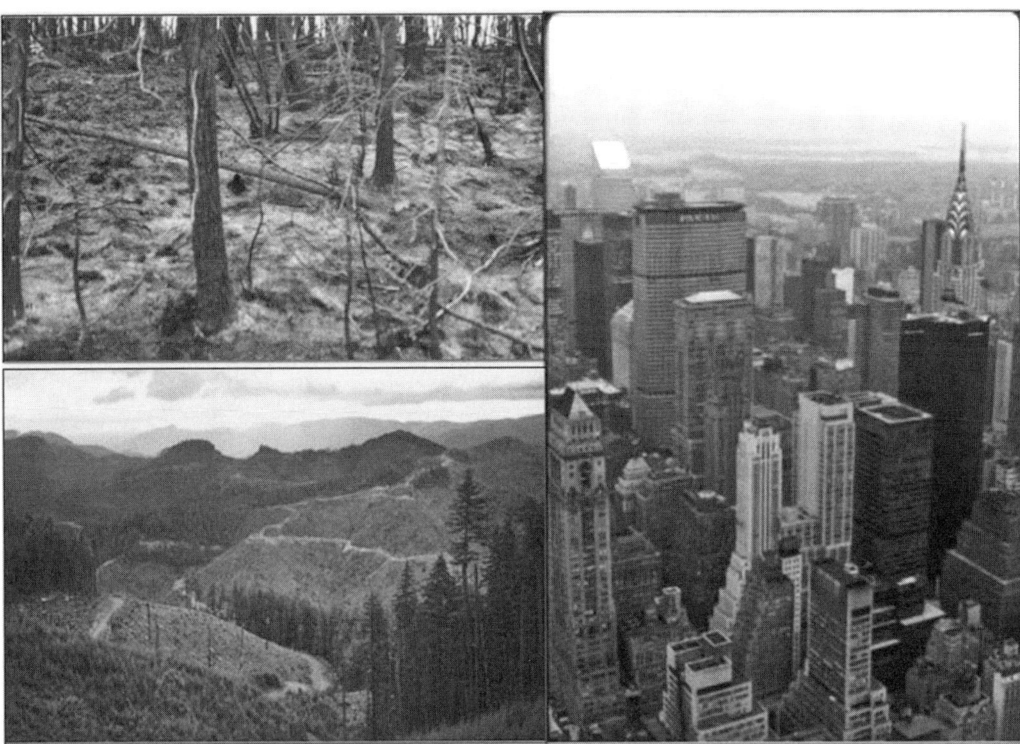

FIGURE 1.6: Examples of permanent perturbations factors. Fires, such as this one in the boreal forest of central Alaska (top left) are natural perturbation factors that have changed habitats for hundreds of millions of years. Some habitats are dependent upon fires to maintain the ecosystem. However, owing to anthropogenic activities, fires are occurring more frequently and in greater intensity, modifying habitats permanently. Urbanization (right-hand panel) changes natural habitat forever, and almost all of the former inhabitants have disappeared. Other human activities, including exploitation of natural resources such as clear-cutting forests, can also permanently alter the habitat. Clear cuts in Western Washington State (lower left panel) are vulnerable to rain erosion, altering soils so that the forest that regenerates may not be the same or is degraded. Permanent perturbation factors such as these may be tolerable if they are not too frequent and allow habitats to persist elsewhere (a form of sustainability) and to coexist with human activities. However, all too often these perturbations become far too widespread for sustainability. Again, coping mechanisms of animals in these areas are critical.

All photos by J. C. Wingfield.

affected by the original event. As global change continues, perturbation factors will occur at greater frequency and intensity. Coping mechanisms will be critical.

Although there has been selection for coping mechanisms for perturbation factors probably for a billion years, most of the time life has been on Earth, some perturbations are so strong that massive mortality results (Gessaman and Worthen 1982, Figure 1.6). Huge numbers of seabirds die of starvation and wash up on beaches (Figure 1.7) during El Niño Southern Oscillation (ENSO) events that decrease food supply. Vast numbers of fish recently died following a hypoxia event in southern Louisiana, not to mention large populations of mammals, birds, marine reptiles, fish, and many marine organisms that died following the Gulf of Mexico oil spill in 2010. Mass mortality does happen, certainly, but rarely are whole populations eliminated. In those that do survive, there has undoubtedly been selection for coping mechanisms, probably with common themes across vertebrates. These coping mechanisms form the positive aspects of stress.

C. Life-History Stages

Transitions in morphology, physiology, and behavior in relation to predictable changes in the

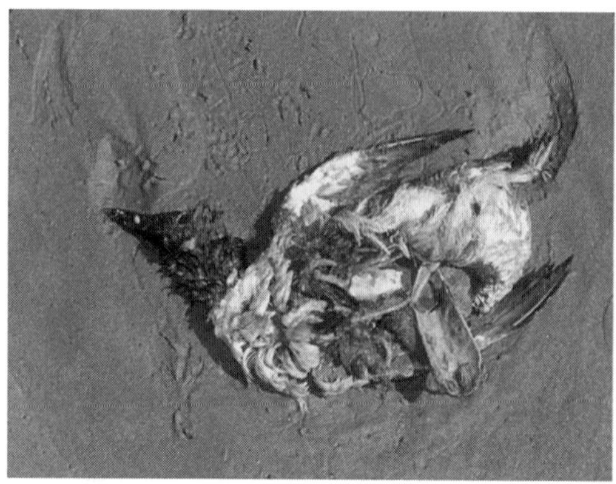

FIGURE 1.7: The carcass of a common murre lies on a beach on the Pacific coast of Oregon in March 1998. This species is particularly vulnerable to direct labile perturbation factors such as El Niño Southern Oscillation events that change the distribution of food (e.g., fish populations). As a result, these seabirds fail to breed and may even starve to death. Massive mortality does occur in response to perturbations, and this likely contributes to loss of biodiversity. In other species, in which a few survive to found new populations, there will be selection for coping mechanisms.

Photo by J. C. Wingfield.

Ontogenetic life-history stages	**Adult life-history stages**
Growth Differentiation Sex determination	Growth Differentiation Sex change
Morphological, physiological and behavioral phenotype develops.	Morphological, physiological and behavioral changes from one stage to next
Not repeatable	**Repeatable**

FIGURE 1.8: There are two major classes of life-history stages. During ontogeny, different stages are expressed during growth, differentiation of cells, tissues, and organs, and sex is usually determined. This process, leading to a particular phenotype, is not reversible. In contrast, once an adult, a different set of life-history stages are expressed, especially as annual environmental variation increases. Again, there is growth and differentiation of cells, tissues, and organs, and sex change may also occur in some species. These changes, however, are reversible—phenotypic flexibility.

From Wingfield (2004, 2005a, 2006). Courtesy of Elsevier Press.

environment allow organisms to adjust their state to maximize survival at different times of year. The state of the individual at any point in its life cycle should ideally be perfectly aligned with the demands imposed on that individual from the physical and social environment. Each individual responds as a finite state machine (FSM) consisting of a temporal sequence of life-history stages that serve to maximize lifetime fitness (Jacobs 1996; Jacobs and Wingfield 2000; Wingfield 2005a, 2008a, 2008b). It is important to understand that life-history trajectories involve ontogenetic stages during development from a zygote to an independent adult, at which point there is a transition to cyclic life-history stages (Figure 1.8). Because most vertebrates have life spans of more than one year, the adult life-history stages may be expressed more than once.

During ontogeny, hormones regulate growth and differentiation, including determination of sex, and although there may be many stages, each is expressed only once. Morphological, physiological, and behavioral phenotypes are developed during this process, and these characters are largely irreversible (Arnold and Breedlove 1985). In some cases they can be expressed in a limited number of ways in adults, the relative plasticity model of Moore (1991). Note that in adults, changes of morphology, physiology, and behavior from one stage to the next also involve growth and differentiation (Figure 1.8). Whereas during ontogeny developmental changes are not reversible (Figure 1.9), development associated with adult life-history cycles is reversible and usually cyclic, which is important to bear in mind when considering regulatory mechanisms (Jacobs and Wingfield 2000; Piersma and van Gils 2011; Wingfield 2005a).

Patterns of ontogenetic and adult life-history stages are complex (Figures 1.9 and 1.10), but they are important to consider because how they respond to perturbations of the environment, and potentially stress, is very different and during ontogeny may have profound implications for how that individual copes the rest of its life. Species such as salmonid fish of the genus *Oncorhynchus* have one ontogenetic sequence culminating in reproduction, senescence, and death. This is called a semelparous life cycle (Figures 1.9 and 1.10), in which ontogeny and adult life-history stages have a single sequence. Most vertebrates have a single ontogenetic sequence (examples given in Figures 1.9 and 1.10), but when adult, the life-history stages of most species show cycles that

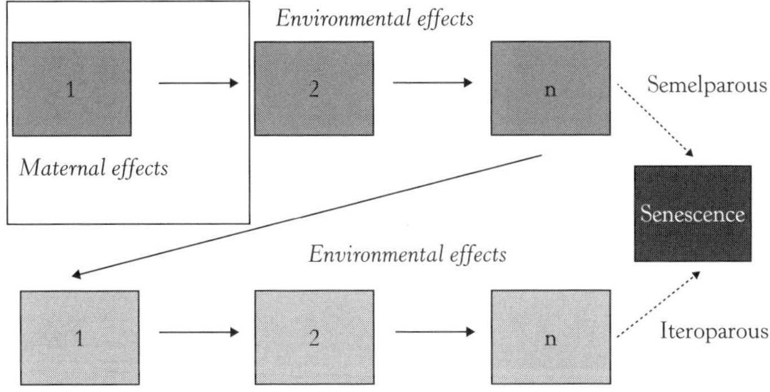

FIGURE 1.9: Ontogenetic stages in these schematic representation can be expressed in multiple ways. Note that maternal (and paternal) effects, as well as environmental effects such as experience and changes in the physical environment, may be important at this time. Ontogenetic stages lead to adult life-history stages or, in the case of semelparity, lead to reproduction and programmed death (in this case the entire life cycle may be made up of ontogenetic stages). In the vast majority of vertebrates, adult life-history stages are often expressed in repeated cycles of about a year with several reproductive periods (iteroparity). These adult stages are strongly influenced by environmental effects.

From Wingfield (2004, 2005a, 2006). Courtesy of Elsevier Press.

can be repeated many times. This is called an iteroparous life cycle, in which the adult life-history stages are repeated for as many years as the individual lives. The transition from ontogeny to adult life-history cycles can involve a metamorphosis, typical of many fish and amphibians, or it can be more gradual with, for example, onset of adult life-history stages occurring at puberty. Compare, for example, the sequences of adult life-history stages for an amphibian, reptile, or bird, and mammals including humans in Figures 1.10 and 1.11.

Each life-history stage, whether ontogenetic or adult, has a characteristic set of substages, such as specific behavioral traits appropriate for that life-history stage, homeostatic mechanisms for the environment the individual is occupying at that time, or morphologies such as energy stores, muscle development, color pattern, and so on. Different combinations of substages are expressed, depending on local environmental conditions. These define the state of the individual at that time in the life cycle (Jacobs and Wingfield 2000; Wingfield 2005a, 2008a, 2008b; Wingfield and Jacobs 1999). Changes in social status, body condition, disease, and so on, are also important in determining the combination of substages to be expressed (Wingfield 2006). Because there is a fixed number of adult life-history stages and characteristic substages, there is a finite number of states an individual can express through its life cycle (Jacobs 1996; Wingfield 2005a; Wingfield and Jacobs 1999), hence the term "finite state machine." It is possible to define a life-history stage at many different levels. Here we define it as a syndrome (Sih et al. 2004) of morphological, physiological, and behavioral traits that allow an individual to best cope with environmental conditions at that time. Examples of such life-history stages include outward and return migrations, reproduction, molting, non-breeding, and hibernation. Others may subdivide these into further life-history stages (Piersma and van Gils 2011). Whatever definition one decides upon, it is important to be consistent so that the framework can then be applied across the vertebrate spectrum.

Examples of diverse sequences of life-history stages (Figure 1.11) reveal some important implications for control mechanisms. Each box in Figure 1.11 represents a distinct life-history stage; in species with more than two, the temporal sequence must progress forward and cannot be reversed. For example, in a migratory bird it is not possible to revert to vernal migration after the breeding season. The sequence of life-history stages must move on to the next stage, in this case pre-basic molt (Figure 1.11). Therefore all life-history stages must be expressed in the correct temporal sequence before vernal migration is again attained, and they occur on a schedule

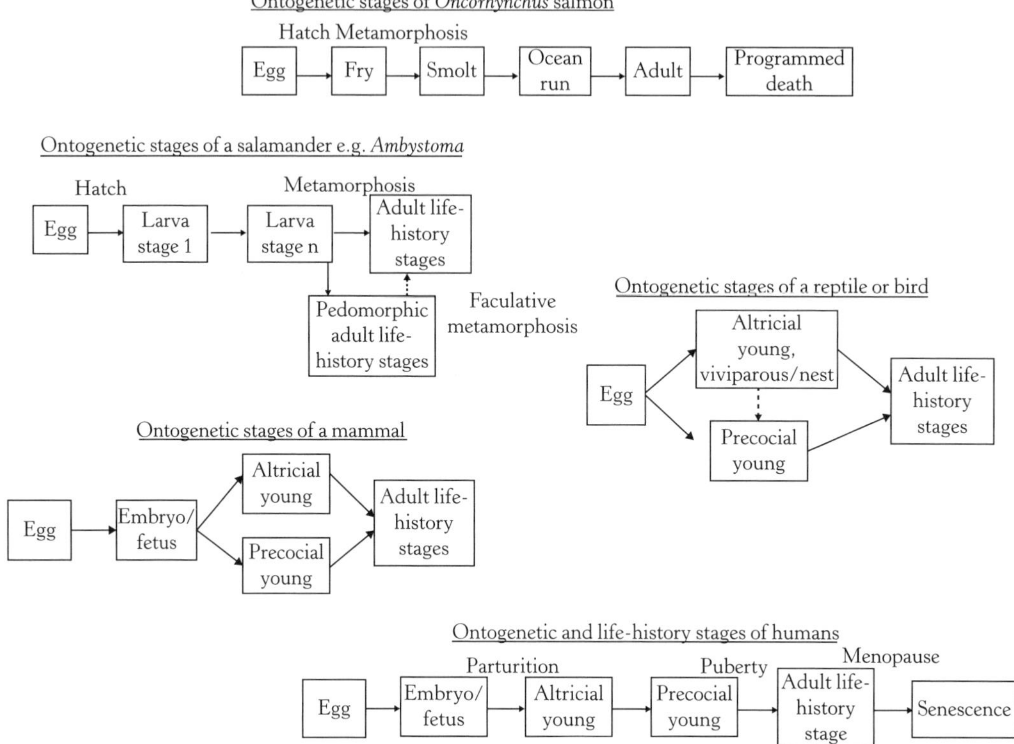

FIGURE 1.10: Some examples of ontogenetic life-history stages from a semelparous species (*Oncorhynchus* salmon) and several iteroparous species, including humans. Beginning with a fertilized egg, several (many) stages may be expressed with some alternative stages (such as altricial versus precocial young). All eventually give rise to the adult life-history stages. Humans represent an interesting situation in which there is only one adult life-history stage (see discussion later in this chapter), but some life cycle events such as menopause occur in an extended ontogenetic progression. Humans are not semelparous, but because they have one adult life-history stage the entire life cycle is ontogenetic and not reversible.

From Wingfield (2004, 2005a, 2006). Courtesy of Elsevier Press.

determined by the changing seasons (Wingfield and Jacobs 1999). Furthermore, the combination of substages expressed within a life-history stage includes factors in the extended phenotype, such as a territory, presence of a mate, and social status within a group (Dawkins 1982). These, along with other factors, such as body condition, disease, pollution, and so on, determine how an individual acclimates to fluctuations in its environment (Wingfield and Jacobs 1999).

There are three phases in the expression of a life-history stage that are important in terms of regulatory mechanisms (Figure 1.12). First, there is a development phase, when characteristic morphology and physiology of that stage is acquired. Behavioral traits that may also be characteristic are also activated. The development phase culminates in "mature capability" in which a number of substages can then be activated and the actual life-history stage can be expressed. The third phase involves termination of the life-history stage, and there is overlap with the development phase of the next life-history stage (Jacobs and Wingfield 2000; Wingfield and Jacobs 1999). Obviously, an organism cannot make an instantaneous transition from one life-history stage to another; there must be some overlap, termed a "super-state" (Jacobs 1996; Jacobs and Wingfield 2000), that may be energetically demanding, but is usually brief. Substages allow specific events to occur within the life-history state, usually in response to signals from the social and physical environment. Although these substages are not expressed randomly, there is much greater flexibility in sequences and timing. For example, the sexual and parental phases of breeding can be turned on and off quickly. Another example is the rapid switch between refueling and flying in migration.

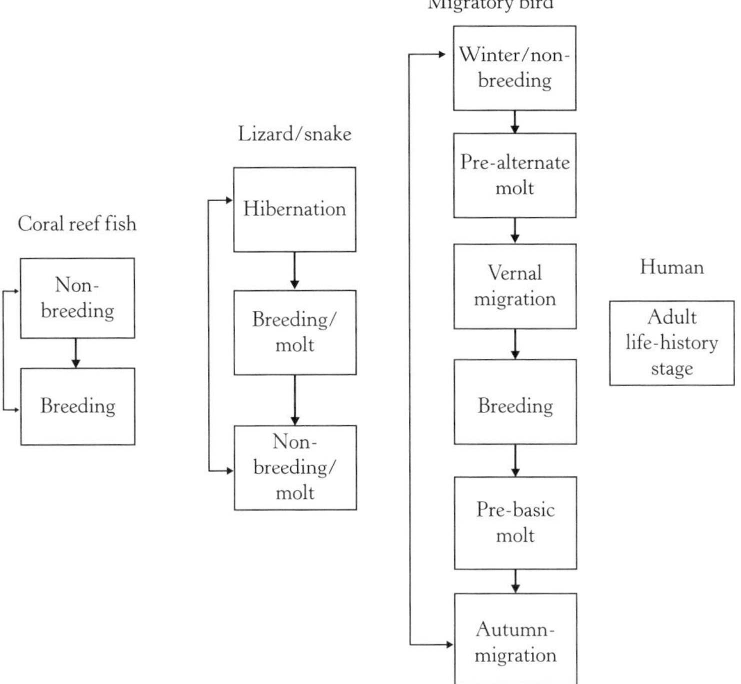

FIGURE 1.11: Examples of adult life-history stages from selected vertebrates. Some, such as coral reef fish and humans, live in environments with little annual variation in environmental conditions and thus need one or two life-history stages. This results in much flexibility in timing, but tolerance of environmental variation will be low. In others (e.g., migratory birds), much greater environmental variation results in up to six or even seven life-history stages. This allows acclimation to greater ranges of annual environmental variation, but because each stage requires time to develop, to be expressed, and then to terminate, flexibility in timing is reduced. Intermediate conditions, in which there are three life-history stages (e.g., for a lizard or snake), may provide greater flexibility in the timing of life-history stages, as well as tolerance of intermediate variation in annual environmental conditions.

From Wingfield (2004, 2006). Courtesy of Elsevier Press.

D. Phenotypic Flexibility

There is variation in the number of life-history stages that some species may have compared with others, and some life-history stages may have more complex sets of substages (Piersma and van Gils 2011). A coral reef fish (Figure 1.11) has two obvious life-history stages, breeding and non-breeding. In contrast, others, such as many temperate-zone lizards and snakes, have three (Figure 1.11). Migratory birds have as many as six distinct life-history stages (Jacobs and Wingfield 2000; Wingfield and Jacobs 1999). At the opposite end of the spectrum, humans have only one adult life-history stage (Figure 1.11). The boundaries of the temporal sequence of life-history stages can be defined at many levels, such as day, month, tidal fluctuation, length of wet/dry seasons, a year, or longer (Jacobs and Wingfield 2000). However, in vertebrates the time taken to pass through the development, mature capability, and termination phases takes at least a month, thus limiting the number of life-history stages an individual can express in one year (Wingfield 2008a, 2008b). The duration of each life-history stage can be measured from field observations. In migratory birds (Figure 1.13), breeding condition may be maintained for 1–3 months, whereas pre-basic molt can be as short as 1 month (Wingfield and Jacobs 1999). In coral reef fish, the two life-history stages of breeding and non-breeding may be interchangeable (Figure 1.13). Life-history stages can overlap mature capability for varying periods, as seen in migratory birds (Figure 1.13). Some life-history stages, such as winter (non-breeding) and molt, may be more compatible for overlap, whereas others (e.g., migration and breeding) are mutually exclusive because it is not possible to build a nest and incubate eggs while covering long distances on migration. On the other hand, it is possible for some fish and mammals to be pregnant during migration.

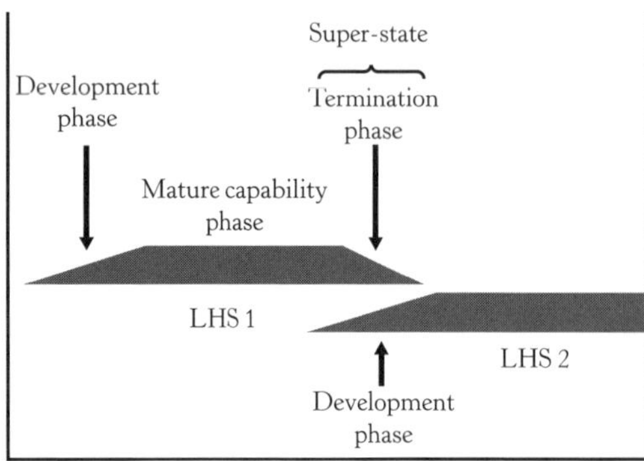

FIGURE 1.12: Each life-history stage (LHS) has three phases. The development phase is when characteristic morphology, physiology, and behavior are expressed. This culminates in the "mature capability" phase, when substages of the LHS can be expressed. An example is development of the reproductive system, which must occur before actual onset of breeding. Finally, the LHS is terminated. All three phases involve varying degrees of regulation of gene expression. Note also that the termination phase of one LHS overlaps with development of the next (i.e., a super-state). See Jacobs and Wingfield (2000); Wingfield and Jacobs (1999); Wingfield (2005a, 2008a, 2008b).

Courtesy of Elsevier Press.

The numbers of life-history stages expressed can allow an organism to acclimate to a wider range of environmental conditions. Breeding and non-breeding stages coupled with migrations, hibernation, and so on, mean that extremes of environment (e.g., seasons) can be tolerated. Those with fewer life-history stages (e.g., breeding and non-breeding) can tolerate only a narrower range of environmental conditions, as might be found in mesic and tropical/oceanic habitats (Wingfield 2005a, 2008a, 2008b). This flexibility of the phenotype (Piersma and Drent 2003) has been termed "finite stage diversity" (FSD) and is an indication to what extent an organism may be able to acclimate to wide ranges of environmental conditions (Wingfield 2005a, 2008a, 2008b). Wingfield (2008b) has suggested several hypotheses that could be tested to explore finite stage diversity:

A. Because of frequently conflicting physiology and behavior, and the energetic costs of maintaining morphological characters, there are limits to the number of life-history stages that can be expressed simultaneously.
B. More life-history stages (finite state diversity) means less flexibility in timing because the development and termination periods are time dependent and must be expressed in the correct temporal sequence. This is turn determines how specific control mechanisms of an individual respond to environmental cues used to pace the life cycle.
C. Life-history stages cannot be omitted completely, thus reducing finite stage diversity, but the expression of substages at "mature capability" may be suppressed (e.g., onset of breeding or migration).

In other words, it is suggested that there is a classic trade-off between the ability to tolerate a wide range of environmental conditions and flexibility in the timing of life-history stages. This may have important implications for how organisms adjust to climate change (Wingfield 2008a, 2008b). It also is important for how organisms may then respond to perturbations of the environment, as will be discussed in later chapters.

The simplest finite state machine is a single adult life-history stage. This is rare in vertebrates, but it is arguable that humans have only one adult life-history stage (Figures 1.11 and 1.13). Once adult, reproductive ability can be constant, we do not molt, nor do we show regular migration patterns that exclude other functions. Seasonal patterns in births are well established in human populations, tending to be most obvious in regions with summer heat or at extreme latitude. At first, this may give the impression of breeding and non-breeding life-history stages; however, as far as we are aware, there are no reports of humans going through periods of gonadal regression (reverse puberty) and subsequent recrudescence (second puberty), as one sees in more seasonal breeding vertebrates. This suggests that differences in birth rates are adjustments of substages, not separate life-history stages (Wingfield 2005a). In men, semen quality changes seasonally but only by ±10% over a year (Dabbs 1990; Levine 1994), consistent with substage changes, or even environmental stress, but not with transition to a different life-history stage.

Considering the concept of finite stage diversity, the single adult life-history stage of humans indicates that we have ultimate flexibility in the timing of reproduction and other things we do. On the other hand, the trade-off is that we can only tolerate a very narrow range of environmental conditions. So, how have we been able to colonize

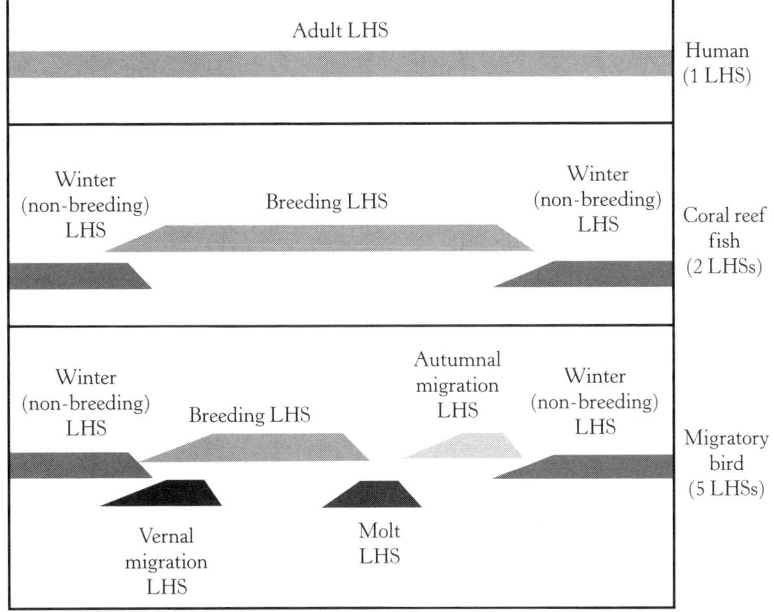

FIGURE 1.13: By arranging adult life-history stages according to time of year, it is clear that the more life-history stages expressed (e.g., lower panel with six stages in migratory birds), the less flexibility there is in timing. Note that the developmental phase of a life-history stage overlaps with the termination phase of the previous stage. Humans (top panel) and coral reef fish (middle panel) have the greatest flexibility, but their tolerance of environmental variation is low.

After Ramenofsky and Wingfield (2006); Wingfield (2008a); courtesy of Elsevier Press and the Royal Society, London.

all regions on the planet regardless of severity of the climate? Short (1994) suggested that because our ancestors were of tropical origin and only recently, in terms of geological time, colonized higher latitudes, a large brain and social skills, including communication, enabled us to solve the problems of severe environments. For example, we developed clothing, houses, heating, agriculture, food storage, and so on, allowing us to breed year round and independently of strong photoperiodism (Short 1994). Furthermore, we have the unique ability to create our own microenvironments, and maintain them anywhere, allowing us to colonize virtually all regions on earth (Farhi 1987). In other words, an Inupiaq Eskimo hunting seals on the Arctic Ocean ice maintains a subtropical environment at the skin level using clothing and can be comfortable despite extreme low temperatures and high winds. By these artificial means, we can survive with a single life-history stage, and have great flexibility in the timing of reproduction, and so on, in extremely variable environments. This does not mean that we are resistant to unpredictable stressful events. Indeed, perturbation factors may temporarily interrupt reproductive function, as well as our normal daily routines.

E. The Emergency Life-History Stage

We have seen how life-history characteristics of the predictable life cycle are organized and expressed, and we now address what happens in response to unpredictable events, the perturbation factors. Unpredictable events can occur at any time in the predictable progression of life-history stages (Figure 1.14). If the perturbation is severe enough, then the individual must temporarily abandon daily routines characteristic of the normal life-history stage and enter a coping state called the "emergency life-history stage" (ELHS; Wingfield 2003; Wingfield et al. 1998). It can be expressed at any time in the life cycle with similar physiological and behavioral responses that thus far appear to be remarkably well conserved across all vertebrates studied to date (Wingfield 2003, 2005a).

The emergency life-history stage serves to direct the individual into a survival mode and then allows it to return to the normal life-history stage once the perturbation factor passes. Substages such as the "flight-or-flight" response are well-known reactions to sudden perturbations, such as attack by a predator, sudden social strife, an accident, and so on. There are different physiological and behavioral strategies that individuals may take to cope with sudden perturbations (e.g., Koolhaas et al. 1999; Figure 1.14). Reactive strategies tend to be used by individuals that are less bold and avoid the perturbation, whereas proactive individuals tend to be much bolder, directly confronting a social challenge, predator, and so on. One or the other strategy has a genetic basis but also can be modified by learning, experience, and age. These extremes are not absolute, and many individuals fall somewhere along the continuum from reactive to proactive (Koolhaas et al. 1999). Injury and potential infection frequently accompany exposure to perturbations and trigger the immune system to respond. Fever and sickness behavior can result, allowing the individual to recover following the perturbation (e.g., Hart 1988; Figure 1.14). There is a fourth substage, much less well understood

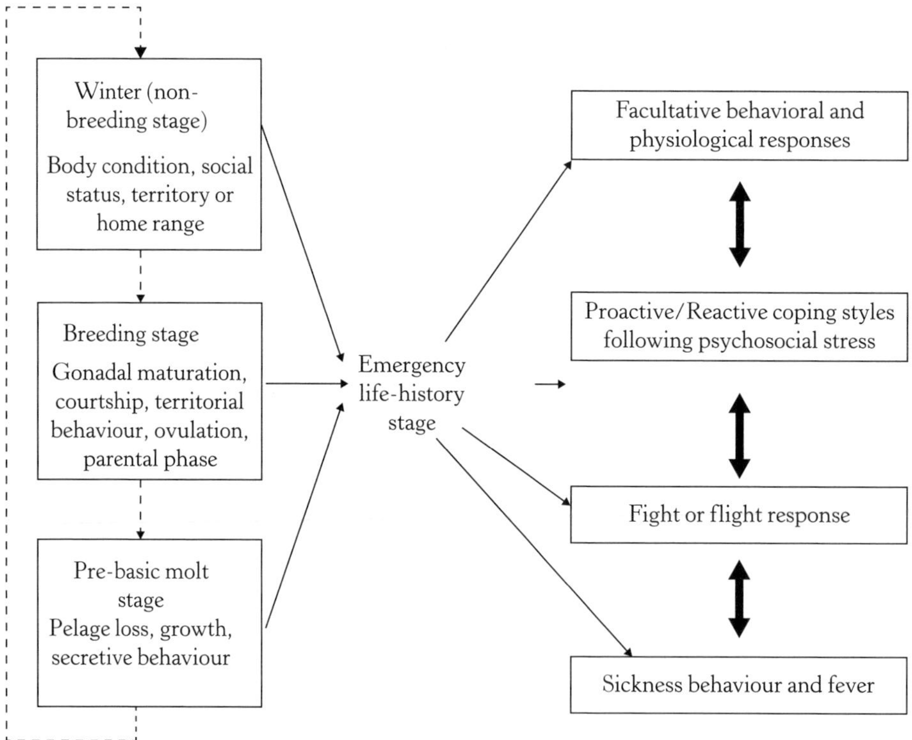

FIGURE 1.14: A scheme showing examples of life-history stages (LHSs) on the left and the emergency life-history stage on the right. In, for example, a non-migratory bird, LHSs include breeding, non-breeding, and molt stages. Each has a unique set of substages. The progression of LHSs is one way, with each cycle taking a year. The temporal progression of normal LHSs is regulated by the predictable annual cycle of seasons. Superimposed upon this predictable life cycle are unpredictable events such as severe storms, predator pressure, human disturbance, and so on. These "labile perturbation factors" have the potential to trigger the emergency life-history stage (ELHS), which redirects the individual away from the normal LHSs into survival mode. Once the perturbation passes, the individual can then return to an LHS appropriate for that time of year. The ELHS has four characteristic components or substages. The "fight-or-flight response" is typical of very rapid responses to, for example, sudden attack by a predator. If the perturbation is an infection, or wounding following an attack by a predator, then sickness behavior and fever may result. Responses to other less acute LPFs, such as a severe storm, trigger facultative behavioral and physiological responses. Individuals may respond to the same perturbation in very different ways, with a reactive strategy at one extreme and a proactive strategy at the other extreme. Note that the four substages can be expressed independently or in varying combinations. See Jacobs and Wingfield (2000); Wingfield and Romero (2001).

From Wingfield (2003), courtesy of Elsevier Press.

than the other three. This involves behavioral and physiological components that make up the facultative responses to perturbation factors (Figure 1.14) as the individual maximizes its survival in the face of long-term disruptions—the direct labile perturbation factors (Wingfield and Ramenofsky 1999). These have been characterized as follows:

1. Following a direct labile perturbation factor, an individual abandons its current life-history stage and leaves its home range or territory to seek shelter or alternate habitat. This is the "leave it" strategy.
2. Alternatively, an individual may remain in its home range or territory and switch to an alternate set of energy-conserving behavioral and physiological traits. This is the "take it" strategy. Note that the individual has still abandoned its normal life-history stage.
3. An individual may first remain on the home range or territory and switch to an energy-conserving mode. Later it can then move away if conditions do not improve. This is the "take at first and then leave it" strategy.
4. Once a "strategy" has been adopted, stored energy must be mobilized from sources such as fat and protein to fuel enduring the perturbation factor while sheltering in a refuge, or to move away.
5. Finally, as the direct labile perturbation factor passes, the individual can resume its life-history stage, or if the individual has moved away, then it must settle in alternate habitat once an appropriate site is identified, or return to the original site and then resume the normal sequence of life-history stages. These dramatic changes in behavior and physiology can occur within minutes to hours of exposure to a direct labile perturbation factor and have been the subject of many experiments to determine the mechanisms underlying them (Wingfield and Kitaysky 2002; Wingfield and Ramenofsky 1999). Recovery from the emergency life-history stage is also an important topic that deserves further attention.

The substages of the emergency life-history stage can be expressed singly or in various combinations (Figure 1.15). Immune systems tend to be activated because responses to sudden attack and the resulting fight-or-flight response frequently result in injury and potentially infection. Furthermore, several mediators of the fight-or-flight response also enhance immune function. A wounded animal needs to heal in order to survive. A reactive or proactive personality may determine if and when an individual stays ("take it" strategy), or abandons its home range ("leave it" strategy). Curiously, as far as we can tell, the temporal sequence, duration and timing, of normal life-history stages continues even if the life-history cycle is interrupted by an unpredictable event. During this interruption an emergency life-history stage is expressed (see Wingfield et al. 1998; Wingfield and Jacobs 1999) and mature capabilities of other life-history stages are suppressed so that, for example, migration or reproduction are interrupted. Once the perturbation passes, the life-history stage appropriate for that time of year will be assumed, suggesting that the mechanisms by which the predictable life-history stages are timed continues unaffected. Interactions of biological clocks with environmental perturbations remain to be explored in detail.

The concept of permanent versus labile perturbation actors may have relevance to the question of acute versus chronic stress. The latter is common in human society, and in agricultural and aquacultural settings, possibly because permanent perturbation factors are common, resulting in chronic stress. However, in nature most perturbations are temporary (labile), and acute stress is common. When permanent perturbations do occur and organisms are unable to cope because the emergency life-history stage is not designed to be a permanent state, then death results before we see manifestations of chronic stress, as are prevalent in human society.

Finally, most of us would regard the emergency life-history stage and its components as different types of stress responses. This is a reasonable conclusion. But, given that the different components of the emergency life-history stage allow an individual to cope with the perturbation, perhaps they should be called "anti-stress responses"! Furthermore, as pointed out by Carr and Summers (2002), stress is something more than just a disease; initial stress responses are designed to help us acclimate and cope with considerable environmental perturbation. When the stress becomes chronic and we cannot cope, then disease becomes a threat.

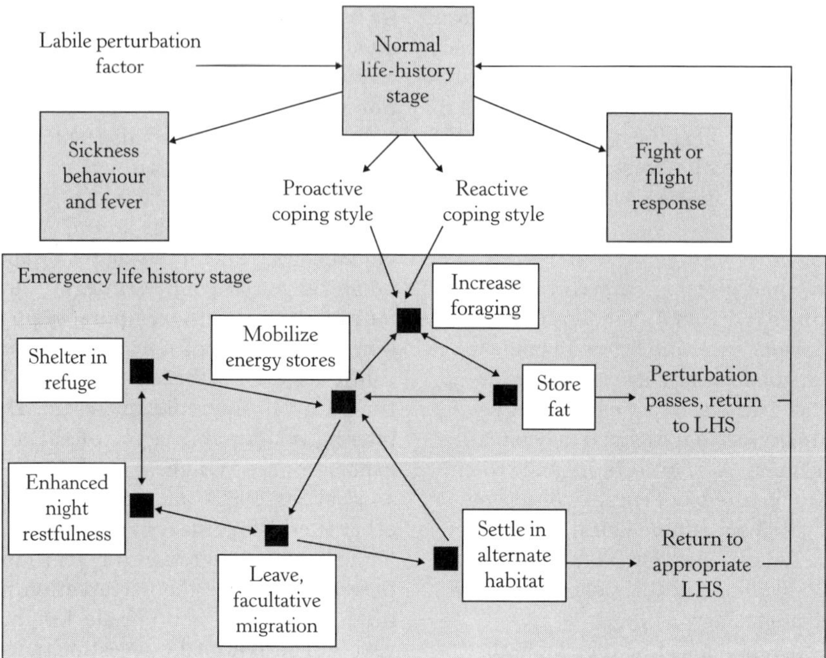

FIGURE 1.15: The emergency life-history stage (ELHS) can be divided into several substages: the fight-or-flight response, facultative behavioral and physiological responses (such as seeking a refuge, leaving the area, or mobilization of energy), and sickness behavior and fever. All of these substages are interconnected and can be expressed sequentially or simultaneously depending upon circumstances. Indirect labile perturbation factors are usually very rapid and do not necessarily interrupt the normal sequence of life-history stages. Thus, they only trigger fight-or-flight responses. However, if wounding or infection resulted from this perturbation, then sickness behavior and fever may follow (upper part of figure). Direct perturbation factors have the potential to disrupt the sequence of life-history stages and also may trigger a fight-or-flight response in some circumstances. Once again, wounding or infection would then trigger sickness behavior and fever. These substages allow the individual to tailor the expression of an emergency life-history stage precisely to the circumstances and type of labile perturbation factor experienced.
Redrawn from Wingfield (2003); Wingfield (2005a). Courtesy of Elsevier Press.

IV. SUMMARY

The answer to the question posed at the beginning of this chapter—what is stress?—is clearly not simple. It requires an idea of what environmental changes animals must cope with, knowledge of different life-history stages, and an understanding of how animals initiate an emergency life-history stage in order to cope with labile perturbation factors. One take-home message is that the stress response, or the emergency life-history stage, is part of a continuum of how animals cope with a changing environment. The focus of this book is on the specific physiological, hormonal, and behavioral responses to labile perturbation factors, but we must always keep in mind that the ultimate goal of each and every stress response is to return the animal to its appropriate life-history stage.

REFERENCES

Arnold, A. P., Breedlove, S. M., 1985. Organizational and activational effects of sex steroids on brain and behavior: A reanalysis. *Horm Behav* 19, 469–498.

Babcock, L. E., Zhang, W., Leslie, S. A., 2001. The Chengjiang Biota: Record of the Early Cambrian diversification of life and clues to exceptional preservation of fossils. *GSA Today* 11, 4–9.

Cannon, W. B., 1932. *The Wisdom of the body.* W.W. Norton, New York.

Carr, J. A., Summers, C. H., 2002. Stress more than a disease? A comparative look at the adaptativeness of stress. *Integ Comp Biol* 42, 505–507.

Dabbs, J. M., 1990. Age and seasonal variation in serum testosterone concentration among men. *Chronobiol Int* 7, 245–249.

Dawkins, R., 1982. *The extended phenotype: The gene as the unit of selection.* W. H. Freeman, Oxford.

de Wilde, J., 1978. Seasonal states and endocrine levels in insects. In: Assenmacher, I., Farner, D. S. (Eds.), *Environmental endocrinology.* Springer-Verlag, Berlin, pp. 10–19.

DiMichele, W. A., Pfefferkorn, H. W., Gastaldo, R. A., 2001. Response of Late Carboniferous and Early Permian plant communities to climate change. *Ann Rev Earth Pl Sci* 29, 461–487.

Falcon-Lang, H. J., Kvacek, J., Ulicny, D., 2001. Fire-prone plant communities and palaeoclimate of a Late Cretaceous fluvial to estuarine environment, Pecinov quarry, Czech Republic. *Geol Mag* 138, 563–576.

Farhi, L. E., 1987. Exposure to stressful environments, strategy of adaptive responses. In: Dejours, P. (Ed.) *Comparative physiology of environmental adaptations*, vol. 2. Karger, Basel, pp. 1–14.

Fraiser, M. L., Bottjer, D. J., 2004. The non-actualistic early triassic gastropod fauna: A case study of the lower triassic sinbad limestone member. *Palaios* 19, 259–275.

Gage, J. D., Tyler, P. A., 1991. *Deep sea biology.* Cambridge University Press, Cambridge.

Gessaman, J. A., Worthen, G. L., 1982. *The effect of weather on avian mortality.* Utah State University Printing Services, Logan, Utah.

Glasspool, I. J., 2003. Hypautochthonous-allochthonous coal deposition in the Permian, South African, Witbank Basin No. 2 seam: A combined approach using sedimentology, coal petrology and palaeontology. *Int J Coal Geol* 53, 81–135.

Harper, D. A. T., Doyle, E. N., 2003. A silurian (Llandovery) Eoplectodonta shell bed in Western Ireland: The role of opportunism, storms and sedimentation rates in its formation. *Irish J Earth Sci* 21, 105–114.

Hart, B. L., 1988. Biological basis of the behavior of sick animals. *Neurosci Biobehav Rev* 12, 123–137.

Hendry, J. P., Perkins, W. T., Bane, T., 2001. Short-term environmental change in a Jurassic lagoon deduced from geochemical trends in aragonite bivalve shells. *Geol Soc Am Bull* 113, 790–798.

IPCC, 2001. *Climate change 2001: impacts, adaptations and vulnerability.* Contribution of working group II to the third assessment report of the Intergovernmental Panel on Climate Change. Cambridge University Press, Port Chester, New York.

Ivany, L. C., Patterson, W. P., Lohmann, K. C., 2000. Cooler winters as a possible cause of mass extinctions at the eocene/oligocene boundary. *Nature* 407, 887–890.

Jacobs, J., 1996. Regulation of life history stages within individuals in unpredictable environments. Ph.D. Thesis, Department of Zoology, University of Washington, Seattle.

Jacobs, J. D., Wingfield, J. C., 2000. Endocrine control of life-cycle stages: A constraint on response to the environment? *Condor* 102, 35–51.

Koolhaas, J. M., Korte, S. M., De Boer, S. F., Van Der Vegt, B. J., Van Reenen, C. G., Hopster, H., De Jong, I. C., Ruis, M. A. W., Blokhuis, H. J., 1999. Coping styles in animals: Current status in behavior and stress-physiology. *Neurosci Biobehav Rev* 23, 925–935.

Levine, R. J., 1994. Male factors contributing to the seasonality of human reproduction In: Campbell, K. L., Wood, J. W. (Eds.), Human reproductive ecology: Interactions of environment, fertility, and behavior. New York Academy of Sciences, New York, vol. 709, pp. 29–45.

Levine, S., Ursin, H., 1991. What is stress? In: Brown, M. R., Koob, G. F., Rivier, C. (Eds.), Stress: Neurobiology and neuroendocrinology, Marcel Dekker, New York, pp. 3–21.

McIver, E. E., 2002. The paleoenvironment of Tyrannosaurus rex from southwestern Saskatchewan, Canada. *Can J Earth Sci* 39, 207–221.

Moore, M. C., 1991. Application of organization activation theory to alternative male reproductive strategies: A review. *Horm Behav* 25, 154–179.

Ozanne, C. R., Harries, P. J., 2002. Role of predation and parasitism in the extinction of the inoceramid bivalves: An evaluation. *Lethaia* 35, 1–19.

Paul, G. S., 1997. Migration. In: Currie, P. J., Padian, K. (Eds.), *Encyclopedia of dinosaurs.* Academic Press, San Diego, pp. 444–446.

Piersma, T., Drent, J., 2003. Phenotypic flexibility and the evolution of organismal design. *Trends Ecol Evol* 18, 228–233.

Piersma, T., van Gils, J. A., 2011. *The flexible phenotype: A body-centred integration of ecology, physiology, and behavior.* Oxford University Press, Oxford.

Poiner, G., Poiner, R., 2008. *What bugged the dinosaurs? Insects, disease and death in the Cretaceous.* Princeton University Press, Princeton, NJ.

Poulson, T. L., 1964. Animals in aquatic environments: animals in caves. In: Dill, D. B., Adolf, E. F., Wilber, C. G. (Eds.), *Handbook of physiology,* Section 4, Chapter 47, American Physiological Society, Washington, DC.

Ramenofsky, M., Wingfield, J. C., 2006. Behavioral and physiological conflicts in migrants: The transition between migration and breeding. *J Ornithol* 147, 135–145.

Selye, H., 1946. The general adaptation syndrome and the diseases of adaptation. *J Clin Endocrinol* 6, 117–230.

Short, R. V., 1994. Human reproduction in an evolutionary context In: Campbell, K. L., Wood, J. W. (Eds.), *Human reproductive ecology: Interactions of environment, fertility, and behavior.* New York

Academy of Sciences, New York, vol. 709. pp. 416–425.

Sih, A., Bell, A., Johnson, J.vC., 2004. Behavioral syndromes: An ecological and evolutionary overview. *Trends Ecol Evol* 19, 372–378.

Soreghan, G. S., 2004. Deja-vu all over again: Deep time (climate) is here to stay. *Palaios* 19, 1–2.

Steuber, T., 1999. Isotopic and chemical intra-shell variations in low-Mg calcite of rudist bivalves (Mollusca-Hippuritacea): Disequilibrium fractionations and late Cretaceous seasonality. *Int J Earth Sci* 88, 551–570.

Tokaryk, T. T., Bryant, H. N., 2004. The fauna from the *Tyrannosaurus rex* excavation, Frenchman Formation (late Maastrichtian), Saskatchewan. *Saskatchewan Geological Survey, Summary of Investigations* 2004, 1, 1–12.

Travis, J. M. J., 2003. Climate change and habitat destruction: A deadly anthropogenic cocktail. *Proc R Soc Lond B* 270, 467–473.

Wingfield, J. C., 1984. Influence of weather on reproduction. *J Exp Zool* 232, 589–594.

Wingfield, J. C., 1985a. Influences of weather on reproductive function in female Song sparrows, *Melospiza melodia*. *J Zool, Lond* 205, 545–558.

Wingfield, J. C., 1985b. Influences of weather on reproductive function in male Song sparrows, *Melospiza melodia*. *J Zool, Lond* 205, 525–544.

Wingfield, J. C., 2003. Control of behavioural strategies for capricious environments. *Anim Behav* 66, 807–815.

Wingfield, J. C., 2004. Allostatic load and life cycles: Implications for neuroendocrine mechanisms. In: Schulkin, J. (Ed.), *Allostasis, Homeostasis and the Costs of Physiological Adaptation*, Cambridge University Press, Cambridge, pp. 302–342.

Wingfield, J. C., 2005a. The concept of allostasis: Coping with a capricious environment. *J Mammal* 86, 248–254.

Wingfield, J. C., 2005b. Modulation of the adrenocortical response to acute stress in breeding birds. In: Dawson, A., Sharp, P. J. (Eds.), *Functional avian endocrinology*. Narosa Publishing House, New Delhi, India, pp. 225–240.

Wingfield, J. C., 2006. Communicative behaviors, hormone-behavior interactions, and reproduction in vertebrates. In: Neill, J. D. (Ed.) *Physiology of reproduction*, Academic Press, New York, pp. 1995–2040.

Wingfield, J. C., 2008a. Comparative endocrinology, environment and global change. *Gen Comp Endocrinol* 157, 207–216.

Wingfield, J. C., 2008b. Organization of vertebrate annual cycles: Implications for control mechanisms. *Philos Trans Roy Soc BBiol Sci* 363, 425–441.

Wingfield, J. C., Jacobs, J. D., 1999. The interplay of innate and experiential factors regulating the life history cycle of birds. In: Adams, N., Slotow, R. (Eds.), *Proceedings of the 22nd International Ornithological Congress*, Birdlife South Africa, Johannesburg, pp. 2417–2443.

Wingfield, J. C., Kitaysky, A. S., 2002. Endocrine responses to unpredictable environmental events: Stress or anti-stress hormones? *Integ Comp Biol* 42, 600–609.

Wingfield, J. C., Maney, D. L., Breuner, C. W., Jacobs, J. D., Lynn, S., Ramenofsky, M., Richardson, R. D., 1998. Ecological bases of hormone-behavior interactions: The "emergency life history stage." *Integ Comp Biol* 38, 191.

Wingfield, J. C., Moore, M. C., Farner, D. S., 1983. Endocrine responses to inclement weather in naturally breeding populations of white-crowned sparrows (*Zonotrichia leucophrys pugetensis*). *Auk* 100, 56–62.

Wingfield, J. C., Ramenofsky, M., 1999. Hormones and the behavioral ecology of stress. In: Balm, P. H. M. (Ed.), *Stress Physiology in Animals*, Sheffield Academic Press, Sheffield, U.K., pp. 1–51.

Wingfield, J. C., Romero, L. M., 2001. Adrenocortical responses to stress and their modulation in free-living vertebrates. In: McEwen, B. S., Goodman, H. M. (Eds.), *Handbook of physiology*; Section 7: *The endocrine system*; Volume IV: *Coping with the environment: neural and endocrine mechanisms*. Oxford University Press, New York, pp. 211–234.

Wingfield, J. C., Sapolsky, R. M., 2003. Reproduction and resistance to stress: When and how. *J Neuroendocrinol* 15, 711.

Wright, V. P., Taylor, K. G., Beck, V. H., 2000. The paleohydrology of Lower Cretaceous seasonal wetlands, Isle of Wight, Southern England. *J Sediment Res* 70, 619–632.

2

Mediators of Stress

I. INTRODUCTION

Homeostatic processes, social systems, growth, reproduction, migration, and so on, require major adjustments of morphological, physiological, and behavioral functions in response to environmental demands. These functions vary in complex ways over the temporal sequence of life history events in a manner unique to a population or individual. Both the correct temporal sequence and the timing of each event must be regulated to maximize overall fitness. Moreover, coping with perturbations of the environment and the potential for stress must also be integrated into the predictable life cycle. How is this done? Environmental signals that are used as indicators for transitions of state required in the near or immediate future can be used to trigger appropriate responses of the individual as follows:

1. Orchestrate development of organisms and respond to environmental changes that require adjustment of developmental trajectories.
2. Regulate when adjustments of homeostasis are to be made in advance of predictable changes in the environment.
3. Signal when alternate behavioral and physiological patterns should be triggered in response to unpredictable and disruptive events.
4. Adjust social interactions to maximize an individual's ability to gain access to shelter, food resources, territories, mates, and so on.

Responses to environmental change, especially perturbations, can involve direct cell effects such as heat shock protein expression, activation of DNA repair mechanisms, and amelioration of oxidative damage. Heat shock proteins (HSPs) are widespread in plants and animals and are expressed in all cells within an organism. They have multiple roles, including chaperoning the folding and unfolding of proteins, and the assembly of protein complexes. Moreover, HSPs have important roles in transporting proteins within cells, cell signaling, and protection and recovery from stress (e.g., Li and Srivastava 2004). They may also play a role in immune responses such as antigen presenting. They are expressed by all cells in response to heat and other stresses, and they also respond to signals not associated with the stress response (Feder and Hofmann 1999). Furthermore, patterns of HSP expression can be associated with resistance to stress and vary markedly among species (Feder and Hofmann 1999). As such, HSPs are key for cellular responses to stress.

Free radicals that are byproducts of aerobic metabolism can damage nuclear and mitochondrial DNA (Richter et al. 1988). Although cells have developed enzyme and non-enzyme systems to control and repair the effects of free radicals, sometimes high levels of aerobic metabolism overwhelm these systems, resulting in damage to proteins, lipids, and nucleic acids. This damage may be permanent or transient, contributing to aging and diseases. Enzyme systems exist to excise damaged sequences (lesions), and others assist repair (Wood 1996). Although the cellular aspects of responses to stress are important and widespread, we will focus in this book on the hormonal responses that orchestrate physiological and behavioral coping mechanisms.

Many rapid changes in physiology and behavior are controlled by the central and autonomic nervous systems (CNS and ANS). Other changes in response to the environment involve chemical messengers, including hormones that are secreted from cells within the organisms or into the environment (pheromones). We refer the reader to classic textbooks on endocrinology and behavior by Norris (2007) and Nelson (2011) and here we will give sufficient introduction for readers unfamiliar with the neural-endocrine system. There are short distance (local) messengers such as neurotransmitters and neuromodulators within the CNS and ANS. Others act over longer distances (i.e., organ to organ). Autocrine secretions are ultra-local signals and feedback on the cell that secreted it and similar nearby cells. Paracrine secretions are also locally acting, but the chemical messenger acts on neighboring, often dissimilar, cells (e.g., in the CNS, gastrointestinal tract). Endocrine secretions, from the Greek meaning "secrete within," are short- to long-distance chemical messengers secreted into blood or cerebrospinal fluid. These chemical messengers are called hormones—from a Greek verb meaning "to excite." Neuroendocrine secretions (i.e., neurons secreting hormones into blood) represent a critical link between the CNS and the perception of environmental signals, the responses of neural and non-neural tissues, and morphological, physiological, and behavioral outcomes.

Hormones each have a target tissue or tissues and act through interaction with a receptor molecule or molecules transducing the signal into cellular processes. The receptor molecule at the target cell determines the response to a hormone. Cells may have more than one type of receptor and can respond to different hormones that trigger responses as appropriate.

There is a complex cascade of events involved in the perception, integration, and transduction of environmental signals into chemical signals, which then initiate appropriate morphological, physiological, and behavioral adjustments (Wingfield 2006):

1. Specialized receptors (often sensory and very different from receptors for hormones) for specific external environmental signals transduce them into neural events.
2. Neural pathways from the specialized receptors project to target areas in the brain that integrate the environmental information in relation to internal physiological state (biological clock, social status, nutritional state, disease, etc.).
3. These target areas of the brain then signal specific neurons in the hypothalamus to release neurosecretions that initiate a hormonal cascade that in turn triggers appropriate adjustments of morphology, physiology, and behavior.
4. Neurosecretions and enzymes within the CNS can have separate regulatory effects on neuroendocrine secretions from the posterior pituitary into the blood circulation. Note also that internal signals (from the biological clock, social status, nutritional state, disease, etc.) may also act at the level of neurosecretions within the CNS.
5. Peripheral, blood-borne hormones (especially steroids) may feed back to act on the brain and alter responsiveness to environmental signals at the receptor,

target brain area, or neurosecretory
neuron levels. These effects may be further regulated by the biological clock, social status, nutritional state, disease, and so on.

Neural pathways for environmental signals can be very different among the types of signal (e.g., food, temperature, social etc.). Furthermore, these neural pathways may not always be stimulatory. Some may inhibit neurosecretion; others may release an inhibition rather than stimulate directly. An almost limitless spectrum of interconnected receptors, neural pathways, and neuromodulator mechanisms exist, but we still know very little about these critical first steps in response to environmental signals. Signals affecting the neuroendocrine/endocrine systems emanating from other individuals (social interactions) are also perceived by sensory receptors and are transduced by areas of the CNS that are very different from physical environmental signals.

Exactly how an organism perceives relevant environmental signals, and the influences those signals have, can be classified in two major ways. First, the effects may be directly on cells that respond with a physiological or morphological response (e.g., gut cells responding to changes in food composition) or are signalized through the CNS (e.g., de Wilde 1978; Wingfield 2006). In addition to external cues, internal signals also have important influences on the neuroendocrine and endocrine systems. Examples are classic homeostatic states, including plasma levels of amino acids, free fatty acids, sugars, vitamins, and so on. Other examples are osmoregulatory functions (salt/water balance), the immune system and disease, endogenous rhythms ("internal clock") and aging. However, the sensory receptors by which such signals are perceived are not completely known.

II. THE ENDOCRINE SYSTEM

The endocrine system is highly conserved among vertebrates, from fishes to humans (Gorbman et al. 1983; Norris 2007), with up to 85% similarity in types of hormones secreted (Wingfield 2006). Components of this system have similarly conserved anatomy that will be briefly described next.

A. The Hypothalamo-Pituitary Unit

Almost all integration and transduction of external and internal signals into neuroendocrine secretions occurs in the hypothalamus, which lies at the base of the brain just posterior to the optic lobes and optic chiasm (Figure 2.1). Neurons project to the base of the hypothalamus and terminate in two neurohemal secretory regions (Figures 2.1, 2.2, and 2.3): the *median eminence* and *pars nervosa* (or neurohypophysis, posterior pituitary gland). The third ventricle of the brain projects ventrally and posteriorly into the pars nervosa. Neurons projecting here have terminal fields that secrete hormones directly into the peripheral circulation (Figures 2.2 and 2.3). The median eminence also has terminal fields, but these release hormones into capillaries that coalesce into a specialized blood portal system that vascularizes the *anterior pituitary* (Figures. 2.2 and 2.3). In some species (e.g., birds) there is evidence of point-to-point circulation, that is, the anterior median eminence releases hormones into the anterior portal system that vascularizes the anterior, or cephalic, lobe of the anterior pituitary. There may be medial and posterior portal systems, too (Figure 2.3). This is the *hypothalamo-hypophysial portal system*. Releasing and inhibiting hormones can have rapid (i.e., release of hormones) and long-term (i.e., tropic) actions on endocrine cells in the anterior pituitary.

The hypothalamo-hypophysial unit is found throughout tetrapod vertebrates (i.e., median eminence plus the pars nervosa, portal system, and entire anterior pituitary). In osteichthyeans, especially the teleost fishes (Figure 2.4), the hypothalamo-hypophysial portal system is absent (or vestigial). Here both the pars nervosa and what would be the median eminence are in direct contact with the anterior pituitary, interdigitating with the tissues of the anterior pituitary. Thus neurohypophysial hormones are released directly into blood here, or releasing and inhibiting hormones are secreted into extra-vascular space to have paracrine actions on cells of the anterior pituitary. In Chondrichthyeans (sharks and rays) an intermediate situation is found. Here the pars nervosa is distinct from the anterior pituitary and there is a median eminence (see Kobayashi et al. 1987). The beginnings of a hypothalamo portal system can be found, and there is some very limited interdigitiation of the anterior pituitary by hypothalamic neurons. In the Agnatha (lampreys and hagfishes) what is perhaps the primitive (ancestral) condition is found. In lampreys the base of the hypothalamus and the pars nervosa are separated from the anterior pituitary by a layer of connective tissue (Kobayashi et al. 1987). This is even more pronounced in the hagfish (Kobayashi et al. 1987; Figure 2.5). It is thought that secretions

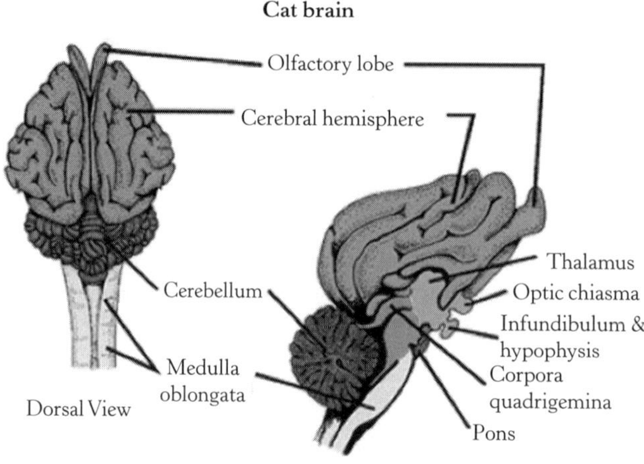

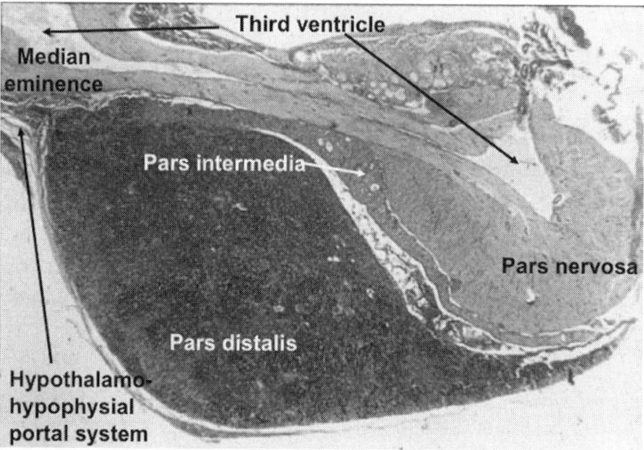

FIGURE 2.1: Section through cat pituitary showing typical mammalian hypothalamo-pituitary unit. Note two parts of the adenohypophysis (large *pars distalis* [darker area], and thin *par intermedia* [half darker area]), neurohypophysis with the *third ventricle* of brain.

of the pars nervosa enter the peripheral blood, as in all vertebrates, but that releasing and inhibiting hormones from hypothalamic neurons reach the anterior pituitary by diffusion across the connective tissue barrier, or through the peripheral blood circulation (Gorbman 1999).

Much has been written on how the association of the hypothalamus, pars nervosa, and anterior pituitary came to be (summarized in Gorbman et al. 1983; Gorbman 1999). The hypothalamus, pars nervosa, and median eminence are brain structures, but the anterior pituitary is derived from the pharynx. It is generally thought that the separation of the anterior pituitary from the hypothalamus is the ancestral scenario and that the fishes in general evolved an interdigitation of the anterior pituitary by hypothalamic neurons. Control of the anterior pituitary secretions is by direct neural input and paracrine secretions (Figure 2.4). However, some fish groups also had rudiments of a blood vascular system connecting part of the base of the hypothalamus with the anterior pituitary. The Sarcopterygeans (lung fish and Coelacanth) and tetrapods evolved the blood portal system as the major link between the hypothalamus and the anterior pituitary (Figure 2.2). This hypothalamo-pituitary blood portal system becomes particularly well developed in birds and mammals.

The pars distalis of the anterior pituitary (adenohypophysis) is a complex gland that produces at least six hormones. They have wide-ranging effects and also regulate the secretion of other endocrine glands, so much so that the anterior

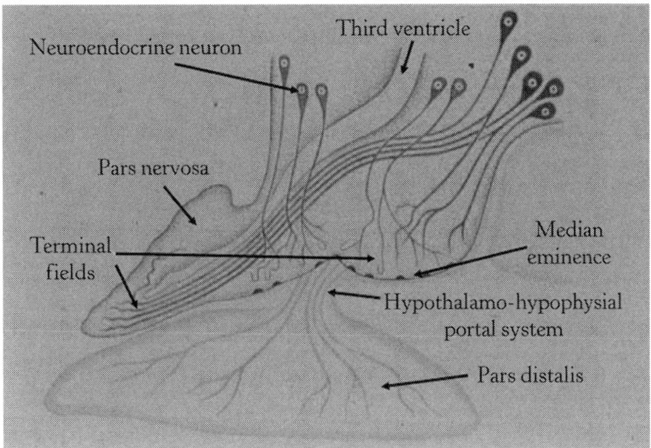

FIGURE 2.2: Diagram of an avian pituitary, showing the tracts of neurosecretory cells to the median eminence and the neurohypophysis. Note the third ventricle of the brain penetrating the neurohypophysis and the hypothalamo-hypophysial portal system connecting the median eminence with the adenohypophysis (anterior pituitary).

From Oksche and Farner (1974).

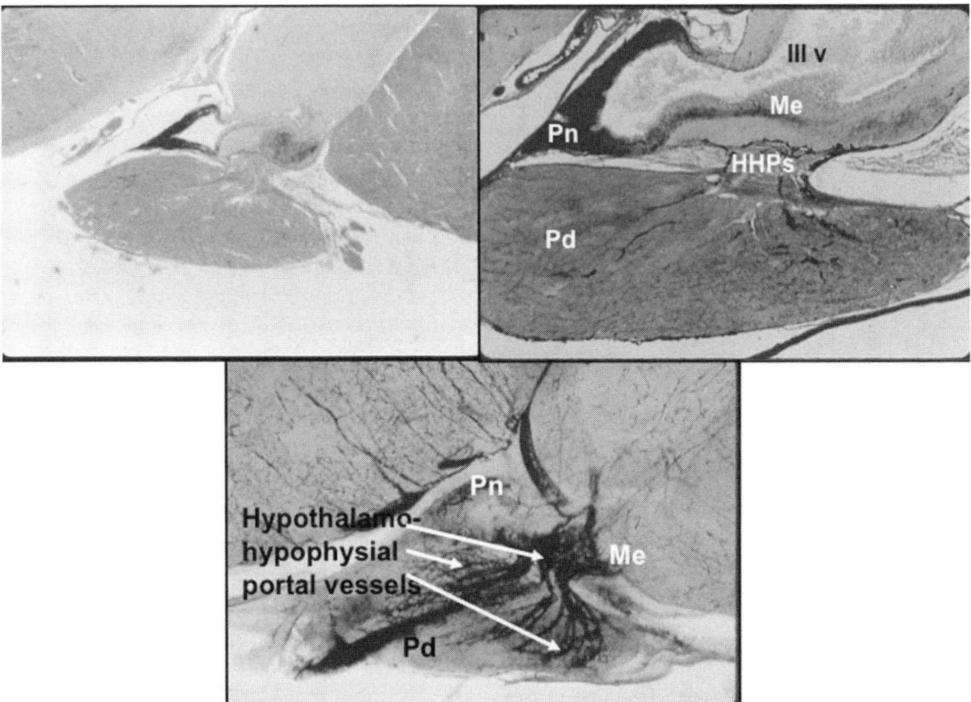

FIGURE 2.3: Diagram of areas of neurosecretory cells in a bird hypothalamo-hypophysial unit (low magnification upper left and higher magnification upper right). Note the vascular bed which forms the neurohemal organ in the neurohypophysis. Black/purple staining shows neurosecretory substances. Note the dark staining in both the median eminence and neurohypophysis (pointed dark stained object). You can also see the pink stained hypothalamo-hypophysial portal system. Lower panel is a section of the hypothalamo-hypophysial unit in a preparation in which blood vessles have been stained with India ink to show blood vessels. The hypothalamo-hypohysial portal vessels can be seen clearly. Orientation of the section is identical to the stained sections above.

Pd = pars distalis, or adenohypophysis (anterior pituitary); Pn = pars nervosa (posterior pituitary); Me = median eminence; IIIv = third ventricle; HHPs = hypothalamo-hypophysial portal system.

From Mikami et al. (1970). Courtesy of Springer-Verlag.

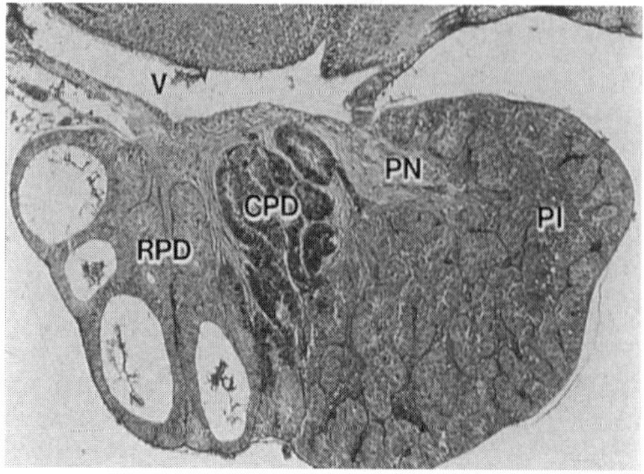

FIGURE 2.4: Section of a teleost (trout) hypothalamo-pituitary unit. Note direct innervation of the adenohypophysis by the hypothalamus, and lack of a portal system. Also note that the pars nervosa is intermingled with the pars intermedia, forming a neurointermediate lobe.

RPD = Rostral pars distalis; CPD = Caudal pars distalis; PI = pars intermedia; PN = pars nervosa; V = third ventricle.

From Kobayashi et al. (1987). Courtesy of Kodansha Lyd., Tokyo.

pituitary is often referred to as the "master gland." Hypophysectomy (surgical removal of the anterior pituitary) has very severe and multiple effects on the vertebrate organism. This experimental approach indicated three major families of anterior pituitary hormones:

1. Growth hormone and prolactin (polypeptides).
2. Glycoproteins: thyroid-stimulating hormone (TSH), luteinizing hormone (LH), and follicle-stimulating hormone (FSH). All are glycoproteins assembled as dimers in which one subunit is common to all.
3. Pro-opiomelanocortin (POMC) hormones: adrenocorticotropin (ACTH), melanocyte-stimulating hormone (MSH), and endorphin. All are peptides cleaved off the POMC precursor molecule.

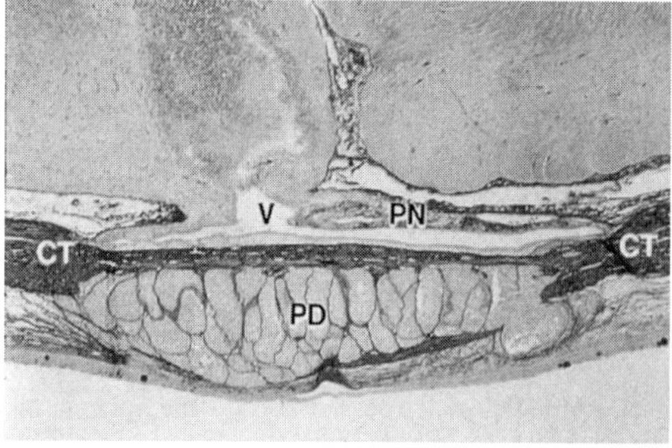

FIGURE 2.5: Section of hagfish (Agnathan) pituitary. Note: no portal system or median eminence. Cartilage (CT) separates pars distalis (PD) from brain.

PN = pars nervosa; V = third ventricle; ME = median eminence.

From Kobayashi et al. (1987). Courtesy of Kodansha Lyd., Tokyo.

Later, immunocytochemical techniques and in situ hybridization showed that some cells may secrete more than one hormone in a gene family, but each cell does not synthesize and release more than one family of hormones.

B. The Pro-opiomelanocortin (POMC) Derived Hormones: Endogenous Opiates (Endorphins), Adrenocorticotropin (ACTH), and the Adrenal Cortex, Alpha-Melanocyte-Stimulating Hormone (α-MSH)

Endorphins are a group of 10 neurosecretory peptides that activate opiate receptors. They are composed of chains of amino acids between five and several dozen members long. Since the discovery of the endorphins in 1975, researchers have hypothesized that they are released into synapses when the body encounters stress. Endorphins also appear in cerebrospinal fluid and can be released into blood, suggesting that they can have paracrine and endocrine actions. After physical injury, endorphins activate opiate receptors and produce an analgesic effect, alleviating severe pain. During times of emotional stress, endorphins are released in the limbic system of the brain and produce a euphoria that lessens anxiety and melancholy.

Recently, scientists have hypothesized that the release of endorphins is the neurochemical cause for the feeling of pleasure. For example, a marathon runner's "high," which has been compared to the "rush" following opioid use, is the product of endorphin release. Unlike synthetic or plant opioids, the body's endorphins are not addicting. When endorphins are not activating receptors, no withdrawal symptoms are felt. Enzymes break down endorphins as soon as they act at receptors, so they are never in contact with receptors long enough to form tolerance or dependency.

Endorphins also interact with dopamine (a neurotransmitter) involved in reward and reinforcement processes, and the nucleus accumbens (NAc) is a brain region involved in mediating alcohol's positive reinforcing effects. Beta endorphin (β-EP) is a neurotransmitter

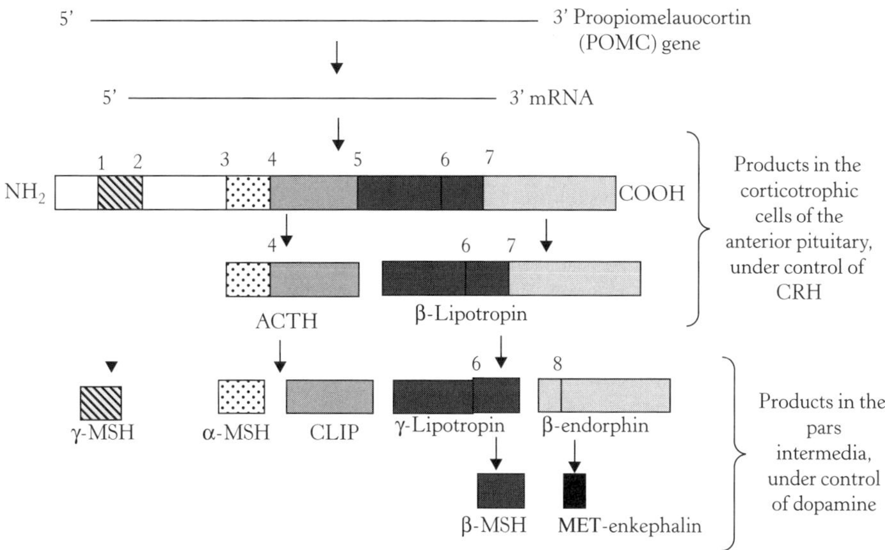

FIGURE 2.6: Pro-opio-melanocortin (POMC) is expressed in corticotroph cells of the vertebrate anterior pituitary. Endopeptidases in corticoptroph cells can cleave POMC to give various peptide fragments (as indicated by block colors). Some of these endopeptidases are under the control of corticotrophin-releasing hormone (CRH) from the hypothalamus, resulting in the production of adrenocorticotropic hormone (ACTH) and beta-lipotropin. In the pars intermedia (e.g., of some mammals) dopamine results in cleavage of POMC to give a further variety of peptides such as melanocyte-stimulating hormone (MSH) and endorphin and MET-enkephalin. In species that lack a pars intermedia, endorphin is cleaved in the corticotroph. CLIP is a fragment of unknown function. The major peptides of interest in this chapter are ACTH, endorphin, enkephalin, and alpha-MSH.

produced in the arcuate nucleus of the hypothalamus (ArcN) by nerve cells (i.e., neurons) that extend to other brain regions, including the ventral tegmental area (VTA) and the NAc. β-EP can stimulate dopamine release in the NAc through two mechanisms. First, it can interfere with (i.e., inhibit) neurons in the VTA that produce gamma-aminobutyric acid (GABA), a neurotransmitter that normally inhibits the dopamine-producing neurons in the VTA. Inhibition of GABA production leads to increased dopamine production and release in the NAc. Second, β-EP can directly stimulate (i.e., excite) dopamine-producing neurons in the NAc. Alcohol stimulates β-EP release in both the VTA and NAc. Classically there are three major receptor types for opiate peptides—mu, delta, and kappa, each linked to G proteins. Mu and delta receptors mediate many actions of endogenous opiates as well as synthetic and plant opiates, whereas the kappa receptor is less well known. Nalaxone is used widely as an antagonist of β-endorphin in experimental studies.

Some cells of the pars distalis and pars intermedia express α-melanocyte-stimulating hormone (α-MSH), β-MSH, and γ-MSH cleaved from the POMC precursor (Figure 2.6). CLIP, a cleavage product from ACTH when α-MSH is formed, has no known biological function (Figure 2.6). These MSHs form the melanocortin group. They have a spectrum of effects including pigment formation and dispersion in skin of lower vertebrates, and effects on fever in the brain. The well-known role of α-MSH in the control of pigment in lower vertebrates involves the capacity to change color rapidly—in minutes to hours. Mammals and birds can also change color, but this requires days to weeks and often a molt or development of special pigmented skin.

α-MSH may mimic ACTH, especially in the mammalian fetus. This is not surprising because it is the same as the first 13 amino acids of ACTH. α-MSH also can increase memory retention as a brain peptide, but this source of MSH is probably central (i.e., the arcuate nucleus of the hypothalamus) rather than from the pars distalis or pars intermedia. In lizards there is evidence for a thermoregulatory role of α-MSH; for example, in the lizard *Sceloporus*, individuals are dark in the morning (to absorb heat from the sun), but much paler during the heat of the day. There is evidence that α-MSH may also regulate temperature—especially fever—in mammals, although again this MSH may be of central origin, acting as a brain peptide.

Another action of α-MSH found in the brain is to suppress appetite. Some cases of extreme obesity have been traced to mutations in the brain receptor for α-MSH. Presumably these people are unable to respond to the appetite-suppressing effect of their α-MSH. There is growing evidence that α-MSH has many additional effects, especially in the brain, that are a probable result of central expression and autocrine/paracrine actions.

Adrenocorticotropin (ACTH) is a 39 amino sequence cleaved off the POMC molecule (Figure 2.6). Amino acids 1–24 are essential for biological action and are highly conserved across vertebrate classes. ACTH release is regulated by several brain peptides (Figures 2.7 and 2.8). One of these, corticotropin-releasing hormone (CRH), is released from the median eminence and acts through G-protein receptors on corticotroph cells in the anterior pituitary. Increased cAMP levels result in rapid cleavage of ACTH from POMC and its secretion into the general bloodstream via exocytosis (Figure 2.8). The other peptides, arginine vasopressin (AVP) and oxytocin in mammals, arginine vasotocin (AVT) and mesotocin in other vertebrates, may also influence the secretion of ACTH. Note that CRH also can regulate gene transcription of POMC. The primary action of ACTH is on the adrenal cortex to produce glucocorticosteroids (see further discussion later in this chapter).

The adrenal glands are always associated with the kidneys. In mammals they are distinct glands (Figure 2.9), just anterior to the kidney, with a distinct cortex separate from a medulla (Figure 2.9). The cortex secretes corticosteroids, whereas the medulla is totally separate and secretes catecholamines under sympathetic nervous control (see further discussion later in this chapter). The mammalian adrenal cortex is arranged in zones of cells (Figure 2.10). The outer zone, or *zona glomerulosa*, consists of whorls of cells (Figure 2.10) that secrete aldosterone (the mineralocorticosteroid). Next is the *zona fasiculata* with columnar cells secreting glucocorticosteroids. The inner layer is the *zona reticularis* (Figure 2.10), formed of a network of cells also secreting steroids and possibly sex steroids in some species. This zones lies next to the medulla (Figure 2.10).

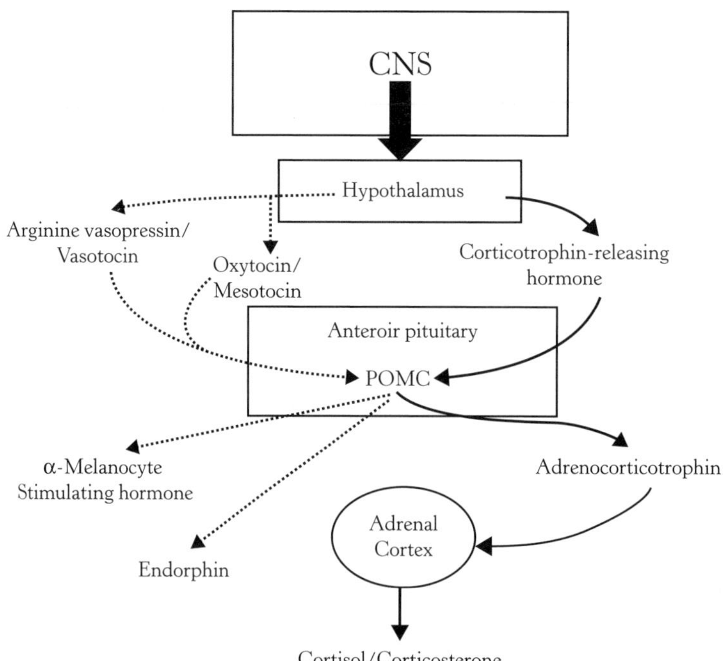

FIGURE 2.7: Schematic diagram of the hormone cascade in the hypothalamo-pituitary-adrenal cortex of vertebrates.

From (Wingfield 2005), courtesy of Elsevier Press.

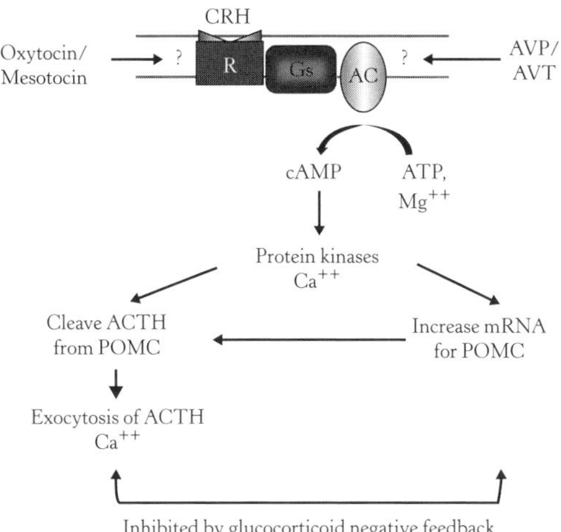

FIGURE 2.8: Actions of corticotropin-releasing hormone (CRH) in a corticotroph of the anterior pituitary. CRH binds to its membrane receptor (R), and activates a stimulatory G protein (Gs). This in turn activates adenylyl cyclase (AC), which results in conversion of ATP to cyclic AMP (magnesium ions required). cAMP activates protein kinases, which through phosphorylation and presence of Ca ions can have rapid effects to cleave ACTH from POMC and later effects to increase gene transcription for the POMC molecule. ACTH is released by exocytosis into the blood (Ca ions required). All these processes can be inhibited by negative feedback from glucocorticoids.

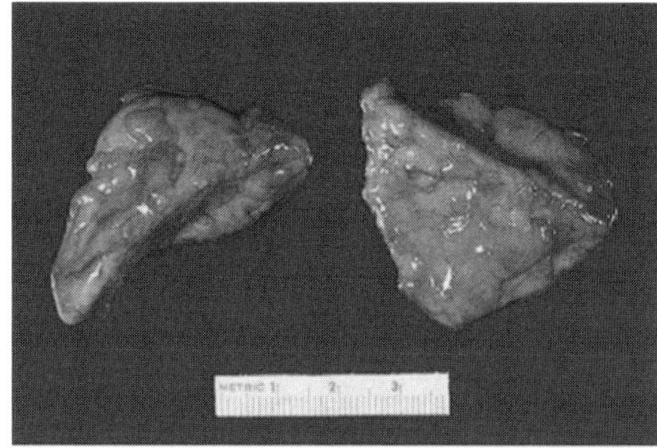

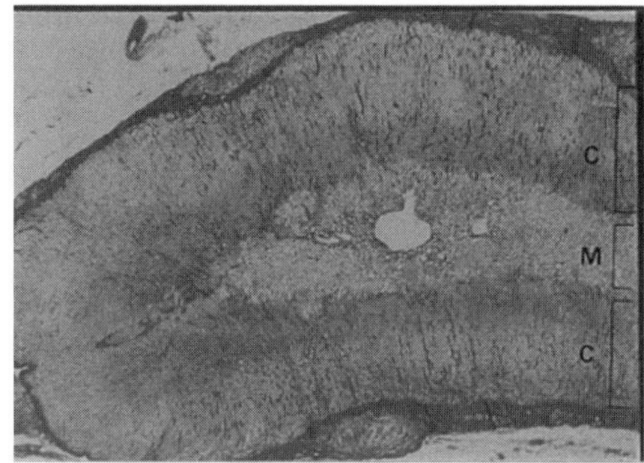

FIGURE 2.9: Normal human adrenal glands (top panel). Each adult adrenal gland weighs from 4 to 6 grams. They are located just anterior to the kidney, hence the name "ad-renal." Cross section of mouse adrenal (lower panel) reveals two major components, the cortex (C), and medulla (M).

The adrenal glands of vertebrates show great variation in structure (Figures 2.10 and 2.11). In mammals the glands are always paired and lie at the anterior end of the kidney. The shape and ratio of cortical cells to medulla may vary (Figure 2.10). In birds, the adrenals are also paired (Figure 2.10); the separation of a cortex and medulla in two different glands is not found. Groups of adrenocortical and medullary cells are found mixed throughout the gland. Since the medullary cells are no longer forming a true medulla, they are known as chromaffin (although they have exactly the same function as mammalian medullary cells). The adrenocortical cells may show some simple zonation, and recent work suggests that this may have functional significance, too (i.e. one zone secretes aldosterone, the other corticosterone; Carsia et al. 1987). In reptiles, adrenocortical cells may be more separate from chromaffin cells but not in the mammalian way (Figure 2.10). Other species show varying degrees of mixing. The adrenal is associated with the mesonephric kidney in anuran amphibians, and is usually on the dorsal surface. Again, adrenocortical and chromaffin tissues are mixed. In urodeles there may be irregular accumulations on the ventral surface of the kidney, between, or even embedded in the kidney itself. In the latter case it is called an interrenal gland (i.e., within the kidney). In bony fish (Osteichthys) adrenocortical and chromaffin tissues are associated with lymphatic tissue in the head kidney (Figure 2.11). In cartilaginous fish adrenocortical cells are associated with the mesonephric kidney, but chromaffin cells are still interrenal (Figure 2.11). The agnathans have catecholaminergic cells along the large veins of the peritoneal cavity and in the heart. Putative adrenocortical cells are found in the head kidney and walls of the cardinal vein, although it is still not clear whether they produce significant quantities of corticosteroids (Figure 2.11).

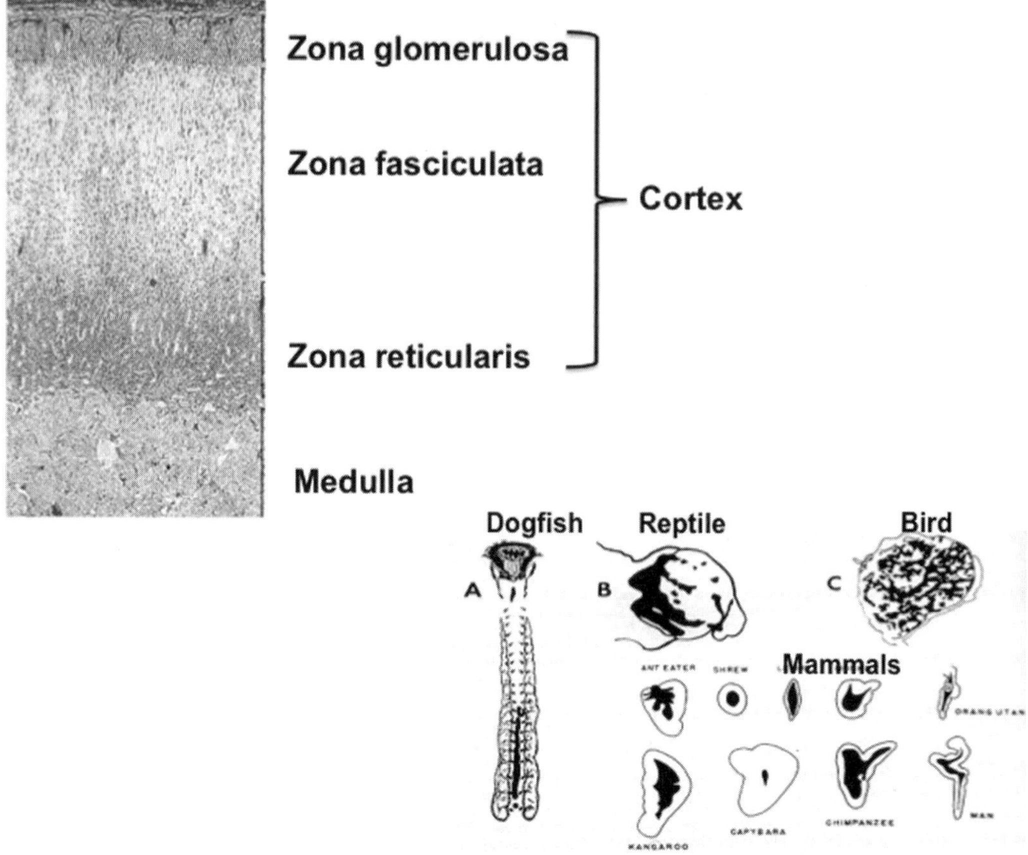

FIGURE 2.10: Higher magnification of the zonation of the mammalian adrenal gland showing the locations of specific zones (top panel). Distribution of adrencortical and medullary (chromaffin) tissue in the adrenal (interrenal) glands of vertebrates (lower panel).

From von Euler and Heller (1963). Courtesey of Academic Press.

III. THE HYPOTHALAMO-PITUITARY- ADRENAL CORTEX AXIS AND THE GLUCOCORTICOID RESPONSE

Circulating levels of glucocorticoids have become perhaps the most common index of stress. In fact, many researchers have used a working definition that a stressor is a stimulus that causes an increase in glucocorticoid release. In many ways this makes sense. Noxious and threatening stimuli almost invariably lead to glucocorticoid release, and much of the pathology associated with stress is a result of glucocorticoid excess. Furthermore, since the middle of the last century, the vast majority of research on stress has focused on the glucocorticoids and has virtually ignored the sympathetic response. In this section we will review the glucocorticoid arm of the stress response, including how glucocorticoids are released, how they exert their effects, and their broad physiological role in orchestrating day-to-day metabolism, as well as the response to stress.

The major glucocorticoids present in vertebrates (Table 2.1) include cortisol as the primary glucocorticoid in all major taxa of osteichthyean fish and in most mammals, including humans. Corticosterone is the primary glucocorticoid in all other vertebrate taxa, including reptiles, amphibians, birds, and many rodents, with the one exception of 1α-hydroxycorticosterone found in chondrichthyean fish such as sharks and rays (Idler 1972). The glucocorticoids (Figure 2.12) are steroid hormones synthesized from cholesterol (Figure 2.13), with P-450_{c11} as the final synthetic enzyme for both steroids (Norris 1997). Note that biologically active steroids have

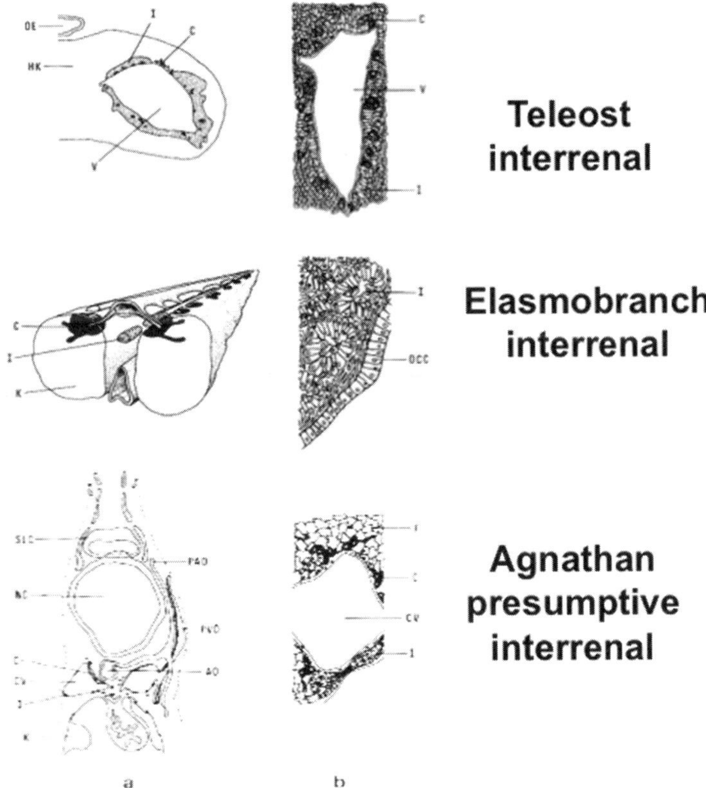

FIGURE 2.11: Diagram of the distribution of interrenal and chromaffin tissue in fishes.
C = chromaffin, HK = head kidney, I = interrenal, K = kidney, V = vein.
From Chester-Jones and Phillips (1986). Courtesey of Academic Press.

a similar structure and an international convention on nomenclature (Figure 2.12). Metyrapone is a drug that interferes with P-450_{c11} and consequently has been used in many experiments to decrease cortisol and corticosterone production. Unfortunately, metyrapone has a side effect of making many animals lethargic and appear sick (personal observations). Dexamethasone is a synthetic glucocorticoid that has been used in a number of recent experiments in free-living animals (Table 2.1).

TABLE 2.1: EXAMPLES OF CORTICOSTEROIDS

Major Corticosteroids	Taxa
Cortisol	Fish, mammals (except some rodents)
Corticosterone	Reptiles, amphibians, birds, rodents
Dexamethasone	Synthetic

Glucocorticoid release is the culmination of an endocrine cascade that begins in the brain (Figure 2.14). Many stressors, especially the psychological stressors, require a cognitive assessment of the stimulus to determine whether it is a stressor. Clearly, there must be decision circuits in the brain that act as gatekeepers that determine which raw sensory information coming from visual, olfactory, and aural systems gets passed on to initiate an endocrine response. There has been substantial work trying to identify these "stress circuits," and even though progress has been hampered by the stressor-specific nature of the neurocircuits (Day 2005), a consensus is building that in mammals much of this gatekeeping function is performed by the amygdala (Labar and Ledoux 2001) and the hippocampus (McEwen 2001). Both of these structures are part of the limbic system. The amygdala helps regulate fear and emotion (Labar and Ledoux 2001),

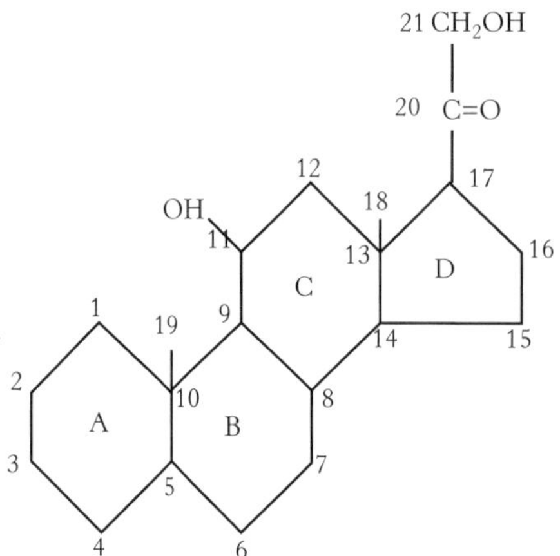

FIGURE 2.12: Structure of a glucocorticosteroid showing the convention of nomenclature for ring structures and carbon atoms. Note that all biologically active glucocorticoids have a hydroxyl group at carbon 11 and a "side chain" at carbon 17. This example is corticosterone. Cortisol has an additional hydroxyl group at carbon 17, and elasmobranchs have a unique glucocorticoid with a hydroxyl group at carbon 1 (1α-hydroxy-corticosterone). However, all must have a hydroxyl at carbon 11. These glucocococorticoids are deactivated if the hydroxyl at carbon 11 is changed to a ketone group. Cells in target tissues, liver, and so on, have enzymes (11β-hydroxysteroid dehydrogenases) that regulate this conversion and may represent additional important foci of regulation for glucocorticoid action.

and the hippocampus is a main site for memory storage (McEwen 2001). It makes intuitive sense that both would be involved in interpreting stimuli. In both structures, an important neurotransmitter for the gatekeeper function appears to be corticotropin-releasing factor (CRF). As we have already seen, CRF is also an important hormone in the neuroendocrine-endocrine cascade (Figures 2.6–2.8). This suggests that CRF plays a central role in regulating the stress response at multiple levels. Interestingly, however, the neurotransmitter function of CRF in the brain is mediated by a different receptor (the CRF type II receptor) than the endocrine function of CRF (the CRF type I receptor) (Weninger and Majzoub 2001). Because CRF serves a neurotransmitter role (as well as other roles in the immune system, etc.) and not just a hormone role, it was recently proposed that CRF was a better nomenclature than corticotropin-releasing hormone (i.e., CRH; Hauger et al. 2003).

Once the hippocampus and amygdala decide that the stimulus is, in fact, a stressor, a neuronal signal is sent to the hypothalamus. The primary neurotransmitters involved in relaying this signal appear to be the catecholamines, epinephrine and norepinephrine (Goldstein and Pacak 2001), again showing that there is considerable cross-talk between the fight-or-flight and the HPA responses. The region of the hypothalamus that is activated is the paraventricular nucleus, so named because of its proximity to the third ventricle, part of the system of open spaces (ventricles) in the brain that contain cerebrospinal fluid (CSF). Many of the physiological functions of the paraventricular nucleus have been delineated by injecting various drugs into the third ventricle (e.g., Maney and Wingfield 1998). The paraventricular nucleus has three important cell types for the classical stress response: those that synthesize CRF; those that synthesize arginine vasopressin (AVP); and those that synthesize both CRF and AVP (Whitnall 1993). AVP is present in mammals, and arginine vasotocin (AVT) serves the same function in birds, reptiles, and amphibians (e.g., Carsia et al. 1987) Although these neurons have their cell bodies in the paraventricular nucleus, they send their axons to the median eminence and they store their CRF and/or AVP in secretory vesicles in the terminals of these axons.

Upon receiving the appropriate signal, the cells in the paraventricular nucleus release their CRF and/or AVP into the blood of the hypothalamic-pituitary portal vasculature (Figures 2.2 and 2.3). The portal vasculature contains three structures. First, a capillary plexus in the median eminence collects the released CRF and AVP. Second, this plexus drains into short portal veins that traverse the pituitary stalk that connects the pituitary to the hypothalamus. Finally, the portal vessels form a second capillary plexus in the pars distalis of the pituitary (Figures 2.2 and 2.3). The purpose of this system is to deliver the hypothalamic releasing factors to the pituitary in locally high concentrations. Delivery of CRF seems to be inhibited by having a CRF-binding protein (CRF-BP) that prevents CRF from binding to its receptors in the pituitary (Turnbull and Rivier 1997). In fish, because of the direct anatomical connection between the hypothalamus and the pituitary (Kobayashi et al. 1987), CRF reaches the pituitary via paracrine means (Figure 2.4). In agnathans (Figure 2.5) a direct anatomical connection from the hypothalamus to the pars distalis is lacking, and presumably CRF reaches the pituitary via the peripheral circulation and/or by diffusion (Gorbman 1999). However, CRF-BP appears to

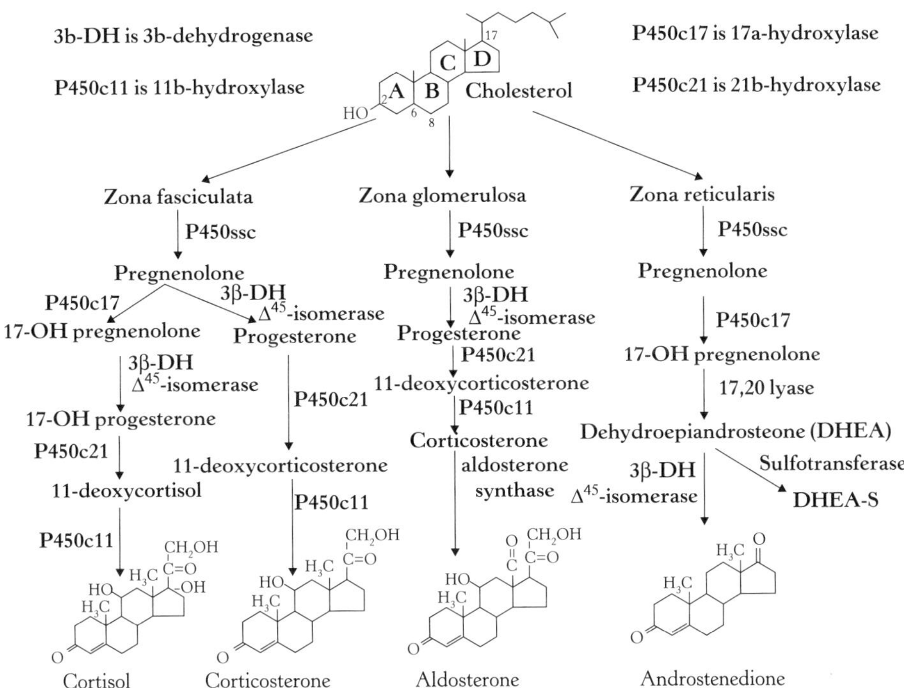

FIGURE 2.13: The formation of adrenal cortical steroids by zone. The glucocorticoids are synthesized in the *zona fasiculata*. The principal enzymes involved are named at the top of the figure. The *zona glomerulosa* is the site of synthesis of the mineralocorticoid, aldosterone. The *zona reticularis* of mammals is a source of weak androgens such as androstenedione and dehydroepiandrosterone. Note also that progesterone is an intermediary product that may also be secreted by the adrenal of some species.

be highly conserved and present in fish as well (Huising et al. 2004).

Once CRF and AVP reach the pituitary (Figure 2.8), they stimulate ACTH release from the corticotropes (CRF and AVP are collectively called secretagogs because they stimulate the secretion of ACTH). Consequently, the next product in the endocrine cascade is the release of ACTH. CRF binds to the CRF type I receptor (Rivier et al. 2003) and stimulates ACTH release via a cAMP pathway (Antoni 1993). AVP binds to the V_1 receptor and stimulates ACTH release via an IP_3 pathway (Antoni 1993). CRF is the most potent secretagog in most mammals (Vale et al. 1981), although AVP is more potent in some mammals, such as sheep (Minton 1994). In most mammals AVP is a weak secretagog for ACTH, but AVP can synergize with CRF and produce a stronger ACTH response than a simple addition of the two secretagogs (Antoni 1993). As a consequence, CRF is generally thought to provide the "scaffolding" for the ACTH response, whereas AVP often fine-tunes the response. Other hormones have been implicated as ACTH secretagogs, but evidence for a physiological role for most of them is sparse. The one possible exception is oxytocin (OT), which may play a significant role in some species (Romero and Sapolsky 1996), but it is not presently clear how taxonomically widespread is the use of OT (or the non-mammalian congener mesotocin).

Although these mechanisms have primarily been elucidated in rats, the few studies that have examined these details in non-mammalian vertebrates have largely confirmed the generality of these results. In birds, the HPA axis architecture is similar to mammals, with pituitary ACTH controlling adrenal glucocorticoid release (Mikami and Yamada 1984; Mikami 1986). CRF, arginine vasotocin (AVT), and mesotocin (MT) are present in the median eminence of the hypothalamus (Mikami and Yamada 1984; Mikami 1986; Ball et al. 1989) and are known to control ACTH secretion (Carsia et al. 1986; Castro et al. 1986), presumably via the hypothalamic-pituitary portal blood. AVT and MT appear to play similar roles in ACTH secretion in birds as AVP and OT do in mammals (Castro et al. 1986). Similar work in reptiles (reviewed by Tokarz and Summers 2011) has confirmed this general pattern, although

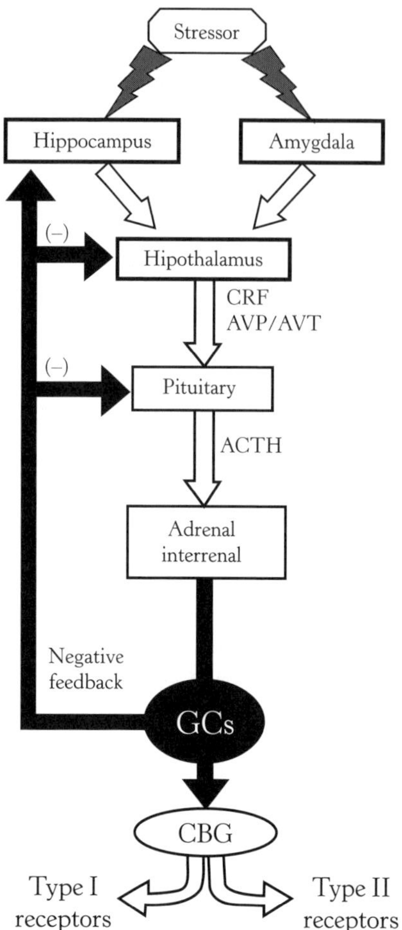

FIGURE 2.14: The main components of the hypothalamic-pituitary-adrenal (HPA) axis involved in stress. The axis begins with a stressor being detected by the brain, and after a cascade of steps, results in glucocorticoids (GCs) being released into the plasma.

CRF = corticotropin releasing factor; AVP = arginine vasopressin; AVT = arginine vasotocin; ACTH = adrenocorticotropin hormone; CBG = corticosteroid binding globulin.

recent data suggest that natriuretic peptides play an inhibitory role in ACTH release (Carsia and John-Alder 2006). In fish CRF also plays a central role in ACTH release (Flik et al. 2006). Furthermore, the molecular regulation of CRF function appears to be highly conserved across taxa (Yao and Denver 2007).

One exception to the centrality of CRF in the HPA axis is that AVP and/or AVT may be the most potent secretagog in some species. In sheep (e.g., Familari et al. 1989) and many bird species (e.g., Castro et al. 1986; Carsia et al. 1987; Carsia 1990; Rich and Romero 2005), CRF is a weaker secretagog. The specific structure of CRF can vary by species, so that some of these results may come from the native CRF receptors having a lower affinity for the specific CRF administered (currently only ovine, porcine, and rat/human CRFs are commercially available). However, recent work suggests that CRFs can be conserved (for example, chicken CRF is identical in structure to rat/human CRF (Vandenborne et al. 2005a), and both in vitro (Carsia et al. 1987) and in vivo (Rich and Romero 2005) studies in birds can show a stronger secretagog function for AVP. What it means physiologically for a species to have a lower secretagog function for CRF is not currently known, but it has some potentially interesting ramifications for glucocorticoid negative feedback (see discussion later in this chapter).

One major question in the early study of the hypothalamic-pituitary portion of the HPA pathway was why more than one hypothalamic-releasing hormone existed for ACTH. Historically, CRF was the last of the hypothalamic-releasing hormones to be discovered and isolated (Vale et al. 1981), in part because other hormones, particularly AVP but also OT and epinephrine (Epi), also showed ACTH secretagog properties. It is now clear that the relative contribution of each secretagog to releasing ACTH depends upon the stressor. Different stressors elicit different mixtures of CRF and AVP by stimulating different subsets of the CRF, AVP, or CRF + AVP containing paraventricular nucleus neurons (Plotsky 1991; Antoni 1993). Other secretagogs may play a role as well (Romero and Sapolsky 1996). There appear to be three major advantages for using multiple secretagogs, even though the end result in all cases is ACTH release. First, both CRF and AVP have functions other than as ACTH secretagogs, and the relative mix might facilitate these other functions. Second, the differences in potency between the secretagogs means that the relative mix can fine-tune ACTH release. Since glucocorticoid responses are proportional to the severity of the stressor (see Chapter 3), this could be a mechanism to produce graded glucocorticoid responses. Additionally, an enhanced use of AVP could protect against excessive negative feedback. Glucocorticoid negative feedback primarily decreases CRF release. AVP is relatively insensitive to the feedback signal (Scaccianoce et al. 1991; Degoeij et al. 1992; Bartanusz et al. 1993). Consequently, by preferentially releasing AVP, ACTH can continue to be released, despite a strong negative feedback signal. This response can have important consequences. Imagine an animal that has recently survived a predation attempt, has released massive amounts of glucocorticoids, and has now shut down the HPA axis via negative feedback. Without a mechanism to circumvent negative feedback, that animal would be unable to mount another rapid response if it were attacked again. Removing AVP from the negative feedback loop plays the vital role of allowing an animal to maintain a glucocorticoid response for long periods and to ignore the negative feedback signal.

As should be clear from the preceding discussion, the pituitary is a major integrative point in the HPA axis. Several signals are integrated at the pituitary, and the end result is ACTH release. Several other POMC products (Figure 2.6), especially α-MSH and β-endorphins, have been reported to be released concurrently with ACTH (e.g., Tonon et al. 1986; Kjaer et al. 1992). Although potential roles for these peptides in the stress response are not well studied, α-MSH has been implicated in stimulation of cortisol release during chronic stress in some fish species (Metz et al. 2005; Flik et al. 2006). In rats acute restraint stress (Kant et al. 1986) and prolonged stress (1.5 cm of water in cages) resulted initially in elevated mRNA for POMC in the pars intermedia and an increase in plasma levels of α-MSH (Ogawa et al. 2009). Later the melanotrophs showed signs of degeneration, possibly as a result of decreased dopamine release from the hypothalamus, suggesting that chronic stress can result in a breakdown of α-MSH responses. Centrally acting α-MSH reduces stress-induced sickness behavior associated with infection in guinea pig pups (Schiml-Webb et al. 2006) that presumably would be reversed in chronic stress (Ogawa et al. 2009). Intra-peritoneal administration of α-MSH had no effect on sickness behavior (Schiml-Webb et al. 2006). In fish such as the carp, α-MSH is secreted along with ACTH and cortisol in stressed larvae (Stouthart et al. 1998) and adults (Metz et al. 2005). Furthermore, α-MSH receptors (melanocortin 2 and 5) were expressed in adrenocortical cells in carp (Metz et al. 2005). Moreover, Sumpter et al. (1985) found significant increases in α-MSH levels following a combination of thermal shock and handling stress in brown trout. The role of α-MSH in the stress response may appear to be widespread in non-mammalian vertebrates, but is much less well studied than in mammals.

The major roles of endorphins in the stress response appear to be behavioral through neuromodulatory actions (e.g., Amir et al. 1980). Blood levels of endorphin increased in stress situations (e.g., inexperienced parachutists), whereas levels of other brain peptides such as substance P did not (Schedlowski et al. 1995). There were also marked increases in plasma levels of endorphins in rats (Kant et al. 1986), and brown trout exposed to handling, confinement, and thermal shock showed elevations in ACTH and cortisol (Sumpter et al. 1985). Comparative aspects of endorphin responses to stress remain unclear.

Once released, ACTH travels to the adrenal tissue via the peripheral blood circulation. The targets of ACTH are corticosteroidogenic cells of the adrenal. However, there is growing evidence that ACTH can have effects independent of corticosteroids and that they are sometimes regulated independently (Bornstein et al. 2008). The lack of a distinct adrenal gland in many lower vertebrates (Figures 2.9–2.11) removes one of the powerful techniques in the endocrinologists' arsenal—the extirpation/replacement experiment. Mammalian stress physiologists have taken full advantage of removing the adrenals (adrenalectomy) and using various replacement regimens to understand glucocorticoid functions at various concentrations. Adrenalectomy is clearly impossible in other vertebrates because removing all the corticosteroidogenic cells would require removing the kidneys (Figures 2.9–2.11), which would prove lethal. There have been several attempts to perform chemical adrenalectomies, using drugs to destroy the corticosteroidogenic cells, including the use of metyrapone (see earlier discussion) and mitotane (Breuner et al. 2000), but these drugs have their own problems and have not been widely used.

ACTH binds to a membrane-bound receptor (Figure 2.15) on the steroidogenic cell and initiates both cAMP and Ca^{2+} second messenger systems (Hall 2001). ACTH increases corticosteroid synthesis in two ways (Hall 2001). The initial response is a rapid (within seconds to minutes) increase in the transport of cholesterol, the initial building block of all steroids, to the corticosteroid synthetic enzymes. This results in the release of corticosteroids into the veins of the adrenal within approximately one minute. Corticosteroids are not stored, so that increases in plasma concentrations are a direct result of increases in steroid synthesis. With long-term ACTH stimulation (days to weeks), ACTH stimulates an increase in corticosteroidogenic cells, leading to adrenal hypertrophy, and an increase in each cell's production of the four P-450 enzymes (Figure 2.13) that comprise the steroidogenic pathway. Initially, increasing concentrations of ACTH result in increasing release of glucocorticoids. However, as shown in

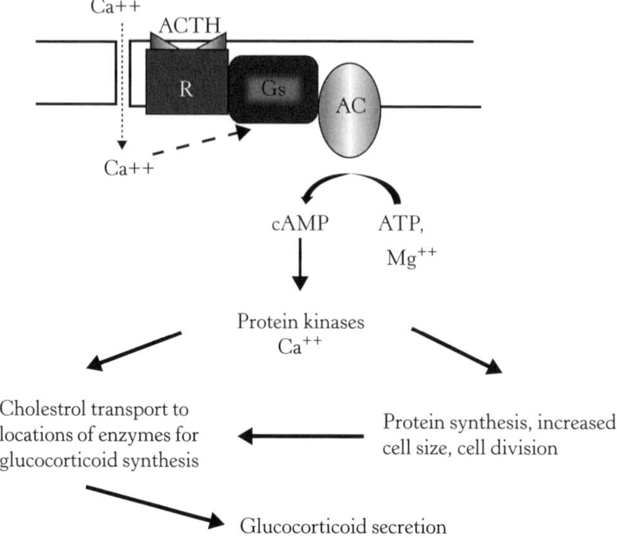

FIGURE 2.15: Adrenocorticotropin (ACTH) binds to its membrane receptor (R) on a zona fasiculata cell in the adrenal cortex, resulting in opening of calcium ion channels and activation of a stimulatory G protein (Gs). This in turn activates adenylyl cyclase (AC), which converts ATP to cyclic AMP (Mg ions required). cAMP activates protein kinases and through phosphorylations and Ca ions rapidly triggers the transport of cholesterol from stores in lipid droplets to locations (smooth endoplasmic reticulum and specialized mitochondria with tubular cristae) where enyzmes result in biosynthesis of glucocortoids. Glucocorticoids such as cortisol and corticosterone are released immediately (i.e., they are not stored—only cholesterol is stored in lipid droplets). Through a slower process, phosphorylations can result in the activation of a gene transcription factor CREB to promote protein synthesis for the transport of cholesterol and biosynthetic enzymes, as well as an increase in cell size, activity, and cell division (e.g., hypertrophy of the adrenal in chronic stress).

Figure 2.16, the response is quickly saturated, and higher ACTH concentrations serve to lengthen rather than augment glucocorticoid release (Dallman et al. 1987).

There are other inputs to the adrenal tissue that can modulate corticosteroid release. Natriuretic peptides, hormones produced by the heart and the brain whose main role is in the regulation of fluid balance, appear to directly inhibit corticosteroid release at the adrenal. Natriuretic peptides inhibited corticosteroid release from lizard adrenal cells maintained in vitro, even in conjunction with moderate amounts of ACTH (Carsia and John-Alder 2006). However, it is not clear yet whether the natriuretic peptides play a physiological role in regulating corticosteroid release in vivo.

There is also evidence that corticosteroid concentrations can decrease rapidly in some contexts. Perhaps the best-known example is from rats trained to drink for only a short period during the day. When they are provided water at the accustomed time, corticosterone concentrations decrease in less than 5 minutes (e.g., Romero et al. 1995). This time span is far too short to result from a simple decrease in ACTH stimulation (Wotus and Engeland 2003). Instead, AVP can regulate corticosteroid release directly from the adrenal (Wotus et al. 2003). In addition, input from the vagus nerve can increase the sensitivity of adrenal cells to ACTH (Ulrich-Lai and Engeland 2002), so that decreases in nerve input could also help reduce corticosteroid release.

A. Circadian Release

Corticosteroid release shows a distinct diurnal rhythm that has been shown to be circadian in all species where it has been examined (Dallman et al. 1993). The rhythm is partially driven by diurnal changes in ACTH release (Dallman et al. 1987) and partially by diurnal differences in the splanchnic nerve modulating adrenal sensitivity to ACTH (Engeland and Arnhold 2005; Ulrich-Lai et al. 2006). In general, the circadian peak occurs just prior to the active period, so the peak is in the early evening in nocturnal species

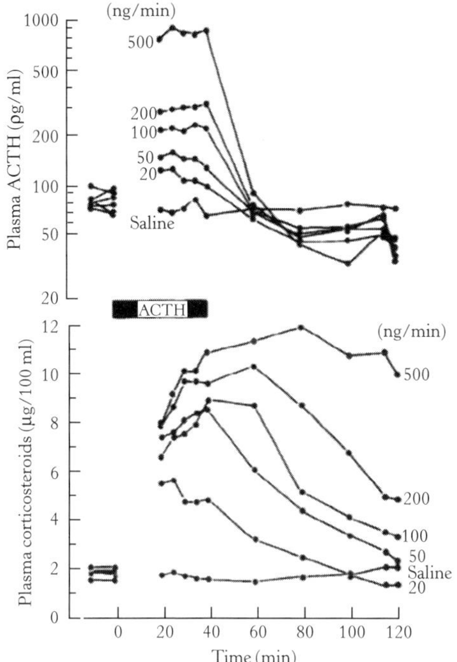

FIGURE 2.16: Mean plasma ACTH and corticosteroid concentrations in dogs infused with 6 doses (20–1500 ng/min) of ACTH or saline from 0 to 40 minutes. ACTH infusion rate (ng/min) and saline infusion are indicated next to each line.

Reprinted with permission from Keller-Wood et al. (1983). Courtesy of Amercian Physiological Society.

such as rats (Dallman et al. 1987) and in the early morning in diurnal species such as humans (Dallman et al. 1987), and in the early morning just prior to lights-on in several bird species (Breuner et al. 1999; Romero and Remage-Healey 2000; Rich and Romero 2001). However, the peak in corticosteroid release can be shifted to coincide with food consumption both under laboratory (e.g., Romero et al. 1995; Dallman et al. 2004) and field conditions. In an example of the latter, free-living Galapagos marine iguanas forage on a tidal cycle, and the diurnal corticosteroid peak occurs just prior to the high tide each day (Woodley et al. 2003).

The source of the diurnal rhythm appears to be a pulsatile release of corticosteroids. In laboratory rats, corticosteroids are released in a series of pulses with a mean interval of approximately 50 minutes (e.g., Windle et al. 1998a; Windle et al. 1998b). The pulses do not appear to be generated at the adrenal, but instead come from pulsatile release of ACTH resulting from the interplay of feedforward and feedback loops (Walker et al. 2010). In the laboratory, the timing of stressor application during the pulse cycle has an important influence on the resulting corticosteroid release (e.g., Windle et al. 1998a; Windle et al. 1998b), but the importance of pulsatile corticosteroid release for free-living animals has not yet been demonstrated.

B. Glucocorticoid Transport

Once released, the glucocorticoids travel to their target tissues via the peripheral circulation. However, steroids are highly hydrophobic and are usually transported through the blood attached to protein globulins. These globulins have glucocorticoid-specific binding sites with low capacity but high affinity and so have consequently been named corticosteroid-binding globulins, or CBG (Hammond 1990). CBG is a very large protein that is produced primarily by the liver. It is usually present in sufficient amounts that little corticosteroid is floating free in the plasma, with estimates that under normal physiological conditions, approximately 90% of corticosteroids are bound to CBG (Siiteri et al. 1982). However, it is only this free, unbound, fraction that is believed to be available for diffusion into tissues (Rosner 1990).

CBG's physiological role in regulating corticosteroid function is a topic of hot debate. Arguments about CBG's role can be summarized by three hypotheses. The first hypothesis has been called the "free hormone hypothesis" (Rosner 1990), but we like to call it the "buffer hypothesis." Because only unbound steroid can diffuse into tissues, and thus have biological activity, CBG acts as buffer to limit corticosteroid effects. In essence, CBG is acting like a giant corticosteroid sponge in the plasma, sopping up all the "excess" corticosteroids, thereby buffering tissues from high corticosteroid concentrations. The analogy of a sponge might be apt in another way. Some researchers have proposed that rapid and regulated changes in CBG binding could provide a quick increase in free corticosteroids during stress (Rosner 1990; Breuner and Orchinik 2002). This would rapidly augment the biological activity of the already-present corticosteroids independent of HPA axis activation. In a sense, the CBG "sponge" could be "wrung out" to provide access to a reserve pool of corticosteroids. CBG binding can decrease rapidly during stress in some, but not all, bird species (Breuner et al. 2006), which has been interpreted as increasing the free hormone fraction and thus is predicted to increase biological activity.

The second competing hypothesis is the "carrier hypothesis" (Rosner 1990). With this hypothesis, CBG acts as a transport molecule to get corticosteroids to their target tissues. Free steroids are still thought to be the biologically active fraction in the plasma, but high hydrophobicity of corticosteroids may require a transport molecule. Diffusion gradients at the target tissues could then increase corticosteroids' dissociation from CBG, with the subsequent diffusion of free steroid into the cell. Although an analogy for the buffer hypothesis is a sponge, an analogy for the carrier hypothesis is hemoglobin. Oxygen also travels poorly in plasma unattached to a carrier molecule, but only free oxygen is available to cells. Without hemoglobin, there would be insufficient oxygen available to tissues, and similarly for corticosteroids, the carrier hypothesis posits that without CBG, there would be insufficient corticosteroids delivered to tissues to stimulate the desired physiological effects.

The carrier hypothesis might also have a twist. CBG might not be simply a carrier, but a partner in initiating a physiological response. The CBG-corticosteroid complex appears to have its own membrane-bound receptor that activates a cAMP intracellular signaling system (Nakhla et al. 1988; Strelchyonok and Avvakumov 1991), although other data suggest that the receptor may only bind CBG when not bound to the steroid (Maitra et al. 1993). The physiological impact of this receptor and its binding is not well studied. CBG would in essence be acting as a carrier to transport the CBG:steroid complex to the receptor (Malisch and Breuner 2010).

The third hypothesis is that CBG's role is to increase the biological effects of corticosteroids by decreasing clearance rates (Shultz and Kitaysky 2008). CBG not only prevents corticosteroids from binding to their receptors, it also prevents corticosteroids from being taken up by the liver, metabolized, and excreted. In other words, CBG is increasing corticosteroid half-life in the plasma (Figure 2.17). As a result, elevations in CBG would increase the biological half-life, decrease corticosteroid clearance, and lead to an augmented physiological effect. Similarly, decreases in CBG would lead to decreases in physiological effect.

At this point it is unclear which hypothesis best fits the available data, and each is not necessarily mutually exclusive. As with many competing hypotheses of this sort in biology, the truth is that probably all three roles are important in at least some circumstances. Notice, however, that the buffer hypothesis makes opposite predictions to both the carrier hypothesis and the clearance hypothesis. If the buffer hypothesis were correct, elevated CBG concentrations would decrease corticosteroids' physiological effects. Furthermore, the fraction of steroid unbound to CBG would be of far more physiological relevance than the total corticosteroid concentrations in the blood. On the other hand, if either the carrier or clearance hypothesis were correct, elevated CBG

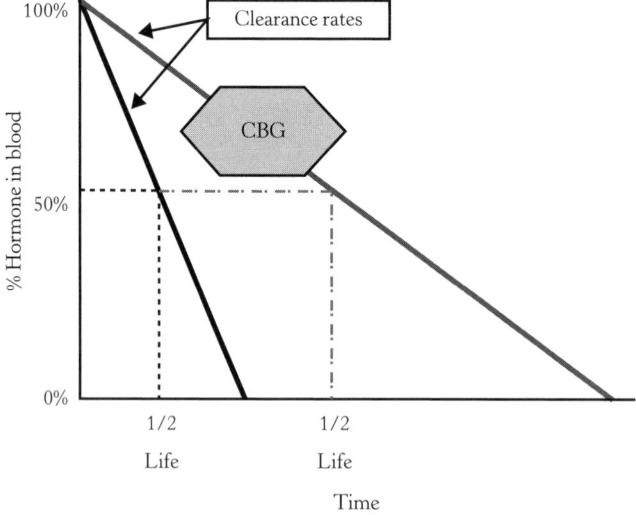

FIGURE 2.17: The effect of CBG on the clearance rates, and thus biological half-life, of corticosteroids in the blood. Because corticosteroids are removed from the plasma by the liver, and the liver only takes up unbound steroid, binding to CBG decreases clearance rate and increases half-life.

concentrations would enhance corticosteroids' physiological effects. Measurements of total corticosteroid concentrations would be more relevant because CBG would be regulating transport and/or clearance, rather than tissue availability.

Currently, the available evidence appears to slightly favor the carrier hypothesis. Perhaps the strongest support is that genetically mutated knockout mice that lack the ability to make CBG show a decrease in some physiological effects of glucocorticoids, such as glucocorticoid-induced increases in gluconeogenic enzymes (Petersen et al. 2006). On the other hand, rapid release of CBG from the liver binds corticosteroids during the acute rise after a stressor so that the tissue concentrations match the free hormone, not the total hormone, concentrations (Qian et al. 2011). However, work in this area has been significantly inhibited by a lack of a robust corticosteroid bioassay. The environmental context associated with a stressor is so critical in determining what physiological or behavioral effect will be elicited (see Chapter 3) that it is difficult to measure any of the corticosteroid effects discussed in the following chapters and unambiguously determine whether changes in CBG result in increases or decreases in physiological impact. In one of our laboratories, we have tried to manipulate CBG concentrations in European starlings by either injecting isolated human CBG or injecting a steroid-free plasma that presumably contains unoccupied CBG. We then monitored changes in blood glucose levels. Unfortunately, the results were inconclusive.

In many ways, the distinction between the free-hormone and carrier hypotheses may only be a difference in the time course. Even though the hormone must be free to interact with its receptor, the lengthy period of a stress response means that the hormone bound to CBG will act as a reservoir. As the corticosteroids are used, or excreted, more hormone from this pool will become available. In this case, measures of free and bound hormone are both important, but just at different time scales.

One final intriguing hypothesis for the function of CBG is that the most important pool of CBG is contained in the interstitial spaces, not in the plasma (Malisch and Breuner 2010). In this hypothesis, the CBG that is surrounding cells act as a shuttle to move corticosteroids from the blood to the target cells. This might explain why there is a receptor for CBG (Maitra et al. 1993) or the CBG:steroid complex (Nakhla et al. 1988; Strelchyonok and Avvakumov 1991) that can activate intracellular signaling pathways, or alternatively may facilitate corticosteroids entering cells (Hammes et al. 2005). To our knowledge, this hypothesis has not yet been tested.

CBG is present in wide variety of vertebrates, including amphibians (e.g., Orchinik et al. 2000; Ward et al. 2007), birds (e.g., Wingfield et al. 1984; Breuner and Orchinik 2001), some (e.g., Jennings et al. 2000), but not all (e.g., Ikonomopoulou et al. 2006), reptiles, and fish (e.g., Idler and Freeman 1968; Fostier and Breton 1975). Even though function is widely conserved, sequence is not (reviewed by Breuner and Orchinik 2002). However, this wide taxonomic distribution suggests that, whatever CBG's physiological role, that role is important to the ultimate function of the corticosteroids. Consequently, there has been a recent vibrant research effort to determine the dynamics of CBG regulation in wild species under natural conditions. Most of this work so far has been done on wild birds.

There are two overwhelming conclusions from the research to date. First, the dynamics of CBG action are complicated and may even vary from species to species. For instance, CBG-binding capacities can change rapidly (within 60 minutes) in some species but not in others (Breuner et al. 2006). Given the large size of CBG and how long it must take to create de novo large amounts of this protein, these rapid changes suggest that CBG can be stored by the liver and rapidly released (Qian et al. 2011), or there may be some interesting mechanisms directly in the plasma that regulate corticosteroid binding. Furthermore, the rapid changes in binding capacity suggest that CBG can dynamically regulate corticosteroid function during an acute stress response in some species. The implications of this are still unclear. However, the time frame for altered CBG-binding capacity after initiation of a stressor can be much longer (on the order of a day) in some species (Lynn et al. 2003), and CBG binding does not change in response to an acute stress at all in other species (Breuner et al. 2006; Shultz and Kitaysky 2008). The large species differences in the dynamics of CBG-binding capacity has greatly complicated the forming of robust hypotheses on what all these changes mean physiologically.

The second conclusion from this research is that any deeper understanding of the connections between CBG and the broad life-history characteristics of a species are greatly hampered by an inability to distinguish between the three hypotheses for CBG function detailed earlier. Fundamentally, we still do not know if the total amount of corticosteroids in the plasma or only the corticosteroids unbound to CBG (free fraction) better represent the physiologically active amount of corticosteroids. This is a critical problem because measures of total and free corticosteroids often are poorly correlated. For example, although CBG-binding capacity varies over the course of the day in many species (e.g., Ottenweller et al. 1979; Meaney et al. 1992), different species show different daily patterns (with some showing bimodal and others unimodal responses) that do not closely coincide with the daily pattern of corticosteroid release. In a second example, both corticosteroid concentrations and CBG-binding capacities vary seasonally in many species (reviewed by Romero 2002). In general, total corticosteroid concentrations show seasonal differences and are usually highest during the breeding season (see Chapter 10). CBG, however, also can vary seasonally. When both CBG-binding capacity and total corticosteroid concentrations are known, the free corticosteroid concentrations can be estimated. When the seasonal variation in total and free steroid concentrations are compared, the two patterns can remain the same (e.g., Romero et al. 1998), can disappear (e.g., Monamy 1995; Breuner and Orchinik 2001), or the pattern can change entirely (Romero et al. 2006).

CBG capacity does change with some intriguing life-history differences, and it would be important to determine what these changes mean physiologically. For example, testosterone can increase CBG capacity (e.g., Klukowski et al. 1997; Deviche et al. 2001; Zysling et al. 2006), but does this enhance (carrier hypothesis) or decrease (buffer hypothesis) the ultimate impact of corticosteroids? In another example, differences in CBG are correlated with the length of the breeding season in three populations of white-crowned sparrows, resulting in population-level differences in free corticosterone, even though there are no differences in total corticosterone (Breuner et al. 2003). This was an exciting paper because it was the first to correlate changes in CBG capacity with life-history traits. And yet, without being able to distinguish between the buffer and carrier hypotheses, we are left with little idea of *why* CBG capacity might change. Unfortunately, until the question of buffer versus carrier versus clearance is solved, documenting changes in CBG capacity is unlikely to provide much explanatory power.

C. Glucocorticoid Receptors: Intracellular

Once corticosteroids reach target tissues, they mediate their effects through two major intracellular receptors and possibly one membrane-bound receptor. The two intracellular receptors are highly conserved across species (Stolte et al. 2006) and share many structural and functional characteristics (Bhargava and Pearce 2004). Work on the membrane-bound receptor is just beginning (see discussion later in this chapter) and it is unknown how conserved it is across species.

The two intracellular receptors are perhaps the best-studied receptors in all of biology. A search on Google Scholar found over 112,000 hits for "glucocorticoid receptor" and a similar search on Medline found over 1,400 reviews. There are several reasons for the prodigious amount of work on these receptors, but perhaps surprisingly, it has little to do with the importance of glucocorticoid effects. Glucocorticoid receptors form part of the gene transcription apparatus of the cell. Therefore, their primary function is to initiate gene transcription (see discussion later in this chapter). It turns out that glucocorticoid receptors became one of the primary models for understanding gene transcription. Consequently, there has been an enormous amount of work that was not interested in glucocorticoid receptors per se, but that was interested in these receptors as tools to understand gene transcription. Furthermore, this knowledge became a springboard to use glucocorticoid receptors as an important tool in modern molecular genetics. A popular technique is to insert the DNA target (GRE—see following discussion) near the gene of interest and thereby create a gene whose transcription can be induced at will. Because of all this work, glucocorticoid receptors are understood at an incredible level of detail. What follows below is a brief outline of what they are and how they function.

The glucocorticoid receptors are present in the cytoplasm of target cells (Figure 2.18). Corticosteroids diffuse across the plasma membrane and bind to the ligand-binding domain of the receptor. Once binding occurs, three important events take place. First, a series of molecular chaperones that were binding to the receptor fall off. These chaperones are the heat-shock proteins (HSP), so named because their production increases dramatically if the cell is stressed by an increase in temperature, although their increase appears to be more a general response to cellular stressors (Kregel 2002). The dissociation of the HSPs exposes the DNA-binding region of the receptor (Norris 2007). Notice that the HSPs form a link between the cellular response to stress and the organismal response to stress (Figure 2.18). Several research groups have attempted to exploit this link by using increases in HSPs as a marker

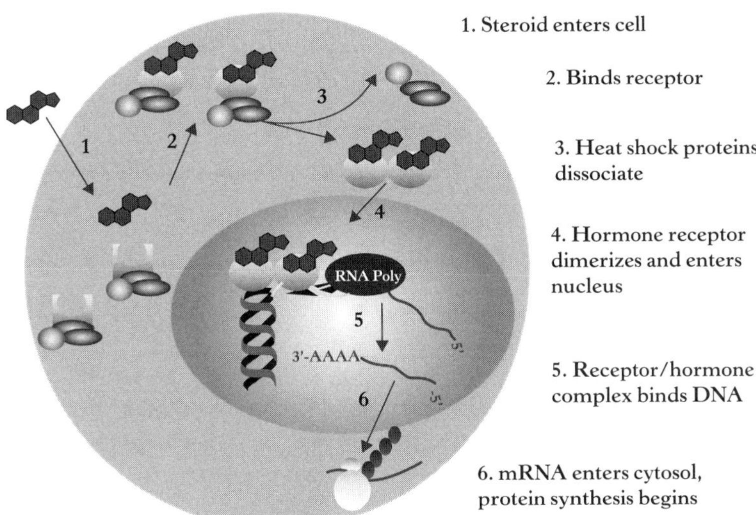

FIGURE 2.18: Glucocorticoids act on target tissues through type 1 intracellular receptors that are of two types, MR (mineralocorticoid type) and GR (glucocorticoid type).

(1) Glucocorticoid (dark) enters the cell passively and binds to an intra-cellular receptor (MR or GR). (2) It binds to the receptor, which results in dissociation of a complex of heat shock proteins (3) that have been shielding the DNA-binding domain of the receptor. The receptor can now also form a homodimer (4) that is now a gene transcription factor. Once translocated to the nucleus, the dimer binds DNA (5), resulting in gene transcription, mRNA production, and eventually protein synthesis (6). MR has the highest affinity for glucocorticoids and is saturated at relatively low circulating levels. GR has a lower affinity and is saturated at higher concentrations of glucocortioids. Thus different circulating levels of glucocorticoids activate different receptor types and thus transcription of different sets of genes.

for an organism-level stress response (Basu et al. 2001; Garamszegi et al. 2006; Martinez-de la Puente et al. 2007), although it is not yet clear that this will be a profitable approach.

The second important event induced by ligand binding is the translocation of the receptor from the cytoplasm to the nucleus. This allows the receptor to associate with a variety of intra-nuclear proteins that together will form the mature transcription apparatus. However, before the transcription apparatus is complete, two ligand-receptor complexes must associate together (dimerize, Figure 2.18). The third important event initiated by corticosteroid binding, therefore, is the dimerization of two receptors (Norris 2007). This is an important step, because the dimerized receptor-ligand complex creates protein domains (zinc finger regions) that recognize specific sequences of DNA in the genome. These DNA sequences are called glucocorticoid response elements (GRE—or MRE for mineralocorticoid response element) and serve as markers for which genes will be transcribed by the newly formed glucocorticoid receptor transcription apparatus (Norris 2007). GREs are ubiquitous throughout the genome, which would certainly explain why corticosteroids can have such profound effects in so many physiological systems.

As mentioned earlier, there are two intracellular receptors. The first is called the Type I, or mineralocorticoid, receptor. Type I receptors have high affinity but low capacity for corticosteroids. In tissues such as the kidney, another steroid hormone, aldosterone, is the primary ligand for this receptor. Aldosterone helps alter fluid balance by regulating sodium concentrations in the kidney, hence its classification as a mineralocorticoid. The binding of aldosterone to this receptor was the genesis of naming it the mineralocorticoid receptor, or MR. However, fish lack aldosterone, and so cortisol plays the mineralocorticoid role. In any event, glucocorticoids bind to the Type I receptor with higher affinity than aldosterone and are also present in higher circulating concentrations, so in most tissues the Type I receptor does not appear to serve a mineralocorticoid function (see discussion later in this chapter on how aldosterone binds to its receptor when there is an excess of corticosteroids).

The second receptor is called the Type II, or glucocorticoid, receptor (GR). Type II receptors have a much lower affinity for corticosteroids, but have a much higher capacity. Type II receptors are present in many tissues throughout the brain and body (Ballard et al. 1974; Oakley and Cidlowski 2011), including the same cells which express MR. However, MR interacts with a different DNA sequence (the MRE) than the Type II receptors (the GRE) so that they initiate transcription of different genes.

Both Type I and Type II glucocorticoid receptors are gene transcription regulators. This means that in order to exert a biological effect, the receptors have to induce sufficient production of new protein. This requires receptor binding, translocation to the nucleus, binding to the DNA, initiating transcription, and completing translation. This entire process is believed to take at least 15 minutes (Haller et al. 2008) and there is the additional time between detecting the stressor and increasing corticosteroid release. This time lag between stressor and genomic effects has a profound impact on our current thinking about corticosteroids' role in surviving stressors (see discussion later in this chapter).

Because Type I receptors have higher affinity than Type II receptors, corticosteroids bind to them first (Figure 2.19). Type I receptors are thought to act primarily in the brain to regulate the circadian variation of corticosteroids. However, Type I receptors have low capacity (i.e., there are few receptors overall) so that they become completely bound relatively quickly. In fact, Type I receptor binding is believed to be completely saturated at peak circadian concentrations (i.e., the peak of the basal range). Once Type I receptors become fully bound, corticosteroids begin to bind to Type II receptors. The lower affinity of Type II receptors ensures that they will bind corticosteroids only after Type I receptors are saturated, but their higher capacity (there are more Type II receptors overall) means that they will bind to a higher range of corticosteroid concentrations (Figure 2.19). Type II receptors are only bound when corticosteroid concentrations are high (i.e., after a stressor) and are believed to regulate the classic functions of corticosteroids (see later chapters in this volume). Consequently, the physiological actions of corticosteroids result from a balance of Type I and Type II binding, with each receptor mediating different physiological and behavioral consequences (de Kloet et al. 1993b; Sousa et al. 2008).

This brings up an important issue of what is the best way to report changes in corticosteroids in response to a stressor. Although the majority of papers in the literature report actual corticosteroid concentrations, it is also common to see papers report a "change from baseline" (defined as peak concentrations minus basal concentrations) or a

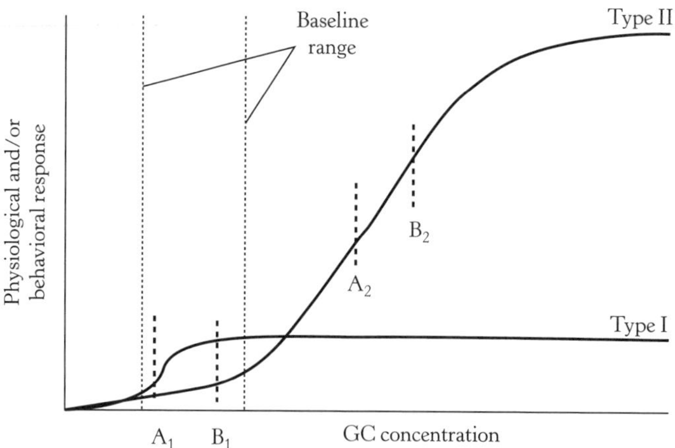

FIGURE 2.19: Biological effects of corticosteroids depend upon the interaction between the hormone and the affinities and capacities of its two receptors. Type I receptors (MR) are saturated first, but have low capacity, and as GC concentrations continue to increase binding shifts to type II receptors (GR). The range for baseline reflects circadian variation. Two hypothetical examples of baseline and stress-induced samples are also included. A_1 and B_1 represent two different baseline concentrations, and A_2 and B_2 represent the respective stress-induced concentrations. Note that examples A and B have similar increases from baseline (and A has a higher percent change due to a lower baseline), but the stress-induced concentrations of A have a lower biological effect than the stress-induced concentrations from B.

Reprinted with modification from (Romero 2004), with permission. Courtesy of Cell Press.

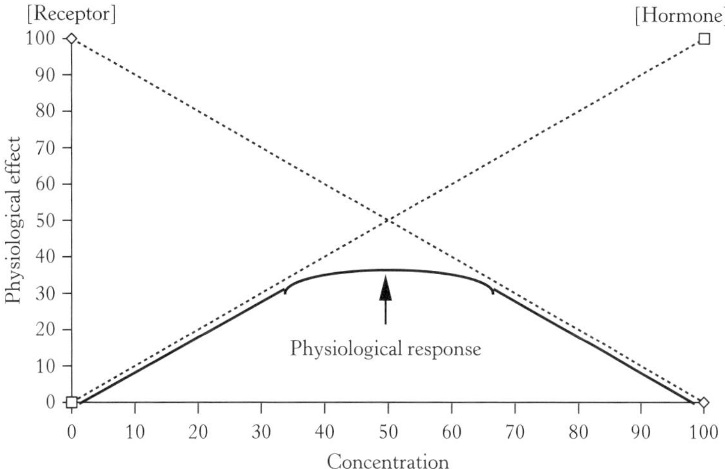

FIGURE 2.20: Theoretical physiological response when increasing hormone concentrations regulate a decrease in the number of is own receptors. Consequently, the physiological response is limited by hormone concentrations when hormone concentrations are low, and by receptor numbers when receptor numbers are low. Absolute numbers on both axes are hypothetical and used only for illustrative purposes (see Table 4.2).

Figure adapted from Munck and Náray-Fejes-Tóth (1992). Courtesy of Elsevier.

"percentage increase" (defined as peak response divided by basal concentrations). The rationale for these transformations is that animals often differ in their basal concentrations, either because of inter-individual variation or because they were sampled at different times of the circadian cycle. However, we propose that reporting the actual concentrations (i.e., not doing either transformation) is far superior. Because basal and stress-induced corticosteroid concentrations interact with different receptors, reporting a change from baseline makes little biological sense. As the examples in Figure 2.19 illustrate, biological effect may be the opposite from what is predicted from percentage changes. Knowing receptor numbers might help determine physiological and behavioral effects, but until these studies are done, absolute concentrations are more likely to provide better interpretations of biological effect.

Unfortunately, the corticosteroid/receptor dynamics are not static. The reason is that corticosteroids must interact with a receptor in order to have a physiological effect, and corticosteroids directly influence receptor numbers (Sapolsky 1992). As hormone concentrations rise, receptor numbers fall. This relationship holds both during the acute stress response (as corticosteroids increase, they bind to receptors, making fewer receptors available) and during chronic increases in corticosteroids (the number of receptors that are produced decreases in the long term in an attempt to compensate for corticosteroid concentrations that the body interprets as too high). Plotting this relationship indicates that the physiological effects resulting from corticosteroid release are not linear, but rather form a bell-shaped curve with increasing hormone concentrations (Figure 2.20; Munck and Náray-Fejes-Tóth 1992). Arbitrarily assigning numbers to these curves will indicate why reporting percent change from baseline makes little sense. Table 2.2 presents corticosteroid concentrations from three hypothetical

TABLE 2.2: CORTICOSTEROID CONCENTRATIONS IN THREE HYPOTHETICAL POPULATIONS

Population	Baseline Corticosteroids	Stress-induced Corticosteroids	Total Increase	% Increase
A	5	25	20	500
B	20	40	20	200
C	40	80	40	200

populations. Although populations A and B have identical increases from baseline, and population A has a dramatically higher percent change from baseline, stress-induced concentrations in population B clearly have a greater physiological effect. Similarly, even though populations B and C have an equivalent percent increase in GC concentrations, their responses to stress have very different physiological effects that are opposite from that suggested by percent increase.

These examples highlight the importance of knowing receptor numbers for the populations under study. Each population could have different overall numbers of receptors, thereby producing different curves. Unfortunately, very few studies have measured receptor numbers in free-living populations (see discussion later in this chapter), and a curve similar to Figure 2.20 has not yet been generated for any free-living species. However, although the absolute values for the curve in Figure 2.20 are hypothetical, the relationship is not. Acute increases in corticosteroid concentrations are known to decrease the number of available receptors, and long-term administration of corticosteroids (as little as 4 days) from either exogenous steroids or chronic stress has been used as a technique to permanently reduce the number of both Type I and Type II receptors in the brains of laboratory rats (e.g., Sapolsky and McEwen 1985).

Research on measuring corticosteroid receptors in free-living species is just beginning. Much of this work to date has focused on corticosteroid receptors in the brain (e.g., Breuner and Orchinik 2001; Breuner and Orchinik 2009), but other tissues have been examined as well (e.g., Schmidt et al. 2010). For example, Type II receptor densities in toad testes were found to not change seasonally (Denari and Ceballos 2006), even though corticosterone titers do (Romero 2002). Future studies that monitor changes in receptor numbers during different life-history stages are likely to provide a fruitful approach in understanding the role of glucocorticoid signaling.

Interestingly, there is some evidence that reductions in densities of Type I and not Type II receptors occur after long-term exposure to stress, either through selection for high corticosterone responders (Hodgson et al. 2007), or in birds exposed to chronic stress (Dickens et al. 2009). Some studies have also tried to infer receptor function using various receptor antagonists (e.g., Koch et al. 2002; Landys et al. 2004a; Landys et al. 2004b). Given the difficulty and time involved in measuring receptor densities or capacities directly, this technique holds considerable promise for addressing questions of receptor function.

D. 11β-Hydroxysteroid Dehydrogenase

There is another mechanism for regulating corticosteroid action that has attracted interest over the years. There are two enzymes present in cells that can either activate or deactivate corticosteroids prior to interaction with a receptor. One enzyme, 11β-hydroxysteroid dehydrogenase type 1, is believed to activate corticosteroids, thereby enhancing receptor activation (reviewed by Tomlinson et al. 2004). To our knowledge, there has not been any work on this enzyme in a non-clinical context, although other enzymes that prevent corticosteroid metabolism may augment corticosteroid function in semelparous fish (Barry et al. 2010). The other enzyme, 11β-hydroxysteroid dehydrogenase type 2 (11-HSD), almost irreversibly deactivates corticosteroids (reviewed by White et al. 1997). In other species, 20-hydroxy-dehydrogenase may play a similar role (Vylitova et al. 1998). Isolation of 11β-HSD solved a major puzzle in aldosterone physiology. Since glucocorticoids have both a higher affinity for the MR (type I) receptor and are present at higher concentrations in the plasma than aldosterone, it was initially unclear how aldosterone ever got access to its own receptor. In other words, why weren't the corticosteroids, not aldosterone, the primary mineralocorticoids? Current thinking is that 11β-HSD deactivates glucocorticoids in certain tissues (especially the kidney), thereby protecting type I receptors in those tissues from binding glucocorticoids and allowing aldosterone to bind (White et al. 1997). Interestingly, licorice can inhibit 11β-HSD function and allows greater glucocorticoid binding to type I receptors.

Even though 11β-HSD function was originally elucidated in the kidney, it is clear that activity is present in many tissues in the body, including the brain, that have no need for a classic aldosterone effect (White et al. 1997). Consequently, 11β-HSD activity may serve a more generalized function in regulating corticosteroid binding (Wyrwoll et al. 2011). A few studies have begun to test this hypothesis outside human medicine. We know that chickens (Kucka et al. 2006; Katz et al. 2008) and several fish species (Baker 2004) have 11β-HSDs that are postulated to alter corticosterone binding. Additionally, toads (Denari and Ceballos 2005), rainbow trout (Kusakabe et al. 2003), and the Japanese eel (Ozaki et al. 2006) have 11β-HSD present in the testes that could potentially modulate corticosteroid binding. This might protect the testes and allow breeding to continue despite high circulating concentrations of corticosteroids (see Chapter 10). However, very little work has been done to study this potentially important regulator of corticosteroid signaling in natural contexts.

E. Glucocorticoid Receptors: Polymorphisms

There is growing evidence that the process of transcription and translation in the production of both MR and GR results in multiple variants (DeRijk and de Kloet 2008; Gross and Cidlowski 2008; Oakley and Cidlowski 2011). These splice variants can dramatically change the binding kinetics to corticosteroids as well as the binding affinities to MRE and GREs. The result can be profound changes in corticosteroid physiology, and there is speculation that human splice variants underlie individual susceptibility to stress-related disease. The importance to wild animals, however, is not yet clear. Characterizing the primary MR and GR is just beginning for many species, much less the search for splice variants. However, one study that investigated MR and GR in house sparrow brains at two different times of the year did not find differences in binding affinity, even though binding capacity changed (Breuner and Orchinik 2001), suggesting that house sparrows were not producing different splice variants seasonally.

F. Glucocorticoid Receptors: Membrane

There is considerable physiological evidence that corticosteroids interact with a membrane-bound receptor as well (Borski 2000; Losel et al. 2003; Tasker et al. 2005). The initial evidence came from studies in rough-skinned newts that showed that corticosterone had an ability to rapidly inhibit reproductive behavior through a G-protein-linked receptor localized in the cell membranes of neurons (Orchinik et al. 1991). Part of the receptor mechanism that links corticosteroid binding to changes in behavior appears to involve endocannabinoids (Denver 2007). Although the receptor that is believed to regulate these rapid effects has been isolated and partially characterized in amphibians and may be linked to opioid activity (Evans et al. 2000), it has not yet been isolated from any other species, and there is some evidence that a modified type II receptor may also associate with neuronal membranes (Losel et al. 2003). However, rapid corticosteroid effects (on the order of seconds to minutes) have been shown in many different species, including fish, amphibians, birds, and mammals (reviewed by Dallman 2005). Since the rapid time course of these effects is far too fast to be explained by changes in gene transcription (Borski 2000), it is likely that most, if not all, vertebrate species have these receptors. In fact, given that the intracellular steroid receptors are apparently unique to vertebrates, the membrane receptor may represent the original ancestral corticosteroid receptor (Dallman 2005).

Although clinical interest in the membrane receptor has stimulated a significant amount of investigation, work to understand the role that these receptors play in natural contexts is just beginning. Results to date, however, clearly indicate that rapid behavioral effects of glucocorticoids could form an important component of the overall stress response. For example, Gulf toadfish exposed to the hunting sounds of bottlenose dolphins rapidly suppress reproductive behavior (especially vocalizations) via a mechanism that appears to be a rapid effect of cortisol on neuronal firing (Remage-Healey and Bass 2006). It seems obvious that curtailing singing to attract a mate when dolphins are hunting in the area would increase these fishes' chances of survival. Similar studies have also shown rapid inhibition of reproductive behavior by corticosterone in a variety of amphibians (reviewed by Moore et al. 2005). In a second example, exogenous corticosterone rapidly increases spontaneous activity in white-crowned sparrows (Breuner et al. 1998). Increased activity would also be a beneficial response to some stressors. Moreover, corticosteroids have a number of effects that are not linked to specific genomic actions. They include direct actions on membrane fluidity, binding to membrane proteins, and potentially indirect effects mediated by proteins (e.g., heat shock proteins) dissociated from the ligand-receptor complex (Haller et al. 2008). Many of these mechanisms are currently being studied, and it is not yet known how much relevance they will have for biomedicine, much less wild animals.

G. Integrating Receptor Signaling

In sum, corticosteroids exert their physiological effects through multiple pathways. Most is known about their genomic effects, although the interplay between type I and type II receptors, as well as the reciprocal relation between these receptors and corticosteroid concentrations, makes the corticosteroid regulation of transcription a complex process. Furthermore, the presence of 11β-HSD can modulate which receptors are bound, and at what amounts, which can ultimately determine whether genes associated with MREs or GREs get transcribed. With all of these factors, it becomes very difficult to predict what an individual cell or tissue's response will be to an increase in corticosteroids. In fact, there is growing evidence that sensitivity to corticosteroids varies by tissue, by individual, and by previous experience (Rohleder et al. 2003). Corticosteroids could sidestep the entire genomic transcription apparatus by binding directly to membrane receptors. Although membrane receptors are primarily implicated in rapid behavioral changes, there is no reason that they are not functioning in somatic tissues, such as liver, as well. One dogma of endocrinology is that physiological effect flows from both an increase in hormone concentration and an interaction with a receptor. In other words, you need both a signal and something to listen to the signal. As an analogy, a telephone is only useful as a signal transfer device if there is someone on the other end to answer the call. In the case of corticosteroid signaling, the question of who is listening (i.e., which cells/tissues have which available receptors) and what they do when they hear that signal (i.e., what responses those cells/tissues initiate) is not always clear-cut.

H. Glucocorticoid Negative Feedback

Corticosteroid secretion must end at the termination of an acute stressor. For example, once an animal has escaped from a predator, or has resolved a fight with a conspecific, a stress response is no longer required, and it is time to turn off the response. For the corticosteroids, the major feedback signal is the corticosteroids themselves. Through multiple regulatory points throughout the HPA axis (Figure 2.14), negative feedback serves to shut off corticosteroid secretion.

The multiple negative feedback loops operate at different speeds. The three primary feedback loops occur at the pituitary, the paraventricular nucleus of the hypothalamus (PVN), and the hippocampus (Keller-Wood and Dallman 1984; Jacobson and Sapolsky 1991; Herman et al. 1992). At the pituitary, corticosteroids rapidly inhibit ACTH release (Keller-Wood and Dallman 1984), POMC synthesis, and the rate of POMC mRNA transcription (Mains and Eipper 2001). This is the strongest site for negative feedback. At the PVN, corticosteroids rapidly inhibit CRF release (Dallman and Bhatnagar 2001). This appears to occur by corticosteroids binding to CRF-producing neurons, initiating endocannabinoid release, and the endocannabinoids then acting in a retrograde fashion to inhibit the stimulatory inputs to the CRF neuron (Tasker and Herman 2011). Furthermore, endocannabinoid signaling from two other brain regions, the prefrontal cortex and the amygdala, appear to play an important role in negative feedback (Hill et al. 2010; Hill et al. 2011). Both PVN and pituitary pathways are considered fast feedback loops because decreases in CRF and ACTH release occur on the order of minutes. Although it isn't entirely clear, fast feedback appears to be mediated by the membrane rather than the type I or II receptors (Dallman 2005; Tasker and Herman 2011). On a longer time scale (on the order of hours), corticosteroids bind to type II receptors in the hippocampus. The hippocampus then sends a signal to the PVN, which results in decreases in CRF release (Jacobson and Sapolsky 1991). Because type I receptors are generally fully saturated when circulating corticosteroid concentrations reach the circadian peak, type II receptors are believed to play the major role in regulating the negative feedback signal (de Kloet et al. 1993a). Each of these feedback loops serves to inhibit continued corticosteroid release after initiation of a stressor. However, there is also a role for direct neural shutoff of corticosteroid release. ACTH levels decrease after a stressor, even in adrenalectomized rats (Jacobson et al. 1988; Herman et al. 1996), indicating that corticosteroids are not necessary for negative feedback to function.

The strength of corticosteroid negative feedback, however, depends heavily on the context in which feedback is occurring. For example, the strength of the feedback signal shows a daily rhythm (reviewed by Keller-Wood and Dallman 1984). In addition, there is a great difference between endogenous and exogenous corticosteroids in their ability to stimulate negative feedback. Exogenous corticosteroids, when given in concentrations mimicking stress-induced increases, can blunt endogenous secretion (presumably through negative feedback; Dallman et al. 1987; Dallman et al. 1992), but stress-induced glucocorticoid release is resistant to feedback effects. This suggests that negative feedback is not simply the result of circulating corticosteroids. Other aspects of the stress response can short-circuit the negative feedback loops when necessary.

Normally, corticosteroid release decreases due to negative feedback, even if a stressor continues. However, what happens if a new stressor occurs and the animal needs another surge of corticosteroids? In fact, when a subsequent stressor occurs when corticosteroids are low due to negative feedback, a new tide of corticosteroids is released. This is thought to occur through facilitation of the glucocorticoid response so that glucocorticoid release continues despite what would normally be a robust feedback signal (Graessler et al. 1989; Dallman et al. 1992). The mechanism underlying this facilitation is not fully understood (Dallman and Bhatnagar 2001). However, there is evidence that AVP is more resistant to negative feedback than CRF (Scaccianoce et al. 1991; Degoeij et al. 1992; Bartanusz et al. 1993). This would suggest that corticosteroid release is maintained in the face of negative feedback by shifting the secretory pathway. When corticosteroid concentrations are low, CRF is the primary hypothalamic secretagog driving ACTH release. When corticosteroid concentrations are high (i.e., after a stressor and during negative feedback), AVP becomes the primary secretagog. A recent study in chickens indicated that feedback primarily inhibited CRF release in this species as well (Vandenborne et al. 2005b), which has interesting implications if, as in other birds, AVT seems to be the primary secretagog (Carsia 1990).

The efficacy of negative feedback also varies in different species. For example, prairie voles (DeVries et al. 1997; Taymans et al. 1997), brown lemmings (Romero et al. 2008), and several bat species (Widmaier and Kunz 1993; Widmaier et al. 1994) have naturally high corticosteroid concentrations—high enough to be lethal in other species. Furthermore, these concentrations are resistant to negative feedback (Taymans et al. 1997; Romero et al. 2008). This suggests that the high corticosteroid concentrations in these species may be maintained by an alteration of the feedback mechanism that prevents such high levels in other vertebrates.

One underappreciated aspect of glucocorticoid physiology is that the duration and the magnitude of corticosteroid release are often both as important. The total amount of corticosteroids released in response to a stressor (the integrated response) is the important variable, not the maximum amount released (Dallman and Bhatnagar 2001). This is because the biological effect results from hormone/receptor interactions that occur over the entire course of the stress response, not just at the peak of corticosteroid release. The total amount released is, at its simplest, a function of the maximum released and the duration of the response.

Deficits in negative feedback efficacy can be a significant problem for the animal since elevated corticosteroids are present for a much longer period (Figure 2.21). Poorly regulated negative

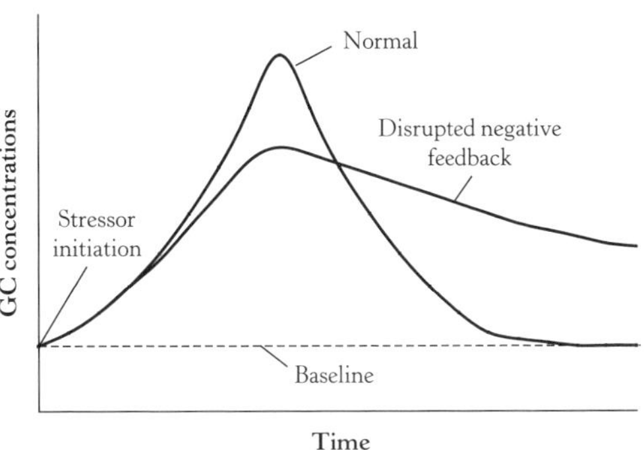

FIGURE 2.21: Corticosteroid responses to a stressor in animals with normal physiology and in animals with disrupted negative feedback. Note that even though one response produces a lower maximal response, the disrupted negative feedback results in more corticosteroids being secreted over time. This response has been demonstrated in dominant and subordinate wild free-living olive baboons (Sapolsky 1993). However, the maximal response could also be equivalent or higher than normal in animals with disrupted negative feedback, in which case the total GCs released will be even higher. The baseline can also be different in animals with disrupted negative feedback.

Reprinted with modification from Romero (2004), with permission.

feedback can be a major factor in human depression (Sapolsky 1992; Erickson et al. 2003) and in problems associated with subordinate status in many species (Sapolsky 2001). For example, subordinate free-living olive baboons had lower maximal cortisol responses to a stressor than did dominant baboons, but their reduced negative feedback efficacy resulted in significantly more cortisol being released over time (Sapolsky 1993). The greater overall cortisol response was then linked to cardiovascular problems in subordinate baboons (Sapolsky and Share 1994). Clearly, the duration of cortisol release can be an important variable (Romero 2004).

One consequence of potential deficits in negative feedback is that higher stress-induced corticosteroid concentrations do not necessarily indicate an animal in poorer health (Figure 2.21). Furthermore, the stress response evolved to help individuals survive, so that lacking a sufficient stress response can often result in an inability to cope with a stressor (e.g., Hontela 1998; Norris et al. 1999). In such cases, assessing negative feedback would provide a clearer picture of which animals might be unable to cope (Romero 2004; Romero and Wikelski 2010).

Researchers have used two ways to monitor the efficacy of negative feedback in free-living animals. One is to monitor changes in corticosteroids over long periods of time (e.g., Knapp and Moore 1995), and the other is to test negative feedback directly. In the later approach, dexamethasone (DEX), a synthetic glucocorticoid, is injected immediately at capture to artificially stimulate negative feedback. An inability to respond to DEX (called DEX resistance) indicates disruption of negative feedback (e.g., Sapolsky and Altmann 1991; Astheimer et al. 1994).

IV. ADRENAL MEDULLA AND CATECHOLAMINES

The adrenal medulla of mammals, and its equivalent—chromaffin tissue—of non-mammalian vertebrates (so named because of its reaction to a stain containing chromium salts (Young and Landsberg 2001)), secrete three major catecholamines that have roles in metabolism (glucose mobilization), muscle contraction, and rapid responses to stress. The major catecholamines in vertebrates are epinephrine, norepinephrine, and dopamine.

Medullary cells have a special relationship to the nervous system related to their origin and function (Figure 2.22). These cells arise in the embryo from neural crest ectoderm that migrates into the region and differentiates. Consequently, cells of the medulla and cortex have different fetal origins (Hammer et al. 2005). As we discussed earlier, the mammalian adrenal gland has two distinct parts: the cortex that secretes corticosteroids, and the medulla (Figure 2.9) that is derived from neural crest. The adrenal medulla is richly innervated by preganglionic sympathetic fibers (Figure 2.22). Additionally, small numbers of sympathetic ganglion cells are commonly observed in the medulla. Ganglion cells are round or polygonal with prominent nuclei. The chromaffin tissue is essentially a modified sympathetic ganglion (Goldstein 1987; Norris 2007) in which each secretory cell is a neuron without an axon. Chromaffin cells in the medulla form two distinct cell populations: those that secrete epinephrine, and those that secrete norepinephrine, with both species and age differences in their relative abundances (Young and Landsberg 2001). The cells in the adrenal medulla do not have their own arterial blood supply (Figure 2.22). The venous drainage from the sinusoids in the cortex trickles down through the medulla and there is a common outflow. Because blood flow is from the outer cortex of the adrenal toward the center, the adrenal medulla is bathed by blood enriched with corticosteroids.

Most non-mammalian species, however, lack an encapsulated adrenal gland and thus do not have a well-defined adrenal medulla (Young and Landsberg 2001). In these species, chromaffin tissue is dispersed, and much of it is embedded in the wall of the kidneys (Figures 2.10 and 2.11). In addition, because phenylethanolamine N-methyltransferase (PNMT; involved in the synthesis of epinephrine) is regulated by corticosteroids that are not as anatomically close as

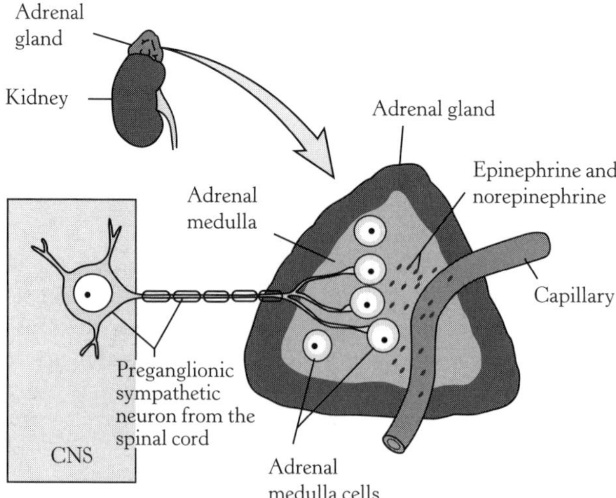

FIGURE 2.22: Adrenal medulla cells are modified postganglionic sympathetic neurons that synthesize and release catecholamines. Epinephrine and norepinephrine are released directly into the blood as circulating hormones.
From Sherwood (2008).

they are in species with distinct adrenals, these species tend to release more norepinephrine than epinephrine (Axelrod and Reisine 1984) and often have lower circulating catecholamine concentrations in general (Hart et al. 1989).

Differentiated medullary cells have developed the secretory function of neurons to the exclusion of the conduction function, so they have no axons and do not resemble neurons (Figure 2.22). Nevertheless, they retain a good deal of their neuronal properties and, in particular, they retain the ability to respond to neuronal signals. Nerve fibers from the sympathetic side of the autonomic nervous system synapse directly with the cells of the adrenal medulla, and when these neurons fire, the medullary cells respond (Figure 2.22). Instead of sending out a neural signal, however, they respond by secretion of the hormone epinephrine.

A. Catecholamine Synthesis

Catecholamines are characterized by a catechol backbone of two hydroxyl groups attached to a six-carbon ring (Figure 2.23). The specific catecholamine is determined by the type of amine attached to this backbone (Norris 2007). Their production is regulated by a suite of enzymes: tyrosine hydroxylase (the rate-limiting enzyme for norepinephrine production); aromatic-L-amino acid decarboxylase; dopamine β-hydroxylase; and phenylethanolamine N-methyltransferase (PNMT), the enzyme regulating epinephrine production (reviewed by Axelrod and Reisine 1984; Young and Landsberg 2001). Synthesis begins with the amino acid tyrosine, progresses through two intermediates (including dopamine), and ends with the production of norepinephrine (Young and Landsberg 2001). PNMT then converts norepinephrine into epinephrine. Epinephrine and norepinephrine are the two primary catecholamines involved in the fight-or-flight response. They are also called adrenaline and noradrenaline ("epinephrine" and "norepinephrine" are the names used in the United States; the terms "adrenaline" and "noradrenaline" are used in Europe). From a historical perspective, it is interesting to note that the first hormone to have its structure determined was epinephrine (Young and Landsberg 2001). Tyrosine hydroxylase activity and production are primarily under the control of sympathetic innervation, whereas PNMT activity and production are primarily regulated by corticosteroids (reviewed by Axelrod and Reisine 1984; Young and Landsberg 2001).

B. Nerve Terminals

Although norepinephrine is also released from adrenal chromaffin tissue, another major source is nerve terminals of the sympathetic nervous system (reviewed by Stanford 1993; Goldstein and Eisenhofer 2001). This provides the anatomical foundation for how different stressors could secrete different ratios of epinephrine and norepinephrine.

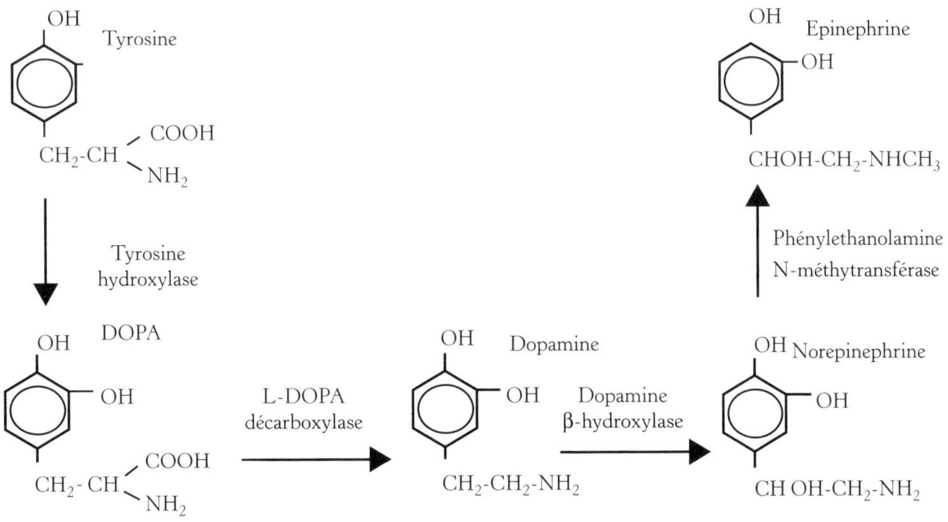

FIGURE 2.23: Biosynthetic pathway and chemical structures of catcholamines. Epinephrine is the hormone released from adrenal medulla. Norepinephrine acts both as a neurotransmitter and a hormone released from adrenal medulla. Dopamine is a precursor of norepinephrine but is also present in some cells. The plasma half-life averages 1 minute.

Once the brain finishes its discrimination/determination function and determines that a stressor exists, a set of neurons in the brainstem (Jansen et al. 1995) initiates and orchestrates the sympathetic nervous system response (Figure 2.22). Both epinephrine and norepinephrine are stored in secretory vesicles. Upon the onset of a stressor, epinephrine and norepinephrine are released from the adrenal medulla and norepinephrine is released from the sympathetic nerve terminals. The speed of release can be explained by the anatomy—both catecholamines are essentially being released by nervous tissue. The ratio of epinephrine to norepinephrine release can depend upon a number of factors, including the type of stressor (Axelrod and Reisine 1984). Release is also facilitated by a positive feedback of catecholamines stimulating increased blood flow to the adrenal medulla (Young and Landsberg 2001).

Catecholamines are extremely potent. They can orchestrate the entire fight-or-flight response with approximately the contents of a single chromaffin cell (Crivellato et al. 2006). Release of more catecholamines is often fatal. Consequently, animals can titrate the amount of epinephrine and norepinephrine released, depending upon the severity of the stressor (Young and Landsberg 2001). Sympathetic activation is not an all-or-nothing response. Like most physiological systems, the strength of the response can be modulated to the needs of the moment.

Once released, resupply is accomplished through both the sympathetic nervous system and corticosteroids up-regulating catecholamine biosynthesis, primarily by stimulating increased activity of synthetic enzymes (Axelrod and Reisine 1984). The primary target is tyrosine hydroxylase activity and production, the rate-limiting step (Young and Landsberg 2001).

C. Adrenergic Receptors

There are two basic receptors for catecholamines, the α- and β-receptors (Figures 2.24 and 2.25), which both come in two subforms (α_1 and α_2, β_1,

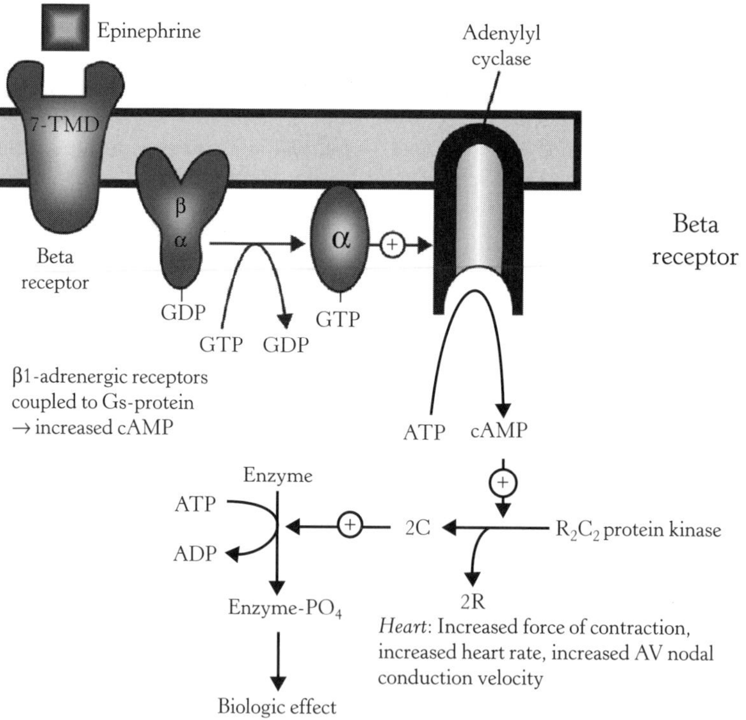

FIGURE 2.24: Adrenergic receptors. The physiological effect observed depends on the nature of involved receptor (α or β type). Beta receptor action is shown here, α and β adrenergic receptors often antagonize one another. When epinephrine binds to β–receptors (in this case a β-1 adrenergic receptor with 7 transmembrane domains, 7-TMD) it activates a stimulatory G protein (Gs) that in turn activates adenylyl cyclase and conversion of ATP to cAMP. GDP and GTP are involved in dissociation of subunits of the G protein prior to activation of adenylyl cyclase. cAMP activates protein kinases, which in turn activate enzymes involved in the biological response. In this example, the β-1 receptor in heart tissue results in increased force of contraction of cardiac muscle, elevated heart rate, and AV nodal conduction velocity.

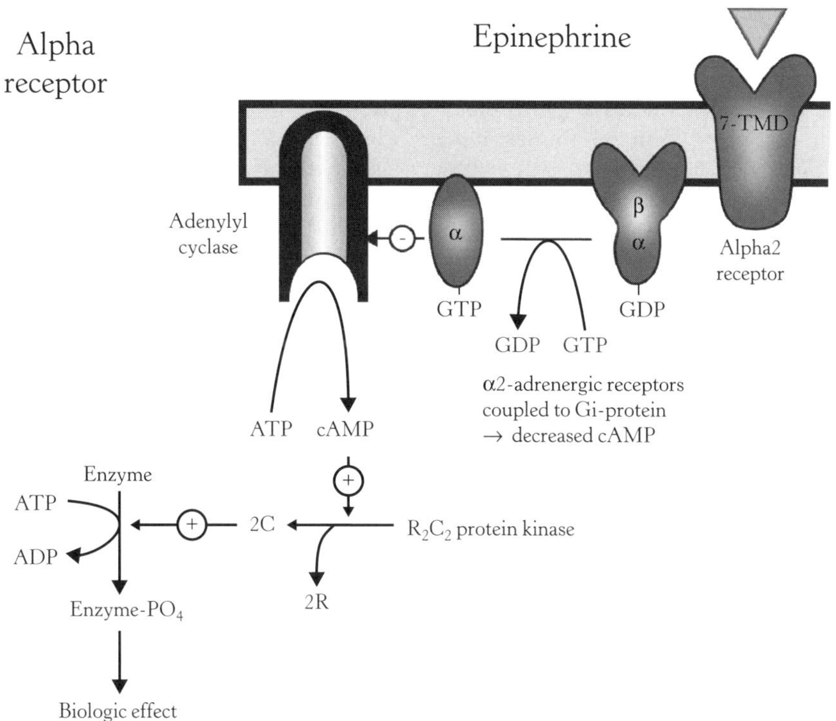

FIGURE 2.25: Action of an α-receptor. In this example, epinephrine binds to an α-2 adrenergic receptor (with 7 transmembrane domains, 7 TMD) that activates an inhibitory G protein (Gi). This in turn deactivates adenylyl cyclase, thus reducing production of cAMP, which would then tend to antagonize the effects of epinephrine via a β-1 receptor in Figure 2.24.

and β_2). The α- and β-receptors receptors have higher affinity for epinephrine and norepinephrine and weaker affinity for the other catecholamines (Norris 2007). α- and β-receptors tend to antagonize one another (G-protein types) and as such have different functions (Figures 2.24 and 2.25). For example, in arteries α_1-receptors mediate vasoconstriction, whereas β_2-receptors mediate vasodilation (reviewed by Bohus and Koolhaas 1993).

D. Functions: Cardiovascular System

The catecholamines initiate several major classes of responses. The first, and probably best known, are changes in the cardiovascular system. Work dating from the beginning of the previous century has identified a number of effects that catecholamines have on the cardiovascular system. As summarized by Herd (1991), they include increased cardiac output (e.g., increased heart rate and stroke volume), increased blood pressure, vasodilation of arteries in skeletal muscle, vasoconstriction of arteries in the kidney, gut, and skin, and vasoconstriction of veins in general. The general result of these changes is to shunt the delivery of nutrients, especially glucose and oxygen, to the brain, heart, lungs, and skeletal muscles, at the cost of peripheral tissues (Goldstein 1987). An exception to this general response is when an animal freezes rather than initiates fight-or-flight. In this case, there is a decrease in heart rate and general vasoconstriction (Fisher 1991; Sapolsky et al. 2000). Together, all of these cardiovascular changes constitute a large component of the fight-or-flight response.

A number of individual variables that could potentially modulate the cardiovascular responses to a stressor have been studied in the laboratory. Interestingly, the fight-or-flight response appears to be remarkably consistent across individuals. Variables such as age, sex, diet, and physical conditioning have, at best, modest impacts on the cardiovascular response (Herd 1991; Goldstein and Eisenhofer 2001). The one factor in humans that does appear to influence the magnitude of cardiovascular responses is a family history of hypertension (Herd 1991). Those with hypertension consistently show greater increases in heart rate and blood pressure.

E. Functions: Respiratory System

In one sense, the major goal of the cardiovascular responses to stress is delivering to tissues the oxygen and nutrients necessary to compensate for the increased demand (Fisher 1991). Catecholamines also help to ensure that those nutrients are available. For example, as discussed previously, catecholamines stimulate the lungs to dilate air passages and initiate hyperventilation (Goldstein 1987).

F. Functions: Metabolism

The second major function of the catecholamines is to increase glucose delivery to the tissues that need it. One major target is the liver (Nonogaki 2000). Both circulating catecholamines (mostly epinephrine) and catecholamines released directly by sympathetic nerve terminals (mostly norepinephrine) stimulate the liver to initiate both glycogen breakdown (glycogenolysis) and production of new glucose (gluconeogenesis) (Goldstein 1987). Glycogen is a short-term storage molecule that can be quickly broken down to glucose that, in the liver, is released into the bloodstream for delivery to other tissues. In skeletal muscle, glycogen breakdown produces glucose that can be directly shuttled into the glycolytic pathway. The end result is that both epinephrine and norepinephrine—although primarily epinephrine (Nonogaki 2000)—rapidly stimulate glycogen breakdown to get a quick burst of glucose. Once glycogen stores have been depleted, the catecholamines begin to stimulate gluconeogenesis in order to sustain glucose release from the liver. To help in both of these functions, epinephrine also inhibits insulin release (Nonogaki 2000).

A second major metabolic target of the catecholamines is fat cells—probably predominant in birds. There are two major types of fat cells. White adipose tissue (WAT) is an important energy storage tissue in vertebrates. Catecholamines, but most likely epinephrine, stimulate lipid breakdown in WAT (Nonogaki 2000). This leads to free fatty acids being released into the circulation, where they can be taken up by the liver and converted to glucose. Brown adipose tissue (BAT) is an important tissue for non-shivering thermogenesis. In these tissues, the electron transport chain can be uncoupled so that glucose metabolism results in heat rather than ATP production. Both epinephrine and norepinephrine, but likely primarily norepinephrine, stimulate heat production in BAT (Nonogaki 2000).

The ultimate purpose of the metabolic effects of catecholamines is to increase the available energy to the muscles and brain, especially after glucose is rapidly consumed during a fight or when fleeing. Once extra glucose becomes available in the bloodstream, the final step in this process is to get the glucose into the cells that need it. Catecholamines also stimulate increased glucose uptake in these cells (Nonogaki 2000). Consequently, we see that the fight-or-flight response helps provide a short-term burst in energy (via glycogen breakdown) and the subsequent sustained resupply of glucose (via gluconeogenesis and fat breakdown) needed to initiate and sustain the responses orchestrated by the other functions of catecholamines.

G. Functions: Skin

Catecholamines also initiate a third set of responses in the skin, along with vasoconstriction (summarized by Goldstein 1987). Anyone who has ever had sweaty palms when undergoing a stressful experience will appreciate the role that catecholamines play in stimulating sweating. This sweat is in addition to sweating for thermoregulatory purposes, which is also initiated by catecholamine signaling. Catecholamines also induce piloerection, the standing up of hairs in their follicles. Piloerection may serve two purposes: to enhance heat retention, and to make the animal appear larger and fiercer to rivals and predators. There is also some evidence that facultative changes in skin color, especially to hide from predators, can be mediated by catecholamines. For example, norepinephrine appears to mediate skin blanching in a fish, the red porgy, exposed to a white background (Fanouraki et al. 2007). Finally, catecholamines activate platelets, presumably to limit hemorrhage in case of wounding.

H. Functions: Nervous System

The nervous system is also a major target for catecholamines (summarized by Goldstein 1987). Catecholamines increase attention and alertness. This leads to increased performance on cognitive tasks, as well as a decrease in muscular and psychological fatigue. These last two effects were presumably the primary desired effects by athletes before catecholamines were banned during competitions. There is also indirect evidence that catecholamines stimulate behavioral changes associated with the fight-or-flight response. In anesthetized cats, when hypothalamic areas involved in both defense and flight behavior were artificially activated, there was a concurrent release of epinephrine and norepinephrine (Stoddard et al. 1986b; Stoddard et al. 1986a).

I. Functions: Other Systems

Finally, catecholamines cause dilation of the pupils, which aids in distance vision, and there is recent evidence that catecholamines can activate parts of the immune system (Karalis et al. 1999; Johnson et al. 2005). Other effects on saliva secretion and loss of gut/urine control (shock defense) are also known.

J. Summary

The details of catecholamine synthesis, release, and functions, as summarized in the preceding sections, are highly conserved among vertebrates. Although there are differences in some of the details, especially in terms of absolute concentrations secreted into the plasma both at baseline and in response to stress, the broad outlines presented here are present in every species examined, from fish to mammals (Hart et al. 1989; Reid et al. 1998). This should highlight how central the fight-or-flight response is for survival and especially the key roles played by epinephrine and norepinephrine.

V. OTHER MEDIATORS: PROLACTIN, HYPOTHALAMO-PITUITARY- THYROID AXIS, CYTOKINES OF THE IMMUNE SYSTEM

We have already mentioned some components of the endocrine system, other than glucococorticoids and catecholamines, that have been implicated in the generalized "stress response." There are many others that will be mentioned, but three groups of these, the polypeptide pituitary hormones such as prolactin, the thyroid hormones, and the cytokines deserve separate explanation.

A. Prolactin

Discovered by Oscar Riddle in 1928, this hormone was termed "prolactin" because pituitary extracts induced lactation in pseudopregnant rabbits. The molecules of growth hormone (GH) and prolactin (PRL) are very similar, both consisting of single peptide chains containing 190–200 amino acids. Prolactin is found in both sexes but its function is better understood in females than in males. It is synthesized as a prohormone in the so-called lactotrophs of the anterior pituitary and is released by exocytosis. Despite the name, over three hundred different actions have been reported for prolactin in various species. Its major effects can be organized into five major types (e.g., Gorbman et al. 1983):

1. Actions related to reproduction
2. Somatotropic effects (e.g., growth)
3. Osmoregulation
4. Actions on the integument and its derivatives
5. Interactions with steroid hormones.

Many of the actions of prolactin may be as a "co-hormone," explaining at least some of the complex differences in actions across vertebrates (e.g., Polzonetti-Magni et al. 1995; Manzon 2002; Sakamoto and McCormick 2006).

The regulation of prolactin release from the anterior pituitary in mammals is primarily inhibitory. Pituitary stalk disconnection, or transplant of the pituitary to an ectopic site such as the kidney capsule, results in an increase in secretion of prolactin. Positive regulators of PRL release include vasoactive intestinal polypeptide (VIP), estrogen, and thyrotropin-releasing hormone (TRH), while negative regulators include dopamine and thyroid hormone. VIP exerts its effects by the G-protein-mediated activation of adenyl cyclase and its downstream effectors cAMP and protein kinase A, culminating in the subsequent release of prolactin. On the other hand, TRH induces PRL expression through activation of the phospholipase C (PLC) signaling pathway and activation of diacylglycerol (DAG) and inositol-1,4,5-trisphosphate (IP_3), which regulates intracellular Ca^{2+} from the endoplasmic reticulum. Dopamine binds to the D_2 dopamine receptor and decreases adenyl cyclase activity. Estrogen directly stimulates the prolactin promoter and can overcome the inhibitory effect of dopamine. Thyroid hormone also directly inhibits the promoter. In birds, prolactin-releasing activity predominates, with VIP the prime candidate. VIP is present in several hypothalamic nuclei that project to the median eminence. Serotonin also increases prolactin secretion in birds. It appears that prolactin has a modulatory role in several aspects of immune function, but is not strictly required for these responses.

The prolactin receptor (PRL-R), which is a member of the hematopoietin/cytokine receptor superfamily, is widely expressed—perhaps in virtually all cells. In rats, stressors such as restraint, foot shock, and so on, result in an increase in prolactin secretion (Kant et al. 1983; Kant et al. 1986; Severino et al. 2004). Social stress has a similar result (Henry 1992). In other species an increase in growth hormone may be more apparent (e.g., humans; Desborough 2000). Generally prolactin tends to increase in response to stress in mammals (Balcombe et al. 2004), but in non-mammalian vertebrates, responses of prolactin to stress are much less clear. In birds, acute stress usually does not result in an increase in prolactin (e.g., Maney et al. 1999), and in breeding birds results in a decrease of prolactin (e.g., Angelier and Chastel 2008).

B. The Glycoprotein Hormones, Hypothalamo-Pituitary-Thyroid Axis

There are three glycoprotein hormones secreted by the pars distalis of the anterior pituitary gland. All have both early and late (trophic) cell responses. They are as follows:

Luteinizing hormone (LH), which regulates sex steroid production as well as ovulation;

Follicle stimulating hormone (FSH), which regulates spermatogenesis and ovarian follicle maturation. It also is involved with secretion of a protein inhibin from the gonads, that feeds back negatively to regulate FSH secretion.

Thyroid-stimulating hormone (TSH; also known as thyrotropin), which regulates thyroid hormone synthesis and secretion.

All three hormones share the characteristic structure of two subunits, α– and β–. The α subunit is composed of 92 amino acids and carries two oligosaccharides. It is shared by all three hormones, whereas the β subunit is specific to each hormone. For example, it is possible to recombine an FSH α subunit with, say, a TSH β subunit and still get good TSH biological activity (Gorbman et al. 1983). However, the association of α and β subunits is essential for binding to receptor and biological action. We will not consider LH and FSH further here.

The two subunits of TSH are attached to each other, and then glycosylation increases the biological activity and the breakdown rate of the hormone. Thyrotropin-releasing hormone (TRH), released by the hypothalamus, stimulates thyrotropes in the anterior pituitary to synthesize and release TSH. TSH binds with membrane-bound TSH receptors on the cells of the thyroid gland, which in turn regulate synthesis of thyroxine (T4). T4 then is modified further by the enzyme monodeiodinase to give tri-iodothyronine (T3). TSH synthesis and release from the anterior pituitary is also controlled by the concentrations of thyroid hormones (especially T3) through negative feedback (Gorbman et al. 1983). The hypothalamus also releases somatostatin and dopamine, which inhibit TSH release from the anterior pituitary. It is believed that both somatostatin and dopamine act through a Gi-coupled signal membrane receptor transduction system. Somatostatin is released by the hypothalamus during hyperthyroidism (high serum T3 and T4), which decreases TSH release. In birds and amphibians, CRH is also a potent releaser of TSH. In reptiles, CRH, vasoactive intestinal peptide (VIP), and TRH regulate TSH release.

Activation of the hypothalamo-hypophysial-thyroid axis often involves a decrease in temperature. This primary neural event (i.e., perception of the temperature change and transduction by neurotransmitters) results in the release of TRH from the median eminence into the portal system. TRH binding to a thyrotrope receptor in the anterior pituitary results in release of TSH by exocytosis.

The thyroid gland is a single lobed gland in some species but may be paired in other species. Cross section of the human trachea shows the thyroid gland almost surrounding it. The shape of the thyroid in mammals varies with species, but is usually fused into a single gland. In amphibians, reptiles, and birds, it can either be a single gland or paired, but is always located in the neck (pharyngeal region), often associated with major blood vessels such as the jugular vein. In fish the thyroid gland is usually, but not always, scattered in small groups of follicles within the walls of the pharynx. The functional component of the thyroid gland is a ring of cells (cuboidal epithelium) surrounding a lumen filled with colloidal material. The cuboidal cells are always a single layer containing lipid droplets and many mitochondria. Capillaries are in close association with the follicles and may form globular networks around follicles before draining into veins.

The TSH receptor is a seven-transmembrane-spanning protein, and a G-protein-coupled signal transduction pathway activates adenylyl cyclase and phosphotidylinositol systems in the cells when bound to TSH. The increased cytosolic cAMP concentrations mediated by the adenylyl cyclase system increase iodine uptake by follicular cells of the thyroid, and the increased cytosolic Ca2+ concentrations mediated by the PIP2 system increase iodination of thyroglobulin. TSH also increases the transcription of mRNA for thyroglobulin and thyroidal peroxidase (TPO), and increases the formation and activity of lysosomes, which will hydrolyze the iodinated thyroglobulin to form thyroid hormones. There is also increased activity in 5′-deiodinase, which helps to conserve iodine in the thyroid. Rapid cell responses include increased iodine incorporation into thyroglobulin; increased oxygen consumption and glucose uptake by cuboid epithelium for the peroxidase cycle; and increased pinocytosis of colloid. Late cell responses are mediated through TSH-stimulated transcription factors to increase synthesis of thyroglobulin, increased epithelial cell height, and synthetic machinery for producing thyroid hormones (colloid tends to be used up when TSH activity is high); elevated iodine pump and peroxidase levels; and increased activity, growth, and mitosis of thyroid hormone secreting cells. TSH also increases the metabolic rate of the thyroid cells, as well as DNA and RNA synthesis.

T3 and T4 have three major types of action: growth and development, thermogenesis, and permissive actions. Because many vertebrates (mostly birds and mammals, but also some other vertebrates) maintain a body temperature above (or below) that of the environment, heat must be generated or dissipated. Thyroid hormones increase mitochondrial oxygen consumption and production of ATP. Also, they increase the number of membrane sodium pumps that use up to 20% or 45% of total cell energy supplies (ATP). Inhibition of Na^+/K^+ATPase activity by, for example, ouabain, reduces the action of thyroid hormones on heat production and oxygen consumption. Earlier it was thought that thyroid hormones acted on heat production by uncoupling oxidative phosphorylation within mitochondria.

Generation of heat by increasing activity of Na^+/K^+ATPase activity in mitochondria is especially important for seasonal adjustments of thermogenesis (e.g. increased during winter). However, under conditions of sudden heat loss, shivering thermogenesis is important in many mammals and birds. As body temperature is lowered, the autonomic nervous system triggers rapid muscle twitches (shivering) that generate heat from ATP use for muscle contractions. Some mammals utilize a different system—non-shivering thermogenesis—by metabolizing fat from brown adipose tissue (BAT) or brown fat. BAT is a red-brown adipose tissue so colored because of its rich blood supply and high concentration of cytochromes. The fat in BAT tissue is contained in several cytoplasmic droplets, whereas white adipose tissue (WAT) has only one huge droplet of fat taking up most of the cell volume. BAT cells have large numbers of mitochondria. Lipolysis in BAT is stimulated by β-adrenergic (norepinephrine from nerve terminals or epinephrine in blood, see earlier discussion), resulting in the liberation of non-esterified fatty acids (NEFA) leading to an uncoupling of oxidative phosphorylation with mitochrondria. NEFA displaces the nucleotide GDP from a protein thermogenin (about 32 K-Daltons) on the inner mitochondrial membrane so that protons (H^+) generated during electron transport can re-enter the mitochondrion and be oxidized, releasing heat. Thermogenesis thus occurs through an oxidation of fatty acids without production of ATP. The BAT system is important in neonates (including humans), rodents, and some hibernating species.

Thyroid hormones can have permissive actions. In synergy with corticosteroids, they can elevate growth hormone secretion and increase lipolysis. However, they have antagonistic actions on prolactin and growth and vice versa. In teleosts, thyroid hormones are essential for gonadal development and thus may have permissive actions for gonadotropins.

Thyroid hormones interact with several forms of receptors and transport proteins. Transport proteins may be important not only for transferring T3 and T4 into cells but also in trafficking hormone to appropriate receptors. Thyroid hormone receptors and transporters (amino acid transporters) interact to modulate thyroid hormone uptake into target tissues and are important sites of controlling thyroid hormone delivery to the cell nucleus. Thyroid hormones mostly mediate their actions via nuclear receptors and act as hormone-induced transcription factors. The T3 nuclear receptor is a member of the steroid-receptor gene super family, forming a hetero-dimer with retinoic acid receptor and then DNA binding. Actions of thyroid hormones at the genomic level are generally slow (hours to days) and may provide the permissive functions. Actions at the membrane receptor level can be fast (minutes).

C. Cytokines of the Immune System

The immune system operates throughout the body as individual cells in blood, lymph, and cerebrospinal fluid, as well as at central lymphoid tissue (bone marrow, thymus) and peripheral lymphoid tissue (lymph nodes, spleen, mucosa-associated lymphoid tissue). Many immune cells secrete proteins, cytokines, that act as classical chemical messengers in autocrine, paracrine, and endocrine ways. These hormones of the immune system are highly complex, and we summarize only a few here—particularly in relation to stress.

Hormones of the immune system interact at all levels with neural, endocrine, and neuroendocrine systems. Two major types of immune system hormones will be reviewed briefly here—lymphokines and monokines. The lymphokines and monokines "qualify" as hormones in that they act locally and can also be blood borne, having actions distant from their source of release. Those that have been characterized act through high affinity membrane receptors, and are secreted in response to stress in the form of infection or tissue damage. They are intimately involved in the regulation of immune and inflammatory responses. These compounds are secreted by monocytes (monokines) or lymphocytes (lymphokines). Cytokines are basically polypeptide hormones, but the term is often used to denote those molecules that are the products of cells of the immune system or that act upon such cells. A few of them will be summarized next.

Today more than 20 interleukins (IL-1—IL-22) have been determined to play an important role in anti-tumor growth. The name "interleukin" was originally coined to describe soluble mediators of communication between leucocytes, but their role is not confined to leucocytes. A number of the cytokines important in natural immunity also play a major role in acquired immunity.

IL-1 appears to act on the fever center of the hypothalamus and mimics (may be identical to) endogenous pyrogen (EP). In addition, it may be the trigger molecule that initiates the synthesis of proteins following tissue injury, inflammation, or infection. IL-2, the primary T cell growth factor (autocrine), also stimulates B cell growth. A product of T lymphocytes, IL-2 appears to provide the key signal for proliferation of antigen-activated T cells and thus is essential for clonal expansion that follows the initial antigen-recognition phase of the normal immune response. Physiological doses of glucocorticoids inhibit production of IL-2 by activated T lymphocytes. Note, however, that although glucocorticoids can inhibit IL-1 and IL-2, this action only prevents clonal expansion of activated T cells early in the sequence. High steroid levels later in the immune response are ineffective since clonal expansion has already occurred.

IL-4 is an important B cell growth factor and has a key role in T cell differentiation (see following discussion). It is required for IgE synthesis. The principal role of IL-5 is in eosinophil activation and maturation. It is important in response to helminths. In addition to its systemic effects (noted earlier), IL-6 is a major growth factor for differentiated B cells/pre-plasma cells. IL-10 acts on macrophages in an inhibitory fashion and is antagonistic to interferon gamma (IFN-g).

Interferons are a family of proteins identified over 30 years ago for their anti-viral actions. IFN-g is a product of antigen-activated T lymphocytes. Mononuclear phagocytes (monocytes and macrophages) have surface receptors that specifically bind the Fc portion of immunoglobulin G (IgG). These receptors are important for recognition by macrophages of particulate antigens that have been antibody-tagged (opsonized) and thus are involved in the clearance of immune complexes, bacterial pathogens (and during the course of autoimmune disease, they clear antibody tagged host cells). They may also guide mononuclear phagocytes in the destruction of tumor cells, in stimulation of immunoglobulin production, and in the release of inflammatory mediators. IFN-g produces up to a 10-fold increase in the number of Fc receptors on normal human monocytes. Glucocorticoids inhibit production of IFN-g. The production of this group of cytokines is stimulated non-specifically by viruses or microbial pathogens. The group includes type I interferon (IFNalpha, IFNbeta), which is produced by lymphocytes and fibroblasts in response to viral infection and stimulates intrinsic defense against virus infection in a wide range of cell types. Interferons and interleukins interact to trigger specific transduction cascades. Molecular interactions among cytokines and cytokine receptors form the basis of many cell-signaling pathways relevant to immune function.

Colony stimulating factor (CSF) is another lymphokine (also called "granulocyte macrophage colony stimulating factor") produced by T lymphocytes. It is a growth factor (or factors) that stimulates production of granulocytes and macrophages from immature progenitor cells in culture. Again, glucocorticoids inhibit production of CSF. Colony stimulating factors are glycoproteins that are required for the survival, proliferation, and differentiation of hematopoietic progenitor cells of myeloid and erythroid linkage. Granulocyte-macrophage colony stimulating factor (GM-CSF) stimulates the growth and differentiation of hematopoietic precursor cells from various lineages, including granulocytes, macrophages, erythrocytes, and eosinophils.

Tumor necrosis factor (TNF) is a lymphokine whose activity is associated with a subpopulation of normal lymphocytes. A large peptide, its activity is measured by the ability of cells to spontaneously lyse certain tumor cell targets. It appears that TNF activity is involved in resistance to tumor growth and may be a primary mechanism of immune surveillance. TNF activity is suppressed by glucocorticoids. TNFα is primarily produced by macrophages. Stimulated by bacteria (LPS), it has a very wide range of biological effects; activation of neutrophils, upregulation of adhesion molecules, and stimulation of IL-1 production (by monocytes) and acute phase proteins (by liver, in synergy with IL-1 and IL-6). Overproduction of TNF causes toxic shock and death. TNF can bind three receptor chains (as a trimer) to initiate a cascade of inflammatory cytokines.

Endogenous pyrogen stimulates the acute phase response (with IL-6 and TNF). IL-6 is also produced by macrophages. It has a key role in inducing an acute phase protein response by the liver. IFN-g, a potent activator of macrophages stimulating secondary release of TNFa, IL-1, and so forth, and critical in inducing secondary killing mechanisms vital to eliminating intracellular pathogens, has a wide variety of other effects; it is a potent antiviral, it up-regulates MHC class I and induces class II on a wide range of cells (monocytes, endothelial cells, epithelial cells, etc.), and it is a major differentiation factor for T and B cells.

VI. SUMMARY

To conclude, this chapter provides an introduction to the major components of the neuroendocrine/endocrine systems that have roles as mediators of stress—or rather, the responses to stress. For the rest of the book we will focus primarily on the hypothalamo-pituitary-adrenal cortex axis and the glucocorticoids that are secreted as a result; and on the catecholamines from the adrenal medulla: epinephrine and norepinephrine. With this introduction in mind, we now go on to discuss the responses to stress and the comparative biology of those responses.

REFERENCES

Amir, S., Brown, Z. W., Amit, Z., 1980. The role of endophins in stress: Evidence and speculations. *Neurosci Biobehav Rev 4*, 77–86.

Angelier, F., Chastel, O., 2008. Stress, prolactin and parental investment in birds: A review. In: *9th International Symposium on Avian Endocrinology*, Leuven, Belgium, pp. 142–148.

Antoni, F. A., 1993. Vasopressinergic control of pituitary adrenocorticotropin secretion comes of age. *Front Neuroendocrinol 14*, 76–122.

Astheimer, L. B., Buttemer, W. A., Wingield, J. C., 1994. Gender and seasonal differences in the adrenocortical response to ACTH challenge in an Arctic passerine, *Zonotrichia leucophrys gambelii*. *Gen Comp Endocrinol 94*, 33–43.

Axelrod, J., Reisine, T. D., 1984. Stress hormones: Their interaction and regulation. *Science 224*, 452–459.

Baker, M. E., 2004. Evolutionary analysis of 11 beta-hydroxysteroid dehydrogenase-type 1, -type 2, -type 3 and 17 beta-hydroxysteroid dehydrogenase-type 2 in fish. *Febs Letters 574*, 167–170.

Balcombe, J. P., Barnard, N. D., Sandusky, C., 2004. Laboratory routines cause animal stress. *Cont Topics Lab Animal Sci 43*, 42–51.

Ball, G. F., Faris, P. L., Wingfield, J. C., 1989. Immunohistochemical localization of corticotropin-releasing factor in selected brain areas of the European starling (*Sturnus vulgaris*) and the song sparrow (*Melospiza melodia*). *Cell Tissue Res 257*, 155–161.

Ballard, P. L., Baxter, J. D., Higgins, S. J., Rousseau, G. G., Tomkins, G. M., 1974. General presence of glucocorticoid receptors in mammalian tissues. *Endocrinology 94*, 998–1002.

Barry, T. P., Marwah, A., Nunez, S., 2010. Inhibition of cortisol metabolism by 17 alpha, 20 beta-P: Mechanism mediating semelparity in salmon? *Gen Comp Endocrinol 165*, 53–59.

Bartanusz, V., Jezova, D., Bertini, L. T., Tilders, F. J. H., Aubry, J. M., Kiss, J. Z., 1993. Stress-induced increase in vasopressin and corticotropin-releasing factor expression in hypophysiotrophic paraventricular neurons. *Endocrinology 132*, 895–902.

Basu, N., Kennedy, C. J., Hodson, P. V., Iwama, G. K., 2001. Altered stress responses in rainbow trout following a dietary administration of cortisol and β-napthoflavone. *Fish Physiol Biochem 25*, 131–140.

Bhargava, A., Pearce, D., 2004. Mechanisms of mineralocorticoid action: Determinants of receptor specificity and actions of regulated gene products. *Trends Endocrinol Metab 15*, 147–153.

Bohus, B., Koolhaas, J. M., 1993. Stress and the cardiovascular system: central and peripheral physiological mechanisms. In: Stanford, S. C., Salmon, P., Gray, J. A. (Eds.), *Stress: From synapse to syndrome*. Academic Press, Boston, MA, pp. 75–117.

Bornstein, S. R., Engeland, W. C., Ehrhart-Bornstein, M., Herman, J. P., 2008. Dissociation of ACTH and glucocorticoids. *Trends Endocrinol Metab 19*, 175–180.

Borski, R. J., 2000. Nongenomic membrane actions of glucocorticoids in vertebrates. *Trends Endocrinol Metab 11*, 427–436.

Breuner, C. W., Greenberg, A. L., Wingfield, J. C., 1998. Noninvasive corticosterone treatment rapidly increases activity in Gambel's white-crowned sparrows (*Zonotrichia leucophrys gambelii*). *Gen Comp Endocrinol 111*, 386–394.

Breuner, C. W., Jennings, D. H., Moore, M. C., Orchinik, M., 2000. Pharmacological adrenalectomy with mitotane. *Gen Comp Endocrinol 120*, 27–34.

Breuner, C. W., Lynn, S. E., Julian, G. E., Cornelius, J. M., Heidinger, B. J., Love, O. P., Sprague, R. S., Wada, H., Whitman, B. A., 2006. Plasma-binding globulins and acute stress response. *Horm Metab Res 38*, 260–268.

Breuner, C. W., Orchinik, M., 2001. Seasonal regulation of membrane and intracellular corticosteroid receptors in the house sparrow brain. *J Neuroendocrinol 13*, 412–420.

Breuner, C. W., Orchinik, M., 2002. Beyond carrier proteins: Plasma binding proteins as mediators of corticosteroid action in vertebrates. *J Endocrinol 175*, 99–112.

Breuner, C. W., Orchinik, M., 2009. Pharmacological characterization of intracellular, membrane, and plasma binding sites for corticosterone in house sparrows. *Gen Comp Endocrinol 163*, 214–224.

Breuner, C. W., Orchinik, M., Hahn, T. P., Meddle, S. L., Moore, I. T., Owen-Ashley, N. T., Sperry, T. S., Wingfield, J. C., 2003. Differential mechanisms for regulation of the stress response across latitudinal gradients. *Am J Physiol 285*, R594–R600.

Breuner, C. W., Wingfield, J. C., Romero, L. M., 1999. Diel rhythms of basal and stress-induced corticosterone in a wild, seasonal vertebrate, Gambel's white-crowned sparrow. *J Exp Zool 284*, 334–342.

Carsia, R. V., 1990. Hormonal control of avian adrenocortical function: Cellular and molecular aspects. In: Epple, A., Scanes, C. G., Stetson, M. H. (Eds.), *Progress in comparative endocrinology*. Wiley-Liss, New York, pp. 439–444.

Carsia, R. V., John-Alder, H. B., 2006. Natriuretic peptides are negative modulators of adrenocortical cell function of the eastern fence lizard (*Sceloporus undulatus*). *Gen Comp Endocrinol 145*, 157–161.

Carsia, R. V., Scanes, C. G., Malamed, S., 1987. Polyhormonal regulation of avian and mammalian corticosteroidogenesis in vitro. *Comp Biochem Physiol 88A*, 131–140.

Carsia, R. V., Weber, H., Perez, F. M. J., 1986. Corticotropin-releasing factor stimulates the release of adrenocorticotropin from domestic fowl pituitary cells. *Endocrinology 118*, 143–148.

Castro, M. G., Estivariz, F. E., Iturriza, F. C., 1986. The regulation of the corticomelanotropic cell activity in Aves. II. Effect of various peptides on the release of ACTH from dispersed, perfused duck pituitary cells. *Comp Biochem Physiol 83A*, 71–75.

Chester-Jones, I., Phillips, J. G., 1986. The adrenal and interrenal glands. In: Pang, P. K. T., Schreibman, M. P. (Eds.), *Vertebrate endocrinology; Vol. I: Fundamentals and biomedical implications*, Academic Press, San Diego, CA, pp. 319–349.

Crivellato, E., Nico, B., Ribatti, D., Nussdorfer, G. G., 2006. Catecholamine release by chromaffin cells: A lesson from mast cells. *Gen Comp Endocrinol 146*, 69–73.

Dallman, M. F., 2005. Fast glucocorticoid actions on brain: Back to the future. *Front Neuroendocrinol 26*, 103–108.

Dallman, M. F., Akana, S. F., Cascio, C. S., Darlington, D. N., Jacobson, L., Levin, N., 1987. Regulation of ACTH secretion: Variations on a theme of B. *Rec Prog Horm Res 43*, 113–173.

Dallman, M. F., Akana, S. F., Scribner, K. A., Bradbury, M. J., Walker, C.-D., Strack, A. M., Cascio, C. S., 1992. Stress, feedback and facilitation in the hypothalamo-pituitary-adrenal axis. *J Neuroendocrinol 4*, 517–526.

Dallman, M. F., Bhatnagar, S., 2001. Chronic stress and energy balance: role of the hypothalamo-pituitary-adrenal axis. In: McEwen, B. S., Goodman, H. M. (Eds.), *Handbook of physiology; Section 7: The endocrine system; Vol. IV: Coping with the environment: Neural and endocrine mechanisms*. Oxford University Press, New York, pp. 179–210.

Dallman, M. F., la Fleur, S. E., Pecoraro, N. C., Gomez, F., Houshyar, H., Akana, S. F., 2004. Minireview: Glucocorticoids—food intake, abdominal obesity, and wealthy nations in 2004. *Endocrinology 145*, 2633–2638.

Dallman, M. F., Strack, A. M., Akana, S. F., Bradbury, M. J., Hanson, E. S., Scribner, K. A., Smith, M., 1993. Feast and famine: Critical role of glucocorticoids with insulin in daily energy flow. *Front Neuroendocrinol 14*, 303–347.

Day, T. A., 2005. Defining stress as a prelude to mapping its neurocircuitry: No help from allostasis. *Prog Neuro-Psychopharmacol Biol Psychiatry 29*, 1195.

de Kloet, E. R., Oitzl, M. S., Joels, M., 1993a. Functional implications of brain corticosteroid receptor diversity. *Cell Mol Neurobiol 13*, 433–455.

de Kloet, E. R., Oitzl, M. S., Joëls, M., 1993b. Functional implications of brain corticosteroid receptor diversity. *Cell Mol Neurobiol 13*, 433–455.

de Wilde, J., 1978. Seasonal states and endocrine levels in insects. In: Assenmacher, I., Farner, D. S. (Eds.), *Environmental endocrinology*. Springer-Verlag, Berlin, pp. 10–19.

Degoeij, D. C. E., Dijkstra, H., Tilders, F. J. H., 1992. Chronic psychosocial stress enhances vasopressin, but not corticotropin-releasing factor, in the external zone of the median-eminence of male-rats: Relationship to subordinate status. *Endocrinology 131*, 847–853.

Denari, D., Ceballos, N. R., 2005. 11β-Hydroxysteroid dehydrogenase in the testis of *Bufo arenarum*: Changes in its seasonal activity. *Gen Comp Endocrinol 143*, 113–120.

Denari, D., Ceballos, N. R., 2006. Cytosolic glucocorticoid receptor in the testis of *Bufo arenarum*: Seasonal changes in its binding parameters. *Gen Comp Endocrinol 147*, 247–254.

Denver, R. J., 2007. Endocannabinoids link rapid, membrane-mediated corticosteroid actions to behavior. *Endocrinology 148*, 490–492.

DeRijk, R. H., de Kloet, E. R., 2008. Corticosteroid receptor polymorphisms: Determinants of vulnerability and resilience. *Eur J Pharmacol 583*, 303–311.

Desborough, J. P., 2000. The stress response to trauma and surgery. *Brit J Anaesth 85*, 109–117.

Deviche, P., Breuner, C., Orchinik, M., 2001. Testosterone, corticosterone, and photoperiod interact to regulate plasma levels of binding globulin and free steroid hormone in Dark-eyed Juncos, *Junco hyemalis. Gene Compar Endocrinol 122*, 67–77.

DeVries, A. C., Gerber, J. M., Richardson, H. N., Moffatt, C. A., Demas, G. E., Taymans, S. E., Nelson, R. J., 1997. Stress affects corticosteroid and immunoglobulin concentrations in male house mice (*Mus musculus*) and prairie voles (*Microtus ochrogaster*). *Comp Biochem Physiol 118A*, 655–663.

Dickens, M., Romero, L. M., Cyr, N. E., Dunn, I. C., Meddle, S. L., 2009. Chronic stress alters glucocorticoid receptor and mineralocorticoid receptor mRNA expression in the European starling (*Sturnus vulgaris*) brain. *J Neuroendocrinol 21*, 832–840.

Engeland, W. C., Arnhold, M. M., 2005. Neural circuitry in the regulation of adrenal corticosterone rhythmicity. *Endocrine 28*, 325–331.

Erickson, K., Drevets, W., Schulkin, J., 2003. Glucocorticoid regulation of diverse cognitive functions in normal and pathological emotional states. *Neurosci Biobehav Rev 27*, 233–246.

Evans, S. J., Murray, T. F., Moore, F. L., 2000. Partial purification and biochemical characterization of a membrane glucocorticoid receptor from an amphibian brain. *J Steroid Biochem Mol Biol 72*, 209–221.

Familari, M., Smith, A. I., Smith, R., Funder, J. W., 1989. Arginine vasopressin is a much more potent stimulus to ACTH release from ovine anterior pituitary cells than ovine corticotropin-releasing factor. *Neuroendocrinol 50*, 152–157.

Fanouraki, E., Laitinen, J. T., Divanach, P., Pavlidis, M., 2007. Endocrine regulation of skin blanching in red porgy, *Pagrus pagrus. Ann Zool Fenn 44*, 241–248.

Feder, M. E., Hofmann, G. E., 1999. Heat-shock proteins, molecular chaperones, and the stress response: Evolutionary and ecological physiology. *Ann Rev Physiol 61*, 243–282.

Fisher, L. A., 1991. Stress and cardiovascular physiology in animals In: Brown, M. R., Koob, G. F., Rivier, C. (Eds.), *Stress: Neurobiology and neuroendocrinology.* Marcel Dekker, New York, pp. 463–474.

Flik, G., Klaren, P. H. M., Van Den Burg, E. H., Metz, J. R., Huising, M. O., 2006. CRF and stress in fish. *Gen Comp Endocrinol 146*, 36.

Fostier, A., Breton, B., 1975. Binding of steroids by plasma of a teleost: the rainbow trout, Salmo gairdnerii. *J Steroid Biochem 6*, 345–351.

Garamszegi, L. Z., Merino, S., Torok, J., Eens, M., Martinez, J., 2006. Indicators of physiological stress and the elaboration of sexual traits in the collared flycatcher. *Behav Ecol 17*, 399–404.

Goldstein, D. S., 1987. Stress-induced activation of the sympathetic nervous system *Baillieres Clin Endocrinol Metabol 1*, 253–278.

Goldstein, D. S., Eisenhofer, G., 2001. Sympathetic nervous system physiology and pathophysiology in coping with the environment. In: McEwen, B. S., Goodman, H. M. (Eds.), *Handbook of physiology; Section 7: The endocrine system; Vol. IV: Coping with the environment: Neural and endocrine mechanisms.* Oxford University Press, New York, pp. 21–43.

Goldstein, D. S., Pacak, K., 2001. Catecholamines in the brain and responses to environmental challenges. In: McEwen, B. S., Goodman, H. M. (Eds.), *Handbook of physiology; Section 7: The endocrine system; Vol. IV: Coping with the environment: Neural and endocrine mechanisms.* Oxford University Press, New York, pp. 45–60.

Gorbman, A., 1999. Brain-Hatschek's pit relationships in amphioxus species. *Acta Zoologica 80*, 301–305.

Gorbman, A., Dickhoff, W. W., Vigna, S. R., Clark, N. B., Ralph, C. L., 1983. *Comparative endocrinology.* Wiley and Sons, New York.

Graessler, J., Kvetnansky, R., Jezova, D., Dobrakovova, M., van Loon, G. R., 1989. Prior immobilization stress alters adrenal hormone responses to hemorrhage in rats. *Am J Physiol 257*, R661–R667.

Gross, K. L., Cidlowski, J. A., 2008. Tissue-specific glucocorticoid action: a family affair. *Trends Endocrinol Metab 19*, 331–339.

Hall, P. F., 2001. Actions of corticotropin on the adrenal cortex: Biochemistry and cell biology. In: McEwen, B. S., Goodman, H. M. (Eds.), *Handbook of physiology; Section 7: The endocrine system; Vol. IV: Coping with the environment: Neural and endocrine mechanisms.* Oxford University Press, New York, pp. 61–84.

Haller, J., Mikics, E., Makara, G. B., 2008. The effects of non-genomic glucocorticoid mechanisms on bodily functions and the central neural system: A critical evaluation of findings. *Front Neuroendocrinol 29*, 273–291.

Hammer, G. D., Parker, K. L., Schimmer, B. P., 2005. Minireview: Transcriptional regulation of adrenocortical development. *Endocrinology 146*, 1018–1024.

Hammes, A., Andreassen, T. K., Spoelgen, R., Raila, J., Hubner, N., Schulz, H., Metzger, J., Schweigert, F. J., Luppa, P. B., Nykjaer, A., Willnow, T. E., 2005. Role of endocytosis in cellular uptake of sex steroids. *Cell 122*, 751–762.

Hammond, G. L., 1990. Molecular properties of corticosteroid binding globulin and the sex-steroid binding proteins. *Endocr Rev 11*, 65–79.

Hart, B. B., Stanford, G. G., Ziegler, M. G., Lake, C. R., Chernow, B., 1989. Catecholamines: Study of interspecies variation. *Crit Care Med 17*, 1203.

Hauger, R. L., Grigoriadis, D. E., Dallman, M. F., Plotsky, P. M., Vale, W. W., Dautzenberg, F. M., 2003. International union of pharmacology. XXXVI. Current status of the nomenclature for receptors for corticotropin-releasing factor and their ligands. *Pharmacol Rev 55*, 21–26.

Henry, J. P., 1992. Biological basis of the stress response: Address upon accepting the Hans Selye Award from the American Institute of Stress in Montreux, Switzerland, February 1991. *Integ Physiol Behav Sci 27*, 66–83.

Herd, J. A., 1991. Cardiovascular response to stress. *Physiol Rev 71*, 305–330.

Herman, J. P., Cullinan, W. E., Young, E. A., Akil, H., Watson, S. J., 1992. Selective forebrain fiber tract lesions implicate ventral hippocampal structures in tonic regulation of paraventricular nucleus corticotropin-releasing hormone (CRH) and arginine vasopressin (AVP) mRNA expression. *Brain Res 592*, 228–238.

Herman, J. P., Prewitt, C. M. F., Cullinan, W. E., 1996. Neuronal circuit regulation of the hypothalamo-pituitary-adrenocortical stress axis. *Crit Rev Neurobiol 10*, 371–394.

Hill, M. N., McLaughlin, R. J., Bingham, B., Shrestha, L., Lee, T. T. Y., Gray, J. M., Hillard, C. J., Gorzalka, B. B., Viau, V., 2010. Endogenous cannabinoid signaling is essential for stress adaptation. *Proc Natl Acad Sci USA 107*, 9406–9411.

Hill, M. N., McLaughlin, R. J., Pan, B., Fitzgerald, M. L., Roberts, C. J., Lee, T. T. Y., Karatsoreos, I. N., Mackie, K., Viau, V., Pickel, V. M., McEwen, B. S., Liu, Q. S., Gorzalka, B. B., Hillard, C. J., 2011. Recruitment of prefrontal cortical endocannabinoid signaling by glucocorticoids contributes to termination of the stress response. *J Neurosci 31*, 10506–10515.

Hodgson, Z. G., Meddle, S. L., Roberts, M. L., Buchanan, K. L., Evans, M. R., Metzdorf, R., Gahr, M., Healy, S. D., 2007. Spatial ability is impaired and hippocampal mineralocorticoid receptor mRNA expression reduced in zebra finches (*Taeniopygia guttata*) selected for acute high corticosterone response to stress. *Proc R Soc Lond B 274*, 239–245.

Hontela, A., 1998. Interrenal dysfunction in fish from contaminated sites: in vivo and in vitro assessment. *Environ Toxicol Chem 17*, 44–48.

Huising, M., Metz, J. R., van Schooten, C., Taverne-Thiele, A. J., Hermsen, T., Verburg-van Kemanade, B. M. L., Flik, G., 2004. Structural characterisation of a cyprinid (*Cyprinus carpio L.*) CRH, CRH-BP and CRH-R1, and the role of these proteins in the acute stress response. *J Mol Endocrinol 32*, 627–648.

Idler, D. R., 1972. *Steroids in nonmammalian vertebrates.* Academic Press, New York.

Idler, D. R., Freeman, H. C., 1968. Binding of testosterone, 1alpha hydroxy corticosterone and cortisol by plasma proteins of fish. *Gen Comp Endocrinol 11*, 366–372.

Ikonomopoulou, M. P., Bradley, A. J., Whittier, J. M., Ibrahim, K., 2006. Identification and properties of steroid-binding proteins in nesting *Chelonia mydas* plasma. *J Comp Physiol B 176*, 775–782.

Jacobson, L., Akana, S. F., Cascio, C. S., Shinsako, J., Dallman, M. F., 1988. Circadian variations in plasma corticosterone permit normal termination of adrenocorticotropin responses to stress. *Endocrinology 122*, 1343–1348.

Jacobson, L., Sapolsky, R., 1991. The role of the hippocampus in feedback regulation of the hypothalamic-pituitary-adrenocortical axis. *Endocr Rev 12*, 118–134.

Jansen, A. S. P., Van Nguyen, X., Karpitskiy, V., Mettenleiter, T. C., Loewy, A.D., 1995. Central command neurons of the sympathetic nervous system: Basis of the fight-or-flight response. *Science 270*, 644–646.

Jennings, D. H., Moore, M. C., Knapp, R., Matthews, L., Orchinik, M., 2000. Plasma steroid-binding globulin mediation of differences in stress reactivity in alternative male phenotypes in tree lizards, *Urosaurus ornatus. Gen Comp Endocrinol 120*, 289–299.

Johnson, J. D., Campisi, J., Sharkey, C. M., Kennedy, S. L., Nickerson, M., Greenwood, B. N., Fleshner, M., 2005. Catecholamines mediate stress-induced increases in peripheral and central inflammatory cytokines. *Neuroscience 135*, 1295–1307.

Kant, G. J., Bunnell, B. N., Mougey, E. H., Pennington, L. L., Meyerhoff, J. L., 1983. Effects of repeated stress on pituitary cyclic-AMP, and plasma prolactin, corticosterone and growth hormone in male rats. *Pharmacol Biochem Behav 18*, 967–971.

Kant, G. J., Mougey, E. H., Meyerhoff, J. L., 1986. Diurnal variation in neuroendocrine response to stress in rats: Plasma ACTH, beta-endorphin, beta-LPH, corticosterone, prolactin and pituitary cyclic-AMP responses. *Neuroendocrinol 43*, 383–390.

Karalis, K. P., Kontopoulos, E., Muglia, L. J., Majzoub, J. A., 1999. Corticotropin-releasing hormone deficiency unmasks the proinflammatory effect of epinephrine. *Proc Natl Acad Sci USA 96*, 7093–7097.

Katz, A., Heiblum, R., Meidan, R., Robinzon, B., 2008. Corticosterone oxidative neutralization by 11-[beta] hydroxysteroid dehydrogenases in kidney and colon of the domestic fowl. *Gen Comp Endocrinol 155*, 814–820.

Keller-Wood, M. E., Dallman, M. F., 1984. Corticosteroid inhibition of ACTH secretion. *Endocr Rev 5*, 1–24.

Keller-Wood, M. E., Shinsako, J., Dallman, M. F., 1983. Integral as well as proportional adrenal responses to ACTH. *Am J Physiol 245*, R53–R59.

Kjaer, A., Knigge, U., Bach, F. W., Warberg, J., 1992. Histamine-induced and stress-induced secretion of acth and beta-endorphin: Involvement of corticotropin-releasing hormone and vasopressin. *Neuroendocrinol 56*, 419–428.

Klukowski, L. A., Cawthorn, J. M., Ketterson, E. D., Nolan, V. J., 1997. Effects of experimentally elevated testosterone on plasma corticosterone and corticosterone-binding globulin in dark-eyed juncos (*Junco hyemalis*). *Gen Comp Endocrinol 108*, 141–151.

Knapp, R., Moore, M. C., 1995. Hormonal responses to aggression vary in different types of agonistic encounters in male tree lizards, *Urosaurus ornatus*. *Horm Behav 29*, 85–105.

Kobayashi, H., Gorbman, A., Wake, K., Mori, T., Matsumoto, A., 1987. *Atlas of endocrine organs*. Kodansha, Tokyo.

Koch, K. A., Wingfield, J. C., Buntin, J. D., 2002. Glucocorticoids and parental hyperphagia in ring doves (*Streptopelia risoria*). *Horm Behav 41*, 9–21.

Kregel, K. C., 2002. Molecular biology of thermoregulation: Invited review: Heat shock proteins: Modifying factors in physiological stress responses and acquired thermotolerance. *J Appl Physiol 92*, 2177–2186.

Kucka, M., Vagnerova, K., Klusonova, P., Miksik, I., Pacha, J., 2006. Corticosterone metabolism in chicken tissues: Evidence for tissue-specific distribution of steroid dehydrogenases. *Gen Comp Endocrinol 147*, 377.

Kusakabe, M., Nakamura, I., Young, G., 2003. 11 beta-Hydroxysteroid dehydrogenase complementary deoxyribonucleic acid in rainbow trout: Cloning, sites of expression, and seasonal changes in gonads. *Endocrinology 144*, 2534–2545.

Labar, K. S., Ledoux, J. E., 2001. Coping with danger: the neural basis of defensive behavior and fearful feelings. In: McEwen, B. S., Goodman, H. M. (Eds.), *Handbook of physiology; Section 7: The endocrine system; Vol. IV: Coping with the environment: Neural and endocrine mechanisms.* Oxford University Press, New York, pp. 139–154.

Landys, M. M., Piersma, T., Ramenofsky, M., Wingfield, J. C., 2004a. Role of the low-affinity glucocorticoid receptor in the regulation of behavior and energy metabolism in the migratory red knot *Calidris canutus islandica*. *Physiol Biochem Zool 77*, 658–668.

Landys, M. M., Ramenofsky, M., Guglielmo, C. G., Wingfield, J. C., 2004b. The low-affinity glucocorticoid receptor regulates feeding and lipid breakdown in the migratory Gambel's white-crowned sparrow *Zonotrichia leucophrys gambelii*. *J Exp Biol 207*, 143–154.

Li, Z., Srivastava, P., 2004. Heat-shock proteins. *Current protocols in immunology, 58*:1T:A.1T.1-A.1T.6.

Losel, R. M., Falkenstein, E., Feuring, M., Schultz, A., Tillmann, H. C., Rossol-Haseroth, K., Wehling, M., 2003. Nongenomic steroid action: Controversies, questions, and answers. *Physiol Rev 83*, 965–1016.

Lynn, S. E., Breuner, C. W., Wingfield, J. C., 2003. Short-term fasting affects locomotor activity, corticosterone, and corticosterone binding globulin in a migratory songbird. *Horm Behav 43*, 150–157.

Mains, R. E., Eipper, B. A., 2001. Proopiomelanocortin synthesis and cell-specific processing. In: McEwen, B. S., Goodman, H. M. (Eds.), *Handbook of physiology; Section 7: The endocrine system; Vol. IV: Coping with the environment: Neural and endocrine mechanisms.* Oxford University Press, New York, pp. 85–101.

Maitra, U. S., Khan, M. S., Rosner, W., 1993. Corticosteroid-binding globulin receptor of the rat hepatic membrane: Solubilization, partial characterization, and the effect of steroids on binding. *Endocrinology 133*, 1817–1822.

Malisch, J. L., Breuner, C. W., 2010. Steroid-binding proteins and free steroids in birds. *Mol Cell Endocrinol 316*, 42–52.

Maney, D. L., Schoech, S. J., Sharp, P. J., Wingfield, J. C., 1999. Effects of vasoactive intestinal peptide on plasma prolactin in passerines. *Gen Comp Endocrinol 113*, 323–330.

Maney, D. L., Wingfield, J. C., 1998. Neuroendocrine suppression of female courtship in a wild passerine: Corticotropin-releasing factor and endogenous opioids. *J Neuroendocrinol 10*, 593.

Manzon, L. A., 2002. The role of prolactin in fish osmoregulation: A review. *Gen Comp Endocrinol 125*, 291–310.

Martinez-de la Puente, J., Merino, S., Moreno, J., Tomas, G., Morales, J., Lobato, E., Garcia-Fraile, S., Martinez, J., 2007. Are eggshell spottiness and colour indicators of health and condition in blue tits *Cyanistes caeruleus*? *J Avian Biol 38*, 377–384.

McEwen, B. S., 2001. Neurobiology of interpreting and responding to stressful events: paradigmatic role of the hippocampus. In: McEwen, B. S., Goodman, H. M. (Eds.), *Handbook of physiology; Section 7: The endocrine system; Vol. IV: Coping with the environment: Neural and endocrine mechanisms*. Oxford University Press, New York, pp. 155–178.

Meaney, M. J., Aitken, D. H., Sharma, S., Viau, V., 1992. Basal acth corticosterone and corticosterone-binding globulin levels over the diurnal cycle and age-related changes in hippocampal type I and type II corticosteroid receptor binding capacity in young and aged handled and nonhandled rats. *Neuroendocrinol 55*, 204–213.

Metz, J. R., Geven, E. J. W., van den Burg, E. H., Flik, G., 2005. ACTH, alpha-MSH, and control of cortisol release: Cloning, sequencing, and functional expression of the melanocortin-2 and melanocortin-5 receptor in Cyprinus carpio. *Am J Physiol 289*, R814–R826.

Mikami, S., 1986. Immunocytochemistry of the avian hypothalamus and adenohypophysis. *Int Rev Cytol 103*, 189–248.

Mikami, S., Yamada, S., 1984. Immunohistochemistry of the hypothalamic neuropeptides and anterior pituitary cells in the Japanese quail. *J Exp Zool 232*, 405–417.

Mikami, S. I., Oksche, A., Farner, D. S., Vitums, A., 1970. Fine structure of vessels of hypophysial portal system of white-crowned sparrow, *Zonotrichia leucophrys gambelii. Z Zellforsch Mik Anat 106*, 155–174.

Minton, J. E., 1994. Function of the hypothalamic-pituitary-adrenal axis and the sympathetic nervous system in models of acute stress in domestic farm animals. *J Animal Sci 72*, 1891.

Monamy, V., 1995. Ecophysiology of a wild-living population of the velvet-furred rat, *Rattus lutreolus velutinus* (Rodentia: Muridae), in Tasmania. *Aust J Zool 43*, 583–600.

Moore, F. L., Boyd, S. K., Kelley, D. B., 2005. Historical perspective: Hormonal regulation of behaviors in amphibians. *Horm Behav 48*, 373–383.

Munck, A., Náray-Fejes-Tóth, A., 1992. The ups and downs of glucocorticoid physiology: Permissive and supressive effects revisited. *Mol Cell Endocrinol 90*, C1–C4.

Nakhla, A. M., Khan, M. S., Rosner, W., 1988. Induction of adenylate cyclase in a mammary carcinoma cell line by human corticosteroid-binding globulin. *Biochem Biophys Res Comm 153*, 1012.

Nelson, R. J., 2011. *An introduction to behavioral endocrinology*, 4th Edition. Sinauer Associates, Sunderland, MA.

Nonogaki, K., 2000. New insights into sympathetic regulation of glucose and fat metabolism. *Diabetologia 43*, 533–549.

Norris, D. O., 1997. *Vertebrate endocrinology*. Academic Press, Boston.

Norris, D. O., 2007. *Vertebrate endocrinology*. Academic Press, Boston.

Norris, D. O., Donahue, S., Dores, R. M., Lee, J. K., Maldonado, T. A., Ruth, T., Woodling, J. D., 1999. Impaired adrenocortical response to stress by brown trout, *Salmo trutta*, living in metal-contaminated waters of the Eagle River, Colorado. *Gen Comp Endocrinol 113*, 1–8.

Oakley, R. H., Cidlowski, J. A., 2011. Cellular processing of the glucocorticoid receptor gene and protein: New mechanisms for generating tissue-specific actions of glucocorticoids. *J Biol Chemi 286*, 3177–3184.

Ogawa, T., Shishioh-Ikejima, N., Konishi, H., Makino, T., Sei, H., Kiryu-Seo, S., Tanaka, M., Watanabe, Y., Kiyama, H., 2009. Chronic stress elicits prolonged activation of alpha-MSH secretion and subsequent degeneration of melanotroph. *J Neurochem 109*, 1389–1399.

Oksche, A., Farner, D. S., 1974. Neurohistological studies on the hypothalamo-hyphophysial system of *Zonotrichia leucophrys gambelii* (Aves Passeriformes), with special attention to its role in the control of reproduction. *Ergebn Anat 48*(4), 1–136.

Orchinik, M., Matthews, L., Gasser, P. J., 2000. Distinct specificity for corticosteroid binding sites in amphibian cytosol, neuronal membranes, and plasma. *Gen Comp Endocrinol 118*, 284–301.

Orchinik, M., Murray, T. F., Moore, F. L., 1991. A corticosteroid receptor in neuronal membranes. *Science 252*, 1848–1851.

Ottenweller, J. E., Meier, A. H., Russo, A. C., Frenzke, M. E., 1979. Circadian rhythms of plasma corticosterone binding activity in the rat and the mouse. *Acta Endocrinol (Copenh) 91*.

Ozaki, Y., Higuchi, M., Miura, C., Yamaguchi, S., Tozawa, Y., Miura, T., 2006. Roles of 11 beta-hydroxysteroid dehydrogenase in fish spermatogenesis. *Endocrinology 147*, 5139–5146.

Petersen, H. H., Andreassen, T. K., Breiderhoff, T., Brasen, J. H., Schulz, H., Gross, V., Grone, H. J., Nykjaer, A., Willnow, T. E., 2006. Hyporesponsiveness to glucocorticoids in mice genetically deficient for the corticosteroid binding globulin. *Mol Cell Biol 26*, 7236–7245.

Plotsky, P. M., 1991. Pathways to the secretion of adrenocorticotropin: A view from the portal. *J Neuroendocrinol 3*, 1.

Polzonetti-Magni, A., Carnevali, O., Yamamoto, K., Kikuyama, S., 1995. Growth hormone and prolactin in amphibian reproduction. *Zool Sci 12*, 683–694.

Qian, X. X., Droste, S. K., Gutierrez-Mecinas, M., Collins, A., Kersante, F., Reul, J., Linthorst, A. C. E., 2011. A rapid release of corticosteroid-binding globulin from the liver restrains the glucocorticoid hormone response to acute stress. *Endocrinology 152*, 3738–3748.

Reid, S. G., Bernier, N. J., Perry, S. F., 1998. The adrenergic stress response in fish: control of catecholamine storage and release. *Comp Biochem Physiol C 120*, 1–27.

Remage-Healey, L., Bass, A. H., 2006. A rapid neuromodulatory role for steroid hormones in the control of reproductive behavior. *Brain Res 1126*, 27–35.

Rich, E. L., Romero, L. M., 2001. Daily and photoperiod variations of basal and stress-induced corticosterone concentrations in house sparrows (*Passer domesticus*). *J Comp Physiol B 171*, 543–547.

Rich, E. L., Romero, L. M., 2005. Exposure to chronic stress downregulates corticosterone responses to acute stressors. *Am J Physiol 288*, R1628–R1636.

Richter, C., Park, J. W., Ames, B. N., 1988. Normal oxidative damage to mitochondrial and nuclear DNA is extensive. *Proc Natl Acad Sci USA 85*, 6465–6467.

Rivier, C. L., Grigoriadis, D. E., Rivier, J. E., 2003. Role of corticotropin-releasing factor receptors type 1 and 2 in modulating the rat adrenocorticotropin response to stressors. *Endocrinology 144*, 2396.

Rohleder, N., Wolf, J. M., Kirschbaum, C., 2003. Glucocorticoid sensitivity in humans-interindividual differences and acute stress effects. *Stress 6*, 207–222.

Romero, L. M., 2002. Seasonal changes in plasma glucocorticoid concentrations in free-living vertebrates. *Gen Comp Endocrinol 128*, 1–24.

Romero, L. M., 2004. Physiological stress in ecology: Lessons from biomedical research. *Trends Ecol Evol 19*, 249–255.

Romero, L. M., Cyr, N. E., Romero, R. C., 2006. Corticosterone responses change seasonally in free-living house sparrows (*Passer domesticus*). *Gen Comp Endocrinol 149*, 58–65.

Romero, L. M., Levine, S., Sapolsky, R. M., 1995. Adrenocorticotropin secretagog release: stimulation by frustration and paradoxically by reward presentation. *Brain Res 676*, 151–156.

Romero, L. M., Meister, C. J., Cyr, N. E., Kenagy, G. J., Wingfield, J. C., 2008. Seasonal glucocorticoid responses to capture in wild free-living mammals. *Am J Physiol 294*, R614-R622.

Romero, L. M., Remage-Healey, L., 2000. Daily and seasonal variation in response to stress in captive starlings (*Sturnus vulgaris*): Corticosterone. *Gen Comp Endocrinol 119*, 52–59.

Romero, L. M., Sapolsky, R. M., 1996. Patterns of ACTH secretagog secretion in response to psychological stimuli. *J Neuroendocrinol 8*, 243–258.

Romero, L. M., Soma, K. K., Wingfield, J. C., 1998. Hypothalamic-pituitary-adrenal axis changes allow seasonal modulation of corticosterone in a bird. *Am J Physiol 274*, R1338–R1344.

Romero, L. M., Wikelski, M., 2010. Stress physiology as a predictor of survival in Galapagos marine iguanas. *Proc R Soc Lond B 277*, 3157–3162.

Rosner, W., 1990. The functions of corticosteroid-binding globulin and sex hormone-binding globulin: Recent advances. *Endocr Rev 11*, 80–91.

Sakamoto, T., McCormick, S. D., 2006. Prolactin and growth hormone in fish osmoregulation. *Gen Comp Endocrinol 147*, 24–30.

Sapolsky, R. M., 1992. *Stress, the aging brain, and the mechanisms of neuron death*. MIT Press, Cambridge, MA.

Sapolsky, R. M., 1993. Endocrinology alfresco: Psychoendocrine studies of wild baboons. *Recent Prog Horm Res 48*, 437–468.

Sapolsky, R. M., 2001. Physiological and pathophysiological implications of social stress in mammals. In: McEwen, B. S., Goodman, H. M. (Eds.), *Handbook of physiology; Section 7: The endocrine system; Vol. IV: Coping with the environment: Neural and endocrine mechanisms*. Oxford University Press, New York, pp. 517–532.

Sapolsky, R. M., Altmann, J., 1991. Incidence of hypercortisolism and dexamethasone resistance increases with age among wild baboons. *Biol Psych 30*, 1008–1016.

Sapolsky, R. M., McEwen, B. S., 1985. Down-regulation of neural corticosterone receptors by corticosterone and dexamethasone. *Brain Res 339*, 161–165.

Sapolsky, R. M., Romero, L. M., Munck, A. U., 2000. How do glucocorticoids influence stress-responses? Integrating permissive, suppressive, stimulatory, and preparative actions. *Endocr Rev 21*, 55–89.

Sapolsky, R. M., Share, L. J., 1994. Rank-related differences in cardiovascular function among wild baboons: Role of sensitivity to glucocorticoids. *Am J Primatol 32*, 261–275.

Scaccianoce, S., Muscolo, L. A. A., Cigliana, G., Navarra, D., Nicolai, R., Angelucci, L., 1991. Evidence for a specific role of vasopressin in sustaining pituitary-adrenocortical stress response in the rat. *Endocrinology 128*, 3138–3143.

Schedlowski, M., Fluge, T., Richter, S., Tewes, U., Schmidt, R. E., Wagner, T. O. F., 1995. Beta-endorphin but not substance-P, is increased by acute stress in humans *Psychoneuroendocrinology 20*, 103–110.

Schiml-Webb, P. A., Deak, T., Greenlee, T. M., Maken, D., Hennessy, M. B., 2006. Alpha-melanocyte stimulating hormone reduces putative stress-induced sickness behaviors in isolated guinea pig pups. *Behav Brain Res 168*, 326–330.

Schmidt, K. L., Malisch, J. L., Breuner, C. W., Soma, K. K., 2010. Corticosterone and cortisol binding sites in plasma, immune organs and brain of developing zebra finches: Intracellular and membrane-associated receptors. *Brain Behav Immun 24*, 908–918.

Severino, G. S., Fossati, I. A. M., Padoin, M. J., Gomes, C. M., Trevizan, L., Sanvitto, G. L., Franci, C. R., Anselmo-Franci, J. A., Lucion, A. B., 2004. Effects of neonatal handling on the behavior and prolactin stress response in male and female rats at various ages and estrous cycle phases of females. *Physiol Behav 81*, 489–498.

Shultz, M. T., Kitaysky, A. S., 2008. Spatial and temporal dynamics of corticosterone and corticosterone binding globulin are driven by environmental heterogeneity. *Gen Comp Endocrinol 155*, 717–728.

Siiteri, P. K., Murai, J. T., Hammond, G. L., Nisker, J. A., Raymoure, W. J., Kuhn, R. W., 1982. The serum tranport of steroid hormones. *Rec Prog Horm Res 38*, 457–510.

Sousa, N., Cerqueira, J. J., Almeida, O. F. X., 2008. Corticosteroid receptors and neuroplasticity. *Brain Res Rev 57*, 561–570.

Stanford, S. C., 1993. Monoamines in response and adaptation to stress. In: Stanford, S. C., Salmon, P., Gray, J. A. (Eds.), *Stress: From synapse to syndrome*. Academic Press, San Diego, CA, pp. 281–331.

Stoddard, S. L., Bergdall, V. K., Townsend, D. W., Levin, B. E., 1986a. Plasma catecholamines associated with hypothalamically-elicited defense behavior. *Physiol Behav 36*, 867–874.

Stoddard, S. L., Bergdall, V. K., Townsend, D. W., Levin, B. E., 1986b. Plasma catecholamines associated with hypothalamically-elicited flight behavior. *Physiol Behav 37*, 709–715.

Stolte, E. H., Verburg van Kemenade, B. M. L., Savelkoul, H. F. J., Flik, G., 2006. Evolution of glucocorticoid receptors with different glucocorticoid sensitivity. *J Endocrinol 190*, 17–28.

Stouthart, A., Lucassen, E., van Strien, F. J. C., Balm, P. H. M., Lock, R. A. C., Bonga, S. E. W., 1998. Stress responsiveness of the pituitary-interrenal axis during early life stages of common carp (*Cyprinus carpio*). *J Endocrinol 157*, 127–137.

Strelchyonok, O. A., Avvakumov, G. V., 1991. Interaction of human CBG with cell-membranes. *J Steroid Biochem Mol Biol 40*, 795–803.

Sumpter, J. P., Pickering, A. D., Pottinger, T. G., 1985. Stress-induced elevation of plasma alpha-MSH and endorphin in brown trout, *Salmo trutta L. Gen Comp Endocrinol 59*, 257–265.

Tasker, J. G., Di, S., Malcher-Lopes, R., 2005. Rapid central corticosteroid effects: Evidence for membrane glucocorticoid receptors in the brain. *Integ Comp Biol 45*, 665–671.

Tasker, J. G., Herman, J. P., 2011. Mechanisms of rapid glucocorticoid feedback inhibition of the hypothalamic–pituitary–adrenal axis. *Stress 14*, 398–406.

Taymans, S. E., DeVries, A. C., DeVries, M. B., Nelson, R. J., Friedman, T. C., Castro, M., Detera-Wadleigh, S., Carter, C. S., Chrousos, G. P., 1997. The hypothalamic-pituitary-adrenal axis of prairie voles (*Microtus ochrogaster*): Evidence for target tissue glucocorticoid resistance. *Gen Comp Endocrinol 106*, 48–61.

Tokarz, R. R., Summers, C. H., 2011. Stress and reproduction in reptiles. In: David, O. N., Kristin, H. L. (Eds.), *Hormones and reproduction of vertebrates*. Academic Press, London, pp. 169–213.

Tomlinson, J. W., Walker, E. A., Bujalska, I. J., Draper, N., Lavery, G. G., Cooper, M. S., Hewison, M., Stewart, P. M., 2004. 11β-Hydroxysteroid dehydrogenase type 1: A tissue-specific regulator of glucocorticoid response. *Endocr Rev 25*, 831–866.

Tonon, M. C., Cuet, P., Lamacz, M., Jegou, S., Cote, J., Gouteux, L., Ling, N., Pelletier, G., Vaudry, H., 1986. Comparative effects of corticotropin-releasing factor, arginine vasopressin, and related neuropeptides on the secretion of ACTH and alpha-MSH by frog anterior-pituitary-cells and neurointermediate lobes in vitro *Gen Comp Endocrinol 61*, 438–445.

Turnbull, A. V., Rivier, C., 1997. Corticotropin-releasing factor (CRF) and endocrine responses to stress: CRF receptors, binding protein, and related peptides. *Proc Soc Exper Biol Med 215*, 1–10.

Ulrich-Lai, Y. M., Arnhold, M. M., Engeland, W. C., 2006. Adrenal splanchnic innervation contributes to the diurnal rhythm of plasma corticosterone in rats by modulating adrenal sensitivity to ACTH. *Am J Physiol 290.*

Ulrich-Lai, Y. M., Engeland, W. C., 2002. Adrenal splanchnic innervation modulates adrenal cortical responses to dehydration stress in rats. *Neuroendocrinol 76*, 79–92.

Vale, W., Spiess, J., Rivier, C., Rivier, J., 1981. Characterization of a 41-residue ovine hypothalamic peptide that stimulates secretion of corticotropin and B-endorphin. *Science 213*, 1394–1397.

Vandenborne, K., De Groef, B., Geelissen, S. M. E., Boorse, G. C., Denver, R. J., Kuhn, E. R., Darras, V. M., Van der Geyten, S., 2005a. Molecular cloning and developmental expression of corticotropin-releasing factor in the chicken. *Endocrinology 146*, 301–308.

Vandenborne, K., De Groef, B., Geelissen, S. M. E., Kuhn, E. R., Darras, V. M., Van der Geyten, S., 2005b. Corticosterone-induced negative feedback mechanisms within the hypothalamo-pituitary-adrenal axis of the chicken. *J Endocrinol 185*, 383–391.

von Euler, U. S., Heller, H., 1963. *Comparative endocrinology. Vol. 1: Glandular hormones*. Academic Press, New York.

Vylitova, M., Miksik, I., Pacha, J., 1998. Metabolism of corticosterone in mammalian and avian intestine. *Gen Comp Endocrinol 109*, 315–324.

Walker, J. J., Terry, J. R., Lightman, S. L., 2010. Origin of ultradian pulsatility in the hypothalamic-pituitary-adrenal axis. *Proc R Soc Lond B 277*, 1627–1633.

Ward, C. K., Fontes, C., Breuner, C. W., Mendonça, M.T., 2007. Characterization and quantification of corticosteroid-binding globulin in a southern toad, *Bufo terrestris*, exposed to coal-combustion-waste. *Gen Comp Endocrinol 152*, 82–88.

Weninger, S. C., Majzoub, J. A., 2001. Regulation and actions of corticotropin-releasing hormone. In: McEwen, B. S., Goodman, H. M. (Eds.), *Handbook of physiology; Section 7: The endocrine system; Vol. IV: Coping with the environment: Neural and endocrine mechanisms*. Oxford University Press, New York, pp. 103–124

White, P. C., Mune, T., Agarwal, A. K., 1997. 11{beta}-hydroxysteroid dehydrogenase and the syndrome of apparent mineralocorticoid excess. *Endocr Rev 18*, 135–156.

Whitnall, M. H., 1993. Regulation of the hypothalamic corticotropin-releasing hormone neurosecretory system. *Prog Neurobiol 40*, 573–629.

Widmaier, E. P., Harmer, T. L., Sulak, A. M., Kunz, T. H., 1994. Further characterization of the pituitary-adrenocortical responses to stress in Chiroptera. *J Exp Zool 269*, 442–449.

Widmaier, E. P., Kunz, T. H., 1993. Basal, diurnal, and stress-induced levels of glucose and glucocorticoids in captive bats. *J Exp Zool 265*, 533–540.

Windle, R. J., Wood, S. A., Lightman, S. L., Ingram, C. D., 1998a. The pulsatile characteristics of hypothalamo-pituitary-adrenal activity in female Lewis and Fischer 344 rats and its relationship to differential stress responses. *Endocrinology 139*, 4044–4052.

Windle, R. J., Wood, S. A., Shanks, N., Lightman, S. L., Ingram, C. D., 1998b. Ultradian rhythm of basal corticosterone release in the female rat: Dynamic interaction with the response to acute stress. *Endocrinology 139*, 443–450.

Wingfield, J. C., 2005. The concept of allostasis: Coping with a capricious environment. *J Mammal 86*, 248–254.

Wingfield, J. C., 2006. Communicative behaviors, hormone-behavior interactions, and reproduction in vertebrates. In: Neill, J.D. (Ed.) *Physiology of reproduction*. Academic Press, New York, pp. 1995–2040.

Wingfield, J. C., Matt, K. S., Farner, D. S., 1984. Physiologic properties of steroid hormone-binding proteins in avian blood. *Gen Comp Endocrinol 53*, 281–292.

Wood, R. D., 1996. DNA repair in eukaryotes. *Ann Rev Biochem 65*, 135–167.

Woodley, S. K., Painter, D. L., Moore, M. C., Wikelski, M., Romero, L. M., 2003. Effect of tidal cycle and food intake on the baseline plasma corticosterone rhythm in intertidally foraging marine iguanas. *Gen Comp Endocrinol 132*, 216–222.

Wotus, C., Engeland, W. C., 2003. Differential regulation of adrenal corticosteroids after restriction-induced drinking in rats. *Am J Physiol 284*.

Wotus, C., Osborn, J. W., Nieto, P. A., Engeland, W. C., 2003. Regulation of corticosterone production by vasopressin during water restriction and after drinking in rats. *Neuroendocrinol 78*, 301.

Wyrwoll, C. S., Holmes, M. C., Seckl, J. R., 2011. 11 beta-Hydroxysteroid dehydrogenases and the brain: From zero to hero, a decade of progress. *Front Neuroendocrinol 32*, 265–286.

Yao, M., Denver, R. J., 2007. Regulation of vertebrate corticotropin-releasing factor genes. *Gen Comp Endocrinol 153*, 200–216.

Young, J. B., Landsberg, L., 2001. Synthesis, storage, and secretion of adrenal medullary hormones: physiology and pathophysiology. In: McEwen, B. S., Goodman, H. M. (Eds.), *Handbook of physiology; Section 7: The endocrine system; Vol. IV: Coping with the environment: Neural and endocrine mechanisms*. Oxford University Press, New York, pp. 3–19.

Zysling, D. A., Greives, T. J., Breuner, C. W., Casto, J. M., Demas, G. E., Ketterson, E. D., 2006. Behavioral and physiological responses to experimentally elevated testosterone in female dark-eyed juncos (*Junco hyemalis carolinensis*). *Horm Behav 50*, 200–207.

3

Models of Stress

I. INTRODUCTION

Most research on stress has muddled along with a poor and often vague definition of stress. This has greatly hampered progress in the field, but there has been a growing consensus about many of the parameters. On the other hand, field investigations of how free-living organisms respond physiologically and behaviorally to acute perturbations of the environment have revealed new insights into the comparative biology of coping (Chapter 1). How all these concepts can be reconciled, if at all, will be the topic of this chapter, and we will present different, yet related, ways to think of stress. The first, which we call the "Traditional Model," is the framework that most biomedical researchers have been using for the past few decades. The second, the "Life-History Model," has raised many issues, such as habituation in the context of an organism in its natural world. The third is a combination of recent models, "Allostasis and Reactive Scope," which attempts to provide a framework to solve the stress quagmire. Each model has pluses and minuses, and we will explore these in depth.

II. THE TRADITIONAL MODEL

The traditional way to view an animal is as an organism at dynamic equilibrium (Figure 3.1A). Another term for dynamic equilibrium is "homeostasis," although that is a more limited term because it tends to only imply physiological processes. Dynamic equilibrium, on the other hand, can imply both physiological and psychological processes. The term "dynamic equilibrium" also encompasses an important concept—short-term adaptation to change. Part of the process of life, of course, is coping with changes in the environment. Many of these changes are highly predictable, such as changes between day and night or seasonal changes, and most animals are exquisitely adapted to prepare for these changes. In fact, daily rhythms, seasonal rhythms, preparation for pregnancy or migration, and so on, are normal physiological and behavioral processes during which an animal maintains equilibrium. For example, even though mammalian pregnancy requires a large increase in the amount of energy consumed and utilized, healthy female mammals easily adjust their metabolism, food intake, and so on, to maintain their equilibrium.

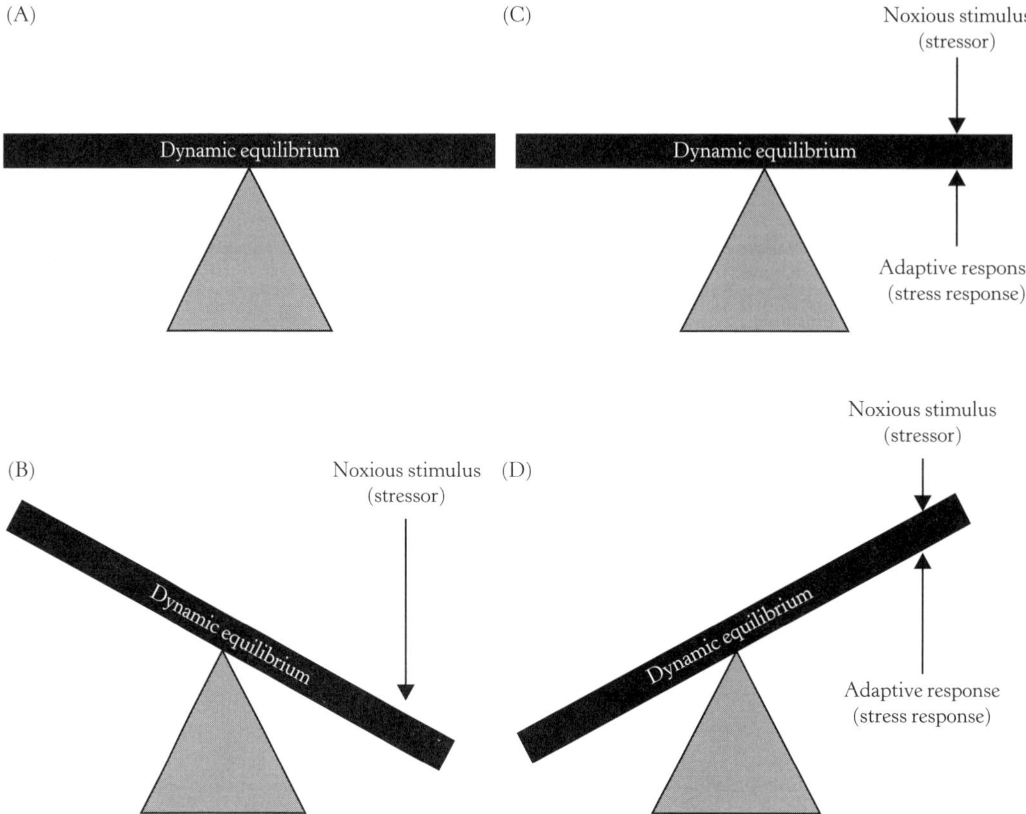

FIGURE 3.1: The traditional model of stress.

This concept might be best illustrated with the classic example of homeostasis—the thermostat in your house. You set the thermostat to a comfortable temperature and the heater adjusts its output to maintain that temperature. The preferred comfortable temperature, however, can change. One modern method of saving energy is to decrease the set temperature of your house at night. The heater then adjusts its output to maintain the lowered temperature. What follows is a daily rhythm of temperature regulation. This illustrates the classic definition of homeostasis (Cannon 1932). Homeostatic mechanisms maintain physiological systems (such as body temperature) in a stable range appropriate to the circumstances such as time of day, season, and so on. An important point here is that physiological changes in response to daily or seasonal environmental fluctuations, or changes in response to normal life events such as pregnancy, are subsumed under dynamic equilibrium. These changes are not stress, regardless of how energetically expensive they are.

In distinct contrast, however, are unpredictable changes in the environment. These changes are almost always noxious and serve to disrupt the dynamic equilibrium (Figure 3.1B). These stimuli are termed "stressors" because they elicit a stress response from the animal and can be either physical or psychological in nature. If the animal does not quickly re-establish its dynamic equilibrium, it will soon be in trouble and will likely die. The various physiological, behavioral, and endocrine response mechanisms that serve to re-establish the dynamic equilibrium have been collectively termed the "stress response" (Figure 3.1C). These are the responses that ultimately allow an animal to survive a stressor. Note, however, that inherent in the definition of dynamic equilibrium is that stressors require emergency reactions. If an animal can adequately predict a future event (i.e., winter), coping will occur through homeostatic mechanisms and the event will not be a stressor. These responses are generally called the "acute stress response" because the emergency is quickly dealt with and the animal returns to a state of dynamic equilibrium. Anyone who has visited a physician to discuss stress will immediately notice that this is not the topic of discussion. Instead of an emphasis on stress helping you survive, the emphasis is on stress causing disease. In this case, the stress response has essentially overcompensated for the stressor and itself causes a disruption in the dynamic equilibrium (Figure 3.1D). This is the concept that most laypeople attach to the word "stress" and is the subject of the vast majority of biomedical research. In the biomedical literature, this is termed "chronic stress."

The four panels of Figure 3.1 summarize the various historical approaches to studying stress. Psychologists have focused on the nature of stressful stimuli; what stimuli elicit a stress response and under what contexts do they do so (Figure 3.1B). Clinical physiologists have focused on the stress responses themselves, with an almost exclusive emphasis on how they cause disease (Figure 3.1D). Finally, field endocrinologists and ecologists have similarly focused on the stress responses, but with a heavy emphasis on how they help wild animals to survive in their natural habitats (Figure 3.1C). None of these approaches is mutually exclusive, of course, but experimental designs are heavily influenced by the background and training of researchers from these three traditions. The last approach is the topic of this book, but we will borrow heavily from the other approaches as well.

The early history of studying stress in wild animals focused on the acute stress response, and this is the subject for much of the remainder of the book. Until very recently, we both would have argued that chronic stress is not a particularly important concept for free-living animals. Except for a few documented cases from highly social species such as primates (e.g., Sapolsky 1993), we generally thought that a chronically stressed animal (i.e., one where the stress response itself was disrupting the dynamic equilibrium) was a dead animal. The pathology associated with chronic stress from the biomedical literature would quickly make the animal a target for either disease or predation. We did not expect to see many examples of chronic stress in the wild, and if we did see it, we expected it to be associated with massive mortality, which certainly happens from time to time (see Gessaman and Worthen 1982). Our thinking has recently changed, however. Chronic stress may be more prevalent than we initially thought (e.g., Kitaysky et al. 1999; Romero and Wikelski 2001) and those that survive a period of chronic stress may be the precise individuals that have a disproportionate impact on the next generation (i.e., evolution). Chronic stress is becoming an increasing focus of work in wild animals, especially in a conservation context (see Chapters 12 and 13).

A. Nature of Stressors and Stimulus Specificity

If we are going to use the traditional model to understand stress responses in wild animals, we need to know when and how a stress response is elicited. The biomedical literature can provide some foundational principles that we can use to guide us. Many laboratory studies have indicated that a stress response is both stimulus specific and context specific.

It seems intuitive that stress responses should be stressor specific. After all, an attack by a predator is a very different stressor and would require a very different response than an attack by a disease organism or lack of food. An important point, therefore, is that not all stressors are equivalent. This is a point often forgotten when researchers try to reconcile apparently anomalous findings. This point is also contrary to the history of studying stress. Selye (1946) originally proposed the General Adaptation Syndrome to describe stress in which he highlighted a common response to all stressors. This thinking dominated the stress field for many years until it was finally shown that, even though they share many common pathways, different stressors do elicit different responses.

The evidence for this is quite extensive. For example, a hemorrhage elicits a massive release of vasopressin to cope with the loss of blood volume, but this response does not occur for other stressors (reviewed by Sapolsky et al. 2000). Although the specificity of responses appears to begin in the brain, there has not been much success identifying a "stress circuit" (Day 2005), presumably because there are multiple stress circuits depending upon the stressor (e.g., Figueiredo et al. 2003). In fact, the brain encodes stressors differently. Evidence indicates that different stressors initiate different endocrine pathways, even when those endocrine pathways converge on the same overall response (Romero and Sapolsky 1996). Consequently, both the central (brain) and peripheral responses appear to depend upon the nature of the specific stressor. Selye's General Adaptation Syndrome seems to be general only in the broadest strokes. (However, there are some common responses to stress, perhaps the best known being glucocorticoid secretion).

The severity of a stressor is also an important factor. In general, the more severe the stressor, the stronger the stress response. Figure 3.2 is a classic example (Hennessy et al. 1979) in which

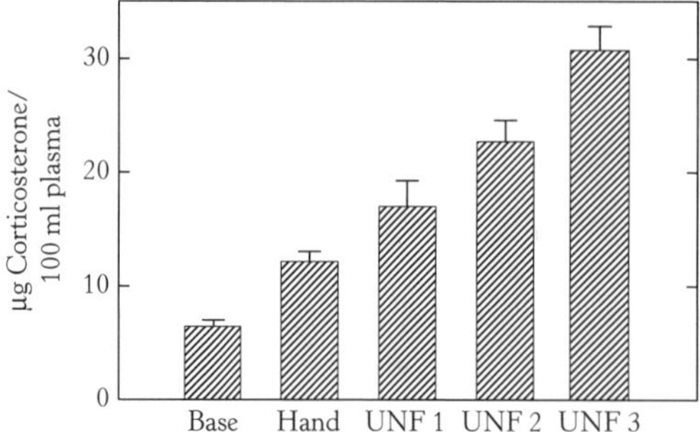

FIGURE 3.2: Corticosterone responses in rats to graded intensities of stress.

Reprinted with permission from Hennessy et al. (1979). Courtesy of Elsevier.

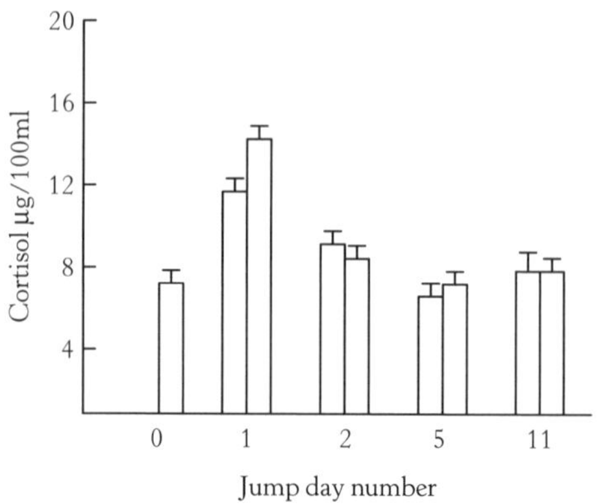

FIGURE 3.3: Cortisol responses in humans paratrooper trainees on different days of jump training.

Reprinted with permission from Levine (1978). Courtesy of Academic Press.

experiments showed that the strength of the stress response was measured as the amount of corticosterone (one of the classic stress hormones; see Chapter 4) released by laboratory rats. The "Base" refers to naïve rats at rest and "Hand" refers to rats that are picked up and handled. The rats were then exposed to three increasingly unfamiliar environments (Unf1–Unf3). The more unfamiliar the environment, the greater the corticosterone response. Graded responses to different severities of stressors are a feature of most stress responses, and indicate that animals can fine-tune their stress responses to cope with the specific stressor that faces them. This makes intuitive sense. For a wild animal, the object is to mount a stress response sufficient to cope with the stressor (i.e., Figure 3.1C), not too little a response (i.e., Figure 3.1B) or too strong a response (i.e., Figure 3.1D).

B. Context Specific

The context of when a stressor occurs turns out to have an incredibly important role in whether a stress response is even expressed. The exact same stressor can elicit very different responses depending upon when the animal experiences it. There are many examples from the literature (e.g., Dobrakova and Kvetnansky 1993), but a good illustration (Figure 3.3) is from a classic study on Norwegian paratrooper trainees (Levine 1978). This study monitored the stress response by measuring salivary cortisol concentrations (another of the classic stress hormones; see Chapter 4). The day before beginning training (Day 0), the trainees had moderate levels of cortisol. The trainees were then taken to the top of the jump tower and essentially pushed off. Not surprisingly, their cortisol concentrations nearly doubled. These soldiers clearly were uncomfortable during this training and consequently mounted a robust stress response. Already by Day 2, however, the cortisol response was greatly diminished, and by Day 5 was completely absent. One way to interpret these data is that after five days of training, these soldiers learned that they were not going to die or be injured jumping off the training tower. Notice that the stimulus was the same—they were still jumping from the tower. The context, however, had changed. The trainees were now comfortable with the training exercise, the experience was no longer noxious, and they consequently had no stress response. Although the authors in the original study did not continue, we're sure that the data in Figure 3.3 were repeated when the trainees started to jump out of airplanes instead of the training tower. Their perception of the danger associated with the exercise would again have changed.

The idea of perception is a powerful principle in determining whether a stress response will occur. Although Berlyne identified three states that will produce psychological stress in an animal: novelty, uncertainty, and conflict (reviewed by Levine et al. 1989), the most important factors are unpredictability and uncertainty, with novelty being a combination of the two. When either unpredictability, uncertainty, or both are present, the animal will initiate a stress response. Notice that the previous two examples, rats exposed to new environments (Figure 3.2) and paratroopers in training (Figure 3.3), are both examples of novelty. Both the rats and soldiers were placed in new environments where there was an unknown risk of danger—hence a stress response. The soldiers subsequently reduced their stress response because the training exercise was no longer novel. In general, animals can reduce a stress response in three other ways: control the stressor, predict the timing of the stressor's occurrence, and learn that the stressor can be avoided (Levine et al. 1989).

The classic examples of how control of a stressor and predicting the timing of a stressor can decrease the stress response were experiments conducted by Weiss and colleagues in the 1960s and 1970s. In one set of experiments, two rats were given identical electrical shocks (Weiss 1968). One rat was given a lever to press, which terminated the shock for both rats. The rat that controlled the lever had dramatically lower corticosterone titers than did the rat that did not have access to the lever. Therefore, even though both rats received identical shocks, the rat that could control the amount of shock had a lower stress response. Other experiments showed that simply knowing when a stressor will occur is sufficient to reduce the stress response (Weiss 1972). In a similar experimental design, two rats are given identical shocks. One rat, however, was given a tone that signaled when the shock would be given. Although the rat that got the warning had a higher stress response than did a non-shocked control, its stress response was dramatically lower than the rat that was not given a warning. As a consequence, the rats given a warning had fewer ulcers (Weiss 1972; Goymann and Wingfield 2004) and higher weight gain (Figure 3.4; Weiss 1970). Clearly, the context is very important—identical stressors elicit different responses solely based on the cognitive feeling of being able to control the stressor or at least being able to predict its onset. Sense of control, or lack thereof, is key to the psychological definition of stress (e.g., Lazarus and Folkman 1984). This helps explain why individuals with low self-esteem, who think of themselves as not having control, do not habituate to stressors (Kirschbaum et al. 1995).

The cognitive role in eliciting a stress response points to an inherent property in both unpredictability and uncertainty. Animals must compare the current situation with expectations and previous experience. In essence, the animal must have a template of what it expects to occur. Any deviation from that template induces uncertainty and unpredictability. There is strong experimental evidence that animals do, in fact, perform this "matching-to-template." The best illustrative example might be that stressors do not necessarily have to be noxious in order to initiate a stress response—even

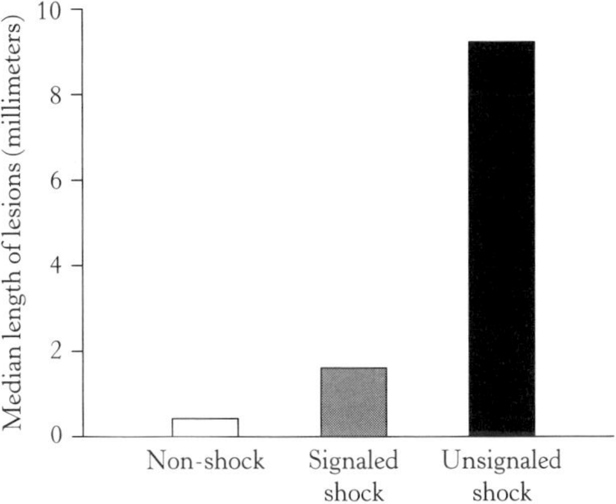

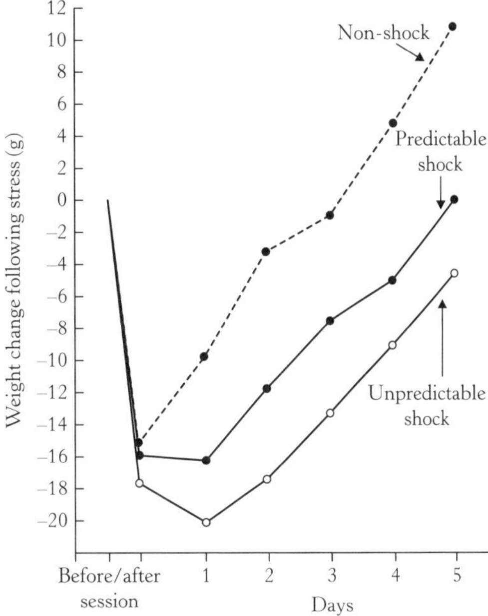

FIGURE 3.4: The effect of predictability of stressor presentation in rats on ulcer formation (upper panel) and weight gain (lower panel).

Reprinted with permission from Weiss (1970, 1972). Courtesy of Wolters Kluwer and Nature Publishing.

seemingly benign environmental changes can suffice. Figure 3.5 (Levine et al. 1972) indicates that a rat trained to press a lever 20 times to get a reward (Fixed Rate [FR] 20) has no higher corticosterone concentrations than an untrained (Pre) rat. If you then shift the reward rate so that every press of the lever results in a food reward (FR20-CRF), corticosterone concentrations decrease. In other words, the rat has compared the new reward schedule to the old reward schedule, concluded that conditions have improved, and reduced its stress. Not all changes are interpreted as being substantially

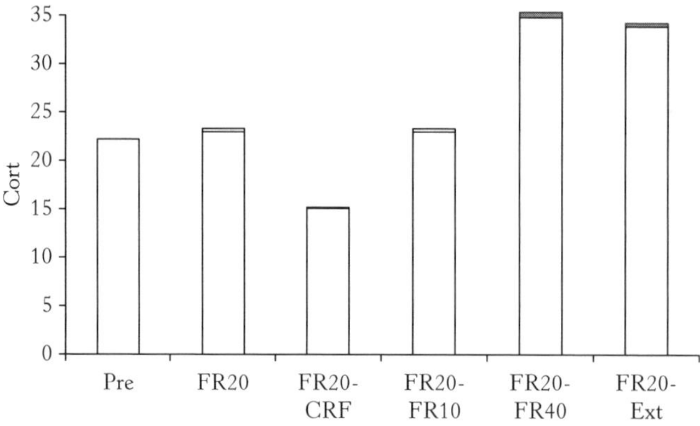

FIGURE 3.5: Corticosterone responses in rats trained to press levers for a reward.

FR = fixed rate with the number indicating the number of lever presses required for reward, CRF = constant rate reinforcement, and Ext = extinction (no reward).

Reprinted with permission from Levine et al. (1972). Courtesy of Associated Scientific Publishers.

better, however, since a shift from a reward every 20 presses to a reward every 10 presses (FR20-FR10) has no effect. In contrast, abruptly ending the reward payout, a process called extinction (Ext), results in a dramatic increase in corticosterone. The rat has compared the new conditions, concluded that it is worse off, and mounted a stress response. The really surprising aspect of this study, however, is that shifting the reward schedule from 20 lever presses per food reward to 40 presses per food reward (FR20–FR40) elicits an identical stress response as does extinction. Even though the rat continues to get a food reward, the longer reward cycle is interpreted as just as bad as if the rat were receiving no reward at all. Context is everything.

Another example of eliciting a stress response when expectations are not met is an experimental paradigm termed "frustration" (Levine and Coover 1976; Coe et al. 1983). In these experiments, rats are trained to receive a water bottle for one hour each day, but always at the same time. Providing an empty rather than a full water bottle (i.e., omitting the expected reward) produces a rapid and robust stress response. An example is given in Figure 3.6, where the stress response was measured as ACTH and corticosterone (CORT) release (Romero et al. 1995). Interestingly, Figure 3.6 also shows that providing the expected reward can result in a rapid down-regulation of the stress response. The mechanism for this is still

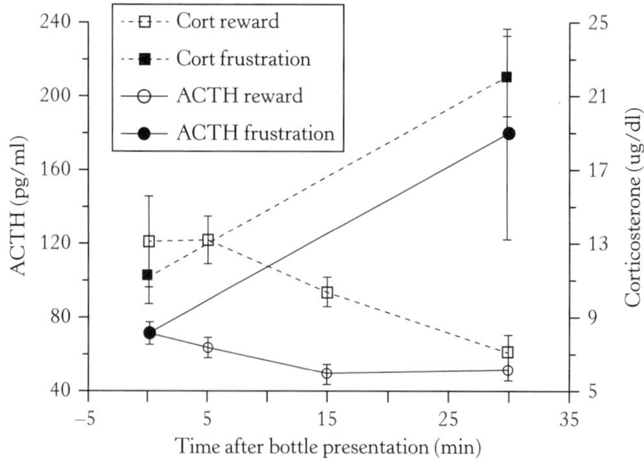

FIGURE 3.6: The effects of reward and frustration on ACTH and corticosterone release (two hormones important in the stress response) in laboratory rats.

Reprinted with permission from Romero et al. (1995). Courtesy of Elsevier.

not entirely clear, but appears to involve a rapid loss of direct stimulation of corticosterone release by vasopressin (Wotus et al. 2003) and does not appear to be due to increased corticosterone clearance after drinking (Wotus and Engeland 2003). The take-home message from these experiments is that the stress response is flexible enough to rapidly increase if expectations are not met, and to rapidly decrease if expectations are met.

In many species, the social context is a major factor in determining whether a stimulus becomes a stressor. Both social stimuli and a lack of social stimuli can be stressors for many species. Studies have shown that dominance ranks can induce stress in several species of primates (e.g., Sapolsky 1982; Schiml et al. 1996; Strier et al. 1999; Pride 2005), several species of mammalian social carnivores (e.g., Creel et al. 1996; Hofer and East 2003; Creel 2005), rabbits (e.g., Eiserman 1992), geese (e.g., Kotrschal et al. 1998; Ely et al. 1999), several passerine bird species (e.g., Hegner and Wingfield 1987; Schwabl et al. 1988; Pravosudov et al. 1999), and potentially even between sibling bird chicks in the nest (e.g., Ramos-Fernandez et al. 2000; Kitaysky et al. 2001; Vallarino et al. 2006). In fact, intraspecific dominance interactions may be the most common stressor in social species (Creel 2001) and can easily be modeled in the laboratory in many species (reviewed for mammals by Tamashiro et al. 2005). Referring to the beginning of this chapter, many authors have argued that for modern Western humans, social stressors are the only stressors (e.g., Sapolsky 1994).

One important aspect of social stress is that individual animals react differently to the same social stressors. Early work on this topic was done on rats that were housed in a visible burrow system (Blanchard et al. 1995). In this experimental paradigm, multiple male rats are housed in a large enclosure with food and water available in only one area. One male quickly monopolizes the resource area and becomes the dominant individual. The subordinate rats, however, form two groups. The majority of subordinates show all the classic symptoms of chronic stress and especially show very high concentrations of the stress hormones. About 20%–30% of subordinates, however, fail to show elevated stress hormones. Ongoing work is attempting to show why subordinates will fall into one group or the other and to determine the underlying pathophysiological mechanisms (reviewed in Tamashiro et al. 2005). The existence of high and low hormonal responders to stressors has been demonstrated in a variety of other species, including turkeys (Brown and Nestor 1973), chickens (Gross and Siegel 1985), Japanese quail (Satterlee and Johnson 1988), foxes (Krass et al. 1979), and rainbow trout (Øverli et al. 2005). Individual differences in hormonal release are akin to different coping styles to social stressors and are often termed "personalities."

There is a rich literature on human personalities and coping styles, for example the so-called type A and type B personalities. There is also good experimental evidence that other species have personalities and different coping styles (Koolhaas et al. 2007). In other words, artificial selection for high and low hormonal responders (cited earlier) is not only for physiological differences, but also for psychological differences, between individuals. Examples include work on birds (reviewed by Groothuis and Carere 2005) and fish (Øverli et al. 2004), but perhaps the best example is illustrated in Figure 3.7 for free-ranging baboons (Sapolsky 1990; Ray and Sapolsky 1992). In these studies, male baboons were observed interacting and subsequently were captured by anesthetic (delivered by a dart) in order to measure cortisol. Different personalities between male baboons were evident, and these personalities were linked to individual endocrine responses to the social stressor. If a male could differentiate between a threatening or neutral interaction with another male, could initiate a fight with a threatening rival that he won, and could tell whether he won or lost the fight, that male had lower cortisol concentrations (Figure 3.7). Furthermore, if that male displaced his aggression after losing a fight by initiating a fight with a lower ranked baboon, he also had lower cortisol concentrations (as might be expected, this response by the male increases the stress in the rest of the baboon troop [Engh et al. 2006]). Note that the personality that resulted in higher cortisol neatly illustrates the definition from the beginning of this section of what causes stress: being unable to decide whom to fight and when to fight increases uncertainty and unpredictability.

There is one final important concept on how the context of a stressor influences the resulting stress response. The example of the Norwegian paratroopers in Figure 3.3 shows acclimation to a prior stressor—the animal no longer responds in the same robust manner to repeated or chronic stressors. However, the opposite can often happen (Dallman et al. 1992). In a process called facilitation, animals that have acclimated to one stressor often show enhanced responses to novel stressors compared to naïve controls that had not acclimated to a prior stressor (Dallman and Bhatnagar 2001; Bhatnagar and Vining 2003).

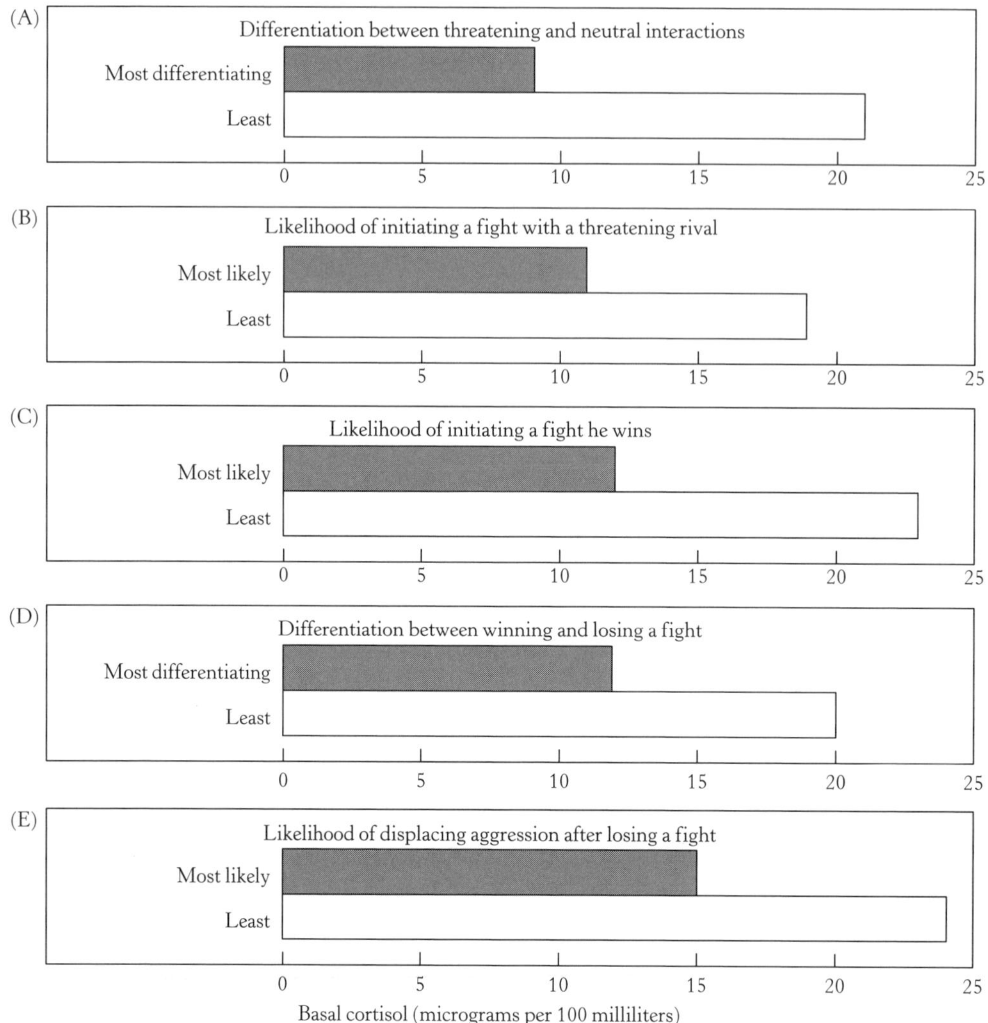

FIGURE 3.7: Personalities in baboons that determine the individual's response to social stressors.
Reprinted with permission from Sapolsky (1990). Courtesy of Nature Publishing.

Two examples of facilitation are given in Figures 3.8 and 3.9. In one classic study shown in Figure 3.8 (Dallman and Jones 1973), plasma corticosterone concentrations in rats were measured at 9:00 p.m., 15 minutes after using injection as a stressor. The only difference in treatment groups was what occurred at 9:00 a.m. Injecting saline alone induced a stress response (rise in corticosterone) compared to un-injected rats, but the response was greatly enhanced if the animals were subjected to restraint in the morning. This effect was not the result of the corticosterone released in the morning in response to restraint, because an injection of corticosterone (abbreviated as "B"; see Chapter 4) had the opposite effect and damped the response (via negative feedback). In this case, the acclimation process primed the animals to have an enhanced response to a different stressor. In the second example in Figure 3.9 (L. M. Romero and N. E. Cyr, unpublished data), chronic stress was induced by exposing European starlings to four to five different mild stressors each day for 14 days. Similar to the non-hormonal responders in the visible burrow system (Tamashiro et al. 2005), these birds down-regulated the increase in heart rate in response to the stressors. When the chronically stressed birds were injected (a stressor not used when inducing chronic stress), however, the birds showed a heightened response. Although acclimation and facilitation do not occur for all stressors, especially those that are relatively severe (Dallman and Bhatnagar 2001),

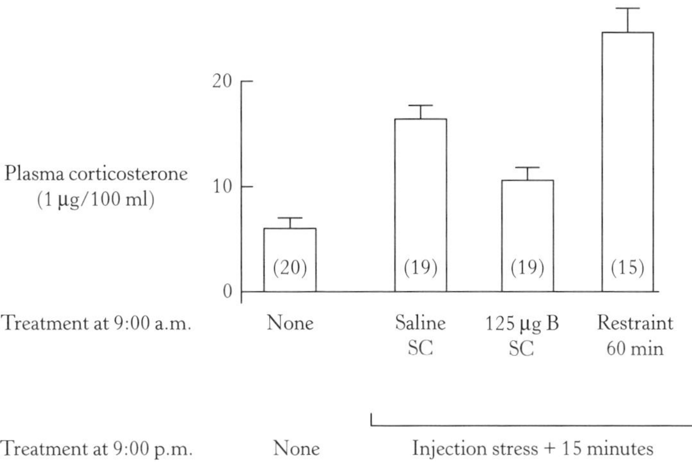

FIGURE 3.8: Example of facilitation in laboratory rats. B is an abbreviation for corticosterone stress hormone. A prior stressor (restraint), but not prior saline or corticosterone injection, primed the animal for a stronger response to a stressor (injection) 12 hours later.

Reprinted with permission from Dallman and Jones (1973). Courtesy of the Endocrine Society.

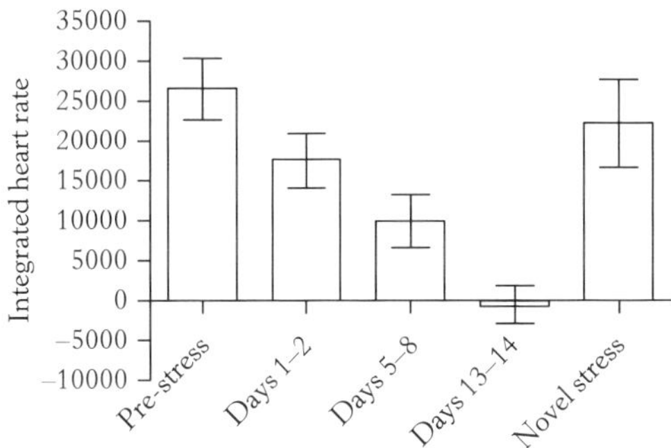

FIGURE 3.9: Example of facilitation in European starlings. Integrated heart rate (the change in heart rate over 15 minutes) decreases when birds are exposed to 13–14 days of chronic stress, but the pre-stress response was duplicated after the novel stressor of a saline injection.

Unpublished data from Cyr and Romero.

these examples illustrate that recent exposure to a stressor can alter the response to subsequent stressors. The mechanism regulating facilitation is not presently known. (Note that this process is different from exposure to stressors during development—a topic that will be discussed in Chapter 11.)

The traditional model of stress has many strengths. By defining stress as a disruption from a dynamic equilibrium, both actual and perceived threats (physical and psychological) to that dynamic equilibrium become stressors. That physical stressors, such as a wound, can disrupt an animal's dynamic equilibrium is self-evident. Determining whether a psychological stimulus becomes a stressor, however, requires a cognitive decision by the animal about whether it is better or worse off than it was before the stimulus. These cognitive decisions often create the majority of stressors in many species and are subject to individual differences such as personalities and different coping styles. In addition, using the concept of a dynamic equilibrium places emphasis on emergency reactions. Normal daily, seasonal, and life-history stage changes do not disrupt the dynamic equilibrium and thus do not elicit a stress response. Consequently, the traditional model meshes nicely with the natural history of stress and the emergency life-history stage (Chapter 1).

The traditional model, however, has two major weaknesses. The first relates to the three major concepts encompassed by Figure 3.1. Traditional use of the term "stress" includes references to the stressors themselves, the stress response, and the pathological consequences of chronic stress (Romero 2004; Le Moal 2007)—three very different concepts. Much of this problem can be resolved through rigorous use of "stressor," "stress response," and "chronic stress" and the avoidance of the use of "stress" itself. However, few people are that disciplined. Instead, most uses of the word "stress" remain ambiguous. The second major weakness derives from an inability to rigorously define these three concepts. When is a stimulus a stressor? In theory it should be easy to predict which stimuli become stressors. An animal should classify as a stressor any physical stimulus that causes or threatens to cause physical harm and any psychological stimulus that is interpreted at placing or threatening to place the animal in a worse condition. In practice, however, it is quite difficult for researchers to make these determinations a priori. Consequently, the working definition of what is a stressor is that which causes a stress response. But what behavioral and physiological responses are stress responses? A typical answer is that a physiological or behavioral response is considered a stress response if it is initiated in response to a stressor, and the problem is compounded when trying to determine when a presumably beneficial stress response becomes pathological. This circular definition is clearly unsatisfactory and a major reason for the periodic calls to abandon the traditional model.

III. HABITUATION

Hormonal, physiological, and behavioral responses to a repeated stressor often wane over time. Stated in a different way, the magnitude of a response lessens at each subsequent exposure to the stressor. There are multiple reasons for the waning of the response, but the most frequently invoked mechanism is habituation. In fact, many researchers use the waning of a response to define habituation.

A recent review provided a brief summary of the history of defining habituation (Cyr and Romero 2009). Much of the early work on habituation originated in the field of physiology and often specifically applied to neural responses (Harris 1943). The focus was on response decrements to repeated stimulations with the subsequent recovery of the responses. Further work refined ideas about when the intensity of response should recover after a period when the stimulus is not applied (e.g., Sharpless and Jasper 1956; Thorpe 1963). What emerged from this work was a set of guiding principles used to determine if habituation was occurring (e.g., Thompson and Spencer 1966). These principles included the ideas that responses must decrease with repeated exposure to the stimulus, that the response should spontaneously recover when the stimulus ends, that particularly strong stimuli may not result in habituation, and that presentation of a different stimulus will override the habituation (called dishabituation).

Notice that the early focus on neural responses resulted in the lack of a direct inclusion of learning and ignored the process whereby an animal perceives that the stressor has become less stressful over time. Although not all researchers agree that learning should be a component of habituation, the term "habituation" usually implies a change in the discrimination decision in the brain that determines that a stimulus is a stressor. An important concept is that the individual becomes familiar with the stressor, learns that the stressor is not harmful, and thus no longer perceives the stressor to be, in fact, a stressor (e.g., Gray 1987; Willner 1993). Consequently, under this formulation habituation is not simply a mechanical change in the response, but rather a perceptual change leading to different decisions of what constitutes a stressor.

We should point out that there will be considerable disagreement with the preceding definition of habituation among many researchers. The concept of habituation seems to be much like the concept of stress—it means different things to different people. Often these differences are linked to an individual researcher's field, be it physiology, psychology, or neuroscience. Our goal here is not to attempt to reconcile all these different definitions of habituation, but rather to propose a definition of habituation that can be useful when studying wild animals under natural contexts. The earliest definitions of habituation were most appropriate for responses of single neurons. Given that free-living animals must integrate extensive information from their environment before determining whether a stimulus is a stressor, we propose that it would be most useful to extend the definition of habituation to describe a situation in which an individual learns to ignore innocuous stimuli, so that habituated animals are those that have changed their categorization of a stimulus from stressor to innocuous (e.g., McCarty et al. 1992; Domjan 1996; Dubovicky and Jezova 2004).

Defining habituation in this way for free-living animals has the advantage of excluding several other reasons that hormonal and physiological responses to stressors attenuate over time. Changes during chronic stress are one example. A substantial minority of studies report either no change or a decrease in responses due to chronic stress (reviewed in Dallman and Bhatnagar 2001). For example, in a laboratory-based social stress model involving dominant and subordinate rodents, there are two classes of subordinates: those that show elevated corticosteroid concentrations and those that do not, yet both classes show evidence of stress-related disease (Blanchard et al. 1995). Clearly both classes of subordinates continue to interpret their subordinate status as stressful, even though one group shows an attenuated response. Notwithstanding these empirical data, habituation is the typical interpretation for any reduced response in many field studies. This leads many researchers to equate reduced stress responses to habituation, and a further conclusion that the animals are no longer chronically stressed (Willner 1993). But there are other possibilities. For example, there could be exhaustion of the response. In this case, the individual has not learned that the stressor is actually innocuous, but simply can no longer respond to the stressor. If exhaustion does occur, it would have separate physiological mechanisms and consequences than habituation. The important concept is that a habituated individual is not considered stressed; if it is stressed, it cannot have habituated to the stressor regardless of any decline in response.

A. Habituation in Free-Living Animals

Cyr and Romero (2009) presented three alternative explanations to habituation that may play important roles in declining responses to repeated exposures to stressors in free-living animals (Table 3.1). As discussed earlier in this chapter, the vertebrate stress response is activated by real and/or perceived stressors. However, wild animals may perceive an event as a stressor only at certain times of the year (e.g., Nelson et al. 2002; Romero 2002). Many species seasonally modulate their responses to stress (Romero 2002). In other words, the physiological responses to a stressor change in magnitude depending upon the time of year, presumably due to different life-history demands. As Landys et al. (2006) persuasively argue, changes that are part of the normal progression of life-history stages should not be misconstrued as indicating stress. In fact, Wingfield and Sapolsky (2003) presented six different life-history contexts in which individuals would be predicted to not have a robust response to a stressor, even though they would be expected to respond to those same stressors at other life-history stages.

A more specific example would be seasonal differences in responses to inclement weather. In nature, animals must learn to adapt to adverse weather conditions. Corticosteroid concentrations increase during storms, theoretically to facilitate survival (Wingfield et al. 1983; Rogers et al. 1993; Smith et al. 1994; Astheimer et al. 1995). Animals frequently exposed to adverse weather may elevate corticosteroid concentrations each time or may habituate, especially if the conditions are only moderately severe. One might assume that a reduced corticosteroid response to repeated inclement weather signifies habituation, but that may not necessarily be the case. In several bird species, inclement weather did not stimulate corticosteroid release during the breeding season even though the birds were exquisitely sensitive to weather conditions later in the year (Romero et al. 2000). This decrease in sensitivity to weather during breeding may be a regulated process to avoid the negative impact of chronic corticosteroid concentrations in disrupting breeding, an important life-history stage (Wingfield 1994). Because responses to stressors are specific to each life-history stage, comparisons of responses in order to diagnose habituation

TABLE 3.1: POTENTIAL REASONS THAT A FREE-LIVING ANIMAL DECREASES ITS RESPONSE TO A STRESSOR

Explanation	Characteristics
1. Seasonal/life-history changes	A natural shift in perception of a stressor such that the animal perceives a given stimulus as noxious at certain times of the year, and thus activates the stress response. However, the animal does not perceive that same stimulus as stressful at other times of the year, and therefore does not activate the stress response.
2. Physiological desensitization without habituation	With repetition, the response to the stimulus decreases, but the animal *does not* learn to adapt to the stimulus. The animal, thus, perceives the stimulus as a stressor even with repetition.
3. Exhaustion	There is a breakdown of the physiological system such that the animal is too fatigued to maintain a stress response with repetition of a stimulus.
4. Habituation	At first, the animal perceives a given stimulus as a stressor. With repetition, the animal learns to perceive that stimulus as innocuous, and thus reduces the intensity of response to that particular stimulus.

Modified with permission from Cyr and Romero (2009).

must be made within, not among, life-history stages. Although this may seem a trivial point, it would clearly be inappropriate to compare responses from two different life-history stages and conclude that the lower response reflected habituation. Consequently, the evidence suggests that the reduced sensitivity to weather conditions during breeding compared to other times of the year is not due to habituation.

B. Desensitization of the Physiological Response

Exposure to either long-term chronic stress or severe stressors often results in attenuated responses to repeated stimulations, but there is good evidence that these decreases are accompanied by changes in the entire stress physiology of the animal (e.g., Tache et al. 1976; Marti and Armario 1998; Marti et al. 1999; Rich and Romero 2005). This appears to be what is occurring in the subordinate rodents that don't show a stress response (discussed earlier). In these cases, attenuation occurs because physiological responses have adjusted to a continued or repeated challenge, even though the animals continue to perceive the stimulus as a stressor. Learning has not taken place, only a desensitization of the physiological systems. Desensitization could result from physiological changes, such as decreases in receptor numbers, decreases in activity of synthetic pathways, decreases in production or release of important stress mediators, and so on. These changes are likely necessary to prevent deleterious side effects of the repeated stimulation of the stress response.

One example of physiological desensitization comes from our work using rotated and varying intermittent stressors to induce chronic stress in birds. We found attenuation in several physiological responses in both the laboratory (Rich and Romero 2005; Cyr et al. 2009) and the field (Cyr and Romero 2007). These attenuated responses cannot be explained by habituation for four reasons. First, the birds never learned that the stressors were innocuous. Second, the dynamics of corticosteroid release (Rich and Romero 2005) and heart rate regulation (Cyr et al. 2009) changed so that the original responses were no longer possible. Third, there were decreases in basal corticosteroid titers and increases in resting heart rate, even though there should not be basal changes if stressors were no longer being interpreted as being stressful. Fourth, in the field the attenuated responses were associated with decreased nesting success (Cyr and Romero 2007), even though habituated birds would not be expected to show a loss of fitness. The conclusion from these data is that the diminished responses over time are better explained by physiological desensitization rather than habituation.

A second example of physiological desensitization is a growing body of work studying ecotourism. The effect of tourism as an anthropogenic stressor on wild species has been investigated extensively (e.g., Fowler 1999; Yorio et al. 2001; Romero and Wikelski 2002; Mullner et al. 2004; Walker et al. 2005; Walker et al. 2006). Many of these species show an attenuated stress response to humans, but two lines of evidence suggest that this attenuation is not a result of habituation. First, there is little evidence for dishabituation (i.e., facilitation). If habituation to tourist visits were occurring, then a different stressor should evoke a response equivalent to non-visited animals (a dishabituated response). This does not occur. Instead, tourist-visited animals also have an attenuated response to subsequent capture and handling. Second, similar to the chronic stress described earlier, the dynamics of the stress response change in the visited animals (e.g., Walker et al. 2006). Consequently, the data suggest that the stress responses of tourist-exposed animals have physiologically desensitized, but that the animals have not fully habituated to humans (i.e., they still categorize human visitation as a stressor).

C. Exhaustion of the Physiological Response

Hans Selye (1946) proposed a concept of physiological exhaustion wherein stress responses decrease because they can no longer be maintained. In other words, the attenuated response resulted not from habituation, but from the breakdown of the physiological systems. This was part of his three-stage model of the stress response, where in the final stage the individual is so fatigued that it is impossible to maintain a stress response and all mediators decrease in their concentrations. There has been very little support for Selye's exhaustion hypothesis and the idea has been largely abandoned (e.g., Sapolsky 1992). However, recent work on several stress-related medical conditions, including fibromyalgia, chronic fatigue syndrome, and post-traumatic stress disorder (PTSD) indicate that these patients often have lower basal and sometimes lower stress-induced corticosteroid concentrations (McEwen 1998), at least during certain times of the day (Miller et al. 2007). More important for our purposes, exhaustion of the physiological systems may play an important role in wild animals in one specific situation—toxic physiological changes resulting from pollution.

Chronic exposure to contaminants can have profound impacts on stress physiology, and especially corticosteroid physiology (e.g., Hontela 1998; Norris et al. 1999; Franceschini et al. 2008). A particularly illuminating example is shown by Norris et al.'s (1997, 1999) work on brown trout living in metal-contaminated water. These fish appeared healthy and had been living in contaminated waters for many years. However, when subjected to capture and handling, contaminated trout initiated an identical corticosteroid response yet failed to sustain that corticosteroid response (i.e., had an attenuated response) compared to uncontaminated controls. Furthermore, all the contaminated fish died during the procedure, whereas none of the controls died. These contaminated animals lacked sufficient ability to mount a stress response to the acute stressor of capture and handling to prevent death. It is unlikely that anyone would make the mistake of concluding that the attenuated corticosteroid response in contaminated fish represented habituation. However, the concern is for field studies where there is hidden contamination (contamination unbeknownst to the researchers). If this had been the case, Norris et al. (1999) could potentially have concluded that some of the fish (the contaminated ones) had habituated (especially if they had not subsequently died). However, Norris et al. did not make that conclusion because the contaminated fish clearly could not sustain a corticosteroid response, akin to Selye's concept of exhaustion of the physiological system. Although it is unclear how prevalent toxic effects leading to physiological exhaustion might be, there may not be a single habitat left on Earth that has not been exposed to some pollution. Consequently, exhaustion derived from hidden toxic effects may be an important alternative explanation to habituation.

D. Criteria for Habituation in Field Studies

As a result of the three potential alternatives to habituation presented in the preceding text, Cyr and Romero (2009) proposed six criteria for determining whether hormonal responses had habituated in field studies. These six criteria were proposed as an "operational definition" of habituation for use in the field. For habituation to be the interpretation in field studies, the response must show the following criteria:

1. The response to the same stressor must decrease over time.
2. The decreased response should not generalize to other stimuli (dishabituation).
3. The decreased response should result from learned, not physiological, changes (the capacity to respond should not be reduced).
4. The decreased response should not lead to decreases in health or fitness.
5. The decrease should be in response to the stimulus, not in the pre-stimulus state (learning that a stimulus is innocuous should return basal mediator levels to the original pre-stimulus state).
6. The decreased response should be compared to responses within a single life-history stage.

E. Diagnostic Tests for Evaluating Habituation in Field Studies

The previous criteria led Cyr and Romero (2009) to propose four diagnostic tests for determining whether habituation has occurred to a stressor or set of stressors in field studies (Table 3.2). It is not always possible to observe the entire process of habituation in the field. For example, if one is interested in learning whether a population of animals has habituated to tourism, the animals may already show an attenuated stress response to human presence, such that the researcher has missed the process of gradual decline in that response. Together, these four diagnostic tests will help to distinguish habituation from other explanations for an observed decrease in response intensity to a repeated stressor or set of repeated stressors in field studies.

Dishabituation takes advantage of the process of facilitation discussed in the traditional model. Because an animal that has habituated to a repeated stressor shows a normal or exaggerated response to a different (novel) stressor (Dallman and Bhatnagar 2001), habituation is not a generalized response; it is a reduced response to one specific stimulus. Therefore, a diagnostic test for habituation is the attenuation to a specific stimulus, combined with the lack of a generalized attenuation.

Dishabituation results from no longer responding to a repeated stimulus after learning that the

TABLE 3.2: DIAGNOSTIC TESTS TO BE USED IN A FREE-LIVING ANIMAL TO DETERMINE WHETHER HABITUATION IS OCCURRING

Test	Description	Which Alternative Explanations Can Be Distinguished from Habituation
Dishabituation	Expose the animal to a novel stressor and look for a normal or exaggerated stress response.	Habituation is a specific response to a repeated stimulus, so exposure to a new stimulus should result in the stress response functioning normally. If the response was generalized and the stress response continued to be blunted during a novel stressor, it would be consistent with either physiological desensitization or exhaustion, not habituation.
Health and fitness	Monitor the health and fitness of individuals. For example, compromised immune responses, survival, reproductive function and/or success.	Animals that exhibit physiological desensitization or exhaustion are likely to experience failing health or fitness costs because they are chronically stressed. Habituated animals have learned to ignore the stimulus and are not stressed; thus habituated animals are not expected to incur health and fitness costs associated with chronic stress.
Changes in baseline stress physiology	Monitor potential changes in the baseline (i.e., pre-stimulus) stress physiology.	Habituated animals reduce their stress response to a repeated stimulus, but baseline physiology should not be altered. An increase in baseline levels indicates an active stress response and a decrease suggests physiological desensitization.
Control for Life-History Stage	1. Compare responses within life-history stages. 2. Compare responses over different times of the year/day/life-history stage.	Comparisons of separate populations (or the same population under different environmental conditions at different times) should be made within the same life-history stage to control for seasonal/life-history changes. Alternatively, multiple measurements during different life-history stages will also control for seasonal/life-history changes.

Modified with permission from Cyr and Romero (2009).

stimulus is not harmful, but continuing to perceive a novel stimulus as potentially harmful and thus mounting a normal stress response. Importantly, the physiological responses should continue to function normally when presented with a novel acute stressor. If, however, the animal has not habituated to the repeated stressor yet still shows an attenuated response, as in the case of physiological desensitization or exhaustion, the introduction of a novel stressor should not cause dishabituation. In the case of exhaustion, the system is too fatigued to respond, and in the case of physiological desensitization, adding a new stressor should not alter the animal's state (i.e., chronic stress) and the stress response should remain attenuated.

F. Health and Fitness

Animals that exhibit physiological desensitization or exhaustion are likely to show changes in weight, as well as other indicators of failing health. Examples include, but are not limited to, decreased immune function, reproductive failure, lethargy, decreased body condition, increased parasite load, behavioral alterations (e.g., anxiety), energy dysregulation, and hypertension. Long-term exposure to repeated stressors is also likely to incur fitness costs, such as compromised survival or reproductive success (although other factors not related to chronic stress can also decrease reproductive success). Consequently, reduced health and/or fitness would suggest that the animal has failed to habituate to the specific stimulus in question.

If we accept that habituation results from learning that the repeated stimulus was not a stressor, baseline (i.e., pre-stimulus, or initial conditions) stress physiology should not be affected. There are three possibilities regarding initial conditions: (1) either baseline physiology is elevated, (2) baseline physiology is equivalent, or (3) baseline physiology is reduced compared to a non-stressed animal. Elevated baseline levels indicate that an animal is currently mounting a stress response, and consequently has not habituated. Baseline levels equivalent to a non-stressed animal suggest that the animal may have habituated, but a final determination depends upon the response to the repeated stimulus, that is, the definition of habituation still requires that the stress response be attenuated compared to a naïve (non-habituated) animal. Baseline levels lower than a non-stressed animal indicate physiological desensitization or exhaustion. If an animal has truly habituated, it has learned that the stimulus is innocuous so that baseline stress physiology should be identical to a non-stressed animal. Consequently, monitoring baseline stress physiology is an excellent diagnostic test for habituation.

G. Control for Life-History Stage

For those stressors that are of relatively short duration (e.g., inclement weather, predator attacks, ecotourism, etc.; but repeated acute stresses could be a problem), physiological responses to repeated stimuli should only be compared within a life-history stage. Otherwise, physiological changes resulting from different life-history demands would be a potential confounding variable. For long-term stressors (e.g., famine, social instability, anthropogenic changes, etc.), or where life-history stage cannot be controlled, the response to a repeated stressor should be compared multiple times over the course of the year or during different life-history stages to control for natural variation in stress responses caused by life-history demands.

Habituation is an important concept in the field of stress, but there is no standard definition of habituation for wild animals. Typical laboratory definitions of habituation are less useful for field studies because other factors might cause a decrease in response intensity (Table 3.2). An animal with an attenuated stress response is not necessarily habituated and thus not being stressed. Furthermore, because the stress response is thought to be adaptive in that it helps an animal survive stressors, an inability to mount a proper stress response would presumably decrease survival and perhaps fitness. Clearly, a proper diagnosis of habituation using unambiguous criteria would greatly help in interpreting how changing stress responses impact wild animals. Cyr and Romero's six diagnostic criteria and four diagnostic tests should provide a starting point for making these interpretations.

IV. THE ALLOSTASIS MODEL

Notwithstanding the progress made in understanding stress that was encompassed in the traditional model, many researchers remained deeply dissatisfied with its overall usefulness. The weaknesses made it difficult to use the concept of stress in a predictive manner. Instead, stress was often invoked only in a post hoc fashion to attempt to explain some physiological and psychological diseases. The difficulty of making predictions led Sterling and Eyer (1988) to propose a new way to think about stress. They, and a number of researchers who came after (e.g., McEwen 2000; Schulkin 2003), proposed that stress could best be understood as a change in allostasis, or the maintenance of constancy (homeostasis) through change. As dynamic equilibrium is maintained through the day or across seasons (migrations, breeding seasons, etc.), the energy required to sustain that equilibrium increases. The mediators required to provide energy also increase and are cumulatively called allostatic load (McEwen and Wingfield 2003).

Allostasis was originally conceived and applied in a biomedical context. It took a number of years to consider its utility in understanding stress in an ecological context. The first attempt to meld biomedical and ecological research was the "Allostasis Model" proposed by McEwen and Wingfield (2003). They emphasized that allostasis is the process of maintaining stability (homeostasis) through change in both environmental stimuli and physiological mechanisms. Allostasis then accounts for daily and seasonal physiological adjustments (termed "allostatic state") that maintain physiological parameters, such as blood glucose, within narrow life-sustaining ranges. With these definitions, homeostasis refers to the maintenance of these physiological parameters, whereas allostasis refers to the physiological mechanisms that maintain that homeostasis (via allostatic mediators). As a consequence, there is a difference between the physiological variables that are kept constant and those mediators that vary in order to maintain constancy. Furthermore, many organisms anticipate changes in life-history stage and environmental conditions and make physiological and behavioral adjustments in anticipation of change, rather than as a reaction to current conditions.

Environmental changes, such as storms or winter conditions, and life-history changes, such as pregnancy, could make the animal work harder to maintain the stability of these physiological parameters. Importantly, environmental and life-history changes can be additive so that an animal would have to work even harder if there were multiple changes, such as a storm occurring during pregnancy. McEwen and Wingfield (2003) termed this increase in workload "allostatic load" and proposed that it could be measured with overall energy expenditure. McEwen and Wingfield then identified two instances in which an animal could get into physiological trouble. The first they termed "allostatic overload type 1," which occurs when the animal's energy demand for maintaining homeostasis exceeds the energy the animal can obtain from its environment. Allostatic overload type 1 then initiates an emergency life-history stage whereby the animal adjusts its behavior and physiology to decrease allostatic load. The second they termed allostatic overload type 2, which occurs when allostatic load is too high for too long but does not exceed the energy available in the environment to fuel it. As a consequence, the prolonged activation of the physiological systems that mediate allostasis start to create pathological problems themselves, despite the presence of adequate energy. Building on Sterling and Eyer's (1988) allostasis concept, McEwen and Wingfield proposed that allostasis, allostatic load, and allostatic overload could provide a framework for understanding how an animal copes with unpredictable challenges, in addition to increased energetic demands of the predictable life cycle (reproduction, migration, etc.). The framework can be tested rigorously by evaluating energy budgets, although such testing has not been reported to date. The allostatic model, if supported, could then replace the concept of stress.

A. Allostasis: A Framework for Assessing Daily/Seasonal Routines and Unpredictable Events

Fieldwork on free-living vertebrates provides an opportunity to investigate morphological, physiological, and behavioral changes and their control throughout the year. Opportunistically, it is also possible to record responses to unpredictable events such as predator attacks, inclement weather, and other perturbations of the environment (Chapter 1). Sometime these perturbations (labile perturbation factors [LPFs]; Chapter 1) disrupt the normal life cycle and daily routines (dynamic equilibrium) and sometimes they do not (Romero et al. 2000; Wingfield 2004), raising the possibility that the disruption of daily and seasonal routines by a given LPF is not only dependent upon intensity and duration (stimulus specificity and context, see earlier discussion) but also on individual characteristics such as gender, age, social status (proactive/reactive), body condition, parasite load, and so on (e.g., Wingfield 2004; Korte et al. 2005).

A framework, in an ecological context, for modeling LPF intensity, duration, and frequency in relation to life-history stages of the predictable life cycle has been elusive, and an approach that is applicable to all life-history stages but that also takes into account individual differences is needed in order to integrate the demands and wear and tear of daily and seasonal routines with the extra demands imposed by environmental perturbations. Over the last two decades, various concepts have been proposed that work toward the development of such a framework with wide relevance to organisms in their natural environment (Wingfield 2004) and the control mechanisms underlying individual differences (Williams 2008). But first, some basic concepts must be articulated so that links can be made among individuals responding to a LPF and the mechanisms underlying that response.

B. Homeostasis in a Changing World and Physiological State Levels

Separation of the energetically demanding aspects of life-history stages in the predictable life cycle from demands imposed by labile perturbation factors that have the potential to be stressful is difficult because they tend to form a continuum, and each individual may respond differently. Furthermore, glucocorticoid secretion increases in response to the demands of daily and seasonal routines as well as to perturbations of the environment (e.g., Romero 2002; Landys et al. 2006). This led to the concept of three state levels (Figure 3.10; Wingfield 2003; Landys et al. 2006): level A, the physiological state required to simply maintain life (basic homeostasis); level B, the change in physiological state (homeostatic set-points) during daily and annual routines (i.e., the predictable life cycle); and level C, facultative adjustments of physiology to adjust to perturbations of the environment in addition to demands of the predictable life cycle. Note that the dynamic equilibrium that we discussed earlier is maintained through levels A and B as part of the reaction norm of that individual through time and life-history stages. The equilibrium becomes disrupted at level C, that is, outside the reaction norm (McEwen and Wingfield 2003;

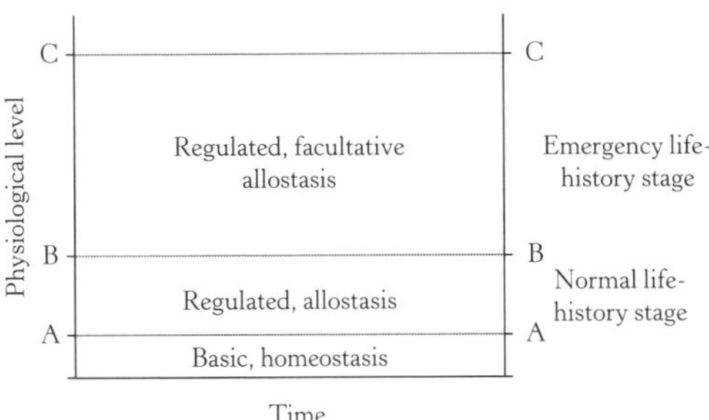

FIGURE 3.10: A summary of the three levels of physiological function. Level A represents basic homeostatic mechanisms required for simple existence of an organism. As the organism goes about its daily routine, or changes life-history stage (LHS) on a seasonal basis, physiological function varies. These processes require change in homeostatic mechanisms as environmental needs and LHS requirements change. These occur on a predictable basis and can be regulated in anticipation of environmental change within level B. There have been several terms coined to describe these changes, including "poikilostasis" (Kuenzel et al. 1999), "homeorhesis" (Bauman 2000), and "rheostasis" (Mrosovsky 1990). Superimposed on this predictable component of the life cycle is the unpredictable. The latter includes storms, predator pressure, human disturbance, disease, injury, and so on. These have been termed "labile perturbation factors" (LPFs; Wingfield et al. 1998; Wingfield and Romero 2001) and can occur at any time in the life cycle and during any LHS. In response to LPFs is a complex suite of physiological and behavioral events that allow the individual to adjust to the challenge. This could be termed regulated, facultative poikilostasis operating from levels B to level C. Following the concepts of Sterling and Eyer (1988), McEwen et al. (1999) and Schulkin (2003), this complex terminology can be unified as allostasis—stability through change.

From Wingfield (2004). Courtesey of Cambridge University Press.

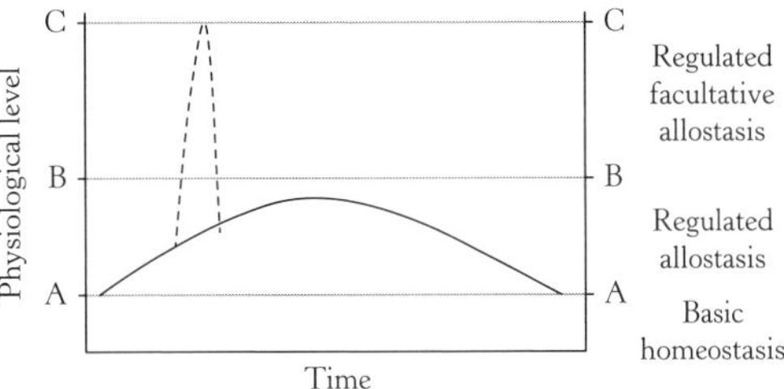

FIGURE 3.11: Basic homeostasis is still important for simple existence (level A), and regulated allostasis includes the predictable life cycle and changes in physiological function within level B. Unpredictable events in the environment trigger regulated, facultative allostasis from Levels B to C.

From Wingfield (2004). Courtesey of Cambridge University Press.

Wingfield 2004; Landys et al. 2006). Potentially, high energetic demand life-history stages such as reproduction and migration could result in greater sensitivity of an individual to labile perturbation factors, but how can we integrate these otherwise different processes through levels A, B, and C?

Allostasis is developing as a framework to integrate metabolic demands along the continuum from the predictable life cycle to the effects of labile perturbation factors, including anticipation of environmental change. Classical homeostasis results in adjustments of physiology and behavior after the environment has changed or as it changes (acclimation). On the other hand, responses to labile perturbation factors, although part of this continuum, must by definition happen during or after the event. Moreover, because labile perturbation factors are relatively short-lived, changes in physiological state (and behavior) are only needed as long as the perturbation persists (Figure 3.11).

Physiological state varies on a predictive cycle within levels A and B as projected by the reaction norm for daily/seasonal routines (lower section of Figure 3.11). When a labile perturbation factor triggers a transitory change in physiological state to level C (upper section of Figure 3.11) involving sudden disruption of dynamic equilibrium (i.e., beyond the reaction norm), coping mechanisms (i.e., the emergency life-history stage) are activated until the perturbation passes (Figure 3.10). Mechanisms maintaining level A are termed "basic homeostasis," those regulating A–B are called "regulated allostasis," and within level C, "facultative allostasis" (Figure 3.12; Wingfield 2004; Landys et al. 2006). Homeostatic set-points must change from one level to another (Figure 3.12) and within level B (Figure 3.13), suggesting that regulatory mechanisms (the mediators of allostasis) are probably different at each level (McEwen and Wingfield 2003; Wingfield 2004; Landys et al. 2006).

There have been several earlier reports that define these adjustments within life-history stages (e.g., rheostasis, homeorhesis, and poikilostasis), but the more recent concept of allostasis incorporates them all (reviewed in McEwen and Wingfield 2003; Wingfield 2004; Korte et al. 2005). Additionally, no individual experiences the environment in exactly the same way as another, territories differ in quality and physical

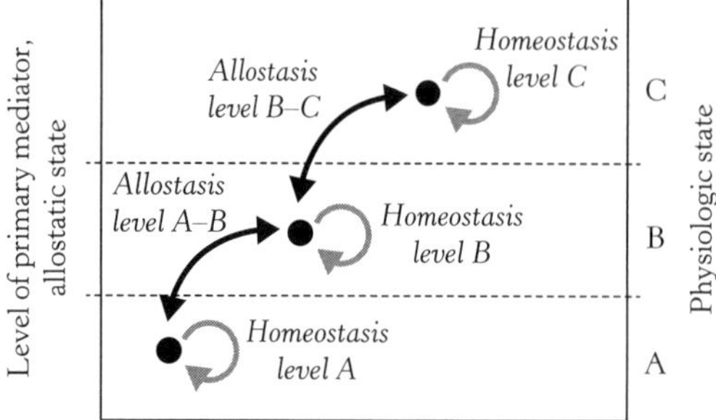

FIGURE 3.12: An explanation of the terms "homeostasis," "allostasis," and "physiological state." Action of primary mediators (i.e., action of hormones, elements of the immune system, and/or neural responses; defined as an allostatic state) tune critical internal variables to specific set-points as appropriate to existing environmental conditions and life-history demands (McEwen and Wingfield 2003). "Allostasis" is defined as the process of adjusting critical internal variables among such set-points. In contrast, we refer to "homeostasis" as the process of maintaining internal variables within a given set-point. The physiological and behavioral characteristics of a specific set-point can be described by three increasingly complex physiological states—A, B, and C (after Wingfield et al. 1997; Wingfield and Ramenofsky 1999). Physiological state A is characterized by basic physiological and behavioral processes fundamental for simple existence. Physiological state B is representative of processes associated with increased but predictable or manageable demands in the environment or in life history. Physiological state C is characterized by facultative responses (e.g., the emergency life-history stage) associated with unpredictable and life-threatening events. The physiological states A, B, and C are paralleled by allostatic states that maintain processes at given set-points through the action of primary mediators.

From Landys et al. (2006). Courtesy of Elsevier.

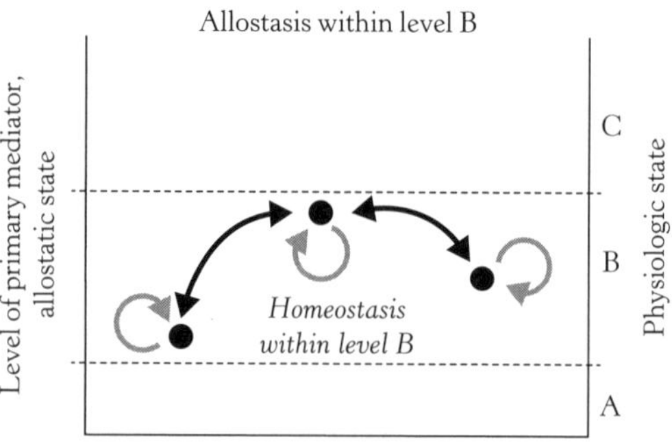

FIGURE 3.13: Following from Figure 3.12, allostasis within level B results in homeostatic changes that do not involve allostatic overload. The individual can cope with the energetic demands of daily/seasonal routines of the predictable life cycle and local perturbations.

structure; social status differs and parasite load, old injuries, and so on, may be present in some but not all. An individual in one territory may be more susceptible to predators or a pathogen that reduces food supply. The allostasis concept thus goes beyond classical homeostasis and acclimation and allows us to integrate all the experiences of an individual, predictable and unpredictable, with the potential for stress, rather than treating them as separate issues. This framework will be critical for understanding the complex behavioral and physiological responses to perturbations in the natural world.

Using the concept of physiological state, it is possible to apply levels A, B, and C to mediators of allostasis, particularly hormone responses (Figure 3.14, from Wingfield 2003, 2004). Many hormones are secreted constitutively (level A), that is, a small amount of hormone is released in small pulses or continuously to maintain level A physiological state. Within level B, hormones are secreted in a regulated fashion as a function of time of day or season. In response to a perturbation, hormone secretion can show a transitory elevation into level C, associated with responses of physiological state and behavior, to cope with the perturbation. As with physiological state (Figure 3.11), this surge is transitory and returns to level B when the perturbation passes. Different suites of hormones mediating allostasis can be secreted at each level, providing specificity of regulation. However, in some cases the same hormone, such as a glucocorticoid, may increase through each level, having different effects as concentrations increase (Figure 3.15; Sapolsky et al. 2000; Wingfield and Romero 2001; Wingfield 2003, 2004; Landys et al. 2006). It is important to remember, however, that mediators of allostasis, such as autonomic, endocrine, and immune mediators, influence each other in complex ways. Note that in Figure 3.15, glucocorticoid levels cycle within level B (the predictable life cycle) but surge to level C following perturbations of the environment (Landys et al. 2006). Because the same hormone has different effects at different levels, this means that receptor types and numbers in target tissues also vary (see Chapter 4). These concepts will become very important in later chapters when we discuss hormonal mechanisms

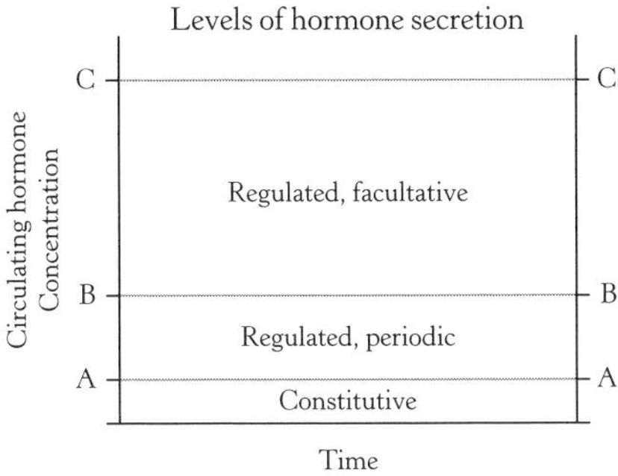

FIGURE 3.14: The concept of levels A–C can be extended to levels of hormone secretion that actually regulate different physiological levels in basic homeostasis, and regulated and facultative allostasis. At level A (hormone levels regulating basic homeostasis), secretion may be constitutive. However, some regulation may be possible. At level B, hormone secretion is regulated according to needs as a function of endogenous rhythms (e.g., circadian, episodic), or in response to environmental signals transduced through neural and neuroendocrine pathways. From level B to C, regulated facultative secretion is controlled exclusively by environmental signals. Depending upon environmental and social contexts, different hormones may operate at each level. In many cases, the same hormone may act at two or all three levels. The latter scenario raises important issues in terms of mechanisms of action of a hormone at more than one level.

From Wingfield (2004). Courtesey of Cambridge University Press.

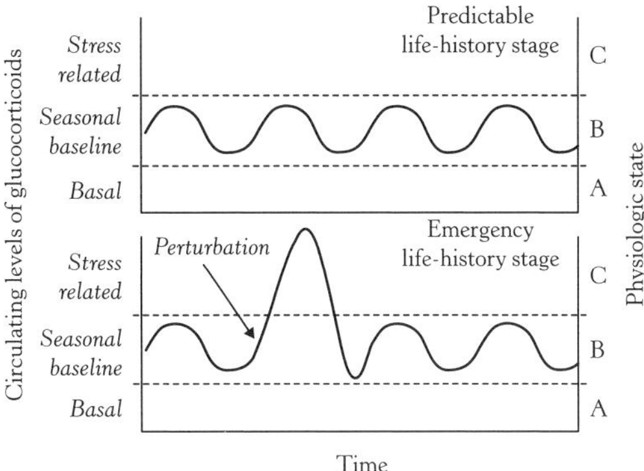

FIGURE 3.15: Variability of physiological glucocorticoid levels in a free-living animal (adapted from Wingfield et al. 1997). Basal levels of glucocorticoids maintain basic life processes and are secreted constitutively. In response to demands associated with the predictable life-history cycle, glucocorticoids fluctuate within a seasonal baseline level. Unpredictable and challenging perturbations may cause glucocorticoids to increase above the seasonal baseline to stress related concentrations. Elevations to this level are usually transitory and can cause animals to enter into an emergency life-history stage. If a perturbation is successfully overcome, plasma glucocorticoids return to the level appropriate for a current life-history stage.

From Landys et al. (2006). Courtesey of Elsevier.

underlying physiological and behavioral responses to labile perturbation factors.

C. Allostatic Load and Allostatic Overload

Evidence to date suggests an overarching physiological pathway by which diverse environmental information regulating the life cycle leads to hormone secretions that regulate the response (Wingfield et al. 1998). This is based on a simple energetic theme that also represents a common currency for allostatic load—the cumulative demands of daily/seasonal routines, parasites, social status, habitat quality, and so on (Figure 3.16; McEwen and Wingfield 2003). The term for general energetic requirements (E) of organisms during their life cycle includes, for convenience, all potential requirements for nutrition in general, although essential components of nutrition could also be modeled.

The energy required for basic homeostasis (existence energy) is represented by Ee (Figure 3.16). Additional energy required for the individual to go about its daily routines to find, process, and assimilate food under ideal conditions is Ei. The amount of energy (in food) available in the environment is Eg (McEwen and Wingfield 2003). These components obviously will change in relation to seasons and other factors. For example, we would expect Eg to rise in spring and summer and subsequently to decline through autumn and winter when primary productivity is low (Figure 3.16). Food availability in relation to demands of routine life cycle activities and hormone action is rarely considered (e.g., Kitaysky et al. 2003). Energy required for basic homeostasis (existence energy, Ee) in endothermic vertebrates should be lowest in summer when ambient temperatures are highest, and thus Ei (energy for daily routines under ideal conditions) will vary in parallel with Ee. The sum of Ee plus Ei is allostatic load of daily and seasonal routines of the individual (Figure 3.16; McEwen and Wingfield 2003). Superimposed on this daily routine are additional demands imposed by

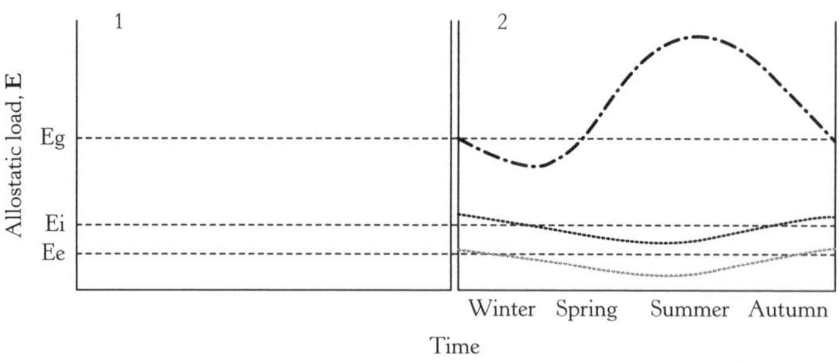

FIGURE 3.16: A framework for modeling energetic requirements (E) of organisms during their life cycle. This energy requirement, E, includes all potential nutritional requirements including energy per se. They are grouped together here for convenience, although essential components of nutrition could also be modeled. Ee represents the energy required for basic homeostasis (i.e., level A). Ei represents the extra energy required for the individual to go out, find, process and assimilate food under ideal conditions (i.e., level B). Eg represents the amount of energy (in food) available in the environment (from Wingfield et al. 1998; Wingfield and Ramenofsky 1999). In panel 1, these requirements are represented as straight lines. In panel 2, the changes in energy levels have been adjusted to represent probable changes in relation to seasons. Eg would be expected to rise dramatically in spring and summer and then decline through autumn and winter when primary productivity is low. Ee would be lowest in summer when ambient temperatures are highest. Ei should be fairly constant (under ideal conditions) and varies in parallel with Ee. Bearing in mind that energy levels will vary in potentially complex ways, Ee and Ei will be held as straight lines for simplicity.

From McEwen and Wingfield (2003). Courtesey of Elsevier.

energy required to reproduce, molt, or migrate. The additional E required to fuel this higher allostatic load must remain below Eg if positive energy balance is to be maintained (Figure 3.17). Similarly, a perturbation (such as a storm) will also increase energetic demand in addition to Ee + Ei. This is Eo and represents the energy required to find food, process it, and assimilate nutrients

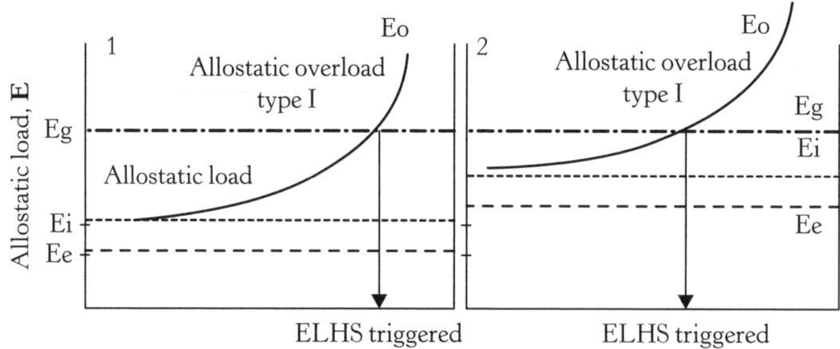

FIGURE 3.17: The effects of labile perturbation factors (LPFs) such as storms, predators, human disturbance, and so forth, on energy requirements in free-living organisms. In this case, Eg is held constant, but as environmental conditions deteriorate, the energy required to go out, obtain food, process and assimilate it increases, and a new line, Eo, can be inserted. As the LPF persists (panel 1), then Eo increases until Ee + Ei + Eo > Eg. At this point, the individual goes into negative energy balance and an emergency life-history stage (ELHS) is triggered. At this point, secretion of glucocorticoids increases dramatically, thus driving the transition to an ELHS (see Wingfield et al. 1998; Wingfield and Romero 2001). Ee can be increased due to low ambient temperature changing basic homeostasis, or due to cumulative allostatic load following infection, injury resulting in permanent disability, and so on (panel 2). In this case, the same LPF would result in the same rise in Eo, but an ELHS would be triggered more quickly. In this way, the energy model can explain individual differences in coping with the environment but keeping the potential mechanisms on a common framework. Note also that when in negative energy balance, the triggering of an ELHS is designed to reduce allostatic load (Ee + Ei + Eo) so that the individual can regain positive energy balance and survive the LPF in the best condition possible. If allostatic load is so high that even an ELHS cannot reduce it sufficiently to gain positive energy balance, then chronic stress will ensue.

From McEwen and Wingfield (2003). Courtesey of Elsevier.

under non-ideal conditions (Figure 3.17). As long as the sum of Ee + Ei + Eo does not exceed Eg, then the individual can tolerate higher allostatic load, at least temporarily (Figure 3.17; McEwen and Wingfield 2003; Wingfield 2004; Korte et al. 2005).

Allostatic load therefore increases further as a direct function of Ee + Ei + Eo, and if it exceeds Eg, then type 1 allostatic overload develops, indicating that the individual is in negative energy balance (Figures 3.17 and 3.18). At this point the individual must begin mobilizing endogenous reserves. The amount of those reserves (e.g., fat stores) determines whether the individual can seek a shelter to endure the perturbation, or if it should trigger an emergency life-history stage to reduce allostatic load in an alternate habitat. In either event, the facultative physiological and behavioral strategies of the emergency life-history stage are triggered to allow the individual to cope. This will result in abandonment of the normal life-history stage with further savings of energy demand. Examples are abandonment of a nest and interruption of reproductive function.

This energy framework allows the visualization of how individuals differ in response to the same perturbation depending upon ecological variables (Figure 3.19). A given perturbation may be tolerated by the scenario in Figure 3.19 panel 1, where Eg is sufficient to allow the organism to go about its daily routines and cope with the perturbation. However, if an individual has a higher Ee + Ei because of injury or other handicap, then the same perturbation would result in allostatic overload type 1 and an emergency life-history stage would be activated (Figure 3.19, panel 2). Conversely, if Eg was lower because a territory was poor quality, then once more the same

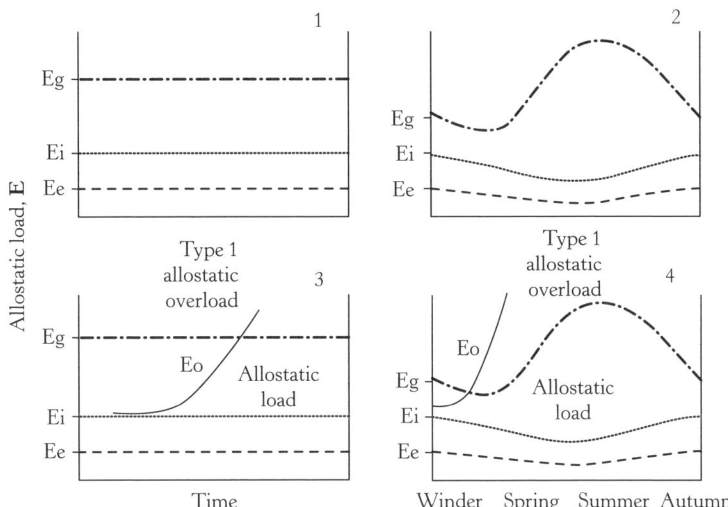

FIGURE 3.18: A framework for modeling energetic requirements (E) of organisms during their life cycle. This energy requirement, E, includes all potential nutritional requirements including energy; Ee represents the energy required for basic homeostasis. Ei represents the extra energy required for the individual to go out, find, process, and assimilate food under ideal conditions. Eg represents the amount of energy (in food) available in the environment (from Wingfield et al. 1998; Wingfield and Ramenofsky 1999). (1) These requirements are represented as straight lines. (2) The changes in energy levels have been adjusted to represent probable changes in relation to seasons. Eg would be expected to rise dramatically in spring and summer and then decline through autumn and winter when primary productivity is low. Ee would be lowest in summer when ambient temperatures are highest. Ei should be fairly constant (under ideal conditions) and varies in parallel with Ee. (3) Bearing in mind that energy levels will vary in potentially complex ways, Ee and Ei are held as straight lines for simplicity. Here we introduce additional costs incurred after a perturbation (such as a storm) that increases costs above Ee + Ei. This line (Eo) represents the energy required to go out and find food, process it, and assimilate nutrients under non-ideal conditions. Allostatic load increases as Eo persists in time. If it exceeds Eg, then type 1 allostatic overload begins, resulting in elevation of plasma glucocorticoid levels. This triggers an emergency life-history stage that results in alternate physiology and behavior intended to reduce allostatic overload. (4) If we then represent the effects of Eo in more naturally fluctuating conditions, then in winter type 1 allostatic overload occurs rapidly.

From McEwen and Wingfield (2003). Courtesey of Elsevier.

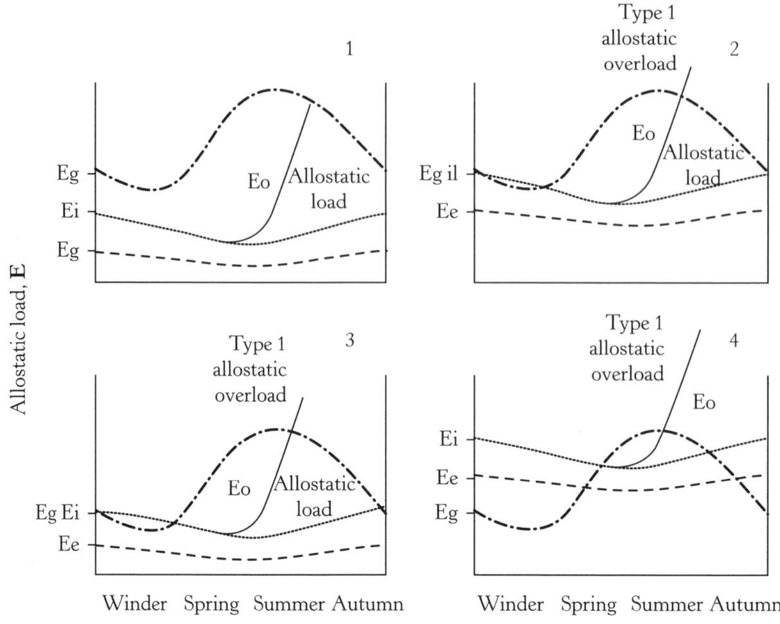

FIGURE 3.19: A schematic representation of the effects of Eo, a line showing an increase in energy costs required to go out and find food, process, and assimilate it under non-ideal conditions. If this occurs in late spring (1), then the seasonal increase in Eg and decreases in Ei and Ee can cover the costs of Eo. (2) A model of the effects if permanent injury, disease, and/or deleterious lifestyle increase Ee + Ei close to resources available (Eg), then the individual may be at type 1 allostatic overload. Through the winter and even in spring and summer, that individual will be susceptible to a perturbation (Eo), resulting in allostatic overload type 1. A perturbation (Eo) occurring in winter, or a time when resources are at low ebb, would result in almost immediate allostatic overload. (3) A scenario in which Eg is reduced dramatically. This can happen in nature as a result of climate change or other perturbation. Additionally, in human society, socioeconomic status reduces resources available (Eg). Then in winter an individual may always be in type 1 allostatic overload, and even in summer Eg does not increase enough to prevent allostatic overload if a perturbation occurs. The same perturbation (Eo) in winter would result in immediate type 1 allostatic overload. (4) If permanent injury, disease, and/or deleterious lifestyle increase Ee + Ei, and an environmental perturbation reduces resources available (Eg), then the individual will be in type 1 allostatic overload through the winter and into spring. Even in summer, susceptibility to a perturbation (Eo) will result in rapid overload.

From McEwen and Wingfield (2003). Courtesey of Elsevier.

perturbation results in allostatic overload type 1 (Figure 3.19, panel 3). A combination of poor territory and a high Ee + Ei would result in immediate allostatic overload (Figure 3.19, panel 4; see also McEwen and Wingfield 2003; Wingfield 2005).

One major assumption of the allostasis model is that circulating levels of glucocorticoids parallel energetic demand of daily routines and responses to perturbations—allostatic load (McEwen and Wingfield 2003; Wingfield 2004; Korte et al. 2005). Higher glucocorticoid secretion in response to elevated allostatic load is supported by an extensive literature (e.g., Sapolsky et al. 2000), activating the emergency life-history stage (Figure 3.20; e.g. Wingfield 2003, 2004). Glucocorticoid levels increase from level A to B as a function of the energetic costs of daily routines of that life-history stage and in response to a perturbation (Eo). If Eo persists, glucocorticoids rise further to level C, where allostatic overload type 1 is likely (Figure 3.20). The emergency life-history stage results in a decrease in Eo, accompanied by a decrease of glucocorticoid levels to avoid chronic stress and associated pathologies (Figure 3.20).

Type 2 allostatic overload is a function of long-term or permanent perturbations resulting from human disturbance, global climate change, and so forth. In this scenario, energetic demand (Eo) of non-ideal conditions increases and remains elevated, but below the amount of energy available as food in the environment (Eg, Figure 3.21). This type of allostatic load represents a permanent increase in Ee + Ei + Eo and has the potential for deleterious effects unless individuals

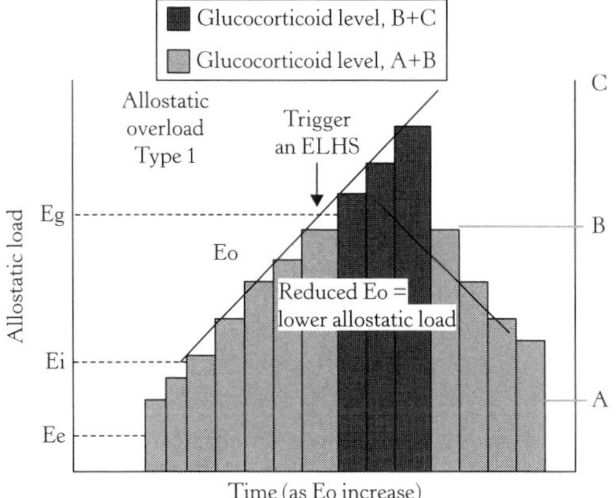

FIGURE 3.20: Summary of type 1 allostatic overload and glucocorticoid secretion. Here Eo increases dramatically, and eventually Eo + Ee + Ei exceeds EG. Increasingly high glucocorticoid secretion then triggers an emergency life-history stage (ELHS). The result is to suppress the expression of other life-history stages, resulting in a net decrease of allostatic load below Eg. The animal can now survive the perturbation in positive energy balance and glucocorticoid secretion subsides, avoiding pathologies associated with chronic high levels. From McEwen and Wingfield (2003). Courtesey of Elsevier.

are able to adjust their life cycles accordingly (McEwen and Wingfield 2003). Increased intensity and frequency of storms as a result of global warming may result in allostatic overload type 2 in the future. Because Eg is not exceeded, the chronic elevation of glucocorticoids leads to an imbalance in other hormones—for example hyper-insulinemia—that can lead to hyperphagia and obesity. The emergency life-history stage is not triggered. In panel 4 of Figure 3.21, type 2 allostatic overload is depicted as a result of permanent increases in Ee and Ei, as in a chronic state of obesity when individuals continue to consume more calories than are needed and enter a state where oxidative stress is elevated, as in type 2 diabetes (Bierhaus et al. 2001). Glucocorticoid secretion parallels this increase, and chronically high levels result in the same pathologies as in Figure 3.21, panel 2.

Gradients of four human diseases as a function of socioeconomic status (from Adler et al. 1993), allostatic overload type 2, are shown in Figure 3.22. These four diseases show gradients across the full range of socioeconomic status and include (a) percentage diagnosed osteoarthritis (Cunningham and Kelsey 1984); (b) relative prevalence of chronic disease (Townsend 1974); (c) prevalence of hypertension; (d) rate of cervical cancer per 100,000 (Devesa and Diamond 1980). Allostatic overload type 2 may be a major cause of such pathologies in human populations, and the extent to which this may also affect wild animal populations remains to be clarified.

Allostasis was conceived originally in the biomedical setting specifically to apply to human health. The concept has great promise in understanding some human diseases and is currently a leading model for understanding the etiology of diseases such as diabetes, obesity, depression, and drug addiction. However, none of these diseases is likely to be important for wild animals attempting to survive in their natural habitats. Allostasis has a number of strengths and weaknesses when applied to more ethologically relevant phenomena. One major strength is that the concept of "constancy through change" incorporates circadian, circannual, and other life-history changes. This allows us to emphasize the importance of regulating the animal's physiological systems at both elevated and reduced levels (Koob and Le Moal 2001; McEwen and Wingfield 2003). This is a key advantage over many earlier uses of the traditional model of stress when applied to wild animals. It indicates that energetically demanding processes, such as pregnancy, increase allostatic load but are not, in themselves, stressful (Landys et al. 2006). By increasing allostatic load, these energetically demanding activities make it more likely that the animal will enter allostatic overload, but as long as energetic stores are sufficient, phrases such as "the stress of reproduction" cease to have much meaning.

A second strength is the introduction of the concept of allostatic load that models the wear and tear on individuals coping with repeated stressors. Further, accumulated allostatic load can indicate how prepared the individual is to cope with future stressors (e.g., McEwen et al. 1999; Figures 3.18 and 3.19) and assumes a threshold for when accumulated allostatic load turns into allostatic overload (Goldstein and McEwen 2002)—in this model, Eg. This threshold allows testable predictions for two related phenomena. First, we can now predict when normal adaptive responses will become insufficient and require new, stronger responses to counteract the stressor. Second, we can now predict when adaptive responses will fail and result in stress-related disease. The ability of the allostasis model to generate testable predictions is an important theoretical advance.

A third strength is the proposed use of energy as both an underlying mechanism and a universal

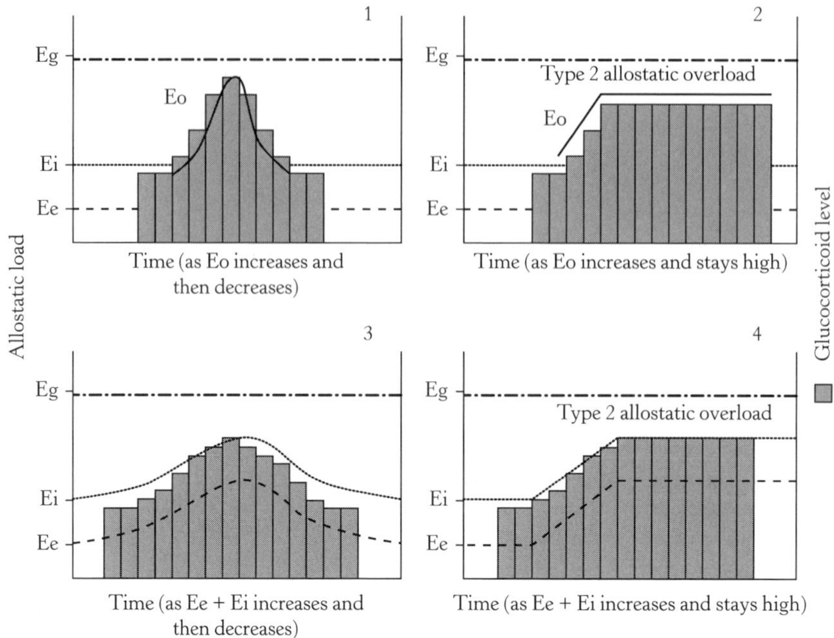

FIGURE 3.21: Glucocorticoids are key biological mediators of both type 1 and type 2 allostatic load and overload, as shown in four different hypothetical scenarios. Depending on the circumstances associated with glucocorticoid elevation other hormones (e.g., insulin and related metabolic hormones) will also be altered. When Eg is not exceeded and individuals are consuming excess calories, obesity, metabolic syndrome, and type 2 diabetes are the result. (1) Normal responses to a challenge when Eg is not exceeded. Eo represents the challenges of daily living in a difficult or challenging environment. In animals in the wild, this would include the demands of finding food and coping with weather. In human terms, this includes the challenges of work and coping with a stressful living environment and interpersonal interactions. Glucocorticoid levels remain low during normal events associated with Ee + Ei. As Eo sets in, glucocorticoid secretion increases in parallel. Eo is transient; when Eo subsides, so do glucocorticoid levels. Because Eg is not exceeded, the individual does not need to trigger an emergency life-history stage (i.e., escape from the situation). (2) Type 2 allostatic overload as a function of permanent perturbations in Eo, which increases and remains high. Glucocorticoid secretion also increases and stays chronically high because of the continuous stress of the living and (in humans) working environment. Because Eg is not exceeded, the chronic elevation of glucocorticoids leads to an imbalance in other hormones (e.g., hyper-insulinemia) that can lead to hyperphagia and obesity. This is type 2 allostatic overload. (3) Increases in allostatic load could be presented as a transitory increase in Ee + Ei, such as is the case when individuals overeat, become obese, and have more weight to carry around. Again glucocorticoid secretion would match this increase and subside as Ee and Ei return to normal, such as after a successful diet and exercise program. Because Eg is never exceeded, then an emergency life-history stage is not needed. In these cases, Ee and Ei are elevated as a result of within-individual changes. Eo is an outside influence, such as social pressure, over and above Ee + Ei. (4) Type 2 allostatic overload as a result of permanent increases in Ee and Ei, as in a chronic state of obesity when individuals continue to consume more calories than are needed and enter a state where oxidative stress is elevated, as in type 2 diabetes (Bierhaus et al. 2001). Glucocorticoid secretion parallels this increase, and chronically high levels result in the same pathologies as in (2).

From McEwen and Wingfield (2003). Courtesey of Elsevier.

metric for allostatic load. Mediators of allostasis influence each other in complex ways, but using energy in this manner allows for integrating diverse physiological responses to get an overall impact on the animal. It also provides, for the first time, a way to predict whether a specific stressor (or series of stressors) would either initiate a stress response or result in the symptoms of chronic stress. The use of energy seems especially useful in ecological studies, and there are examples where using energy and allostatic load can help explain empirical data (e.g., Romero et al. 2000; Romero and Wikelski 2001; Goymann and Wingfield 2004). In addition, the use of energy as a metric

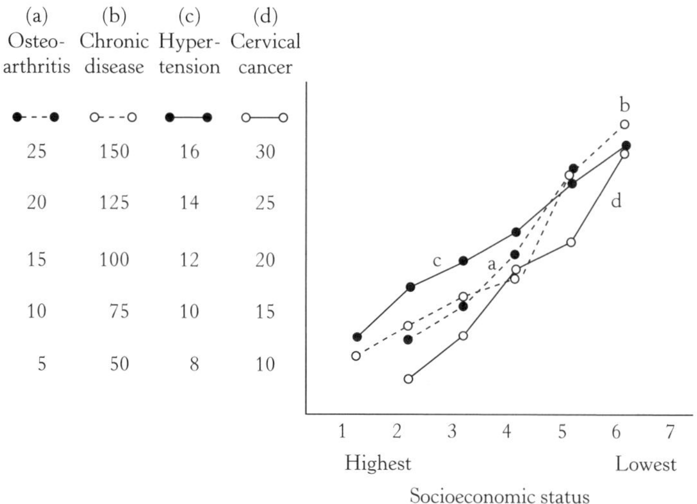

FIGURE 3.22: Gradients of four human diseases as a function of socioeconomic status. These diseases show gradients across the full range of socioeconomic status. Data for the following are shown: (a) Percentage diagnosed osteoarthritis (Cunningham and Kelsey 1984); (b) Relative prevalence of chronic disease (Townsend 1974); (c) Prevalence of hypertension (Kraus et al. 1980); (d) Rate of cervical cancer per 100,000 (Devesa and Diamond 1980).

Republished from Adler et al. (1994) by permission.

From McEwen and Wingfield (2003). Courtesy of Elsevier.

of allostatic load allows mathematical modeling of the impact of stress on individuals and populations (e.g., Fefferman and Romero 2013), something that would have been impossible using only the traditional model of stress. Theoretical mathematical models can then produce novel testable hypotheses.

The original formulation of allostasis, however, had a few weaknesses. One is, ironically, the reliance of allostasis on energy as the mechanism and metric for allostatic load. Energy input and expenditure provide a fantastic framework for understanding allostatic load and the transition to allostatic overload, but in practice these measurements are not always very simple (e.g., Walsberg 2003). The devil is in the details. An animal's energy usage is heavily dependent upon the time frame over which the measurements are made, making it difficult to differentiate changes in energy use resulting from normal consumption (allostasis) from those resulting from increased expenditures (allostatic load). This problem is exacerbated when comparing across species such as endotherms (limited storage capacities in relation to high rates of energy consumption) and ectotherms (subsisting for months between meals).

Furthermore, four examples indicate that not all energy use has the same impact. In the first example, if animals alter the rate rather than the amount of energy consumed during different life-history stages, the connection between energy consumption and allostatic load becomes more difficult to detect. Experiments on common eiders, a large sea duck, provide a good example. The increase in foraging activity prior to migration in these ducks is not accompanied by a concurrent increase in daily heart rate, which is an index of daily energy consumption (Pelletier et al. 2008). In other words, a large increase in allostatic load (foraging effort) is not reflected in increased daily energy consumption. Instead, birds appear to compensate for the increased energy consumption during active foraging by decreasing energy consumption during the inactive period. On the other hand, such potential mechanisms in the allostasis framework suggest the evolution of ways by which organisms can regulate their food intake and energetic costs to cope with potential bottlenecks resulting from climatic events and so on. We expect exciting new developments in this area.

In the second example, not all energy mobilization is equivalent. The problems of acidosis and potential cell damage (allostatic overload) that can accompany glycolysis or gluconeogenesis (conversion of protein to glucose) are not present when converting glycogen to glucose. In other words, the metabolic source of the energy makes a difference in the impact on the animal.

Nonetheless, in the allostasis model, the role of repair mechanisms for oxidative damage comes to the fore, and future research should combine cellular aspects of stress responsiveness and humoral (hormonal) mechanisms.

In the third example, the connection between energy regulation and corticosteroids, a major stress hormone presumed to be one of the prime mediators of energy balance during stress (see Chapter 4), is not as well understood as once thought (see Chapter 5). Although corticosteroids are thought to mobilize energy (specifically glucose) to cope with a stressor (Sapolsky et al. 2000), the foundation for this idea comes from work on fasted animals. Free-living animals are unlikely to be fasting when exposed to a stressor in a natural context, and corticosteroids seem to be ineffective at regulating energy in fed animals (e.g., Remage-Healey and Romero 2001; see Chapter 5). Allostasis loses some of its explanatory power if stress mediators do not consistently regulate energy, but again the framework might prove heuristic in specifically testing at what stage glucocorticoids become gluconeogenic in a free-living animal exposed to a perturbation. Furthermore, ectotherms that can go days (even weeks) between feeding events might prove to be critical research subjects in this regard.

Finally, in the fourth example, not all stress responses culminate in immediate measurable energy expenditure. Primarily this is a result of very rapid acute responses. For example, if robust sympathetic and behavioral responses to moderate psychological stressors are not sustained for sufficient time, they fail to incur significant energy consumption when compared to the 24-hour energy budget (Cyr et al. 2008, Walsberg, 2003). At least in the short term, behavioral responses are sufficiently inexpensive to initiate that they are essentially cost-free in the context of normal daily/weekly energy budgets. As an example, if an animal freezes in the presence of a predator, overall energy expenditure may actually decrease (i.e., it is no longer active). Consequently, a highly relevant behavioral stress response becomes essentially invisible to the allostasis model. To be fair, however, allostasis was not designed to model these very acute stress responses (McEwen and Wingfield 2010). On the other hand, it is critical to understand that although behavioral changes may have minimal energetic costs, they do determine availability of food (access to Eg). The allostasis model must not only consider the energetic costs of allostatic load but also Eg and access to it. If behavioral interactions result in one individual having to work harder to get at Eg, or has restricted access to Eg (e.g., a subordinate), then the same perturbation, Eo, could trigger allostatic overload more quickly (see also Goymann and Wingfield 2004).

The original formulation of the allostasis model does not include a number of concepts typically included in discussions of stress. Examples include developmental effects that alter an individual's responses to stressors later in life (see Chapter 5), cognitive evaluations of a stimulus (e.g., controllability, predictability, and distinguishing stressful from non-stressful stimuli [e.g., Day 2005]), and the virtual omission of short-term responses (see Chapter 4). Especially developmental effects following environmental perturbations, including maternal effects, will determine the phenotype and how the individual will fit into the allostasis framework as an adult. Again, more research is needed in this area (e.g., Korte et al. 2005).

Note, however, that omitting short-term responses might not be an important weakness in the context of free-living animals. Responses to predator attacks clearly have profound consequences on fitness, but predicting the circumstances and the results of these responses is comparatively easy. Acute responses either work (the animal escapes) or they don't (the predator is successful). Neither result provides much explanation for how animals survive over prolonged periods such as seasons or years. What is more interesting and difficult to predict is how effective those acute responses are depending upon time of year (breeding vs. non-breeding), physiological condition (fat vs. lean), immunological status (healthy vs. sick), social rank (dominant vs. subordinate), and so on. In other words, understanding how animals cope throughout their lifetimes requires understanding the impact of allostatic load.

V. THE REACTIVE SCOPE MODEL

This model (Romero et al. 2009) originated as an attempt to modify and extend allostasis to encompass many of the features of a stress response left out of the original attempt to apply the concepts of allostasis to free-living animals. The idea was to move beyond a reliance on energy availability and usage and address the dynamics and regulation of the underlying physiological responses, such as receptor-ligand interactions, as a mechanistic foundation for allostatic load. In this way the reactive scope and allostasis models interface very well, with reactive scope taking a more mechanistic, mediators of allostasis, approach, and the allostasis model taking a model framework approach to explain individual, seasonal, and social differences in how individuals cope with daily/seasonal routines and perturbations (McEwen and Wingfield 2010).

A. The Basic Reactive Scope Model

This model presupposes that researchers are measuring some physiological mediator that is important in the stress response. The goal of the reactive ccope model is to understand how the levels and/or concentrations of those mediators change over time and how the resultant levels and/or concentrations allow the animal to cope with stressors. The emphasis is on when levels/concentrations represent normal functioning (i.e., basal function and an adaptive stress response) and when they represent a situation that has become problematic for the animal (i.e., chronic stress). In this regard the model expands greatly on the state levels concepts described earlier.

The basic model is a graph of the level of some physiological mediator over time. These physiological mediators are part of the processes such as hormones, cytokines, behavior, and cardiovascular regulation, and so forth, that are involved in maintaining physiological variables such as oxygen, glucose, and so on, in a constant state. A number of different names have been used for these processes, including "homeostatic mediators" (McEwen 2003), "allostatic mediators" (McEwen and Wingfield 2003) and more generally, the "stress response" (Sapolsky et al. 2000). The concentration or level of each mediator is placed on the *y* axis to form a graph of the concentration/level of the mediator over time (Figure 3.23; compare with state-level models in Figures 3.10–3.15).

The values of a mediator exist in four ranges, rather than three in the state-level model (Figures 3.10–3.15). The normal circadian and seasonal range

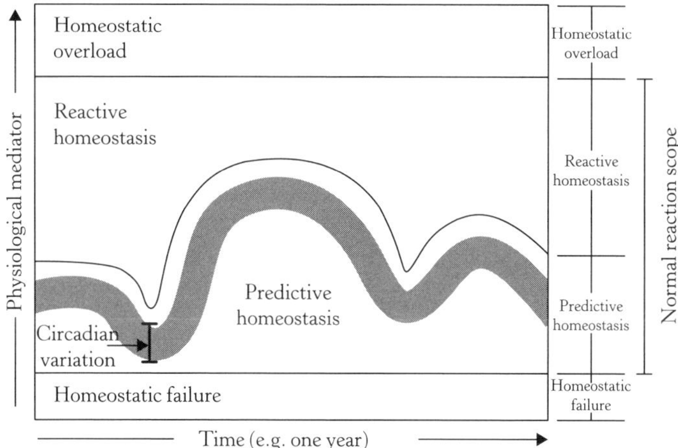

FIGURE 3.23: Graphical model of the concentrations of different physiological mediators on the *y* axis versus time. The range of concentrations or levels of physiological mediators is broken into four ranges. The lowest range depicts concentrations/levels that are too low to maintain homeostasis and is termed homeostatic failure. The minimum required concentration/level forms a threshold that does not change over time. Above this threshold is the predictive homeostasis range that varies according to predictable life-history changes. The circadian variation in concentrations is depicted as a gray bar (with the bottom being the circadian nadir and the top being the circadian peak). The range of predictive homeostasis varies depending upon life-history demands, and thus changes seasonally. The predictive range extends slightly above the circadian peak in each season to encompass predictable daily events such as foraging. Above the predictive homeostasis range is the reactive homeostasis range, which represents concentrations/levels of the physiological mediator necessary to maintain homeostasis following an unpredictable event that threatens homeostasis. The predictive and reactive homeostasis ranges form the normal reactive scope for that physiological mediator. The upper limit of the reactive homeostasis range is the concentration/level where the mediator itself starts to cause damage, and the range above this threshold is termed "homeostatic overload." The threshold between reactive homeostasis and homeostatic overload is presumed to not change on a daily or seasonal basis.

Reprinted with permission from Romero et al. (2009). Courtesy of Elsevier.

frames "predictive homeostasis," a term co-opted from Moore-Ede (1986). Predictive homeostasis encompasses the adjustable range of values associated with challenges predictable by major environmental cues such as photoperiod. Such challenges include, but are not limited to, predictable daily changes in day and night and seasonal life-history stages (daily routines) such as reproduction and migration. These would be equivalent to levels A and B in the allostasis model (Figures 3.10–3.14). The wide gray band represents daily circadian variation that changes seasonally to reflect predictable changes driven by changes in photoperiod. Using the "set-point" metaphor often used to explain homeostasis, the predictive homeostasis range can be thought of as the range of homeostatic set-points (Figure 3.23; compare with Figures 3.12–3.14).

Predictive homeostasis also encompasses slight increases in the mediator associated with normal predictable daily activities, such as foraging. Consequently, predictive homeostasis combines the concepts of Ee and Ei from the allostasis model. The key concept is that predictive homeostasis encompasses responses of the physiological mediator to *predictable* environmental change.

When levels/concentrations of the mediators extend beyond the predictive homeostasis range, they enter the reactive homeostasis range (Figure 3.23). Reactive homeostasis encompasses the range of the physiological mediator during a response to unpredictable changes in the environment. Levels in this range are needed to re-establish homeostasis. This is the scope of responses introduced by Cannon (1932) and Selye (1946) and corresponds both to the stress response in the traditional model and the emergency life-history stage (e.g., Wingfield et al. 1998) (see previous sections in this chapter). The key concept here is that reactive homeostasis refers to *normal* concentrations in response to *unpredictable* environmental change. Reactive homeostasis thus reflects the aspects of unpredictability and uncontrollability at the heart of the traditional model.

Although predictive and reactive homeostasis ranges differ in whether the responses are due to predictable or unpredictable environmental events, both reflect normal responses—rather like levels A, B, and C in the allotasis model (Figures 3.10–3.15). Consequently, these two ranges establish the normal reactive scope for this particular mediator for this individual (Figure 3.23). The normal reactive scope thus defines the normal physiological response to predictable and unpredictable events in the environment in a healthy animal.

Concentrations of a physiological mediator can also be abnormal, however. In other words, the levels can extend outside the normal reactive scope. When this occurs, the animal can no longer successfully cope. The mediator can be outside the normal reactive scope in two directions. If it is below the lower limit of predictive homeostasis, the normal physiological processes that the mediator regulates cannot be maintained, and death usually rapidly follows. This range is termed "homeostatic failure" (Figure 3.23), that is, below level A in Figures 3.10–3.15. The minimum concentration/level of a physiological mediator required to maintain homeostasis constitutes a threshold that current data suggest is constant over time. The level/concentration of a physiological mediator can also exceed the reactive homeostatic range. This extends the physiological mediator past the normal reactive scope, and the animal enters a pathological state termed "homeostatic overload." The physiological mediator can enter homeostatic overload, but cannot be maintained in this range without the mediator causing physiological disruption itself.

Homeostatic overload may appear similar to allostatic overload, but there are major differences. Allostatic overload type 1 results from an animal being in negative energy balance (see previous section). This triggers the emergency life-history stage, which then reduces allostatic load (Figure 3.20) and is within the reactive scope of the animal. In contrast, homeostatic overload results from the mediator itself becoming a problem. Homeostatic overload is thus more closely related to allostatic overload Type 2 (Figure 3.21). Note also that homeostatic overload corresponds to the concept of chronic stress in the traditional model (see earlier section). In the traditional model, chronic stress and thus stress-related disease result from an excessive stress response (Figure 3.1D). Because the allostatic load model addresses animals in their natural environment, homeostatic overload is almost always fatal (massive die-offs do occur; e.g., Gessaman and Worthen 1982), although we will discuss some interesting possible exceptions in later chapters. Homeostatic overload likewise results from an excessive response by the physiological mediator. In both cases, it is an over-exuberant increase in the mediators that causes the problem, leading to chronic stress-like symptoms.

There are numerous examples of how inappropriate levels of mediators can cause disease. One is of glucocorticoids creating tissue damage by breaking down proteins during gluconeogenesis (Sapolsky 1992). A second example is the long-term behavioral and cardiovascular responses to stressors that result in cardiovascular disease (Sapolsky 2001). Mediators in the homeostatic overload range do not result in immediate death, but instead cause disease over time that could eventually result in death. Homeostatic overload, therefore, is different from homeostatic failure. Similar to homeostatic failure, however, current data suggest a threshold between reactive homeostasis and homeostatic overload that does not vary daily or seasonally. However, unlike the threshold for homeostatic failure, the threshold for homeostatic overload and thus the normal reactive scope can differ between individuals and within a single individual (see discussion later in this chapter).

To conclude so far, the allostasis, allostatic load, and allostatic overload model refers to the individual in its environment in relation to resource availability. The model specifically provides a framework to assessing the potential for different components of environmental change, social status, and body condition to increase energetic demand (allostatic load) in relation to available resources, and the extent to which an individual has access to those resources. This framework enables insight into how an individual should respond in terms of hormonal and other physiological mediators—that is, the interface with the reactive scope model. The latter model extends the state-level framework in a highly predictive way and includes the consequences of homeostatic failure and homeostatic overload, which represent the individual in a life-threatening state beyond what it would normally be able to cope with.

The combination of these two models represents a wide-ranging framework to understand how daily routines, resources, body condition, and perturbations add up to affect homeostatic responses. The confusing word "stress" does not have to be invoked and thus allows a more objective assessment of homeostasis across the entire possible ranges of organism-environment interaction.

B. Physiological Mediators

Many physiological mediators are involved in returning an animal to homeostasis in response to unpredictable environmental stimuli. Many of them are discussed in detail in this book. Table 3.3 presents five major systems involved in the stress response and examples of their common mediators. Although the list of mediators is not exhaustive, Table 3.3 contains potential mediators for the *y* axis of the reactive scope model. These are often the very indices of stress used in various studies, and we now have a firm understanding of the functioning of many of these mediators. Furthermore, recent advances in our understanding of allostasis have allowed us to start putting the function of these mediators into the context of changes in life-history stages. For example, seasonal variation can occur in immune function (Nelson et al. 2002), hypothalamic-pituitary-adrenal (HPA) function (Romero 2002), and the size of dendritic trees in hippocampal neurons (Popov and Bocharova 1992; Popov et al. 1992). In each case, different seasons and different life-history stages have different demands and different risks. Preparing physiologically for those predictable changes in demands and risks and adjusting the level/concentration of each mediator forms the foundation for the predictive homeostasis range.

Furthermore, the entire field of stress research has been dedicated to understanding how short-term (acute) increases in these mediators help to counteract stressors (the reactive homeostatic range), how chronic increases can lead to problems including disease (homeostatic overload), and how lack of these mediators can lead to homeostasis failure. A key insight from the previous decades of research on stress is that stress mediators play central roles in both successful adaptation and pathophysiology. This Janus-faced nature of mediators has been one of the major difficulties in understanding stress responses and the source of many arguments about whether a certain mediator was "good" or "bad" for the animal. Assigning the physiological effects of each mediator in each of the four ranges of the reactive scope model provides a solution to this conundrum.

Common examples of the physiological consequences of mediators being in each of these ranges are also given in Table 3.3. Of course, Table 3.3 is overly simplistic. Each system has extensive crosstalk and non-linear interactions that are not represented in the table. However, Table 3.3 provides examples of how what is currently known about stress physiology can be incorporated into the reactive scope model.

C. Responses to Stressors

Acute responses to stressors are easily modeled using the reactive scope model. An unpredictable or uncontrollable environmental stimulus results in a rapid spike in the physiological mediator that

TABLE 3.3: EXAMPLES OF PHYSIOLOGICAL MEDIATORS AND EFFECTS AT DIFFERENT RANGES

Physiological System	Physiological Mediator	Predictive Homeostasis Range	Reactive Homeostasis Range	Homeostatic Overload Range	Homeostatic Failure Range
Immune	Prostaglandin T-cell activation Antibody titers	Seasonal ability to fight infection	Mobilization of immune system	Autoimmune immunosuppression	Immune failure
HPA	Glucocorticoids ACTH	Seasonal life-history needs a. Energetic needs b. Behavioral needs c. Preparative needs	Inhibit immune system Energy mobilization Change behavior Inhibit reproduction Inhibit growth	Immunosuppression Diabetes Muscle breakdown Reproductive failure Decreased survival	Energy disregulation Water balance failure Catecholamine insufficiency Decreased survival
Cardiovascular (Catecholamines)	Heart rate Heart rate variability Blood pressure	Life-history energy needs	Fight-or-flight energy mobilization	Hypertension Myocardial infarction Muscle break down	Hypotension Lethargy Decreased survival
Behavior	Foraging/Feeding Locomotion Migration Conspecific aggression	Life-history changes a. Energy needs b. Energy availability c. Predator presence d. Mate access	Fleeing behavior Freezing behavior Increase/Decrease foraging Increase food intake Increase vigilance	Tonic immobility Obesity Anxiety Fear Violence	
Central Nervous System	Neurogenesis Dendritic arborization Neurotransmitter concentrations	Life-history changes in neural networks Learning & memory	Increase neurotransmission (titers or receptors) Increase learning and memory	Neuronal atrophy/death Depression Decrease learning and memory	Post-traumatic stress disorder

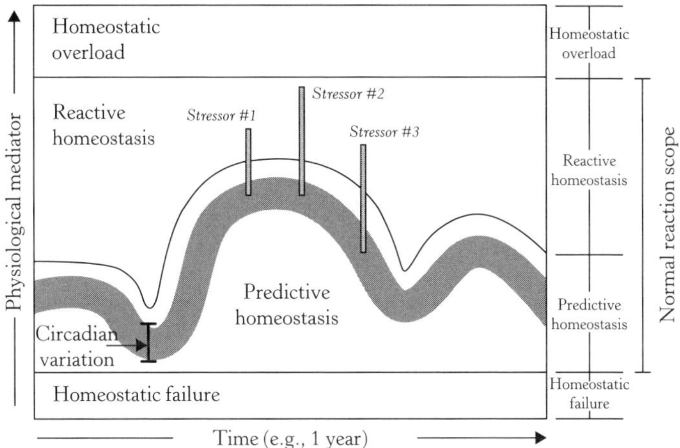

FIGURE 3.24: A graphical depiction of the response to stressors. Each vertical line represents both a rapid spike of the mediator into the reactive homeostasis range in order to maintain homeostasis in the face of a stressor and a rapid decrease in the mediator once the stressor has ended. Stressor #2 is a stronger stressor than #1 and thus requires a stronger response to maintain homeostasis. Stressors #2 and #3 are of equivalent strength, but occur at different times of year. Consequently, the mediator is at different concentrations/levels in the predictive homeostasis range, so that stressor #3 is less likely to elicit a response from the mediator that extends into the homeostatic overload range.

Reprinted with permission from Romero et al. (2009). Courtesy of Elsevier.

moves its level out of the predictive homeostasis range and into the reactive homeostasis range (stressor #1 in Figure 3.24). The mediator then either counteracts the effect of the stressor or allows the impact of the stressor to be avoided. To put this response into the context of the allostasis model, this would represent increasing allostatic load above the daily/seasonal routines (Eo) and would peak when Eg is exceeded and the individual is in negative energy balance. Once the stimulus has been adequately dealt with, the level of the physiological mediator quickly returns to the predictive homeostasis range. Alternatively, if allostatic overload type 1 is reached, then the emergency life-history stage will reduce Eo to a manageable range similar to the predictive homeostasis range.

Responses both in anticipation of a stressor and to an actual stressor evoke indistinguishable responses and are represented as equivalent spikes into the reactive homeostasis range. Note, however, that the mediator remains within the normal reactive scope throughout the response, even in allostatic overload. This corresponds to the stress response in the traditional model adequately rebalancing the dynamic equilibrium of the animal (Figure 3.1C). Another feature of the traditional model can also be incorporated. Stronger stressors evoke stronger responses (Figure 3.2, also as Eo increases) and a mediator can vary in the magnitude of its responses to different stressors (stressors #1 and #2 in Figure 3.24). Note again that different magnitude responses will still remain within the reactive homeostasis range. The same is true of equivalent responses occurring at different times of year (stressors #2 and #3 in Figure 3.24), although in this case the two responses can differ dramatically in how closely they come to the range of homeostatic overload. Therefore, the move into the reactive homeostasis range (the stress response) at each life-history stage, with each stage having its own predictable demands, resulting in different ranges of predictable homeostasis, will have different consequences even though the response of the mediator may appear equivalent. This encompasses the concept of allostatic state from the allostasis model. Animals will be more resistant to entering allostatic overload at some times of the year, specifically when Eg is greater and Ee + Ei is lower. Note that the reactive scope model does not always indicate when an emergency life-history stage will be triggered, whereas the allostasis model does. This point will be taken up again in Chapter 4, when transitions mediated via receptors and enzymes will be discussed. Homeostatic overload, that is, beyond the reactive scope of the individual, will be avoided, as death is likely soon thereafter.

D. Modeling "Wear and Tear" (or Allostatic Load)

With the reactive scope model, allostatic load can be defined as the ease with which an animal maintains mediators in the reactive homeostasis range. There are a number of costs associated with sustaining mediators in the reactive homeostasis range. These costs include direct energy consumption (such as the extra energy needed to drive the heart to sustain an increased heart rate), lost opportunities to perform other tasks (such as basic tissue maintenance), and tissue damage (such as might occur from breaking down tissues for energy). Furthermore, these costs continue to mount for as long as the mediator stays in the reactive homeostasis range. "Wear and tear" refers to the accumulation of these costs. Wear and tear, however, is not the same as the pathology that occurs when mediators enter homeostatic overload. Instead, "wear and tear" refers to the increased likelihood of the mediator causing pathology, and homeostatic overload refers to the mediators themselves causing damage to the animal. One can see also how wear and tear might permanently increase Ee + Ei in the allostasis model, thus making the individual more susceptible to perturbations (a form of allostatic overload type 2, Figure 3.21).

Another way to think of wear and tear is by a gradual decrease in the ability of the animal to cope. The ability of the animal to counteract the stressor diminishes because of the accumulated costs of maintaining the mediators in the reactive homeostasis range. At some point, the costs become so great that they cross a threshold and the mediator itself starts to create problems. For example, direct tissue breakdown, combined with deferred tissue maintenance, will eventually result in degraded tissue function. When this occurs, the mediator will have moved from the reactive homeostasis range to the homeostatic overload range, even though its level/concentration may not have changed. The accumulated damage from the mediator creates the wear and tear and consequently decreases the animal's ability to cope (similar to allostatic overload type 2). Note that the emergency life-history stage may not ameliorate the effect of the mediator, resulting in homeostatic overload. This means that there are two ways to enter homeostatic overload. In the first, the concentration or level of the mediator extends beyond the normal reactive scope—the level is so high that it immediately starts to cause damage. In the second, the concentration or level of the mediator remains in the reactive homeostasis range for an extended period and results in accumulated wear and tear—thereby creating a decrease in the reactive scope. A decrease in the reactive scope is modeled graphically by a gradual decrease in the threshold between the reactive homeostasis range and the homeostatic overload range. Figure 3.25 shows two ways that wear and tear will result in homeostatic overload, one with a sustained elevation of the mediator and the other with multiple increases of the mediator into the reactive scope range. In Gambel's white-crowned sparrows, frequent (3 times a day) but acute pulses of corticosterone (within the reactive homeostasis range for this species) increased overall baseline levels of corticosterone but also blunted the adrenocortical response to handling stress (Busch et al. 2008b), as well as decreased body weight, muscle mass, and delayed onset of molt compared with controls (Busch et al. 2008a). However, fat depot, bile retention in

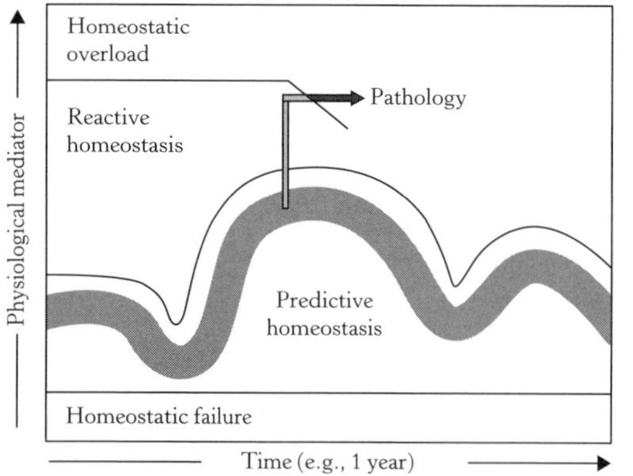

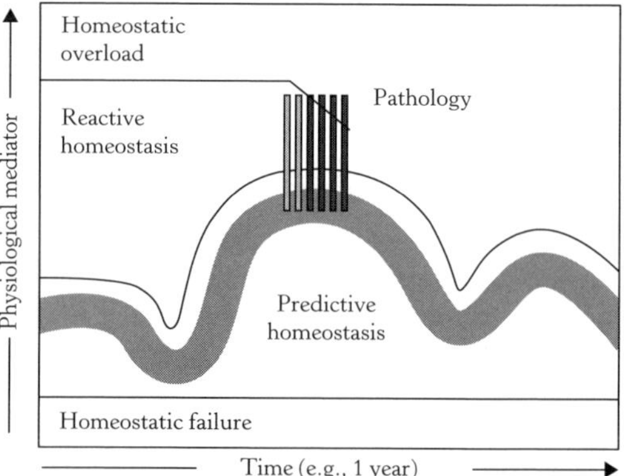

FIGURE 3.25: How wear and tear arising from sustained (left) or repeated (right) elevations of a mediator into the reactive homeostasis range will eventually result in the mediator entering homeostatic overload.

Adapted from Romero et al. (2009). Courtesy of Elsevier.

the gall bladder, and migratory-like restlessness behavior were not affected.

The progressive decrease in the animal's reactive scope (i.e., wear and tear) results from underlying changes in the regulation of mediator activation. All physiological mediators are controlled by networks of underlying regulators. Heart rate, for example, is under the control of two primary regulators—vagal input that decreases heart rate and sympathetic input that increases heart rate (Bohus and Koolhaas 1993; Perini and Veicsteinas 2003). Figure 3.26 represents a stylized network of a mediator controlled by two regulators—a positive regulator

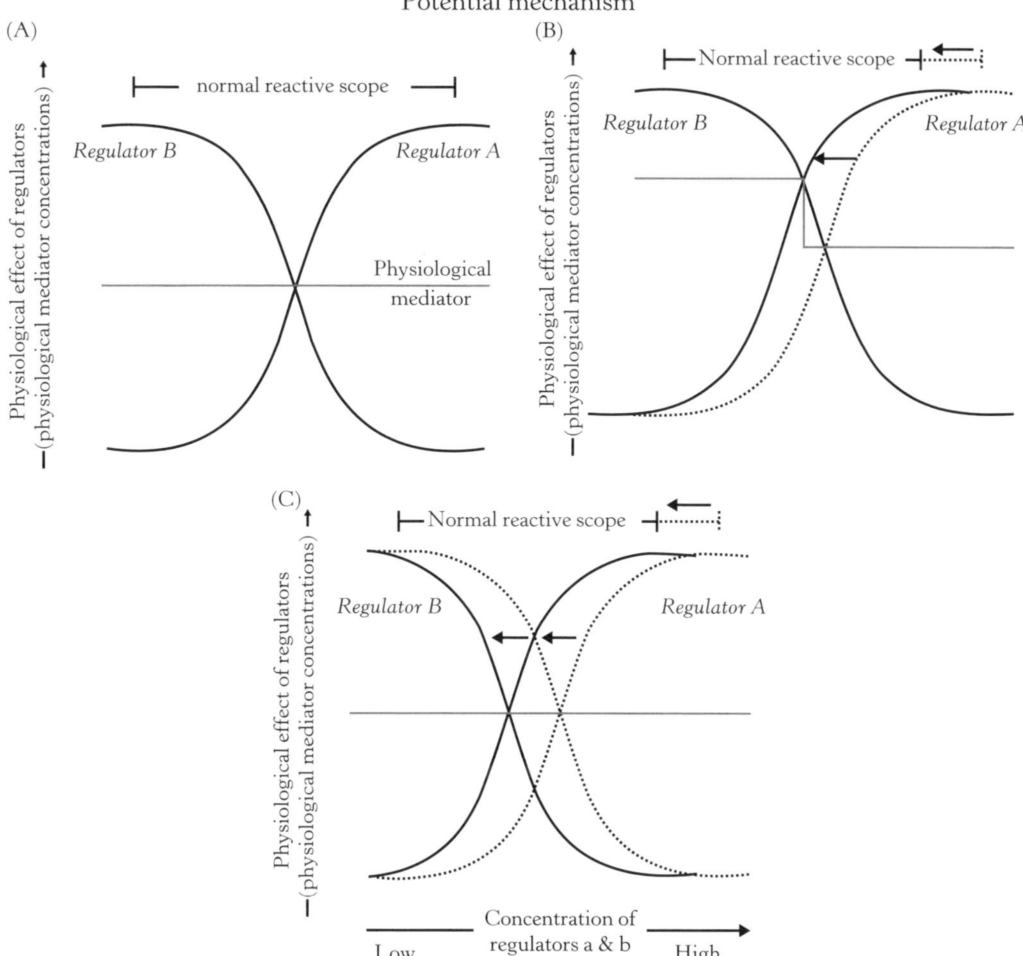

FIGURE 3.26: A. The concentration of the physiological mediator (*y* axis) depends upon the interaction between the concentrations of a positive Regulator A and a negative Regulator B (*x* axis). Normal fluctuations of the level of the mediator (represented by horizontal line) are regulated by changes in the concentrations of both regulators. The *y* axis can also be thought of as the effectiveness of Regulators A and B in driving the level of the physiological mediator. The normal reactive scope for the system is determined by the dose-response curves of the two regulators. B. Long-term increases in the efficacy of Regulator A causes a left-shift in the dose response curve (Regulator A becomes more effective at smaller levels). This results in a shift in the balance between Regulators A and B and a long-term increase in the concentration of the physiological mediator (represented by horizontal lines). C. The original concentration of the physiological mediator can be restored by an equivalent increase in the efficacy of Regulator B, resulting in a left-shift of Regulator B's dose-response curve. In this case, however, the normal reactive scope of the system has narrowed. Note that a similar narrowing of the normal reactive scope would occur if there were a decrease in the efficacies of Regulators A and B (right-shifts to the dose-response curves).

Reprinted with permission from Romero et al. (2009). Courtesy of Elsevier.

(A) and a negative regulator (B). These regulators act in concert to determine the level of the mediator. However, these regulators also have their normal ranges, the sum of which then determines the normal range of the mediator. This means that the normal concentration ranges for the pair of regulators forms the normal reactive scope for the system (i.e., the normal reactive scope in Figure 3.23).

When the physiological mediator is in the predictive homeostasis range, the concentrations of regulators A and B are balanced so that the physiological mediator is maintained at a stable level (Figure 3.26A). When the animal is faced with a stressor, however, the mediator needs to enter the reactive homeostasis range. This is easily accomplished by adjusting the concentrations of the underlying regulators. For example, by increasing the level of regulator A in Figure 3.26A while maintaining (or decreasing) the concentration of regulator B, the level of the mediator increases. You will notice that this acute response is a classic example of the physiological regulation of a system. Furthermore, the dynamic range of these underlying regulators will determine how high or how low the level of the mediator can go—in other words, the reactive scope.

The underlying response is different when the mediator needs to be maintained in the reactive homeostasis range for an extended period (i.e., a long-term response). Instead of simply increasing or decreasing the levels of the regulators, there is an adjustment of the underlying function of the regulators. For example, the function of regulator A can be made more efficient. One mechanism might be an up-regulation in regulator A's receptors. The end result is a shift in the physiological effect curve to the left, as shown in Figure 3.26B. This left-shift generates a greater effect at lower concentrations and drives up the level of the physiological mediator.

There are two possible ways to restore the mediator to its original level. One is for regulator A to return to its original efficacy. The result is a right-shift in the physiological effect curve. In effect, the curve returns to its original position and the original reactive scope is restored. Alternatively, Figure 3.26C shows how regulator B could compensate for the change in regulator A and also become more efficient. This will result in a similar shift in its physiological effect curve to the left. The ultimate result would again be a restoration of the mediator to its original concentration. However, the dynamic ranges of both regulators A and B have now shrunk. Much smaller acute increases in regulator A will now result in robust increases in the mediator. The consequence of this regulation is that the longer a mediator remains in the reactive homeostasis range, the more disrupted the functioning of the underlying regulators becomes. Importantly, the process is dynamic. The decrease in reactive scope (or homeostatic overload threshold) begins and continues until the stressors end. This pushes the system closer to its limits much faster, making it more likely that the regulators will drive the mediator beyond the normal reactive scope and into homeostatic overload. The increased propensity to exceed the normal reactive scope is the mechanism for wear and tear.

Another way to think of wear and tear is with a children's seesaw. Figure 3.27 shows how a seesaw can be perfectly balanced with two small weights or two large weights. However, the seesaw will wear out a lot faster with the large weights—the dynamic range (reactive scope) of the system is narrower because the system is less capable of absorbing more weight. In other words, the closer regulators A and B are to their limits, the less "buffer" there is before the system goes into overload, meaning that there is a decrease in the animal's capacity to cope.

A financial metaphor might help. Assume that you are faced with a financial emergency such as car repairs. This financial emergency requires removing money from savings, but that is easily solved. The initial removal of money represents the animal's short-term acute stress response—you pay off your debts and there is no lasting damage. Long-term problems only arise if the financial emergency is sustained (the car needs to be completely replaced) or further financial emergencies occur too frequently (the car is always breaking down). In these cases, the initial removal of money from savings certainly decreased your ability to cope with the subsequent emergencies. Every emergency requires more money from your savings, and if the situation doesn't improve you will quickly deplete your savings and face financial ruin. For an animal, the counterpart for the depletion of savings is the decrease in the threshold between reactive homeostasis and homeostatic overload (i.e., increased wear and tear, leading to a decrease in reactive scope). If the car payments end before you deplete your savings, however, you can earn more money, replace your savings, and restore your financial health. Likewise, Figure 3.28 indicates that if the stressor ends before the decrease in the homeostatic overload threshold becomes lower than the stress response, then the animal recovers

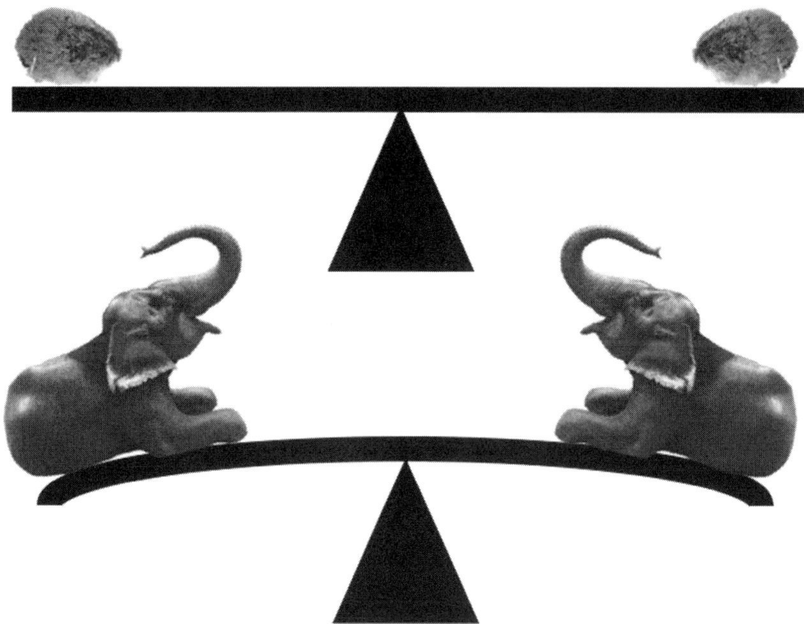

FIGURE 3.27: Wear and tear effects on the reactive scope. The animal's reactive scope (or dynamic equilibrium) can be perfectly balanced with two lemmings or with two elephants, but the elephants make it far more likely that the system will collapse with any additional stressors.

and the homeostatic overload threshold returns to its original state. If, however, the stressors continue after the homeostatic overload threshold becomes lower than the stress response (Figure 3.25), then the animal enters homeostatic overload, and the consequences summarized in Table 3.3 begin to occur.

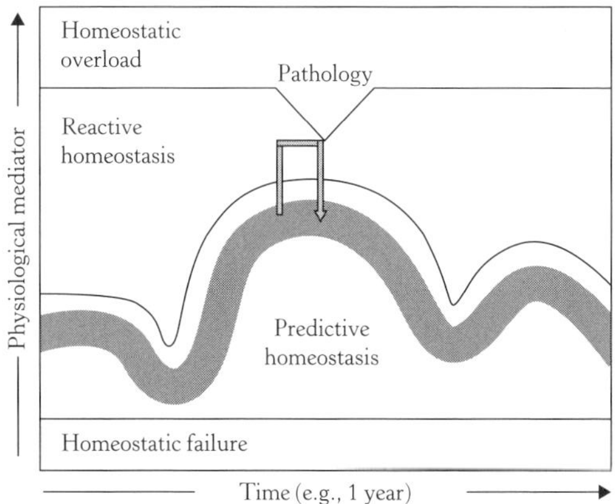

FIGURE 3.28: A sustained stressor causes a decrease in reactive scope, but the stressor ends before it enters homeostatic overload, and the reactive scope returns to its original state.

Adapted from Romero et al. (2009). Courtesy of Elsevier.

The rate at which wear and tear occurs, or in other words, the slope of the decrease in the boundary between reactive homeostasis and homeostatic overload, might be able to be determined empirically. Because the level of the threshold results from the underlying reactive scope of the regulators in Figure 3.26, the peak physiological response in a young, healthy, naïve animal should provide the upper level of the mediator that forms the limit to reactive homeostasis. Then if a moderate stressor that produces a sub-peak response is repeatedly applied, the reactive slope will begin to narrow. The difference between the peak mediator response and the response to the moderate stressor will provide one side of the triangle. When the symptoms of homeostatic overload begin to occur (from Table 3.3), the duration required will provide the second leg of the triangle. The rate of the reduction in reactive scope can then be calculated from the hypotenuse of that triangle. Although this experiment has not yet been attempted, at least in principle the rate of wear and tear on the organism can be determined empirically. The slope of this line undoubtedly will differ depending upon the physiological mediator and the species.

Habituation can also help an animal avoid entering homeostatic overload. As discussed earlier in this chapter, habituation entails reducing the magnitude of a stress response to a stimulus because the animal learns that the stimulus is not actually a stressor. Figure 3.29 shows how this can be modeled using reactive scope. In this case the mediator's responses to the stressor progressively decrease, with the end result that the mediator never enters homeostatic overload. Habituation may also influence allostatic load, particularly if it affects access to Eg.

Homeostatic overload can also be avoided if the stressor occurs when the predictive homeostasis range is lower. Figure 3.30 shows that when predictive homeostasis is lower, there is a bigger buffer for wear and tear. Even when faced with an equivalent stressor, the animal's susceptibility to enter homeostatic overload is dramatically reduced. To return to the financial metaphor, the size of your savings may change over time, providing more or less of a financial buffer.

Figure 3.31 indicates that there are three potential consequences of entering homeostatic overload. The first shows that when the stressors cease, the animal recovers to its original physiological state and suffers no long-term detriments. The animal recovers its original reactive scope. However, an extension of a mediator into the homeostatic overload range can also cause permanent changes to the animal's physiology. There can be a permanent change in the boundary between the reactive homeostasis range and the homeostatic overload range. In this case, the

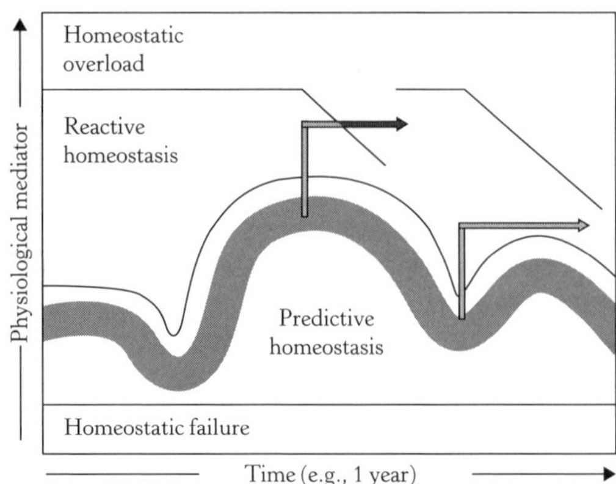

FIGURE 3.30: Consequences differ if a stressor occurs when the initial concentration of the physiological mediator is maintained at different ranges of predictive homeostasis. The wider range of reactive homeostasis in the right-hand response means that the response can be sustained longer, and wear and tear can be accumulated for a longer time, before the mediator crosses the threshold between reactive homeostasis and homeostatic overload.

Adapted from Romero et al. (2009). Courtesy of Elsevier.

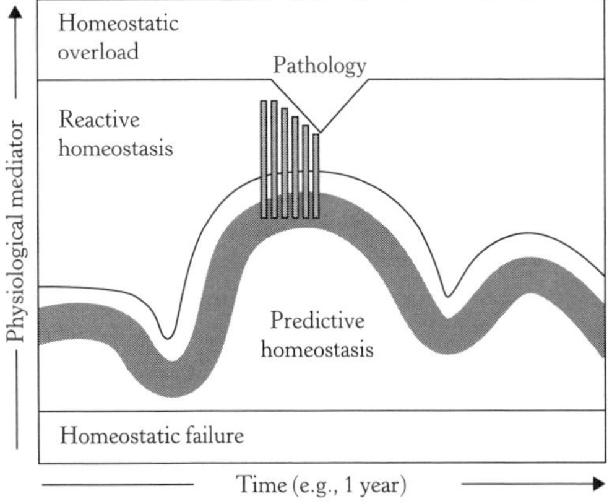

FIGURE 3.29: The animal habituates to a repeated stressor. The response of the physiological mediator to the stressor decreases over time. Even though wear and tear continues to occur, the responses never cross the threshold into homeostatic overload, and pathology does not develop.

Reprinted with permission from Romero et al. (2009). Courtesy of Elsevier.

animal does not return to its original physiological state, even though the stressor ended and the animal survived. In other words, the animal suffers a permanent decrease in its reactive scope. For example, repeated stressors can cause the remodeling of dendritic processes of neurons and a change in synapse densities. This process can be reversible (e.g., Stewart et al. 2005), leading to the scenario in Figure 3.26A, or permanent (e.g. Sapolsky 1992), leading to the scenario in Figure 3.26B. In the later case, the long-term functioning of the brain has changed. The difference between having a recovered or permanently altered reactive scope occurs with a subsequent stress response. A permanently reduced reactive scope leaves the animal more vulnerable to future stressors (Figure 3.31b), whereas an equivalent stress response in an animal that recovers its reactive scope remains inside the reactive homeostasis range (Figure 3.31a).

The final potential consequence of entering homeostatic overload is that the entire system is overwhelmed. Reactive scope continues to shrink as long as the mediator remains in the homeostatic overload range. When the reactive scope narrows to the point that the mediator cannot even remain in the predictive homeostasis range without causing problems, normal homeostasis cannot be maintained. Figure 3.31c shows that

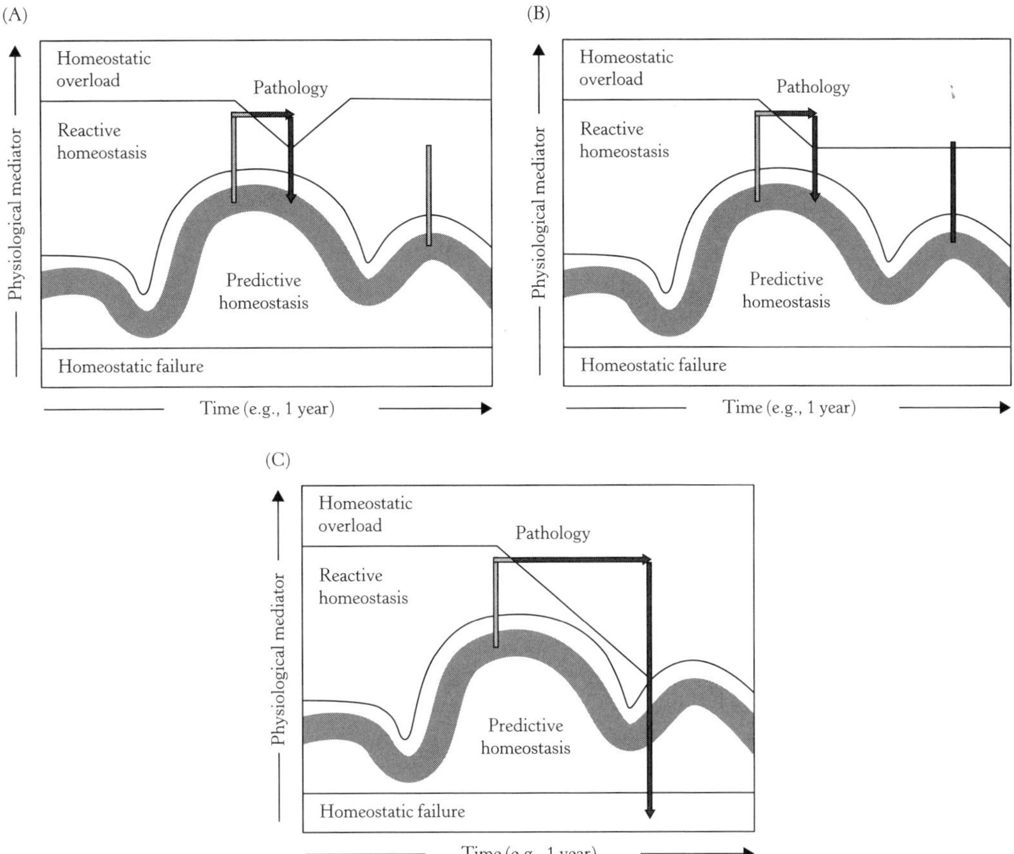

FIGURE 3.31: Three consequences of entering homeostatic overload. (A) Once the stressor ends, the threshold between reactive homeostasis and homeostatic overload (i.e., reactive scope) recovers to its original concentration/level. A future stressor does not extend into homeostatic overload. (B) Even though the stressor eventually ends, the wear and tear become permanent and reactive scope does not recover. A future stressor now immediately enters homeostatic overload. (C) As the mediator remains in the homeostatic overload range, it continues to accumulate wear and tear. When the reactive scope becomes too narrow to sustain the mediator in the predictive homeostasis range, the concentration of the physiological mediator collapses into the homeostatic failure range.

Reprinted with permission from Romero et al. (2009). Courtesy of Elsevier.

homeostatic collapse will occur and the physiological mediator will fall into the homeostatic failure range. Death will soon follow.

VI. INTEGRATING THE ALLOSTASIS AND REACTIVE SCOPE MODELS

The reactive scope model is an attempt to reconcile allostasis with aspects of the traditional model. It was based specifically on allostasis principles, although the reactive scope model refers to the four ranges as homeostatic failure, predictive homeostasis, reactive homeostasis, and homeostatic overload. This nomenclature could easily be changed, however, to allostatic failure, predictive allostasis, reactive allostasis, and allostatic overload. The reactive scope model uses a broad definition of homeostasis that includes daily and seasonal variation—similar to the definition of allostasis. The original nomenclature was chosen to distinguish the ranges from published uses of allostasis, but the four ranges certainly fit with the spirit of allostasis, if not the strict definitions in some papers.

As with allostasis, there are a number of strengths and weaknesses of the reactive scope model. One of the main strengths is a melding of both acute and chronic stress in the same model. Neither of the previous models did this well. The traditional model created a dichotomy between adaptive short-term responses and pathological long-term responses in which chronic stress derived from dysregulation of the stress response. Allostasis was not designed to address short-term responses. In contrast, reactive scope proposes that chronic stress derives from a shrinking of the reactive scope, which is in turn derived from the extension of normal physiological adaptations in the underlying regulators. Chronic stress can thus be thought of as a consequence of the physiological adjustment of regulators when they are forced into extended activation.

A second strength of reactive scope is that it puts the focus directly on the mediators of the stress response. One of the difficulties of the traditional definition of stress was its inherent circular argument. Stressors were defined as those stimuli that increased mediators, and stress mediators were defined as those mediators that increased in response to a stressor. Reactive scope resolves this dilemma by returning to the principles of homeostasis. Any extension of a mediator into the reactive homeostasis realm is a stress response. Reactive scope puts the emphasis on the mediators. This is a distinct advantage because virtually all studies measure changes to these mediators, and reactive scope provides a foundation upon which to interpret these changes. The allostasis model avoids using the terms "stress" and "stress response" because it focuses more on the extended picture of daily/seasonal routines in addition to perturbations that have the potential to be stressful. The reactive scope model looks at these issues in a totally different way by focusing on the mediators and the potential deleterious effects of chronic stress.

Reactive scope provides a mechanism for wear and tear, also part of allostatic load. If allostatic load derives from the underlying regulation of mediator release and/or function, then studies can start to explore how the physiology of the underlying regulation changes under different conditions. The reactive scope model thus provides testable hypotheses about how wear and tear accumulate and what the impact on the animal will be. Furthermore, reactive scope provides testable predictions on the timing of when wear and tear will become so great that pathology starts to occur. In the allostasis model, wear and tear will increase Ee + Ei, and/or change the slope of Eo.

The reactive scope model proposes that chronic stress and thus pathology begin when the threshold between reactive homeostasis and homeostatic overload, that is, the reactive scope, drops below the actual level/concentration of the mediator. The slope of this decrease should be able to be empirically determined, thereby predicting the timing of when different stressors applied at different times of the year will result in homeostatic overload. No previous model has allowed us to make timing predictions, yet understanding how long it takes for accumulated acute stress to become chronic stress is highly desirable.

Another strength of reactive scope is that it can model different stressors and animals in different circumstances, as does the allostasis model. However, a key difference is that reactive scope provides a spectrum of responses of mediators, whereas allostasis predicts environmental situations in which an individual's underlying reactive scope will determine how that individual might fare. Reactive scope, like allostasis, can be modified to model animals subjected to different conditions.

One example of the value of both reactive scope and allostasis is that both provide a framework for understanding the long-term changes in vulnerability associated with different developmental histories. Stress during development can reset an individual's reactive scope (see Chapter 5), which can be easily modeled by increasing or decreasing the animal's initial threshold between reactive homeostasis and homeostatic overload (Romero et al. 2009). This would then adjust the slope of Eo for that individual. Another example is that reactive scope can provide the framework for how animals respond when exposed to different stressors. Starvation requires and elicits a very different response from a predation attempt, yet both stressors are easy to model using reactive scope (Romero et al. 2009). The allostasis model would then provide predictions on how an individual might interact with its environment; that is, does starvation result because of a dramatic decrease in Eg, or does Eg remain unchanged and the presence of predators prevents normal access to Eg (i.e., because Eo is very high)?

A final example is how reactive scope, like allostasis, can provide a framework for understanding how animals respond to different social contexts (Romero et al. 2009). Lifestyle, or how an individual copes with its living conditions, could apply to living in poor neighborhoods, coping with agonistic and antagonistic conspecific encounters, living in a zoo, foraging in a dangerous environment, and so forth. Lifestyle has a profound impact on both the perception of what constitutes a stressor and the anticipation of when that stressor will occur. The consequence is an increase in wear and tear and a reduced reactive scope. Different lifestyles, therefore, will result in different vulnerabilities to further stressors, which is seen in many human studies. The allostasis model would approach these same social issues by considering the allostatic load accrued by individuals in the group (Goymann and Wingfield 2004). The accumulation of wear and tear eventually leads to numerous physiological problems, including, but not limited to, hypertension, a pathogenic cholesterol profile, decreased fertility, immunosuppression, and dendritic atrophy (reviewed by Sapolsky 2005). Note that reactive scope predicts that the accumulated wear and tear (i.e., allostatic load) of a poor lifestyle will result in the mediators causing pathology (i.e., homeostatic overload), and each of the above pathologies is a consequence of excessive stress mediator function. In conclusion, much of reactive scope's value will come from modifying the basic model to accommodate the specifics of the species, the individual, or disease that is being studied. Intriguingly, the reactive scope and allostasis models interface well and potentially provide a very complete picture of how individuals deal with a changing and frequently capricious world.

Reactive scope is relatively new and has yet to be adequately tested. However, a number of weaknesses have already been identified. One is that reactive scope examines only one mediator at a time. The basic model (Figure 3.23) only provides a framework for understanding the functions at different ranges of a single mediator. Actions of other mediators are assumed to be modeled using parallel versions of the basic model tailored for the subsequent mediators. In other words, each mediator is assumed to get its own modified version of the basic model. However, all of the mediators involved in a stress response share extensive crosstalk, no mediator has actions independent of others, and the extent of the crosstalk is often bewildering. The reactive scope model does a poor job of incorporating this crosstalk (McEwen and Wingfield 2010).

Another weakness of reactive scope is that it does not directly address energy available in the environment (McEwen and Wingfield 2010). Clearly, the amount of available energy is a key environmental factor for a wild animal. Without adequate food, physiology itself becomes impossible. Consequently, animals expend considerable effort finding food. Different strategies for doing so result in the wonderful variety of different life-history strategies shown by different species. By focusing so heavily on the underlying mediators, reactive scope minimizes this important feature of the environment. Some of the variation in available energy is incorporated by mediators functioning at the predictive and reactive homeostatic ranges, but the emphasis is far less than in allostasis. Again, the interaction of the two models looks to be highly promising, providing new insights into environmental problems that can be tested in counterintuitive ways.

VII. CONCLUSION

In this chapter we have presented three different models for how to think about stress. We feel that this is an exciting time for our field. Until quite recently, the traditional model provided the only way to place empirical data into a theoretical context. The traditional model provided some help, but its many weaknesses, especially when applied to wild free-living animals, slowed progress considerably. An especially glaring weakness was the poor help that the traditional model provided in generating testable predictions about what stimuli would be stressors to wild animals, what their stress responses would be, and how those stress responses would help wild animals survive in their natural habitats. The lack of testable predictions was especially problematic with the recent focus on anthropogenic stressors and their potential to cause chronic stress and conservation problems (see Chapter 12).

The introduction of allostasis and reactive scope, however, has fostered a huge change in the theoretical underpinnings of stress. These models are better than the traditional model at explaining many empirical data from field studies. Both models also provide testable predictions about how animals will react to various stimuli. Many of these ideas are beginning to be tested, and we both anticipate exciting progress in the near future.

We are sure it has not escaped the reader's attention that your two authors helped create the allostasis and reactive scope models. We also assume that it has not escaped the reader that there are substantial differences between the two models, but that they do interface well in addressing different but interrelated aspects of how organisms deal with a changing environment. At the root of the differences between the two models, however, is a difference in perspective between the two authors in the cause of allostatic/homeostatic overload. One of us (JCW) believes that allostatic/homeostatic overload arises because the animal is in negative energy balance—either because of high energetic costs of coping *or* greatly decreased access to food without a major change in energetic costs. The emergency life-history stage serves to shift behavior toward maintenance activities in order to conserve energy and avoid entering allostatic overload. Pathology occurs because the animal cannot acquire sufficient energy to sustain itself and is a result of the ultimate failure of the emergency life-history stage to adequately compensate for the low available energy. The foundation of this viewpoint is in ecology—the animal's intimate relationship with its environment. As a consequence, although type 2 allostatic overload is independent of energy deficiencies, type 2 allostatic overload is assumed to be relatively unimportant to wild animals existing in their normal habitats. There is good evidence that, although type 2 allostatic overload is critical to human health, it is rare in wild animals. In the few cases when it does occur, it is quickly lethal. As a consequence, type 1 allostatic overload forms the predominant mode by which stress gets animals into trouble.

In contrast, the other of us (LMR) believes that allostatic/homeostatic overload derives from problems with the mediators. It is not the consequences of being in negative energy balance that causes the problems. Rather, homeostatic overload results from a central irony: physiological processes intended to aid health end up undermining health instead. Specifically, the physiological mediators that form the stress response shift from being positive to negative components of health. High levels/concentrations of the physiological mediators themselves cause the symptoms of allostatic/homeostatic overload. The foundation for this viewpoint is in physiology. It builds upon the classic physiological inverted-U dose response curve where low and high concentrations are damaging, but middle concentrations are beneficial. This viewpoint also builds on the traditional model of stress from the first part of the chapter, where stress-related disease is thought to derive from the stress response overcompensating for the stressor and itself disrupting the animal's dynamic equilibrium (i.e., allostasis). The result is that, whereas the key to understanding allostasis is to "follow the energy," the key to understanding reactive scope is to understand the functions of the physiological mediators at different levels/concentrations (Table 3.3). We both note again that the two models are not mutually exclusive and in many ways compliment each other.

The emergency life-history stage is still important in reactive scope, but its primary role is assumed to provide a behavioral mechanism that can lead to a decrease in the concentrations of mediators (decrease wear and tear) rather than to conserve energy. The preceding descriptions of the differences between the two models, however, only focus on the philosophies underlying allostasis and reactive scope. As mentioned earlier, we believe that the two models are not, in reality, that different. Both focus heavily on the underlying physiology and the ecology of the animal. The emphasis on some of the underlying details may be different, but the broad themes of the two models are nearly identical. Indeed, reactive scope would have been impossible without the contributions of allostasis. Much of the perceived difference derives from allostasis tending to focus on ultimate causes and reactive scope tending to focus on physiological mechanisms. As a result, the models are complementary. Of course, it is also clear that combining the two models into one unified theory of coping will be a goal for the future and will require building on empirical data generated by the two current models. We are currently working to mesh the two approaches to create a new model that integrates both approaches. Stay tuned.

REFERENCES

Adler, N. E., Boyce, T., Chesney, M. A., Cohen, S., Folkman, S., Kahn, R. L., Syme, S. L., 1994. Socioeconomic status and health: The challenge of the gradient *Am Psychol 49*, 15–24.

Adler, N. E., Boyce, W. T., Chesney, M. A., Folkman, S., Syme, S. L., 1993. Socioeconomic inequalities in health: No easy solution. *JAMA 269*, 3140–3145.

Astheimer, L. B., Buttemer, W. A., Wingfield, J. C., 1995. Seasonal and acute changes in adrenocortical responsiveness in an arctic-breeding bird. *Horm Behav 29*, 442–457.

Bauman, D. E., 2000. Regulation of nutrient partitioning during lactation: homeostasis and homeorhesis revisited. In: Cronje, P. J. (Ed.) *Ruminant physiology: Digestion, metabolism and growth and reproduction*. CAB Publishing, New York, pp. 311–327.

Bhatnagar, S., Vining, C., 2003. Facilitation of hypothalamic-pituitary-adrenal responses to novel stress following repeated social stress using the resident/intruder paradigm. *Horm Behav 43*, 158–165.

Bierhaus, A., Schiekofer, S., Schwaninger, M., Andrassy, M., Humpert, P. M., Chen, J., Hong, M., Luther, T., Henle, T., Kloting, I., Morcos, M., Hofmann, M., Tritschler, H., Weigle, B., Kasper, M., Smith, M., Perry, G., Schmidt, A. M., Stern, D. M., Haring, H. U., Schleicher, E., Nawroth, P. P., 2001. Diabetes-associated sustained activation of the transcription factor nuclear factor-kappa B. *Diabetes 50*, 2792–2808.

Blanchard, D. C., Spencer, R. L., Weiss, S. M., Blanchard, R. J., McEwen, B., Sakai, R. R., 1995. Visible burrow system as a model of chronic social stress: Behavioral and neuroendocrine correlates. *Psychoneuroendocrinology 20*, 117–134.

Bohus, B., Koolhaas, J. M., 1993. Stress and the cardiovascular system: central and peripheral physiological mechanisms. In: Stanford, S. C., Salmon, P., Gray, J. A. (Eds.), *Stress: From synapse to syndrome.* Academic Press, Boston, MA, pp. 75–117.

Brown, K. I., Nestor, K. E., 1973. Some physiological responses of turkeys selected for high and low adrenal response to cold stress. *Poult Sci 52*, 1948–1954.

Busch, D. S., Sperry, T. S., Peterson, E., Do, C. T., Wingfield, J. C., Boyd, E. H., 2008a. Impacts of frequent, acute pulses of corticosterone on condition and behavior of Gambel's white-crowned sparrow (*Zonotrichia leucophtys gambelii*). *Gen Comp Endocrinol 158*, 224–233.

Busch, D. S., Sperry, T. S., Wingfield, J. C., Boyd, E. H., 2008b. Effects of repeated, short-term, corticosterone administration on the hypothalamo-pituitary-adrenal axis of the white-crowned sparrow (*Zonotrichia leucophrys gambelii*). *Gen Comp Endocrinol 158*, 211–223.

Cannon, W. B., 1932. *The wisdom of the body.* W.W. Norton, New York.

Coe, C. L., Stanton, M. E., Levine, S., 1983. Adrenal responses to reinforcement and extinction: role of expectancy versus instrumental responding. *Behav Neurosci 4*, 654–658.

Creel, S., 2001. Social dominance and stress hormones. *Trends Ecol Evol 16*, 491–497.

Creel, S., 2005. Dominance, aggression, and glucocorticoid levels in social carnivores. *J Mammal 86*, 255.

Creel, S., Creel, N. M., Monfort, S. L., 1996. Social stress and dominance. *Nature 379*, 212.

Cunningham, L. S., Kelsey, J. L., 1984. Epidemiology of musculoskeletal impairments and associated disability. *Am J Public Health 74*, 574–579.

Cyr, N. E., Dickens, M. J., Romero, L. M., 2009. Heart rate and heart rate variability responses to acute and chronic stress in a wild-caught passerine bird. *Physiol Biochem Zool 82*, 332–344.

Cyr, N. E., Romero, L. M., 2007. Chronic stress in free-living European starlings reduces corticosterone concentrations and reproductive success. *Gen Comp Endocrinol 151*, 82–89.

Cyr, N. E., Romero, L. M., 2009. Identifying hormonal habituation in field studies of stress. *Gen Comp Endocrinol 161*, 295–303.

Cyr, N. E., Wikelski, M., Romero, L. M., 2008. Increased energy expenditure but decreased stress responsiveness during molt. *Physiol Biochem Zool 81*, 452–462.

Dallman, M. F., Akana, S. F., Scribner, K. A., Bradbury, M. J., Walker, C.-D., Strack, A. M., Cascio, C. S., 1992. Stress, feedback and facilitation in the hypothalamo-pituitary-adrenal axis. *J Neuroendocrinol 4*, 517–526.

Dallman, M. F., Bhatnagar, S., 2001. Chronic stress and energy balance: role of the hypothalamo-pituitary-adrenal axis. In: McEwen, B. S., Goodman, H. M. (Eds.), *Handbook of physiology; Section 7: The endocrine system; Vol. IV: Coping with the environment: Neural and endocrine mechanisms.* Oxford University Press, New York, pp. 179–210.

Dallman, M. F., Jones, M. T., 1973. Corticosteroid feedback control of ACTH secretion: effect of stress-induced corticosterone secretion on subsequent stress responses in the rat. *Endocrinology 92*, 1367–1375.

Day, T. A., 2005. Defining stress as a prelude to mapping its neurocircuitry: No help from allostasis. *Prog Neuro-Psychopharmacol Biol Psychiatry 29*, 1195.

Devesa, S. S., Diamond, E. L., 1980. Association of breast cancer and cervical cancer incidences with income and education among whites and blacks. *J Natl Cancer Inst 65*, 515–528.

Dobrakova, M., Kvetnansky, R., 1993. Specificity of the effect of repeated handling on sympathetic-adrenomedullary and pituitary-adrenocortical activity in rats. *Psychoneuroendocrinology 18*, 163–174.

Domjan, M., 1996. Habituation and sensitization. In: Knight, V. (Ed.) *The essentials of conditioning and learning.* Brooks/Cole Publishing, Pacific Grove, pp. 23–205.

Dubovicky, M., Jezova, D., 2004. Effect of chronic emotional stress on habituation processes in open field in adult rats. *Annals of the New York Academy of Sciences 1018*, 199–206.

Eiserman, K., 1992. Long-term heart rate responses to social stress in wild european rabbits: predominant effect of rank position. *Physiol Behav 52*, 33–36.

Ely, C. R., Ward, D. H., Bollinger, K. S., 1999. Behavioral correlates of heart rates of free-living greater white-fronted geese. *Condor 101*, 390–395.

Engh, A. L., Beehner, J. C., Bergman, T. J., Whitten, P. L., Hoffmeier, R. R., Seyfarth, R. M., Cheney, D. L., 2006. Female hierarchy instability, male immigration and infanticide increase glucocorticoid levels in female chacma baboons. *Anim Behav 71*, 1227.

Fefferman, N. H., Romero, L. M., 2013. Can physiological stress alter population persistance? A model with conservation implications. *Conserv Physiol 1*, cot012.

Figueiredo, H. F., Bodie, B. L., Tauchi, M., Dolgas, C. M., Herman, J. P., 2003. Stress integration after acute and chronic predator stress: Differential activation of central stress circuitry and sensitization of the hypothalamo-pituitary-adrenocortical axis. *Endocrinology 144*, 5249–5258.

Fowler, G. S., 1999. Behavioral and hormonal responses of Magellanic penguins (*Spheniscus magellanicus*) to tourism and nest site visitation. *Biol Conserv 90*, 143–149.

Franceschini, M. D., Custer, C. M., Custer, T. W., Reed, J. M., Romero, L. M., 2008. Corticosterone stress response in tree swallows, *Tachycineta bicolor*, nesting near PCB and dioxin contaminated rivers. *Environ Toxicol Chem 27*, 2326–2331.

Gessaman, J. A., Worthen, G. L., 1982. *The effect of weather on avian mortality*. Utah State University Printing Services, Logan, Utah.

Goldstein, D. S., McEwen, B., 2002. Allostasis, homeostats, and the nature of stress. *Stress 5*, 55–58.

Goymann, W., Wingfield, J. C., 2004. Allostatic load, social status and stress hormones: the costs of social status matter. *Anim Behav 67*, 591–602.

Gray, J. A., 1987. *The psychology of fear and stress*. 2nd Edition. Cambridge University Press, New York.

Groothuis, T. G. G., Carere, C., 2005. Avian personalities: Characterization and epigenesis. *Neurosci Biobehav Rev 29*, 137.

Gross, W. B., Siegel, P. B., 1985. Selective breeding of chickens for corticosterone response to social stress. *Poult Sci 64*, 2230–2233.

Harris, J. D., 1943. Habituatory response decrement in the intact organism. *Psychol Bull 40*, 385–422.

Hegner, R. E., Wingfield, J. C., 1987. Social status and circulating levels of hormones in flocks of house sparrows, *Passer domesticus*. *Ethology 76*, 1–14.

Hennessy, M. B., Heybach, J. P., Vernikos, J., Levine, S., 1979. Plasma corticosterone concentrations sensitively reflect levels of stimulus intensity in the rat. *Physiol Behav 22*, 821–825.

Hofer, H., East, M. L., 2003. Behavioral processes and costs of co-existence in female spotted hyenas: A life history perspective. *Evol Ecol 17*, 315–331.

Hontela, A., 1998. Interrenal dysfunction in fish from contaminated sites: In vivo and in vitro assessment. *Environ Toxicol Chem 17*, 44–48.

Kirschbaum, C., Prussner, J. C., Stone, A. A., Federenko, I., Gaab, J., Lintz, D., Schommer, N., Hellhammer, D. H., 1995. Persistent high cortisol responses to repeated psychological stress in a subpopulation of healthy men. *Psychosom Med 57*, 468–474.

Kitaysky, A. S., Kitaiskaia, E. V., Piatt, J. F., Wingfield, J. C., 2003. Benefits and costs of increased levels of corticosterone in seabird chicks. *Horm Behav 43*, 140–149.

Kitaysky, A. S., Wingfield, J. C., Piatt, J. F., 1999. Dynamics of food availability, body condition and physiological stress response in breeding black-legged kittiwakes. *Func Ecol 13*, 577–584.

Kitaysky, A. S., Wingfield, J. C., Piatt, J. F., 2001. Corticosterone facilitates begging and affects resource allocation in the black-legged kittiwake. *Behav Ecol 12*, 619.

Koob, G. F., Le Moal, M., 2001. Drug addiction, dysregulation of reward, and allostasis. *Neuropsychopharmacology 24*, 97–129.

Koolhaas, J. M., de Boer, S. F., Buwalda, B., van Reenen, K., 2007. Individual variation in coping with stress: A multidimensional approach of ultimate and proximate mechanisms. *Brain Behav Evol 70*, 218–226.

Korte, S. M., Koolhaas, J. M., Wingfield, J. C., McEwen, B. S., 2005. The Darwinian concept of stress: Benefits of allostasis and costs of allostatic load and the trade-offs in health and disease. *Neurosci Biobehav Rev 29*, 3–38.

Kotrschal, K., Hirschenhauser, K., Moestl, E., 1998. The relationship between social stress and dominance is seasonal in greylag geese. *Anim Behav 55*, 171–176.

Krass, P. M., Bazhan, N. M., Reshetnikov, S. S., Trut, L. N., 1979. Adrenal reactivity to ACTH age changes in silver foxes inheriting different defensive behaviors. *Biol Bull Acad Sci USSR 6*, 306–310.

Kraus, J. F., Borhani, N. O., Franti, C. E., 1980. Socioeconomic status, ethnicity, and risk of coronary heart disease. *Am J Epidemiol 111*, 407–414.

Kuenzel, W. J., Beck, M. M., Teruyama, R., 1999. Neural sites and pathways regulating food intake in birds: A comparative analysis to mammalian systems. *J Exp Zool 283*, 348–364.

Landys, M. M., Ramenofsky, M., Wingfield, J. C., 2006. Actions of glucocorticoids at a seasonal baseline as compared to stress-related levels in the regulation of periodic life processes. *Gen Comp Endocrinol 148*, 132–149.

Lazarus, R. S., Folkman, S., 1984. *Stress, appraisal, and coping*. Springer Verlag, New York.

Le Moal, M., 2007. Historical approach and evolution of the stress concept: A personal account. *Psychoneuroendocrinology 32*, S3-S9.

Levine, S., 1978. Cortisol changes following repeated experiences with parachute training. In: Ursin, H., Badde, E., Levine, S. (Eds.), *Psychobiology of stress: A study of coping men*. Academic Press, New York, pp. 51–56.

Levine, S., Coe, C., Wiener, S. G., 1989. Psychoneuroendocrinology of stress-a psychobiological perspective. In: Brush, F. R., Levine, S. (Eds.), *Psychoendocrinology*. Academic Press, New York, pp. 341–377.

Levine, S., Coover, G. D., 1976. Environmental control of suppression of the pituitary-adrenal system. *Physiol Behav 17*, 35–37.

Levine, S., Goldman, L., Coover, G. D., 1972. Expectancy and the pituitary-adrenal system. *Ciba Found Symp 8*, 281–291.

Marti, O., Andres, R., Armario, A., 1999. Defective ACTH response to stress in previously stressed rats: Dependence on glucocorticoid status. *Am J Physiol 277*, R869–R877.

Marti, O., Armario, A., 1998. Anterior pituitary response to stress: Time-related changes and adaptation. *Int J Devel Neurosci 16*, 241–260.

McCarty, R., Konarska, M., Stewart, R. E., 1992. Adaptation to stress: a learned response? In: Kvetnansky, R., McCarty, R., Axelrod, J. (Eds.), *Stress: Neuroendocrine and molecular approaches, Vol. 2*. Gordon and Breach Science Publishers, Philadelphia, pp. 521–535.

McEwen, B. S., 1998. Protective and damaging effects of stress. *N Engl J Med 338*, 171–179.

McEwen, B. S., 2000. Allostasis and allostatic load: implications for neuropsychopharmacology. *Neuropsychopharmacology 22*, 108–124.

McEwen, B. S., 2003. Interacting mediators of allostasis and allostatic load: Towards an understanding of resilience in aging. *Metabolism 52*, 10–16.

McEwen, B. S., Seeman, T., Anonymous, 1999. Protective and damaging effects of mediators of stress: Elaborating and testing the concepts of allostasis and allostatic load. *Annals of the New York Academy of Sciences, 896*, 30–47.

McEwen, B. S., Wingfield, J. C., 2003. The concept of allostasis in biology and biomedicine. *Horm Behav 43*, 2–15.

McEwen, B. S., Wingfield, J. C., 2010. What is in a name? Integrating homeostasis, allostasis and stress. *Horm Behav 57*, 105–111.

Miller, G. E., Chen, E., Zhou, E. S., 2007. If it goes up, must it come down? Chronic stress and the hypothalamic-pituitary-adrenocortical axis in humans. *Psychol Bull 133*, 25–45.

Moore-Ede, M. C., 1986. Physiology of the circadian timing system: Predictive versus reactive homeostasis. *Am J Physiol 250*, R735–R752.

Mrosovsky, N., 1990. *Rheostasis: The physiology of change*. Oxford University Press, New York.

Mullner, A., Linsenmair, K. E., Wikelski, M., 2004. Exposure to ecotourism reduces survival and affects stress response in hoatzin chicks (*Opisthocomus hoazin*). *Biol Conserv 118*, 549–558.

Nelson, R. J., Demas, G. E., Klein, S. L., Kriegsfeld, L. J., 2002. *Seasonal patterns of stress, immune function, and disease*. Cambridge University Press, Cambridge.

Norris, D. O., Donahue, S., Dores, R. M., Lee, J. K., Maldonado, T. A., Ruth, T., Woodling, J. D., 1999. Impaired adrenocortical response to stress by brown trout, *Salmo trutta*, living in metal-contaminated waters of the Eagle River, Colorado. *Gen Comp Endocrinol 113*, 1–8.

Norris, D. O., Felt, S. B., Woodling, J. D., Dores, R. M., 1997. Immunocytochemical and histological differences in the interrenal axis of feral brown trout, *Salmo trutta*, in metal-contaminated waters. *Gen Comp Endocrinol 108*, 343–351.

Øverli, Ø., Korzan, W. J., Hoglund, E., Winberg, S., Bollig, H., Watt, M., Forster, G. L., Barton, B. A., Øverli, E., Renner, K. J., Summers, C. H., 2004. Stress coping style predicts aggression and social dominance in rainbow trout. *Horm Behav 45*, 235.

Øverli, Ø., Winberg, S., Pottinger, T. G., 2005. Behavioral and neuroendocrine correlates of selection for stress responsiveness in rainbow trout: A review. *Integ Comp Biol 45*, 463–474.

Pelletier, D., Guillemette, M., Grandbois, J. M., Butler, P.J., 2008. To fly or not to fly: High flight costs in a large sea duck do not imply an expensive lifestyle. *Proc R Soc Lond B 275*, 2117–2124.

Perini, R., Veicsteinas, A., 2003. Heart rate variability and autonomic activity at rest and during exercise in various physiological conditions. *Eur J Appl Physiol 90*, 317–325.

Popov, V. I., Bocharova, L. S., 1992. Hibernation-induced structural changes in synaptic contacts between mossy fibres and hippocampal pyramidal neurons. *Neuroscience 48*, 53–62.

Popov, V. I., Bocharova, L. S., Bragin, A. G., 1992. Repeated changes of dendritic morphology in the hippocampus of ground squirrels in the course of hibernation. *Neuroscience 48*, 45–51.

Pravosudov, V. V., Grubb, T. C., Jr., Doherty, P. F., Jr., Bronson, C. L., Pravosudova, E. V., Dolby, A. S., 1999. Social dominance and energy reserves in wintering woodland birds. *Condor 101*, 880.

Pride, R. E., 2005. Optimal group size and seasonal stress in ring-tailed lemurs (Lemur catta). *Behav Ecol 16*, 550.

Ramos-Fernandez, G., Nunez-de la Mora, A., Wingfield, J. C., Drummond, H., 2000. Endocrine correlates of dominance in chicks of the blue-footed booby (*Sula nebouxii*): Testing the Challenge Hypothesis. *Ethol Ecol Evolution 12*, 27–34.

Ray, J. C., Sapolsky, R. M., 1992. Styles of male social behavior and their endocrine correlates among high-ranking wild baboons. *Am J Primatol 28*, 231–250.

Remage-Healey, L., Romero, L. M., 2001. Corticosterone and insulin interact to regulate glucose and triglyceride levels during stress in a bird. *Am J Physiol 281*, R994–R1003.

Rich, E. L., Romero, L. M., 2005. Exposure to chronic stress downregulates corticosterone responses to acute stressors. *Am J Physiol 288*, R1628–R1636.

Rogers, C. M., Ramenofsky, M., Ketterson, E. D., Nolan, V., Jr., Wingfield, J. C., 1993. Plasma corticosterone, adrenal mass, winter weather, and season in nonbreeding populations of dark-eyed juncos (*Junco hyemalis hyemalis*). *Auk 110*, 279–285.

Romero, L. M., 2002. Seasonal changes in plasma glucocorticoid concentrations in free-living vertebrates. *Gen Comp Endocrinol 128*, 1–24.

Romero, L. M., 2004. Physiological stress in ecology: Lessons from biomedical research. *Trends Ecol Evol 19*, 249–255.

Romero, L. M., Dickens, M. J., Cyr, N. E., 2009. The reactive scope model: A new model integrating homeostasis, allostasis, and stress. *Horm Behav 55*, 375–389.

Romero, L. M., Levine, S., Sapolsky, R. M., 1995. Adrenocorticotropin secretagog release: stimulation by frustration and paradoxically by reward presentation. *Brain Res 676*, 151–156.

Romero, L. M., Reed, J. M., Wingfield, J. C., 2000. Effects of weather on corticosterone responses in wild free-living passerine birds. *Gen Comp Endocrinol 118*, 113–122.

Romero, L. M., Sapolsky, R. M., 1996. Patterns of ACTH secretagog secretion in response to psychological stimuli. *J Neuroendocrinol 8*, 243–258.

Romero, L. M., Wikelski, M., 2001. Corticosterone levels predict survival probabilities of Galápagos marine iguanas during El Niño events. *Proc Natl Acad Sci USA 98*, 7366–7370.

Romero, L. M., Wikelski, M., 2002. Exposure to tourism reduces stress-induced corticosterone levels in Galápagos marine iguanas. *Biol Conserv 108*, 371–374.

Sapolsky, R. M., 1982. The endocrine stress-response and social status in the wild baboon. *Horm Behav 16*, 279–287.

Sapolsky, R. M., 1990. Stress in the wild. *Scientific American 262*, 116–123.

Sapolsky, R. M., 1992. *Stress, the aging brain, and the mechanisms of neuron death.* MIT Press, Cambridge, MA.

Sapolsky, R. M., 1993. Endocrinology alfresco: Psychoendocrine studies of wild baboons. *Recent Prog Horm Res 48*, 437–468.

Sapolsky, R. M., 1994. *Why zebras don't get ulcers: A guide to stress, stress-related diseases, and coping.* W. H. Freeman, New York.

Sapolsky, R. M., 2001. Physiological and pathophysiological implications of social stress in mammals. In: McEwen, B. S., Goodman, H. M. (Eds.), *Handbook of physiology; Section 7: The endocrine system; Vol. IV: Coping with the environment: Neural and endocrine mechanisms.* Oxford University Press, New York, pp. 517–532.

Sapolsky, R. M., 2005. The influence of social hierarchy on primate health. *Science 308*, 648–652.

Sapolsky, R. M., Romero, L. M., Munck, A. U., 2000. How do glucocorticoids influence stress-responses? Integrating permissive, suppressive, stimulatory, and preparative actions. *Endocr Rev 21*, 55–89.

Satterlee, D. G., Johnson, W. A., 1988. Selection of Japanese quail for contrasting blood corticosterone response to immobilization. *Poult Sci 67*, 25–32.

Schiml, P. A., Mendoza, S. P., Saltzman, W., Lyons, D. M., Mason, W. A., 1996. Seasonality in squirrel monkeys (*Saimiri sciureus*): social facilitation by females. *Physiol Behav 60*, 1105–1113.

Schulkin, J., 2003. *Rethinking homeostasis: Allostatic regulation in physiology and pathophysiology.* MIT Press, Cambridge, MA.

Schwabl, H., Ramenofsky, M., Schwabl-Benzinger, I., Farner, D. S., Wingfield, J. C., 1988. Social status, circulating levels of hormones, and competition for food in winter flocks of the white-throated sparrow. *Behaviour 107*, 107–121.

Selye, H., 1946. The general adaptation syndrome and the diseases of adaptation. *J Clin Endocrinol 6*, 117–230.

Sharpless, S., Jasper, H., 1956. Habituation of the arousal reaction. *Brain 79*, 655.

Smith, G. T., Wingfield, J. C., Veit, R. R., 1994. Adrenocortical response to stress in the common diving petrel, *Pelecanoides urinatrix. Physiol Zool 67*, 526–537.

Sterling, P., Eyer, J., 1988. Allostasis a new paradigm to explain arousal pathology. In: Fisher, S., Reason, J. (Eds.), *Handbook of life stress cognition and health.* John Wiley and Sons, New York, pp. 629–650.

Stewart, M. G., Davies, H. A., Sandi, C., Kraev, I. V., Rogachevsky, V. V., Peddie, C. J., Rodriguez, J. J., Cordero, M. I., Donohue, H. S., Gabbott, P. L. A., Popov, V. I., 2005. Stress suppresses and learning induces plasticity in CA3 of rat hippocampus: A three-dimensional ultrastructural study of thorny excrescences and their postsynaptic densities. *Neuroscience 131*, 43–54.

Strier, K. B., Ziegler, T. E., Wittwer, D. J., 1999. Seasonal and social correlates of fecal testosterone and cortisol levels in wild male muriquis (*Brachyteles arachnoides*). *Horm Behav 35*, 125–134.

Tache, Y., Duruisseau, P., Tache, J., Selye, H., Collu, R., 1976. Shift in adenohypophyseal activity during chronic intermittent immobilization of rats. *Neuroendocrinol 22*, 325–336.

Tamashiro, K. L. K., Nguyen, M. M. N., Sakai, R. R., 2005. Social stress: From rodents to primates. *Front Neuroendocrinol 26*, 27–40.

Thompson, R. F., Spencer, W. A., 1966. Habituation: A model phenomenon for study of neuronal substrates of behavior. *Psychol Rev 73*, 16–33.

Thorpe, W. H., 1963. *Learning and instinct in animals.* Harvard University Press, Cambridge, MA.

Townsend, P., 1974. Inequality and health service. *Lancet 1*, 1179–1190.

Vallarino, A., Wingfield, J. C., Drummond, H., 2006. Does extra corticosterone elicit increased begging and submissiveness in subordinate booby (*Sula nebouxii*) chicks? *Gen Comp Endocrinol 147*, 297.

Walker, B. G., Boersma, P. D., Wingfield, J. C., 2005. Physiological and behavioral differences in Magellanic Penguin chicks in undisturbed and tourist-visited locations of a colony. *Conserv Biol 19*, 1571–1577.

Walker, B. G., Boersma, P. D., Wingfield, J. C., 2006. Habituation of adult magellanic penguins to human visitation as expressed through behavior and corticosterone secretion. *Conserv Biol 20*, 146–154.

Walsberg, G. E., 2003. How useful is energy balance as a overall index of stress in animals? *Horm Behav 43*, 16–17.

Weiss, J. M., 1968. Effects of coping responses on stress. *J Comp Physiol Psychol 65*, 251–260.

Weiss, J. M., 1970. Somatic effects of predictable and unpredictable shock. *Psychosom Med 32*, 397–408.

Weiss, J. M., 1972. Psychological factors in stress and disease. *Scientific American 226*, 104–113.

Williams, T. D., 2008. Individual variation in endocrine systems: moving beyond the "tyranny of the Golden Mean." *Phil Trans R Soc B 363*, 1687–1698.

Willner, P., 1993. Animal models of stress: An overview. In: Stanford, S. C., Salmon, P., Gray, J. P. (Eds.), *Stress: From synapse to syndrome.* Academic Press, San Diego, pp. 145–165

Wingfield, J. C., 1994. Modulation of the adrenocortical response to stress in birds. In: Davey, K. G., Peter, R. E., Tobe, S. S. (Eds.), *Perspectives in comparative endocrinology.* National Research Council of Canada, Ottawa, pp. 520–528.

Wingfield, J. C., 2003. Control of behavioural strategies for capricious environments. *Anim Behav 66*, 807–815.

Wingfield, J. C., 2004. Allostatic load and life cycles: Implications for neuroendocrine mechanisms. In: Schulkin, J (Ed.), *Allostasis, Homeostasis and the Costs of Physiological Adaptation*, Cambridge University Press, Cambridge, pp. 302–342.

Wingfield, J. C., 2005. Modulation of the adrenocortical response to acute stress in breeding birds. In: Dawson, A., Sharp, P. J. (Eds.), *Functional avian endocrinology*, Narosa Publishing House, New Delhi, India, pp. 225–240.

Wingfield, J. C., Breuner, C., Jacobs, J., 1997. Corticosterone and behavioral responses to unpredicatble events. In: Harvey, S., Etches, R. J. (Eds.), *Perspectives in avian endocrinology.* Journal of Endocrinology Press, Bristol, UK, pp. 267–278.

Wingfield, J. C., Maney, D. L., Breuner, C. W., Jacobs, J. D., Lynn, S., Ramenofsky, M., Richardson, R. D., 1998. Ecological bases of hormone-behavior interactions: The "emergency life history stage." *Integ Comp Biol 38*, 191–206.

Wingfield, J. C., Moore, M. C., Farner, D. S., 1983. Endocrine responses to inclement weather in naturally breeding populations of white-crowned sparrows (*Zonotrichia leucophrys pugetensis*). *Auk 100*, 56–62.

Wingfield, J. C., Ramenofsky, M., 1999. Hormones and the behavioral ecology of stress. *Stress Physiol Animals* 1-51.

Wingfield, J. C., Romero, L. M., 2001. Adrenocortical responses to stress and their modulation in free-living vertebrates. In: McEwen, B. S., Goodman, H. M. (Eds.), *Handbook of physiology; Section 7: The endocrine system; Vol. IV: Coping with the environment: Neural and endocrine mechanisms.* Oxford University Press, New York, pp. 211–234.

Wingfield, J. C., Sapolsky, R. M., 2003. Reproduction and resistance to stress: When and how. *J Neuroendocrinol 15*, 711.

Wotus, C., Engeland, W. C., 2003. Differential regulation of adrenal corticosteroids after restriction-induced drinking in rats. *Am J Physiol 284*, R183–R191.

Wotus, C., Osborn, J. W., Nieto, P. A., Engeland, W. C., 2003. Regulation of corticosterone production by vasopressin during water restriction and after drinking in rats. *Neuroendocrinol 78*, 301–311.

Yorio, P., Frere, E., Gandini, P., Schiavini, A., 2001. Tourism and recreation at seabird breeding sites in Patagonia, Argentina: Current concerns and future prospects. *Bird Conserv Int 11*, 231–245.

4

The Classic Stress Response

I. INTRODUCTION: FOUR MAJOR COMPONENTS OF THE CLASSIC STRESS RESPONSE

To this point we have introduced the concept of stress in the context of the predictable life cycle and responses to unpredictable perturbations. We have also considered the major models of stress that seek to explain the complex ways by which organisms cope with a changing world, and what implications these might have for human populations at a biomedical level and also for coping with global change and environmental catastrophes. There are many mediators involved in coping strategies, and now it is important to discuss the hormonal responses to stress: What are the actions of stress hormones that allow us to cope? As outlined in Chapters 1 and 3, the stress response means many things to different people. Taking an ecological approach, the stress response is considered highly adaptive, allowing organisms to respond to stressful and potentially stressful events with the emergency life-history stage (ELHS). This complex life-history stage serves to redirect an individual from its normal life cycle into an emergency coping mode, promoting survival in the best condition possible. After the perturbation passes, the normal life cycle can be resumed.

Stress responses also mean bad things to many people, especially in the biomedical realm and animal agriculture. As discussed in Chapters 1 and 3, sometimes stress becomes chronic, and then the mediators of the initially adaptive ELHS become destructive, leading to the symptoms of chronic stress and eventually death. Chronic stress does occur in the natural world as well, but it is almost always accompanied by massive mortality. However, some individuals usually survive, suggesting very strong selection for coping mechanisms that avoid the deleterious effects of chronic stress. The ELHS is critical in this regard, but it is a complex life-history stage with four distinct components, as discussed in Chapter 1. These components are the fight-or-flight response (an immediate response to sudden threatening events such as an attack by a predator), reactive/proactive coping strategies (especially in response to social stress), preparations of the immune system for potential injury and infection, and facultative behavioral and physiological responses that potentiate avoidance of chronic stress. The hormonal responses to stress, or perturbations that have the potential to be stressful, are described next, and their biological functions are discussed in subsequent chapters.

II. THE FIGHT-OR-FLIGHT RESPONSE

If a brain were so simple we could understand it, we would be so simple we couldn't.

—LYALL WATSON

One thing that should be clear from the previous two chapters is that there are numerous physiological mediators of a stress response. Arguably the two most important responses, however, are the activation of the sympathetic nervous system concordant with the release of catecholamines (often called the fight-or-flight response) and the release of glucocorticoids (Figure 4.1). The decision to initiate these two responses is under the control of an ill-defined discrimination/determination function in the brain that weighs the contextual factors, as discussed in Chapter 2. Once the determination is made that the stimulus is, in fact, a stressor, signaling to both arms of the stress response (Figure 4.1) is commenced.

The term "fight-or-flight," as described by Cannon (1932), is an excellent succinct encapsulation of sympathetic nervous system activation in many regards. Perhaps the term's greatest strength is that "fight-or-flight" evokes immediacy. There is the sense that something must happen, and is happening, *right now*. Life itself is hanging in the balance. There is no time for fancy discussions of reproductive success, sexual selection, inclusive fitness, and so on, that comprise the overall fitness, in an evolutionary sense, of an individual. Survival is the ultimate arbiter of an animal's success, and the fight-or-flight response is the first-line physiological mechanism for giving an animal its best chance for survival. When you hear "fight-or-flight," you immediately think of an animal that must react quickly, react strongly, and react now, in order to survive. The sympathetic nervous system mediates these reactions.

The types of immediate stressors that could trigger a fight-or-flight response—predators, social interactions, severe but brief weather events (tornadoes, for example), and fire—are all called indirect perturbation factors. The quintessential stressor that initiates a fight-or-flight response, of course, is a predator attack. Predators can exert profound effects on potential prey. They can alter numerous individual behaviors (reviewed by Lima 1998) as well as affect where individual animals choose to live (e.g., Blumstein et al. 2006b; Losos et al. 2004). The threat of predation is sufficiently powerful that animals often react as if there are predators present even when there are none (Creel and Christianson 2008), although these behaviors can be lost when predators disappear (Blumstein

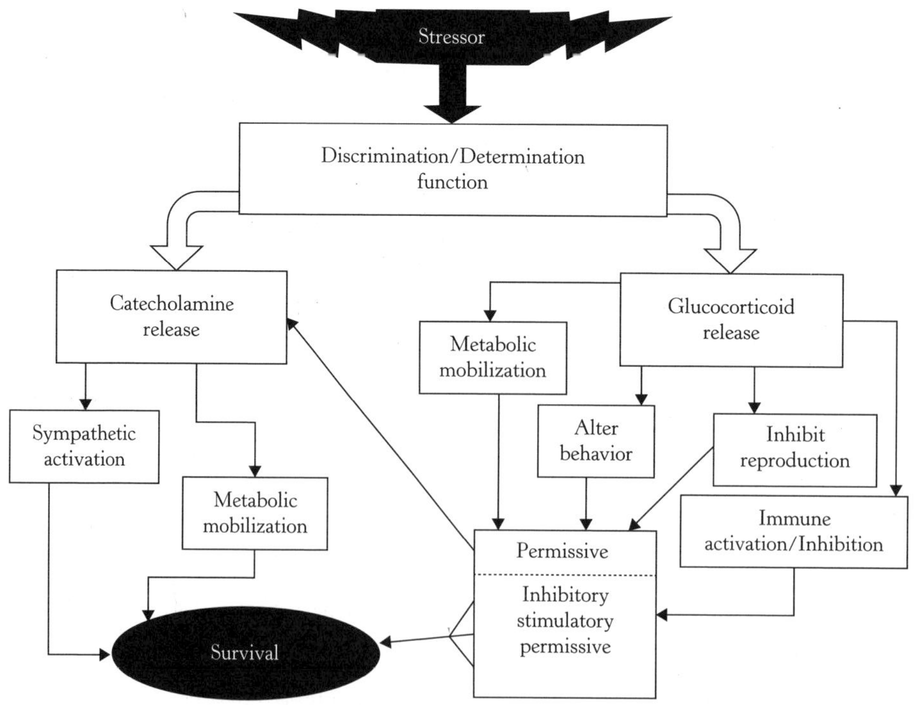

FIGURE 4.1: The two major arms of the stress response that aid in helping an animal survive.

2006; Blumstein et al. 2006a), especially on islands (e.g., Beauchamp 2004; Blumstein et al. 2004; Blumstein and Daniel 2005; Roedl et al. 2007).

Predator-induced changes in behavior have been studied for decades, but the changes in hormonal and physiological systems can also be extensive. For example, predation risk can alter reproductive physiology (Clinchy et al. 2004; Creel et al. 2007; Mateo 2007). In fact, as we elaborate in Chapter 10, successful reproduction under certain contexts may require not responding to predators (Jessop et al. 2004; Wingfield and Sapolsky 2003). Predation risk in some bird species even appears to have led to the evolution of restricting sleep to one hemisphere of the brain at a time, an adaptation thought to allow the bird to literally "keep one eye open" for predators at all times (Rattenborg et al. 1999). The physiological changes associated with predation risk are so powerful that recent laboratory studies have used chronic exposure to predator cues as a model for studying human anxiety (Adamec et al. 2004; Adamec et al. 2006).

Many of the responses to predators are also mediated, at least in part, by either catecholamine or glucocorticoid release. For example, individuals from several species elevate catecholamine levels (e.g., Adamec et al. 2007) and corticosteroid levels (e.g., Breves and Specker 2005; Rogovin et al. 2004; Scheuerlein et al. 2001) when predators are nearby. Even predator calls (Eilam et al. 1999) and odors (Zhang et al. 2003; but see Fletcher and Boonstra 2006) can evoke catecholamine or corticosteroid release. Furthermore, these responses can be long lasting and indirect. For example, loss of a close relative can lead to elevated corticosteroids in baboons (Engh et al. 2006).

The above discussion of the impact of predators points out two weaknesses of the term "fight-or-flight." The first is that not all immediate emergency behaviors can be easily categorized as a fight response or a flight response. "Flight" generally conjures images of animals running/flying/swimming away from a predator, yet moving toward a predator may actually decrease predator success (such as group mobbing of a predator by a flock of birds) (Hochachka 2004; Shifferman and Eilam 2004). In other cases, often the most effective tactic is to freeze and not move at all, a tactic taken to its extreme in those species that feign death. Furthermore, the type of tactic employed by an animal often varies and can be species specific (Eilam et al. 1999; Hendrie et al. 1998). For example, rats flee when faced with a predator if an escape route is available, but they instead freeze and prepare to attack if escape routes are closed (Blanchard and Blanchard 2003). In another example, several closely related whale species react differently to attacking killer whales, with some species fleeing and others fighting (Ford and Reeves 2008). In this case, some species only have a "fight" response, whereas other only have a "flight" response (but note that this might not be true in the face of other immediate threats). The second weakness of the term is that "fight-or-flight" does not obviously encompass the unifying underlying physiological mechanism that regulates and mediates the immediate emergency reactions—the sympathetic nervous system.

Despite these two weaknesses, the strengths of the term "fight-or-flight," especially in emphasizing the speed and immediacy of the response, suggest that it is still useful shorthand for sympathetic activation and the ensuing behavioral and physiological responses. But how does the sympathetic nervous system elicit those responses? Furthermore, how do those responses actually help wild animals to cope with stressors? What follows is a brief overview of what we know about the fight-or-flight response from laboratory studies, and how that information can be used to understand the fight-or-flight response in an ecological context.

A. Changes in Heart Rate

Measuring the strength of the fight-or-flight response, or even determining whether a fight-or-flight response is initiated, is very difficult in wild animals (see Chapter 6). Currently, one of the few techniques available is to use changes in heart rate as an index of catecholamine release. Although resting and stress-induced heart rates differ by species and by taxa (Lillywhite et al. 1999), the basic regulation of cardiac function is common across the vertebrates. Heart rate is regulated both via direct neural connection, wherein epinephrine released from nerve terminals binds to β-receptors on the heart, and via indirect release of epinephrine and norepinephrine from the adrenal medulla (chromaffin). Heart rate is elevated during stress by β-receptor binding, making epinephrine the primary mediator of heart rate during acute stress in mammals. A number of studies have applied this approach to wild animals, both free-ranging and captive. These studies report two major responses—an increase in heart rate (tachycardia) due to most stressors, and a decrease in heart rate (bradycardia) in certain special circumstances. However, heart rate is not exclusively under sympathetic control. The parasympathetic nervous system also participates in regulating heart rate. Assessing heart rate variability is a technique that can distinguish between these two inputs (Billman 2011).

Heart rate is regulated by both negative parasympathetic input from the vagus nerve and positive sympathetic input from epinephrine and norepinephrine (Figure 4.2). Under non-stressed conditions (e.g., exercise), increases in heart rate are primarily driven by decreases in vagal input (Perini and Veicsteinas 2003), which is part of the parasympathetic nervous system. In contrast, the increase in heart rate during the fight-or-flight response is primarily driven by the increased catecholamines of the sympathetic response (Bohus and Koolhaas 1993). Numerous studies have demonstrated a shift from parasympathetic to sympathetic control over heart rate during acute stress in mammals (reviewed by Stauss 2003).

The relative contributions of vagal and sympathetic inputs to regulating heart rate can be determined by monitoring the variation between heart beats, such as the R-R interval of the QRS wave of the electrocardiogram (ECG; Perini and Veicsteinas 2003; Stauss 2003). Vagal input produces variability in the inter-beat frequency (called heart rate variability). The variability results from a number of other functions of the vagus nerve, the most important being the regulation of respiration. Coordinating respiratory and cardiac function apparently results in substantial variability in the signal that goes to the heart and results in the variation between heart beats (see Figure 4.3). In contrast, sympathetic activation produces a more regular beat. The sympathetic signal overrides the variability produced by the vagus nerve and produces a heart that beats like a metronome. Figure 4.3 helps illustrate the difference between changes in heart rate and changes in heart rate variability. In the bottom panel, the heart rate has increased and the inter-beat period is shorter. Which pathway is driving the increase in heart rate? The more regular inter-beat interval indicates that it is an increase in sympathetic input, not a decrease in parasympathetic input. As you can see, the relative contributions of vagal versus sympathetic inputs can be determined from the amount of variability: the less the variability, the greater the sympathetic (i.e., catecholamine) input and the less the vagal input (e.g., Korte et al. 1999; Perini and Veicsteinas 2003). However, the inputs from the two pathways are not synchronized and can function independently (von Borell et al. 2007).

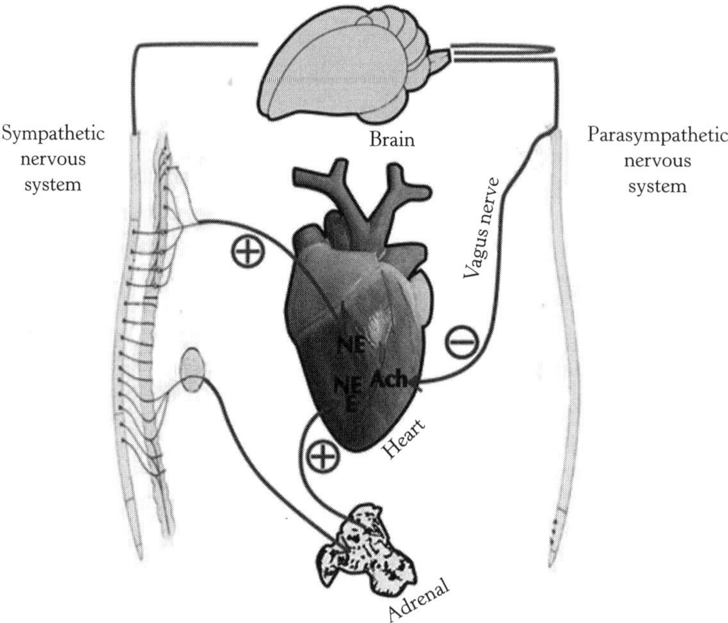

FIGURE 4.2: Heart rate is regulated by two pathways: parasympathetic input from the vagus nerve, and sympathetic input from both direct neural connections and via catecholamine release from the adrenal. Heart rate results from the balance of these two inputs.

Diagram courtesy of M. Dickens.

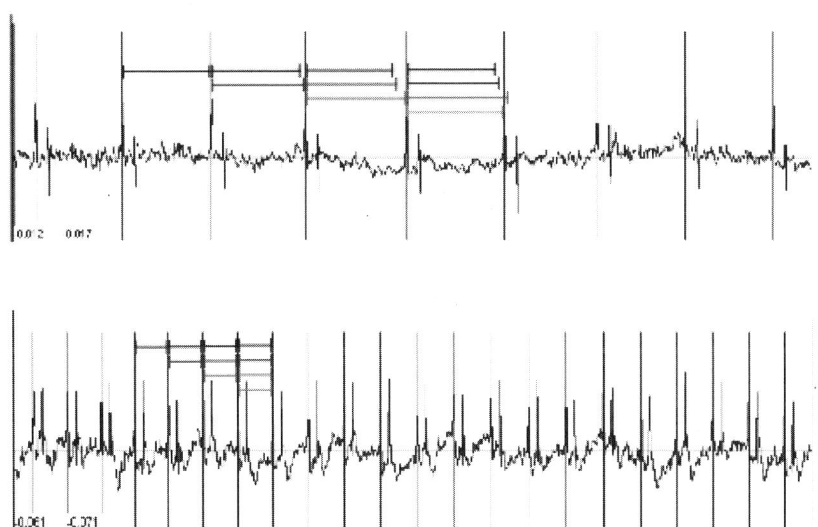

FIGURE 4.3: Inter-beat intervals when an animal is at rest (upper graph) and exposed to a stressor (lower graph). Vertical lines are superimposed on the ECG to emphasize the R portion of the heart beat. Even though the inter-beat intervals are dramatically smaller during the stressor (stress-induced tachycardia), the distance between those beats is much more variable when the heart is under parasympathetic control. The brackets represent an inter-beat interval superimposed on another inter-beat interval to show how closely the distance is duplicated from beat to beat.

Figure courtesy of M. Dickens.

Figure 4.4 shows a schematic of parasympathetic and sympathetic regulation of heart rate and heart rate variability.

Analysis of heart rate variability is commonly used in humans and laboratory mammals to determine the source of cardiac stimulation (reviewed by Stein and Kleiger 1999; Acharya et al. 2006). In general, however, heart rate variability has been used to study long-term, or chronic, changes in parasympathetic/sympathetic balance, especially in terms of chronic disease in humans. For instance, quail selected for high fearfulness show lower heart rate variability than do quail selected for low fearfulness (Valance et al. 2007). These long-term chronic changes are probably what heart rate variability analysis is best for. When heart rate variability is examined in the time frame of a short acute stressor, heart rate variability decreases (Cyr et al. 2009), just as Cannon would have predicted a century ago (Cannon and de la Paz 1911).

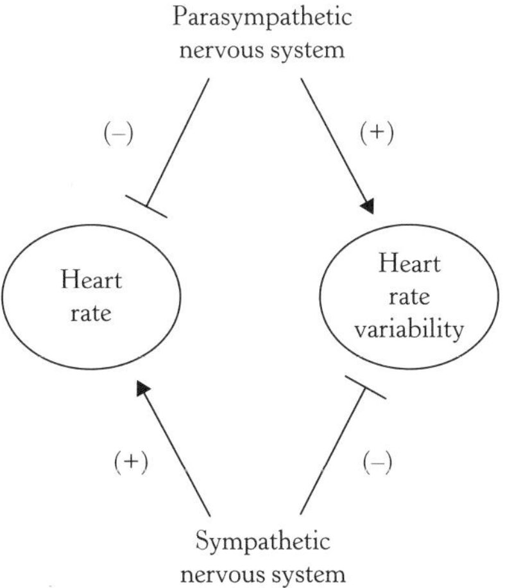

FIGURE 4.4: Scheme for sympathetic and parasympathetic regulation of heart rate and heart rate variability.

There have been a number of methods used to analyze changes in heart rate variability (Acharya et al. 2006; Berntson et al. 1997). These methods can be divided into two major categories—those that directly measure differences between successive beats and those that use spectral analyses to determine beat-to-beat frequencies. Spectral analyses are currently preferred in mammalian research, but many techniques appear to produce adequate results. One problem with the spectral analysis approach is that it requires an extensive period (e.g., > 5 min is recommended [von Borell et al. 2007]) of unbroken ECG recordings. Not only can sufficient unbroken periods be difficult to obtain in free-living animals, it also precludes studying the initiation of the fight-or-flight response. Other techniques (e.g., Cyr et al. 2009) can provide better resolution.

It is important to remember that there can be considerable species differences in how heart rate is regulated that can potentially impact analyses of heart rate variability. We might anticipate, for example, that heart rate variability will differ in birds and mammals because the natural variance in inter-beat frequency could be entirely different, considering that birds and mammals have different respiratory physiologies. Our recent work on European starlings indicated that common techniques for spectral analysis were not possible for these birds, and we relied upon comparing changes in beat-to-beat intervals (Cyr et al. 2009). Furthermore, even though the vertebrate fight-or-flight response is highly conserved, the mechanisms underlying acute stress-induced heart rate may differ among vertebrates. For example, unlike in mammals, in birds both epinephrine and norepinephrine bind preferentially to β-receptors, and in vitro studies have shown that injecting both catecholamines onto avian heart tissue increases heart rate (Smith et al. 2000). However, heart rate variability has been used to study sympathetic activity in chickens (e.g., Korte et al. 1999; Kuo et al. 2001), Atlantic salmon (Altimiras et al. 1996), and mammalian species such as prairie voles (Grippo et al. 2007a), although not, to our knowledge, in a reptile or an amphibian. This work indicates that concurrent analysis of both heart rate and heart rate variability is likely to be a useful index for the activation of the sympathetic nervous system (i.e., the fight-or-flight response) during stress in a number of species.

Finally, although heart rate variability has not yet been used to study stress in free-living animals, the technique has considerable promise. Heart rate variability decreases during psychological stress (Rietmann et al. 2004; Visser et al. 2002) and chronic stress (see discussion later in this chapter) in laboratory settings, so presumably could be used to study sympathetic responses to a number of stressors in the wild.

The short-term increases in heart rate (tachycardia) are driven primarily by the sympathetic nervous system, although a decrease in parasympathetic input can also occur (von Borell et al. 2007). This response can be extremely rapid (Figure 4.5). Because the tachycardia associated with stress is linked to catecholamine release, heart rate responses show many of the same dynamics as catecholamine release. For example, just as both epinephrine and norepinephrine can be modulated to fit the demands of different stressors (Hart et al. 1989), so can heart rate. Figure 4.6 shows that stronger stressors evoke higher increases in heart rate (Nephew et al. 2003).

Few studies have examined heart rate responses to stress in either free-living or captive species. In general, those studies have confirmed what we would have predicted—stressors result in increases in heart rate (but see the following section). Stressors that have been studied include human disturbance in several bird species (Ackerman et al. 2004; Bisson et al. 2009; De Villiers et al. 2006; Ellenberg et al. 2006; Holmes et al. 2005; Nimon et al. 1996; Weimerskirch et al. 2002), social interactions in greylag geese (Wascher et al. 2008b), handling in common eiders (Cabanac and Guillemette 2001) and an iguana (but interestingly, not in two species of frogs [Cabanac and Cabanac 2000]), exercise in toads (Romero et al. 2004), aircraft noise in black ducks (Harms et al. 1997), and trapping stress in European badgers (Schutz et al. 2006). A reduction in the heart rate response to stressors also seems to be one physiological mechanism underlying tameness in island species (Vitousek et al. 2010). In addition, a number of stimuli in captive situations, such as sounds, lighting conditions, novel odors, confinement, and abnormal social groups, are known to stimulate increases in heart rate (reviewed by Morgan and Tromborg 2007) These studies fit nicely into what is known about increases in heart rate due to stress from traditional laboratory species (Goldstein 1987; Sapolsky et al. 2000; Stanford 1993).

One important type of stressor for free-living animals are those associated with social interactions. Laboratory studies on domestic rats indicate that social stressors can elicit very strong increases in heart rate that are accompanied by decreases in heart rate variability (Sgoifo et al. 1998). Rats can habituate their heart rate responses to intermittent social stressors (i.e., decrease their response to equivalent stressors), but interestingly, this only occurs when the animal "wins" the social encounter (Sgoifo et al. 2005). Furthermore, several laboratory species show distinct individual differences in the magnitude of their responses (e.g., Fox et al. 2005; Sgoifo et al. 2005), including humans (e.g., LeBlanc et al. 2004). Although little work has been done on nontraditional species, the few laboratory studies suggest that the work done on rats is likely to reflect responses in many species. For example, using a protocol to induce crowding, European starlings adjust the magnitude of their heart rate responses depending upon

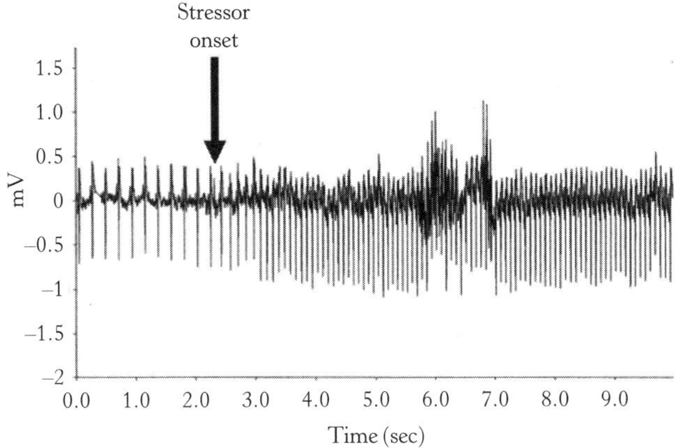

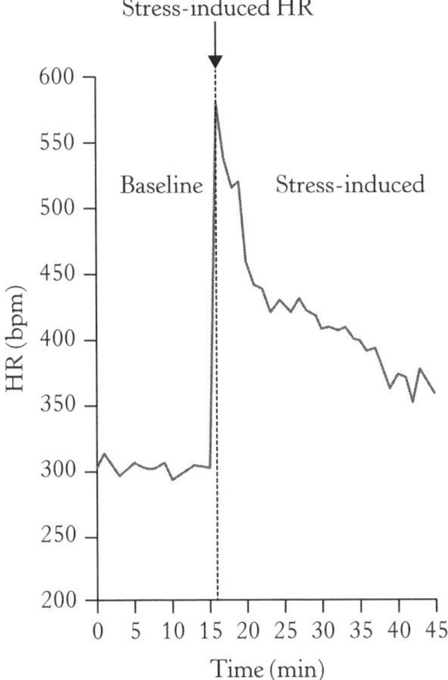

FIGURE 4.5: Upper panel is an ECG trace showing individual QRS waves from a European starling. The bird was exposed to a stressor at the arrow, and stress-induced tachycardia ensued. Lower panel shows 5 sec. running mean heart rates from just before and during exposure to a stressor from a European starling.

Reprinted with permission from Nephew et al. (2003) courtesy of Elsevier. Diagram courtesy of M. Dickens.

the degree of crowding (Figure 4.7; Nephew and Romero 2003).

A few studies have also explored the impact of social stressors in the field. Heart rate increases indicate that little blue penguin chicks can distinguish between familiar and unfamiliar conspecific calls (Nakagawa et al. 2001), an effect also shown in captive European blackbirds (Diehl and Helb 1986), chiffchaffs (Zimmer 1982), and bottlenose dolphins (Miksis et al. 2001). Tamar wallabies increase heart rate when fighting and mating (Dressen and Hendrichs 1992). Finally, free-living greylag geese show robust increases in heart rate in response to agonistic interactions, nearly the equivalent to increases associated with flying (Figure 4.8; Ely et al. 1999; Wascher et al. 2008a). In fact, geese can have robust increases in heart rate by simply watching agonistic interactions by other animals, even though they are not directly involved (Wascher et al. 2008b). Figure 4.9 indicates that social interactions, even those in which the individual is not directly involved, can elicit far more robust responses than other potentially dangerous stimuli. Clearly much more work needs to be done exploring the impact of social stressors on the fight-or-flight response, and it is an exciting avenue for future research.

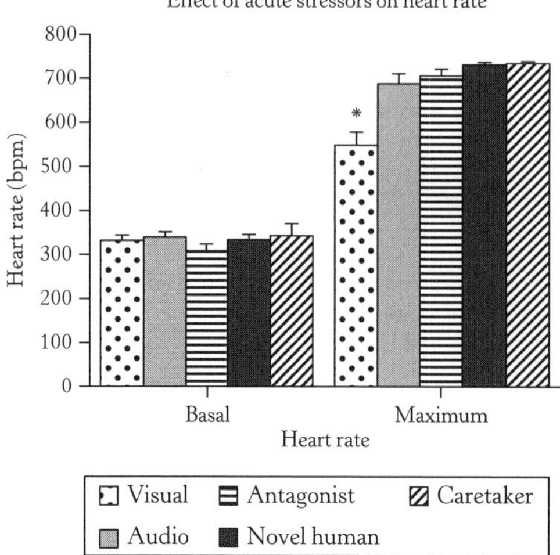

FIGURE 4.6: Graded responses within an individual to different stressors in captive European starlings. Different stressors were presented to the starlings, including a strobe light (visual), a radio (audio), and three different humans, the experimenter (antagonist), a novel human, and the birds' normal caretaker.

Reprinted with permission from Nephew et al. (2003) courtesy of Elsevier.

In many ways, the increase in heart rate is a more sensitive index of a fight-or-flight response than even behavior (Ely et al. 1999; Wascher et al. 2008b), as illustrated by the following anecdote:

> At one point we watched the bird sitting on a telephone pole 100 m away. A child moved toward the bird offering a bit of food. The bird watched, seemingly otherwise unconcerned, but its apprehension was signaled by a heart rate that accelerated from 160 to 440 beats/min and then returned to 200 as the child backed off. (Kanwisher et al. 1978)

Behavior is often used in order to avoid a costly physiological response (consider that when you walk out of the house into the cold without a jacket, your first response is to return indoors, a behavior, rather than initiate shivering thermogenesis, a physiological response), but when it comes to responding to stressors, the behavior and physiological responses are often uncoupled. We have also seen this uncoupling in the laboratory (Nephew et al. 2003). Conversely, behavioral changes may not always reflect an underlying

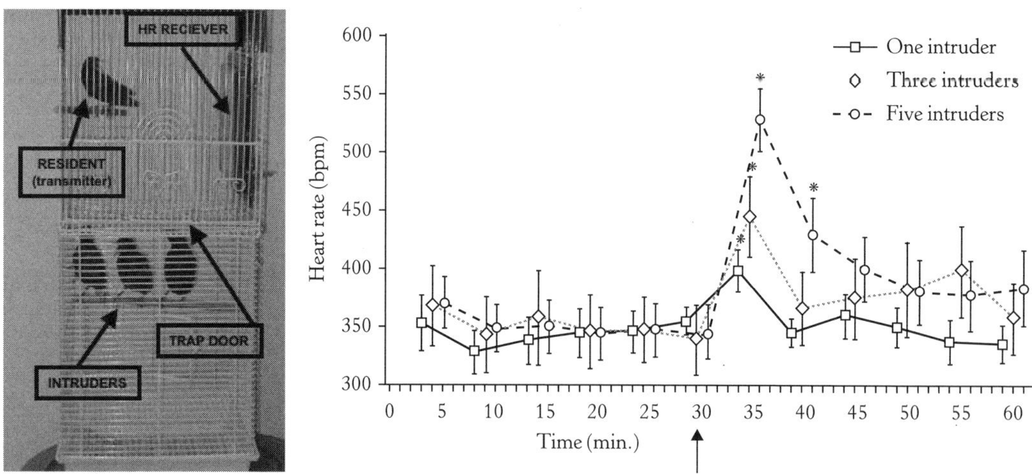

FIGURE 4.7: Use of a crowding, or acute increase in density, social stressor in European starlings. In the left panel, a starling with an implanted radiotransmitter for monitoring heart rate is placed in the upper cage and one, three, or five intruders are placed in the bottom cage. The cages are separated by a closed trap door. The trap door is then opened remotely, the intruders fly up into the resident's cage, and the trap door is closed. This increase in crowding results in an elevation in the resident's heart rate (right panel), where the arrow indicates the opening of the trap door. However, the magnitude of the increase depends upon the degree of crowding, with five intruders inducing a stronger response than three or one intruder.

Photo courtesy of B. Nephew.

Graph reprinted with permission from Nephew and Romero (2003). Courtesy of Elsevier.

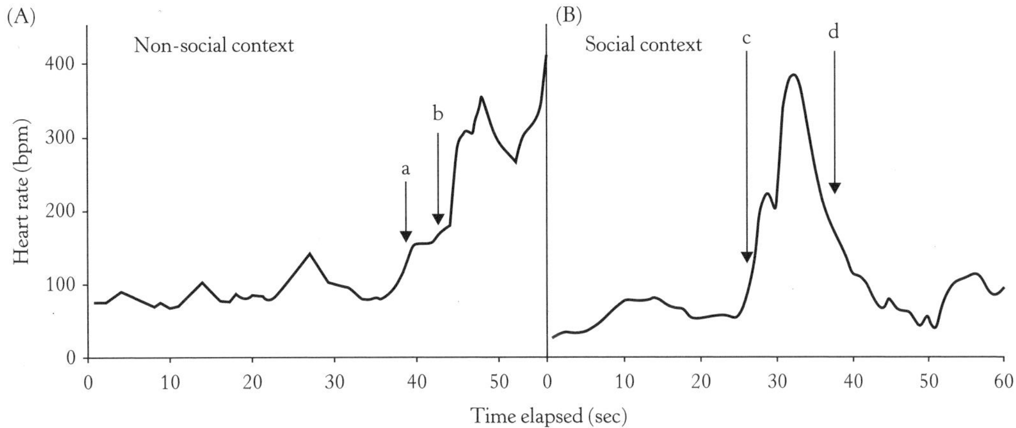

FIGURE 4.8: Single examples of heart rate modulation. (A) Departure event of focal individual 1. At the first arrow (a) behavior changed from head up to preflight synchronization behavior; the second arrow (b) marks the actual departure. Recording ends when the individual had left the recording range. (B) Attack by focal individual 1. The goose showed the behavior head up when interaction of intensity 1 started (marked by arrow c). The end of the interaction is marked by arrow (d).

Reprinted with permission from Wascher et al. (2008a), coutesy of the American Psychological Association.

stress response. We find it likely that not all disturbances will initiate a fight-or-flight response. For example, a bird flying from its perch in order to avoid someone walking nearby does not always result in a fight-or-flight response (Bisson et al. 2009). Evidence is thus building that increases in heart rate are better indicators of an underlying physiological fight-or-flight response than overt changes in behavior.

Finally, it should be remembered that an increase in heart rate, driven by the sympathetic nervous system, can extract a heavy price. For many years we have known that humans can go into sudden cardiac arrest and die due to severe emotional trauma (reviewed by Ziegelstein 2007). Although it is unknown if this occurs in wild animals, it could be the mechanism underlying reports of "trap death," when wild animals spontaneously die for no apparent reason when captured. The fight-or-flight response is clearly necessary to escape from predators, but the increase in heart rate can create its own problems.

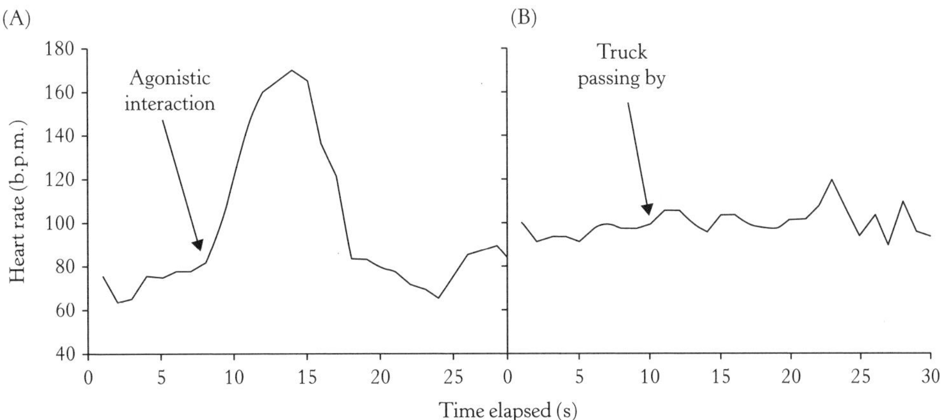

FIGURE 4.9: Examples of a social and a non-social bystander event of one focal individual. (A) The focal individual watched an agonistic interaction at a distance of approximately 5 m. The two interacting individuals were non-affiliated with the focal individual that was resting all the time. (B) A truck passed by, at a distance of approximately 10 m. In this case, the focal individual was vigilant and did not change its behavior in response to the event.

Reprinted with permission from Wascher et al. (2008b). Courtesty of the Royal Society.

On the other hand, heart rate does not always increase during stress. Certain stimuli evoke behavioral immobility rather than hyperactivity. An example would be an animal freezing when detecting a predator. Essentially an animal has two mutually exclusive choices when faced with a predator—to flee immediately or to freeze and hope that it eludes detection (Eilam 2005). Both responses have pluses and minuses. Fleeing immediately works if there is sufficient distance and speed to outrun the predator, but also immediately draws the predator's attention and almost guarantees a chase. Freezing, on the other hand, is useful if the animal is not yet detected or has an asset, such as a nest, that needs to stay hidden, but can allow a predator to get lethally close. The decision whether to freeze or flee is complex, partially dependent upon the individual animal's predilection, its distance from a refuge, and the potential benefit of confusing a predator by being unpredictable (Eilam 2005).

Behavioral immobility is paralleled by a marked bradycardia (reviewed by Bohus and Koolhaas 1993). There are some excellent examples in the literature from a variety of species under field conditions. Female willow ptarmigan show a typical difference in responses (Figure 4.10). When brooding (incubating eggs on the nest), they display freezing behavior and a marked bradycardia in response to a threat (humans approaching the nest), but non-incubating females show the classic tachycardia of a fight-or-flight response (Gabrielsen et al. 1977; Gabrielsen et al. 1985; Steen et al. 1988). Clearly, being tied to a nest, where freezing and remaining motionless is an excellent tactic to avoid predation, requires a different physiological response than fleeing. Similarly in American alligators, marked bradycardia ensued when a canoe passed over the stationary and submerged alligator, but a human approaching a captive alligator always resulted in tachycardia (Smith et al. 1974). There was a similar response in box turtles (Smith and Decarvalho 1985). Freezing accompanied by bradycardia has also been demonstrated in two squirrel species (Smith and Johnson 1984), woodchucks (Smith and Woodruff 1980), beaver (Swain et al. 1988), and little blue penguins (Nakagawa et al. 2001). In a fascinating example, feigned death in the American opossum is also accompanied by bradycardia (Gabrielsen and Smith 1985). It is presently unknown whether bradycardia results from increased vagal or decreased sympathetic input, or both, but determining the mechanism will have interesting implications for the regulation of the fight-or-flight response.

B. The Use of Heart Rate to Estimate Energy Consumption

There have been many studies over the past few decades in which heart rate was measured in free-living animals. However, the goal of most of these studies was to use changes in heart rate to estimate energy consumption (Butler et al. 2004). This work is based upon the strong relationship between heart rate and oxygen consumption, which in turn is a direct measure of oxidative metabolism. An example of this relationship from our work on European starlings is shown in Figure 4.11. Once the correlation between heart rate and oxygen consumption has been generated for the specific species of interest, changes in heart rate can be used to infer the energetic

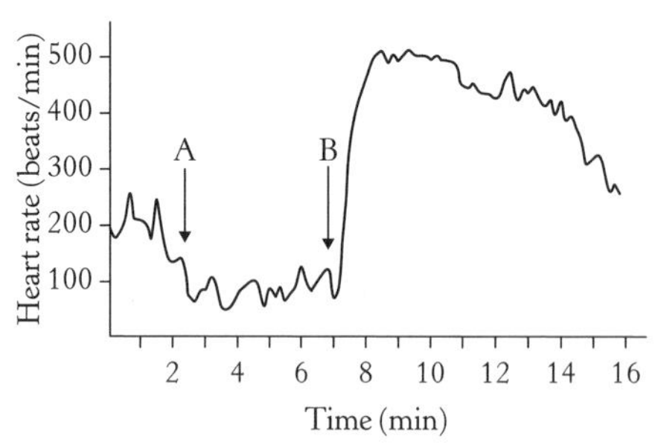

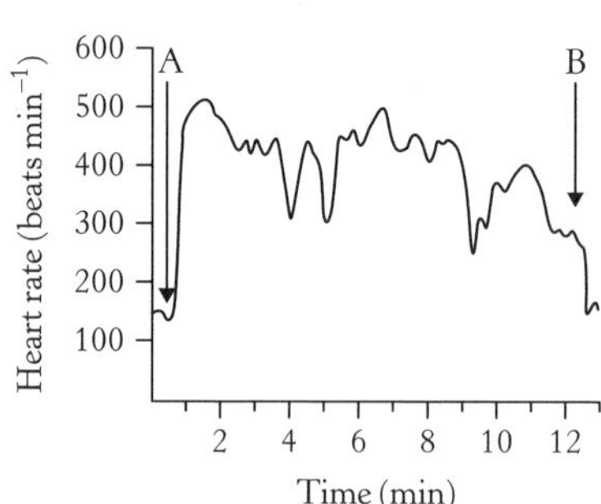

FIGURE 4.10: Heart rate responses in an incubating (left panel) and non-incubating (right panel) willow ptarmigan when approached by one person. Point A is when the hen can see the approaching person and point B is when the same person turns and leaves the area.

Graphs reprinted with permission, left panel from Gabrielsen et al. (1977) and right panel from Steen et al. (1988). Courtesy of Oxford.

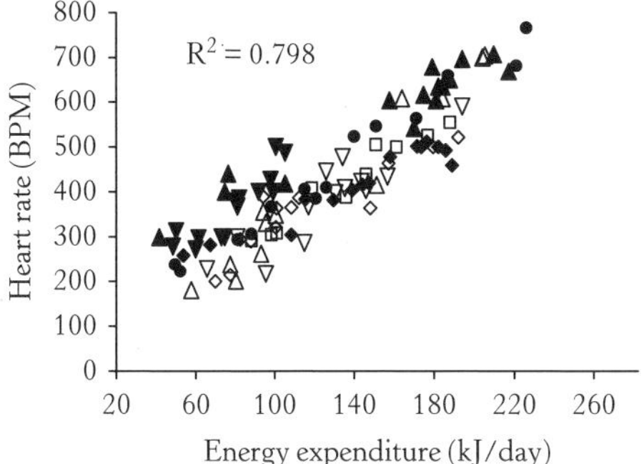

FIGURE 4.11: The relationship between heart rate and energy expenditure, as computed from oxygen consumption in captive European starlings. Each symbol represents different heart rates from an individual animal.

Reprinted with permission from Cyr et al. (2008). Courtesy of University of Chicago.

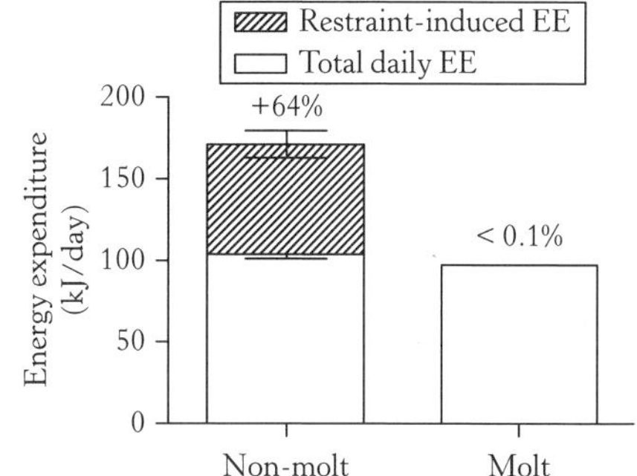

FIGURE 4.12: Using the conversion of heart rate to energy consumption in European starlings from Figure 4.11, the total amount of energy consumed during the day (12 hours) is indicated by the white bars. Captive starlings were tested in two physiological conditions: in molt and in non-molt (the replacing of feathers). Birds were then subjected to 30 min of restraint, and the resultant increase in heart rate was converted to energy consumption and indicated by the shaded bars. There was no increase in heart rate due to restraint during molt.

Reprinted with permission from Cyr et al. (2008). Courtesy of University of Chicago.

requirements of various behaviors and activities (Butler et al. 2004). Decreases in heart rate to save energy can be substantial, especially for species that undergo torpor (e.g., Bartholomew et al. 1962; Schaub and Prinzinger 1999).

Very few of these studies extended their work to measure heart rate responses to acute stressors. The researchers either were not interested in stress per se or were using techniques, such as loggers, that did not allow them to easily monitor acute responses to stressors. However, the melding of these two approaches holds much promise. Converting heart rate responses to energy consumption allows us to estimate the energetic cost of a stress response. For example, Figure 4.12 shows the increase in energy consumption in a starling during a 30-minute restraint. When these birds were not molting, the response to restraint incurred the substantial cost of 64% of the normal daily energy budget. Costs of this magnitude would clearly have profound impacts on the overall energy allocations made to different physiological and behavioral processes. Interestingly, however, a similar 30-minute restraint had no impact on energy consumption when the bird was undergoing molt (Figure 4.12). The molting birds essentially had no fight-or-flight response to restraint, which resulted in no increase in energy consumption. Why this occurred is still not clear, but the lack of response highlights that the magnitude, and perhaps even the presence, of a fight-or-flight response may depend upon the season and/or physiological state of the animal (see further discussion later in this chapter).

Converting heart rate to energy consumption has two potential applications when applied to stress physiology. The first is as a way to test some of the hypotheses generated by the Allostasis Model (see Chapter 3). The foundation of the Allostasis Model is energy usage, so being able to determine the energetic costs of various stress responses will allow specific responses to be placed within the foundation of allostasis (i.e., Figure 4.12). The second application is to use the conversion of heart rate to energy consumption as a potential way to link physiology to ecology. Life-history theory rests on assumptions of trade-offs between different behaviors and activities (Ricklefs and Wikelski 2002). These trade-offs can be mediated by the relative energetic costs. Using heart rate to convert fight-or-flight responses to their energetic costs potentially allows us to fit these stress responses into the overall ecology of the animal.

C. Seasonal Changes in Heart Rate

One of the defining features of a temperate environment is the changing of the seasons. All animals adjust their behavior and physiology to adapt to the changing conditions, and it appears that cardiovascular function is no exception. The few studies that have determined seasonal heart rate changes indicate that resting heart rate is lower during the winter than during the summer. This has been shown in captive and free-ranging deer species (Moen 1978; Price et al. 1993; Theil et al. 2004), captive juvenile green turtles (Southwood et al. 2003), the temperature-resistant green toad (Chapovetsky and Katz 2003), but not in the bullfrog (Rocha and Branco 1998). In general, this seasonal change appears to be linked to energetics, as discussed previously: the lower heart rate in winter reflects the energetic savings of a lower metabolism during the time of year with low energy availability.

However, seasonal changes in heart rate can also reflect seasonal differences in fight-or-flight responses to stressors. Although a study on free-ranging roe deer did not show a seasonal change in heart rate responses when fleeing from human harassment (Theil et al. 2004), a recent study on European starlings indicated that the fight-or-flight response can be modulated depending upon life-history stage (Dickens et al. 2006). In this study, captive starlings were either held on a short-day photoperiod to mimic winter conditions when this species normally forms large single species flocks, or held on a long-day photoperiod to mimic spring breeding conditions when starlings defend breeding territories. Birds implanted with heart rate transmitters were then exposed to acute crowding conditions of one or five intruders using the crowding protocol in Figure 4.7. The differences in heart rate increases due to crowding were dramatic (Figure 4.13). Even though five intruders elicited nearly equivalent responses under both photoperiods, one intruder elicited a markedly lower response when birds were on short days. The differences in response to one intruder may reflect an underlying mechanism for the observed life-history differences in behavior. One intruder elicits a robust fight-or-flight response when the bird is normally territorial and actively excluding rivals, whereas it elicits a greatly attenuated response when birds are tolerating many nearby conspecifics as part of flocking behavior.

A second example occurs in captive starlings during the annual prebasic molt. The avian molt entails the replacement of all flight and body feathers and incurs a substantial energetic cost (King 1981; Lindstrom et al. 1993; Murphy and King 1992). Figure 4.14 indicates that the increased energy requirement is reflected in a robust increase in resting heart rate during the night but that heart rates were not significantly different during the day (Cyr et al. 2008). This appears to support an earlier suggestion that the deposition of new feathers occurs primarily at night (Murphy 1996). Furthermore, Figure 4.14

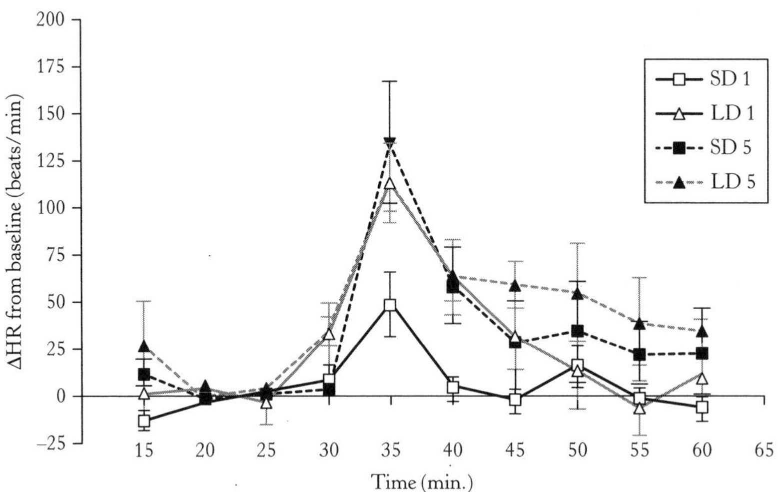

FIGURE 4.13: Change in heart rate (mean baseline heart rate from 15–30 min was subtracted at each time point) in captive European starlings exposed to either one or five intruders using the crowding protocol from Figure 4.7. Birds were held on a short-day photoperiod (SD) mimicking the time of year when starlings form flocks, and on a long-day photoperiod (LD) mimicking the time of year when starlings are territorial. The arrow indicates when the trap door was opened and the intruders entered the resident's cage.

Reprinted with permission from Dickens et al. (2006). Courtesy of University of Chicago.

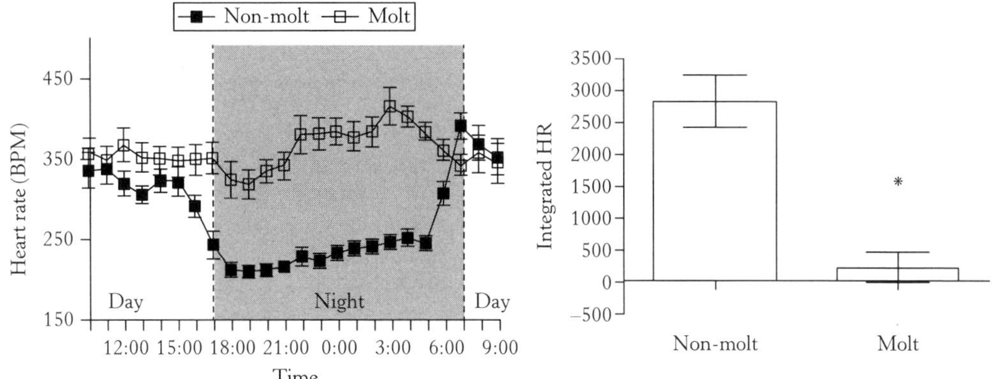

FIGURE 4.14: Changes in heart rate in molting captive European starlings. Left panel presents the daily pattern of resting heart rates in either molting or non-molting birds. Right panel presents the integrated heart rate during restraint stress administered during the day. Integrated heart rate indicates the change in heart rate over the 15 min of restraint and thus integrates both the magnitude of the peak response and the duration of the response. Note that there is essentially no increase in heart rate resulting from restraint during molt.

Reprinted with permission from Cyr et al. (2008). Courtesy of University of Chicago.

indicates that the heart rate response to restraint changed dramatically when the birds were molting. Although the birds responded to restraint with a robust increase in heart rate when not molting, molting birds essentially failed to increase their heart rates. The fight-or-flight response is clearly not activated in these birds during molt.

Although the above starling studies are only two examples, and in only one species, of how fight-or-flight responses might be modulated during different seasons and/or life-history stages, we think this is likely to be an exciting area for future research. The corticosteroid response is also modulated seasonally (see Chapter 10) and there is no reason to suspect that similar modulation is not occurring in sympathetic responses as well. If it does occur, determining how and when sympathetic responses are modulated should provide important insights into the survival benefits of the generalized fight-or-flight response. After all, the prevalence and severity of stressors likely changes throughout the year (as discussed by Nelson et al. 2002; Romero 2002), so it would make sense for animals to fine-tune their fight-or-flight responses in order to maximize effectiveness.

D. Heart Rate and Chronic Stress

Dysregulation of the sympathetic nervous system as a result of chronic stress has been known for decades. For example, long-term psychological stress at the workplace (Aboa-Eboule et al. 2007), as well as a number of other stressors (e.g., Cohen et al. 2007; McEwen et al. 1999), can lead to coronary heart disease in humans, and rank instability can change cardiac function in free-living baboons (Sapolsky and Share 1994). In fact, much of the work on heart rate variability has focused on the long-term changes in the sympathetic/parasympathetic balance in predicting coronary disease (e.g., Lucini et al. 2005). However, little work has been done on long-term changes in heart rate or catecholamine levels during chronic stress (reviewed by Bohus and Koolhaas 1993; Stanford 1993), and even less is known about potential changes in wild animals.

Laboratory experiments indicate a general decrease in the magnitude of heart rate elevations over time in response to a variety of stressors in many studies (reviewed by Bohus and Koolhaas 1993). For example, when mice were allowed aggressive interactions for 15 minutes per day for 15 days, both the dominants and subordinates increased heart rate during the encounter, but the magnitude of the heart rate response decreased over the 15 days (Bartolomucci et al. 2003). Although this decrease is often interpreted as animals habituating to the stressor, this might not be the case. There are significant decreases in the release of epinephrine, and to a lesser extent norepinephrine, during chronic stress (Dobrakovova et al. 1990; Dobrakovova et al. 1993), but this may result from the depletion of catecholamine stores (reviewed by Stanford 1993). If the capacity to release epinephrine and norepinephrine is decreased, the attenuated response over time likely reflects exhaustion of the system rather than habituation (see Chapter 3).

Other work, however, reports long-term increases in heart rate during chronic stress. Rats subjected to social defeat (Sgoifo et al. 2005) and highly social prairie voles subjected to social isolation (Grippo et al. 2007b) show increases in heart rate. Furthermore, in the prairie vole study there was a decrease in heart rate variability, indicating chronic sympathetic overstimulation. It also appears that the magnitude of the heart rate increase to an acute stressor is bigger for chronically stressed rats (Grippo et al. 2003; Grippo et al. 2006). These increases are likely supported by increased synthesis and storage of catecholamines during chronic stress, which is thought to allow the animal to respond appropriately to an unknown or more severe stressor if one is presented (McCarty and Stone 1983). It is currently unknown why some studies show increases and others decreases in heart rates during chronic stress, but there is some evidence that individual differences may play a role (Sgoifo et al. 2005).

It is not clear how relevant the data on laboratory rodents will be for other species or for free-living animals. An example is a study that measured heart rates for 1500 days in European rabbits maintained in outdoor enclosures (Eiserman 1992). The semi-natural conditions allowed the rabbits to develop typical dominance relationships, with some of the rabbits becoming dominant and others becoming subordinate. The presumed chronic stress of long-term subordinate status resulted in chronic increases in heart rate. Furthermore, the heart rate slowly returned to the level of the dominants if the dominant was removed, although the decrease took place gradually over a few weeks. These data match what is commonly believed to be the underlying mechanism for cardiac disease in humans and free-ranging baboons.

In contrast is some recent work on chronic stress in captive European starlings (Cyr et al. 2009; Kostelanetz et al. 2009). Daytime baseline heart rate increased during chronic stress without changes in heart rate variability (Figure 4.15), suggesting that the increased heart rate was not driven by increases in sympathetic activity. Instead, decreases in parasympathetic input appear to regulate this increase. Although the daytime increase in heart rate matches results from some of the mammalian laboratory studies, the presence of parasympathetic regulation is in contrast to many studies. These data also suggest caution in using increases in heart rate as an index of the fight-or-flight response. Increases could potentially indicate decreased parasympathetic rather than elevated sympathetic activity. Figure 4.15 also indicates that the increase in daytime baseline heart rate recovers quickly when the chronic stress ends.

The increase in baseline heart rate during the day, however, is only part of the story. Figure 4.16 shows that baseline heart rate measured in

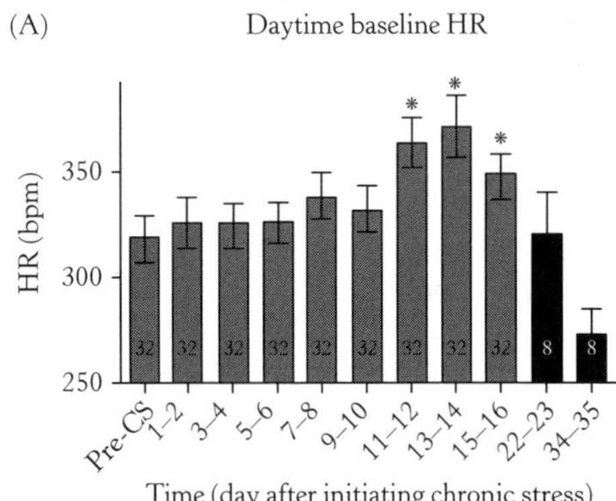

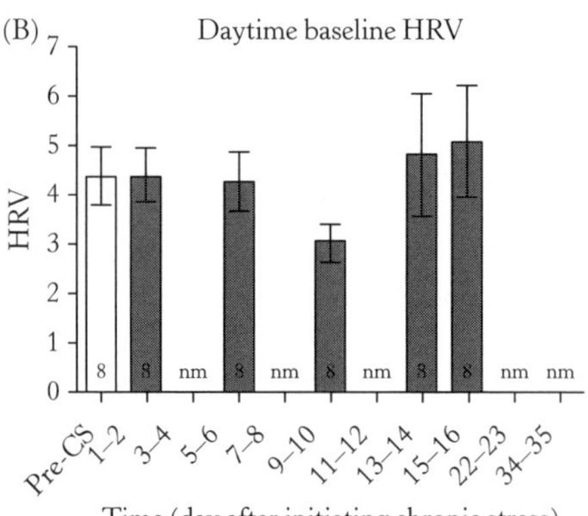

FIGURE 4.15: The change in daytime baseline heart rate (A) and heart rate variability (B) due to chronic stress in European starlings. Chronic stress was induced by applying four different mild psychological stressors per day in a random and rotated sequence for 16 days. Pre-CS stands for prechronic stress and last two bars are following the end of the chronic stress period. Half the birds were measured on each day, so the full data are grouped in two-day increments. Sample sizes are included in each bar, and asterisks indicate significant differences from prechronic stress levels.

Nm = not measured.

Reprinted with permission from Cyr et al. (2009). Courtesy of University of Chicago.

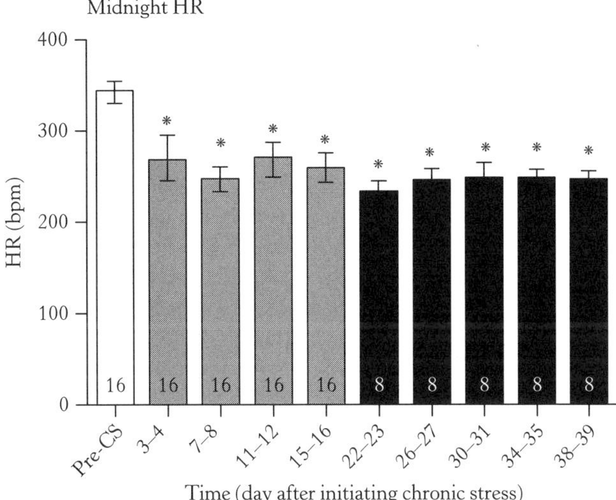

FIGURE 4.16: The change in nighttime baseline heart rate due to chronic stress in European starlings. See caption of Figure 4.15 for details.

Reprinted with permission from Cyr et al. (2009). Courtesy of University of Chicago.

the middle of the night decreases rather than increases. It is not clear why baseline heart rate should be lower at night. One possibility is that, because of the connection between heart rate and energy expenditure, the decrease in heart rate at night compensates for the increase occurring during the day. In effect, the animal is attempting to balance its daily energy budget. Balancing the energy expended when responding to the acute stressors comprising the chronic stress period could also explain why the nighttime decrease occurs much earlier than the daytime increase. Interestingly, the decrease at night appears to be a profound change; it does not recover for many weeks after the end of the chronic stress period and may indicate a long-term change in physiology.

Perhaps the most exciting result from this study is that the starling's ability to respond to restraint was greatly diminished after day 11 of the chronic stress period, although this change recovers quickly (Figure 4.17). This is not simply

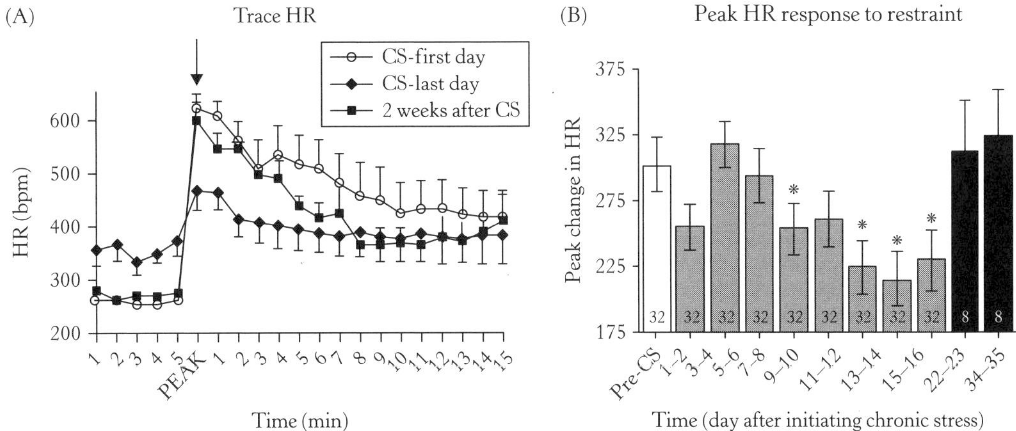

FIGURE 4.17: Chronic stress-induced changes in heart rate responses to acute restraint stress in European starlings. Individual traces at three points during the chronic stress period are in (A) and changes in the peak heart rate response throughout the chronic stress period are in (B). See caption of Figure 4.15 for details.

Reprinted with permission from Cyr et al. (2009). Courtesy of University of Chicago.

a result of a higher baseline heart rate during chronic stress, although that magnifies the lack of a heart rate response. It appears, therefore, that the entire fight-or-flight response is down-regulated during chronic stress. This could have tremendous fitness implications since an appropriate fight-or-flight response is likely to be necessary to survive stressors in the wild. These data suggest that any chronic stress, be it natural or anthropogenic, will greatly impact an animal's potential survival.

E. Conclusions on Heart Rate

Monitoring responses of the sympathetic nervous system and the fight-or-flight response is difficult, but measuring changes in heart rate has considerable promise. There have been a number of studies in wild animals under captive conditions, and it is beginning to be used in the field. Currently there are few options for field studies because there are no commercially available transmitters, but that is likely to change. Current studies have all used custom transmitters. Furthermore, the miniaturization of electronics promises to provide transmitters that can be used on smaller animals, thus expanding the species available for potential studies. We feel that these studies will be very important. The vast majority of studies to date on stress responses in wild animals have focused on the glucocorticoid arm of the stress response. The fight-or-flight response is likely to play a critical role in survival and fitness, and yet our understanding of how and when it is initiated, regulated, and modulated in free-living animals is rudimentary at best.

III. THE GLUCOCORTICOID RESPONSE

Chapter 2 detailed the pathways to corticosteroid secretion, how corticosteroids travel to their target tissues, and, once they reach their targets, how they elicit changes in target cell function. The next, and probably most important, question is, what changes do corticosteroids stimulate? At the mechanistic level, an enormous amount of information is known. For example, we know that in tissue X genes A and B are turned on, in tissue Y genes A and C are turned on, and so forth. What has become clear is that the question of what changes corticosteroids stimulate has multiple answers that depend upon the stimulus, the tissue type, the receptors involved, the context of the cellular milieu, and so on. Unfortunately, forming a coherent picture of corticosteroid function that integrates all these molecular and cellular mechanisms has proven difficult. To use an analogy, if we asked, what does insulin do? we would be able to provide a basic response. Although there are of course many subtleties and exceptions, our answer would be some version of the following: insulin helps regulate both blood glucose levels and cellular glucose uptake in order to regulate the flow of energy throughout the body. In other words, we can put the molecular and cellular functions of insulin into a broader physiological context. A similar answer for the corticosteroids, however, has proven far more elusive. At the physiological (i.e., whole-organism) level, it is far more difficult to answer the question, what do glucocorticoids do?

A. Physiological Roles of Glucocorticoids

A review by Sapolsky et al. (2000) attempted to place the myriad corticosteroid effects into a physiological context. They pointed out that classically three roles have been assigned to the corticosteroids, and went on to propose a fourth. The first, and historically oldest, role was that of a positive mediator of the stress response. Selye (1946) originally conceived of corticosteroids as having a direct stimulatory role in successfully coping with an acute stressor. In his view, corticosteroids help orchestrate a common organismal-level response to stressors. An example would be the corticosteroid-induced rapid mobilization of energy substrates that occurs in response to many stressors (reviewed in Sapolsky et al. 2000). However, a stimulatory role for corticosteroids failed to distinguish between those effects that take place at elevated corticosteroid concentrations from those that take place at basal concentrations. It quickly became clear that low (often called maintenance) concentrations of corticosteroids (levels A and B, predictive homeostasis; see Chapter 3) make other stress-response systems work better, such as helping sustain increased cardiovascular function (Ingle 1952). Corticosteroid concentrations at these low levels were not part of the acute stress response themselves, but instead played a permissive role. In essence, these low concentrations help prime many elements of the first wave of the stress response (i.e. the fight-or-flight response; see Chapter 2 and previous section) so that the animal will be prepared for upcoming stressors.

In hindsight, the dichotomy between stimulatory and permissive corticosteroid effects can be explained easily by the two-receptor system. Permissive effects are generally activated at basal concentrations by the Type I (MR) receptor, whereas stimulatory effects are generally activated at stress-induced concentrations by the Type II (GR) receptor (Dallman and Bhatnagar 2001; Sapolsky et al. 2000). Therefore, basal and stress-induced concentrations of corticosteroids have completely different physiological and behavioral effects and might even be thought of as reflecting two complementary hormonal systems. This has important implications for studying stress under field conditions. Changes in corticosteroid concentrations that remain in the basal range (level A, or predictive homeostasis of Chapter 3) are likely to reflect changes in the permissive actions, whereas changes in concentrations that extend above the basal range are likely to reflect changes in stimulatory, inhibitory, or preparative actions (levels A–B, reactive homeostasis in Chapter 3).

There are other changes initiated by corticosteroids that do not fit into either a stimulatory or a permissive role. There is compelling evidence that, in some cases, corticosteroids actually turn off aspects of the stress response once the acute stressor has been successfully dealt with (Munck et al. 1984). Powerful evidence for this role came from clinical studies showing that corticosteroids were potent inhibitors of the immune system. In fact, this is a major reason that corticosteroids are so important in clinical medicine. In a very influential review, Munck et al. (1984) proposed that corticosteroids are not actually part of the stress response, as Selye suggested, but instead serve as the brake to the stress response. They emphasized that the stress response unleashed powerful physiological forces that, if unchecked, would themselves threaten homeostasis. In a wonderful analogy (published many years earlier but unbeknownst to Munck et al.), a stressor was likened to a fire, the stress response was compared to the fire department's use of water hoses to put out the fire, and glucocorticoids' actions were related to turning off the water at the end to minimize water damage (Tausk 1951 as cited by Sapolsky et al. 2000).

Finally, most of the researchers interested in glucocorticoid physiology were studying it from the perspective of human health. They then chose their animal models to reflect human conditions. Consequently, researchers applied acute stressors such as 30 minutes of handling and restraint, hypoglycemia induced by exogenous insulin injection, electric shock, and so on (Dallman and Bhatnagar 2001). Although these stressors were chosen for their presumed clinical relevance, it was unclear how they related to the stressors experienced by wild freely behaving animals (e.g., Wingfield et al. 1998). Sapolsky et al. (2000) proposed that the "prototypical" stressor (i.e., the stressor that natural selection sculpted the stress response to be able to survive) was a predator attack. Although this proposal is a bit simplistic in that it ignores many other common stressors for free-living animals (see Chapter 1), the use of a predator attack by Sapolsky et al. highlighted another problem for Selye's original idea that the corticosteroids help stimulate the stress response—the time course is all wrong. Since most of the classic functions of glucocorticoids are mediated by Type I and Type II receptors, the expression of these functions must await the new protein produced by these transcription factors (see discussion on receptors in Chapter 2). Consequently, corticosteroid actions generally take 30–60 minutes or so to become manifest (Haller et al. 2008). Clearly, this is far too slow to help in surviving a typical predator attack, which may be over in seconds, but corticosteroid actions would help the individual to adjust to social changes precipitated by losing a member of a social group to the predator, or to adjust to the potential of further attacks in the immediate future.

This slow time course led Sapolsky et al. (2000) to propose that the fourth major physiological function of corticosteroids is preparative. They argued that the occurrence of a stressor often predicts the onset of a subsequent stressor (e.g., an injury sustained in escaping from a predator targets the animal for further predator attacks). Corticosteroids function to prepare the animal for these future stressors. Examples would be shifting energy usage from long-term physiological processes (e.g., reproduction, digestion) in order to mobilize glucose to replace the glycogen used in escaping from the predator, replenishing the catecholamines to aid in mounting another fight-or-flight response, inhibiting inflammation to hide injuries from other predators, and so on. Note that these functions are not helping the animal escape and so cannot be interpreted as helping mediate the stress response, nor are they inhibitory since these functions are clearly not shutting off the stress response. Although they might be thought of as permissive in that they will help other aspects of the stress response work better, perhaps the best interpretation is that they are helping the animal recover from the initial stress response and are preparing the system for a potential repeat performance.

In fact, Sapolsky et al. (2000) proposed that corticosteroids perform all four functions:

stimulatory, permissive, inhibitory, and preparative. They illustrated how all four functions could fit into a coherent physiology with the following analogy:

> In response to the stressor of an invading army, an immediate response would be to shoot at the enemy; this is akin to the actions of the first wave of stress-responsive hormones (catecholamines, CRH, etc.). Among actions that would modulate this response, permissive actions would be those already in place at time of the attack, such as setting up defenses. Stimulating actions enhance the response and are undertaken after the attack, e.g., calling up active combatants from reserves. Suppressive actions, which constrain defense responses, might include calling off an attack to avoid self-destructive friendly fire (friendly fire being an example of defensive "overshoot," akin to autoimmunity). Preparative actions would be, for example, to institute rationing, an action designed not to repel the invader but to set up long-term measures for survival should the conflict continue, or enhance responsiveness to the next invasion (such as designing better systems for detection). (Sapolsky et al. 2000)

Clearly, corticosteroids could have all four functions and thereby orchestrate the stress response of each physiological system reacting to the stressor. For example, corticosteroids could prime the immune system to function better during a stress response (permissive effect), activate the immune system immediately after a stressor (stimulatory effect), inhibit the immune system if the stressor continues to avoid autoimmune problems (inhibitory effect), and inhibit inflammation to hide injuries from potential predators (preparative effect) (Sapolsky et al. 2000). The dominant function depends upon the physiological or behavioral system. For example, acute increases in corticosteroids seem to serve primarily permissive and stimulatory roles in metabolism and behavior, but primarily suppressive roles in the immune system (Sapolsky et al. 2000).

Preparative actions of corticosteroids are not necessarily dependent upon an earlier stressor, and in some cases, might be equivalent to permissive actions. For instance, if an animal could predict that they were more likely to be stressed in the future, even if they were not stressed at that time, they still might increase corticosteroids in order to prepare for the eventuality of that stressor. One of us (LMR) proposed this rationale to explain why corticosteroid concentrations vary seasonally in many species (Romero 2002). Animals might increase their corticosteroids at those times of the year when they are most likely to be exposed to stressors (e.g., when more prone to predation during breeding). This would better prepare them to survive those predation attempts. To expand on the Sapolsky et al. (2000) analogy, what might be the response of a nation if its neighbor started to build its army, even if there was no overt aggression? A prudent nation would start to invest in its military as well. We would argue that this nation has not yet been stressed (no actual attack has either occurred or been threatened), yet it is preparing for that eventuality nonetheless. Similarly, an animal might increase its corticosteroid concentrations in order to prepare for a higher likelihood of stressors, and yet that increase in corticosteroids is not part of a stress response. This has long been the argument to explain why corticosteroids vary in a circadian cycle, with the peak occurring just prior to the beginning of the active period (Dallman and Bhatnagar 2001).

Note that these arguments are different from the allostasis model, which suggests that baseline levels of corticosteroids change according to the allostatic load that an individual experiences during daily routines and across seasons. For example, energetic costs of reproduction, migration, and so on, are greater, resulting in higher allostatic loads that are matched by baseline glucocorticoids (see Chapter 3). However, the allostatic load model (McEwen and Wingfield 2003) predictions are not mutually exclusive from those of preparative changes of baseline glucocorticoids by Sapolsky et al. (2000) and Romero (2002). A combination of field investigations and controlled laboratory "common garden" experiments will indicate to what extent allostatic load and/or preparative functions contribute to changes in baseline glucocorticoids.

B. Acute versus Chronic Corticosteroid Release

The presumed benefits of an acute activation of the HPA axis contrasts with chronic activation. Various deleterious effects of chronic corticosteroid elevation have been documented in many species: suppression of reproductive function and behavior, immune system suppression, muscle wasting, growth suppression, and neuronal cell damage (Sapolsky et al. 2000; Wingfield et al. 1997). Therefore, animals, especially endangered species and captive, domesticated, or hospitalized animals, must avoid chronic stress situations if they are to remain healthy.

In general (but see discussion later in this chapter), chronic activation of the HPA axis occurs when the animal is subjected to a long-term stressor (lasting weeks to months) or a series of repeated mild stressors. The more intense the stressor, the greater the amount of corticosteroid released (Dallman et al. 1987) and the greater the impact. For an acute stressor, corticosteroids return to baseline concentrations once the stimulus ends. If the stressor persists or occurs at regular frequent intervals (i.e., becomes chronic), the entire functioning of the HPA axis changes. The animal may start to show chronic elevations in baseline corticosteroid concentrations that quickly lead to the deleterious effects mentioned earlier. Furthermore, chronic stress is known to decrease CBG concentrations in the blood (Breuner and Orchinik 2002), thereby altering corticosteroid concentrations available to the tissues. Studies of chronically stressed rats, however, indicate that multiple and chronic stressors interact in unpredictable ways to alter corticosteroid release (Dallman et al. 1992). The two primary changes are acclimation and facilitation.

With acclimation, the animal no longer responds in the same robust manner to repeated or chronic stressors. In effect, the psychological context of the stressor has changed, and the animal no longer perceives the stressor to be as noxious. For example, after two weeks of being handled several times a day, the corticosteroid response of adult rats to handling is significantly reduced compared to their initial response (Dobrakova and Kvetnansky 1993). Repeated exposures acclimate these rats to the handling stressor and result in the identical stressor eliciting very different responses. Acclimation, therefore, results in lower corticosteroid responses.

The acclimation process, however, alters HPA axis physiology such that corticosteroid responses to novel stressors are enhanced compared to responses of non-acclimated animals (Bhatnagar and Vining 2003; Dallman and Bhatnagar 2001). This process is called facilitation. In the preceding example, if rats exposed to repeated handling are transferred to a novel environment, or even are handled by a new person, their corticosteroid response is higher than in naïve controls (Dobrakova and Kvetnansky 1993). The acclimation process has primed the animals to have an enhanced response to a different stressor.

Acclimation and facilitation do not occur for all stressors, especially those that are relatively severe (Dallman and Bhatnagar 2001). For relatively severe stressors, corticosteroid responses either do not change over time (no acclimation), become chronically elevated (no acclimation), or there is chronically diminished functioning of the entire HPA axis (no acclimation or facilitation). In the last case, the HPA axis shuts down and becomes incapable of mounting an appropriate response. This results, over time, in lower endogenous baseline corticosteroids, lower or nonexistent endogenous stress-induced corticosteroids, and, most important, lower corticosteroid receptor numbers (Sapolsky 1992). Unfortunately, we are not able at this time to predict which HPA axis response will be manifested during chronic stress.

Facilitation and acclimation can be confounding factors in field studies. The recent experience of an animal is important in determining whether facilitation or acclimation might be occurring, but it can be difficult to obtain. For example, corticosteroid responses to capture and handling will be different in animals chased by predators an hour before capture than in animals quietly foraging before capture (Silverin 1998a). Traditionally, researchers have assumed that most captured animals were unstressed before capture and that any animals that were stressed were distributed evenly among treatment groups (i.e., no systematic bias) so that statistics diluted any potential problems.

Although it is widely assumed that prolonged elevated corticosteroid concentrations indicate chronically stressed individuals (Wingfield et al. 1997), our laboratory data suggest just the opposite. Most "stressed" populations in the wild, however, have been identified as such on the basis of elevated corticosteroid titers, in the context of perturbations of the environment such as inclement weather (Romero et al. 2000), food supply (Romero and Wikelski 2001), the presence of predators, and so on (e.g., Clinchy et al. 2004). But it is not entirely clear whether these situations in the field represent "chronic stress" or are just a manifestation of increased allostatic load but are not sufficient to induce allostatic overload. Laboratory experiments can tease apart possible chronic stress scenarios (e.g., Busch et al. 2008a; Busch et al. 2008b) in which 2–3 physiological doses of corticosteroids per day were sufficient to result in symptoms of chronic stress, suggesting that repeated acute stressors in the field might be interpreted as chronic.

C. Sex Differences

In many species, males and females release different amounts of corticosteroids, both at basal concentrations and in response to stressors. In other words, the HPA axis is sexually differentiated (Levine 2002). For species studied in the laboratory, especially laboratory rodents, females have elevated corticosteroids compared to males. One apparent mechanism is that testosterone inhibits HPA axis function (e.g., Viau et al. 2001), but estrogens also can have an effect. Both basal and stress-induced corticosteroid concentrations vary over the rat estrous cycle (Viau and Meaney 1991). The organizing effects of gonadal steroids are even further implicated because the male-female differences become more apparent after puberty. During puberty, testosterone appears to reorganize HPA axis function, primarily by altering CRF gene regulation in the hypothalamus (e.g., Viau et al. 2005). Consequently, the interplay between the HPA axis and gonadal steroids, especially testosterone, may provide the mechanism underlying sexual differentiation of the HPA axis.

Although the evidence for sex differences in the laboratory is fairly clear, the evidence for sex differences in free-living animals is far more complex. There are often seasonal changes in male-female differences (Romero 2002). In many avian species the sexes have identical corticosterone concentrations outside the breeding season, but the females have lower concentrations than males when breeding (see Chapter 10). This response has been proposed as a mechanism to prevent elevated corticosterone from interfering with breeding (Wingfield 1994). In polyandrous arctic shorebirds (O'Reilly and Wingfield 2001), males provide most, if not all, parental care, and they tend to have lower baseline corticosterone levels than females. In species in which parental duties are split equally, then corticosterone titers tend to be similar (O'Reilly and Wingfield 2001). Understanding why sex differences develop, both at the evolutionary and mechanistic levels, is likely to be important for connecting corticosteroid function with life-history changes. Substantial progress has been made to answer this question at the evolutionary level (see Chapter 10), but to our knowledge, work at the mechanistic level, comparable to what is known for laboratory rodents, has not been attempted.

D. Facultative Behavioral and Physiological Actions

Sapolsky et al. (2000) have provided us with a framework for how to make physiological sense of corticosteroid effects at the organismal level, and application of this framework to diverse taxa in different habitats will be most informative. Typically, reproduction can be interrupted while the individual responds to an environmental perturbation, but the reproductive system remains in a near functional state so that breeding can begin again once the perturbation passes (see Wingfield 1988, 1994). For example, direct labile perturbation factors (LPFs; see Chapter 1) trigger facultative behavioral and physiological responses (ELHS) that appear to be mediated by increases in corticosteroid secretion (Wingfield et al. 1998). There are several components to the ELHS (Wingfield and Ramenofsky 1997, 1999), as follows (see also Chapter 1):

1. Deactivation of the current life-history stage (e.g., territorial behavior, abandonment of current nesting effort).
2. Active response to the LPF. There are two, possibly three options here:
   (a) movements away from the source of the LPF ("leave it" strategy);
   (b) if the individual remains, it will seek a refuge ("take it" strategy);
   (c) seek a refuge first and then move away if conditions do not improve ("take it" at first and then "leave it").
3. Mobilization of stored energy sources such as fat and perhaps protein to fuel the movement, or to provide energy while sheltering in a refuge.
4. Continued movement until suitable habitat is discovered or the perturbation passes.
   Settlement in alternate habitat once an appropriate site is identified, or a return to the original site and resumption of the normal sequence of life-history stages.
5. Recovery of body condition after depletion during the perturbation.

In recent years there have been numerous investigations on the hormonal bases of these facultative behavioral and physiological responses to LPFs, especially in relation to the ecology of animals in their natural environment (Silverin 1997, 1998a, 1998b; Silverin and Wingfield 1998; Wingfield et al. 1998; see later chapters of this volume). It is also clear that the HPA axis plays a major role in concert with central actions of several peptides (reviewed in Wingfield et al. 1998). In fact, the ELHS fits nicely into the stimulating (steps 1–4 above) and the preparative (step 5) actions of corticosteroids. The ELHS can be triggered at any time of year and from any life-history stage (see Chapter 1) and the process involved can occur at all times of year in most species. Immediate responses to LPFs (e.g., the fight-or-flight responses to predators), result in immediate avoidance behavior and possibly an increase in corticosteroids within a few minutes. These responses are generally too short-lived to activate an ELHS (Wingfield and Ramenofsky 1997). In contrast, a longer term LPF (e.g., inclement weather, human disturbance, etc.) may not affect the nest and young directly but can decrease available food, temperature, and so on. As a result, adults may experience allostatic overload. This is a *direct* effect of LPFs that trigger the ELHS via increased secretion of corticosteroids (Wingfield and Ramenofsky 1997; Wingfield et al. 1998). The ELHS is temporary (hours to days), and once the perturbation passes the individual will return to the same life-history stage, or the next if the ELHS was long in duration (Wingfield et al. 1998). This is an intriguing possibility because it appears that the timing mechanisms for expression of life-history stages over the year continue even if that life-history stage is interrupted by a direct LPF and expression of the ELHS.

E. Rapid Recovery after an Indirect Labile Perturbation Factor

Resumption of the normal life-history stage after an indirect LPF represents a recovery component of the overall responses to environmental perturbations. For example, breeding pairs of birds that have lost the nest and young to a storm or predator frequently will renest. Loss of the nest is a considerable disruption to the normal temporal progression of the breeding season. Major reorganization of endocrine function and expression of substages is necessary to coordinate the renest attempt. Because an indirect LPF and the fight-or-flight response can be over very quickly, within minutes, then it is unlikely that an ELHS will be triggered. Thus individuals should return to their normal life-history stage immediately with no prolonged elevation of blood corticosteroids.

In the high-latitude-breeding Gambel's white-crowned sparrow, luteinizing hormone (LH), testosterone, and testis mass increased dramatically after loss of the nest, coincident with elevated LH and estrogens in females, leading to production of a replacement clutch of eggs (Wingfield and Farner 1979). Similarly, in female mallards, after experimental removal of the eggs (Donham et al. 1976), there were rapid increases in reproductive hormones just prior to renesting. It is important to note that in white-crowned sparrows there were also increased concentrations of testosterone when producing a replacement clutch. This is unlike multiple brooding after *successfully* raising young and suggests that different mechanisms may initiate a second clutch in these two ecological contexts (Wingfield and Farner 1993; Wingfield and Moore 1987).

This type of response is interesting because an LPF briefly disrupts a normal life-history stage (breeding) and, except for a brief fight-or-flight response to the predator or event that destroyed the nest, the adult birds involved are no longer stressed per se but must resume breeding as soon as possible. Note that circulating concentrations of testosterone rise when renesting, but not during the egg-laying period of a normal second brood (Wingfield and Farner 1979). Why would this happen? High levels of testosterone, accompanied by increased territorial and "mate-guarding" aggression, are well known and there is considerable evidence that they can interfere with male parental behavior in many socially monogamous species (Hegner and Wingfield 1987; Silverin 1980; Wingfield et al. 1990), resulting in reduced reproductive success (Beletsky et al. 1995; Ketterson et al. 1996). If male birds feed fledglings from the first brood to independence, their chances of survival are greater than for young from later broods (e.g., Perrins 1970), and this may outweigh the advantages of mate-guarding the female to ensure paternity of later clutches. On the other hand, if the eggs or young are lost, an increase of LH and testosterone secretion enhancing aggression in relation to mate-guarding in turn would lead to protection of paternity of the replacement clutch (Wingfield and Moore 1987). These explanations have been examined further in the field (Goymann et al. 2004; Lynn et al. 2005).

Once again, renesting after loss of a clutch or brood to an indirect LPF should not result in a change in corticosteroid release. To test this prediction, blood samples were collected from free-living male and female white-crowned sparrows that lost nests to predators in central Alaska (Wingfield and Farner 1979). In both sexes, plasma levels of corticosterone were similar during the first clutch and when renesting (Figure 4.18). Essentially identical results were obtained experimentally in free-living song sparrows (Wingfield et al. 1989).

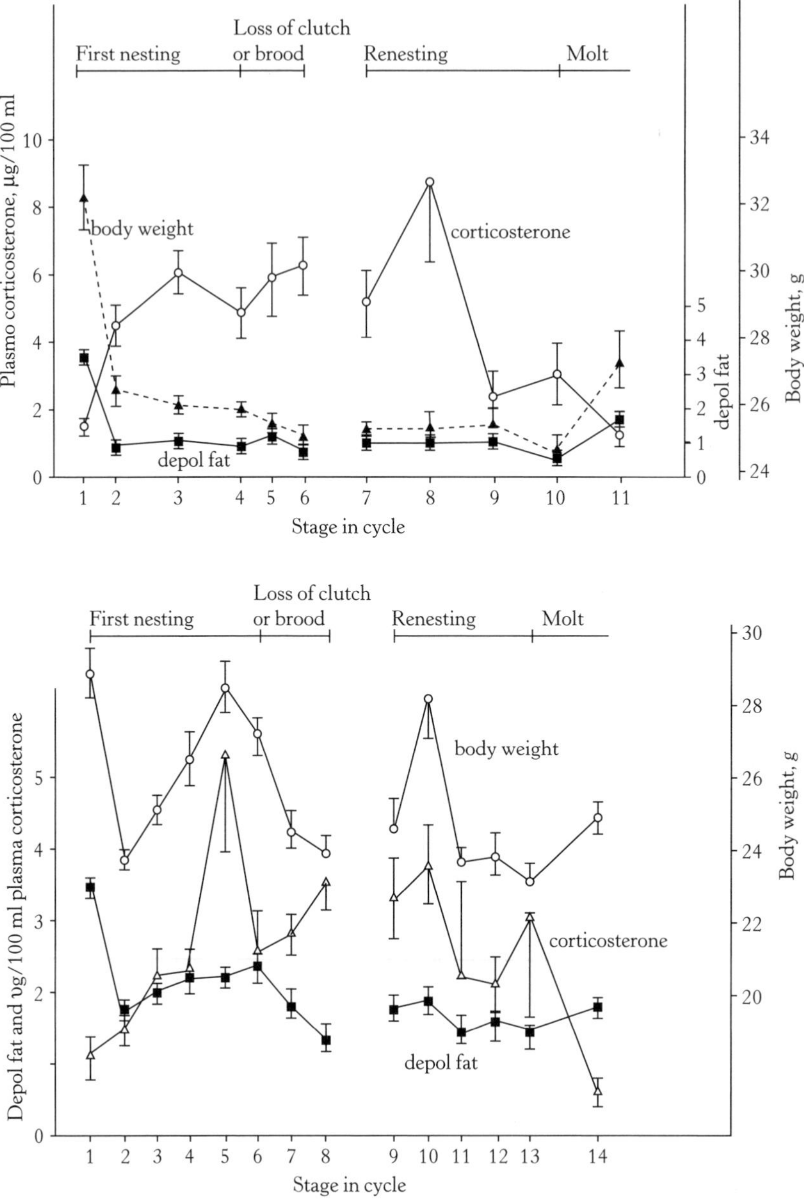

FIGURE 4.18: Changes in body weight, depot fat, and plasma levels of corticosterone during renesting in free-living male (top panel) and female (bottom panel) Gambel's white-crowned sparrows. Data are arranged as to substage in the breeding cycle and spaced in time according to the average interval required for courtship, egg-laying, incubation, etc., (indicated by horizontal lines at the top of each panel; males top panel and females bottom panel). Stages 3 and 5 represent egg-laying time for the first clutch in males and females, respectively. Stages 7 and 9 represent renesting in males and females, respectively. There are no differences in corticosterone titers between laying for the first clutch and renesting in ether males or females as predicted for a response to an indirect labile perturbation factor. From Wingfield and Farner (1979). Courtesy of Elsevier.

F. Allostatic Load, Reactive Scope, and Glucocorticoid Responses to LPFs

To build on earlier summaries in this chapter, (see Figure 4.1), it is useful to integrate further components of the classic stress response with the models of stress outlined in Chapter 3. The relationships among energetic demand (allostatic load), available energy (Eg), and corticosteroid levels (i.e., its reactive scope) in the promotion of physiological states are modeled in Figure 4.19

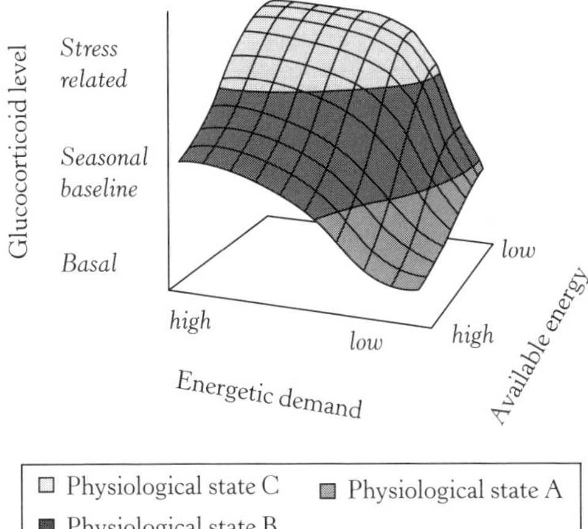

FIGURE 4.19: Relationship between energetic demand (allostatic load), available energy, and glucocorticoid level in the promotion of physiological states. Energetic demand can change with daily activity patterns or with life-history stage, and may also increase as a consequence of challenging perturbations in the environment. Although animals respond to energetic demand by secreting corticosteroids, this response may be attenuated by high energy availability (i.e., abundant food resources and/or internal energy depots). For example, even when energy demand is high, animals that have access to sufficient energy stores may remain within the reaction norm for a particular life-history stage and may not increase plasma corticosteroids above a seasonal baseline. Within seasonal baseline levels, corticosteroids may promote processes representative of physiological state B (predictive homeostasis). However, as energy stores become depleted, corticosteroids may increase to level C, reactive homeostasis, concentrations at which point they support increasingly complex physiological states to allow an individual to cope.

From Landys et al. (2006). Courtesy of Elsevier.

(from Landys et al. 2006). Note that the physiological states (levels A, B, and C) are indicated by shading. These levels are also compatible with the levels of reactive scope (predictive homeostasis and reactive homeostasis; see Chapter 3). Energetic demand changes with daily activity patterns or with life-history stage (Ee + Ei, levels A and B), and can also increase as a consequence of challenging perturbations in the environment (Eo, levels B to C). Although animals respond to energetic demand by secreting glucocorticoids, this response may be attenuated by high energy availability (i.e., abundant food resources and/or internal energy depots [Eg]). For example, even when energy demand is high, animals that have access to sufficient energy stores may remain within the reaction norm for a particular life-history stage and may not increase plasma glucocorticoids above a seasonal baseline (levels A + B). Within seasonal baseline levels, glucocorticoids may promote processes representative of physiological state B (predictive homeostasis). However, as energy stores become unavailable, glucocorticoids may increase to level C concentrations (allostatic or homeostatic overload), at which point they support increasingly complex physiological states to allow an individual to cope (Figure 4.19; Landys et al. 2006).

We can now revisit Figure 2.19, considering all types of glucocorticoid receptors and how they might be important as glucocorticoid levels transition through these state levels. Hypothetical binding curves of the three known adrenal steroid receptors—the genomic mineralocorticoid receptor (MR, type 1 in Figure 2.19), the genomic glucocorticoid receptor (GR, type 2 in Figure 2.19), and the non-genomic, membrane-associated glucocorticoid receptor (mGR)—are shown in Figure 4.20. The MR binds glucocorticoids with a higher affinity than does the GR. At least in birds, the mGR displays the lowest affinity for glucocorticoids (Breuner and Orchinik 2001). These in vitro receptor properties suggest that low glucocorticoid concentrations primarily bind the MR, whereas elevated levels bind the GR and begin to bind the mGR. Thus, differences in the proportion of bound receptor types may provide a mechanism whereby different glucocorticoid concentrations are able to produce specific physiological states. Low glucocorticoid levels that predominantly activate the MR may promote physiological state A (predictive homeostasis). Seasonal elevations in plasma glucocorticoids may support physiological state B through partial binding to the GR and the mGR. As glucocorticoids increase above the seasonal baseline, increased binding of all three receptor types may stimulate the physiological state C (reactive homeostasis, Figure 4.20; from Landys et al. 2006).

Corticosteroid levels can vary as a consequence of allostatic load spanning the reactive scope for this hormone (Figure 4.21; Landys et al. 2006). Receptor number may show seasonal or circadian variation. For example, house sparrows display a greater GR population in the brain during nesting and molt than during winter (Breuner and Orchinik 2001). Thus, receptor number may mediate the ability of plasma corticosteroids to affect behavior and physiology (pers. comm. Todd Sperry). Basic life processes typical of

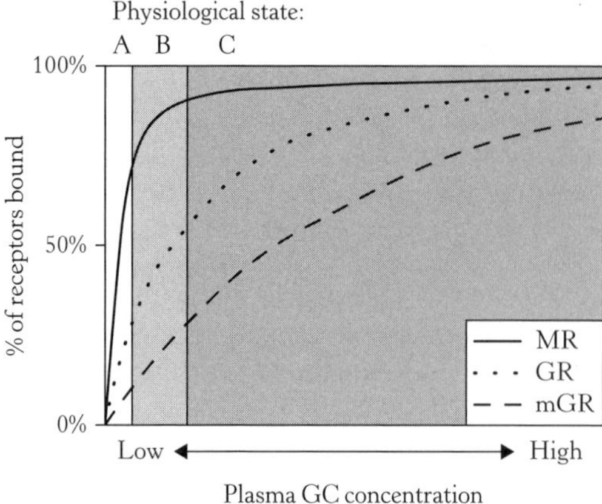

FIGURE 4.20: Hypothetical binding curves of the three known adrenal steroid receptors: the genomic mineralocorticoid receptor (MR, type 1), the genomic glucocorticoid receptor (GR, type 2), and the non-genomic membrane-associated glucocorticoid receptor (mGR). The MR binds corticosteroids with a higher affinity than does the GR. At least in birds, the mGR displays the lowest affinity for corticosteroids (Breuner and Orchinik 2001). These in vitro receptor properties suggest that low corticosteroid concentrations primarily bind the MR, whereas elevated levels bind the GR and may begin to bind the mGR. Thus, differences in the proportion of bound receptor types may provide a mechanism whereby different corticosteroid concentrations are able to produce specific physiological states. Low corticosteroid levels that predominantly activate the MR may promote physiological state A. Seasonal elevations in plasma corticosteroids may support physiological state B through partial binding to the GR and the mGR. As corticosteroids increase above the seasonal baseline, increased binding of all three receptor types may stimulate the physiological state C. Note that physiological states A–B are roughly equivalent to predictive homeostasis of the reactive scope model and physiological states B–C, equivalent to reactive homeostasis (chapter 3, Romero et al. 2009).

From Landys et al. (2006). Courtesy of Elsevier.

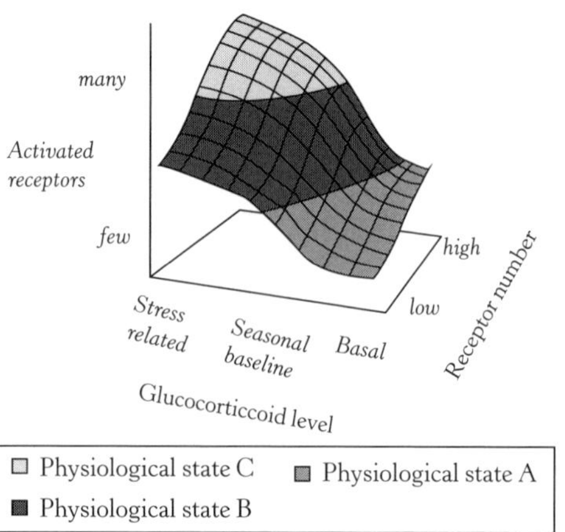

FIGURE 4.21: Effect of glucocorticoid (GC) level and GC receptor number on the formation of activated receptors. GC levels can vary as a consequence of allostatic load. Receptor number may show seasonal or circadian variation. For example, house sparrows display a greater glucocorticoid receptor (GR) population during nesting and molt than during winter (Breuner and Orchinik 2001). Thus, receptor number may mediate the ability of plasma GCs to affect behavior and physiology (pers. comm. T. Sperry). Basic life processes typical of physiological state A may be maintained by only a few activated receptors. As more receptors are activated, behavior and physiology appropriate for physiological state B may be induced. However, the activation of a large population of receptors may induce facultative responses typical of physiological state C. This figure is meant to address the effects of only one receptor type. Note that physiological states A–B are roughly equivalent to predictive homeostasis of the reactive scope model and physiological states B–C equivalent to reactive homeostasis (chapter 3, Romero et al. 2009).

From Landys et al. (2006). Courtesy of Elsevier.

physiological state A may be maintained by only a few activated receptors (Figure 4.21). As more receptors and receptor types are activated, behavior and physiology appropriate for physiological state B may be induced (predictive homeostasis). However, the activation of a large population of receptors of all types may induce facultative responses typical of physiological state C (reactive homeostasis). Note that although Figure 4.21 is meant to address the effects of only one receptor type, modeling all three receptor types (when affinity and capacity are known) with CBG levels and plasma concentrations of corticosteroids will be a challenge, but also highly informative. A combination of modeling and experiments with specific receptor agonists and antagonists will tease apart the cellular mechanisms of action (Landys et al. 2006).

G. Levels of Regulation

It is important here to reflect on the complexity of ways by which responses to environmental perturbations can be regulated. We have already discussed control of the HPA axis leading to secretion of corticosteroids, binding proteins in the blood (CBG) and receptor types and numbers in specific target cells. All these add up to three levels of regulation: secretion, transport, and target cell response (Figure 4.22; Wingfield et al. 2011a). Diverse pathways by which corticosteroids can act in a target cell depend upon the expression of steroidogenic enzymes that modulate how much corticosteroid encounters genomic receptors. There are two isozymes of 11β-hydroxysteroid dehydrogenase (11β-HSD) that play important roles in glucocorticoid metabolism (Holmes et al. 2001). Regulation of 11-βHSD activity involves two gene splices and may regulate local production of corticosteroids in neural tissue, immune system, and skin (i.e., extra-adrenal sources, Schmidt et al. 2008; Taves et al. 2011a; Taves et al. 2011b). Type 1 in vivo acts mostly as a reductase, regenerating active glucocorticoids from 11-ketosteroids. Type 2 acts to inactivate corticosteroids. For example, 11β-HSD knockout mice show signs of hypertension because of activation of MR receptor by corticosteroids in the absence of the protection from the type 2 enzyme (Holmes et al. 2001) and have reduced glucocorticoid-induced processes such as gluconeogenesis when fasting, as well as lower glucose levels in response to obesity or stress (Holmes et al. 2001). Thus it has been proposed that 11β-HSD 2 converts corticosterone to deoxycorticosterone, or cortisol to cortisone, neither of which bind with high affinity to any known corticosteroid receptor. As such, this enzyme can be regarded as a deactivation shunt. 11β-HSD 1 tends to have the opposite effect of enhancing corticosteroids and thus the likelihood of binding to MR or GR. It should be noted that these intracellular mechanisms will likely not affect binding to the membrane corticosteroid receptor unless these enzymes are secreted into the immediate extra-cellular space.

Exciting new evidence suggests that 5a-reductases in cells may also produce metabolites of corticosteroids that can bind to GR type 2 receptors. Two metabolites in particular, 5a-dihydrocortisol and 5a-terahydrocortisol, may have important effects in mammals (Nixon et al. 2012). Actions of such metabolites in other vertebrates and in relation to coping with environmental perturbations remain to be determined.

Co-repressors and co-activators are additional points of regulation for gene transcription

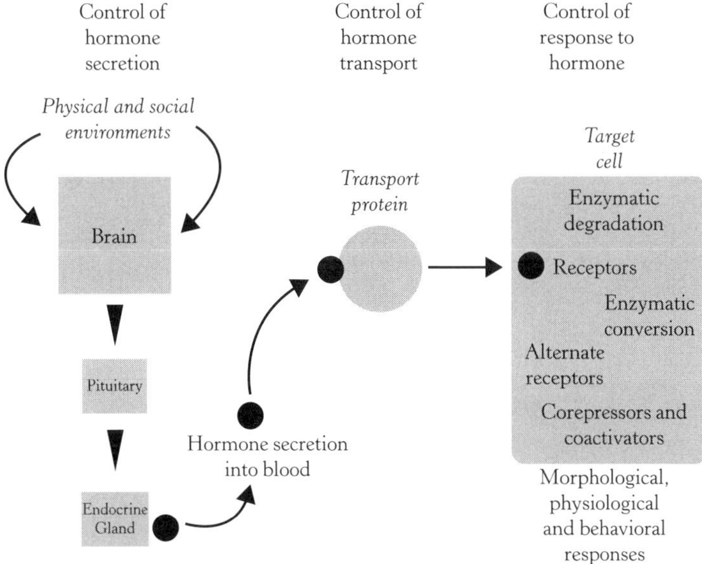

FIGURE 4.22: There are three components of the transduction response, which can be regulated in diverse ways. The left-hand part of the figure shows the perception-transduction-response system triggering the neural, neuroendocrine, and endocrine cascades that result in production of a highly specific signal: hormone secretion. The central part of the figure shows that after secretion into the blood, many hormones (particularly steroids, thyroid hormones, and some peptides) are transported by carrier proteins. Once the hormonal signal reaches the target cell (e.g., a neuron in the brain), it can act in various ways by binding to membrane or intracellular receptors that trigger extremely complex actions in a cell. Note that all three components are sites of regulation that could change daily or seasonally, or vary among individuals, populations, gender, or in response to unique experience of the environment.
From Wingfield et al. (2011a). Courtesy of the Chinese Academy of Sciences.

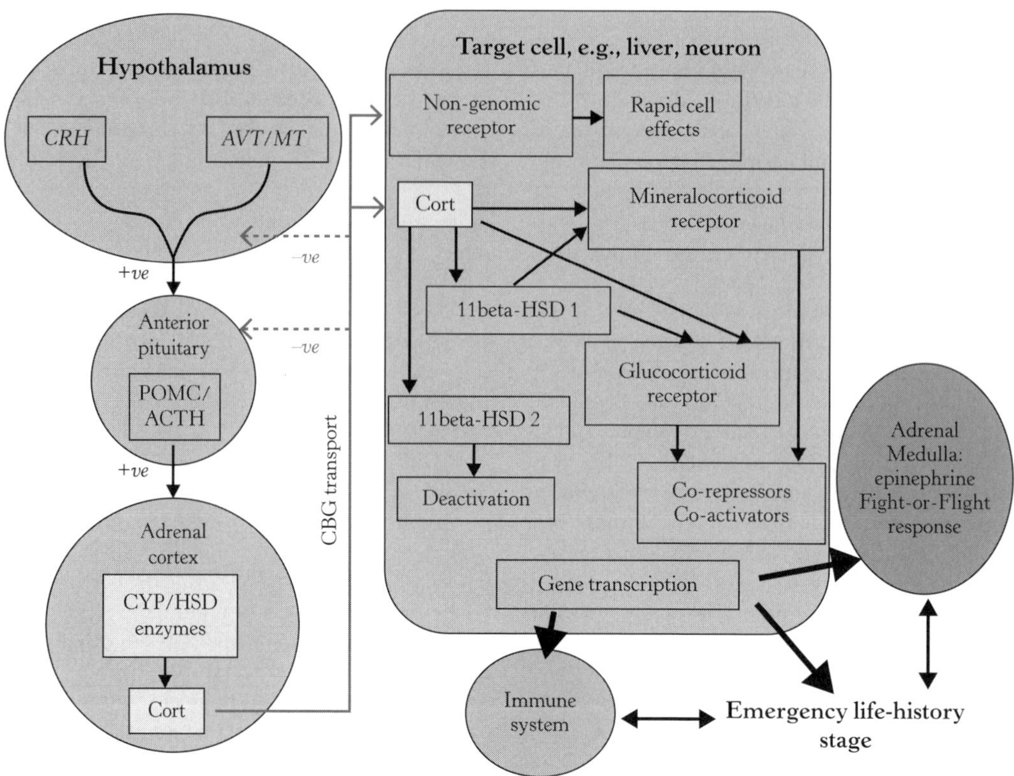

FIGURE 4.23: The three-part regulatory system of secretion control, transport, and hormone responses for the adrenocortical response to acute environmental perturbations that trigger an emergency life-history stage (ELHS). The left-hand part of the figure represents the hormone secretion cascade, in this case the hypothalamo-pituitary-adrenal cortex (HPA) axis. Perturbations of the environment are perceived by sensory modalities, and that information is transduced into neuropeptide secretions such as corticotropin-releasing hormone (CRH), and in birds, for example, arginine vasotocin (AVT) and mesotocin (MT) that regulate expression of a precursor or pro-peptide hormone, pro-opiomelanocortin (POMC), in the anterior pituitary. POMC can be then cleaved to give several peptides, including adrenocorticotropin (ACTH). Release of ACTH from the pituitary gland into the blood is also regulated by CRH and AVT. ACTH acts on adrenocortical cells to activate CYP enzymes, including hydroxysteroid dehydrogenases, that synthesize glucocorticoids such as corticosterone (Cort). Release of Cort into the blood is a major endpoint of the cascade of events that are part of the adrenocortical response to stress. Once in the blood, Cort circulates bound to a carrier protein corticosteroid-binding globulin (CBG), which is part of the transport part of the system (ash lines). Cort provides negative feedback signals for ACTH release from the pituitary as well as CRH release from the hypothalamus. More than 90% of Cort circulating in avian blood is bound by CBG. On reaching target cells, such as liver or neurons in the brain involved in the emergency life-history (coping) stage, it is thought that only Cort unbound to CBG can enter cells. Once inside the cell, there are two types of genomic receptor that can bind Cort and become gene transcription factors. The mineralocorticoid type 1 receptor (MR) binds with high affinity and so can be saturated at low levels of Cort. The glucocorticoid type 2 receptor (GR) has a lower affinity for Cort and is saturated only at higher concentrations of Cort. Thus GR has been proposed as the “stress” receptor. Note also that there is strong evidence for a membrane receptor (non-genomic) that mediates rapid behavioral effects within minutes. The genomic receptors have effects through gene transcription (different genes affected by each receptor type) and thus require up to several hours for biological effects to be manifest. There are also steroidogenic enzymes expressed in target cells that can modulate how much Cort encounters at least genomic receptors. 11β-hydroxysteroid-dehydrogenase (11β-HSD) has two major forms: 1 and 2. 11β-HSD 2 converts corticosterone to deoxycorticosterone, which cannot bind to any known Cort receptor and is a deactivation shunt. 11β-HSD 1 tends to have the opposite effect, enhancing Cort and thus the likelihood of binding to MR or GR. Co-repressors and co-activators also are points of regulation for gene transcription and responses that control the emergency life-history stage and affect the immune system. The adrenal medulla of mammals (medullary cells in birds are called chromaffin) is a key component of the fight-or-flight response (right-hand part of the figure), secreting epinephrine. This neuroendocrine system is also involved in the emergency life-history stage. The three part system, hormone cascade, transport in blood, and response networks in the target cells are also well conserved across vertebrates, but the diversity of ways by which specific components can be regulated to modulate responsiveness to stress is very great.

From Wingfield et al. (2011b). Courtesy of Springer.

and responses that control the ELHS and also the immune system and adrenal medullary (chromaffin) responses (Figure 4.23). This three-part system, hormone cascade, transport in blood, and response networks in the target cells, is conserved across vertebrates. It is intriguing that the diversity of ways by which specific components of this cascade can be regulated to modulate responsiveness to stress is considerable. Evidence is growing for not only the regulation of secretion of corticosteroid at the hypothalamic, pituitary, or adrenal cortex levels, but also for regulation of CBG (e.g., Breuner et al. 2003; Wingfield and Romero 2001). Regulatory mechanisms of enzymes affecting corticosteroid action within target cells await investigation (e.g., Wingfield et al. 2011a; Wingfield et al. 2011b).

REFERENCES

Aboa-Eboule, C., Brisson, C., Maunsell, E., Masse, B., Bourbonnais, R., Vezina, M., Milot, A., Theroux, P., Dagenais, G. R., 2007. Job strain and risk of acute recurrent coronary heart disease events. *JAMA* 298, 1652–1660.

Acharya, U. R., Joseph, K. P., Kannathal, N., Lim, C. M., Suri, J. S., 2006. Heart rate variability: a review. *Med Biol Eng Comput* 44, 1031–1051.

Ackerman, J. T., Takekawa, J. Y., Kruse, K. L., Orthmeyer, D. L., Yee, J. L., Ely, C. R., Ward, D. H., Bollinger, K. S., Mulcahy, D. M., 2004. Using radiotelemetry to monitor cardiac response of free-living tule greater white-fronted geese (Anser albifrons elgasi) to human disturbance. *Wilson Bull* 116, 146–151.

Adamec, R., Head, D., Blundell, J., Burton, P., Berton, O., 2006. Lasting anxiogenic effects of feline predator stress in mice: Sex differences in vulnerability to stress and predicting severity of anxiogenic response from the stress experience. *Physiol Behav* 88, 12.

Adamec, R., Muir, C., Grimes, M., Pearcey, K., 2007. Involvement of noradrenergic and corticoid receptors in the consolidation of the lasting anxiogenic effects of predator stress. *Behav Brain Res* 179, 192–207.

Adamec, R., Walling, S., Burton, P., 2004. Long-lasting, selective, anxiogenic effects of feline predator stress in mice. *Physiol Behav* 83, 401–410.

Altimiras, J., Johnstone, A. D. F., Lucas, M. C., Priede, I. G., 1996. Sex differences in the heart rate variability spectrum of free-swimming Atlantic salmon (Salmo salar L) during the spawning season. *Physiol Zool* 69, 770–784.

Bartholomew, G. A., Hudson, J. W., Howell, T. R., 1962. Body temperature, oxygen consumption, evaporative water loss, and heart rate in the poor-will. *Condor* 64, 117–125.

Bartolomucci, A., Palanza, P., Costoli, T., Savani, E., Laviola, G., Parmigiani, S., Sgoifo, A., 2003. Chronic psychosocial stress persistently alters autonomic function and physical activity in mice. *Physiol Behav* 80, 57–67.

Beauchamp, G., 2004. Reduced flocking by birds on islands with relaxed predation. *Proc R Soc Lond B* 271, 1039–1042.

Beletsky, L. D., Gori, D. F., Freeman, S., Wingfield, J. C., 1995. Testosterone and polygyny in birds. *Curr Ornithol* 1–41.

Berntson, G. G., Bigger, J. T., Eckberg, D. L., Grossman, P., Kaufmann, P. G., Malik, M., Nagaraja, H. N., Porges, S. W., Saul, J. P., Stone, P. H., VanderMolen, M. W., 1997. Heart rate variability: Origins, methods, and interpretive caveats. *Psychophysiology* 34, 623–648.

Bhatnagar, S., Vining, C., 2003. Facilitation of hypothalamic-pituitary-adrenal responses to novel stress following repeated social stress using the resident/intruder paradigm. *Horm Behav* 43, 158–165.

Billman, G.E., 2011. Heart rate variability: A historical perspective. *Front Physiol* 2.

Bisson, I. A., Butler, L. K., Hayden, T. J., Romero, L. M., Wikelski, M. C., 2009. No energetic cost of anthropogenic disturbance in a songbird. *Proc R Soc Lond B* 276, 961–969.

Blanchard, R. J., Blanchard, D. C., 2003. Bringing natural behaviors into the laboratory: A tribute to Paul MacLean. *Physiol Behav* 79, 515–524.

Blumstein, D. T., 2006. The multipredator hypothesis and the evolutionary persistence of antipredator behavior. *Ethology* 112, 209–217.

Blumstein, D. T., Bitton, A., DaVeiga, J., 2006a. How does the presence of predators influence the persistence of antipredator behavior? *J Theor Biol* 239, 460–468.

Blumstein, D. T., Daniel, J. C., 2005. The loss of anti-predator behaviour following isolation on islands. *Proc R Soc Lond B* 272, 1663–1668.

Blumstein, D. T., Daniel, J. C., Springett, B. P., 2004. A test of the multi-predator hypothesis: Rapid loss of antipredator behavior after 130 years of isolation. *Ethology* 110, 919–934.

Blumstein, D. T., Ozgul, A., Yovovich, V., Van Vuren, D. H., Armitage, K. B., 2006b. Effect of predation risk on the presence and persistence of yellow-bellied marmot (Marmota flaviventris) colonies. *J Zool (Lond)* 270, 132–138.

Bohus, B., Koolhaas, J. M., 1993. Stress and the cardiovascular system: Central and peripheral physiological mechanisms. In: Stanford, S. C., Salmon, P., Gray, J. A. (Eds.), *Stress: From synapse to syndrome*. Academic Press, Boston, MA, pp. 75–117.

Breuner, C. W., Orchinik, M., 2001. Seasonal regulation of membrane and intracellular corticosteroid receptors in the house sparrow brain. J *Neuroendocrinol* 13, 412–420.

Breuner, C. W., Orchinik, M., 2002. Beyond carrier proteins: Plasma binding proteins as mediators of corticosteroid action in vertebrates. *J Endocrinol* 175, 99–112.

Breuner, C. W., Orchinik, M., Hahn, T. P., Meddle, S. L., Moore, I. T., Owen-Ashley, N. T., Sperry, T. S., Wingfield, J. C., 2003. Differential mechanisms for regulation of the stress response across latitudinal gradients. *Am J Physiol* 285, R594–R600.

Breves, J. P., Specker, J. L., 2005. Cortisol stress response of juvenile winter flounder (Pseudopleuronectes americanus, Walbaum) to predators. *J Exp Marine Biol Ecol* 325, 1–7.

Busch, D. S., Sperry, T. S., Peterson, E., Do, C. T., Wingfield, J. C., Boyd, E. H., 2008a. Impacts of frequent, acute pulses of corticosterone on condition and behavior of Gambel's white-crowned sparrow (Zonotrichia leucophtys gambelii). *Gen Comp Endocrinol* 158, 224–233.

Busch, D. S., Sperry, T. S., Wingfield, J. C., Boyd, E. H., 2008b. Effects of repeated, short-term, corticosterone administration on the hypothalamo-pituitary-adrenal axis of the white-crowned sparrow (Zonotrichia leucophrys gambelii). *Gen Comp Endocrinol* 158, 211–223.

Butler, P. J., Green, J. A., Boyd, I. L., Speakman, J. R., 2004. Measuring metabolic rate in the field: The pros and cons of the doubly labelled water and heart rate methods. *Func Ecol* 18, 168–183.

Cabanac, A., Cabanac, M., 2000. Heart rate response to gentle handling of frog and lizard. *Behav Process* 52, 89–95.

Cabanac, A. J., Guillemette, M., 2001. Temperature and heart rate as stress indicators of handled common eider. *Physiol Behav* 74, 475–479.

Cannon, W. B., 1932. *The wisdom of the body.* W. W. Norton, New York.

Cannon, W. B., de la Paz, D., 1911. Emotional stimulation of adrenal secretion. *Am J Physiol* 28, 64–70.

Chapovetsky, V., Katz, U., 2003. Effects of season and temperature acclimation on electrocardiogram and heart rate of toads. *Comp Biochem Physiol Part A: Mol Integr Physiol* 134A, 77–83.

Clinchy, M., Zanette, L., Boonstra, R., Wingfield, J. C., Smith, J. N. M., 2004. Balancing food and predator pressure induces chronic stress in songbirds. *Proc R Soc Lond B* 271, 2473–2479.

Cohen, S. P., Janicki-Deverts, D. P., Miller, G. E. P., 2007. Psychological stress and disease. *JAMA* 298, 1685–1687.

Creel, S., Christianson, D., 2008. Relationships between direct predation and risk effects. *Trends Ecol Evol* 23, 194–201.

Creel, S., Christianson, D., Liley, S., Winnie, J. A., Jr., 2007. Predation risk affects reproductive physiology and demography of elk. *Science (Washington DC)* 315, 960.

Cyr, N. E., Dickens, M. J., Romero, L. M., 2009. Heart rate and heart rate variability responses to acute and chronic stress in a wild-caught passerine bird. *Physiol Biochem Zool* 82, 332–344.

Cyr, N. E., Wikelski, M., Romero, L. M., 2008. Increased energy expenditure but decreased stress responsiveness during molt. *Physiol Biochem Zool* 81, 452–462.

Dallman, M. F., Akana, S. F., Cascio, C. S., Darlington, D. N., Jacobson, L., Levin, N., 1987. Regulation of ACTH secretion: Variations on a theme of B. *Rec Prog Horm Res* 43, 113–173.

Dallman, M. F., Akana, S. F., Scribner, K. A., Bradbury, M. J., Walker, C.-D., Strack, A. M., Cascio, C. S., 1992. Stress, feedback and facilitation in the hypothalamo-pituitary-adrenal axis. *J Neuroendocrinol* 4, 517–526.

Dallman, M. F., Bhatnagar, S., 2001. Chronic stress and energy balance: Role of the hypothalamo-pituitary-adrenal axis. In: McEwen, B. S., Goodman, H. M. (Eds.), *Handbook of physiology*; Section 7: *The endocrine system*; Volume IV: *Coping with the environment: Neural and endocrine mechanisms.* Oxford University Press, New York, pp. 179–210.

De Villiers, M., Bause, M., Giese, M., Fourie, A., 2006. Hardly hard-hearted: Heart rate responses of incubating Northern Giant Petrels (Macronectes halli) to human disturbance on sub-Antarctic Marion Island. *Polar Biol* 29, 717–720.

Dickens, M. J., Nephew, B. C., Romero, L. M., 2006. Captive European starlings (Sturnus vulgaris) in breeding condition show an increased cardiovascular stress response to intruders. *Physiol Biochem Zool* 79, 937–943.

Diehl, P., Helb, H. W., 1986. Radiotelemetric monitoring of heart-rate responses to song playback in blackbirds (*Turdus-merula*). *Behav Ecol Sociobiol* 18, 213–219.

Dobrakova, M., Kvetnansky, R., 1993. Specificity of the effect of repeated handling on sympathetic-adrenomedullary and pituitary-adrenocortical activity in rats. *Psychoneuroendocrinology* 18, 163–174.

Dobrakovova, M., Kvetnansky, R., Oprsalova, Z., Jezova, D., 1993. Specificity of the effect of repeated handling on sympathetic-adrenomedullary and pituitary-adrenocortical activity in rats. *Psychoneuroendocrinology* 18, 163–174.

Dobrakovova, M., Kvetnansky, R., Oprsalova, Z., Macho, L., 1990. Effect of chronic stress on the activity of the sympatho-adrenomedullary system. *Bratisl. Lek. Listy* 91, 587–592.

Donham, R. S., Dane, C. W., Farner, D. S., 1976. Plasma luteinizing hormone and development of ovarian follicles after loss of clutch in female

mallards (*Anas platyrhynchos*). *Gen Comp Endocrinol* 29, 152–155.
Dressen, W., Hendrichs, H., 1992. Social behavior and heart rate in tammar wallabies (*Macropodidae, Macropus-eugenii*). *J Zool* 227, 299–317.
Eilam, D., 2005. Die hard: A blend of freezing and fleeing as a dynamic defense—implications for the control of defensive behavior. *Neurosci Biobehav Rev* 29, 1181–1191.
Eilam, D., Dayan, T., Ben-Eliyahu, S., Schulman, I., Shefer, G., Hendrie, C.A., 1999. Differential behavioural and hormonal responses of voles and spiny mice to owl calls. *Anim Behav* 58, 1085–1093.
Eiserman, K., 1992. Long-term heart rate responses to social stress in wild european rabbits: predominant effect of rank position. *Physiol Behav* 52, 33–36.
Ellenberg, U., Mattern, T., Seddon, P. J., Jorquera, G.L., 2006. Physiological and reproductive consequences of human disturbance in Humboldt penguins: The need for species-specific visitor management. *Biol Conserv* 133, 95–106.
Ely, C. R., Ward, D. H., Bollinger, K. S., 1999. Behavioral correlates of heart rates of free-living Greater White-fronted Geese. *Condor* 101, 390–395.
Engh, A. L., Beehner, J. C., Bergman, T. J., Whitten, P. L., Hoffmeier, R. R., Seyfarth, R. M., Cheney, D. L., 2006. Behavioural and hormonal responses to predation in female chacma baboons (Papio hamadryas ursinus). *Proc R Soc Lond B* 273, 707–712.
Fletcher, Q. E., Boonstra, R., 2006. Do captive male meadow voles experience acute stress in response to weasel odour? *Can J Zool* 84, 583–588.
Ford, J. K. B., Reeves, R. R., 2008. Fight or flight: antipredator strategies of baleen whales. *Mammal Rev* 38, 50–86.
Fox, A. S., Oakes, T. R., Shelton, S. E., Converse, A. K., Davidson, R. J., Kalin, N. H., 2005. Calling for help is independently modulated by brain systems underlying goal-directed behavior and threat perception. *Proc Natl Acad Sci USA* 102, 4176–4179.
Gabrielsen, G., Kanwisher, J., Steen, J. B., 1977. "Emotional" bradycardia: a telemetry study on incubating willow grouse (Lagopus lagopus). *Acta Physiol Scand* 100, 255–257.
Gabrielsen, G. W., Blix, A. S., Ursin, H., 1985. Orienting and freezing responses in incubating ptarmigan hens. *Physiol Behav* 34, 925–934.
Gabrielsen, G. W., Smith, E. N., 1985. Physiological responses associaed with feigned death in the American opossum. *Acta Physiol Scand* 123, 393–398.
Goldstein, D. S., 1987. Stress-induced activation of the sympathetic nervous system. *Bailliere Clin Endoc Metab* 1, 253–278.
Goymann, W., Moore, I. T., Scheuerlein, A., Hirschenhauser, K., Grafen, A., Wingfield, J. C., 2004. Testosterone in tropical birds: Effects of environmental and social factors. *Am Nat* 164, 327–334.
Grippo, A. J., Beltz, T. G., Johnson, A. K., 2003. Behavioral and cardiovascular changes in the chronic mild stress model of depression. *Physiol Behav* 78, 703–710.
Grippo, A. J., Beltz, T. G., Weiss, R. M., Johnson, A. K., 2006. The effects of chronic fluoxetine treatment on chronic mild stress-induced cardiovascular changes and anhedonia. *Biol Psych* 59, 309–316.
Grippo, A. J., Lamb, D. G., Carter, C. S., Porges, S. W., 2007a. Cardiac regulation in the socially monogamous prairie vole. *Physiol Behav* 90, 386–393.
Grippo, A. J., Lamb, D. G., Carter, C. S., Porges, S. W., 2007b. Social isolation disrupts autonomic regulation of the heart and influences negative affective behaviors. *Biol Psych* 62, 1162–1170.
Haller, J., Mikics, E., Makara, G. B., 2008. The effects of non-genomic glucocorticoid mechanisms on bodily functions and the central neural system: A critical evaluation of findings. *Front Neuroendocrinol* 29, 273–291.
Harms, C. A., Fleming, W. J., Stoskopf, M. K., 1997. A technique for dorsal subcutaneous implantation of heart rate biotelemetry transmitters in black ducks: Application in an aircraft noise response study. *Condor* 99, 231–237.
Hart, B. B., Stanford, G. G., Ziegler, M. G., Lake, C. R., Chernow, B., 1989. Catecholamines: Study of interspecies variation. *Crit Care Med* 17, 1203.
Hegner, R. E., Wingfield, J. C., 1987. Social status and circulating levels of hormones in flocks of house sparrows, *Passer domesticus*. *Ethology* 76, 1–14.
Hendrie, C. A., Weiss, S. M., Eilam, D., 1998. Behavioural response of wild rodents to the calls of an owl: A comparative study. *J Zool (Lond)* 245, 439–446.
Hochachka, W. M., 2004. Running away may not pay. *J Avian Biol* 35, 97–98.
Holmes, M. C., Kotelevtsev, Y., Mullins, J. J., Seckl, J. R., 2001. Phenotypic analysis of mice bearing targeted deletions of 11 beta-hydroxysteroid dehydrogenases 1 and 2 genes. *Mol Cell Endocrinol* 171, 15–20.
Holmes, N., Giese, M., Kriwoken, L. K., 2005. Testing the minimum approach distance guidelines for incubating Royal penguins *Eudyptes schlegeli*. *Biol Conserv* 126, 339–350.
Ingle, D. J., 1952. The role of the adrenal cortex in homeostasis. *J Endocrinol* 8, 23–37.
Jessop, T., Sumner, J., Lance, V., Limpus, C., 2004. Reproduction in shark-attacked sea turtles is supported by stress-reduction mechanisms. *Proc R Soc Lond B* 271, S91-S94.
Kanwisher, J. W., Williams, T. C., Teal, J. M., Lawson, K. O., 1978. Radiotelemetry of heart rates from free-ranging gulls. *Auk* 95, 288–293.
Ketterson, E. D., Nolan, V., Cawthorn, M. J., Parker, P. G., Ziegenfus, C., 1996. Phenotypic

engineering: Using hormones to explore the mechanistic and functional bases of phenotypic variation in nature. *Ibis* 138, 70–86.

King, J. R., 1981. Energetics of avian molt. *Proc Int Ornithol Cong* 17, 312–317.

Korte, S. M., Ruesink, W., Blokhuis, H. J., 1999. Heart rate variability during manual restraint in chicks from high-and low-feather pecking lines of laying hens. *Physiol Behav* 65, 649–652.

Kostelanetz, S., Dickens, M. J., Romero, L.M., 2009. Combined effects of molt and chronic stress on heart rate, heart rate variability, and glucocorticoid physiology in European Starlings. *Comp Biochem Physiol A* 154, 493–501.

Kuo, A. Y., Lee, J. C., Siegel, P. B., Denbow, D. M., 2001. Differential cardiovascular effects of pharmacological agents in chickens selected for high and low body weight. *Physiol Behav* 74, 573–579.

Landys, M. M., Ramenofsky, M., Wingfield, J. C., 2006. Actions of glucocorticoids at a seasonal baseline as compared to stress-related levels in the regulation of periodic life processes. *Gen Comp Endocrinol* 148, 132–149.

LeBlanc, J., Ducharme, M. B., Thompson, M., 2004. Study on the correlation of the autonomic nervous system responses to a stressor of high discomfort with personality traits. *Physiol Behav* 82, 647–652.

Levine, J. E., 2002. Editorial: Stressing the importance of sex. *Endocrinology* 143, 4502–4504.

Lillywhite, H. B., Zippel, K. C., Farrell, A. P., 1999. Resting and maximal heart rates in ectothermic vertebrates. *Comp Biochem Physiol A* 124, 369–382.

Lima, S. L., 1998. Stress and decision making under the risk of predation: Recent developments from behavioral, reproductive, and ecological perspectives. In: Moller, A.P., Milinski, M., Slater, P.J.B. (Eds.), *Advances in the study of behavior: Stress and behavior.* Academic Press, San Diego, pp. 215–290.

Lindstrom, A., Visser, G. H., Daan, S., 1993. The energetic cost of feather synthesis is proportional to basal metabolic rate. *Physiol Zool* 66, 490–510.

Losos, J. B., Schoener, T. W., Spiller, D. A., 2004. Predator-induced behaviour shifts and natural selection in field-experimental lizard populations. *Nature (London)* 432, 505–508.

Lucini, D., Di Fede, G., Parati, G., Pagani, M., 2005. Impact of chronic psychosocial stress on autonomic cardiovascular regulation in otherwise healthy subjects. *Hypertension* 46, 1201–1206.

Lynn, S. E., Walker, B. G., Wingfield, J. C., 2005. A phylogenetically controlled test of hypotheses for behavioral insensitivity to testosterone in birds. *Horm Behav* 47, 170–177.

Mateo, J. M., 2007. Ecological and hormonal correlates of antipredator behavior in adult Belding's ground squirrels (Spermophilus beldingi). *Behav Ecol Sociobiol* 62, 37–49.

McCarty, R., Stone, E. A., 1983. Chronic stress and regulation of the sympathetic nervous system. In: Usdin, E., Kvetnansky, R., Axelrod, J. (Eds.), *Stress: The role of catecholamines and other neurotransmitters.* Gordon and Breach Science Publishers, New York, pp. 563–576.

McEwen, B. S., Seeman, T., 1999. Protective and damaging effects of mediators of stress: Elaborating and testing the concepts of allostasis and allostatic load. *Annals of the New York Academy of Sciences* 896: 30–47.

McEwen, B. S., Wingfield, J. C., 2003. The concept of allostasis in biology and biomedicine. *Horm Behav* 43, 2–15.

Miksis, J. L., Grund, M. D., Nowacek, D. P., Solow, A. R., Connor, R. C., Tyack, P. L., 2001. Cardiac responses to acoustic playback experiments in the captive bottlenose dolphin (*Tursiops truncatus*). *J Comp Psychol* 115, 227–232.

Moen, A. N., 1978. Seasonal changes in heart rates, activity, metabolism, and forage intake of white-tailed deer. *J Wildlife Manage* 42, 715–738.

Morgan, K. N., Tromborg, C. T., 2007. Sources of stress in captivity. *Appl Anim Behav Sci* 102, 262–302.

Munck, A., Guyre, P. M., Holbrook, N. J., 1984. Physiological functions of glucocorticoids in stress and their relation to pharmacological actions. *Endocr Rev* 5, 25–44.

Murphy, M. E., 1996. Energetics and nutrition of molt. In: Carey, C. (Ed.), *Avian energetics and nutritional ecology.* Chapman & Hall, New York, pp. 158–198.

Murphy, M. E., King, J. R., 1992. Energy and nutrient use during moult by white-crowned sparrows *Zonotrichia leucophrys gambelii. Ornis Scan* 23, 304–313.

Nakagawa, S., Waas, J. R., Miyazaki, M., 2001. Heart rate changes reveal that little blue penguin chicks (*Eudyptula minor*) can use vocal signatures to discriminate familiar from unfamiliar chicks. *Behav Ecol Sociobiol* 50, 180–188.

Nelson, R. J., Demas, G. E., Klein, S. L., Kriegsfeld, L. J., 2002. *Seasonal patterns of stress, immune function, and disease.* Cambridge University Press, Cambridge.

Nephew, B. C., Kahn, S. A., Romero, L. M., 2003. Heart rate and behavior are regulated independently of corticosterone following diverse acute stressors. *Gen Comp Endocrinol* 133, 173–180.

Nephew, B. C., Romero, L. M., 2003. Behavioral, physiological, and endocrine responses of starlings to acute increases in density. *Horm Behav* 44, 222–232.

Nimon, A. J., Schroter, R. C., Oxenham, R. K. C., 1996. Artificial eggs: Measuring heart rate and effects of disturbance in nesting penguins. *Physiol Behav* 60, 1019–1022.

Nixon, M., Upreti, R., Andrew, R., 2012. 5 alpha-Reduced glucocorticoids: a story of natural selection. *J Endocrinol* 212, 111–127.

O'Reilly, K. M., Wingfield, J. C., 2001. Ecological factors underlying the adrenocortical response to capture stress in arctic-breeding shorebirds. *Gen Comp Endocri*nol 124, 1–11.

Perini, R., Veicsteinas, A., 2003. Heart rate variability and autonomic activity at rest and during exercise in various physiological conditions. *Eur J Appl Physiol* 90, 317–325.

Perrins, C. M., 1970. Timing of birds breeding seasons. *Ibis* 112, 242.

Price, S., Sibly, R. M., Davies, M. H., 1993. Effects of behavior and handling on heart rate in farmed red deer. *Appl Anim Behav Sci* 37, 111–123.

Rattenborg, N. C., Lima, S. L., Amlaner, C. J., 1999. Half-awake to the risk of predation. *Nature* 397, 397–398.

Ricklefs, R. E., Wikelski, M., 2002. The physiology/life-history nexus. *Trends Ecol Evol* 17, 462–468.

Rietmann, T. R., Stuart, A. E. A., Bernasconi, P., Stauffacher, M., Auer, J. A., Weishaupt, M. A., 2004. Assessment of mental stress in warmblood horses: Heart rate variability in comparison to heart rate and selected behavioural parameters. *Appl Anim Behav Sci* 88, 121–136.

Rocha, P. L., Branco, L. G. S., 1998. Seasonal changes in the cardiovascular, respiratory and metabolic responses to temperature and hypoxia in the bullfrog, *Rana catesbeiana*. J Exp Biol 201, 761–768.

Roedl, T., Berger, S., Romero, L. M., Wikelski, M., 2007. Tameness and stress physiology in a predator-naive island species confronted with novel predation threat. *Proc R Soc Lond B* 274, 577–582.

Rogovin, K., Randall, J. A., Kolosova, I., Moshkin, M., 2004. Predation on a social desert rodent, *Rhombomys opimus*: Effect of group size, composition, and location. *J Mammal* 85, 723–730.

Romero, L. M., 2002. Seasonal changes in plasma glucocorticoid concentrations in free-living vertebrates. *Gen Comp Endocrinol* 128, 1–24.

Romero, L. M., 2004. Physiological stress in ecology: Lessons from biomedical research. *Trends Ecol Evol* 19, 249–255.

Romero, L. M., Dickens, M. J., Cyr, N. E., 2009. The reactive scope model: A new model integrating homeostasis, allostasis, and stress. *Horm Behav* 55, 375–389.

Romero, L. M., Reed, J. M., Wingfield, J. C., 2000. Effects of weather on corticosterone responses in wild free-living passerine birds. *Gen Comp Endocrinol* 118, 113–122.

Romero, L. M., Wikelski, M., 2001. Corticosterone levels predict survival probabilities of Galápagos marine iguanas during El Niño events. *Proc Natl Acad Sci USA* 98, 7366–7370.

Romero, S. M. B., Pereira, A. F., Garofalo, M. A. R., Hoffmann, A., 2004. Effects of exercise on plasma catecholamine levels in the toad, *Bufo paracnemis*: Role of the adrenals and neural control. *J Exp Zool A: Comp Exp Biol* 301A, 911–918.

Sapolsky, R. M., 1992. *Stress, the aging brain, and the mechanisms of neuron death*. MIT Press, Cambridge, MA.

Sapolsky, R. M., Romero, L. M., Munck, A. U., 2000. How do glucocorticoids influence stress-responses? Integrating permissive, suppressive, stimulatory, and preparative actions. *Endocr Rev* 21, 55–89.

Sapolsky, R. M., Share, L. J., 1994. Rank-related differences in cardiovascular function among wild baboons: role of sensitivity to glucocorticoids. *Am J Primatol* 32, 261–275.

Schaub, R., Prinzinger, R., 1999. Long-term telemetry of heart rates and energy metabolic rate during the diurnal cycle in normothermic and torpid African blue-naped mousebirds (Urocolius macrourus). *Comp Biochem Physiol* A 124, 439–445.

Scheuerlein, A., Van't Hof, T. J., Gwinner, E., 2001. Predators as stressors? Physiological and reproductive consequences of predation risk in tropical stonechats (*Saxicola torquata axillaris*). *Proc R Soc Lond B* 268, 1575.

Schmidt, K. L., Pradhan, D. S., Shah, A. H., Charlier, T. D., Chin, E. H., Soma, K. K., 2008. Neurosteroids, immunosteroids, and the Balkanization of endocrinology. *Gen Comp Endocrinol* 157, 266–274.

Schutz, K. E., Agren, E., Amundin, M., Roken, B., Palme, R., Morner, T., 2006. Behavioral and physiological responses of trap-induced stress in European badgers. *J Wildlife Manage* 70, 884–891.

Selye, H., 1946. The general adaptation syndrome and the diseases of adaptation. *J Clin Endocrinol* 6, 117–230.

Sgoifo, A., Costoli, T., Meerlo, P., Buwalda, B., Pico'Alfonso, M. A., De Boer, S., Musso, E., Koolhaas, J., 2005. Individual differences in cardiovascular response to social challenge. *Neurosci Biobehav Rev* 29, 59–66.

Sgoifo, A., Stilli, D., de Boer, S. F., Koolhaas, J. M., Musso, E., 1998. Acute social stress and cardiac electrical activity in rats. *Aggressive Behav* 24, 287–296.

Shifferman, E., Eilam, D., 2004. Movement and direction of movement of a simulated prey affect the success rate in barn owl *Tyto alba* attack. *J Avian Biol* 35, 111–116.

Silverin, B., 1980. Effects of long-acting testosterone treatment on free-living pied flycatchers, *Ficedula hypoleuca*, during the breeding period. *Anim Behav* 28, 906–912.

Silverin, B., 1997. The stress response and autumn dispersal behaviour in willow tits. *Anim Behav* 53, 451–459.

Silverin, B., 1998a. Behavioural and hormonal responses of the pied flycatcher to environmental stressors. *Anim Behav* 55, 1411–1420.

Silverin, B., 1998b. Territorial behavioural and hormones of pied flycatchers in optimal and suboptimal habitats. *Anim Behav* 56, 811.

Silverin, B., Wingfield, J. C., 1998. Adrenocortical responses to stress in breeding Pied Flycatchers Ficedula hypoleuca: Relation to latitude, sex and mating status. *J Avian Biol* 29, 228.

Smith, E. N., Allison, R. D., Crowder, W. E., 1974. Bradycardia in a free ranging American alligator. *Copeia* 770–772.

Smith, E. N., Decarvalho, M.C., 1985. Heart rate response to threat and diving in the ornate box turtle, *Terrapene-ornata*. *Physiol Zool* 58, 236–241.

Smith, E. N., Johnson, C., 1984. Fear bradycardia in the eastern fox squirrel, Sciurus-niger, and eastern grey squirrel, *Sciurus-carolinesis*. *Comp Biochem Physiol A* 78, 409–411.

Smith, E. N., Woodruff, R. A., 1980. Fear bradycardia in free-ranging woodchucks, *Marmota-monax*. *J Mammal* 61, 750–753.

Smith, H. M., West, N. H., Jones, D. R., 2000. The cardiovascular system. In: Whittow, G. C. (Ed.), *Sturkie's avian physiology*. Academic Press, San Diego, pp. 141–223.

Southwood, A. L., Darveau, C. A., Jones, D. R., 2003. Metabolic and cardiovascular adjustments of juvenile green turtles to seasonal changes in temperature and photoperiod. *J Exp Biol* 206, 4521–4531.

Stanford, S. C., 1993. Monoamines in response and adaptation to stress. In: Stanford, S. C., Salmon, P., Gray, J. A. (Eds.), *Stress: From synapse to syndrome*. Academic Press, San Diego, CA, pp. 281–331.

Stauss, H. M., 2003. Heart rate variability. *Am J Physiol* 285, R927-R931.

Steen, J. B., Gabrielsen, G. W., Kanwisher, J. W., 1988. Physiological aspects of freezing behavior in willow ptarmigan hens. *Acta Physiol Scand* 134, 299–304.

Stein, P. K., Kleiger, R. E., 1999. Insights from the study of heart rate variability. *Ann Rev Med* 50, 249–261.

Swain, U. G., Gilbert, F. F., Robinette, J. D., 1988. Heart rates in the captive, free-ranging beaver. *Comp Biochem Physiol A* 91, 431–435.

Tausk, M., 1951. Hat die Nebenniere tatsächlich eine Verteidigungsfunktion? *Das Hormon (Organon, Holland)* 3, 1–24.

Taves, M. D., Gomez-Sanchez, C. E., Soma, K. K., 2011a. Extra-adrenal glucocorticoids and mineralocorticoids: Evidence for local synthesis, regulation, and function. *Am J Physiol* 301, E11–E24.

Taves, M. D., Ma, C., Heimovics, S. A., Saldanha, C. J., Soma, K. K., 2011b. Measurement of steroid concentrations in brain tissue: methodological considerations. *Front Endocrinol* 2, 1–13.

Theil, P. K., Coutant, A. E., Olesen, C. R., 2004. Seasonal changes and activity-dependent variation in heart rate of roe deer. *J Mammal* 85, 245–253.

Valance, D., Boissy, A., Despres, G., Constantin, P., Leterrier, C., 2007. Emotional reactivity modulates autonomic responses to an acoustic challenge in quail. *Physiol Behav* 90, 165–171.

Viau, V., Bingham, B., Davis, J., Lee, P., Wong, M., 2005. Gender and puberty interact on the stress-induced activation of parvocellular neurosecretory neurons and corticotropin-releasing hormone messenger ribonucleic acid expression in the rat. *Endocrinology* 146, 137–146.

Viau, V., Meaney, M. J., 1991. Variations in the hypothalamic-pituitary-adrenal response to stress during the estrous cycle in the rat. *Endocrinology* 129, 2503–2511.

Viau, V., Soriano, L., Dallman, M. F., 2001. Androgens alter corticotropin releasing hormone and arginine vasopressin mRNA within forebrain sites known to regulate activity in the hypothalamic-pituitary-adrenal axis. *J Neuroendocrinol* 13, 442–452.

Visser, E. K., van Reenen, C. G., van der Werf, J. T. N., Schilder, M. B. H., Knaap, J. H., Barneveld, A., Blokhuis, H. J., 2002. Heart rate and heart rate variability during a novel object test and a handling test in young horses. *Physiol Behav* 76, 289–296.

Vitousek, M. N., Romero, L. M., Tarlow, E., Cyr, N. E., Wikelski, M., 2010. Island tameness: An altered cardiovascular stress response in Galapagos marine iguanas. *Physiol Behav* 99, 544–548.

von Borell, E., Langbein, J., Despres, G., Hansen, S., Leterrier, C., Marchant-Forde, J., Marchant-Forde, R., Minero, M., Mohr, E., Prunier, A., Valance, D., Veissier, I., 2007. Heart rate variability as a measure of autonomic regulation of cardiac activity for assessing stress and welfare in farm animals: A review. *Physiol Behav* 92, 293–316.

Wascher, C. A. F., Amold, W., Kotrschal, K., 2008a. Heart rate modulation by social contexts in greylag geese (Anser anser). *J Comp Psychol* 122, 100–107.

Wascher, C. A. F., Scheiber, I. B. R., Kotrschal, K., 2008b. Heart rate modulation in bystanding geese watching social and non-social events. *Proc R Soc Lond B* 275, 1653–1659.

Weimerskirch, H., Shaffer, S. A., Mabille, G., Martin, J., Boutard, O., Rouanet, J. L., 2002. Heart rate and energy expenditure of incubating wandering albatrosses: Basal levels, natural variation, and the effects of human disturbance. *J Exp Biol* 205, 475–483.

Wingfield, J. C., 1988. Changes in reproductive function of free-living birds in direct response to environmental perturbations. In: Stetson, M. H. (Ed.) *Processing of environmental information in vertebrates*. Springer-Verlag, Berlin, pp. 121–148.

Wingfield, J. C., 1994. Modulation of the adrenocortical response to stress in birds. In: Davey, K. G., Peter, R. E., Tobe, S. S. (Eds.), *Perspectives in comparative endocrinology*. National Research Council of Canada, Ottawa, pp. 520–528.

Wingfield, J. C., Farner, D. S., 1979. Some endocrine correlates of renesting after loss of clutch or brood in the white-crowned sparrow, *Zonotrichia leucophrys gambelii*. *Gen Comp Endocrinol* 38, 322–331.

Wingfield, J. C., Farner, D. S., 1993. The endocrinology of wild species. In: Farner, D. S., King, J. R., Parkes, K. C. (Eds.), *Avian biology*, vol. 9. Academic Press, New York, pp. 163–327.

Wingfield, J. C., Hegner, R. E., Dufty, A. M. Jr., Ball, G. F., 1990. The "challenge hypothesis": Theoretical implications for patterns of testosterone secretion, mating systems, and breeding strategies. *Am Nat* 136, 829–846.

Wingfield, J. C., Hunt, K., Breuner, C., Dunlap, K., Fowler, G. S., Freed, L., Lepson, J., 1997. Environmental stress, field endocrinology, and conservation biology. In: Clemmons, J. R., Buchholz, R. (Eds.), *Behavioral approaches to conservation in the wild*. Cambridge University Press, Cambridge, pp. 95–131.

Wingfield, J. C., Kelley, J. P., Angelier, F., 2011a. What are extreme environmental conditions and how do organisms cope with them? *Curr Zool* 57, 363–374.

Wingfield, J. C., Kelley, J. P., Angelier, F., Chastel, O., Lei, F. M., Lynn, S. E., Miner, B., Davis, J. E., Li, D. M., Wang, G., 2011b. Organism-environment interactions in a changing world: a mechanistic approach. *J Ornithol* 152, 279–288.

Wingfield, J. C., Maney, D. L., Breuner, C. W., Jacobs, J. D., Lynn, S., Ramenofsky, M., Richardson, R. D., 1998. Ecological bases of hormone-behavior interactions: The "emergency life history stage." *Integ Comp Biol* 38, 191.

Wingfield, J. C., Moore, M. C., 1987. Hormonal, social, and environmental factors in the reproductive biology of free-living birds. In: Crews, D. (Ed.) *Psychobiology of reproductive behavior: An evolutionary perspective*. Prentice Hall, Englewood Cliffs, NJ, pp. 149–175.

Wingfield, J. C., Ramenofsky, M., 1997. Corticosterone and facultative dispersal in response to unpredictable events. *Ardea* 85, 155–166.

Wingfield, J. C., Ramenofsky, M., 1999. Hormones and the behavioral ecology of stress. *Stress Physiol Animals* 1–51.

Wingfield, J. C., Romero, L.M., 2001. Adrenocortical responses to stress and their modulation in free-living vertebrates. In: McEwen, B. S., Goodman, H. M. (Eds.), *Handbook of physiology*; Section 7: *The endocrine system*; Vol. IV: *Coping with the environment: Neural and endocrine mechanisms*. Oxford University Press, New York, pp. 211–234.

Wingfield, J. C., Ronchi, E., Goldsmith, A. R., Marler, C., 1989. Interactions of sex steroid hormones and prolactin in male and female song sparrows, *Melospiza melodia*. *Physiol Zool* 62, 11–24.

Wingfield, J. C., Sapolsky, R. M., 2003. Reproduction and resistance to stress: When and how. *J Neuroendocrinol* 15, 711.

Zhang, J.-X., Cao, C., Gao, H., Yang, Z.-S., Sun, L., Zhang, Z.-B., Wang, Z.-W., 2003. Effects of weasel odor on behavior and physiology of two hamster species. *Physiol Behav* 79, 549–552.

Ziegelstein, R. C., 2007. Acute emotional stress and cardiac arrhythmias. *JAMA* 298, 324–329.

Zimmer, U. E., 1982. Birds react to playback of recorded songs by heart rate alteration. *Zeitschrift Tierpsychol-J Comp Ethology* 58, 25–30.

5

Impacts on Physiological and Behavioral Systems

I. INTRODUCTION

Responses to perturbations of the environment, with the potential for stress, are extremely complex and involve suites of neural and hormonal reactions. In earlier chapters we discussed the contexts of stress responses and the major models, and next we discuss impacts of the mediators of stress on physiology and behavior. Doing justice to all the mechanisms of neural and hormonal mediators of stress responses could fill several volumes and is beyond the scope of this book. Nonetheless, it is important to acknowledge this diversity before we go on to focus on the two most common and ubiquitous mediators: corticosteroids and catecholamines. Cytokines of the immune system are also essential when injury and infection are involved. However, if the nature of the stressor involves temperature extremes, osmoregulatory adjustments, adaptation to hypoxia, and so on, then it comes as no surprise that other hormone systems are involved.

The stress response varies depending upon the stressor. For example, a number of studies suggest that the degree of corticosteroid response of an individual varies as a function of the stressful stimulus. In stonechats, capture and caging followed by exposure to a predator (an owl) induced a greater corticosterone increase in blood than capture and restraint alone (Canoine et al. 2002). It is also very important to bear in mind that the hormonal responses to stress can also vary markedly in terms of the suite of hormones released or inhibited, depending on the type of stressor. We do not attempt to provide a full account of the vertebrate endocrine system here and we refer the reader to excellent textbooks addressing biomedical endocrinology (Norman and Litwack 1997; Larsen et al. 2003) and comparative endocrinology (Norris 2007; Nelson 2011). We do provide some examples in this chapter to illustrate this point, but it is important to emphasize that for an extremely broad spectrum of stressors, corticosteroids and catecholamines are the common mediators and other hormones can provide specific context.

Many direct labile perturbation factors (LPFs) involve extremes of temperature or wind chill factors that require major metabolic adjustments as diverse as increased metabolism to maintain constant body temperature or decreased metabolic rate, as many ectotherms do. This can also include torpor and estivation in endotherms (see later chapters). Changes in metabolism are driven by hormones such as insulin, glucagon, leptin, adiponectins, thyroid hormones, and prolactin. Some of these we will consider in this chapter. Osmoregulatory stresses, such as transitions between fresh and salt water, droughts and water conservation, hemorrhage, and so on, involve the renin-angiotensin-aldosterone system, arginine vasopressin/vasotocin, prolactin, and atrial natriuretic factor, to name a few of the hormones involved. A third example includes hypoxia associated with migration at altitude, high-altitude breeding, dead zones in oceans, and involves erythropoietin and hypoxia-induced transcription factors. One can imagine many other scenarios where combinations of environmental stress can include metabolic changes as well as osmotic and hypoxic extremes. Clearly such complex environmental perturbations require responses of complex suites of neural and hormonal input, but because corticosteroids and catecholamines are common to all these scenarios, we focus on their impacts on stress.

II. METABOLISM

Many of the remaining chapters in this book will discuss the types of emergency responses that are mediated by stress. These include both internal physiological responses, such as increasing heart rate or mobilizing the immune system, and behavioral responses directed at external events such as fleeing from a predator or fighting with a rival. Initiating an emergency response requires energy. Consequently, one of the fundamental requirements of a successful stress response is the mobilization of energy stores to make extra energy available to those tissues (e.g., brain and muscles) that need to ramp up their consumption. Not surprisingly, both catecholamines and corticosteroids play major roles in energy mobilization.

The role of corticosteroids especially in regulating metabolism and energy flow has been of long-standing interest to the biomedical community. The central role that corticosteroids play in glucose regulation was the impetus for putting the "gluco" into the name "glucocorticoids." As we will see later in this chapter, corticosteroids regulate glucose trafficking in the body. Dysregulation of these processes has been implicated in a number of human diseases such as obesity and diabetes (e.g., Dallman et al. 2003; Friedman 2003). However, the role of glucocorticoids in energy trafficking in wild and free-living animals appears to be far more complicated, and laboratory results have not always translated to field conditions. It is also important to establish at the outset that not every metabolic action of corticosteroids is related to a response to a stressor. Several researchers have argued that not all activity that requires extra energy is a stressor (e.g., Sapolsky et al. 2000; Landys et al. 2006). There are many normal life-history events that require a substantial increase in energy consumption, including reproduction, lactation, active foraging, migration, and others. Animals plan for these activities by storing fat and/or restricting these activities to bountiful periods during the annual cycle (Wingfield 2004; Korte et al. 2005). They do not constitute an emergency use of energy. To return to Chapter 3, energetically costly normal life-history stages serve to increase allostatic load, or to place the animal near the upper limit of predictive homeostasis. In other words, as long as the animal is energetically prepared, these normal events will not constitute stressors. Confusion can occur because low concentrations of corticosteroids can still be involved in mobilizing energy in these cases, but as we will see, the physiological dynamics are very different from emergency responses.

A. Glucose Mobilization and Metabolism

Catecholamines and corticosteroids initiate a suite of metabolic changes. With coordination worthy of a symphony, they orchestrate a number of pathways that convert energy stored in various forms into glucose, a universal energy molecule for transport to tissues throughout the body. Figure 5.1 summarizes the major pathways for glucose metabolism, but bear in mind that other molecules such as fatty acids, glycerol, ketone bodies can also be primary energy molecules (Ramenofsky 1990; Dallman et al. 1993). As discussed in Chapter 4, catecholamines are released within seconds once an animal determines that a given stimulus is a stressor (e.g., an indirect LPF). One of the major functions of catecholamines, especially epinephrine, is to rapidly stimulate glycogenolysis (the breakdown of glycogen into glucose) in both muscles and liver (Nonogaki 2000). Glycogen is broken down to glucose-6-phosphate. In the liver, glucose-6-phosphate is converted to glucose, which can then leave the liver, leading to a burst of glucose hitting the bloodstream within minutes (Sapolsky et al. 2000). Glucose derived from the liver primarily supports nervous system function (Taborsky and Porte 1991; Cherrington

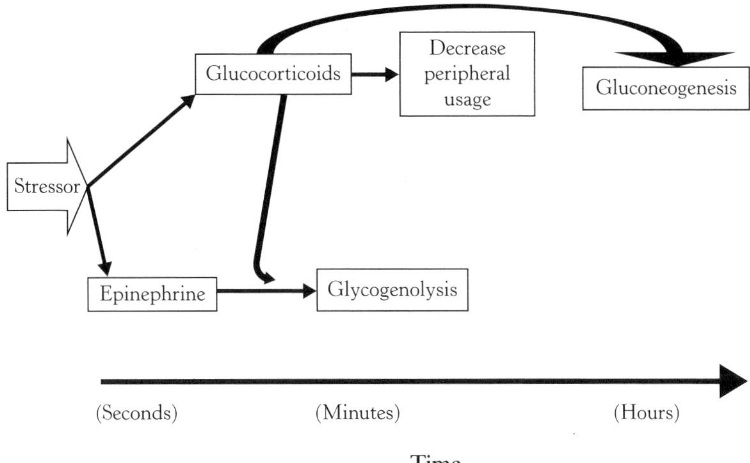

FIGURE 5.1: Schematic of the major pathways leading to increased blood glucose concentrations during stress.

1999). In muscles, however, glucose-6-phosphate is not converted to glucose, cannot leave the cell, and thus directly enters the glycolytic pathway and provides energy.

Catecholamines also increase blood glucose via two indirect mechanisms. First, they inhibit insulin release from the pancreas, thereby decreasing the ability of insulin to clear the glucose that has just been released from the liver (Taborsky and Porte 1991). Second, they initiate the mobilization of fat that can be used by the liver to sustain glucose production (Cherrington 1999), primarily by preferentially stimulating visceral fat depots that drain directly to the liver (Wajchenberg et al. 2002).

For stressors such as predator attacks, the speed at which catecholamines are released and subsequently act to convert glycogen makes this the preeminent pathway for delivering new energy to working muscles and neurons. However, the short-term nature of catecholamine actions makes them poor mediators for providing sustained glucose provisioning required to either maintain a fight-or-flight response or provide the replenishment of energy stores once the stressor has ended. Corticosteroids play this role.

The glucose regulatory function of corticosteroids has been studied for many years and continues to be a major focus of research. One of the early studies demonstrating that corticosteroids increase blood glucose concentrations is presented in Figure 5.2. Although increases in blood glucose concentrations are the integrated physiological consequence, corticosteroids accomplish this by initiating three major mechanistic pathways (Figure 5.1). The first is in a permissive role (see Chapter 4) to sustain catecholamine-induced glycogenolysis (Taborsky and Porte 1991)—primarily by increasing the number of active catecholamine receptors (Davies and Lefkowitz 1984). Although corticosteroids do not appear to stimulate glycogen breakdown themselves, when they are present prior to the onset of a stressor they allow catecholamines to convert glycogen for a longer time.

The second pathway involves altering the cellular trafficking of glucose transporters. Glucose must be actively transported across cell membranes using a transmembrane protein (Norris 2007). This transport protein shuttles glucose across the membrane using concentration gradients. When the glucose concentration is lower inside the cell, such as a neuron that is metabolically active, glucose flows inward. When the glucose concentration is higher inside the cell, such as a liver cell converting glycogen, the glucose flows out into the blood. Cells regulate the flow of glucose by controlling the number of glucose transporters on the external cell membranes. If a cell needs less glucose, a section of membrane is pinched off (using clathrin-coated pits) and internalized, forming a free-floating vesicle inside the cell that contains glucose transporters (among other membrane-bound proteins). If a cell needs more glucose, the cell either makes new transporters or replaces the previously invaginated vesicle containing transporters back into the membrane. Corticosteroids alter this system in two ways: by stimulating the sequestration of extant glucose transporters (Horner et al. 1987; Dimitriadis et al. 1997), and by decreasing the transcription of new

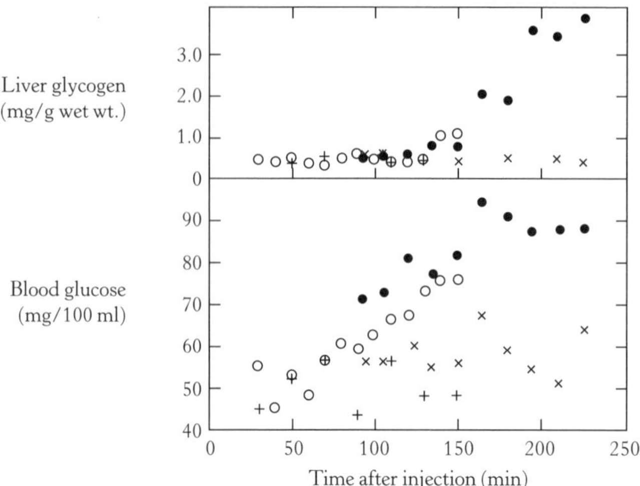

FIGURE 5.2: An early experiment indicating that corticosterone increases liver glycogen and blood glucose concentrations in laboratory rats. Each symbol represents an independent experiment, with the circles indicating animals injected with corticosterone and the + and x indicating controls.

Reprinted with permission from Munck and Koritz (1962). Courtesy of Elsevier.

transporters (Garvey et al. 1989) over the course of days. Corticosteroids stimulate sequestration by initiating the transcription of a protein that stimulates the formation and invagination of the vesicles—a process that takes approximately 8–12 hours (Sapolsky 1992).

The physiological consequences of corticosteroids internalizing glucose transporters are profound. Plasma glucose concentrations increase because cells are no longer using as much glucose (Munck 1971; Munck et al. 1984). Essentially, some of the hyperglycemia during stress, at least after glycogenolysis in the liver has slowed, is a side effect of decreasing cellular metabolism throughout the body. Furthermore, this implies that the excess glucose in the blood may not correspond to an increase in glucose available to target tissues (Sapolsky 1992). This is opposite from the common-sense interpretation that the hyperglycemia indicates and reflects increased cellular metabolism. However, certain tissues either may be resistant to glucocorticoid effects (such as some tumors; Romero et al. 1992) or may be able to compensate for the decreased glucose transporters, either of which will result in a diversion of glucose to those tissues that need it (Sapolsky et al. 2000).

We should remember, however, that our understanding of corticosteroid effects on glucose transporters has been derived primarily from mammalian tissues. Although it is likely that these mechanisms are important across vertebrate taxa, there may be subtle differences in non-mammalian species. For example, recent evidence suggests that insulin has a weaker impact on glucose uptake in house sparrow muscles (Sweazea and Braun 2005), possibly as a result of a lack of insulin-dependent glucose transporters (Sweazea and Braun 2006; Sweazea et al. 2006). Although to our knowledge no one has yet examined glucose transporter sensitivity to corticosteroids in a non-mammalian species, the evidence from insulin sensitivity in birds suggests caution in extrapolating across taxa.

The third major pathway that corticosteroids initiate is gluconeogenesis. In order to continue fueling recovery from the emergency response, fats and proteins are converted to glucose in the liver (Dallman et al. 1993). Fat mobilization occurs from fat depots throughout the body, but subcutaneous fat depots are a primary target (Dallman et al. 2004). Corticosteroids also inhibit the uptake of new fat by adipose tissues. The end result is an increase in free fatty acids in the blood, which are then transported to the liver and converted to glucose.

A similar process occurs with proteins. Corticosteroids initiate the breakdown of muscle proteins into their constituent amino acids (e.g., Bowes et al. 1996; Schakman et al. 2008). Corticosteroids also inhibit the formation of new proteins (e.g., Dong et al. 2007) by inhibiting both RNA synthesis and translation (Umpleby and RussellJones 1996). The process can be so

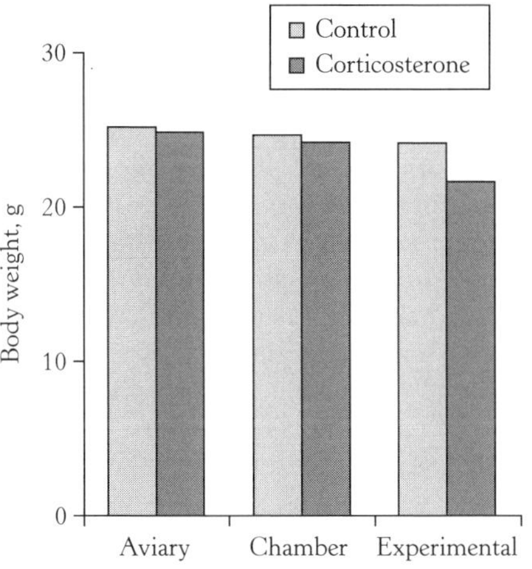

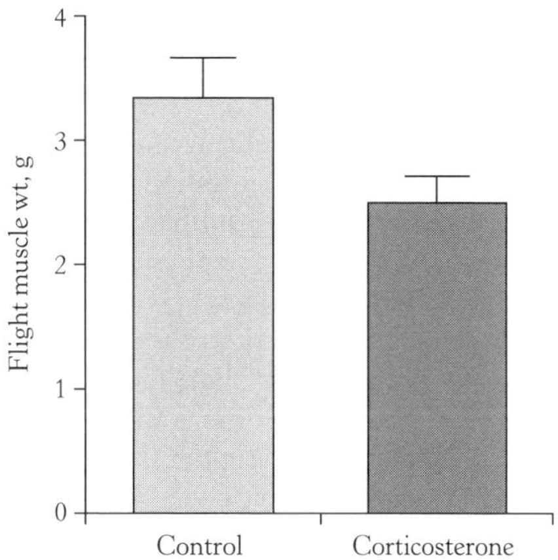

FIGURE 5.3: Effects of corticosterone on body weight of house sparrows. In the left-hand panel, birds in aviaries and after transfer to experimental chambers and before treatment had identical body weight. After treatment with a corticosterone implant or empty implant as control, body weight declined. Weight of the pectoralis muscles were reduced also with corticosterone treatment (right-hand panel).

From Honey (1990). Unpublished Ph.D. Thesis.

powerful that severe muscle atrophy and weakness can result (Schakman et al. 2008). The net result is a release of amino acids into the blood. These amino acids are then transported to the liver and are converted to glucose (Goldstein et al. 1993). In wild species, corticosteroids have been shown to decrease body weight, such as in house sparrows (Figure 5.3), including a decrease in weight of the pectoralis major (huge flight muscle), suggesting that the loss of body mass was through mobilization of protein for gluconeogenesis (Honey 1990).

The glucose produced through gluconeogenesis is then released into the bloodstream and is available to other tissues. However, this process takes hours to days, a time frame much too long to help provide energy during the initial phases of responding to a stressor (Sapolsky et al. 2000). Instead, the primary role for gluconeogenesis presumably is to replace the glycogen consumed earlier in the stress response. In other words, gluconeogenesis is a prime example of a recovery and/or preparative role for corticosteroids (see Chapter 4). Consequently, one major function of corticosteroids is to promote gluconeogenesis in order to orchestrate the mobilization of energy from long-term storage sites.

The gluconeogenic effects of corticosteroids appear to be conserved across taxa. For example, corticosterone stimulates proteolysis and gluconeogenesis in chickens (Lin et al. 2004a; Lin et al. 2004b). Protein catabolism is also evident in pigeons undergoing sustained flight (Bordel and Haase 2000), which is presumably regulated by corticosteroid increases resulting from the exercise. Corticosterone also increases lipid metabolism in several other bird species (Bray 1993; Latour et al. 1996; Kern et al. 2005). In addition, protein restriction can cause changes in the HPA axis in several species (Carsia and Weber 1988; Carsia et al. 1988; Carsia and McIlroy 1998; Carsia and Weber 2000a; Carsia and Weber 2000b), suggesting that an animal's body condition can alter whether corticosteroids are preferentially mobilizing lipids or proteins (Heath and Dufty 1998).

Finally, corticosteroids help in the replacement of even these long-term stores. The urge to consume food, or appetite, is an incredibly complex process regulated by a multitude of neural, neuroendocrine, and endocrine factors (Schwartz et al. 2000), including peptides of the CRF family (e.g., Heinrichs and Richard 1999; la Fleur 2005). Corticosteroids are important players in that they help stimulate appetite (Dallman and Bhatnagar 2001; Dallman et al. 2003; Dallman 2005; Nieuwenhuizen and Rutters 2008) and in many cases, influence what kinds of food are sought (Dallman et al. 2003; Dallman et al. 2004). Corticosteroids stimulate the preference for sweet and high-fat foods in what appears to be a rapid non-genomic mechanism involving endocannabanoids (Dallman et al. 2004). Given the current epidemic in obesity in Western societies, it is not surprising that the corticosteroid role in appetite has attracted considerable attention. Current theories have focused on the complex interplay between corticosteroids and insulin (Dallman et al. 1993; Dallman et al. 2003), although corticosteroid interactions with other peptides such as NPY and leptin are currently being actively studied. At low or sustained moderate concentrations, corticosteroids tend to synergize with insulin to promote fattening. This occurs both at the physiological level (glucose uptake into adipocytes) and at the behavioral level (stimulating appetite). These concentrations typically occur during short-term fasts and near the end of a stress response, and are thought to interact with the type I receptor. Consequently, low to moderate corticosteroid concentrations help regulate the body's normal daily energy flux, aid in the recovery from a stressor, and help the animal prepare for a future stressor.

Corticosteroid replacement of energy is not simple, however. Stress, presumably via a corticosteroid mechanism, appears to make glucose absorption from the intestines more efficient (e.g., Boudry et al. 2007). Corticosteroids also mediate the redistribution of energy into different types of fat so that calories are preferentially stored in abdominal fat (Dallman et al. 2004). This process has also been shown in other animal species provided long-term corticosteroid implants (e.g., Gray et al. 1990). Although this can be a serious problem in human health, where high levels of abdominal fat are associated with numerous diseases such as diabetes and cardiovascular disease, it is unclear what role this rearranging of fat storage plays in wild animals. However, it is becoming increasingly clear that not all fat depots are created equally. For example, mesenteric and abdominal fat depots secrete different hormones, such as leptin, and appear to play very different roles in calorie storage (Wajchenberg et al. 2002). It would not be surprising to learn that corticosteroids have different impacts on different fat depots, especially since mesenteric and subcutaneous fat stores have different abundances of corticosteroid receptors (e.g., Leibel et al. 1989; Pedersen et al. 1992; Sjogren et al. 1994; Wajchenberg et al. 2002). Furthermore, subcutaneous fat breakdown preferentially travels to the liver for immediate conversion into glucose (Cherrington 1999; Dallman et al. 2004). If such differences in fat depots are widespread taxonomically, it would have clear ramifications on how wild animals are using stored energy during emergencies. Such studies would be a fruitful avenue for future research.

The corticosteroid synergy with insulin led Dallman et al. (1993) to propose an intriguing hypothesis. They predicted that corticosteroids would play a major role in regulating the severe hyperphagia (overeating) and fat accumulation required in the fall by many mammalian hibernators. A seasonal increase in corticosteroids would interact with insulin to promote increased energy acquisition through feeding and increased energy storage in adipocytes. A recent test of this prediction did not support their hypothesis. Corticosteroid concentrations were lower in the fall than in the spring in a species that relies upon endogenous fat stores to survive the winter, but concentrations were higher in the fall for a species that caches food and does not rely upon fat stores (Romero et al. 2008). This result was exactly opposite of what Dallman et al. (1993) predicted, suggesting that the interplay between insulin and corticosteroids may be different in hibernators, or potentially that the interplay is more complex in free-living animals.

In contrast to low to moderate concentrations of corticosteroids, high concentrations inhibit insulin function. One major function of insulin is to promote synthesis of glucose transporters as well as mobilization of internalized transporters back to the cell surface. High corticosteroid concentrations mediate "insulin resistance" by inhibiting both of these functions (Dimitriadis et al. 1997). Furthermore, high corticosteroid concentrations decrease appetite, perhaps indirectly via CRF release (Carr 2002). The combination of these effects, especially insulin resistance, can lead to devastating effects on human health. Elevated corticosteroids are a major component leading to a disease termed "metabolic syndrome," which is typified by obesity, type II diabetes, altered metabolism in multiple organ systems, and cardiac disease (e.g., Qi and Rodrigues 2007; Roberge et al. 2007).

This biphasic nature of corticosteroid function makes sense—inhibit insulin function and decrease appetite when you are in the height of a stress response (i.e., when corticosteroid concentrations are high), and switch to promoting food acquisition and storage to promote recovery and prepare for a subsequent stressor after the original stressor has passed (i.e., low to moderate corticosteroid concentrations). Unfortunately, this biphasic response can make it difficult to isolate and study the different corticosteroid functions experimentally.

In birds, it appears that corticosterone and other components of the HPA axis have mixed effects on food intake (e.g., Astheimer et al. 1992; Ramenofsky et al. 1992). In Gambel's

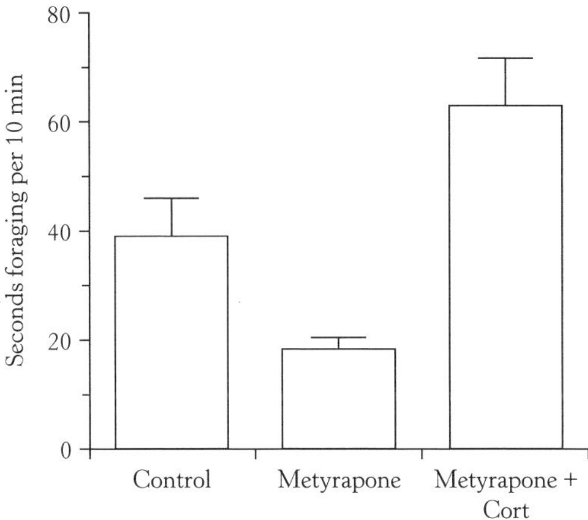

FIGURE 5.4: Effects of a corticosteroid synthesis inhibitor, metyrapone, on feeding rate in captive white-crowned sparrows. Replacement therapy of corticosterone treatment to metyrapone treated birds increased feeding compared to metyrapone treated birds but not above controls.

From Wingfield (1994). Courtesey of Cambridge University Press.

white-crowned sparrows held in captivity, an inhibitor of corticosterone synthesis, metyrapone, decreased rate of food intake (but not significantly), but replacement therapy of metyrapone-treated birds with corticosterone significantly increased food intake but not above controls (Figure 5.4; Wingfield 1994). On the other hand, corticosterone implants into captive Gambel's white-crowned sparrows had mixed and mostly non-significant effects on food intake (Figures 5.5 and 5.6; Astheimer et al. 1992). Similar results were found in corticosterone-treated dark-eyed juncos (Astheimer et al. 1992). On the other hand, corticosterone implants did increase food intake in Gambel's white-crowned sparrows after a period of fasting, suggesting a significant role for corticosterone in recovery after a stressful event (Figure 5.5; Astheimer et al. 1992).

Experiments in birds have shown that peptides of the HPA axis also can affect food intake. Beta-endorphin injected into the third ventricle of male Gambel's white-crowned sparrows increased the number of feeding bouts and time spent feeding in a dose-dependent manner, whereas latency to feed decreased, also in a dose dependent manner (Figure 5.7; Maney and Wingfield 1998a). Nalaxone, a beta-endorphin receptor antagonist, had the opposite effects, again in a dose-dependent manner (Figure 5.8; Maney and Wingfield 1998a).

When these pathways are integrated, we see an emerging picture of how energy is mobilized during a stressor (Figure 5.1). Epinephrine is released immediately and mobilizes energy from short-term storage depots (glycogen). Shortly thereafter, corticosteroids act to extend this response and to decrease glucose transport into tissues, thereby making the newly released energy

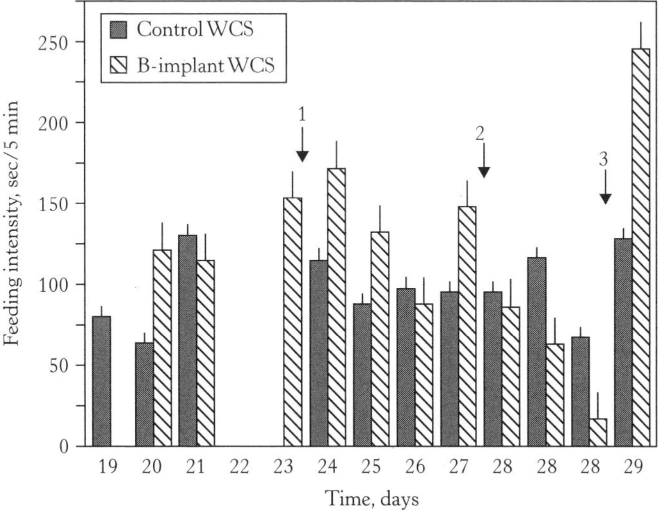

FIGURE 5.5: Daily feeding intensity of caged white-crowned sparrows (mean + s.e.m. of 10 min observations for each bird) under conditions of 8L 16D. Arrows indicate: 1 = date of implant (evening of January 23); 2 = beginning of the fast; 3 = end of the fast and beginning of refeeding. All observations were made between 0900 and 1100 hours with the exception of the last set of observations made on the fast day (January 28), which were made between 1400 and 1530 hours.

Astheimer et al. (1992). Courtesey of Ornis Scandinavica.

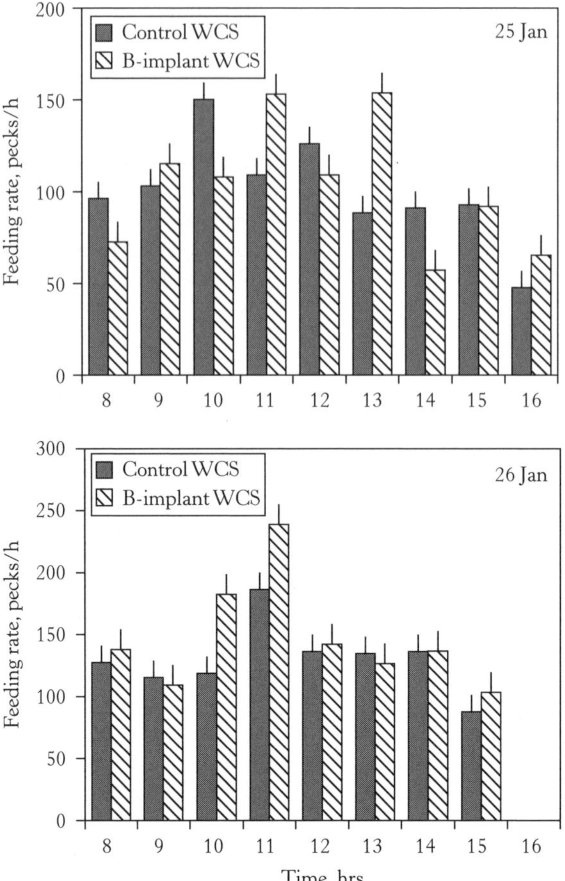

FIGURE 5.6: Hourly feeding rates (mean + s.e.m.) for white-crowned sparrows with empty (control) or corticosterone implants during consecutive days 2 and 3 following implantation.

Astheimer et al. (1992). Courtesey of Ornis Scandinavica.

preferentially available to tissues that need it. On a longer time scale, corticosteroids extend the period of energy provisioning by orchestrating the shift to utilizing long-term storage depots (gluconeogenesis). Finally, corticosteroids, and perhaps peptides of the HPA axis, help mediate the replacement of lost energy by stimulating both appetite and new fat deposition. The overall impression is of corticosteroids as the maestro, overseeing and directing the complex metabolic dance necessary for provisioning cells with energy during and following an emergency.

B. Metabolic Rate

Stress can obviously have a large impact on metabolic rate. After all, activation of the sympathetic nervous system will require substantial increases in metabolic fuel consumption, and any exercise appears to result in increased catecholamine and corticosteroid release (Jimenez et al. 1998; de Graaf-Roelfsema et al. 2007). But do the later phases of the stress response, and especially the corticosteroids, also increase metabolic rates?

In ectotherms, corticosterone can have a profound effect on metabolic rate. Corticosterone injection into lizards (DuRant et al. 2008) or maintaining geckos on short-term corticosterone implants (Preest and Cree 2008) results in a sustained elevation in oxygen consumption (Figure 5.9). In contrast, long-term corticosterone implants can have an opposite effect, resulting in a lower metabolic rate (Miles et al. 2007). The short-term increases in metabolic rate due to corticosterone appear to be in addition to the impact of epinephrine on muscle metabolism (Gleeson et al. 1993). In fact, most of corticosteroids' impact on metabolic rate may be occurring directly at the level of muscle. There is an increase

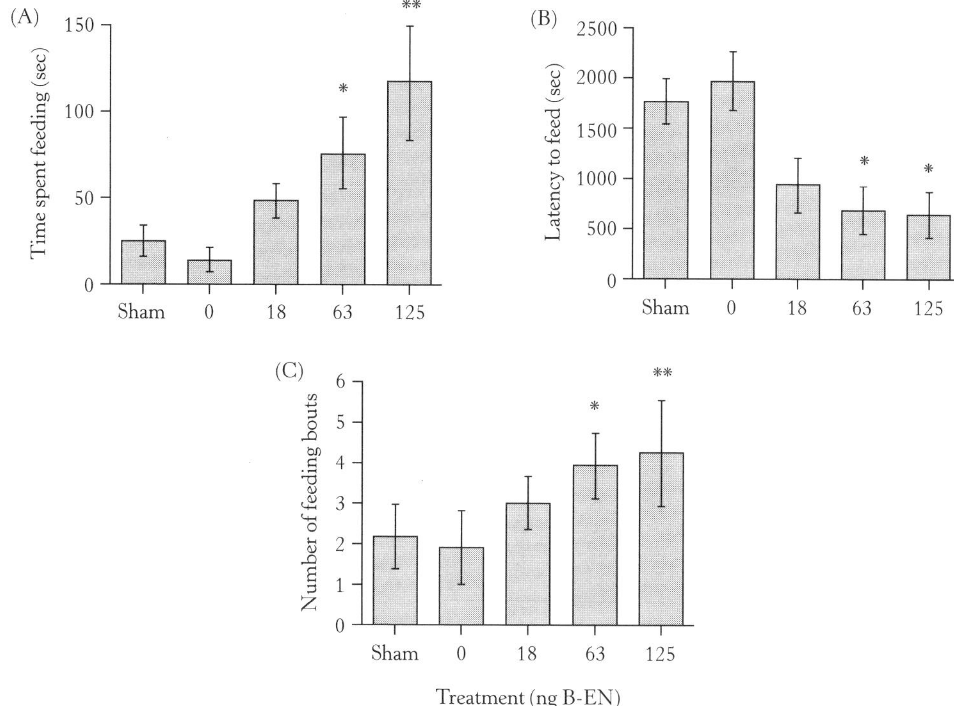

FIGURE 5.7: Effects of intraventricular b-EN on feeding behavior for 45 min after treatment. Asterisks denote a significant difference from saline. (A) Amount of time subjects spent pecking at or manipulating food. (B) Latency to feed after treatment. (C) Number of feeding bouts.

From Maney and Wingfield (1998a). Courtesy of Elsevier.

in mitochondria mass and changes in mitochondria function in skeletal muscle tissues, at least in mammals (Weber et al. 2002; Arvier et al. 2007; Manoli et al. 2007). The increased energy consumption is compensated for by an increase in food intake that leads to an overall increase in survival (Cote et al. 2006).

The impact of corticosteroids on metabolic rate is less well studied in endotherms. There have been a few studies in birds. On the other hand, there does seem to be an impact on the variability of nighttime metabolic rate within an individual. Corticosterone administration to white-crowned sparrows and pine siskins decreased the variability associated with measuring an individual's metabolic rate resulting in approximately 20% energy savings overnight (Buttemer et al. 1991). Wikelski et al. (1999) found no effect of corticosterone on metabolic rate in white-crowned sparrows during the day, but in both white-crowned sparrows and pine siskins sampled at night, corticosterone also had no effect on minimum metabolic rate but did decrease extended metabolic rate overnight (Figures 5.10 and 5.11; Buttemer et al. 1991; Astheimer et al. 1992). Furthermore, in both pine siskins and white-crowned sparrows, fasting reduced extended metabolic rate in controls, but if corticosterone implants were combined with a fast (which may be common during direct LPFs in the wild), extended metabolic rate was not significantly reduced further (Figure 5.12; Buttemer et al. 1991; Astheimer et al. 1992). Thus corticosterone treatment has similar effects to reduce nocturnal extended metabolic rate at night rather like in control birds that are fasted. This may have important implications during a response to a direct LPF; longer-term conservation of energy will be important during the night, which can then be invested in coping during the day. In contrast, corticosterone administration to juvenile zebra finches increased the variability in metabolic rate (Spencer and Verhulst 2008). What makes these studies different is not clear, although the results from the juvenile zebra finches may also incorporate growth effects.

Although the preceding studies have measured metabolic rate using various measures of oxygen consumption or carbon dioxide emission,

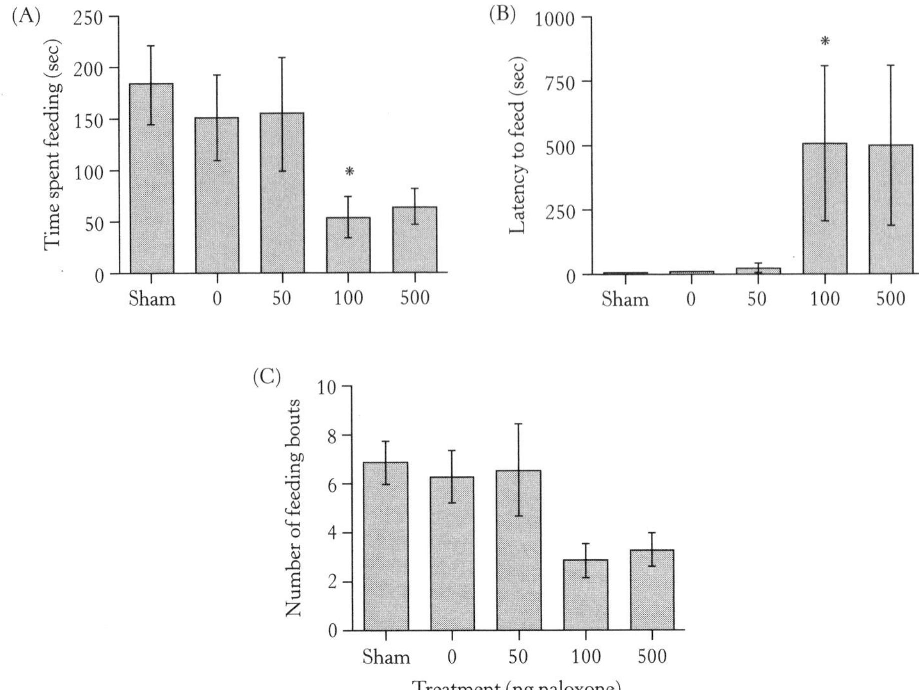

FIGURE 5.8: Effects of intraventricular naloxone on feeding behavior in food-deprived subjects for 45 minutes after treatment. Asterisks denote a significant difference from saline. (A) Amount of time subjects spent pecking at or manipulating food. (B) Latency to feed after treatment and return of food. (C) Number of feeding bouts.

From Maney and Wingfield (1998a). Courtesey of Elsevier.

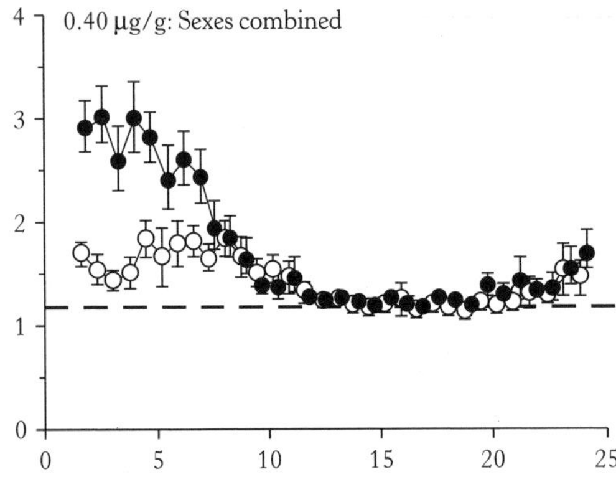

FIGURE 5.9: Oxygen consumption rates (ml/hr) of *Sceloporus occidentalis* before (open circles) and after (closed circles) injection with 0.4 ug/g corticosterone measured over 24 hours. Dashed lines indicate the average standard metabolic rate (SMR) of lizards during the pre-treatment respirometry trial.

Reprinted with permission from DuRant et al. (2008). Courtesy of Elsevier.

a number of studies have used the correlation between heart rate and oxygen consumption to infer changes in metabolic rate from changes in heart rate (e.g., Butler et al. 2002; Cyr et al. 2008; Bisson et al. 2009). These studies have indicated that the connection between stress and metabolic rates can be complex. Cyr et al. (2008) showed that different stressors can have different metabolic impacts, and the same stressor can have a different metabolic impact during different physiologic states (Figure 5.13). Furthermore, some stressors, such as human disturbance, which evoke strong stress responses in the laboratory, fail to evoke similar responses under natural conditions (Bisson et al. 2009; Bisson et al. 2011). These data suggest that the impact of a stressor is heavily dependent upon the severity of the stressor (see also Canoine et al. 2002) and the physiological state of the animal when the stressor is encountered. Consequently, these data provide strong support to the allostasis and reactive scope models presented in earlier chapters.

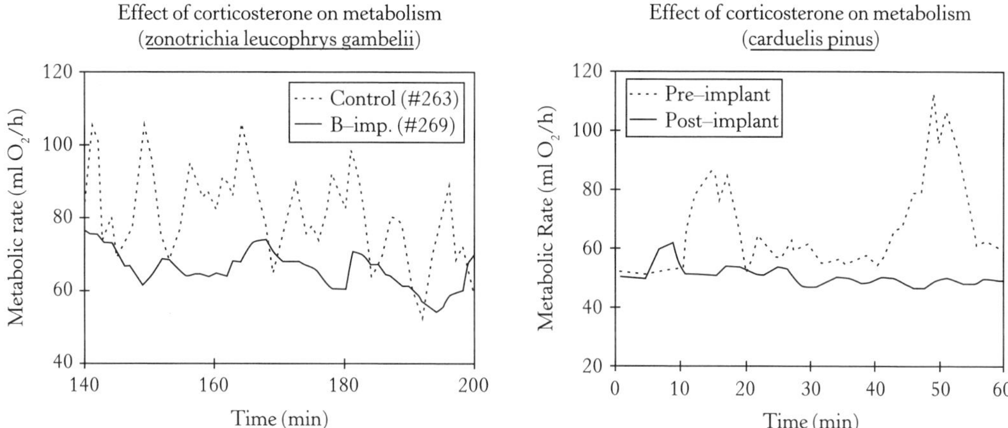

FIGURE 5.10: Effects of corticosterone of extended metabolic rate in white-crowned sparrows and pine siskins.

From Buttemer et al. (1991). Courtesey of Springer.

C. Recovery from Stress

Earlier in this chapter, we discussed the normal biphasic corticosteroid response. Corticosteroids inhibit insulin function and decrease appetite at the height of a stress response, but switch to promoting food acquisition and storage to promote recovery and prepare for a subsequent stressor after the original stressor has passed. Remember that recovery from a stressor and preparation for subsequent stressors are two important roles for corticosteroids (Chapter 4; see also Sapolsky et al. 2000). As an example of this switch in function, Figure 5.14 indicates that corticosterone had no effect or a slight stimulatory effect on feeding before a fast in caged white-crowned sparrows. Feeding time (or rather trying to feed) during the fast was greatly decreased, as expected. However, when food was returned, corticosterone-treated birds had greatly elevated feeding times, suggesting a role in recovery from a perturbation (Astheimer et al. 1992). We have discussed the initial response in the preceding sections, but do the recovery and preparation functions play an important role in free-living animals?

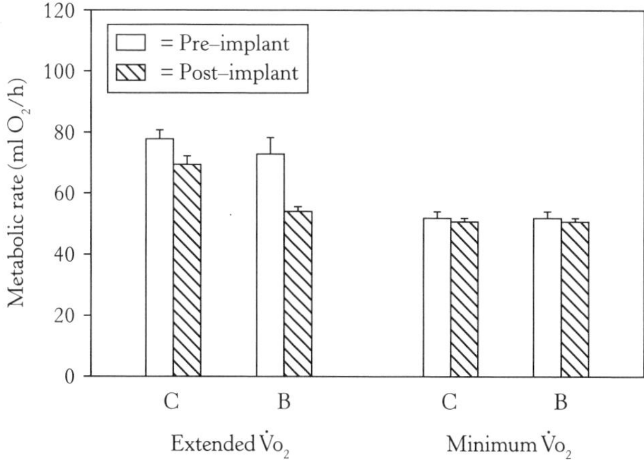

FIGURE 5.11: Extended and minimum (basal) metabolic rates (mean + s.e.m.) for pine siskins before and after birds were given control or corticosterone implants.

From Astheimer et al. (1992). Similar data for white-crowned sparrows are reported in Buttemer et al. (1991). Courtesey of Ornis Scandinavica and Springer.

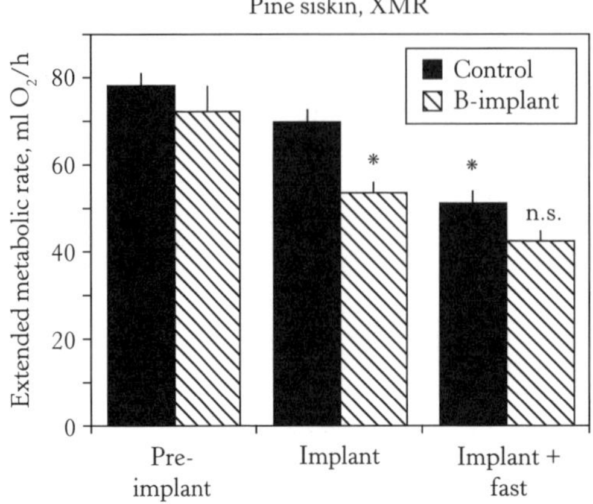

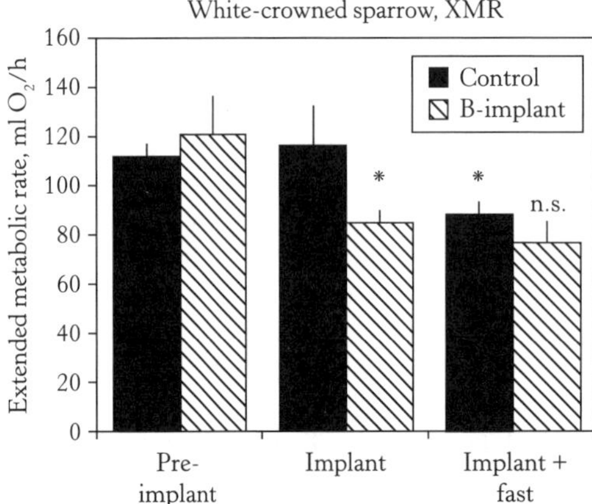

FIGURE 5.12: Extended metabolic rates (mean + s.e.m.; XMR) for pine siskins (upper panel) and white-crowned sparrows (lower panel) before and after control or corticosterone implants, and during a 24-hour fast. Significant differences ($p < 0.05$) occur between corticosterone-implanted and control, and between control fed and control fasted XMR in both species (asterisk, Tukey's test). Difference between control and corticosterone implanted fasted birds was not significant. From Astheimer et al. (1992. Courtesey of Ornis Scandinavica.

One line of evidence suggests that recovery from a stressor is a prime function for corticosteroids, including the time course of metabolic changes. As discussed earlier, corticosteroids often do not have an impact on plasma glucose concentrations when the animal is fed. However, even in fed animals a prolonged stressor will start to elevate plasma glucose. For example, although capture itself may not increase glucose concentrations, 2–4 hours of handling and transport can result in elevated levels (Grutter and Pankhurst 2000).

Long-term corticosterone implants in a lizard can result in several features of enhancing recovery. When these lizards are exposed to exhaustive exercise, they show better stamina and faster recovery times compared to controls (Miles et al. 2007). However, the interplay between corticosterone and other hormones is undoubtedly complicated because blocking endogenous corticosterone synthesis in another study had no impact on recovery (Scholnick et al. 1997).

Another line of evidence that corticosteroids can help in recovery comes from the metabolic studies in birds. Buttemer et al. (1991) interpreted the decrease in the variability of metabolic measurements at night in birds as promoting night restfulness. Even though there was no overall change in minimum nighttime metabolic rate, they suggested that decreasing the variability reduced the responsiveness to external stimuli, stabilized metabolism, and resulted in energy savings (see Figures 5.10–5.12). If this interpretation is correct, corticosteroids may be helping shift daily energy metabolism such that the energetic costs of coping with a stressor during the active period are compensated for by saving energy during the inactive period. The overall energetic cost of a stressor, therefore, would be ameliorated, if not negligible. Unfortunately, this idea has not yet been rigorously tested, but the results to date are mixed. Two studies with similar data are not supportive, although neither was a definitive test. Chicks, with likely a different metabolism than adults, showed the opposite result with increases in variability in metabolic rate (Spencer and Verhulst 2008), and inferring metabolic rate from changes in heart rate showed no nighttime compensation for daytime stressors (Cyr et al. 2008). In contrast, administering corticosterone to rufous hummingbirds increased the duration of overnight torpor (Hiebert et al. 2000). Corticosteroid-mediated shifting of energy consumption is an intriguing hypothesis with important fitness ramifications and so deserves more attention.

Finally, the behavioral effects of corticosteroids can also potentially influence metabolic rates. Corticosteroids are thought to elicit either a "wait it out" or a "leave" strategy (Wingfield and Ramenofsky 1997). Part of the "wait it out" strategy is to carefully select a suitable microhabitat. Use of microclimates can dramatically alter the amount of energy that is needed (Blem 1990). For example, during heavy snowfall, the area underneath trees will have much less snow and may be 7°–10°C warmer than other nearby

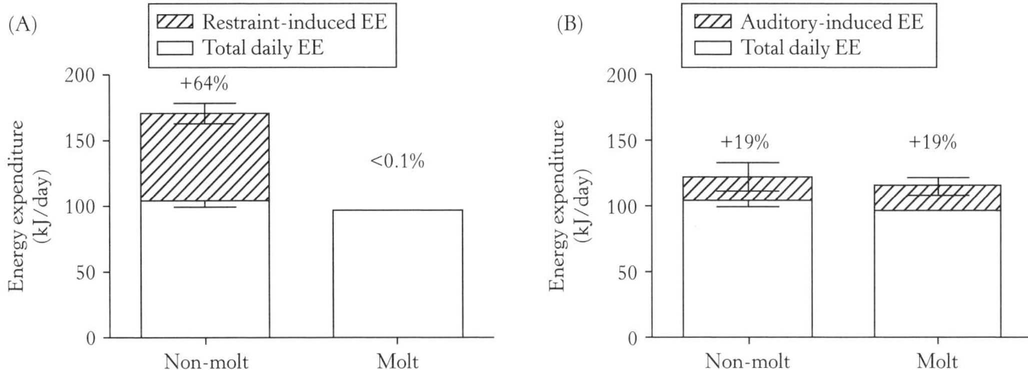

FIGURE 5.13: Increase in the rate of energy expenditure during restraint (A) and an auditory stressor (B—a loud radio). The white bars indicate the mean energy expenditure (± SE) during the daytime (lights on) for molting and non-molting starlings. The bars with diagonal lines represent the percentage of the normal daytime energy expenditure that was additionally expended during the 30-minute stressor. Values were calculated by subtracting the baseline energy expenditure prior to the stressor from the energy expenditure during the stressor.

EE = energy expenditure.

Reprinted with permission from Cyr et al. (2008). Courtesy of University of Chicago Press.

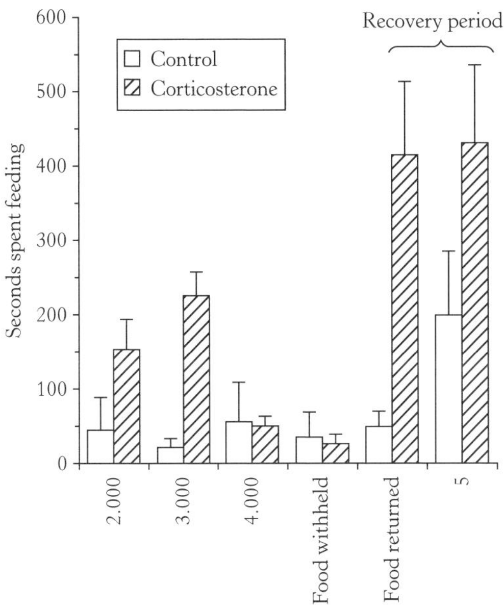

FIGURE 5.14: Effects of corticosterone on time spent feeding both before and after a fast in caged white-crowned sparrows. Corticosterone had no effect or a slight stimulatory effect on feeding before a fast. Feeding time (or rather trying to feed) during the fast was greatly decreased as expected. However, when food was returned, corticosterone-treated birds had greatly elevated feeding times, suggesting a role in recovery from a perturbation.

From Astheimer et al. (1992). Courtesey of Ornis Scandinavica.

locations (Wingfield and Ramenofsky 1997), meaning that an animal seeking refuge in this microhabitat will require significantly less energy to maintain body temperature. The opposite can also be true. Geckos implanted with corticosterone maintained an elevated metabolic rate that was at least partially mediated by the selection of a warmer microhabitat and thus increased body temperature (Preest and Cree 2008). The selection of microhabitats is likely to be a major underappreciated way in which stress has an impact on metabolic rates.

III. IMMUNE SYSTEM

Perhaps no aspect of stress has created more confusion, puzzlement, and sustained controversy than the corticosteroid effects on the immune system. In many ways the controversy continues today. The interaction between corticosteroids and the immune system has a sordid history. Selye (1946) originally conceived of the corticosteroids as being immuno-enhancing. He proposed that excess corticosteroids would make autoimmune diseases worse, and might even be the causative agent for these diseases. However, corticosteroids quickly became the preeminent drug in clinical medicine for inhibiting the immune system—exactly the opposite of what Selye proposed! The spectacular failure of Selye's proposal led to the extended abandonment of trying to make sense of the integrated physiology of corticosteroids (documented in Munck et al. 1984; Sapolsky et al. 2000).

Everything changed in 1984 with the publication of a seminal review paper by Munck and colleagues (Munck et al. 1984). Relying heavily on data from corticosteroid effects on the immune system, Munck et al. proposed that corticosteroids were essentially inhibitory regulators during the stress response. Munck et al. essentially flipped the prevailing view on the role of corticosteroids. Instead of conceiving of corticosteroids as forming part of the stress response, Munck et al, suggested that corticosteroids' major role was in turning off stress-induced responses, especially stress-induced immune responses. Left unchecked, the activated immune system would run amok, so failure to shut off the immune system could be catastrophic. In this view, corticosteroids serve as the brakes to the stress-activated immune system. This proposal had great appeal, especially given the preeminence of corticosteroids in clinical practice in inhibiting inflammation.

Partially in response to Munck et al.'s (1984) review, Sapolsky et al. (2000), proposed a more nuanced view of corticosteroid actions that encompassed activating, inhibitory, permissive, and preparatory functions (see Chapter 4). In their analysis of different physiological systems, Sapolsky et al. retained the conclusion that corticosteroids were broadly immunosuppressive. However, new evidence was appearing, suggesting that even this view was too simplistic. Starting in the late 1990s, studies started to show that corticosteroids, under some circumstances, might activate the immune system after all. The difference was in the time course: corticosteroids appeared to enhance immune function in the short term but become immunosuppressive in the long term (e.g., Dhabhar and McEwen 1999). Part of this re-evaluation of corticosteroids' effects on immune function also derived from focusing on the functions of corticosteroids at endogenous, rather than exogenous (e.g., clinical treatment), concentrations (Spencer et al. 2001).

The current hypothesis of corticosteroid actions in immunity is a melding of the earlier views. Corticosteroids are now thought to have a biphasic response; they enhance immune responses immediately after exposure to a stressor, but inhibit immune responses as the corticosteroid response continues and extends into chronic release. This modern conception fits nicely into the allostasis and reactive scope models of stress (see Chapter 3). With allostasis, the corticosteroid-mediated enhancement of immune function primes the body to fight a potential infection, but concurrently increases allostatic load. If there is no infection, corticosteroids then inhibit the immune response in order to reduce allostatic load and allocate resources to other systems. However, if the inhibition continues, there will be a decrease in the reactive scope, making it more likely that corticosteroids will end up harming the animal by preventing adequate immune responses in the future.

Given the enormous importance of corticosteroids in clinical medicine, we have extensive knowledge of corticosteroid impacts on the immune system at the cellular and molecular level. This information could fill several books in their own right and are beyond the scope of this chapter. What follows is a broad outline of corticosteroid effects, focusing especially on how corticosteroids might affect the overall efficacy of an immune response.

A. Corticosteroids Enhance Immunity and Inflammation

Two types of stressors initiate an immune response—injury and infection. Although injury (i.e., tissue damage) seems different from infection, injury (especially wounding) often results in infection. Research on corticosteroid/immune interactions tends to focus on infectious stressors, but corticosteroid effects during injury are similar (Yeager et al. 2004).

At the onset of a stressor, especially one with a disease component, the initial immune system activation is called the acute phase response. Immune cells, especially macrophages, congregate at the primary trauma site and initiate the release of cytokines (see Chapter 2). Cytokines are generic chemical messengers of the immune system. The only real difference between cytokines and hormones is that cytokines are released preferentially by immune tissues, although the more we study cytokines, the more this distinction breaks down. The primary cytokines involved in the acute phase response are interleukins 1 and 6 (IL-1 and IL-6), and their job is to help initiate and maintain the acute phase response. Two primary functions of corticosteroids are to stimulate the production of acute phase proteins and to enhance IL-1 and IL-6 function (Bulloch 2001; Spencer et al. 2001).

The acute phase response sets the stage for the later phases of the immune response. Immune responses specific to the emergency are initiated, with both B and T lymphocytes flooding to the injury and/or infection site. This appears

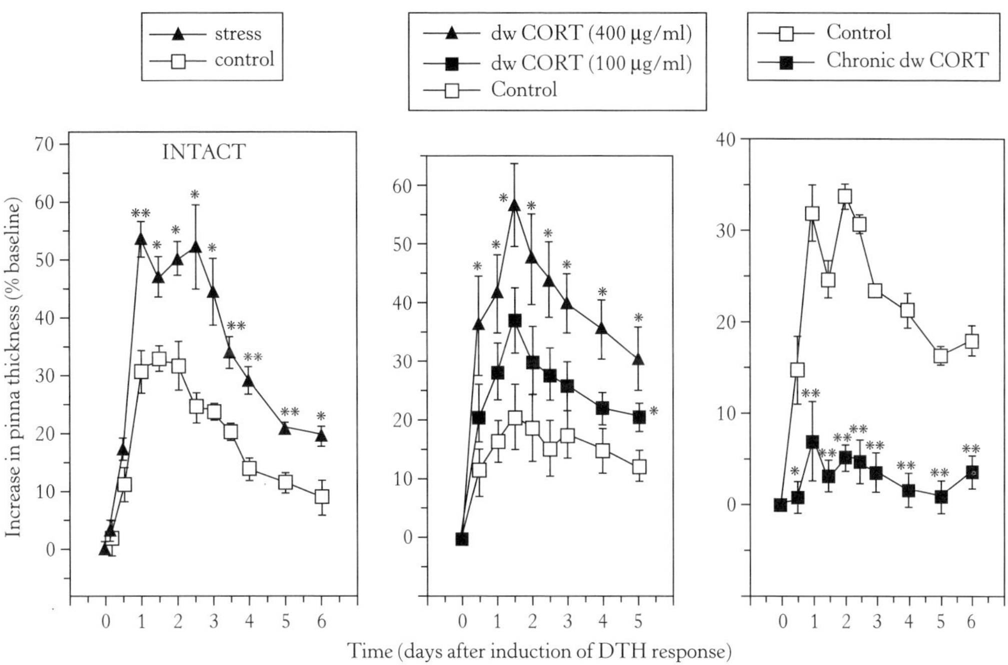

FIGURE 5.15: The effect of stress (left panel) on immune responses. Pinna (the external part of the ear) increases in thickness due to inflammation during delayed type hypersensitivity (DTH). DTH refers to an inflammatory response mediated by macrophages and T-helper leukocytes. The middle panel indicates that the increased inflammation is likely mediated by acute increases in corticosterone. In contrast, the right panel indicates that chronic exposure to corticosteroids inhibits the inflammation.

Reprinted with permission from Dhabhar and McEwen (1999). Courtesy of the National Academy of Sciences.

to be another major role for corticosteroids. Corticosteroids increase neutrophil function and stimulate lymphocyte migration to the infection site (Spencer et al. 2001). Essentially, corticosteroids are mediating a redistribution of lymphocytes from their surveillance sites (peripheral blood) to their active sites (sites of infection). If corticosteroid concentrations continue to be elevated, however, they quickly begin to suppress immune function. Figure 5.15 illustrates the differences between acute and chronic corticosteroid responses.

Corticosteroids also play a permissive role in immune function. Immature immune cells in the thymus have greater sensitivity to corticosteroids, and corticosteroids can be produced locally in the thymus (all the corticosterone synthetic apparatus is present in the thymus), suggesting an important role for corticosteroids in lymphocyte maturation (Spencer et al. 2001).

There is also extensive crosstalk between the HPA axis and the activated immune system. A number of different cytokines stimulate the HPA (Turnbull and Rivier 1999), either through stimulation of CRF release or directly at the pituitary to stimulate ACTH release. This means that the initial phase of an infection involves a feed-forward loop—cytokines stimulate corticosteroid release (Figure 5.16), which in turn makes the cytokines more effective. In addition, neutrophils may be able to elicit increased corticosteroid concentrations directly at the site of infection. Neutrophils secrete enzymes that degrade proteins, and one target of these proteases might be CBG. CBG is especially sensitive to these proteases, and when degraded by them, releases its bound corticosteroids (Hammond 1990). This potentially allows the immune system to target specific tissues for the enhancing effects of corticosteroids.

Although trauma and infection share many elements, corticosteroids are also critical for two other important pathways for surviving trauma (Yeager et al. 2004). The first is that corticosteroids help support the cardiovascular changes necessary to cope with the hemorrhage from the wound. Second, corticosteroids play a key role in moderating the tissue damage due to a lack of blood flow arising from vasoconstriction. These two pathways

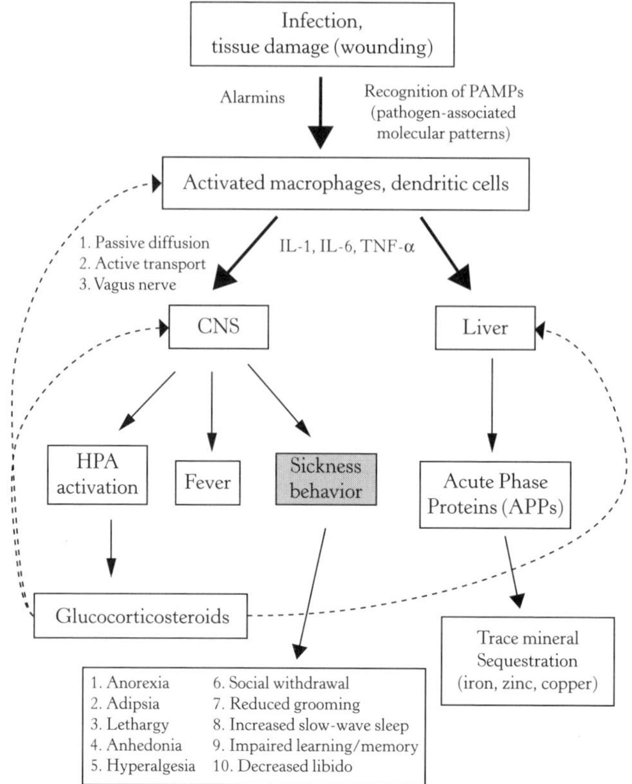

FIGURE 5.16: Schematic of the neuroendocrine-immune circuit for activating sickness behavior. Recognition of infection or injury triggers the release of cytokines, which activates a suite of physiological and behavioral responses that include sickness behavior, fever, acute phase protein (APP) production from the liver, and activation of the hypothalamo-pituitary-adrenal (HPA) axis and subsequent release of glucocorticoids. These hormones will initially stimulate immune function, but later provide negative feedback at multiple levels to the overall circuit. Dotted and continuous lines represent inhibitory and stimulatory actions, respectively.

From Ashley and Wingfield (2012). Courtesey of Oxford University Press.

then combine with corticosteroids, helping to stimulate the initial phases of the acute phase response for a coordinated response to a wound.

There is also excellent evidence that corticosteroids can enhance immune function prior to an infection (Dhabhar 2006; Dhabhar 2009). Acute release of corticosteroids directs lymphocytes to the skin prior to a wound or an infection. Because the skin is the major front-line defense against pathogens, and because many stressors such as agonistic encounters can raise the chances of injury and subsequent infection, the movement of lymphocytes to "battle stations" in the skin can enhance the ability of the immune system to fight infection. An interesting consequence, however, is that the movement of lymphocytes to the skin produces a transient decrease in lymphocytes in the blood. Historically, this decrease was interpreted as stress-induced immunosuppression. Current thinking, however, is that examination of immune function at the most likely site of wounding or infection (i.e., the skin rather than the blood) reveals immune enhancement rather than suppression (Dhabhar 2009).

B. Corticosteroids Inhibit Immunity and Inflammation

There is little doubt that prolonged stress can greatly inhibit immune function. Our favorite example comes from the human literature. One way to study the effects of psychological stress on immune function is to give humans a disease. This is essentially what vaccinations do. There is strong evidence that individuals exposed to psychological stress at the time of vaccination (such as students taking exams) show weaker induced immunity (Pedersen et al. 2009), an effect likely due directly to corticosteroids (Cohen et al. 2001).

After the initial "call to arms," corticosteroids help mediate a profound system-wide suppression of immune function (Sapolsky et al. 2000). They do this in a number of direct and indirect ways. At the molecular level, corticosteroids suppress the transduction of many genes involved in the initiation and maintenance of an immune response (Spencer et al. 2001). Examples include decreasing cytokine production (especially IL-1 and IL-6), inhibiting the synthesis of matrix proteins important in wound healing, inhibiting neutrophil and other leukocyte infiltration at the site of inflammation, and turning off production of a number of factors important in inflammation (e.g., eicosanoids, nitric oxide synthase, and cell adhesion molecules; Spencer et al. 2001). Especially in inflammation, corticosteroids have three generalized molecular effects: they suppress the production of inflammatory proteins; they stimulate the production of anti-inflammatory proteins; and they activate anti-inflammatory proteins (Rhen and Cidlowski 2005; Beck et al. 2009).

Corticosteroids also inhibit the function of numerous immune cells. Among the most potent effects are on lymphocyte activity, specifically by killing both T and B lymphocytes through either direct cell death (lysis) or through initiating programmed suicide, apoptosis (Spencer et al. 2001). Corticosteroids also exert profound effects on the thymus. Historically, shrinking of the thymus was one of the first diagnostic criteria of stress (Selye 1946). The reduction in the size of the thymus appears to be predominantly a result of corticosteroid-induced apoptosis of immature T-lymphocytes (Spencer et al. 2001). Although this clearly will result in long-term immunosuppression, there is some evidence that the corticosteroids may be "pruning" T cell function by removing those T cells that target the animal's own tissue or that do not target anything at all. Similar effects appear to occur in antibody production from B-lymphocytes, where mature B-cells are more resistant to corticosteroid effects (Spencer et al. 2001).

Suppressive effects of corticosteroids are generally mediated by GR type II receptor binding. Most immune tissues have very high levels of type II receptors, but very few MR type I receptors. This suggests that those immune cells that do express type I receptors will be affected by corticosteroids at much smaller concentrations (Spencer et al. 2001). Furthermore, the relative expression of corticosteroid receptors in different immune cells is thought to underlie why some cell types (e.g., lymphocytes) respond more strongly to a corticosteroid signal than other cell types (e.g. neutrophils; Spencer et al. 2001).

Interestingly, the inhibitory effects on the immune system occur despite a likely down-regulation of corticosteroid receptors in immune tissues (Spencer et al. 2001). Similar to other non-immune tissues, there is evidence that extended exposure to corticosteroids results in a reduction in the number of receptors in various immune cells (Bauer 2005). Cytokines may also modulate corticosteroid receptor levels and/or function (Spencer et al. 2001), and immune cells may switch to producing a type II receptor variant with decreased binding affinity for corticosteroids (DeRijk and de Kloet 2008). The reduction in receptor numbers then leads to desensitization to the corticosteroid signal. Despite desensitization, however, corticosteroids continue to exert profound immunosuppressive effects.

Corticosteroid feedback on immune function is one of the primary stop signals that ends the acute phase response, generally in 24–48 hours (Bulloch 2001). Failure of corticosteroid shutdown of the acute phase response is an important cause of chronic inflammation (Bulloch 2001) and appears to lead to reduced survival after exposure to acute inflammatory stimuli (Spencer et al. 2001). This effect was one of the main features of corticosteroid function that led to corticosteroids being classified as inhibiting the immune system to prevent a dangerous overshoot of immune function. In fact, patients with Addison's disease (those who lack corticosteroids) require corticosteroid supplementation during infections to prevent excessive inflammatory responses (Rhen and Cidlowski 2005).

C. Integration of Inhibiting and Enhancing Effects

The previous discussion indicates that corticosteroids have a biphasic response on mediating effects. First comes immuno-enhancement. This makes sense in the context of wild animals. Just as corticosteroids help prime the fight-or-flight system for an upcoming predator attack, so do corticosteroids help prime the immune system for an upcoming immune challenge (Dhabhar 2009). Both effects fit nicely into the role corticosteroids have for preparing the animal for future stressors (Chapter 4). Priming the immune system will be invaluable if an immune challenge does occur.

Can we make similar sense of the second half of the biphasic response? Although it might seem counterintuitive for corticosteroids to be immunosuppressive (after all, pathogens are likely to be a major stressor in wild animals), this too might make ecological sense. In an analogy presented by Sapolsky et al. (2000), a bigger immediate danger might be predation. Considerable evidence suggests that predators preferentially target animals showing signs of sickness or injury. Think of a zebra with a puffy red inflamed ear. It would certainly stand out from the herd. If this zebra wishes to avoid a predatory attack, it would make sense to inhibit the inflammatory symptoms so that it blends better into the herd. Consequently, corticosteroids might initially prime the immune system to fight the initial infection, then quickly inhibit the inflammation to reduce the chances of being targeted for predation. Notice that, under this scenario, corticosteroid anti-inflammatory effects also prepare the animal for a future stressor.

Alternatively, the activating/deactivating dichotomy of corticosteroid effects on immune function might make sense in the context of allostasis and reactive scope. An infection stimulates an immune response, which in turn stimulates corticosteroid release. This produces a large allostatic load on the organism and decreases the animal's reactive scope to cope with further stressors. Without further stressors, the immune system does its job, the corticosteroids help constrain the inflammatory response, and the animal recovers. If, however, the animal is faced with additional stressors concurrent to infection, the increased allostatic load and reduced reactive scope make the animal more likely to enter allostatic overload and it is more likely for the corticosteroids to begin to have counterproductive effects on the immune response.

The function of catecholamines in immune function is not well studied. In general, catecholamines appear to mimic the effects of corticosteroids. Adrenergic receptors are present on a number of immune cells and stimulate both shifts in cytokine production (Padgett and Glaser 2003) and redistribution of lymphocytes to the skin (Dhabhar and McEwen 1999). This suggests that at least acute catecholamine exposure is immuno-enhancing. Catecholamines also have more direct effects on the immunity through the sympathetic nervous system, which in turn connects to a number of immune tissues, including the bone marrow and the thymus. In the bone marrow, epinephrine appears to stimulate the production of immature immune cells (Bulloch 2001). This suggests an interesting possibility during chronic stress. Since chronic stress often results in lower catecholamine responses to new stressors, decreased stimulation of immune tissues may be another way in which chronic stress inhibits immune function. In contrast, the sympathetic nervous system appears to be inhibitory for immune function in both the thymus and the lymph nodes (Bulloch 2001), thereby inhibiting maturation and activity of lymphocytes. Many studies also indicate that stress-induced increases in corticosteroids cannot account for all the immunosuppressive effects of stress (Spencer et al. 2001). Catecholamine secretion is an obvious candidate mechanism for non-corticosteroid-mediated immunosuppression.

D. Sickness Behavior and Fever

There is another potential connection between stress and the immune system. Stress appears to activate immune parameters in order to promote sickness behaviors (Deak 2007). Stress stimulates the release of inflammatory cytokines not only at the site of infection or injury, but also centrally in the brain. Centrally released cytokines in turn can alter behavior, inducing malaise, lack of appetite, and so on. (Figure 5.16). These are the familiar behavioral symptoms of illness (e.g., Hart 1988; Ashley and Wingfield 2012) and also include reduced social behavior, increased sleep, reduced libido, and failure to groom/preen, resulting in poor self-maintenance. Furthermore, cytokines released during the acute phase response (i.e., IL-1, IL-6, and TNF) stimulate prostaglandin release, which in turn leads to fever (Spencer et al. 2001). The conclusion is that acute stress produces a suite of behaviors nearly identical to the suite of behaviors elicited by acute infections.

Why would acute stress make an animal act as if it were sick? The solution may be in how we perceive sickness behavior. Traditionally, sickness behavior was thought to be reactionary—a result of the raging battle between immune system and pathogen. Recent thinking, however, is that sickness behavior is proactive—a way for the animal to conserve energy (e.g., malaise results in decreased foraging) to promote recovery (Deak 2007). If sickness behavior is proactive, then sickness behaviors elicited by acute stress would fit into the broad concept of preparing the animal for future stressors.

IV. BEHAVIORAL EFFECTS

The behavioral effects of corticosteroids have been the subject of decades of study, especially in biomedicine. In humans, the majority of stressors derive from psycho-social pressures, and stress-related disease often manifests itself in various psychological (i.e., behavioral) pathologies. Consequently, the role of stress, and specifically corticosteroids, in altering these behaviors has been the focus of entire subfields of psychology (e.g., Gray 1987). In general, we know that corticosteroids do not directly induce behaviors. Instead, they alter the strength of various neural pathways to make certain behaviors more or less likely (Korte 2001). This means that studies have increasingly focused on the neurological underpinnings of behavior. The types of behavior thought to be most affected by corticosteroids include fear, anxiety, aggression, and brain function in memory and cognition, although the specific impact of corticosteroids on each of these classes of behavior depends upon a bewildering array of factors, including context, age, specific behavioral test, corticosteroid titers, and other factors (e.g., Korte 2001; Lupien et al. 2009). Detailing these responses would fill numerous volumes and is beyond the scope of this book. Furthermore, the psychopathologies important in biomedicine are unlikely to pose a major problem for wild free-living animals (although clearly might be a concern for captive animals in the laboratory or zoo). Consequently, we will focus the remainder of this section on corticosteroid impacts on behaviors likely to be important to free-living animals.

Looking back at Chapter 1, we discussed how the emergency life-history stage (ELHS) comprises a potentially broad spectrum of physiological and behavioral responses, all tailored to allow the individual to cope with a perturbation of the environment. In this section we review some of the more common behavioral effects in which glucocorticoids play important regulatory roles. Many others will be reviewed in later chapters in relation to responses to specific environmental events.

A. Survival/Coping Behavior

Glucocorticoids play major roles in orchestrating complex behavioral response patterns to unpredictable environmental events (Wingfield and Ramenofsky 1997, 1999; Silverin 1998; Wingfield and Silverin 2002, 2009). In a laboratory experiment Astheimer et al. (1992) showed how elevation of corticosterone levels in captive white-crowned sparrows resulted in decreased activity (perch hopping) if the birds had ad libitum food (Figure 5.17). This is consistent with the "take it" strategy (chapter 1, Wingfield and Ramenofsky 1997, 1999), in which a bird may seek a refuge while waiting for a stressful event to pass, thus saving energy. However, if food was removed, simulating a temporary loss of resources as happens frequently under natural conditions, then all birds showed dramatically increased perch-hopping

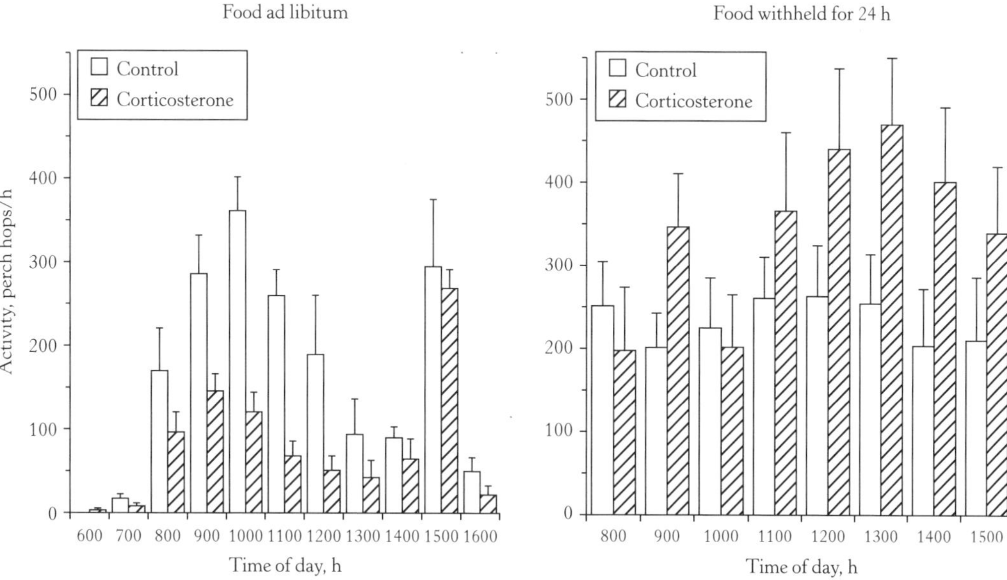

FIGURE 5.17: Hourly perch-hopping activity (mean + s.e.m.) for white-crowned sparrows during 2 days before a fast (left-hand panel) and during the fast (right-hand panel). With food ad libitum, corticosterone implants resulted in reduced activity, whereas if food was removed all birds became more active, but corticosterone-implanted birds even more so.

From Astheimer et al. (1992). Courtesey of Ornis Scandinavica.

activity. However, corticosterone-treated white-crowned sparrows had the highest levels of activity (Figure 5.17; Astheimer et al. 1992). These results are consistent with the "leave it" strategy (chapter 1, Wingfield and Ramenofsky 1997, 1999) and resemble escape behavior of a bird trying to get away from a labile perturbation factor in the field. This initial response is consistent with the "take it" strategy, followed later (when food was removed) by the "leave it" strategy. In an example from field studies, observations on free-living birds such as Lapland longspurs breeding on the North Slope of Alaska, revealed that exposure to a prolonged snowstorm did not result in abandonment of their nests until after two to three days. After eventually abandoning their nests, baseline corticosterone levels were low but sensitivity to additional stress was greatly enhanced (Astheimer et al. 1995).

The impact of corticosteroids on behavior can be very sensitive to concentrations. Free-living pied flycatchers breeding in Scandinavia showed a tri-phasic response. When they had a slight increase in circulating corticosterone, the parents increased feeding frequency of nestlings but showed only minor effects on body weights (Silverin 1986). On the other hand, moderate elevations of corticosterone led to reduced feeding frequency of the nestlings and subsequent high mortality of those nestlings. However, body weights of the adults remained constant during this period. Finally, very high levels of corticosterone, similar to those seen after severe stress, led to territories and nests being abandoned, with 100% mortality of nestlings (Silverin 1986). This time the parents actually increased their body weight, potentially promoting survival to breed at another time when conditions are more benign. These data indicate a shifting behavioral strategy with progressively increasing circulating levels of corticosterone, ultimately redirecting behavior away from reproduction to survival (Silverin 1986).

The short-term effects of corticosteroids, that is, within hours to days, regulate many facets of the facultative behavioral and physiological responses typical of an ELHS. Nonetheless, the different behavioral effects in corticosterone-treated white-crowned sparrows in relation to access to food suggest that additional factors are involved, at least in regulating activity (Figure 5.17). It is possible that neuropeptides such as CRF and beta-endorphin may also be involved. There is considerable experimental evidence that CRF increases activity in many vertebrate species (Bale and Vale 2004). In captive white-crowned sparrows, intra-cerebroventricular injection of CRF increased perch-hopping activity in a dose-related manner, whereas beta-endorphin did not (e.g., Figure 5.18; Maney and Wingfield 1998a, 1998b; Wingfield et al. 1998). Similarly, in free-living white-crowned sparrows, intra-cerebroventricular injection of CRF decreased territorial defense, consistent with redirecting behavior away from reproductive behaviors (Romero et al. 1998). It is possible that circulating corticosterone interacts and combines in complex ways with multiple brain peptides to redirect the individual away from the normal life-history stage and thus maximizes survival until the perturbation passes.

There is also growing evidence that very rapid actions of corticosterone may also influence activity (Figure 5.19). Breuner et al. (1998) injected mealworms with corticosterone in DMSO and fed them to captive white-crowned sparrows. These birds showed a surge of circulating corticosterone between 5 and 20 minutes after eating the worm, compared to controls that consumed mealworms injected with DMSO only. The surge in corticosterone was followed by increases in activity within 7–15 minutes of ingesting the mealworm, suggesting a biological action via a rapid-acting, membrane-like receptor mechanism (Figure 5.19; Breuner et al. 1998). An action through classical genomic receptors would take at least 30 minutes, and probably hours. Thus, an additional mechanism through rapid action membrane receptors may also interact with brain peptides to regulate complex behaviors during the perturbation of the environment. A similar experiment in free-living white-crowned sparrows also resulted in behavioral changes, in this case an increase in overall activity and a decrease in propensity to return to an abandoned territory (Breuner and Hahn 2003). It is interesting to note that this rapid action of corticosterone on activity in captive birds only works when birds are held on long days and in reproductive condition. Corticosterone does not appear to increase activity during short days mimicking winter (Breuner and Wingfield 2000).

Field and laboratory experiments using corticosterone implants also have dramatic effects on the behavior of seabirds such as black-legged kittiwakes and a close relative the red-legged kittiwake of the northern Pacific Ocean and the Bering Sea. Evidence reveals important implications for elevated corticosterone while raising chicks, in both young and adults (e.g., Kitaysky et al. 1999a; Kitaysky et al. 1999b; Kitaysky et al. 2003). Black-legged kittiwake chicks respond to food shortages while in the nest by increasing

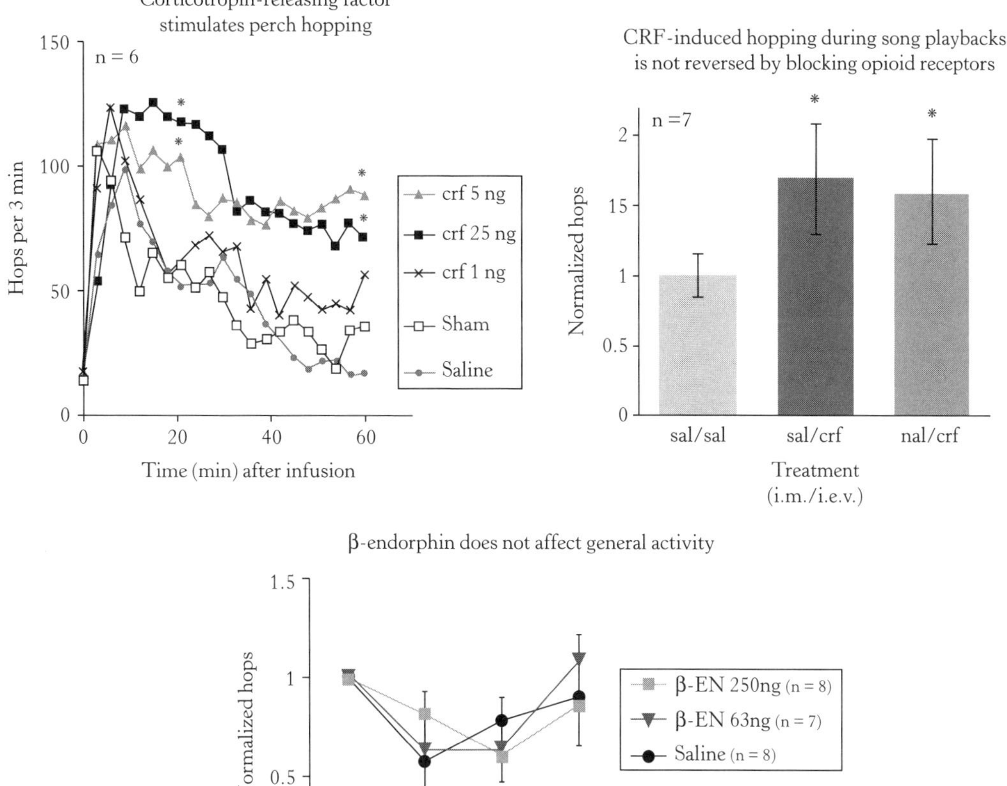

FIGURE 5.18: Top panel, effects of intra-cerebroventricular injection of CRF on activity in white-crowned sparrows. ICV injection of beta-endorphin had no effects on activity (lower panel).

From Maney and Wingfield (1998b). Courtesey of Elesevier.

corticosterone secretion (Figure 5.20). Implants of corticosterone into black-legged kittiwake chicks elevated baseline levels, but within a physiological range equivalent to those in food-restricted chicks (top right panel of Figure 5.20; Kitaysky et al. 1999a). Elevated corticosterone resulted in chicks begging for food more than control-implanted birds (Figure 5.20), and this behavior may have been responsible for altering behavioral responses of the parents of these chicks. Parents increased the feeding rate of corticosterone-implanted chicks and embarked on more foraging trips (Figure 5.21; Kitaysky et al. 1999a; Kitaysky et al. 1999b). Note also that implants of corticosterone into hand-raised red-legged kittiwake chicks in the laboratory also increase begging for food (Figure 5.26). Taken together, these data suggest the remarkable conclusion that poor foraging conditions result in an increase in corticosterone in kittiwake chicks, which in turn results in an increase in begging behavior. This triggers a behavioral cascade, and adults increase foraging rate and feeding rates in response—even though the parents were never exposed to elevated corticosterone. These data also suggest that parents must respond to reduce the potential for nutritional stress on growing chicks that might be deleterious during their development.

Black-legged kittiwake parents also respond to food shortages by increasing corticosterone secretion (Figure 5.22; Kitaysky et al. 1999b). Implants into breeding adults elevated baseline levels of corticosterone to those similar to times of food shortage. This led to high-corticosterone parents allocating more time to foraging, but with the potential cost of chicks of high-corticosterone parents spending more time unattended and

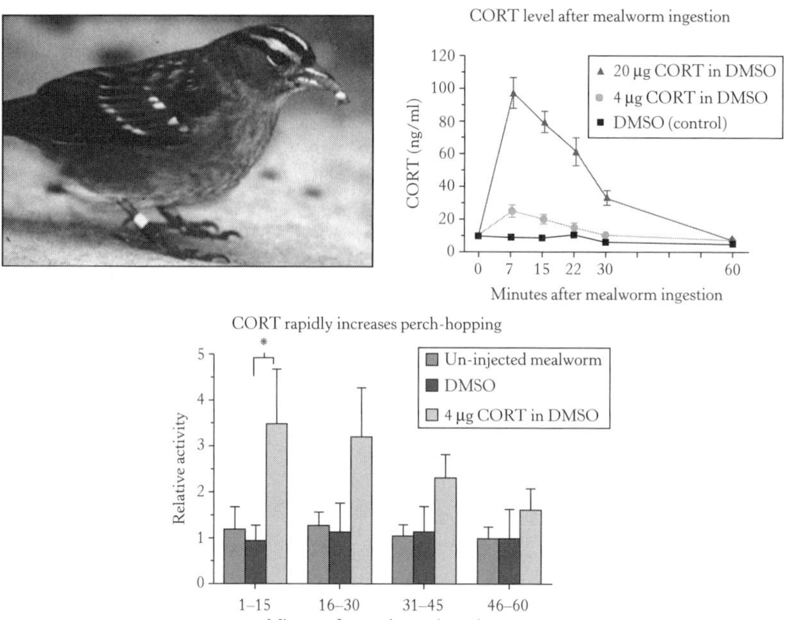

FIGURE 5.19: Rapid actions of ingested corticosterone on activity are not consistent with the time scale for genomic actions and probably represent action through a membrane-like, non-genomic receptor. The top left panel shows a white-crowned sparrow eating a mealworm injected with corticosterone in dimethylsulfoxide (DMSO—a non-polar solvent) at two doses. The top right panel shows the increase in plasma corticosterone (CORT) following mealworm ingestion compared with controls (ingestion of a mealworm injected with DMSO alone). Corticosterone levels in the blood show a large increase 5–20 mins after ingestion that are physiological and represent responses to a labile perturbation factor. Corticosterone titers returned to control levels between 30 and 60 mins. Administration of corticosterone in this way increased activity significantly within 7 mins of ingestion.

From Breuner et al. (1998). Courtesey of Elsevier.

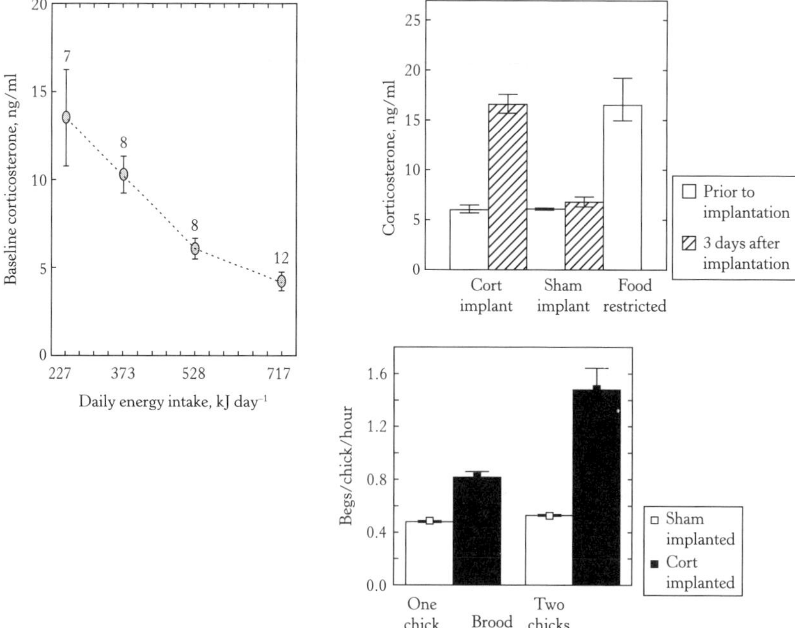

FIGURE 5.20: Black-legged kittiwake chicks respond to food shortages by increasing corticosterone secretion (top left panel). Implants of corticosterone into chicks in Alaska elevated baseline levels but within a physiological range equivalent to those in food restricted chicks (top right panel). Elevated corticosterone increases chick begging rates (bottom right panel).

From Kitaysky et al. (1999a); Kitaysky et al. (2001). Courtesey of Wiley, and Behav. Ecol.

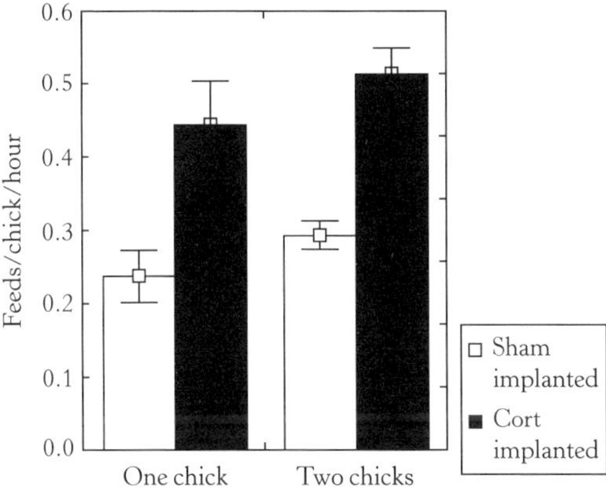

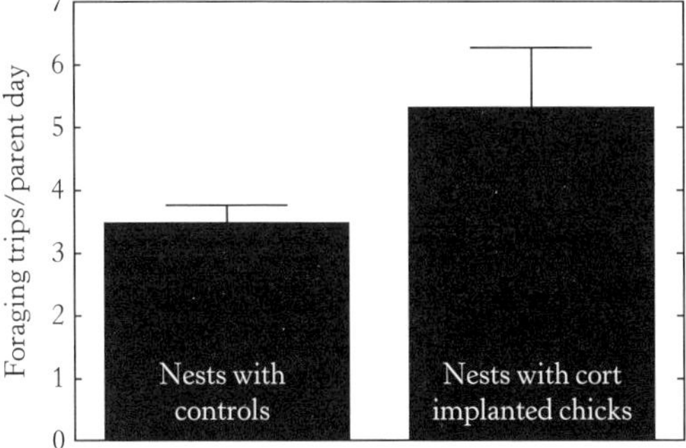

FIGURE 5.21: Black-legged kittiwake parents feed high corticosterone (implanted) chicks at a higher rate (top panel) and increase frequency of foraging trips (lower panel).

From (Kitaysky et al. 1999a; 1999b). Courtesy of Elsevier.

possibly exposed to predators (Figure 5.22; Kitaysky et al. 1999b). Curiously, although parents spent more time foraging, they did not bring more food to the chicks, suggesting that chick behavior is indeed important (Kitaysky et al. 1999b; Kitaysky et al. 2001). These data led to a laboratory experiment to tease apart what deleterious effects high corticosterone levels in chicks might have once they reach independence. Both species of kittiwakes are pelagic feeding gulls, and after the chicks fledge they have to find fish and catch them without any apparent help from their parents. Thus learning abilities may be blunted in chicks developing with high corticosterone levels.

To test this hypothesis, fertile eggs of red-legged kittiwakes were transported in mobile incubators to the University of Washington, where they were hatched (Figure 5.23). Chicks were housed in a light- and temperature-controlled chamber until they were able to thermoregulate independently (Figure 5.23). At this time they were transferred to outdoor aviaries and were placed in a simulated seabird colony consisting of wire nest baskets attached to the wall (Figure 5.24; Kitaysky et al. 2003). All chicks were fed fish (herring) using a model head and neck of the adult to avoid chicks imprinting on human caregivers (Figure 24). Chicks fledge by jumping from the nest to the floor of the aviary, where they had unlimited access to tubs of seawater and were able to feed themselves on fish (Figure 5.24). Growing chicks were then given either a control, one, or two subcutaneous implants of corticosterone for about a week from approximately 7 days of age. Treatment had mild, if any, effects on physiology. Corticosteroid implants had only very slight effects on growth rate (Figure 5.25), and sped up fledging time, but only by two days (Figure 5.25; Kitaysky et al. 2003). It is not clear whether a reduced fledging time of two days has any potential deleterious effects. In contrast, there were dramatic behavioral effects of corticosterone treatment. Corticosterone-treated chicks increased begging behavior, as seen in the field in black-legged kittiwake chicks, and curiously, showed higher aggression when competing with a control chick for access to a piece of herring offered by the investigator (Figure 5.26; Kitaysky et al. 2003). This is intriguing because other studies show that corticosterone tends to decrease aggression in other contexts (see discussion later in this chapter).

After fledging, at the time when free-living chicks would be learning to find fish on their own, experiments were conducted to test the learning abilities of chicks exposed to corticosterone treatment during development in the nest. Compared with control-implanted birds, the transitory peak of corticosterone during development impaired learning ability. Kitaysky et al. (2003) gave the fledged chicks petri dishes with a piece of food (herring) and they had to learn to remove the lid to get at that food (step 1 in Figures 5.27 and 5.28). Then they had to learn to distinguished between black petri dishes that contain food and opaque white dishes that never contain food (Figures. 5.27 and 5.28). Increasing complexity of arrays tested how well treated chicks and controls could find food (Figure 5.28). In Figure 5.27, a bird easily finds food and opens all the black dishes and ignores white dishes. Note also that Kitaysky et al. (2003) were careful to coat all dishes with fish odor to avoid olfactory means of identifying food dishes (Figure 5.27). Treated birds took significantly longer to open dishes than did controls, and two birds treated with two implants of corticosterone never did learn how to open a dish (Figure 5.29; Kitaysky et al. 2003). Furthermore,

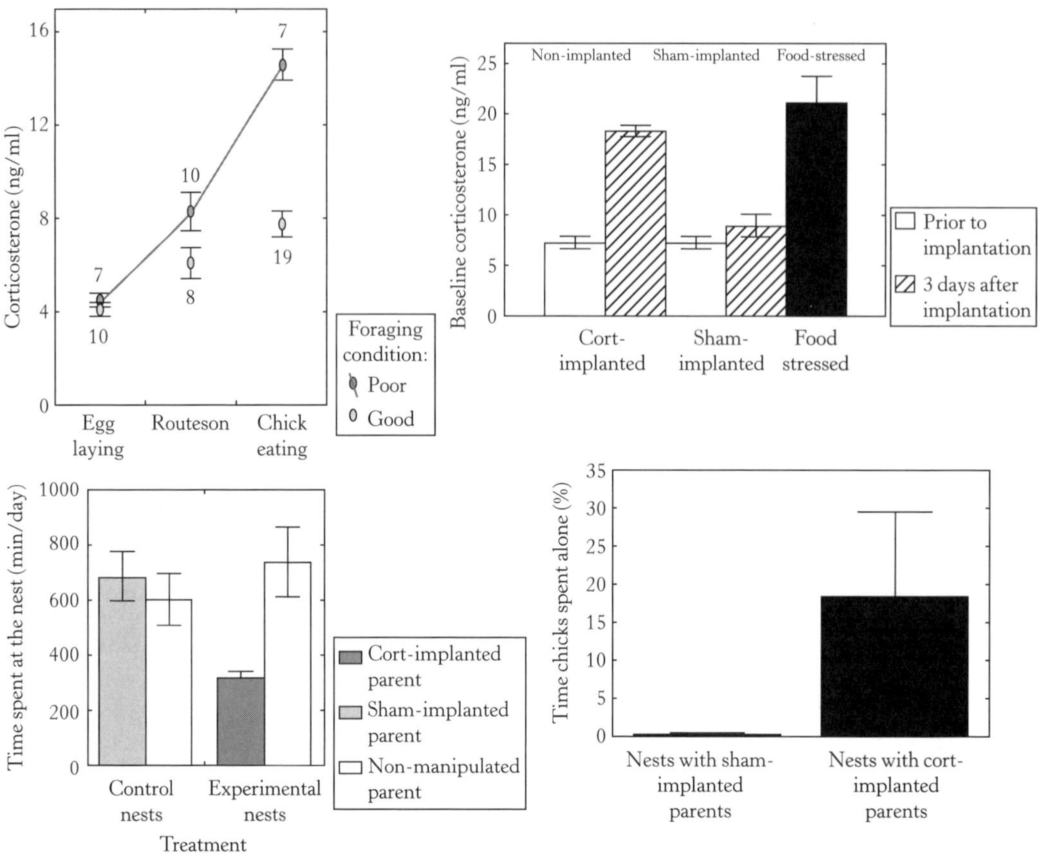

FIGURE 5.22: Black-legged kittiwake parents respond to food shortages by increasing corticosterone secretion (Kitaysky et al. 1999b). Implants elevated baseline levels of corticosterone to those similar to times of food shortage. High-CORT parents allocate more time to foraging, but chicks of high-CORT parents spent more time unattended.

treated birds never reached the number of dishes successfully opened by controls (Figure 5.30).

Taken together, these remarkable data indicate that seabirds are very sensitive to foraging conditions but will try to compensate if chicks beg for more food by increasing foraging rate. This may be a mechanism by which the adults reduce potential learning deficits in their offspring after they fledge. What costs this may have for adults will be discussed in later chapters on glucocorticoids and fitness.

B. Aggression/Submission

It is well known that hormone secretions may suppress expression of aggression and promote other behaviors such as submission (for review, see Wingfield 2005). However, it is important to keep in mind that aggression can be divided into offensive and defensive aggression, and, at least in the laboratory, these two types of aggression are regulated by very different hormonal and neurotransmitter mechanisms (Blanchard and Blanchard 2005). In free-living birds, elevated levels of corticosterone inhibit territorial aggression including singing, as well as sexual and parental behavior (e.g., Silverin 1986; Wingfield and Silverin 1986). Similar inhibitory effects of corticosteroids on reproductive behavior have been established in reptiles and amphibians (Moore and Miller 1984; Moore et al. 2001). High circulating titers of corticosteroids following stress inhibit the reproductive system, resulting in a decrease of circulating LH and testosterone (for reviews, see Greenberg and Wingfield 1987; Sapolsky 2001; Moore and Jessop 2003). As a result, the expression of behaviors, especially territorial aggression activated by testosterone, is reduced. However, after acute elevation of corticosteroid secretion such as during labile perturbation factors, a more direct suppression of reproductive behaviors, independent of inhibition of the reproductive system itself, has been demonstrated (Wingfield

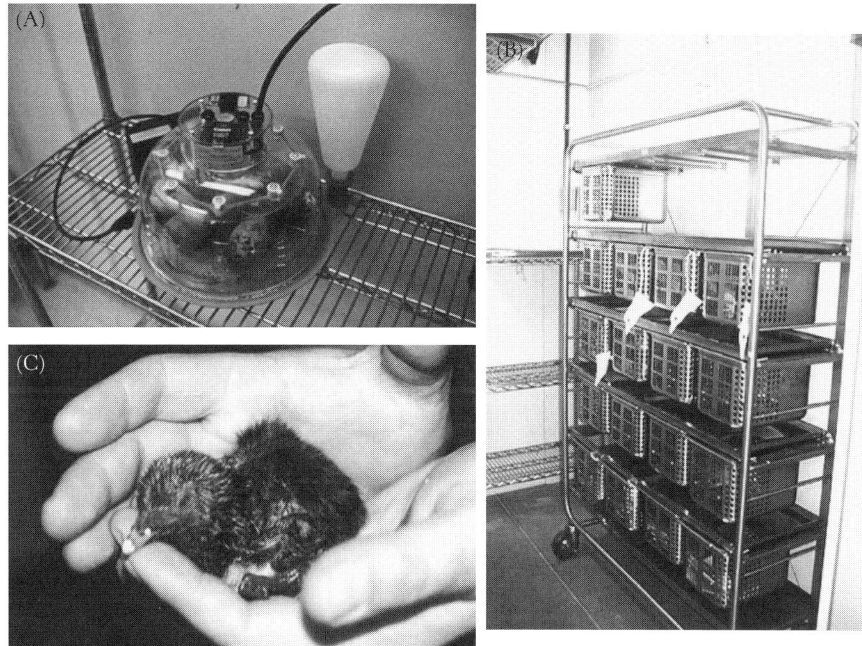

FIGURE 5.23: Eggs of red-legged kittiwakes were collected in Alaska and transported in mobile incubators to the University of Washington, Seattle (Kitaysky et al. 2003). Panel A, eggs were incubated until hatching (panel C). Chicks were housed in temperature and light controlled chambers (panel B) until they were able to regulate their own body temperature.

Photos by J. C. Wingfield.

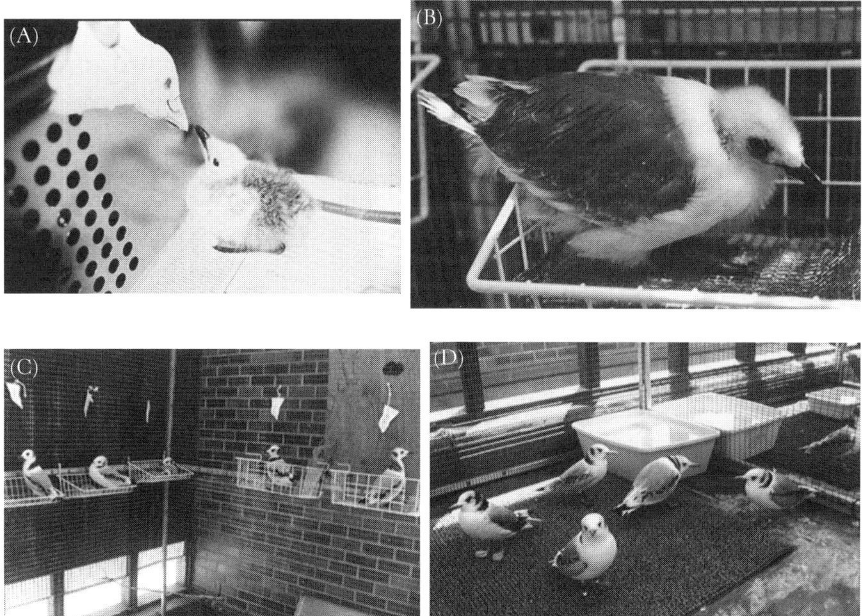

FIGURE 5.24: Red-legged kittiwake chicks were fed using a model head and neck of an adult to avoid chicks imprinting on human caregivers (Panel A, Kitaysky et al. 2003). After chicks were able to regulate their own body temperature they were transferred to artificial wire nests (Panel B) mounted on the wall of outdoor aviaries (Panel C) to simulate a nesting colony on a cliff. Chicks fledge by jumping out of the nest to the floor of the aviary where they had constant access to tubs of seawater (Panel D).

Photos by J. C. Wingfield.

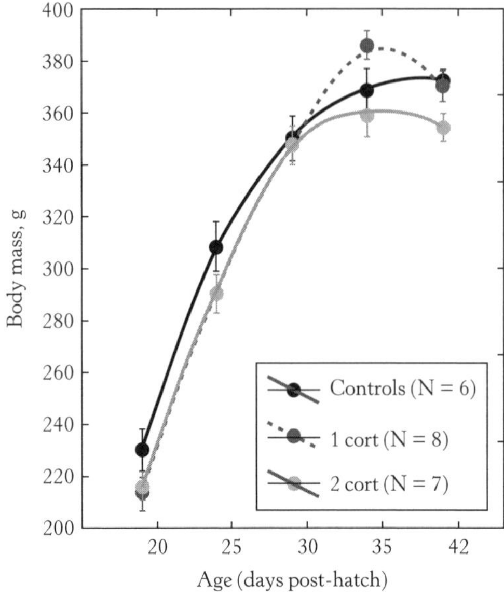

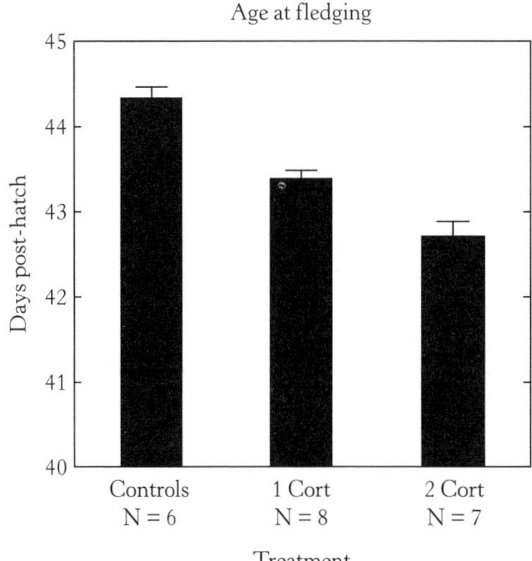

FIGURE 5.25: Subcutaneous implants of corticosterone were given to red-legged kittiwake chicks during development (days 7–14 post hatch). Compared to controls, corticosterone treatment only had slight effects on growth (top panel) and speeded up fledging by two days. 1 CORT = 1 corticosterone implant, 2 CORT = 2 corticosterone implants.

From Kitaysky et al. (2003). Courtesey of Elsevier.

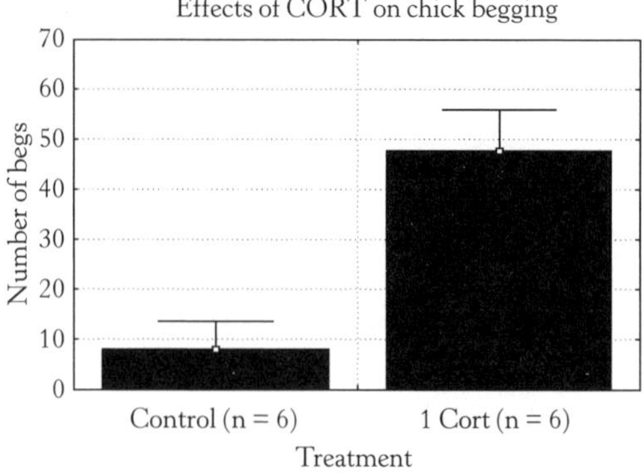

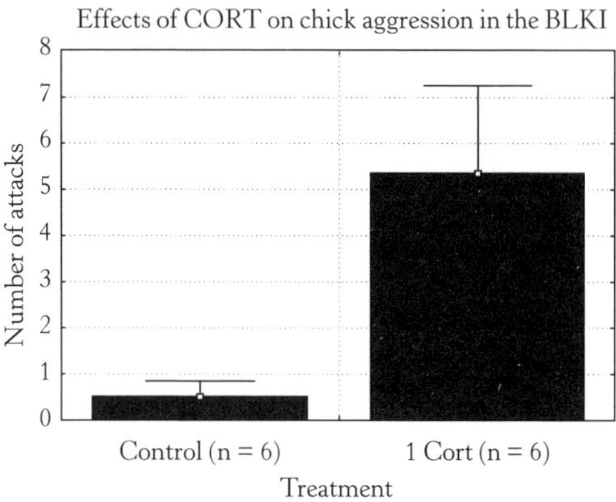

FIGURE 5.26: Corticosterone treatment of red-legged kittiwake chicks increased begging behavior and elevated aggression when competing for food with a control-implanted chick.

From Kitaysky et al. (2003). Courtesey of Elsevier.

and Silverin 1986). For example, subcutaneous corticosterone implants decreased expression of inter-male aggression in the side-blotched lizard. When these males were subsequently exposed to females made sexually receptive by implants of estradiol, courtship and copulation behavior were not affected (DeNardo and Licht 1993). Furthermore, simultaneous implants of corticosterone and testosterone also suppressed expression of aggression, indicating that corticosterone was not acting solely by the inhibition of testosterone secretion (DeNardo and Licht 1993). Whether or not the actions of corticosterone are at the level of testosterone-sensitive neurons or through different mechanisms remains to be determined. Moreover, a role for brain peptides must be borne in mind, as central injection of CRF suppressed territorial aggression in the high-latitude breeding white-crowned sparrow (Romero et al. 1998). Other peptides such as vasopressin/vasotocin and vasoactive intestinal peptide (VIP) may also be involved (e.g., Goodson and Bass 2001; Goodson 2005), but their interactions with stress and corticosterone are largely unknown (e.g., Wingfield et al. 2005).

An intriguing alternate mechanism by which behavior, especially in potentially stressful

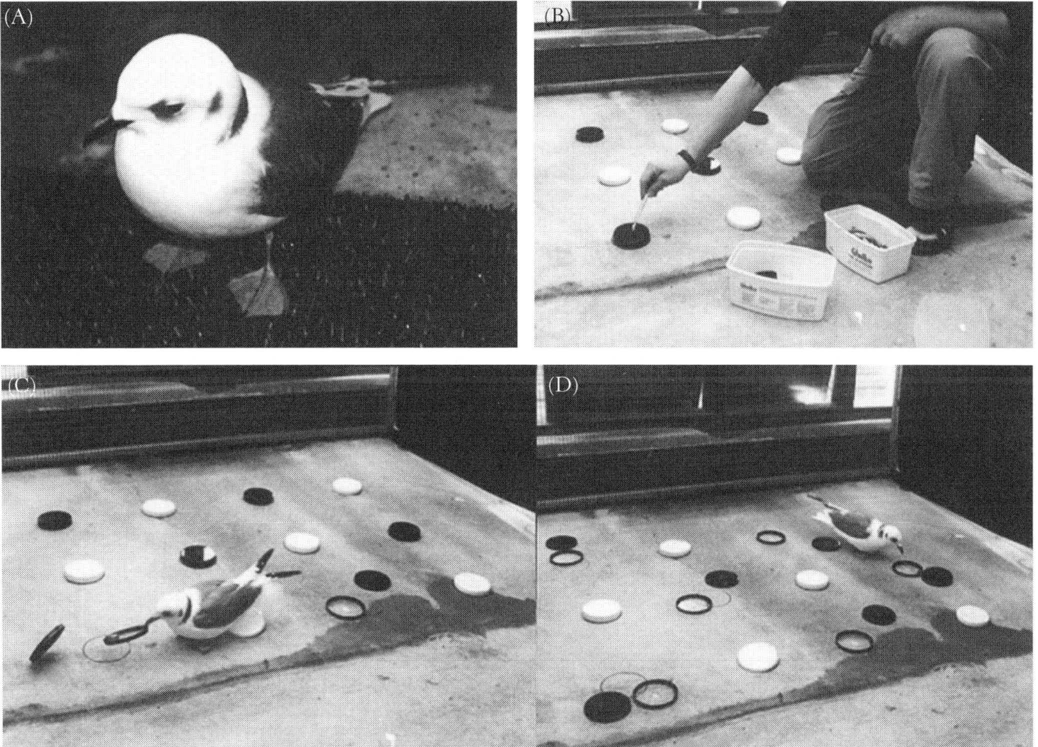

FIGURE 5.27: Fledged red-legged kittiwake chicks in an outdoor aviary (Panel A, Kitaysky et al. 2003), learned how to open a petri dish with a piece of herring inside. Next they were tasked to learn to discriminate between white petri dishes with no food and black petri dishes with food. All dishes were swabbed with fish oil (Panel B) to avoid odor discrimination. Kitiwakes quickly learned to open the petri dishes (Panel C) and furthermore soon learned that only black dishes contained food. They ignored white dishes (Panel D).

All photos by J. C. Wingfield.

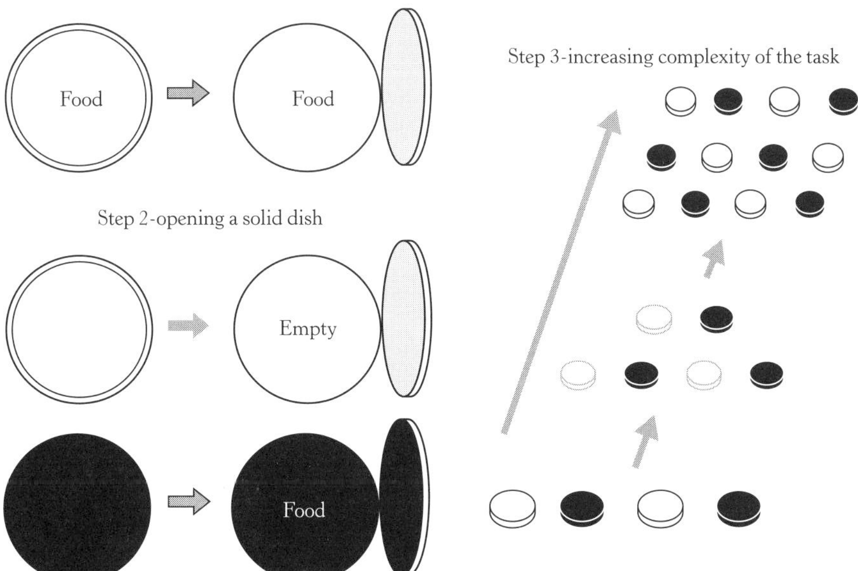

FIGURE 5.28: Captive red-legged kittiwakes, post-fledging, were taught to open petri dishes containing food (herring, step 1). Then they learned that black petri dishes contain food, and white dishes with opaque lids do not (step 2). Then they were asked to find food in increasingly complex arrays of black or white petri dishes and effects of corticosterone implants were tested.

From Kitaysky et al. (2003). Courtesey of Elsevier.

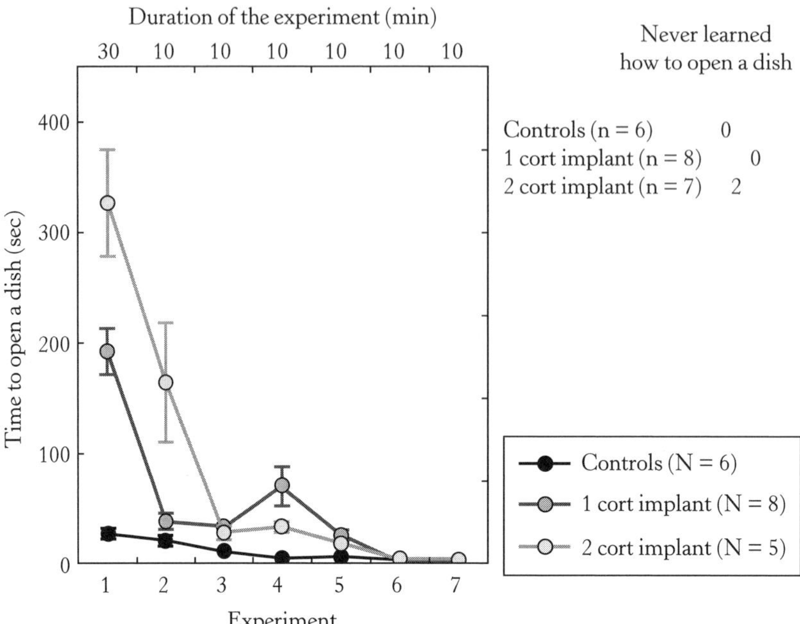

FIGURE 5.29: Effects of corticosterone treatment for 7–10 days while in the nest on the ability of red-legged kittiwake chicks to open petri dishes containing food (herring). Treated birds took significantly longer to open dishes than did controls, and two birds treated with two implants of corticosterone never did learn how to open a dish.

From Kitaysky et al. (2003). Courtesey of Elsevier.

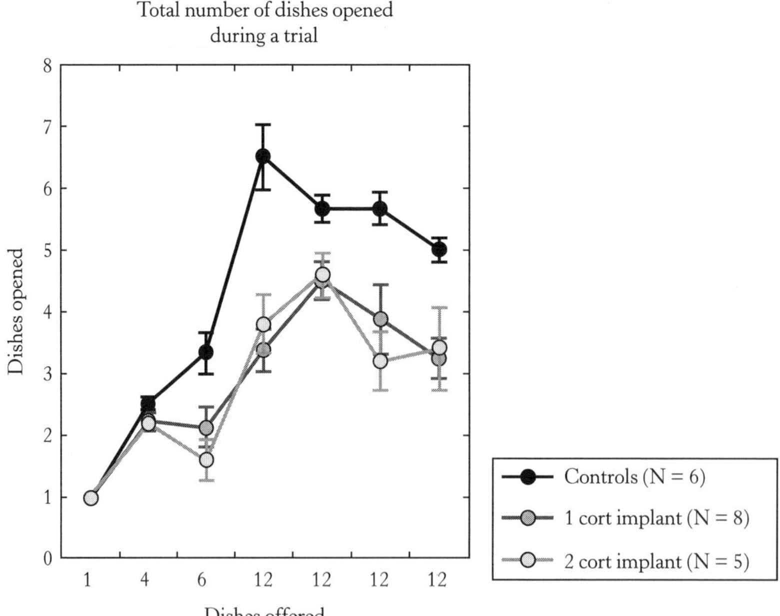

FIGURE 5.30: Effects of corticosterone treatment for 7–10 days while in the nest on total number of food dishes opened after fledging. Treated birds never reached the number of dishes successfully opened by controls.

From Kitaysky et al. (2003). Courtesey of Elsevier.

situations, is regulated involves the activation of behavioral patterns that override the expression of others. Corticosterone treatment activates submissive behavior in agonistic encounters among mice (Leshner 1978; Leshner and Politch 1979), and the simultaneous decrease of testosterone secretion was not required. This effect of corticosterone on submission may be critical for behavioral modulation in response to social stress. It is possible that androgens and corticosteroids may "polarize" the direction of agonistic behavior toward dominance or submission (Leshner 1981) and if so, it is also possible that as corticosteroid levels increase, such as following defeat by a conspecific, then expression of submissive behaviors could take precedence. Both winning and losing male rats undergo increases in plasma corticosterone after agonistic encounters, but the effect was greater in losers and they took longer to return to a baseline level (Schuurman 1980). Moreover, corticosterone treatment had little effect on the submissiveness of male mice in an aggressive encounter (Leshner et al. 1980) unless that treatment followed the experience of defeat. These critical roles for corticosterone regulating stress behavior are clearly complex, and involve other mediators such as catecholamines, brain peptides, and probably cytokines. Natural scenarios of responses to labile perturbation factors will likely be important to tease apart such complex interrelationships.

V. REPRODUCTIVE EFFECTS

Stress in general inhibits reproductive function, delays puberty, and interferes with ongoing breeding attempts in seasonally breeding species (e.g., Sapolsky et al. 2000). For example, heat stress reduces LH pulse amplitude in cattle but did not affect responsiveness to GnRH treatment (Gilad et al. 1993). Cortisol treatment did not reduce GnRH pulses but did suppress LH pulses from the pituitary (Breen et al. 2004). In ovariectomized sheep, psychosocial stress-induced corticosteroids suppress LH pulses. This action appears to be at the level of pituitary gonadotrope responsiveness to GnRH pulses and is mediated via type 2 glucocorticoid receptors (Wagenmaker et al. 2009). Modulation of GnRH pulses during psychosocial stress also appears to be independent of type 2 receptor activation (Wagenmaker et al. 2009). In rats, corticosteroids suppress GnRH synthesis via type 2 receptors on a subset of GnRH neurons (Ahima and Harlan 1992; Chandran et al. 1994; Defranco et al. 1994), decrease the activity of the GnRH pulse generator (Dubey and Plant 1985), and suppress the responsiveness of gonadotropes to GnRH (Baldwin et al. 1991). However, more recent evidence suggests that dexamethasone results in elevated transcription of the GnRH receptor promoter (Maya-Nunez and Conn 2003).

Despite extensive evidence that stress-induced levels of corticosteroids suppress reproductive function, probably through type 2 receptor-induced regulation of gene expression, additional components of the HPA axis such as CRF, arginine vasopressin, and ACTH have all been shown to inhibit GnRH release from the hypothalamus and gonadotropin release from the anterior pituitary (e.g., Maeda and Tsukamura 2006). Evidence from Matsuwaki et al. (2003, 2004, 2006) is convincing that corticosteroids may also play a protective role for gonadotropin secretion and reproductive function during stress. Their model proposes that stress-induced suppression of the hypothalamo-pituitary-gonad axis is mediated through prostaglandin production in the brain and that corticosteroids during stress suppress cyclo-oxygenase (COX2) activity, reducing prostaglandin synthesis and maintaining gonadotropin secretion (Matsuwaki et al. 2006). By decreasing prostaglandin synthesis, corticosteroids also counteract the suppressive actions of tumor necrosis factor-alpha on LH secretion (Matsuwaki et al. 2004).

It has long been known that elevated corticosteroids also suppress testosterone secretion (e.g., Schaison et al. 1978; Greenberg and Wingfield 1987; Sapolsky 2001; Moore and Jessop 2003). This action could be through the suppression of GnRH and LH secretion, as noted earlier, but there is also evidence for the direct action of corticosteroids on testosterone secretion (e.g., Monder et al. 1994). Furthermore, the enzyme 11β-hydroxysteroid dehydrogenase (11β-HSD) in rat Leydig cells may determine whether corticosteroids are inhibitory to testosterone secretion. Studies on rats suggest that 11β-HSD may play a protective role against corticosteroid suppression of testosterone secretion by converting corticosteroids to inactive metabolites (Monder et al. 1994). A decrease in 11β-HSD could then result in the suppression of testosterone secretion. On the other hand, corticosteroids have been shown to decrease testosterone production in rats by decreasing receptors for LH on Leydig cells (Bambino and Hsueh 1981). In vitro studies with Leydig cells from pigs showed that dexamethasone suppressed gonadotropin-induced testosterone production, but natural corticosteroids were much less effective (Bernier et al. 1984).

In contrast, estrogens and corticosteroids may interact positively rather than suppressing estrogen synthesis. Rather, corticosteroids inhibit reproductive functions at the level of the hypothalamus and pituitary gonadotropin secretion and uterine growth. For example, in ovariectomized rats, corticosterone treatment inhibited estrogen-mediated uterine growth (Rabin et al. 1990). In contrast in rats, estradiol increases baseline and stress-induced increases in corticosteroids, but these effects are less clear in humans.

Taken together, corticosteroid secretion in response to acute stress has the potential to disrupt reproductive function and redirect behavior away from breeding. These responses may be key for explaining the abandonment of breeding in response to weather (see Chapters 7 and 8). Corticosteroids also can alter the timing of reproduction (e.g., Yajurvedi and Menon 2005; Schoech et al. 2009). The potential protective effects of corticosteroids and 11β-HSD on responsiveness of the reproductive system to stress are intriguing and deserve further study in the context of organism-environment interaction. Much work remains to be done to clarify these issues.

Over the past decade, since a hypothalamic RFamide was discovered that inhibited LH secretion in a dose-dependent manner in vitro in quail (Tsutsui et al. 2000), extensive research has confirmed that this peptide can inhibit gonadotropin secretion both at the levels of the pituitary and centrally by inhibiting GnRH and GnRH-regulated sexual behavior (Osugi et al. 2004; Bentley et al. 2006; Tsutsui et al. 2007). This gonadotropin-inhibiting hormone (GnIH) and its orthologues in other vertebrates may play a major role in regulating the onset of breeding once the reproductive system is mature, and in regulating transitions between the sexual and parental phases of the breeding cycle (Bentley et al. 2007; Calisi et al. 2008; Kriegsfeld et al. 2010; Tsutsui et al. 2010). The GnIH receptor is also distributed on GnRH neurons, as well as in the median eminence and gonads (Yin et al. 2005; Bentley et al. 2008), all potential sites of inhibition of gonadotropin secretion and expression of sexual behavior, although the roles of GnIH gene expression and its receptor are not entirely clear at present.

As GnIH has the ability to suppress LH secretion as well as inhibit sexual behavior (at least in female birds) it is possible that GnIH might also be involved in the stress-induced inhibition of reproductive function. Recent evidence from rats (Kirby et al. 2009) and house sparrows (Calisi et al. 2008) showed that acute handling stress enhanced GnIH expression, which could potentially inhibit reproduction. This exciting result opens the door for many roles of GnIH in stress-induced suppression of breeding, but a direct link between corticosteroids and GnIH expression remains to be clarified.

VI. DEVELOPMENTAL EFFECTS

Most of the book to this point has focused on how adults detect and cope with stressors. However, two things are becoming increasingly clear. First, young individuals show many differences from adults, both in what they consider to be stressors and in the physiological responses they make. Some of these differences are clearly developmental, but others result from the different needs of young vis-à-vis adults. In other words, age produces a contextual lens through which stressors are interpreted. Second, growing evidence indicates that many stressors, when experienced during development, can leave a lifelong imprint on the individual. These imprints appear to have profound fitness consequences and collectively have been termed "maternal effects." Maternal effects have been of intense interest to biomedical researchers and have recently started to attract considerable interest among ecologists.

In this section we will present some of the data on how young vertebrates are exposed to, cope with, and are changed by different stressors. We have divided the evidence somewhat arbitrarily by progressing through development from the zygote to the adult. We start with stressors affecting developing fetuses, progress to stressors affecting neonates (young post-birth/hatch but prior to becoming young adults), and finish with what are currently known or suspected to be long-term and often permanent consequences. It is important to remember, however, that conception to death is a continuum; it would be remarkable if disturbances to a fetus or a neonate *did not* result in long-term changes. This means that there will be extensive crosstalk between the sections of this chapter. Just because long-term consequences are discussed separately does not imply that prenatal and neonatal stress does not impact the other systems presented in this chapter.

A. Development of the Hypothalamo-Pituitary-Adrenal Axis (HPA)

A zygote obviously does not have an HPA axis or a sympathetic nervous system. Development of these systems has to take place before a stress response can be initiated by the animal. However, maternal corticosteroids can be passed into eggs (see later discussion), with potential consequences for the offspring. Most of the work delineating the ontogeny of the stress response has been done in mammals, but the broad outlines are assumed to be similar across vertebrate taxa. The general pattern that emerges is that the HPA architecture is produced rather late in development and begins to function a short period before birth.

Development of the cell bodies in the paraventricular nucleus (PVN), the area of the hypothalamus that regulates HPA activity, occurs rather late in gestation, yet precedes the development of other components in the brain (Walker et al. 2001). For instance, the projections of the PVN to the median eminence occur later, as does the first production of CRF and AVP (Walker et al. 2001). In fact, CRF receptors do not assume their adult numbers or distribution until well after birth (Insel et al. 1988). In contrast, catecholamine receptors are functional much earlier in development (Walker et al. 2001), suggesting that the sympathetic system might develop prior to the HPA.

The hypothalamic-pituitary portal vasculature starts to develop about the same time as the PVN neurons, but can take longer to complete. A fully functioning portal system is not completed until after birth (Walker et al. 2001). However, the pituitary secretes ACTH, stimulated by hypothalamic CRF and AVP, before birth, even if full regulatory control by the hypothalamus continues to mature.

The adrenal gland is also functional before birth. Although a substantial fetal zone (primarily involved in producing androgens) is present in many mammals (Norris 2007), both the cortex and medulla are present and functioning (Walker et al. 2001). However, ACTH receptors are first detected fairly late in development (Chatelain et al. 1989), approximately at the time that ACTH begins to be secreted by the pituitary. The full development of the HPA negative feedback system continues until well after birth. Negative feedback functioning at the level of the hippocampus especially requires substantial development. Neonatal mammals do not show a fully functioning negative feedback system, and thus show delayed shutoff of corticosteroid release (Walker et al. 2001).

It would be a mistake, however, to assume that the growing embryo and fetus are not affected by stress simply because the HPA is not yet fully functional. Corticosteroids can easily pass between mother and fetus, either through the placenta or via steroids deposited in the yolk (see later discussion). In addition, corticosteroid receptors are present in the brain much earlier than the maturation of the HPA axis (Walker et al. 2001). For example in the rat, corticosteroid receptors are present approximately two-thirds through gestation, although type I and II receptor distributions develop at different rates (Kapoor et al. 2006). Consequently, the embryo would appear to be sensitive to a corticosteroid signal before it can generate that signal on its own. Presumably that signal is anticipated as coming from the mother. The potential functional role of receiving a corticosteroid signal from the mother is discussed later in this section.

Another aspect of adrenal development involves the sympathetic nervous system and the adrenal medulla. The adrenal medulla begins to form at approximately the same time as the adrenal cortex, with secretory vesicles containing catecholamines evident shortly thereafter. However, at least in rats, neural control of the medulla is not completed until after birth. Although this would suggest that the fight-or-flight response is not functional until the neural connections are completed, catecholamines are released in response to stressors before this time, presumably via a non-neuronal mechanism (Walker et al. 2001).

B. Parturition

Corticosteroids play a major role in mammalian birth. For successful birth to take place, two critical functions must occur. First, the uterus has to expel the fetus, and second, the fetus has to be prepared to survive outside the uterus. Corticosteroids play a role in both processes.

The primary endocrine regulation of uterine contraction in most mammalian species is a coordinated decrease in progesterone and increase in prostaglandins (Challis et al. 2000). Both of these events appear to be orchestrated by an increase in activation of the fetal HPA axis with an assist from the mother (for detailed reviews, see Challis et al. 2000; Walker et al. 2001). Just prior to birth, the fetus initiates CRF secretion. This occurs both from the hypothalamus and from a large increase in CRF generated from the fetal portion of the placenta. The placental CRF stimulates both the embryonic and maternal HPA axes. The resultant increase in circulating corticosteroids is accompanied by a decrease in the efficacy of negative feedback, facilitated by a decrease in corticosteroid receptors both in the pituitary and in CRF neurons of the PVN. The end result is a large increase in corticosteroids stimulated by the embryo and a substantial increase in corticosteroids crossing from the mother to the fetus just prior to birth.

The elevated corticosteroids act on the placenta to inhibit the production of progesterone (Challis et al. 2000) and to increase the production of prostaglandins (Challis et al. 2000; Whittle et al. 2001). Uterine contractions then commence. The fetus, therefore, controls the timing of its own birth. In fact, transplant studies between breeds with different gestation periods indicate that the gestational duration depends upon the fetal, not the maternal, genotype (reviewed by Challis et al. 2000).

Elevated corticosteroid concentrations also are believed to be a major regulator of organ maturation, especially of the lungs. In fact, the highest densities of corticosteroid receptors just after birth are in the liver and lungs (Walker et al. 2001). Corticosteroids stimulate a number of molecular changes in the lung, but the primary end result seems to be the production of surfactant (Liggins 1994; Grier and Halliday 2004). Surfactant allows alveoli to inflate, and stimulating its production is a major goal of corticosteroid therapy in preterm human infants (Kapoor et al. 2008).

However, fetal control can be short-circuited. Maternal stress during pregnancy can also shut off progesterone production in the placenta, presumably via corticosteroid secretion, which leads to premature pregnancy termination (Arck et al. 2007). In humans, higher cortisol concentrations lead to a higher risk of preterm birth (Giurgescu 2009). Corticosteroid regulation of the gestation period may be evolutionarily conserved. For example, corticosteroid administration to lizard eggs can lead to early hatching (Weiss et al. 2007), corticosteroid administration to chickens decreases laying rate (Cook et al. 2009), and increased corticosteroids in quail results in lower hatching rates (Schmidt et al. 2009). Clearly the mechanisms for regulating premature hatching and premature birth must be different, considering that most lizards and all birds lack a placenta and a uterus, but it is intriguing that corticosteroids should regulate such similar endpoints in such diverse vertebrates.

Pregnancy can also have profound effects on the mother. Given the potent effects that corticosteroids have in stimulating preterm births, one would expect a relative damping of the mother's HPA axis function. In fact, this is exactly what occurs. CRF secretion from the hypothalamus is decreased, circadian rhythms in HPA function are disrupted, and there is attenuated sensitivity to various stressors (Brunton et al. 2008). The end result is a global damping of corticosteroid release. Furthermore, increased placental production of 11β-hydoxysteroid dehydrogenase helps prevent maternal corticosteroids from crossing the blood/placenta barrier (Challis et al. 2000; Kapoor et al. 2006). As described earlier, a severe stressor can override this attenuation and lead to premature birth, but the changes during the later part of pregnancy in general do a good job of buffering the growing embryo from exposure to maternal corticosteroids.

C. Prenatal Effects (Maternal)

Despite the buffering capacity of the placenta described in the previous section, there is substantial evidence that maternal corticosteroids can affect the growing embryo. Not only can the increase in maternal corticosteroids overwhelm the buffering capacity and let corticosteroids across the placental barrier, but chronic stress can decrease the buffering ability by decreasing the placental production of 11β-hydoxysteroid dehydrogenase (Mairesse et al. 2007). Corticosteroid receptors are present prior to birth/hatch, although the timing of the emergence and creation of mature receptor distributions depends upon both the type of receptors (i.e., type 1 vs. type 2) and the degree of brain maturity at birth (Kapoor et al. 2006). Species that show relatively greater brain maturity at birth/hatch also have relatively earlier production of corticosteroid receptors.

Prenatal exposure is not limited to mammals. Evidence is building that all vertebrates can potentially be exposed to prenatal corticosteroids (see later discussion in this chapter). The transport of corticosteroids across the placenta is the mechanism in mammals, but corticosteroids can also be deposited in the egg in species with external incubation (Hayward and Wingfield 2004). Once the corticosteroids are deposited in the egg, there are similar impacts on the growing embryos.

Both stressors applied to the mother and exogenous corticosteroid application can have profound effects on HPA development and function in the offspring (Kapoor et al. 2006). One common stressor in mammalian studies is providing mothers with restricted nutrition (Kapoor et al. 2006; Chadio et al. 2007), although the presence or degree of HPA changes can depend upon sex, species, and timing of the restricted nutrition. In general, prenatal stress results in elevated HPA function in offspring (Kapoor et al. 2006).

Elevated corticosteroids during early brain development can have profound consequences. Corticosteroids can alter a number of features of growing neurons. These include neuron growth, maturation, and distribution throughout the brain; function of individual neurons, including myelinization patterns and what types of neurotransmitters are produced; production of receptors, especially corticosteroid receptors; the connectivity between neurons across the brain via dendrite formation; and in some cases, elevated corticosteroids can lead to the death of growing neurons (Sapolsky 1992; McEwen 2001; Walker et al. 2001). In sum, excess corticosteroids can disrupt many features of normal brain maturation. Likely as a result, corticosteroid secretion is highly regulated during peak periods of neuron growth. Changes in corticosteroid receptor distribution especially are thought to underlie many of the lifelong changes in HPA axis function that result from prenatal stress (see later discussion in this chapter).

Corticosteroids can have dramatic impacts on the growing offspring throughout early life. Viability itself can be compromised, with evidence indicating that elevated cortisol concentrations in the first three weeks of pregnancy in humans results in higher rates of spontaneous abortions (Nepomnaschy et al. 2006).

Maternal stress can also stimulate fetal catecholamine release. For example, the catecholamine release resulting from a mother's fight-or-flight response can lead to placental vasoconstriction, fetal hypoxia, and ultimately fetal HPA activation (Kapoor et al. 2006). Being exposed to prenatal stressors can also alter catecholamine function. Exposure of the mother to stress can alter the normal development of the adrenal medulla (Molendi-Coste et al. 2009) so that, upon weaning, circulating catecholamines can be elevated by as much as 50% (Molendi-Coste et al. 2006). Presumably, this increase results from long-term increases in activity of phenylethanolamine N-methyl transferase (PNMT), the rate-limiting enzyme in catecholamine production, in the adrenal medulla (Roussel et al. 2005). Whether or not these adrenal medulla changes result in alterations to the fight-or-flight response is not currently known, and any effects might be indirect (Woods 2006).

D. Neonatal Effects

Once born, the neonatal laboratory rodent proceeds to attenuate the reactivity of its HPA axis. This period is called the stress hyporesponsive period, or SHRP. The SHRP is a refractory period and does not reflect HPA maturation (Sapolsky and Meaney 1986) because the HPA is already fully active to support birth. The existence of an SHRP is believed to protect growing neurons from the adverse effects of corticosteroids, especially during the initial rapid growth phase immediately after birth (Sapolsky and Meaney 1986; Caldji et al. 2001).

The SHRP is only an attenuation of HPA activity. Moderate stressors that elicit robust corticosteroid responses in adults (e.g., handling, Walker et al. 2001) elicit almost no response in the first few days of life. The SHRP was originally called the stress nonresponsive period (SNRP), but severe stressors can elicit a response. For example, extended maternal separation (60+ min; Plotsky and Meaney 1993) or inducing illness (Shanks et al. 1995) will result in a robust increase in corticosteroids, and the response is resistant to negative feedback (Caldji et al. 2001). Because severe stressors do elicit a response, the terminology was changed to the "hypo-responsive period."

The SHRP appears to be regulated in two primary ways. During this period there is a buildup of CRF and AVP in the median eminence, suggesting that there is decreased release of ACTH secretagogs from the hypothalamus (Walker et al. 2001; Okimoto et al. 2002). Second, the adrenal has a reduced sensitivity to ACTH (Walker et al. 2001). Consequently, the blunted corticosteroid release results from decreased signal originating from the brain, and a reduced efficacy of what signal does get released.

Exposure to corticosteroids during the SHRP, either through severe stressors or through exogenous corticosteroids, can have a variety of long-term consequences (see next section). Although an SHRP is a robust phenomenon in laboratory rodents, and SHRPs have been demonstrated in several other species (rabbits, guinea pigs, and dogs) and hinted at in others (e.g., horses; Wong et al. 2009), their existence in many species has yet to be determined (Walker et al. 2001).

Interestingly, there is some evidence that an SHRP can be achieved socially rather than physiologically (Gunnar and Quevedo 2007). Human children show a reduced corticosteroid response to stress during the first year, but unlike rodents, this decrease depends heavily on the quality of care the infant receives from the caregiver (Gunnar and Donzella 2002). When exposed to a stressor, infants with a strong attachment to their caregiver fail to secrete corticosteroids, whereas infants without a strong attachment show a robust response (reviewed by Gunnar and Donzella 2002). In effect, the strength of the infant's attachment to the caregiver can act as a buffer to ameliorate corticosteroid release. Similar effects might occur in other social species. Although few species have yet to be tested, there is some evidence in ravens (Stöwe et al. 2008).

E. Long-Term Consequences

Early exposure to stress, either prenatally or postnatally, appears to profoundly alter both HPA axis and catecholamine function as these individuals age and become adults. Many of these changes appear to be lifelong and permanent. Two major changes include hyperactivity of HPA activity and disruption of the normal corticosteroid circadian rhythm (Darnaudery and Maccari 2008). Both changes lead to elevated basal and stress-induced corticosteroid concentrations. One primary underlying mechanism is disruption of the corticosteroid negative feedback system. An appropriate circadian rhythm is thought to depend in part on negative feedback. and turning off corticosteroid secretion when a stressor ceases is an important feature of the overall stress response (see Chapter 2). The inability to turn off corticosteroid secretion is what often leads to sustained overexposure to corticosteroids during stress later in life. Negative feedback, in turn, depends upon proper function and activity of the corticosteroid receptors. Unsurprisingly, exploration of the next underlying mechanistic layer has focused on receptor changes.

Recent evidence now points to epigenetic changes as the mechanism for the long-term changes to an individual's stress phenotype. Epigenetic changes refer to long-lasting changes in the regulation of gene transcription that do not entail changes to the DNA sequence (Tsankova et al. 2007). Gene transcription is altered through a complex dance of methylation and acetylation of both the histones packaging DNA and the DNA itself. The pattern of acetylation and methylation determines whether a specific gene is accessible to the transcription apparatus and thus is able to be transcribed (Tsankova et al. 2007). Although not permanent, these patterns of methylation and acetylation are very stable and can last a long time (throughout the life of an organism). In fact, epigenetic changes can extend past the current generation and alter HPA function in offspring. For example, reproductive output can be reduced in prenatally stressed females, and the offspring they succeed in producing can show reduced basal and stress-induced corticosteroid levels (Kapoor et al. 2006). Whether or not such changes occur in offspring catecholamine responses is currently unknown.

In the case of HPA function, stress during early development is associated with methylation of the corticosteroid receptor promoter (Szyf et al. 2005; Tsankova et al. 2007). This methylation results in down-regulation of corticosteroid receptor transcription, and thus fewer overall corticosteroid receptors. It is this decrease in overall receptor number that is thought to underlie the reduction in the efficacy of negative feedback.

In contrast, mild stimuli applied to the neonate can be beneficial. For example, mild handling (thought to mimic maternal grooming) of neonatal rats results in long-term increases in type II (GR) corticosteroid receptors, specifically in the hippocampus. The mechanism appears to be epigenetic changes at the corticosteroid receptor promoter that are the opposite of the methylation changes that occur during more severe stressors (Szyf et al. 2005). These methylation changes are linked to differences in maternal care, whereby mothers that provide more maternal care (usually quantified as licking the pup) induce less methylation and thus more corticosteroid receptor transcription (Szyf et al. 2005). The resultant increase in receptors then leads to increased efficacy of negative feedback, which in turn means that individuals are exposed to less corticosteroid exposure during a stressful stimulus later in life (Kapoor et al. 2006). There are also enormous differences in CRF signaling in the brain (Cameron et al. 2005), including a decrease in stimulation of CRF release and suppression of CRF expression (Korosi et al. 2010). A key implication from this work is that normal variation in adult stress responses may have its genesis in normal variation in maternal care (Cameron et al. 2005; Gunnar and Quevedo 2007). Furthermore, given that an attentive mother will produce daughters that have less reactive HPA responses, who in turn are likely to produce daughters with less reactive HPA responses (and visa versa), these variations in maternal care can propagate through generations (Cameron et al. 2005). Because differences in maternal care can result in epigenetic changes in methylation patterns, there is enormous potential to create long-term stable variation in stress responses that will appear to be genetically based, even though the mechanisms do not involve changes in allelic frequencies.

Long-term changes resulting from stress during early development are not, however, limited to epigenetic changes. Early stress is associated with changes in gross brain architecture, leading some brain areas to become enlarged and others to shrink (Teicher et al. 2005; Spinelli et al. 2009). How these gross morphological changes impact behavior, however, is not well understood. In contrast, considerable evidence indicates that neuronal connections in the brain (de Kloet et al. 2005), especially in the hippocampus and the amygdalla (McEwen 2001), are also altered. There are marked changes in the number of dendrites and the number of connections those dendrites make. These dendritic changes can lead to changes in behavioral responses.

For example, the amygdala is an important region of the brain that regulates fear and anxiety. Corticosteroids are important regulators of the developmental onset of both amygdala function and of the fear response to predator cues (Moriceau et al. 2004), and the mechanism appears to be a corticosteroid-induced increase in dendritic density (Mitra and Sapolsky 2008). Consequently, when stress alters dendritic density (McEwen 2001; Fenoglio et al. 2006), it implies that the behaviors regulated by those neurons will also be altered. Changes in dendrites can occur quite quickly, such as in the time frame of the few hours of the arousal period during hibernation (Popov and Bocharova 1992; Popov et al. 1992), as well as longer term, such as after prenatal stress (McEwen 2001). Neuronal changes, therefore, may be another underlying mechanism explaining profound long-term behavioral changes found in individuals exposed to stress during early development.

Regardless of the specific mechanism, the long-term consequences of these epigenetic and neuronal changes can be profound. Behavior appears to be especially sensitive (Braastad 1998). Early stress can enhance an adult individual's level of fear (Lukkes et al. 2009) and change the perception of pain (Butkevich et al. 2009), both of which could dramatically alter the ultimate behavioral response of an animal in the wild. Early stress can also produce higher anxiety levels (e.g., Richardson et al. 2006) and increases in neophobia (Fone and Porkess 2008), depression-like behavior (Weinstock 2008), decreased sexual behavior (Wang et al. 2006), sleep disturbances (Darnaudery and Maccari 2008), and altered memory performance (Weinstock 2008). Furthermore, prenatal exposure to corticosteroids in humans has been associated with disrupted HPA regulation (e.g., Entringer et al. 2009), and disrupted HPA regulation with a number of physiological and psychiatric problems. Physiological problems include altered growth, altered immune responses, changes in metabolism, disrupted reproductive physiology, and cardiovascular disease (reviewed by de Kloet et al. 2005; Kapoor et al. 2008). Psychological problems include depression, anxiety, drug abuse, memory problems, and childhood behavioral problems (reviewed by de Kloet et al. 2005; Darnaudery and Maccari 2008; Kapoor et al. 2008). Many of these changes have been documented, and extensively studied, in laboratory rodents (in fact, much of what we understand about human health is extrapolated from these rodent models). Dysregulation of the HPA axis has also been shown for a number of agriculturally important species (e.g., Osadchuk et al. 2001; Osadchuk et al. 2003).

In conclusion of this section, the emerging picture is that significant variation in individual differences in stress responses can be "programmed" early in life. This programming primarily occurs through epigenetic and neuronal changes resulting from the balance of noxious and beneficial stimuli experienced by the individual during early development. Although this picture primarily arises from laboratory studies, it is widely assumed to reflect what occurs in wild animals as well. The extension of this work to an ecological context is a growing field (see Chapter 11).

VII. GROWTH AND VISCERAL ACTIVITY

Growth is a process intimately tied to metabolism, so it makes sense to briefly cover the topic here. Corticosteroids can exert profound impacts on growth. There appear to be several interrelated mechanisms. First, corticosteroids block the secretion of growth hormone from the pituitary, probably by stimulating neuropeptide Y (NPY) activity. NPY in turn inhibits growth hormone release by suppressing growth hormone releasing hormone (GHRH) secretion (Deltondo et al. 2008). Second, corticosteroids decrease the sensitivity of target cells to growth hormone. Third, corticosteroids inhibit protein synthesis (related to corticosteroid-stimulated gluconeogenesis from protein catabolism; Sapolsky 1992). Fourth, corticosteroids can inhibit release of thyroid hormones and alter deiodinase function (Pamenter and Hedge 1980; Rubello et al. 1992). Finally, corticosteroids induce osteoporosis, both directly via receptor-mediated alterations of osteoblast and osteoclast function, and indirectly by decreasing vitamin D-induced calcium uptake from the gut and possibly by increasing calcium mobilization from bone by enhancing parathyroid hormone release and function (Adler and Rosen 1994; Mazziotti et al. 2006). Corticosteroid-induced osteoporosis is an important human clinical problem, especially with therapeutic administration, and also may play a function in certain conditions in wild animals. Galápagos marine iguanas shrink during severe El Niño events (Wikelski and Thom 2000). Shrinkage appears to be a consequence of bone resorption, which may be regulated by the increase in corticosteroids during the El Niño–induced starvation. In general, however, growth inhibition is transient during acute stress and, because growth is a long-term process, appears to have little impact on overall growth. Prolonged exposure to corticosteroids, however, can dramatically inhibit growth. Growth inhibition is likely an example of corticosteroids shifting resources away from processes that can be postponed in order to use those resources to cope with an emergency.

A. Stress-Induced Dwarfism

One important, although rare, syndrome in human clinical medicine is stress-induced dwarfism, or psychogenic dwarfism (Green et al. 1984). In this syndrome, stress (presumably via corticosteroid release but also potentially via catecholamines) inhibits growth hormone release, thereby stunting growth. Sapolsky (1994) provides an excellent and approachable description of the causes and effects of this process in both humans and laboratory animal models.

It is clear from the literature that stress-induced dwarfism is the result of profound and lengthy chronic stress and is a classic example of homeostatic overload. Consequently, it is difficult to imagine that this is an important problem in free-living wildlife—individuals who experience this much chronic stress likely do not survive very long. However, there has been a suggestion that a population of small sperm whales living in the Gulf of Mexico might represent a case of stress-induced dwarfism in a wild population (Wright et al. 2007). Sperm whales in the Gulf of Mexico are significantly smaller than others elsewhere in the world (Jaquet 2006). Because of the history of extensive human exploitation of the Gulf ever since the discovery of the Mississippi River, including potential stressors such as noise, shipping, offshore drilling, fishing, and pollution, Wright et al. (2007) speculated that the apparent dwarfism in the resident sperm whales might be a symptom of these stressors. Although genetic differences and other factors cannot be excluded, the suggestion is intriguing.

VIII. OSMOREGULATION

Corticosteroids have profound influences on salt balance, probably through the regulation of ion channels such as Na/K ATPase (e.g. Norris 2007). These effects may be particularly important in animals that move among habitats with varying degrees of osmotic stress.

A. Euryhaline Fish

A good example are fishes that move from salt water to fresh (anadromous) at some stage in their life cycle and others that move in the opposite direction (catadromous). Yet others are amphidromous and can move repeatedly between fresh and salt water, but on a predictable schedule associated with migration and reproduction. In these cases, corticosteroids and prolactin play a key role in preparing the gill epithelium of fish (where most osmoregulation takes place) for either fresh-water or salt-water conditions (Wendalaar Bonga 1997; Schreck et al. 2001; Norris 2007). Some organisms, however, are able to move among aqueous habitats with varying degrees of salinity—completely fresh to brackish and full salt water. Such conditions prevail in estuaries, in the inter-tidal zone where hot days may concentrate pools and rain dilute them; and in ephemeral pools where after rainfall, the pool dries up and concentrates salts. Such animals that can cope with varying degrees of salinity are called euryhaline. These movements tend to be less predictable in nature and thus these organisms must respond immediately and frequently to salinity changes. In fishes, stress responses in general are very similar to those of other vertebrates, with acute stress of many types increasing corticosteroid and catecholamine levels (Schreck et al. 2001). Ion concentrations in water, as well as pH, are strong releasers of corticosteroids in fishes and act through type 1 (MR)- and type 2 (GR)-like receptor responses (Wendalaar Bonga 1997).

B. Droughts

Hormonal responses of animals to drought conditions in nature are not well known (see Chapters 7 and 8), although behavioral responses such as migration to wetter areas, abandonment of reproduction, and so on, are well documented. It is likely that hormones involved in water balance, such as arginine vasopressin and arginine vasotocin from the posterior pituitary, which regulate water retention, and the renin-angiotensin-aldosterone system, which regulates salt retention (Schulkin

2005), are involved. Corticosteroids are also probably involved at least in their capacity to regulate ion channels (Norris 2007).

IX. HYPOXIA

Lowered oxygen availability occurs in air as altitude increases, or reduced oxygen can occur in water (fresh and salt) as a result of prolonged heat or concentration of salts and organic material. Both scenarios result in hypoxia and can have profound implications for migrating birds at altitude, other animals moving up and down altitudinal gradients in mountains, and fish that depend on dissolved oxygen in water (Dipnoans, lung fish, notwithstanding).

Hypoxic conditions, or dead zones, occur seasonally in shallow coastal seas, estuaries, and brackish lagoons as a result of high temperatures and increasing salt concentrations that decrease oxygen content. These conditions result in mortality of marine life, or movement away from the area in, for example, fish (e.g., Pihl et al. 1991; Engle et al. 1999; Joyce 2000; Rabalais and Turner 2001; Thomas et al. 2006; Thomas et al. 2007). In the northern Gulf of Mexico, seasonal moderate hypoxia may affect up to 30% of the region's shallow coastal waters in late summer (Engle et al. 1999). Increased eutrophication of coastal waters due to agricultural use of fertilizers rich in nitrogen and raw sewage has resulted in expansion by 2–10-fold of seasonal hypoxic zones and the development of new hypoxic areas (Diaz and Rosenberg 1995; Joyce 2000; Rabalais and Turner 2001; Thomas et al. 2006, 2007). These dead zones likely will result in major changes in coastal ecosystems and represent a major perturbation for many marine plants and animals (Joyce 2000). It is important to note that natural states of hypoxia occur seasonally, and so many organisms in this region can prepare for these extreme conditions. However, an increased area of hypoxic zones and the development of new zones represent an unpredictable source of perturbation that could be particularly devastating locally.

Until recently, very little was known about how fish cope with hypoxic conditions. Initially, hypoxia-tolerant fish increase capacity to deliver oxygen to tissue and reduce aerobic metabolism and oxygen demand (Hochachka and Somero 2002). In addition, hypoxia-induced gene expression inhibits reproductive function in Atlantic croaker. This species also appears to shift distribution and possibly decreases metabolism at times of the year when hypoxic zones usually occur naturally (Eby and Crowder 2002; Bell and Eggleston 2005). This suggests that mild to moderate hypoxia may signal changes in metabolic, behavioral, and reproductive functions to cope with seasonal hypoxia.

In the croaker from an estuary in Florida, exposure to moderate hypoxia resulted in significant reduction of ovarian and testicular development. Hypoxia-induced gene expression accompanied a decrease of serotonin content in the hypothalamus through the inhibition of tryptophan hydroxylase, an enzyme critical for the synthesis of serotonin. Experimental replacement of serotonin restored reproductive function, suggesting that this mechanism may be adaptive in regulating reproduction in response to unfavorable conditions (Thomas et al. 2006, 2007). These authors point out that because the intensity and extent of hypoxic zones is increasing, then the metabolic, behavioral, and reproductive changes triggered by hypoxia may severely disrupt the life cycle of this fish and other organisms.

In the channel catfish, another estuarine fish, low oxygen content of the water resulted in a significant increase in plasma cortisol levels, which then declined within 30 minutes when fish were returned to normal oxygen concentrations in sea water (Tomasso et al. 1981). In parrotfishes from Caribbean Islands, experimental exposure to hypoxia increased corticosteroid metabolite levels in feces of these aquarium adapted fish (Turner et al. 2003). Indeed there is growing evidence that corticosteroids may play a major role in responses to and acclimatization to hypoxic conditions in vertebrates in general (Kodama et al. 2003). In mammals, hypoxia-inducible transcription factor (HIF-1) is up-regulated by corticosteroids acting through type 2 receptors (Kodama et al. 2003).

Rainbow trout subjected to severe hypoxia showed marked increases in blood cortisol and catecholamines during the trial period (Swift 1981; vanRaaij et al. 1996). About 60% of the fish did not survive recovery after the trial, probably because their behavioral response to hypoxia included bursts of activity and strenuous avoidance behavior. Those fish that survived showed much less activity and conservation of energy with reduced oxygen demand. Non-surviving fish had higher levels of catecholamines, but lower cortisol (vanRaaij et al. 1996). The physiological and behavioral responses to unpredictable hypoxic conditions deserve more study to clarify coping strategies.

X. CONCLUSIONS

This chapter focused on the major effects of corticosteroids and catecholamines during a stress response. The emphasis was on how these effects are understood from biomedical studies. These mechanisms will form the foundation for our further exploration of stress responses in free-living animals. As you will see in the following chapters, the responses are often quite different in free-living animals than in captive animals, and especially different from the highly inbred laboratory species from which the bulk of our knowledge was gathered. Although the responses from this chapter will provide the major themes in later chapters, it is the variations on these themes that has made the study of stress responses under natural conditions so fascinating.

REFERENCES

Adler, R. A., Rosen, C. J., 1994. Glucocorticoids and osteoporosis. *Endocrinol Metabol Clin N Am 23*, 641–654.

Ahima, R. S., Harlan, R. E., 1992. Glucocorticoid receptors in LHRH neurons. *Neuroendocrinol 56*, 845–850.

Arck, P., Hansen, P. J., Jericevic, B. M., Piccinni, M. P., Szekeres-Bartho, J., 2007. Progesterone during pregnancy: Endocrine-immune cross talk in mammalian species and the role of stress. *Am J Reproduct Immunol 58*, 268–279.

Arvier, M., Lagoutte, L., Johnson, G., Dumas, J. F., Sion, B., Grizard, G., Malthiery, Y., Simard, G., Ritz, P., 2007. Adenine nucleotide translocator promotes oxidative phosphorylation and mild uncoupling in mitochondria after dexamethasone treatment. *Am J Physiol 293*, E1320–E1324.

Ashley, N. T., Wingfield, J. C., 2012. Sickness behavior in vertebrates. In: Demas, G. E., Nelson, R. J. (Eds.), *Ecoimmunology*. Oxford University Press, New York, pp. 45–91.

Astheimer, L. B., Buttemer, W. A., Wingfield, J. C., 1992. Interactions of corticosterone with feeding, activity and metabolism in passerine birds. *Ornis Scan 23*, 355–365.

Astheimer, L. B., Buttemer, W. A., Wingfield, J. C., 1995. Seasonal and acute changes in adrenocortical responsiveness in an arctic-breeding bird. *Horm Behav 29*, 442–457.

Baldwin, D. M., Srivastava, P. S., Krummen, L. A., 1991. Differential actions of corticosterone on luteinizing hormone and follicle-stimulating hormone biosynthesis and release in cultured rat anterior pituitary cells: Interactions with estradiol. *Biol Reprod 44*, 1040–1050.

Bale, T. L., Vale, W. W., 2004. CRF and CRF receptors: Role in stress responsivity and other behaviors. *Ann Rev Pharmacol Toxicol 44*, 525–557.

Bambino, T. H., Hsueh, A. J. W., 1981. Direct inhibitory effect of glucocorticoids upon testicular luteinizing hormone receptor and steroidogenesis invivo and invitro. *Endocrinology 108*, 2142–2148.

Bauer, M. E., 2005. Stress, glucocorticoids and ageing of the immune system. *Stress 8*, 69–83.

Beck, I. M. E., Berghe, W. V., Vermeulen, L., Yamamoto, K. R., Haegeman, G., De Bosscher, K., 2009. Crosstalk in inflammation: The interplay of glucocorticoid receptor-based mechanisms and kinases and phosphatases. *Endocr Rev 30*, 830–882.

Bell, G. W., Eggleston, D. B., 2005. Species-specific avoidance responses by blue crabs and fish to chronic and episodic hypoxia. *Marine Biol 146*, 761–770.

Bentley, G. E., Jensen, J. P., Kaur, G. J., Wacker, D. W., Tsutsui, K., Wingfield, J. C., 2006. Rapid inhibition of female sexual behavior by gonadotropin-inhibitory hormone (GnIH). *Horm Behav 49*, 550–555.

Bentley, G. E., Perfito, N., Ubuka, T., Ukena, K., Osugi, T., O'Brien, S., Tsutsui, K., Wingfield, J. C., 2007. Gonadotropin-inhibitory hormone in seasonally-breeding songbirds: neuroanatomy and functional biology. *J Ornithol 148*, S521–S526.

Bentley, G. E., Ubuka, T., McGuire, N. L., Chowdhury, V. S., Morita, Y., Yano, T., Hasunuma, I., Binns, M., Wingfield, J. C., Tsutsui, K., 2008. Gonadotropin-inhibitory hormone and its receptor in the avian reproductive system. *Gen Comp Endocrinol 156*, 34–43.

Bernier, M., Gibb, W., Collu, R., Ducharme, J. R., 1984. Effect of glucocorticoids on testosterone production by porcine leydig cells in primary culture. *Can J Physiol Pharmacol 62*, 1166–1169.

Bisson, I. A., Butler, L. K., Hayden, T. J., Kelley, P., Adelman, J. S., Romero, L. M., Wikelski, M. C., 2011. Energetic response to human disturbance in an endangered songbird. *Anim Conserv 14*, 484–491.

Bisson, I. A., Butler, L. K., Hayden, T. J., Romero, L. M., Wikelski, M. C., 2009. No energetic cost of anthropogenic disturbance in a songbird. *Proc R Soc Lond B 276*, 961–969.

Blanchard, D. C., Blanchard, R. J., 2005. Stress and aggressive behaviors. In: Nelson, R. J. (Ed.), *Biology of aggression*. Oxford University Press, New York, pp. 275–291

Blem, C. R., 1990. Avian energy storage. In: Power, D. (Ed.), *Current ornithology*. Plenum, New York, pp. 59–113.

Bordel, R., Haase, E., 2000. Influence of flight on protein catabolism, especially myofilament breakdown, in homing pigeons. *J Comp Physiol B 170*, 51–58.

Boudry, G., Cheeseman, C. I., Perdue, M. H., 2007. Psychological stress impairs Na+-dependent glucose absorption and increases GLUT2 expression in the rat jejunal brush-border membrane. *Am J Physiol 292*, R862–R867.

Bowes, S. B., Jackson, N. C., Papachristodoulou, D., Umpleby, A. M., Sonksen, P. H., 1996. Effect of corticosterone on protein degradation in isolated rat soleus and extensor digitorum longus muscles. *J Endocrinol 148*, 501–507.

Braastad, B. O., 1998. Effects of prenatal stress on behaviour of offspring of laboratory and farmed mammals. *Appl Anim Behav Sci 61*, 159–180.

Bray, M. M., 1993. Effect of ACTH and glucocorticoids on lipid metabolism in the Japanese quail, *Coturnix coturnix japonica*. *Comp Biochem Physiol A 105*, 689–696.

Breen, K. M., Stackpole, C. A., Clarke, I. J., Pytiak, A. V., Tilbrook, A. J., Wagenmaker, E. R., Young, E. A., Karsch, F. J., 2004. Does the type II glucocorticoid receptor mediate cortisol-induced suppression in pituitary responsiveness to gonadotropin-releasing hormone? *Endocrinology 145*, 2739–2746.

Breuner, C. W., Greenberg, A. L., Wingfield, J. C., 1998. Noninvasive corticosterone treatment rapidly increases activity in Gambel's white-crowned sparrows (*Zonotrichia leucophrys gambelii*). *Gen Comp Endocrinol 111*, 386–394.

Breuner, C. W., Hahn, T. P., 2003. Integrating stress physiology, environmental change, and behavior in free-living sparrows. *Horm Behav 43*, 115–123.

Breuner, C. W., Wingfield, J. C., 2000. Rapid behavioral response to corticosterone varies with photoperiod and dose. *Horm Behav 37*, 23.

Brunton, P. J., Russell, J. A., Douglas, A. J., 2008. Adaptive responses of the maternal hypothalamic-pituitary-adrenal axis during pregnancy and lactation. *J Neuroendocrinol 20*, 764–776.

Bulloch, K., 2001. Regional neural regulation of immunity: Anatomy and function. In: McEwen, B. S., Goodman, H. M. (Eds.), *Handbook of physiology*; Section 7: *The endocrine system*; Vol. IV: *Coping with the environment: Neural and endocrine mechanisms*. Oxford University Press, New York, pp. 353–379.

Butkevich, I., Mikhailenko, V., Semionov, P., Bagaeva, T., Otellin, V., Aloisi, A. M., 2009. Effects of maternal corticosterone and stress on behavioral and hormonal indices of formalin pain in male and female offspring of different ages. *Horm Behav 55*, 149–157.

Butler, P. J., Frappell, P. B., Wang, T., Wikelski, M., 2002. The relationship between heart rate and rate of oxygen consumption in Galapagos marine iguanas (*Amblyrhynchus cristatus*) at two different temperatures. *J Exp Biol 205*, 1917–1924.

Buttemer, W. A., Astheimer, L. B., Wingfield, J. C., 1991. The effect of corticosterone on standard metabolic rates of small passerine birds. *J Comp Physiol B 161*, 427–431.

Caldji, C., Liu, D., Sharma, S., Diorio, J., Francis, D., Meaney, M. J., Plotsky, P. M., 2001. Development of individual differences in behavioral and endocrine responses to stress: role of the postnatal environment. In: McEwen, B. S., Goodman, H. M. (Eds.), *Handbook of physiology*; Section 7: *The endocrine system*; Vol. IV: *Coping with the environment: Neural and endocrine mechanisms*. Oxford University Press, New York, pp. 271–292.

Calisi, R. M., Rizzo, N. O., Bentley, G. E., 2008. Seasonal differences in hypothalamic EGR-1 and GnIH expression following capture-handling stress in house sparrows (*Passer domesticus*). *Gen Comp Endocrinol 157*, 283–287.

Cameron, N. M., Champagne, F. A., Parent, C., Fish, E. W., Ozaki-Kuroda, K., Meaney, M. J., 2005. The programming of individual differences in defensive responses and reproductive strategies in the rat through variations in maternal care. *Neurosci Biobehav Rev 29*, 843–865.

Canoine, V., Hayden, T. J., Rowe, K., Goymann, W., 2002. The stress response of European stonechats depends on the type of stressor. *Behaviour 139*, 1303–1311.

Carr, J. A., 2002. Stress, neuropeptides, and feeding behavior: A comparative perspective. *Integ Comp Biol 42*, 582–590.

Carsia, R. V., McIlroy, P. J., 1998. Dietary protein restriction stress in the domestic turkey (*Meleagris gallopavo*) induces hypofunction and remodeling of adrenal steroidogenic tissue. *Gen Comp Endocrinol 109*, 140–153.

Carsia, R. V., Weber, H., 1988. Protein malnutrition in the domestic fowl induces alterations in adrenocortical cell adrenocorticotropin receptors. *Endocrinology 122*, 681–688.

Carsia, R. V., Weber, H., 2000a. Dietary protein restriction stress in the domestic chicken (*Gallus gallus domesticus*) induces remodeling of adrenal steroidogenic tissue that supports hyperfunction. *Gen Comp Endocrinol 120*, 99–107.

Carsia, R. V., Weber, H., 2000b. Remodeling of turkey adrenal steroidogenic tissue induced by dietary protein restriction: The potential role of cell death. *Gen Comp Endocrinol 118*, 471–479.

Carsia, R. V., Weber, H., Lauterio, T. J., 1988. Protein malnutrition in the domestic fowl induces alterations in adrenocortical function. *Endocrinology 122*, 673–680.

Chadio, S. E., Kotsampasi, B., Papadomichelakis, G., Deligeorgis, S., Kalogiannis, D., Menegatos, I., Zervas, G., 2007. Impact of maternal undernutrition on the hypothalamic-pituitaryadrenal axis responsiveness in sheep at different ages postnatal. *J Endocrinol 192*, 495–503.

Challis, J. R. G., Matthews, S. G., Gibb, W., Lye, S. J., 2000. Endocrine and paracrine regulation of birth at term and preterm. *Endocr Rev 21*, 514–550.

Chandran, U. R., Attardi, B., Friedman, R., Dong, K. W., Roberts, J. L., Defranco, D. B., 1994. Glucocorticoid receptor-mediated repression of gonadotropin-releasing-hormone promoter activity in GT1 hypothalamic cell lines. *Endocrinology 134*, 1467–1474.

Chatelain, A., Durand, P., Naaman, E., Dupouy, J. P., 1989. Ontogeny of ACTH(1-24) receptors in rat adrenal glands during the perinatal period. *J Endocrinol 123*, 421–428.

Cherrington, A. D., 1999. Control of glucose uptake and release by the liver in vivo. *Diabetes 48*, 1198–1214.

Cohen, S., Miller, G. E., Rabin, B. S., 2001. Psychological stress and antibody response to immunization: A critical review of the human literature. *Psychosom Med 63*, 7–18.

Cook, N. J., Renema, R., Wilkinson, C., Schaefer, A. L., 2009. Comparisons among serum, egg albumin and yolk concentrations of corticosterone as biomarkers of basal and stimulated adrenocortical activity of laying hens. *Brit Poultry Sci 50*, 620–633.

Cote, J., Clobert, J., Meylan, S., Fitze, P. S., 2006. Experimental enhancement of corticosterone levels positively affects subsequent male survival. *Horm Behav 49*, 320–327.

Cyr, N. E., Wikelski, M., Romero, L. M., 2008. Increased energy expenditure but decreased stress responsiveness during molt. *Physiol Biochem Zool 81*, 452–462.

Dallman, M. F., 2005. Fast glucocorticoid actions on brain: Back to the future. *Front Neuroendocrinol 26*, 103–108.

Dallman, M. F., Bhatnagar, S., 2001. Chronic stress and energy balance: role of the hypothalamo-pituitary-adrenal axis. In: McEwen, B. S., Goodman, H. M. (Eds.), *Handbook of physiology*; Section 7: *The endocrine system*; Vol. IV: *Coping with the environment: Neural and endocrine mechanisms*. Oxford University Press, New York, pp. 179–210.

Dallman, M. F., la Fleur, S. E., Pecoraro, N. C., Gomez, F., Houshyar, H., Akana, S. F., 2004. Minireview: glucocorticoids—food intake, abdominal obesity, and wealthy nations in 2004. *Endocrinology 145*, 2633–2638.

Dallman, M. F., Pecoraro, N., Akana, S. F., la Fleur, S. E., Gomez, F., Houshyar, H., Bell, M. E., Bhatnagar, S., Laugero, K. D., Manalo, S., 2003. Chronic stress and obesity: A new view of "comfort food." *Proc Natl Acad Sci USA 100*, 11696–11701.

Dallman, M. F., Strack, A. M., Akana, S. F., Bradbury, M. J., Hanson, E. S., Scribner, K. A., Smith, M., 1993. Feast and famine: Critical role of glucocorticoids with insulin in daily energy flow. *Front Neuroendocrinol 14*, 303–347.

Darnaudery, M., Maccari, S., 2008. Epigenetic programming of the stress response in male and female rats by prenatal restraint stress. *Brain Res Rev 57*, 571–585.

Davies, A. O., Lefkowitz, R. J., 1984. Regulation of beta-adrenergic receptors by steroid hormones. *Ann Rev Physiol 46*, 119–130.

de Graaf-Roelfsema, E., Keizer, H. A., van Breda, E., Wijnberg, I. D., van der Kolk, J. H., 2007. Hormonal responses to acute exercise, training and overtraining: A review with emphasis on the horse. *Veterinary Quarterly 29*, 82–101.

de Kloet, E. R., Joels, M., Holsboer, F., 2005. Stress and the brain: From adaptation to disease. *Nature Rev Neurosci 6*, 463–475.

Deak, T., 2007. From classic aspects of the stress response to neuroinflammation and sickness: implications for individuals and offspring. *Int J Comp Psychol 20*, 96–110.

Defranco, D. B., Attardi, B., Chandran, U. R., 1994. Glucocorticoid receptor-mediated repression of GnRH gene expression in a hypothalamic GnRH-secreting neuronal cell line. *Annals of the New York Academy of Science, 746*, 473–475.

Deltondo, J., Por, I., Hu, W., Merchenthaler, I., Semeniken, K., Jojart, J., Dudas, B., 2008. Associations between the human growth hormone-releasing hormone—and neuropeptide-Y-immunoreactive systems in the human diencephalon: A possible morphological substrate of the impact of stress on growth. *Neuroscience 153*, 1146–1152.

DeNardo, D. F., Licht, P., 1993. Effects of corticosterone on social behavior of male lizards. *Horm Behav 27*, 184–199.

DeRijk, R. H., de Kloet, E. R., 2008. Corticosteroid receptor polymorphisms: Determinants of vulnerability and resilience. *Eur J Pharmacol 583*, 303–311.

Dhabhar, F. S., 2006. Stress-induced changes in immune cell distribution and trafficking: Implications for immunoprotection versus immunopathology. In: Welsh, C. J., Meagher, M. W., Sternberg, E. M. (Eds.), *Neural and neuroendocrine mechanisms in host defense and autoimmunity*, Springer, New York, pp. 7–25.

Dhabhar, F. S., 2009. A hassle a day may keep the pathogens away: The fight-or-flight stress response and the augmentation of immune function. *Integ Comp Biol 49*, 215–236.

Dhabhar, F. S., McEwen, B. S., 1999. Enhancing versus suppressive effects of stress hormones on skin immune function. *Proc Natl Acad Sci USA 96*, 1059–1064.

Diaz, R. J., Rosenberg, R., 1995. Marine benthic hypoxia: A review of its ecological effects and the behavioural responses of benthic macrofauna. In: Ansell, A. D., Gibson, R. N., Barnes, M. (Eds.), *Oceanography and marine biology: An annual review*, U.C.L. Press, London, *vol. 33*, pp. 245–303.

Dimitriadis, G., Leighton, B., ParryBillings, M., Sasson, S., Young, M., Krause, U., Bevan, S., Piva, T., Wegener, G., Newsholme, E. A., 1997. Effects of glucocorticoid excess on the sensitivity of glucose transport and metabolism to insulin in rat skeletal muscle. *Biochem J 321*, 707–712.

Dong, H., Lin, H., Jiao, H.C., Song, Z. G., Zhao, J. P., Jiang, K. J., 2007. Altered development and protein metabolism in skeletal muscles of broiler chickens (*Gallus gallus domesticus*) by corticosterone. *Comp Biochem Physiol A 147*, 189–195.

Dubey, A. K., Plant, T. M., 1985. A suppression of gonadotropin secretion by cortisol in castrated male rhesus monkeys (*Macaca mulatta*) mediated by the interruption of hypothalamic gonadotropin-releasing hormone release. *Biol Reprod 33*, 423–431.

DuRant, S. E., Romero, L. M., Talent, L. G., Hopkins, W. A., 2008. Effect of exogenous corticosterone on respiration in a reptile. *Gen Comp Endocrinol 156*, 126–133.

Eby, L. A., Crowder, L. B., 2002. Hypoxia-based habitat compression in the Neuse River Estuary: Context-dependent shifts in behavioral avoidance thresholds. *Can J Fish Aquat Sci 59*, 952–965.

Engle, V. D., Summers, J. K., Macauley, J. M., 1999. Dissolved oxygen conditions in northern Gulf of Mexico estuaries. *Environ Monitor Assess 57*, 1–20.

Entringer, S., Kumsta, R., Hellharnmer, D. H., Wadhwa, P. D., Wust, S., 2009. Prenatal exposure to maternal psychosocial stress and HPA axis regulation in young adults. *Horm Behav 55*, 292–298.

Fenoglio, K. A., Brunson, K. L., Baram, T. Z., 2006. Hippocampal neuroplasticity induced by early-life stress: Functional and molecular aspects. *Front Neuroendocrinol 27*, 180–192.

Fone, K. C. F., Porkess, M. V., 2008. Behavioural and neurochemical effects of post-weaning social isolation in rodents: Relevance to developmental neuropsychiatric disorders. *Neurosci Biobehav Rev 32*, 1087–1102.

Friedman, J. M., 2003. A war on obesity, not the obese. *Science 299*, 856–858.

Garvey, W. T., Huecksteadt, T. P., Lima, F. B., Birnbaum, M. J., 1989. Expression of a glucose transporter gene cloned from brain in cellular models of insulin resistance: Dexamethasone decreases transporter messenger RNA in primary cultured adipocytes. *Mol Endocrinol 3*, 1132–1141.

Gilad, E., Meidan, R., Berman, A., Graber, Y., Wolfenson, D., 1993. Effect of heat stress on tonic and GnRH-induced gonadotropin secretion in relation to concentration of estradiol in plasma of cyclic cows. *J Reprod Fertil 99*, 315–321.

Giurgescu, C., 2009. Are maternal cortisol levels related to preterm birth? *Jognn 38*, 377–390.

Gleeson, T. T., Dalessio, P. M., Carr, J. A., Wickler, S. J., Mazzeo, R. S., 1993. Plasma catecholamine and corticosterone and their in vitro effects on lizard skeletal muscle lactate metabolism *Am J Physiol 265*, R632–R639.

Goldstein, R. E., Wasserman, D. H., McGuinness, O. P., Lacy, D. B., Cherrington, A. D., Abumrad, N. N., 1993. Effects of chronic elevation in plasma cortisol on hepatic carbohydrate metabolism. *Am J Physiol 264*, E119–E127.

Goodson, J. L., 2005. The vertebrate social behavior network: Evolutionary themes and variations. *Horm Behav 48*, 11–22.

Goodson, J. L., Bass, A. H., 2001. Social behavior functions and related anatomical characteristics of vasotocin/vasopressin systems in vertebrates. *Brain Res Rev 35*, 246–265.

Gray, J. A., 1987. *The psychology of fear and stress*, 2nd Edition. Cambridge University Press, New York.

Gray, J. M., Yarian, D., Ramenofsky, M., 1990. Corticosterone, foraging behavior, and metabolism in dark-eyed juncos, *Junco hyemalis. Gen Comp Endocrinol 79*, 375–384.

Green, W. H., Campbell, M., David, R., 1984. Psychosocial dwarfism: A critical review of the evidence. *J Am Acad Child Psychiatry 23.*

Greenberg, N., Wingfield, J., 1987. Stress and reproduction: reciprocal relationships. In: Norris, D. O., Jones, R. E. (Eds.), *Hormones and reproduction in fishes, amphibians, and reptiles.* Plenum Press, New York, pp. 461–503.

Grier, D. G., Halliday, H. L., 2004. Effects of glucocorticoids on fetal and neonatal lung development. *Treat Respir Med 3*, 295–306.

Grutter, A.S., Pankhurst, N.W., 2000. The effects of capture, handling, confinement and ectoparasite load on plasma levels of cortisol, glucose and lactate in the coral reef fish *Hemigymnus melapterus. J Fish Biol 57*, 391–401.

Gunnar, M., Quevedo, K., 2007. The neurobiology of stress and development. *Ann Rev Psychol 58*, 145–173.

Gunnar, M. R., Donzella, B., 2002. Social regulation of the cortisol levels in early human development. *Psychoneuroendocrinology 27*, 199–220.

Hammond, G. L., 1990. Molecular properties of corticosteroid binding globulin and the sex-steroid binding proteins. *Endocr Rev 11*, 65–79.

Hart, B. L., 1988. Biological basis of the behavior of sick animals. *Neurosci Biobehav Rev 12*, 123–137.

Hayward, L. S., Wingfield, J. C., 2004. Maternal corticosterone is transferred to avian yolk and may alter offspring growth and adult phenotype. *Gen Comp Endocrinol 135*, 365–371.

Heath, J. A., Dufty, A. M., 1998. Body condition and the adrenal stress response in captive American kestrel juveniles. *Physiol Zool 71*, 67–73.

Heinrichs, S. C., Richard, D., 1999. The role of corticotropin-releasing factor and urocortin in the modulation of ingestive behavior. *Neuropeptides 33*, 350–359.

Hiebert, S. M., Salvante, K. G., Ramenofsky, M., Wingfield, J. C., 2000. Corticosterone and nocturnal torpor in the rufous hummingbird (*Selasphorus rufus*). *Gen Comp Endocrinol 120*, 220–234.

Hochachka, P. W., Somero, G. N., 2002. *Biochemical adaptation: Mechanisms and process in physiological adaptation*. Oxford University Press, Oxford.

Honey, P. K., 1990. *Avian flight muscle* Pectoralis major *as a reserve of proteins and amino acids*. Department of Zoology, Ph.D. Thesis, University of Washington, Seattle.

Horner, H. C., Munck, A., Lienhard, G. E., 1987. Dexamethasone causes translocation of glucose transporters from the plasma membrane to an intracellular site in human fibroblasts. *J Biol Chem 262*, 17696–17702.

Insel, T. R., Battaglia, G., Fairbanks, D. W., Desouza, E. B., 1988. The ontogeny of brain receptors for corticotropin-releasing factor and the development of the their functional association with adenylate-cyclase. *J Neurosci 8*, 4151–4158.

Jaquet, N., 2006. A simple photogrammetric technique to measure sperm whales at sea. *Marine Mammal Sci 22*, 862–879.

Jimenez, M., Hinchcliff, K. W., Farris, J. W., 1998. Catecholamine and cortisol responses of horses to incremental exertion. *Vet Res Comm 22*, 107–118.

Joyce, S., 2000. The dead zones: Oxygen-starved coastal waters. *Environ Health Perspect 108*, A120–A125.

Kapoor, A., Dunn, E., Kostaki, A., Andrews, M. H., Matthews, S. G., 2006. Fetal programming of hypothalamo-pituitary-adrenal function: Prenatal stress and glucocorticoids. *J Physiol 572*.

Kapoor, A., Petropoulos, S., Matthews, S. G., 2008. Fetal programming of hypothalamic-pituitary-adrenal (HPA) axis function and behavior by synthetic glucocorticoids. *Brain Res Rev 57*, 586–595.

Kern, M., Bacon, W., Long, D., Cowie, R. J., 2005. Blood metabolite and corticosterone levels in breeding adult pied flycatchers. *Condor 107*, 665–677.

Kirby, E. D., Geraghty, A.C., Ubuka, T., Bentley, G. E., Kaufer, D., 2009. Stress increases putative gonadotropin inhibitory hormone and decreases luteinizing hormone in male rats. *Proc Natl Acad Sci USA 106*, 11324–11329.

Kitaysky, A. S., Kitaiskaia, E. V., Piatt, J. F., Wingfield, J. C., 2003. Benefits and costs of increased levels of corticosterone in seabird chicks. *Horm Behav 43*, 140–149.

Kitaysky, A. S., Piatt, J. F., Wingfield, J. C., Romano, M., 1999a. The adrenocortical stress-response of black-legged kittiwake chicks in relation to dietary restrictions. *J Comp Physiol B 169*, 303–310.

Kitaysky, A. S., Wingfield, J. C., Piatt, J. F., 1999b. Dynamics of food availability, body condition and physiological stress response in breeding black-legged kittiwakes. *Func Ecol 13*, 577–584.

Kitaysky, A. S., Wingfield, J. C., Piatt, J. F., 2001. Corticosterone facilitates begging and affects resource allocation in the black-legged kittiwake. *Behav Ecol 12*, 619.

Kodama, T., Shimizu, N., Yoshikawa, N., Makino, Y., Ouchida, R., Okamoto, K., Hisada, T., Nakamura, H., Morimoto, C., Tanaka, H., 2003. Role of the glucocorticoid receptor for regulation of hypoxia-dependent gene expression. *J Biol Chem 278*, 33384–33391.

Korosi, A., Shanabrough, M., McClelland, S., Liu, Z. W., Borok, E., Gao, X. B., Horvath, T. L., Baram, T. Z., 2010. Early-life experience reduces excitation to stress-responsive hypothalamic neurons and reprograms the expression of corticotropin-releasing hormone. *J Neurosci 30*, 703–713.

Korte, S. M., 2001. Corticosteroids in relation to fear, anxiety and psychopathology. *Neurosci Biobehav Rev 25*, 117–142.

Korte, S. M., Koolhaas, J. M., Wingfield, J. C., McEwen, B. S., 2005. The Darwinian concept of stress: Benefits of allostasis and costs of allostatic load and the trade-offs in health and disease. *Neurosci Biobehav Rev 29*, 3–38.

Kriegsfeld, L. J., Gibson, E. M., Williams, W. P., Zhao, S., Mason, A. O., Bentley, G. E., Tsutsui, K., 2010. The roles of RFamide-related peptide-3 in mammalian reproductive function and behaviour. *J Neuroendocrinol 22*, 692–700.

la Fleur, S.E., 2005. The effects of glucocorticoids on feeding behavior in rats. In: *3rd Food summit meeting on making sense of food*, Wageningen, Netherlands, pp. 110–114.

Landys, M. M., Ramenofsky, M., Wingfield, J. C., 2006. Actions of glucocorticoids at a seasonal baseline as compared to stress-related levels in the regulation of periodic life processes. *Gen Comp Endocrinol 148*, 132–149.

Larsen, P. R., Kronenberg, H. M., Melmed, S., Polonsky, K. S., Wilson, J. D., Kronenberg, H. M., Foster, D. W., 2003. *Williams textbook of endocrinology*. Saunders, Philadelphia.

Latour, M. A., Laiche, S. A., Thompson, J. R., Pond, A. L., Peebles, E. D., 1996. Continuous infusion of adrenocorticotropin elevates circulating lipoprotein cholesterol and corticosterone concentrations in chickens. *Poult Sci 75*, 1428–1432.

Leibel, R. L., Edens, N. K., Fried, S. K., 1989. Physiologic basis for the control of body-fat distribution in humans. *Ann Rev Nutrition 9*, 417–443.

Leshner, A. I., 1978. *An introduction to behavioral endocrinology*. Oxford University Press, New York.

Leshner, A. I., 1981. The role of hormones in the control of submissiveness. In: Brain, P. F., Benton, D.

(Eds.), *Multidisciplinary approaches to aggression research*. Elsevier/North Holland, Amsterdam, pp. 309–322.

Leshner, A. I., Korn, S. J., Mixon, J. F., Rosenthal, C., Besser, A. K., 1980. Effects of corticosterone on submissiveness in mice: Some temporal and theoretical considerations. *Physiol Behav 24*, 283–288.

Leshner, A. I., Politch, J. A., 1979. Hormonal control of submissiveness in mice: Irrelevance of the adrogens and relevance of the pituitary-adrenal hormones. *Physiol Behav 22*, 531–534.

Liggins, G. C., 1994. The role of cortisol in preparing the fetus for birth. *Reprod Fertil Devel 6*, 141–150.

Lin, H., Deculypere, E., Buyse, J., 2004a. Oxidative stress induced by corticosterone administration in broiler chickens (*Gallus gallus domesticus*). 2. Short-term effect. *Comp Biochem Physiol B 139*, 745–751.

Lin, H., Decuypere, E., Buyse, J., 2004b. Oxidative stress induced by corticosterone administration in broiler chickens (*Gallus gallus domesticus*). 1. Chronic exposure. *Comp Biochem Physiol B 139*, 737–744.

Lukkes, J. L., Mokin, M. V., Scholl, J. L., Forster, G. L., 2009. Adult rats exposed to early-life social isolation exhibit increased anxiety and conditioned fear behavior, and altered hormonal stress responses. *Horm Behav 55*, 248–256.

Lupien, S. J., McEwen, B. S., Gunnar, M. R., Heim, C., 2009. Effects of stress throughout the lifespan on the brain, behaviour and cognition. *Nature Rev Neurosci 10*, 434–445.

Maeda, K., Tsukamura, H., 2006. The impact of stress on reproduction: Are glucocorticoids inhibitory or protective to gonadotropin secretion? *Endocrinology 147*, 1085–1086.

Mairesse, J., Lesage, J., Breton, C., Breant, B., Hahn, T., Darnaudery, M., Dickson, S.L., Seckl, J., Blondeau, B., Vieau, D., Maccari, S., Viltart, O., 2007. Maternal stress alters endocrine function of the feto-placental unit in rats. *Am J Physiol 292*, E1526–E1533.

Maney, D. L., Wingfield, J. C., 1998a. Central opioid control of feeding behavior in the white-crowned sparrow, *Zonotrichia leucophrys gambelii*. *Horm Behav 33*, 16–22.

Maney, D. L., Wingfield, J. C., 1998b. Neuroendocrine suppression of female courtship in a wild passerine: Corticotropin-releasing factor and endogenous opioids. *J Neuroendocrinol 10*, 593.

Manoli, I., Alesci, S., Blackman, M. R., Su, Y. A., Rennert, O. M., Chrousos, G. P., 2007. Mitochondria as key components of the stress response. *Trends Endocrinol Metab 18*, 190–198.

Matsuwaki, T., Kayasuga, Y., Yamanouchi, K., Nishihara, M., 2006. Maintenance of gonadotropin secretion by glucocorticoids under stress conditions through the inhibition of prostaglandin synthesis in the brain. *Endocrinology 147*, 1087–1093.

Matsuwaki, T., Suzuki, M., Yamanouchi, K., Nishihara, M., 2004. Glucocorticoid counteracts the suppressive effect of tumor necrosis factor-alpha on the surge of luteinizing hormone secretion in rats. *J Endocrinol 181*, 509–513.

Matsuwaki, T., Watanabe, E., Suzuki, M., Yamanouchi, K., Nishihara, M., 2003. Glucocorticoid maintains pulsatile secretion of luteinizing hormone under infectious stress condition. *Endocrinology 144*, 3477–3482.

Maya-Nunez, G., Conn, P. M., 2003. Transcriptional regulation of the GnRH receptor gene by glucocorticoids. *Mol Cell Endocrinol 200*, 89–98.

Mazziotti, G., Angeli, A., Bilezikian, J. P., Canalis, E., Giustina, A., 2006. Glucocorticoid-induced osteoporosis: An update. *Trends Endocrinol Metab 17*, 144–149.

McEwen, B. S., 2001. Neurobiology of interpreting and responding to stressful events: paradigmatic role of the hippocampus. In: McEwen, B. S., Goodman, H. M. (Eds.), *Handbook of physiology*; Section 7: *The endocrine system*; Vol. IV: *Coping with the environment: Neural and endocrine mechanisms*. Oxford University Press, New York, pp. 155–178.

Miles, D. B., Calsbeek, R., Sinervo, B., 2007. Corticosterone, locomotor performance, and metabolism in side-blotched lizards (*Uta stansburiana*). *Horm Behav 51*, 548–554.

Mitra, R., Sapolsky, R. M., 2008. Acute corticosterone treatment is sufficient to induce anxiety and amygdaloid dendritic hypertrophy. *Proc Natl Acad Sci USA 105*, 5573–5578.

Molendi-Coste, O., Grumolato, L., Laborie, C., Lesage, J., Maubert, E., Ghzili, H., Vaudry, H., Anouar, Y., Breton, C., Vieau, D., 2006. Maternal perinatal undernutrition alters neuronal and neuroendocrine differentiation in the rat adrenal medulla at weaning. *Endocrinology 147*, 3050–3059.

Molendi-Coste, O., Laborie, C., Scarpa, M. C., Montel, V., Vieau, D., Breton, C., 2009. Maternal perinatal undernutrition alters postnatal development of chromaffin cells in the male rat adrenal medulla. *Neuroendocrinol 90*, 54–66.

Monder, C., Sakai, R. R., Miroff, Y., Blanchard, D. C., Blanchard, R. J., 1994. Reciprocal changes in plasma corticosterone and testosterone in stressed male rats maintained in a visible burrow system: Evidence for a mediating role of testicular 11-beta-hydroxysteroid dehydrogenase. *Endocrinology 134*, 1193–1198.

Moore, F. L., Miller, L. J., 1984. Stress-induced inhibition of sexual behavior: corticosterone inhibits courtship behaviors of a male amphibian. *Horm Behav 18*, 400–410.

Moore, I. T., Greene, M. J., Mason, R. T., 2001. Environmental and seasonal adaptations of the adrenocortical and gonadal responses to capture stress in two populations of the male garter snake, *Thamnophis sirtalis*. *J Exp Zool 289*, 99–108.

Moore, I. T., Jessop, T. S., 2003. Stress, reproduction, and adrenocortical modulation in amphibians and reptiles. *Horm Behav 43*, 39–47.

Moriceau, S., Roth, T. L., Okotoghaide, T., Sullivan, R. M., 2004. Corticosterone controls the developmental emergence of fear and amygdala function to predator odors in infant rat pups. *Int J Devel Neurosci 22*, 415–422.

Munck, A., 1971. Glucocorticoid inhibition of glucose uptake by peripheral tissues: Old and new evidence, molecular mechanisms, and physiological significance *Perspect Biol Med 14*, 265.

Munck, A., Guyre, P. M., Holbrook, N. J., 1984. Physiological functions of glucocorticoids in stress and their relation to pharmacological actions. *Endocr Rev 5*, 25–44.

Munck, A., Koritz, S. B., 1962. Studies on the mode of action of glucocorticoids in rats. I. Early effects of cortisol on blood glucose and on glucose entry into muscle, liver and adipose tissue. *Biochim Biophys Acta 57*, 310–317.

Nelson, R. J., 2011. *An introduction to behavioral endocrinology*, 4th Edition. Sinauer Associates, Sunderland, MA.

Nepomnaschy, P. A., Welch, K. B., McConnell, D.S., Low, B. S., Strassmann, B. I., England, B. G., 2006. Cortisol levels and very early pregnancy loss in humans. *Proc Natl Acad Sci USA 103*, 3938–3942.

Nieuwenhuizen, A. G., Rutters, F., 2008. The hypothalamic-pituitary-adrenal-axis in the regulation of energy balance. *Physiol Behav 94*, 169–177.

Nonogaki, K., 2000. New insights into sympathetic regulation of glucose and fat metabolism. *Diabetologia 43*, 533–549.

Norman, A. W., Litwack, G., 1997. *Hormones*. Academic Press, Boston.

Norris, D. O., 2007. *Vertebrate endocrinology*. Academic Press, Boston.

Okimoto, D. K., Blaus, A., Schmidt, M., Gordon, M. K., Dent, G. W., Levine, S., 2002. Differential expression of c-fos and tyrosine hydroxylase mRNA in the adrenal gland of the infant rat: Evidence for an adrenal hyporesponsive period. *Endocrinology 143*, 1717–1725.

Osadchuk, L. V., Braastad, B. O., Hovland, A. L., Bakken, M., 2001. Handling during pregnancy in the blue fox (*Alopex lagopus*): The influence on the fetal pituitary-adrenal axis. *Gen Comp Endocrinol 123*, 100–110.

Osadchuk, L. V., Braastad, B. O., Hovland, A. L., Bakken, M., 2003. Reproductive and pituitary-adrenal axis parameters in normal and prenatally stressed prepubertal blue foxes (*Alopex lagopus*). *Anim Sci 76*, 413–420.

Osugi, T., Ukena, K., Bentley, G. E., O'Brien, S., Moore, I. T., Wingfield, J. C., Tsutsui, K., 2004. Gonadotropin-inhibitory hormone in Gambel's white-crowned sparrow (*Zonotrichia leucophrys gambelii*): cDNA identification, transcript localization and functional effects in laboratory and field experiments. *J Endocrinol 182*, 33–42.

Padgett, D. A., Glaser, R., 2003. How stress influences the immune response. *Trends Immunol 24*, 444–448.

Pamenter, R. W., Hedge, G. A., 1980. Inhibition of thyrotropin secretion by physiological levels of corticosterone. *Endocrinology 106*, 162–166.

Pedersen, A. F., Zachariae, R., Bovbjerg, D. H., 2009. Psychological stress and antibody response to influenza vaccination: A meta-analysis. *Brain Behav Immun 23*, 427–433.

Pedersen, S. B., Borglum, J. D., Mollerpedersen, T., Richelsen, B., 1992. Characterization of nuclear corticosteroid receptors in rat adipocytes: Regional variations and modulatory effects of hormones. *Biochim Biophys Acta 1134*, 303–308.

Pihl, L., Baden, S. P., Diaz, R. J., 1991. Effects of periodic hypoxia on distribution of demersal fish and crustaceans. *Marine Biol 108*, 349–360.

Plotsky, P. M., Meaney, M. J., 1993. Early, postnatal experience alters hypothalamic corticotropin-releasing factor (CRF) mRNA, median eminence CRF content and stress-induced release in adult rats. *Mol Brain Res 18*, 195–200.

Popov, V. I., Bocharova, L. S., 1992. Hibernation-induced structural changes in synaptic contacts between mossy fibres and hippocampal pyramidal neurons. *Neuroscience 48*, 53–62.

Popov, V. I., Bocharova, L. S., Bragin, A. G., 1992. Repeated changes of dendritic morphology in the hippocampus of ground squirrels in the course of hibernation. *Neuroscience 48*, 45–51.

Preest, M. R., Cree, A., 2008. Corticosterone treatment has subtle effects on thermoregulatory behavior and raises metabolic rate in the new Zealand common gecko, Hoplodactylus maculatus. *Physiol Biochem Zool 81*, 641–650.

Qi, D., Rodrigues, B., 2007. Glucocorticoids produce whole body insulin resistance with changes in cardiac metabolism. *Am J Physiol 292*, E654–E667.

Rabalais, N. N., Turner, R. E., 2001. Hypoxia in the northern Gulf of Mexico: Description, causes and change. In: Rabalais, N. N. (Ed.), *Coastal and estuarine sciences*, Vol 58: *Coastal hypoxia: Consequences for living resources and ecosystems*, NOAA Coastal Ocean Program, Silver Spring, MD, pp. 1–36.

Rabin, D. S., Johnson, E. O., Brandon, D. D., Liapi, C., Chrousos, G. P., 1990. Glucocorticoids inhibit estradiol-mediated uterine growth: Possible role of the uterine estradiol receptor. *Biol Reprod 42*, 74–80.

Ramenofsky, M., 1990. Fat storage and fat metabolism in relation to migration. In: Gwinner, E. (Ed.), *Bird migration: Physiology and ecophysiology*. Springer-Verlag, Berlin, pp. 214–231.

Ramenofsky, M., Gray, J. M., Johnson, R. B., 1992. Behavioral and physiological adjustments of birds living in winter flocks. *Ornis Scan 23*, 371–380.

Rhen, T., Cidlowski, J. A., 2005. Antiinflammatory action of glucocorticoids: New mechanisms for old drugs. *N Engl J Med 353*, 1711–1723.

Richardson, H. N., Zorrilla, E. P., Mandyam, C. D., Rivier, C. L., 2006. Exposure to repetitive versus varied stress during prenatal development generates two distinct anxiogenic and neuroendocrine profiles in adulthood. *Endocrinology 147*, 2506–2517.

Roberge, C., Carpentier, A. C., Langlois, M. F., Baillargeon, J. P., Ardilouze, J. L., Maheux, P., Gallo-Payet, N., 2007. Adrenocortical dysregulation as a major player in insulin resistance and onset of obesity. *Am J Physiol 293*, E1465–E1478.

Romero, L. M., Dean, S. C., Wingfield, J. C., 1998. Neurally-active stress peptide inhibits territorial defense in wild birds. *Horm Behav 34*, 239–247.

Romero, L. M., Meister, C. J., Cyr, N. E., Kenagy, G. J., Wingfield, J. C., 2008. Seasonal glucocorticoid responses to capture in wild free-living mammals. *Am J Physiol 294*, R614–R622.

Romero, L. M., Raley-Susman, K. M., Redish, D. M., Brooke, S. M., Horner, H. C., Sapolsky, R. M., 1992. Possible mechanism by which stress accelerates growth of virally derived tumors. *Proc Natl Acad Sci USA 89*, 11084–11087.

Roussel, S., Boissy, A., Montigny, D., Hemsworth, P. H., Duvaux-Ponter, C., 2005. Gender-specific effects of prenatal stress on emotional reactivity and stress physiology of goat kids. *Horm Behav 47*, 256–266.

Rubello, D., Sonino, N., Casara, D., Girelli, M.E., Busnardo, B., Boscaro, M., 1992. Acute and chronic effects of high glucocorticoid levels on hypothalamic-pituitary-thyroid axis in man. *J Endocrinol Invest 15*, 437–441.

Sapolsky, R. M., 1992. *Stress, the aging brain, and the mechanisms of neuron death*. MIT Press, Cambridge, MA.

Sapolsky, R. M., 1994. *Why zebras don't get ulcers: A guide to stress, stress-related diseases, and coping*. W.H. Freeman, New York.

Sapolsky, R. M., 2001. Physiological and pathophysiological implications of social stress in mammals. In: McEwen, B. S., Goodman, H. M. (Eds.), *Handbook of physiology*; Section 7: *The endocrine system*; Vol. IV: *Coping with the environment: Neural and endocrine mechanisms*. Oxford University Press, New York, pp. 517–532.

Sapolsky, R. M., Meaney, M. J., 1986. Maturation of the adrenocortical stress response: neuroendocrine control mechanisms and the stress hyporesponsive period. *Brain Res Rev 11*, 65–76.

Sapolsky, R. M., Romero, L. M., Munck, A. U., 2000. How do glucocorticoids influence stress-responses? Integrating permissive, suppressive, stimulatory, and preparative actions. *Endocr Rev 21*, 55–89.

Schaison, G., Durand, F., Mowszowicz, I., 1978. Effect of glucocorticoids on plasma testosterone in men. *Acta Endocrinologica 89*, 126–131.

Schakman, O., Gilson, H., Thissen, J. P., 2008. Mechanisms of glucocorticoid-induced myopathy. *J Endocrinol 197*, 1–10.

Schmidt, J. B., Satterlee, D. G., Treese, S. M., 2009. Maternal corticosterone reduces egg fertility and hatchability and increases the numbers of early dead embryos in eggs laid by quail hens selected for exaggerated adrenocortical stress responsiveness. *Poult Sci 88*, 1352–1357.

Schoech, S. J., Rensel, M. A., Bridge, E. S., Boughton, R. K., Wilcoxen, T. E., 2009. Environment, glucocorticoids, and the timing of reproduction. *Gen Comp Endocrinol 163*, 201–207.

Scholnick, D. A., Weinstein, R. B., Gleeson, T. T., 1997. The influence of corticosterone and glucagon on metabolic recovery from exhaustive exercise in the desert iguana Dipsosaurus dorsalis. *Gen Comp Endocrinol 106*, 147–154.

Schreck, C. B., Contreras-Sanchez, W., Fitzpatrick, M. S., 2001. Effects of stress on fish reproduction, gamete quality, and progeny. *Aquaculture 197*, 3–24.

Schulkin, J., 2005. *Curt Richter: A life in the laboratory*. Johns Hopkins University Press, Baltimore, MD.

Schuurman, T., 1980. Hormonal correlates of agonistic behavior in adult male rats. *Prog Brain Res 53*, 415–420.

Schwartz, M. W., Woods, S. C., Porte, D., Seeley, R. J., Baskin, D. G., 2000. Central nervous system control of food intake. *Nature 404*, 661–671.

Selye, H., 1946. The general adaptation syndrome and the diseases of adaptation. *J Clin Endocrinol 6*, 117–230.

Shanks, N., Larocque, S., Meaney, M. J., 1995. Neonatal endotoxin exposure alters the development of the hypothalamic-pituitary-adrenal axis: Early illness and later responsivity to stress. *J Neurosci 15*, 376–384.

Silverin, B., 1986. Corticosterone-binding proteins and behavioral effects of high plasma levels of corticosterone during the breeding period in the pied flycatcher. *Gen Comp Endocrinol 64*, 67.

Silverin, B., 1998. Behavioural and hormonal responses of the pied flycatcher to environmental stressors. *Anim Behav 55*, 1411–1420.

Sjogren, J., Weck, M., Nilsson, A., Ottosson, M., Bjorntorp, P., 1994. Glucocorticoid hormone binding to rat adipocytes. *Biochim Biophys Acta Mol 1224*, 17–21.

Spencer, K. A., Verhulst, S., 2008. Post-natal exposure to corticosterone affects standard metabolic rate in the zebra finch (*Taeniopygia guttata*). *Gen Comp Endocrinol 159*, 250–256.

Spencer, R. L., Kalman, B. A., Dhabhar, F. S., 2001. Role of endogenous glucocorticoids in immune system function: regulation and counterregulation. In: McEwen, B., Goodman, H. M. (Eds.), *Handbook of physiology*; Section 7: *The endocrine system*; Vol. IV: *Coping with the environment: Neural and endocrine mechanisms*. Oxford University Press, New York, pp. 381–423.

Spinelli, S., Chefer, S., Suomi, S. J., Higley, J. D., Barr, C. S., Stein, E., 2009. Early-life stress induces long-term morphologic changes in primate brain. *Arch Gen Psychiatry 66*, 658–665.

Stöwe, M., Bugnyar, T., Schloegl, C., Heinrich, B., Kotrschal, K., Möstl, E., 2008. Corticosterone excretion patterns and affiliative behavior over development in ravens (*Corvus corax*). *Horm Behav 53*, 208–216.

Sweazea, K. L., Braun, E. J., 2005. Glucose transport by English sparrow (Passer domesticus) skeletal muscle: Have we been chirping up the wrong tree? *J Exp Zool A: Comp Exp Biol 303A*, 143–153.

Sweazea, K. L., Braun, E. J., 2006. Glucose transporter expression in English sparrows (*Passer domesticus*). *Comp Biochem Physiol B 144*, 263–270.

Sweazea, K.L., McMurtry, J.P., Braun, E.J., 2006. Inhibition of lipolysis does not affect insulin sensitivity to glucose uptake in the mourning dove. *Comp Biochem Physiol B 144*, 387–394.

Swift, D.J., 1981. Changes in selected blood component concentrations of rainbow trout, *Salmo gairdneri*, Richardson, exposed to hypoxia or sublethal concentrations of phenolor ammonia. *J Fish Biol 19*, 45–61.

Szyf, M., Weaver, I. C. G., Champagne, F. A., Diorio, J., Meaney, M. J., 2005. Maternal programming of steroid receptor expression and phenotype through DNA methylation in the rat. *Front Neuroendocrinol 26*, 139–162.

Taborsky, G. J., Porte, D. J., 1991. Stress-induced hyperglycemia and its relation to diabetes mellitis. In: Brown, M. R., Koob, G. F., Rivier, C. (Eds.), *Stress: Neurobiology and neuroendocrinology*. Marcel Dekker, New York, pp. 519–548.

Teicher, M. H., Tomoda, A., Andersen, S. L., 2005. Neurobiological consequences of early stress and childhood maltreatment: Are results from human and animal studies comparable? In: Yehuda, R. (Ed.) *Meeting on psychobiology of post-traumatic stress disorder*. New York, pp. 313–323.

Thomas, P., Rahman, M. S., Khan, I. A., Kummer, J. A., 2007. Widespread endocrine disruption and reproductive impairment in an estuarine fish population exposed to seasonal hypoxia. *Proc R Soc Lond B 274*, 2693–2701.

Thomas, P., Rahman, M. S., Kummer, J. A., Lawson, S., 2006. Reproductive endocrine dysfunction in Atlantic croaker exposed to hypoxia. *Marine Environ Res 62*, S249–S252.

Tomasso, J. R., Davis, K. B., Parker, N. C., 1981. Plasma corticosteroid dynamics in channel catfish, *Ictalurus punctatus* (Rafinesque), during and after oxygen depletion. *J Fish Biol 18*, 519–526.

Tsankova, N., Renthal, W., Kumar, A., Nestler, E. J., 2007. Epigenetic regulation in psychiatric disorders. *Nature Rev Neurosci 8*, 355–367.

Tsutsui, K., Bentley, G. E., Kriegsfeld, L. J., Osugi, T., Seong, J. Y., Vaudry, H., 2010. Discovery and evolutionary history of gonadotrophin-inhibitory hormone and kisspeptin: New key neuropeptides controlling reproduction. *J Neuroendocrinol 22*, 716–727.

Tsutsui, K., Saigoh, E., Ukena, K., Teranishi, H., Fujisawa, Y., Kikuchi, M., Ishii, S., Sharp, J. P., 2000. A novel avian hypothalamic peptide inhibiting gonadotropin release. *Biochem Biophys Res Comm 275*, 661–667.

Tsutsui, K., Ubuka, T., Yin, H., Osugi, T., Ukena, K., Bentley, G. E., Sharp, P. J., Wingfield, J. C., 2007. Discovery of gonadotropin-inhibitory hormone in a domesticated bird, its mode of action and functional significance. *J Ornithol 148*, S515–S520.

Turnbull, A. V., Rivier, C.L., 1999. Regulation of the hypothalamic-pituitary-adrenal axis by cytokines: Actions and mechanisms of action. *Physiol Rev 79*, 1–71.

Turner, J. W., Jr., Nemeth, R., Rogers, C., 2003. Measurement of fecal glucocorticoids in parrotfishes to assess stress. *Gen Comp Endocrinol 133*, 341–352.

Umpleby, A. M., RussellJones, D. L., 1996. The hormonal control of protein metabolism. *Baillieres Clin Endocrinol Metab 10*, 551–570.

vanRaaij, M. T. M., Pit, D. S. S., Balm, P. H. M., Steffens, A. B., vandenThillart, G., 1996. Behavioral strategy and the physiological stress response in rainbow trout exposed to severe hypoxia. *Horm Behav 30*, 85–92.

Wagenmaker, E. R., Breen, K. M., Oakley, A. E., Tilbrook, A. J., Karsch, F. J., 2009. Psychosocial stress inhibits amplitude of gonadotropin-releasing hormone pulses independent of cortisol action on the type II glucocorticoid receptor. *Endocrinology 150*, 762–769.

Wajchenberg, B. L., Giannella-Neto, D., da Silva, M. E. R., Santos, R. F., 2002. Depot-specific hormonal characteristics of subcutaneous and visceral adipose tissue and their relation to the metabolic syndrome. *Horm Metab Res 34*, 616–621.

Walker, C.-D., Anand, K. J. S., Plotsky, P. M., 2001. Development of the hypothalamic-pituitary-adrenal axis and the stress response. In: McEwen, B. S., Goodman, H. M. (Eds.), *Handbook of physiology*; Section 7: *The endocrine system*; Vol. IV: *Coping with the environment: Neural and endocrine mechanisms*. Oxford University Press, New York, pp. 237–270.

Wang, C. T., Shui, H. A., Huang, R. L., Tai, M. Y., Peng, M. T., Tsai, Y. F., 2006. Sexual motivation is demasculinized, but not feminized, in prenatally stressed male rats. *Neuroscience 138*, 357–364.

Weber, K., Bruck, P., Mikes, Z., Kupper, J. H., Klingenspor, M., Wiesner, R. J., 2002. Glucocorticoid hormone stimulates mitochondrial biogenesis specifically in skeletal muscle. *Endocrinology 143*, 177–184.

Weinstock, M., 2008. The long-term behavioural consequences of prenatal stress. *Neurosci Biobehav Rev 32*, 1073–1086.

Weiss, S. L., Johnston, G., Moore, M. C., 2007. Corticosterone stimulates hatching of late-term tree lizard embryos. *Comp Biochem Physiol A 146*, 360–365.

Wendalaar Bonga, S. E., 1997. The stress response in fish. *Physiol Rev 77*, 591–625.

Whittle, W. L., Patel, F. A., Alfaidy, N., Holloway, A. C., Fraser, M., Gyomorey, S., Lye, S. J., Gibb, W., Challis, J. R. G., 2001. Glucocorticoid regulation of human and ovine parturition: The relationship between fetal hypothalamic-pituitary-adrenal axis activation and intrauterine prostaglandin production. *Biol Reprod 64*, 1019–1032.

Wikelski, M., Lynn, S., Breuner, C., Wingfield, J. C., Kenagy, G. J., 1999. Energy metabolism, testosterone and corticosterone in white-crowned sparrows. *J Comp Physiol A 185*, 463.

Wikelski, M., Thom, C., 2000. Marine iguanas shrink to survive El Niño. *Nature 403*, 37–38.

Wingfield, J. C., 1994. Modulation of the adrenocortical response to stress in birds. In: Davey, K. G., Peter, R. E., Tobe, S. S. (Eds.), *Perspectives in comparative endocrinology.* National Research Council of Canada, Ottawa, pp. 520–528.

Wingfield, J. C., 2004. Allostatic load and life cycles: implications for neuroendocrine mechanisms. In: Schulkin, J. (Ed.), *Allostasis, homeostasis and the costs of physiological adaptation*, Cambridge University Press, Cambridge, pp. 302–342.

Wingfield, J. C., 2005. Modulation of the adrenocortical response to acute stress in breeding birds. In: Dawson, A., Sharp, P. J. (Eds.), *Functional avian endocrinology.* Narosa Publishing House, New Delhi, India, pp. 225–240.

Wingfield, J.C., Silverin, B. 2002. Ecophysiological studies of hormone–behavior relations in birds. In: Pfaff, D. W., Arnold, A. P., Etgen, A. M., Fahrbach, S. E., Rubin, R. T. (Eds.), *Hormones, brain, and behavior, vol. 2.* Elsevier Science, Amsterdam, pp. 587–647.

Wingfield, J. C., Maney, D. L., Breuner, C. W., Jacobs, J. D., Lynn, S., Ramenofsky, M., Richardson, R. D., 1998. Ecological bases of hormone-behavior interactions: The "emergency life history stage." *Integ Comp Biol 38*, 191.

Wingfield, J. C., Moore, I. T., Goymann, W., Wacker, D. W., Sperry, T., 2005. Contexts and ethology of vertebrate aggression: implications for the evolution of hormone-behavior interactions. In: Nelson, R. J. (Ed.), *Biology of aggression.* Oxford University Press, New York, pp. 179–210.

Wingfield, J. C., Ramenofsky, M., 1997. Corticosterone and facultative dispersal in response to unpredictable events. *Ardea 85*, 155–166.

Wingfield, J. C., Ramenofsky, M., 1999. Hormones and the behavioral ecology of stress. *Stress Physiol Animals* 1–51.

Wingfield, J. C., Silverin, B., 1986. Effects of corticosterone on territorial behavior of free-living male song sparrows *Melospiza melodia. Horm Behav 20*, 405–417.

Wingfield, J. C., Silverin, B., 2009. Ecophysiological studies of hormone-behavior relations in birds. In: Pfaff, D. W., Arnold, A. P., Etgen, A. M., Fahrbach, S. E., Rubin, R. T. (Eds.), *Hormones, brain, and behavior, vol. 2.* Academic Press, New York, pp. 817–854.

Wong, D. M., Vo, D. T., Alcott, C. J., Stewart, A. J., Peterson, A. D., Sponseller, B. A., Hsu, W. H., 2009. Adrenocorticotropic hormone stimulation tests in healthy foals from birth to 12 weeks of age. *Can J Vet Res73*, 65–72.

Woods, L. L., 2006. Maternal glucocorticoids and prenatal programming of hypertension. *Am J Physiol 291*, R1069–R1075.

Wright, A. J., Aguilar Soto, N., Baldwin, A. L., Bateson, M., Beale, C. M., Clark, C., Deak, T., Edwards, E. F., Fernández, A., Godinho, A., Hatch, L., Kakuschke, A., Lusseau, D., Martineau, D., Romero, L. M., Weilgart, L., Wintle, B., Notarbartolo di Sciara, G., Martin, V., 2007. Anthropogenic noise as a stressor in animals: a multidisciplinary perspective. *Int J Comp Psychol 20*, 250–273.

Yajurvedi, H. N., Menon, S., 2005. Influence of stress on gonadotrophin induced testicular recrudescence in the lizard Mabuya carinata. *J Exp Zool A: Comp Exp Biol 303A*, 534–540.

Yeager, M. P., Guyre, P. M., Munck, A. U., 2004. Glucocorticoid regulation of the inflammatory response to injury. *Acta Anaesthesiol Scand 48*, 799–813.

Yin, H., Ukena, K., Ubuka, T., Tsutsui, K., 2005. A novel G protein-coupled receptor for gonadotropin-inhibitory hormone in the Japanese quail (Coturnix japonica): identification, expression and binding activity. *J Endocrinol 184*, 257–266.

PART II

Coping with a Capricious Environment

6

Field Techniques

Measuring Stress Responses in Wild Animals

I. INTRODUCTION

One hallmark of stress in humans is the great inter-individual variation in responses. People react differently to identical stimuli. What may be terrifying to one person (jumping out of an airplane, for example) might be a recreational activity for others (skydiving). As we discussed in Chapter 3, both the context of the stimulus and how that stimulus is perceived can have an enormous impact on the ultimate behavioral and physiological responses. We also know that people have different coping styles that can influence these responses. For example, a new personality type has recently been described. The "Type D" personality (D stands for distressed) describes a person who both experiences increased negative emotions and who ameliorates those emotions by avoiding social contact with others (Denollet 1998). Recent research indicates that Type D people are associated with increased risk of cardiovascular disease and elevated cortisol concentrations (Pedersen and Denollet 2003; Sher 2005). The clear lesson from this, and similar research, is that individual differences can have profound effects on human health.

Furthermore, there has been substantial research on how various real-world stressors can cause stress in humans. A recent reference work, *The Encyclopedia of Stress*, second edition (Fink 2007), summarized the impact of stressors such as floods, earthquakes, war, terrorism, and accidents. In these types of studies, the impact on the affected population is compared to an unaffected population and the differences are ascribed to impact of the stressor.

However, many of these studies rely upon a simple, yet profound, research technique—they ask the subject questions. The elegance of this approach is perhaps best shown by the work on Type D personalities. An individual is assigned the Type D designation based upon a written series of questions (Denollet 1998). Consequently, feelings of negative emotions are self-reported by the subject. In another example, individuals in a refugee camp were given an oral interview to assess their "sense of coherence" (SOC), defined briefly as a belief that the individual has sufficient resources to handle predictable events and activities and that those activities are important. In this study, the lower the SOC score, the higher the cortisol concentrations in mothers who recently gave birth (Almedom et al. 2005). The conclusion that many clinicians make is that a medical history is currently the best way to diagnose stress in a human (Noble 2002).

Clearly, the oral or written survey technique is successful in that it has provided a basis for distinguishing between people, and the resultant distinguishing traits have a large impact on stress responses and ultimately on health. It is just as clear, however, that this technique is impossible with animals. Researchers might infer depression by observing depression-like behaviors, but we cannot ask the animal if it is depressed. Similarly, researchers can infer that an animal is stressed based upon cardiovascular or hormonal (Chapter 4) changes associated with stressors, but the independent oral or written assessment provided by humans cannot be supplied by animals.

This leaves us with a major question that is not faced by human clinical researchers, nor by most biomedical research on animals, that can be summarized by the following question: What kinds of differences can be profitably studied in wild and free-living animals? To answer this question, we need to know something about the homeostatic mediators involved in responding to stressors. For example, it has long been known that both baseline (Romero 2004) and stimulated (Wingfield 1994) corticosteroid concentrations vary tremendously from individual to individual and from species to species. Such variation makes it difficult to compare the effects of stress in different taxa. On the other hand, changes in adrenocortical responses to acute stress of individuals clearly suggest that modulation of sensitivity of the HPA axis is occurring (Sapolsky 1987; Wingfield 1988; Wingfield 1994; Schwabl 1995; Walker et al. 2001). Which variation has an ecological and/or physiological basis, and which is just physiological noise? We feel that the following four types of variation are excellent targets for field studies of modulation of responses to stress (adapted from Wingfield and Romero 2001):

1. Adaptations to specific habitats: Variation among populations of the same, similar, or other species living in different habitats or similar habitats but different environments (e.g., Wingfield et al. 1992). Comparisons of closely related species decrease the likelihood of phylogenetic differences that may have little physiological significance.
2. Responses to environmental change: Variation from season to season, time of day, weather conditions, predator densities, anthropomorphic disturbance, and so on (e.g., Dauphin-Villemant and Xavier 1987; Romero et al. 2000; Scheuerlein et al. 2001; Romero 2002; Homan et al. 2003b).
3. Facultative changes: Variation in adjusting to repeated stressors within a population, season, and life-history stage. Examples include changes in corticosteroid receptor numbers (Hodgson et al. 2007), adjustments in 11β—HSD (Funder et al. 1988), and responsiveness of the HPA axis to chronic stress (e.g., Astheimer et al. 1995; Cyr and Romero 2007).
4. Individual differences: Variation within a population and season. For example, sensitivity to a stressor may vary as a function of social status (e.g., Schwabl et al. 1988; Creel et al. 1996; Sapolsky 2001), body condition (e.g., Romero and Wikelski 2001), infection (e.g., Dunlap and Schall 1995), sexual dimorphism (e.g., Grassman and Hess 1992), age (e.g., Angelier et al. 2006; Heidinger et al. 2006), and early development (e.g., Walker et al. 2001).

Notice that generating data in each of these four areas depends heavily on the comparative method. Although there are inherent weaknesses in doing fieldwork, chief among them being the difficulty of performing controlled experiments (although these are eminently possible), there are also some major strengths. First, laboratory experiments, by definition, cannot be performed on free-ranging individuals. If the goal is to understand how an animal interacts with its environment, there is little choice but to perform at least the initial studies in the field (Calisi and Bentley 2009). Second, field studies can provide ecologically relevant hypotheses that can be tested in laboratory settings to determine mechanisms underlying the modulation of the HPA axis responses to stress. Third, we feel that data collected from free-living animals is much less likely to represent physiological noise. The consequences of a suboptimal response is likely to be much more severe for a free-living animal than for one housed in a laboratory. Natural selection is likely to act as a powerful force to cull animals that make sub-optimal responses from the population. Finally, the comparative method can provide powerful "natural experiments" that can be as useful, if not more useful, than laboratory studies using modern techniques. For example, the entire area of the roles of vasopressin and oxytocin in affiliative behavior began with studies comparing monogamous and polygamous voles (Young and Wang 2004) and is now thought to represent a common mechanism for all mammals (Curley and Keverne 2005; Lim and Young 2006) and possibly even birds (Goodson 2005).

Caution must be taken, however, when comparing corticosteroid concentrations quantitatively across distantly related species. Corticosteroid concentrations from different taxa can vary over three orders of magnitude (Romero 2004), with concentrations in some species far exceeding lethal concentrations in others. It is not yet clear why concentrations vary so extensively, but differences in other aspects of the HPA axis (such as receptor densities) make attractive hypotheses. Furthermore, reported corticosteroid concentrations can differ among laboratories using different techniques (Wingfield 1994; Bókony et al. 2009). Consequently, qualitative, not quantitative differences between distantly related species are likely to be of more physiological relevance.

In order to study the different types of variation described in the preceding text we need to have techniques to evaluate the function of either or both arms of the stress response (i.e., catecholamines or corticosteroids) in free-living animals. Although there are numerous techniques available for laboratory studies, there are fewer options for field studies. This is primarily a result of the difficulty of capturing wild animals (hence a need to maximize information from low sample sizes) and the even greater difficulty of capturing the same animal multiple times. What follows is a description of the strengths and weaknesses of the major techniques, either currently in use or recently proposed, to evaluate the stress responses of wild animals.

II. THE "CAPTURE STRESS" PROTOCOL

The most widely used technique to assess a wild animal's response to a stressor is to capture an animal and take serial blood samples over time to monitor corticosteroid release. This has commonly been called the "capture stress" or the "stress series" test and was first introduced by two independent papers published in 1982. In one of the papers, Sapolsky (1982) used the stress of darting olive baboons with an anesthetic to follow changes in plasma levels of cortisol. In the other paper, Wingfield and colleagues (1982) caught white-crowned sparrows in mist nets and used the stressor of capture and handling to monitor changes in corticosterone over the next two hours. Since those two pioneering studies, hundreds of other studies, monitoring corticosteroid release from over 200 species, have used this technique (Table 6.1).

A. Strengths of the Capture Stress Protocol

The utility of the capture stress protocol rests upon two core assumptions. The first is that the capture

TABLE 6.1: EXAMPLES OF SPECIES WHERE CORTICOSTEROIDS FROM FREE-LIVING INDIVIDUALS WERE STUDIED USING THE CAPTURE STRESS PROTOCOL

Birds	
Songbirds (passerines)	
White-crowned sparrow (*Zonotrichia leucophrys*)	Romero et al. (1997)
White-throated sparrow (*Zonotrichia albicollis*)	Schwabl et al. (1988)
Savannah sparrow (*Passerculus sandwichensis*)	Holberton and Wingfield (2003)
Black-throated sparrow (*Amphispiza bilineata*)	Wingfield et al. (1992)
American tree sparrow (*Spizella arborea*)	Holberton and Wingfield (2003)
Rufous-collared sparrow (*Zonotrichia capensis*)	Wada et al. (2006)
Dark-eyed juncos (*Junco hyemalis*)	Schoech et al. (1999)
Lapland longspur (*Calcarius lapponicus*)	Romero et al. (1998c)
Chestnut-collared longspur (*Calcarius ornatus*)	Lynn et al. (2003)
Smith's longspur (*Calcarius pictus*)	Meddle et al. (2003)
McCown's longspur (*Calcarius mccownii*)	Lynn et al. (2003)

(*continued*)

TABLE 6.1: CONTINUED	
Birds	
Songbirds (passerines)	
House sparrow (*Passer domesticus*)	Romero et al. (2006a)
North American house finch (*Carpodacus mexicanus*)	Lindstrom et al. (2005)
Zebra finch (*Taeniopygia guttata*)	Perfito et al. (2007)
European starling (*Sturnus vulgaris*)	Remage-Healey and Romero (2001)
Superb starling (*Lamprotornis superbus*)	Rubenstein (2007)
Common redpoll (*Carduelis flammea*)	Romero et al. (1998d)
Cactus wren (*Campylorhynchus brunneicapillus*)	Wingfield et al. (1992)
Curve-billed thrasher (*Toxostoma curvirostre*)	Wingfield et al. (1992)
Abert's towhee (*Pipilo aberti*)	Wingfield et al. (1992)
Yellow-rumped warbler (*Dendroica coronata*)	Holberton et al. (1996b)
Yellow warbler (*Dendroica petechia*)	Wilson and Holberton (2004)
Bush warbler (*Cettia diphone*)	Wingfield et al. (1995a)
Willow warbler (*Phylloscopus trochilus*)	Silverin et al. (1997)
American redstart (*Serophaga ruticilla*)	Marra and Holberton (1998)
Blue tit (*Parus caeruleus*)	Mueller et al. (2006)
Willow tit (*Parus montanus*)	Silverin (1997)
Great tit (*Parus major*)	Cockrem and Silverin (2002)
Stonechat (*Saxicola torquata*)	Scheuerlein et al. (2001)
Dusky flycatcher (*Empidonax oberholseri*)	Pereyra and Wingfield (2003)
Pied flycatcher (*Ficedula hypoleuca*)	Silverin and Wingfield (1998)
Snow bunting (*Plectrophenax nivalis*)	Romero et al. (1998b)
Gray catbird (*Dumetella carolinensis*)	Holberton et al. (1996b)
Hermit thrush (*Catharus guttatus*)	Long and Holberton (2004)
Northern mocking bird (*Mimus polyglottos*)	Sims and Holberton (2000)
Blackbird (*Turdus merula*)	Adams et al. (2011)
Florida scrub-jay (*Aphelocoma coerulescens*)	Boughton et al. (2006)
Eastern bluebird (*Sialia sialis*)	Mayne et al. (2004)
Red crossbill (*Loxia curvirostra*)	Cornelius et al. (2011)
Tree swallow (*Tachycineta bicolor*)	Mayne et al. (2004)
Barn swallow (*Hirundo rustica*)	Jenni-Eiermann et al. (2008)
Shorebirds	
Pectoral sandpiper (*Calidris melanotos*)	O'Reilly and Wingfield (2001)
Semipalmated sandpiper (*Calidris pusilla*)	Mizrahi et al. (2001)
Western sandpiper (*Calidris mauri*)	O'Reilly and Wingfield (2001)
Red phalarope (*Phalaropus fulicaria*)	O'Reilly and Wingfield (2001)
Red knot (*Calidris canutus*)	Reneerkens et al. (2002)
Bar-tailed godwit (*Limosa lapponica*)	Landys-Ciannelli et al. (2002)
Ruddy Turnstone (*Arenaria interpres*)	Perkins et al. (2006)
Ocean birds	
Magellanic penguin (*Spheniscus magellanicus*)	Hood et al. (1998)
Gentoo penguin (*Pygoscelis papua*)	Holberton et al. (1996a)
King penguin (*Aptenodytes patagonicus*)	Holberton et al. (1996a)
Yellow-eyed penguin (*Megadyptes antipodes*)	Ellenberg et al. (2007)
Adelie penguin (*Pygoscelis adeliae*)	Cockrem et al. (2006)
Tufted puffin (*Fratercula cirrhata*)	Kitaysky et al. (2005)
Crested auklet (*Aethia cristatella*)	Douglas et al. (2009)
Least auklet (*Aethia pusilla*)	Benowitz-Fredericks et al. (2008)

TABLE 6.1: CONTINUED

Birds	
Ocean birds	
Thick-billed murre (*Uria lomvia*)	Benowitz-Fredericks et al. (2008)
Common murre (*Uria aalge*)	Kitaysky et al. (2007)
Black-legged kittiwake (*Rissa tridactyla*)	Chastel et al. (2005)
Common eider (*Somateria mollissima*)	Criscuolo et al. (2006)
Blue-footed booby (*Sula nebouxii*)	Wingfield et al. (1999)
Common diving petrel (*Pelecanoides urinatrix*)	Smith et al. (1994)
Snow petrel (*Pagadroma nivea*)	Angelier et al. (2007a)
Grey-faced petrel (*Pterodroma macroptera*)	Adams et al. (2005)
Common tern (*Sterna hirundo*)	Breuner et al. (2006)
Xantus's murrelet (*Synthliboramphus hypoleucus*)	Newman et al. (2005)
Non-Songbirds (terrestrial)	
Pigeons (*Columba livia*)	Romero and Wingfield (2001)
Inca dove (*Scardafella inca*)	Wingfield et al. (1992)
Raptors	
Snowy owl (*Nyctea scandiaca*)	Romero et al. (2006b)
Long-eared owl (*Osio otus*)	Romero et al. (2009)
American kestrel (*Falco sparverius*)	Heath (1997)
Water Birds	
European white stork (*Ciconia ciconia*)	Blas et al. (2007)
Harlequin duck (*Histrionicus histrionicus*)	Perfito et al. (2002)
Reptiles	
Green turtle (*Chelonia mydas*)	Jessop (2001)
Hawksbill turtle (*Eretmochelys imbricata*)	Jessop (2001)
Loggerhead turtle (*Caretta caretta*)	Gregory et al. (1996)
Olive ridley turtle (*Lepidochelys olivacea*)	Valverde et al. (1999)
Kemp's ridley turtle (*Lepidochelys kempii*)	Gregory and Schmid (2001)
Red-eared slider turtle (*Trachemys scripta*)	Cash et al. (1997)
Gopher tortoise (*Gopherus polyphemus*)	Ott et al. (2000)
Tree lizard (*Urosaurus ornatus*)	Moore et al. (1991)
Western fence lizard (*Sceloporus occidentalis*)	Dunlap and Wingfield (1995)
Lizard (*Podarcis sicula*)	Manzo et al. (1994)
Side-blotched lizard (*Uta stansburiana*)	Comendant et al. (2003)
Texas horned lizard (*Phrynosoma cornutum*)	Wack et al. (2008)
Common gecko (*Hoplodactylus maculates*)	Girling and Cree (1995)
Bearded dragon (*Pogona barbata*)	Cree et al. (2000)
Galapagos marine iguana (*Amblyrhynchus cristatus*)	Romero and Wikelski (2001)
Tuatara (*Sphenodon punctatus*)	Tyrrell and Cree (1998)
Viviparous skink (*Egernia whitii*)	Jones and Bell (2004)
Freshwater crocodile (*Crocodylus johnstoni*)	Jessop et al. (2003)
American alligator (*Alligator mississippiensis*)	Elsey et al. (1991)
Red-sided garter snake (*Thamnophis sirtalis parietalis*)	Moore et al. (2000)
Red-spotted garter snake (*Thamnophis sirtalis concinnus*)	Lutterschmidt and Mason (2005)
Brown treesnake (*Boiga irregularis*)	Mathies et al. (2001)

(*continued*)

TABLE 6.1: CONTINUED

Species	Citation
Amphibians	
Spotted salamander (*Ambystoma maculatum*)	Homan et al. (2003a)
Eastern hellbender (*Cryptobranchus alleganiensis*)	Hopkins and DuRant (2011)
Green frog (*Rana esculenta*)	Zerani et al. (1991)
Great plains toad (*Bufo cognatus*)	Leary et al. (2006)
Woodhouse's toad (*Bufo woodhousii*)	Leary et al. (2006)
Cascades frog (*Rana cascadae*)	Belden et al. (2003)
Pacific treefrog (*Hyla regilla*)	Belden et al. (2005)
Mammals	
Olive baboon (*Papio anubis*)	Sapolsky (1982)
Yellow-pine chipmunk (*Tamias amoenus*)	Place and Kenagy (2000)
Brown lemming (*Lemmus trimucronatus*)	Romero et al. (2008)
Golden-mantled ground squirrel (*Spermophilus saturatus*)	Romero et al. (2008)
Belding's ground squirrel (*Spermophilus beldingi*)	Nunes et al. (2006)
Tuco-tuco (*Ctenomys talarum*)	Vera et al. (2011)
Common fruit bat (*Artibeus jamaicensis*)	Klose et al. (2006)
Little brown bat (*Myotis lucifugus*)	Reeder et al. (2004)
Platypus (*Ornithorhynchus anatinus*)	Handasyde et al. (2003)
Spotted hyena (*Crocuta crocuta*)	Van Jaarsveld and Skinner (1992)
Wild dog (*Lycaon pictus*)	De Villiers et al. (1997)
Bottlenose dolphin (*Tursiops truncatus*)	Ortiz and Worthy (2000)
Southern elephant seal (*Mirounga leonina*)	Engelhard et al. (2002)
Impala (*Aepyceros melampus*)	Hattingh et al. (1988)
Fish	
Rainbow trout (*Oncorhynchus mykiss*)	Meka and McCormick (2005); Clements et al. (2002)
Brown trout (*Salmo trutta*)	Norris et al. (1999)
Atlantic salmon (*Salmo salar*)	Poole et al. (2003)
Snapper (*Pagrus auratus*)	Cleary et al. (2000)
Striped bass (*Morone saxatilis*)	Bettinger et al. (2005)
Black bream (*Acanthopagrus butcheri*)	Haddy and Pankhurst (2000)
Tropical labrid (*Hemigymnus melapterus*)	Grutter and Pankhurst (2000)
Spiny damselfish (*Acanthochromis polyacanthus*)	Pankhurst (2001)
Coral trout (*Plectropomus leopardus*)	Frisch and Anderson (2000)
Coral trout (*Plectropomus maculatus*)	Frisch and Anderson (2005)
Red drum (*Sciaenops ocellatus*)	Gallman et al. (1999)
Striped trumpeter (*Latris lineata*)	Morehead (1998)
Kahawai (*Arripis trutta*)	Davidson et al. (1997)
Blue mao mao (*Scorpis violaceus*)	Lowe and Wells (1996)
Golden perch (*Macquaria ambigua*)	Carragher and Rees (1994)

Only one representative citation is provided for each species, even though there may be many studies performed on some species. Citations included here contain data where corticosteroid titers were measured at least twice in the same individual during the same capture event (repeated-measures design) or where different individuals were sampled at different intervals after capture (factorial design) and where the measurements included baseline.

stress protocol is itself a stressor. This seems to be a safe assumption. Capture, handling, and restraint are known to elicit marked increases in circulating corticosteroids (Harvey et al. 1984; Greenberg and Wingfield 1987; Boonstra and Singleton 1993; Gregory et al. 1996). Although acute capture stress appears at first to be highly artificial, it is likely that all individuals regard the procedure as a potential predation attempt (by the investigator) because they all struggle, show elevated respiration rate, defecate profusely, and may give distress vocalizations. The second assumption is that the stressor of capture, handling, and restraint is an equivalent, and specifically maximal, stimulus to all wild animals. Canoine et al. (2002) show that in stonechats capture stress may not increase corticosteroids maximally, but nonetheless the capture stress protocol provides a repeatable and uniform acute stress (Wingfield and Romero 2001). Capture and handling are far from normal occurrences in the lives of free-living animals, which supports this assumption.

If we accept these two assumptions, the capture stress protocol becomes a powerful tool for evaluating the sources of variation in the field as discussed at the beginning of this chapter. All individuals are treated the same way and are provided the identical stressor. Consequently, the capture stress protocol is a measure of responsiveness of the HPA axis in which variation results from physiological constraints rather than changes in the perceived stressfullness of the stimuli (Wingfield 1994; Wingfield et al. 1994a; Wingfield et al. 1995b). The responsiveness of the HPA axis can then be compared across individuals, populations, seasons, and so on. Because the adrenocortical response to stressors is taxonomically widespread and occurs following an extremely wide spectrum of stressors (both acute and chronic), we feel that the dynamics of the subsequent rise of plasma corticosteroid concentrations during the capture stress protocol is a useful indication of the sensitivity of the HPA axis to acute stress in general.

Mimicking predation as a stressor has distinct advantages compared to mimicking other stressors that wild animals might face. Other techniques that more closely resemble potential perturbation factors, such as low or high temperature, food restriction, and so on, tend to vary markedly as a function of season and body condition (Wingfield and Romero 2001). Furthermore, there is some evidence that animals can change their perceptions of the severity of these types of stressors. For example, animals appear to perceive a storm as a stressor only if it persists for several days (Astheimer et al. 1992) or occurs at certain life-history stages (Romero et al. 2000). In either case, the storm is not an equivalent stressor for each individual. In contrast, it is unlikely that a wild animal ever interprets a predation attempt, especially one that appears to have been successful (i.e., they are caught by the researcher), as an event that requires less than the full response that the animal is currently capable of making.

The capture stress protocol can be performed with either a repeated-measures or factorial design, although because of the difficulty in capturing most wild animals, the repeated-measures design is far more common. Briefly, approximately 30 ul of whole blood is collected from an appropriate vein (for example, wing vein for birds, orbital sinus or tail vein for reptiles) as soon as possible after capture (Figure 6.1). Time is noted at capture and again when the first sample is collected. Virtually all samples can be collected within 1–2 minutes. Additional samples can then be collected at intervals post-capture (Figures 6.2 and 6.3). Although samples are typically collected 5, 10, 30, and 60 minutes following capture, the time intervals can be adjusted, especially for species of different sizes (e.g., samples collected at 5, 20, and 60 min after capture in animals weighing less than 15 g). In some cases the 60-minute sample may be omitted—especially in smaller species—to avoid debilitation. Conversely, samples from longer after capture can be collected in order to examine negative feedback. Individuals are then restrained between sample collections. Once the initial sample is collected, plasma concentrations of corticosteroids in subsequent samples will be an indication of the degree and time course of the response to capture, handling, and restraint (Wingfield and Romero 2001). The initial samples can be used to check that time of day of capture is not resulting in variation owing to daily or circadian rhythms (Figure 6.3).

A new version of the capture stress protocol can provide even more information (Romero and Wikelski 2006; Dickens et al. 2009). The typical protocol described in the preceding paragraph provides information about the pre-stressed concentrations (see below), the maximal response to the stressor, and the speed at which that response is mounted. Samples collected at 60 minutes or later can often provide some limited information about negative feedback as well. However, negative feedback efficacy and adrenal capacity can also be tested directly using a modified capture stress protocol. With this technique, the initial sample is taken as before and provides information about the pre-stressed concentrations. A second sample is then collected at 15 or 30 minutes post-capture to assess the corticosteroid response. Immediately after this sample, the animal is injected with dexamethasone (DEX) as part of a DEX suppression test (Carroll et al. 1981). DEX is a synthetic glucocorticoid that binds to type II (GR) receptors and artificially stimulates negative feedback. This results in a decrease in circulating endogenous corticosteroid levels if feedback is functioning normally (see Figure 6.4). This decrease can be monitored since DEX does not bind to the commonly used antibodies in the radioimmunoassays. Further samples can then be taken over the next 30–180 minutes

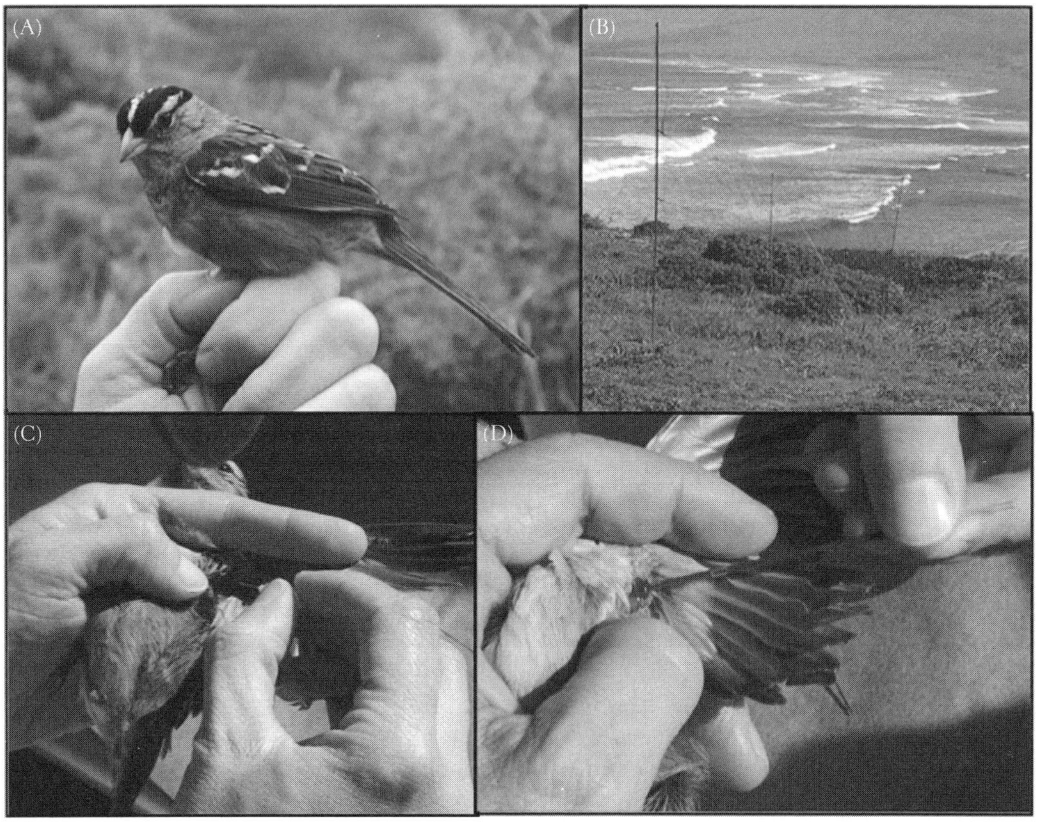

(A) (B) (C) (D)

FIGURE 6.1: This white-crowned sparrow (A) has been caught in a mist net out in the field (B). The bird was removed from the net within 3 minutes of capture and the brachial vein of the wing punctured with a 26-gauge needle (C). Emergent blood can then be collected into heparinized micro-hematocrit tubes (D).

Photos by J. C. Wingfield.

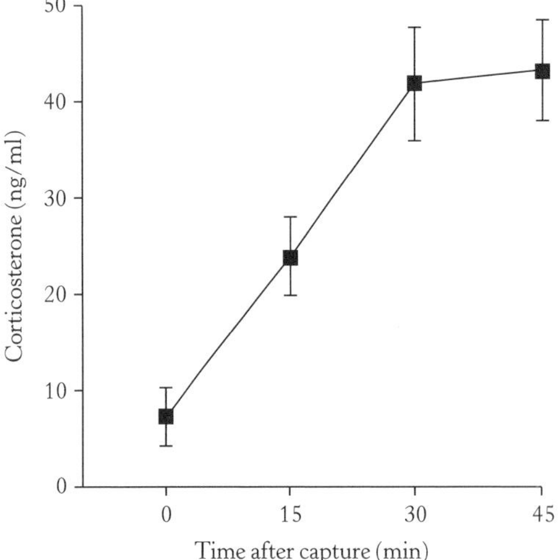

FIGURE 6.2: Corticosterone response to capture, handling, and restraint in wild-caught European starlings.

Reprinted with permission from Remage-Healey and Romero (2001). Courtesy of American Physiological Society.

(depending upon the species) in order to monitor the effectiveness of negative feedback (Sapolsky and Altmann 1991). Finally, after the second-to-last sample, animals can be injected with ACTH. The exogenous ACTH will stimulate the adrenal tissue so that we can ascertain its maximal capacity. Injecting both DEX and ACTH (as well as CRF and AVP—see later discussion) are classic endocrinological tests (Armario 2006). Using this modified protocol, we can collect data from a single individual on (1) pre-stressed titers, (2) normal corticosteroid response, (3) efficacy of negative feedback, and (4) maximal adrenal capacity (Figure 6.4).

There have been a number of studies that have modified the capture stress protocol to directly examine the pituitary and adrenal sensitivities to their respective releasing factors (reviewed by Romero 2001). Immediately following capture, animals are injected with ACTH, CRF, or AVT. These exogenous releasing hormones are intended to stimulate their target glands to ascertain whether or not

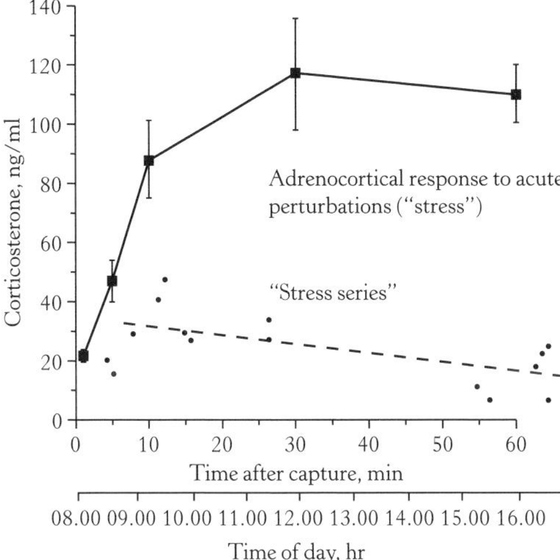

FIGURE 6.3: Plasma levels of corticosterone in free-living white-crowned sparrows following capture, handling, and restraint. The initial blood sample (collected very soon after capture) represents baseline circulating levels of corticosterone. Subsequent samples taken at 5, 10, 30 and 60 minutes after capture (during handling procedures and restraint) show the pattern of increased secretion of corticosterone in response to the acute stress. This is the stress series. Comparisons of baseline corticosterone levels with time of day provide a "control," showing that the increase induced by capture stress is not an artifact of time of day (see also Wingfield 2003).

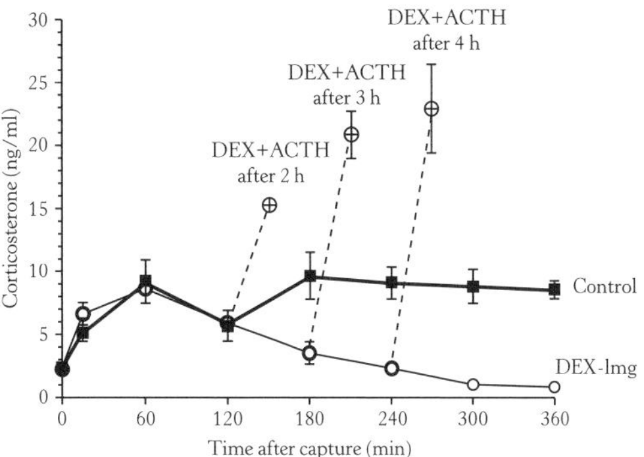

FIGURE 6.4: Corticosterone responses to capture, dexamethasone (DEX) injection 15 minutes after capture, and ACTH injection immediately after 2, 3, or 4 hours of capture in Galapagos marine iguanas. Controls were uninjected.

Reprinted with permission from Romero and Wikelski (2006). Courtesy of Elsevier.

the gland is functioning maximally in response to capture. A second blood sample is collected 30 minutes later to assess the ability of the releasing factor to elevate corticosteroid levels above those from stress alone. The responses to these exogenous releasing factors can then be compared across seasons, sexes, habitats, and so on, providing an indication of whether the underlying physiological regulation of the HPA axis changes under these conditions.

B. Weaknesses of the Capture Stress Protocol: Methodological Concerns

Because this technique has been so widely used for over 30 years (see Table 6.1), there has been substantial work addressing its strengths and weaknesses. Perhaps the biggest strength of the capture stress protocol is that it builds on the understanding of blood-borne corticosteroid physiology and release gained from over 70 years of biomedical and laboratory research (Sapolsky et al. 2000). In fact, much of what we know about corticosteroid physiology has been derived from taking blood samples. Presumably, what we have learned in the laboratory and clinical settings is directly transferable to wild animals under field conditions. This connection to the extensive biomedical literature continues to make collecting blood for corticosteroid analysis an attractive technique. Furthermore, many of the difficulties in interpreting plasma corticosteroid concentrations in wild animals either have been addressed or are currently under study. What follows below is a discussion of many of these methodological concerns.

Collecting the first sample as quickly as possible in order to determine basal concentrations is vital to the successful interpretation of data from the capture stress protocol. The distinction between basal and stress-induced corticosteroid concentrations is important physiologically because corticosteroid effects at these different concentrations are mediated by different receptors. At basal concentrations, corticosteroids are interacting with type I (MR) receptors, and at higher concentrations are interacting with type II (GR) receptors (see Chapter 4). However, basal concentrations are generally defined as concentrations from unstressed animals at rest. Samples can be very difficult to collect from inactive free-living animals, which generally have to be active in order to be captured (in order to encounter the traps, etc.). Consequently, the term "baseline" is more appropriate than "basal" for samples collected from free-living wild animals within a few minutes of capture. A detailed knowledge of a free-living animal's prior activity or exposure to stressors is difficult to ascertain (for example, the animal may have recently been chased by a predator, unbeknownst to the researcher).

One question that is often asked is, "How fast does the first sample need to be collected in order to represent a true baseline concentration and not the beginning of the response to the capture itself?" Corticosteroid release is under the control of ACTH, which is in turn under the control of CRF and AVP/AVT, depending upon the species, which are ultimately under the control of higher brain centers that detect a stimulus, decide that the stimulus is noxious, and send neuronal signals to the CRF and AVP/AVT cell bodies in the hypothalamus (see Chapter 2). This cascade of events, from the animal detecting a stressful stimulus to measurably elevated corticosteroid concentrations in the blood, takes 3–5 minutes in domestic rats (Dallman and Bhatnagar 2001). Consequently, if the animal can be removed from the trap and bled within 3–5 minutes of capture, field researchers have assumed that the corticosteroid concentrations in that sample represent baseline, or pre-stressed, concentrations (Sapolsky et al. 2000; Wingfield and Romero 2001).

The available evidence suggests that a 3–5 minute window might be too long to reflect true baseline concentrations in many free-living animals. Only a few studies have directly tested whether corticosteroid concentrations begin to increase in the first few minutes of capture in free-living animals, and results have been equivocal. Some studies found no increase in the first few minutes (e.g., Wingfield et al. 1982; Schoech et al. 1999), in concordance with laboratory studies, but one study found measurable increases within 1 minute (Dawson and Howe 1983). One recent investigation examined concentrations within the first 3 minutes of nearly 950 individuals from six species and concluded that corticosteroid titers were beginning to increase in the 2–3 minute window (Romero and Reed 2005). These authors concluded that samples collected in under 2 minutes most likely reflected baseline concentrations, and that samples collected in the 2–3 minute window likely reflected "near baseline" concentrations. A similar time frame appears to be functioning in fish as well (Clark et al. 2011). On the other hand, a longer window may be sufficient for several reptile species, where increased corticosterone concentrations are not detectable for 10 minutes (reviewed by Tyrrell and Cree 1998). What is clear from the available evidence is that there is a high degree of confidence that samples collected within 2 minutes of capture represent baseline titers, that for most species samples collected within 2–3 minutes are at or near baseline, and that baseline samples can still be collected after 3 minutes for some species, but this should be verified on an individual species basis.

One other factor that should be considered is that recent evidence indicates that corticosteroid concentrations can differ between blood vessels going to and from the brain. Newman et al. (2008) showed that corticosteroid titers in song sparrow brachial veins (reflecting peripheral titers) differed from titers in the jugular vein (reflecting blood draining the brain), a difference they interpreted as reflecting local corticosteroid synthesis in the brain. The lesson here is that jugular and peripheral blood samples may show different concentrations.

One problem that frequently arises is how to interpret changes in corticosteroid responses between two groups or populations when the baseline titers differ. Here are two versions of the typical dilemma (Figure 6.5): the titers at 15 and 30 minutes are the same between two groups, but the baselines differ; the baseline, 15-, and 30-minute titers are all equivalently elevated in one of the groups. In the first case, is it better to report the actual stress-induced concentrations (no difference) or the change from baseline (weaker response in the group with the elevated baseline)? Similarly, in the second case, reporting the actual titers (elevated response in the group with higher titers) creates a different interpretation than a change from baseline (equivalent responses, Figure 6.5). Which interpretation is the most physiologically relevant for the animal?

The biomedical literature clearly argues for reporting actual titers and not changes from baseline (Romero 2004). The reason is twofold. First, corticosteroids must interact with a receptor to have a physiological or behavioral effect, and the baseline and stress-induced corticosteroid titers generally interact with different receptors and therefore mediate different effects (see Chapter 2). In other words, a change from baseline would only make sense if the higher titer were producing more of the same effect as the lower dose, not if the higher and lower doses were producing entirely different effects. Second, hormone titers influence receptor numbers (Sapolsky 1992). Receptor production decreases in an attempt to compensate for long-term elevations of corticosteroids (typical of chronic stress) and, because there are fewer available receptors, a given concentration of corticosteroids has a diminished biological effect (Sapolsky 2001). Consequently, the actual changes in titers are far more likely to be the physiologically relevant metric.

Despite some weaknesses, the stress series can provide a wealth of information. Using

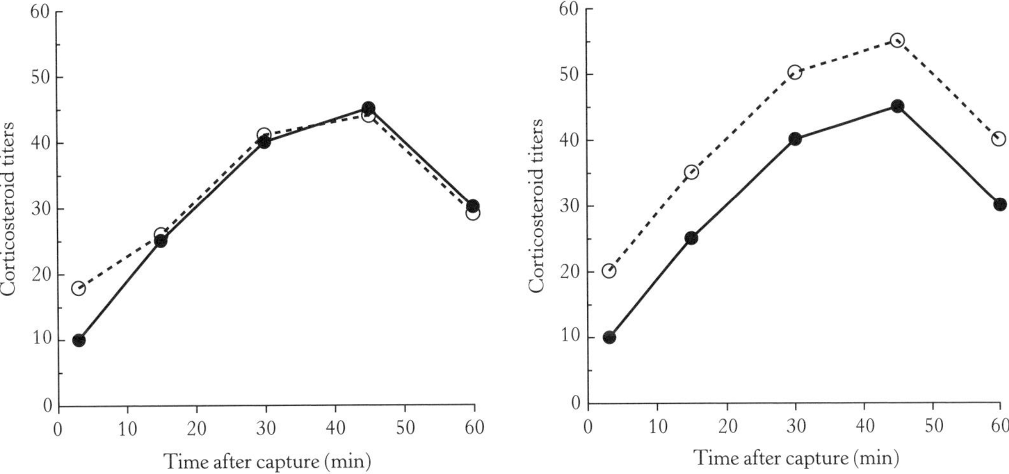

FIGURE 6.5: Two theoretical graphs to illustrate different patterns in the corticosteroid response that could occur when there is a change in baseline titers.

the identical stressor of capture, handling, and restraint provides a standardized method that can be used to compare stress responses. The capture stress protocol has been very successful at exploring sources of variation in the first three categories listed in the introduction to this chapter (i.e., adaptations to specific habitats, responses to environmental change, and facultative changes). The first sample, if collected within 2 minutes, provides a measure of basal levels of corticosteroid prior to capture, and the 30–60-minute sample the maximum level induced by this procedure (Figure 6.6). Additionally, the slope of the increase can indicate rate, and the area under the curve represents a metric of the total amount of corticosteroid the animal has been exposed to during the procedure (Figure 6.6). All of these metrics provide useful information that can be compared over seasons, time of day, with gender, age, body condition, parasite load, weather events, and so on.

The two of us (LMR and JCW) disagree, however, as to how useful the capture stress protocol is for exploring individual variation. JCW believes that the capture stress protocol is an excellent tool for forming hypotheses concerning the sources of individual variation—but the hypotheses need to be tested and not left to correlation only. Figures 6.7 and 6.8 show examples of this type of analysis. In Figure 6.8 the individual snow bunting with a fat score of 0 has the highest corticosterone titer. This individual is on the extreme end of the range of fat scores, which helps identify fat stores as a potential source of individual variation in corticosteroid responses. Data such as these are hypothesis generating in the sense that now we can focus on what made this bird lose its fat stores, why the loss of fat is correlated with a corticosteroid response, and how that corticosteroid response might help the bird survive despite the presumably low energy reserves. Analyses of this sort are becoming more common in the literature

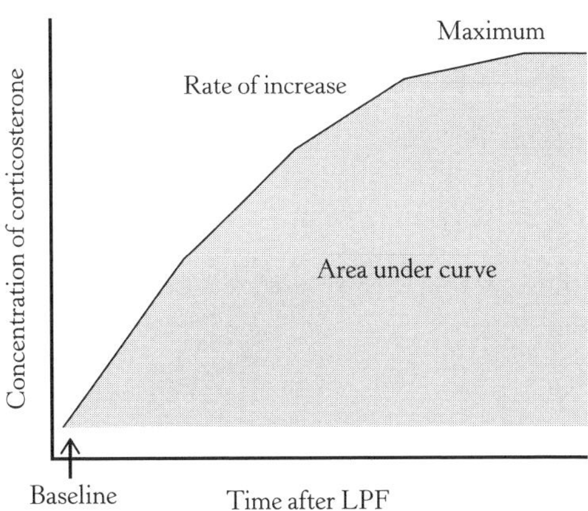

FIGURE 6.6: Types of information that can be gleaned from a stress series after a labile perturbation factor (LPF) such as capture stress. In addition to baseline, we can assess rate of increase and maximal levels of corticosteroids attained, and the area under the curve is a measure of the total amount of corticosteroids that tissues may have been exposed to during the stress series.

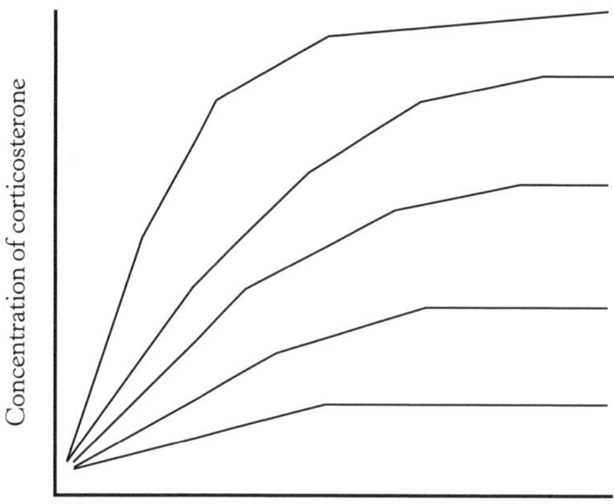

FIGURE 6.7: The patterns of corticosteroid levels in blood following a labile perturbation factor such as a stress series can vary markedly from one individual to another, or within an individual in relation to season, time of day, and other factors. These kinds of analyses of samples collected in the field allow assessment of potential ecological factors modulating the adrenocortical response to stress.

and have been used to assess variation due to such factors as sex (e.g., Romero et al. 2006a), age (e.g., Heidinger et al. 2006; Angelier et al. 2007b), body mass or condition (e.g., Silverin et al. 1997), and parasite load (Wingfield et al. 1999).

On the other hand, analyses such as these require significant caution because there can often be substantial uncertainty associated with isolated measurements of corticosteroid titers. When assessing individual variation, it is assumed, usually implicitly, that the corticosteroid titer measured for an individual represents its true state (i.e., the true endocrine phenotype), so patterns driving individual differences could be discerned if they are biologically significant. In other words, it is assumed that patterns in individual differences found on one sampling occasion would be found consistently across sampling occasions. For example, research specifically on differences among individuals, or where breeding high-corticosteroid and low-corticosteroid lineages is needed as a tool, presumes that single samples are representative of the individuals, and for the latter type of study, that they are heritable (Jones et al. 1994a; Evans et al. 2006). But how true is the assumption that a single sample reflects the true endocrine phenotype of the individual? There have been surprisingly few studies testing this assumption, and the data are mixed. On one hand, four published studies of repeatability, or consistency, within individuals of baseline corticosterone or stress-induced corticosterone under the same conditions and life-history stage found consistent corticosteroid responses (Cockrem and Silverin 2002; Love et al. 2003; Schjolden et al. 2005; Kralj-Fiser et al. 2007), at least for baseline titers within a single season (Ouyang et al. 2011). An example with great tits is shown in Figure 6.9, where corticosterone titers are reasonably consistent over three different sampling periods separated by 10–15 days. Furthermore, there have been a number of artificial selection

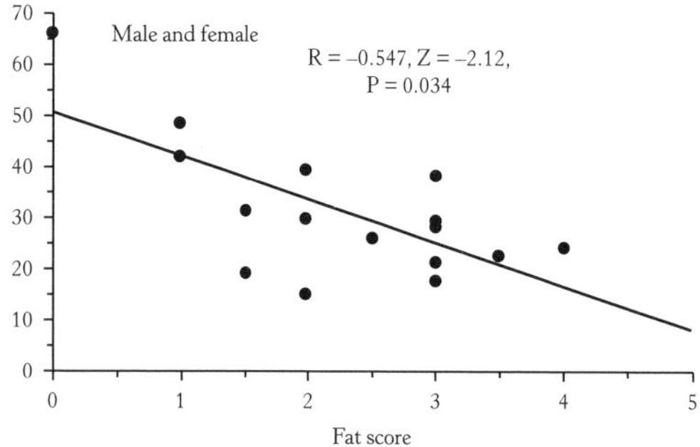

FIGURE 6.8: Correlation between fat score (a visual inspection of furcular and abdominal fat stores graded on a scale of 0 [least] to 5 [most]) and maximal corticosterone titers (ng/ml) during a 60-minute capture stress protocol in male and female snow buntings. Note the one bird with a fat score = 0 and maximal corticosterone titer of approximately 68 ng/ml.

Reprinted with permission from Wingfield et al. (1994b). Courtesy of Elsevier.

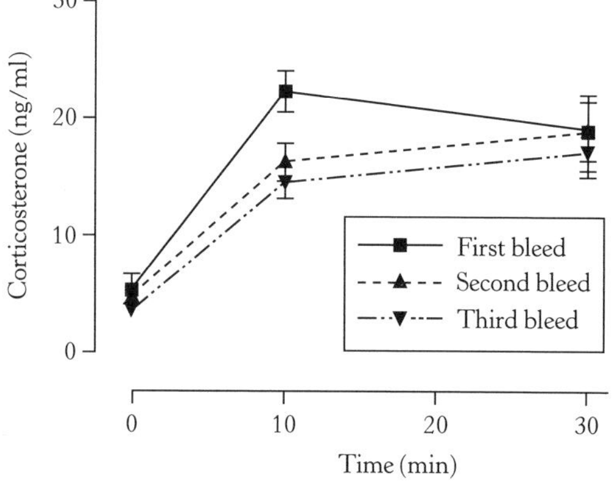

FIGURE 6.9: Mean corticosterone levels in great tits bled on three occasions at intervals of 10–15 days. Data are represented as means +/– SE for 13 birds.

Reprinted with permission from Cockrem and Silverin (2002). Courtesy of Elsevier.

studies that clearly demonstrate that there is a genetic basis for individual corticosteroid titers, at least in some species (e.g., Brown and Nestor 1973; Krass et al. 1979; Gross and Siegel 1985; Satterlee and Johnson 1988; Jones et al. 1994b; Satterlee and Jones 1997; Øverli et al. 2002; Evans et al. 2006). These studies would suggest, therefore, that the individual variation in corticosteroid titers often found in free-living animals (e.g., Wingfield et al. 1992; Wingfield et al. 1997) indicates true inter-individual variation and is not an artifact of random selection of a sample within a wide range of intra-individual variation.

On the other hand, there are a number of reasons, both biological and technical, to be very cautious in assuming that a single titer represents the true endocrine phenotype of the individual. Returning to Figure 6.8, the one individual with a low fat score is driving the entire statistical correlation—if that individual is removed, the regression line is no longer significant. Consequently, the conclusion that fat stores correlate with corticosteroid titers places an enormous weight on one individual. Similar conclusions supported by one or only a few individuals are common in the literature. How confident are we about the accuracy of this data point(s)? What is the justification to remove an individual from the analysis simply because it is at one extreme or another? Both of us agree, however, that correlations of these types should never be endpoints but a springboard for further experimental manipulations to establish cause and effect.

An excellent discussion of many technical concerns is presented in a recent review by Williams (2008). He includes the inherent stochasticity of the radioimmunoassays, although at generally 10%–15% intra-assay variation this is too low to fully explain the magnitude of corticosteroid differences. Extreme values could also be measurement artifacts, which is far more difficult to address since samples are rarely measured more than once.

Of far greater interest, however, are potential confounding variables that are biological in origin. There are two sources for these confounding effects—those that come from the environment and those that come from within the individual animal. Environmental factors primarily result from imperfect knowledge of the individual's recent history. For example, corticosteroid responses to capture and handling will be different in animals chased by predators an hour before capture than in animals quietly foraging before capture (Silverin 1998). In most studies, the activity of the animal just prior to capture, much less hours before capture, is entirely unknown. Traditionally, researchers have assumed that most captured animals were unstressed before capture and that any animals that were stressed were distributed evenly among treatment groups (i.e., no systematic bias) so that statistics diluted any potential problems. However, this only helps if the analysis is on the treatment means. When the analysis is on the individual values, the homogenizing effect of performing statistical tests on group means is lost. Varying environmental factors may explain why stress-induced titers were not consistent between capture events in a recent study (Ouyang et al. 2011).

In contrast to the studies that found consistent corticosteroid responses cited earlier, a recent paper indicated that internal variation within an animal could also obscure its "endocrine phenotype." In some cases there appears to be substantial individual variation in corticosteroid titers over time. An example in house sparrows is given in Figure 6.10 (Romero and Reed 2008). Even birds with the greatest differences in corticosterone means had overlapping samples, such that random selection of single samples could produce the interpretation that a bird with a lower mean had a higher corticosterone titer. Furthermore, other data from that paper showed that an individual bird's mean compared to other birds could shift when sampling changes from day to night, a phenomenon shown in several other species (e.g., Baylé 1980; Breuner et al. 1999). Even more problematic was that in some circumstances an individual's relative rank compared to its cohort during the first collection of a baseline titer had no predictive value for its relative rank compared to the same cohort on subsequent collections of baseline titers (Romero and Reed 2008). For example, if an individual bird had the lowest baseline titer during the first time it was bled, it was unlikely to have the lowest baseline titer during any subsequent sampling.

This discussion is not intended to lead to a conclusion that the capture stress protocol can never be used to study individual variation. There are many studies that have done so successfully. It is only intended to provide caution when using a few, or even a single, sample to support conclusions or form new hypotheses—there is a chance that the corticosteroid titer does not reflect the true endocrine phenotype of that animal. This caution should be even greater when the assumption that an animal is unstressed prior to capture is intentionally disregarded. For example, any

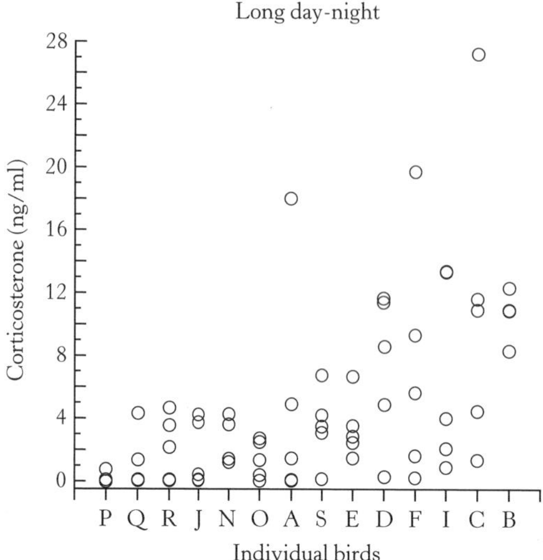

FIGURE 6.10: Corticosterone concentrations in captive house sparrows held on a long-day photoperiod and sampled at night. Each individual bird was sampled at five different times over a six-week period. Circles represent each corticosterone titer for each individual bird. Individual birds are placed on the *x* axis in order of increasing mean corticosterone concentrations from the five bleeds. There was a significant repeatability within the group of birds, such that a bird's relative rank of its corticosterone titers were relatively consistent across samples (e.g., if the bird had a low titer compared to the group, on the first bleed, it tended to be low compared to the group on subsequent bleeds).

Reprinted with permission from Romero and Reed (2008). Courtesy of Elsevier.

study that expressly tests whether individuals, or subpopulations, are exposed to chronic stressors (e.g., conservation studies) directly violates this assumption. Unfortunately, we rarely know what the endocrine phenotype should look like in animals under these conditions, so direct comparisons using the capture stress protocol can be problematic. Nonetheless, if two populations are studied, one assumed to be unstressed and the other stressed, then if samples sizes are reasonable this can be a useful comparison. Only if one population is tested and compared with itself would the assumption be violated.

With the possible exception of some reptiles (e.g., Knapp and Moore 1997; Tyrrell and Cree 1998), every species examined increases circulating corticosteroid titers within a few minutes of capture. Some trapping techniques, however, make it impossible to collect the first plasma sample rapidly enough. Directly measured baseline concentrations are unobtainable in such cases. There are two options available to still collect usable data using the capture stress protocol. The first is to focus exclusively on stress-induced concentrations. Although much of the value of the capture stress protocol is lost (i.e., the baseline, "pre-stress" concentrations and the rate of increase cannot be determined), there is still valuable information available from the stress-induced concentrations. Because baseline and stress-induced concentrations interact with different receptors, these different concentration ranges can almost be thought of as two different hormonal systems. Consequently, all the behavioral and physiological effects accruing from type II (GR) receptor binding remain potentially available for study. On the plus side, type II receptor-mediated effects are often of greater interest for the specific study. Therefore, there must be considerable caution when interpreting stress-induced concentrations when the time of capture is also unknown (see further discussion later in this chapter).

The second option is to focus on negative feedback and physiological constraints of the HPA axis. For example, Boonstra and colleagues have placed all their animals in an equivalent physiological state by waiting a few hours after an approximately known capture time and injecting DEX (Boonstra and Singleton 1993; Boonstra and McColl 2000; Boonstra et al. 2001). DEX stimulates negative feedback and essentially shuts off endogenous corticosteroid release in all animals. Each animal is then injected with exogenous ACTH. Although this protocol was introduced earlier than the modified capture stress protocol described earlier in this section, it is a close relative. The injection of DEX allows the evaluation of the efficacy of negative feedback, and the injection of exogenous ACTH allows the evaluation of a combination of the adrenal sensitivity to ACTH and its corticosteroid synthetic capacity. In other words, injecting ACTH provides the maximal response of which the adrenal tissue is capable. Presumably, one could also inject exogenous CRF and/or AVP/AVT in order to evaluate pituitary sensitivity, although to our knowledge this has not yet been done using this technique.

In contrast, there are a few approaches for attempting to cope with a lack of samples collected within a few minutes of capture that are clearly problematic. Several reports have tried to infer baseline concentrations from stress-induced concentrations, primarily by using linear regression to extrapolate baseline concentrations from samples taken later. This approach rests upon two assumptions: that the rate of increase is linear; and that the rate of increase to handling and restraint does not change when the animal has an extended period in a trap. Both assumptions are potentially flawed. First, the rate of increase is unlikely to be linear. It can take several minutes for corticosteroids to be measurable in the plasma, thereby creating a time lag. Consequently, a linear regression should not extrapolate baseline from the time of capture, and, because the extent of the time lag differs in different species, it is not always clear where the appropriate time would be. In addition, most studies show that the rate of increase is not constant throughout the 60-minute protocol (see Figures 6.2, 6.3, 6.4, and 6.9).

Available evidence also suggests that the second assumption, that an animal's corticosteroid response does not change with time in a trap, is often not true. Those few studies that have left animals in traps before initiating a capture stress protocol have indicated that the trap can induce changes in the response such that longer-term corticosteroid release is different (Romero and Romero 2002; Lynn and Porter 2008; Delehanty and Boonstra 2009). An example is provided in Figure 6.11. However, the time spent in a trap appears to have different effects in different species (Fletcher and Boonstra 2006). These data, combined with nonlinear rates of increase, indicate that estimating baseline concentrations in any manner other than direct measurement is problematic at best.

There are two further serious drawbacks to the capture stress protocol. The first is that plasma measurements provide only a "snapshot" of the endocrine state of the animal. One hallmark of endocrine systems is that hormone titers vary. This is to be expected. Since hormones are regulators of physiological systems (e.g., glucose concentrations), their concentrations must vary in order to maintain the physiological parameter they are regulating within the appropriate range. Corticosteroids are no different. Their titers vary daily, seasonally, and in response to various stressors (see Chapter 4). Consequently, a "point" sample of a particular corticosteroid titer may poorly reflect the overall corticosteroid milieu over a longer time period. This is especially true of baseline titers, but it is also true of the entire response measured by the capture stress protocol. The capture stress protocol only assesses how an animal responds to stress under those specific conditions. Furthermore, researchers often forget that changes to the corticosteroid response to the capture stress protocol do not necessarily indicate that the animal has been exposed

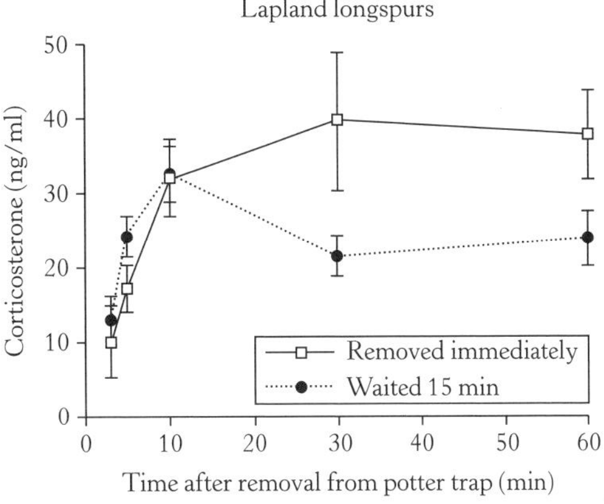

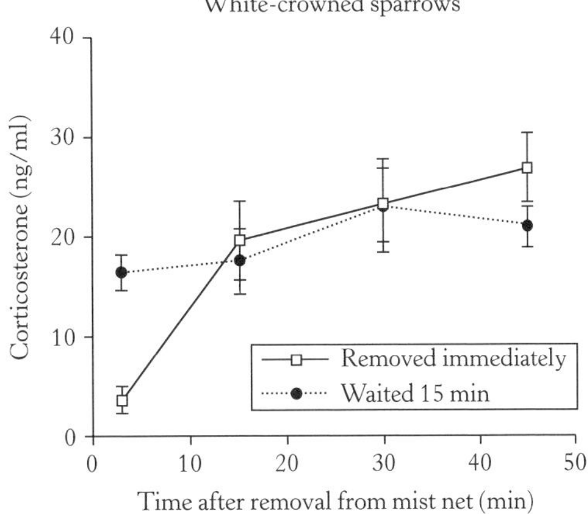

FIGURE 6.11: The effect of leaving a bird in a trap for 15 minutes before initiating a capture stress protocol. Notice that even when the trap had no immediate effect on corticosterone concentrations in the Lapland longspurs, the birds had a different long-term response.

Reprinted with permission from Romero and Romero (2002). Courtesy of the Cooper Ornithological Society.

to a stressor. The capture stress protocol is only measuring the response to a simulated predation attempt. How changes in those responses do or do not reflect underlying chronic stress is still under debate (see Chapter 4).

The second serious drawback of the capture stress protocol is that animals must be captured and handled to acquire the blood samples. This creates two problems. One is that the protocol itself will disrupt normal behavioral and physiological activity, thereby potentially confounding long-term studies. Since previous stressors can alter the responses to future stressors (see Chapter 2), there will always be concern that the subsequent physiology and behavior will be transformed from what would have been observed if the animal had not been exposed to the capture stress protocol (e.g., Lynn et al. 2010). Although factorial experimental designs can alleviate this problem, field studies rarely can generate sufficient sample sizes for this approach and instead usually rely upon repeated measures designs. Brown and Brown (2009) showed that in cliff swallows, collection of blood samples from free-living populations resulted in fewer birds returning in subsequent years compared to birds that were only caught and banded and not sampled. Failure to return might indicate higher mortality, although this cannot be confirmed. However, studies in many other species indicate that taking blood samples is not detrimental (e.g., Sheldon et al. 2008; Voss et al. 2010; Angelier et al. 2011; Redmond and Murphy 2011). Potential mortality leads to yet another problem—endangered species. Many endangered species have both practical and ethical limits to both the number of individuals that can be sampled as well as the invasiveness of that sampling. Consequently, many endangered species are off-limits to the capture stress protocol. Nonetheless, the capture stress protocol is without doubt a powerful technique despite the drawbacks; alternative methods have been developed that are much less invasive, but that must be interpreted in very different ways.

III. FECAL CORTICOSTEROIDS

Many researchers have recognized the drawbacks of the capture stress protocol discussed in the preceding section. The most popular solution is to measure corticosteroid metabolites excreted in the feces. The first papers to use fecal metabolites to monitor stress in wild free-living animals were published in 1997 (Creel et al. 1997; Wasser et al. 1997), although several earlier papers had been published using captive animals (e.g., Miller et al. 1991; Graham and Brown 1996; Palme et al. 1996). From a historical perspective, it is interesting that both of the papers from 1997 measured fecal corticosteroid metabolites in endangered species. Wasser et al. (1997) collected feces from spotted owls in order to assess the impact of habitat disturbance and Creel et al. (1997) used fecal corticosteroids to assess the potential physiological impact of radio collars on African wild dogs. Clearly, the impetus for developing techniques for measuring fecal corticosteroids was an inability or undesirability of capturing and handling specific species. This continues to be a driving force for the majority of fecal corticosteroid studies, as can be seen from Table 6.2. Although over 90 species have been used in fecal corticosteroid studies, only about 40% have been studied under field conditions. In fact, close inspection of Table 6.2

TABLE 6.2: EXAMPLES OF SPECIES WHERE FECAL CORTICOSTEROID METABOLITES HAVE BEEN MEASURED

Birds		
Sandhill crane (*Grus canadensis*)	Ludders et al. (2001)	
Whooping crane (*Grus americana*)	Hartup et al. (2005)	X
Northern bald ibis (*Geronticus eremita*)	Sorato and Kotrschal (2006)	X
Greylag goose (*Anser anser*)	Frigerio et al. (2001)	X
Snow goose (*Chen caerulescens*)	Legagneux et al. (2011)	X
Upland goose (*Chloephaga picta*)	Gladbach et al. (2011)	X
Great hornbill (*Buceros bicornis*)	Crofoot et al. (2003)	
Goshawk (*Accipiter gentiles*)	Dehnhard et al. (2003)	
Peregrine falcon (*Falco peregrinus*)	Staley et al. (2007)	
Golden eagle (*Aquila chrysaetos*)	Staley et al. (2007)	
Northern spotted owl (*Strix occidentalis caurina*)	Wasser et al. (1997)	X
California spotted owl (*Strix occidentalis occidentalis*)	Tempel and Gutierrez (2003)	X
Barred owl (*Strix varia*)	Wasser and Hunt (2005)	
Great horned owl (*Bubo virginianus*)	Wasser and Hunt (2005)	
Red-tailed parrot (*Amazona brasiliensis*)	Popp et al. (2008)	
Common raven (*Corvus corax*)	Selva et al. (2011)	X
Alpine chough (*Pyrrhocorax graculus*)	Jimenez et al. (2011)	X
Red-billed chough (*Pyrrhocorax pyrrhocorax*)	Jimenez et al. (2011)	X

TABLE 6.2: CONTINUED

	Birds	
Carolina chickadee (*Poecile carolinensis*)	Lucas et al. (2006)	X
Stonechat (*Saxicola torquata*)	Goymann et al. (2006)	
Great tit (*Parus major*)	Carere et al. (2003)	
Mourning dove (*Zenaida macroura*)	Washburn et al. (2003)	
European starling (*Sturnus vulgaris*)	Cyr and Romero (2008)	X
Dickcissel (*Spiza americana*)	Wells et al. (2003)	
Black grouse (*Tetrao tetrix*)	Arlettaz et al. (2007)	X
Capercaillie (*Tetrao urogallus*)	Thiel et al. (2005)	X
Greater sage grouse (*Centrocercus urophasianus*)	Jankowski et al. (2009)	X
Adelie penguin (*Pygoscelis adeliae*)	Nakagawa et al. (2003)	
Wilson's storm-petrel (*Oceanites oceanicus*)	Quillfeldt and Möstl (2003)	X
Common tern (*Sterna hirundo*)	Braasch et al. (2011)	X
Greater rhea (*Rhea Americana*)	Leche et al. (2011)	
	Mammals	
Chimpanzee (*Pan troglodytes*)	Whitten et al. (1998)	
Bonobo (*Pan paniscus*)	Dittami et al. (2008)	X
Western lowland gorilla (Gorilla gorilla gorilla)	Peel et al. (2005)	
Chacma baboon (*Papio hamadryas ursinus*)	Weingrill et al. (2004)	X
Yellow baboon (*Papio cynocephalus*)	Gesquiere et al. (2005)	X
Hybrid baboon (*Papio hamadryas anubis & P.h. hamadryas*)	Beehner and Whitten (2004)	X
Gelada baboon (*Theropithecus gelada*)	Beehner and McCann (2008)	X
Barbary macaque (*Macaca sylvanus*)	Wallner et al. (1999)	X
Long-tailed macaque (*Macaca fascicularis*)	Girard-Buttoz et al. (2009)	X
Rhesus macaque (*Macaca mulatta*)	Brent et al. (2011)	X
Japanese macaque (*Macaca fuscata*)	Barrett et al. (2002)	X
Assamese macaque (*Macaca assamensis*)	Ostner et al. (2008)	X
Black howler monkey (*Alouatta pigra*)	Martinez-Mota et al. (2007)	X
Spider monkey (*Ateles geoffroyi*)	Rangel-Negrin et al. (2009)	X
Blue monkey (*Cercopithecus mitis*)	Foerster et al. (2011)	X
Brown capuchin (*Cebus apella*)	Boinski et al. (1999)	
Tufted capuchin (*Cebus apella nigritus*)	Lynch et al. (2002)	X
White-faced capuchin (*Cebus capucinus*)	Carnegie et al. (2011)	X
Muriquis (*Brachyteles arachnoids*)	Strier et al. (1999)	X
Red colobus (*Piliocolobus tephrosceles*)	Chapman et al. (2006)	X
Gray-cheeked mangabey (*Lophocebus albigena*)	Arlet et al. (2009)	X
Common marmoset (*Callihrix jacchus*)	Sousa and Ziegler (1998)	
Ring-tailed lemur (*Lemur catta*)	Cavigelli (1999)	X
Sifaka (*Propithecus verreauxi*)	Brockman et al. (2009)	X
Garnett's bushbaby (*Otolemur* garnettii)	Watson et al. (2005)	
Golden lion tamarin (*Leontopithecus rosalia*)	Bales et al. (2005)	X
African wild dog (*Lycaon pictus*)	Creel et al. (1997)	X
Wolf (*Canis lupus*)	Sands and Creel (2004)	X
Red wolf (*Canis rufus*)	Young et al. (2004)	
Maned wolf (*Chrysocyon brachyurus*)	Vasconcellos et al. (2011)	
Island fox (*Urocyon littoralis*)	Asa et al. (2007)	
Spotted hyena (*Crocuta crocuta*)	Goymann et al. (2003)	X
Cheetah (*Acinonyx jubatus*)	Jurke et al. (1997)	
Clouded leopard (*Neofelis nebulosa*)	Wasser et al. (2000)	
Tiger (*Panthera tigris*)	Dembiec et al. (2004)	

(continued)

TABLE 6.2: CONTINUED

Mammals		
Jaguar (*Panthera onca*)	Morato et al. (2004)	
Couger (*Puma concolor*)	Bonier et al. (2004)	
Pallas' cat (*Otocolobus manul*)	Newell-Fugate et al. (2007)	
Black-footed ferret (*Mustela nigripes*)	Young et al. (2001)	
European pine marten (*Martes martes*)	Barja et al. (2007)	X
Wolverine (*Gulo gulo*)	Dalerum et al. (2006)	
Slender-tailed meerkat (*Suricata suricata*)	Young et al. (2004)	
Northern Atlantic right whale (*Eubalaena glacialis*)	Hunt et al. (2006)	X
Pacific harbor seal (*Phoca vitulina richardii*)	Gulland et al. (1999)	X
Weddell seal (*Leptonychotes weddellii*)	Mellish et al. (2010)	X
Steller sea lion (*Eumetopias jubatus*)	Mashburn and Atkinson (2004)	
Alaskan sea otter (*Enhydra lutris kenyoni*)	Wasser et al. (2000)	
Malayan sun bear (*Helarctos malayanus*)	Wasser et al. (2000)	
Himalayan black bear (*Ursus thibetanus*)	Young et al. (2004)	
Alaskan brown bear (*Ursus arctos horribilis*)	von der Ohe et al. (2004)	X
Giant panda (*Ailuropoda melanoleuca*)	Liu et al. (2006)	
African elephant (*Loxodonta Africana*)	Foley et al. (2001)	X
Black rhinoceros (*Diceros bicornis*)	Linklater et al. (2010)	X
White rhinoceros (*Ceratotherium simum*)	Brown et al. (2001)	
Elk (*Cervus elaphus*)	Creel et al. (2002)	X
Roosevelt elk (*Cervus elaphus roosevelti*)	Wasser et al. (2000)	
Reindeer (*Rangifer tarandus*)	Rehbinder and Hau (2006)	
Musk deer (*Moschus moschiferus*)	Gerlinskaya et al. (2000)	
Roe deer (*Capreolus capreolus*)	Dehnhard et al. (2001)	
White-tailed deer (*Odocoileus virginianus*)	Millspaugh et al. (2002)	
Red deer (*Cervus elaphus*)	Huber et al. (2003)	X
Fallow deer (*Dama dama*)	Konjevic et al. (2011)	X
Pere David's deer (*Elaphurus davidianus*)	Li et al. (2007)	
Pampas deer stag (*Ozotoceros bezoarticus*)	Pereira et al. (2006)	X
Bighorn sheep (*Ovis canadensis*)	Coburn et al. (2010)	
Gerenuk (*Litocranius walleri*)	Wasser et al. (2000)	
Pyrenean chamois (*Rupicapra pyrenaica*)	Dalmau et al. (2007)	X
Scimitar-horned oryx (*Oryx dammah*)	Wasser et al. (2000)	
Grevy's zebra (*Equus grevyi*)	Franceschini et al. (2008)	X
European hare (*Lepus europaeus*)	Teskey-Gerstl et al. (2000)	
Snowshoe hare (*Lepus americanus*)	Sheriff et al. (2009)	
European rabbit (*Oryctolagus cuniculus*)	Monclus et al. (2006)	
Red squirrel (*Tamiasciurus hudsonicus*)	Dantzer et al. (2010)	X
Belding's ground squirrel (*Spermophilus beldingi*)	Mateo and Cavigelli (2005)	X
European ground squirrel (*Spermophilus citellus*)	Aschauer et al. (2006)	
Columbian ground squirrel (*Spermophilus columbianus*)	Bosson et al. (2009)	X
Speckled ground squirrel (*Spermophilus suslicus*)	Kuznetsov et al. (2006)	X
European badger (*Meles meles*)	Schutz et al. (2006)	
Yellow-bellied marmot (*Marmota flaviventris*)	Blumstein et al. (2006)	X
House mouse (*Mus musculus*)	Harper and Austad (2000)	X
Deer mouse (*Peromyscus maniculatus*)	Harper and Austad (2000)	X
Oldfield mouse (*Peromyscus polionotus*)	Good et al. (2003)	
Spiny mouse (*Acomys cahirinus*)	Gutman et al. (2011)	X
Spiny mouse (*Acomys russatus*)	Gutman et al. (2011)	X
Striped mouse (*Rhabdomys*)	Jones et al. (2011)	
Short-tailed singing mouse (*Scotinomys teguina*)	Crino et al. (2010)	

TABLE 6.2: CONTINUED

Mammals		
Red-backed vole (*Clethrionomys gapperi*)	Harper and Austad (2000)	X
Bank vole (*Clethrionomys glareolus*)	Zav'yalov et al. (2003)	
Water vole (*Arvicola terrestris*)	Zav'yalov et al. (2007)	X
Water vole (*Arvicola scherman*)	Charbonnel et al. (2008)	X
Great gerbil (*Rhombomys opimus*)	Rogovin et al. (2003)	X
Mongolian gerbil (*Meriones unguiculatus*)	Scheibler et al. (2004)	X
Common hamster (*Cricetus cricetus*)	Franceschini et al. (2007)	X
Syrian hamster (*Mesocricetus auratus*)	Chelini et al. (2010)	
Degu (*Octodon degu*)	Ebensperger et al. (2011)	X
Tuco-tuco (*Ctenomys sociabilis*)	Woodruff et al. (2010)	X
Chinchilla (*Chinchilla lanigera*)	Ponzio et al. (2004)	
Honey possums (*Tarsipes rostratus*)	Oates et al. (2007)	
Pichis (*Zaedyus pichiy*)	Superina et al. (2009)	X
Tammar wallaby (*Macropus eugenii*)	McKenzie and Deane (2005)	
Wombat (*Lasiorhinus latifrons*)	Hogan et al. (2011)	
Gilbert's potoroo (*Potorous gilbertii*)	Stead-Richardson et al. (2010)	X
Fish		
Parrotfish (*Osteichthyes*)	Turner et al. (2003)	X
Epaulette shark (*Hemiscyllium ocellatum*)	Karsten and Turner (2003)	
Reptiles		
Eastern box turtle (*Terrapene carolina carolina*)	Case et al. (2005)	
Three-toed box turtle (*Terrapene carolina triunguis*)	Rittenhouse et al. (2005)	
Spiny tailed iguana (*Ctenosaura acanthura*)	Suarez-Dominguez et al. (2011)	X

An X in the last column indicates if the study was from free-living individuals or individuals in semi-natural enclosures. Only one representative citation is provided for each species, even though there may be many studies performed on some species. Common domestic species are not included.

indicates a strong bias toward exotic zoo species, where it is desirable to minimize the handling of animals. It is striking that so few of the species overlap between Tables 6.1 and 6.2, which further indicates that the major reason researchers choose fecal measurements rather than the capture stress protocol is to avoid handling the animal.

A. Strengths of the Fecal Steroid Techniques

The ability to measure fecal corticosteroids non-invasively is particularly appealing to conservation biologists and has, in many ways, become the primary technique for assessing stress in conservation studies. This is especially true for endangered mammals (Table 6.2).

Although not as prominent as the work on endangered species, some recent studies using fecal corticosteroids have had the explicit aim of avoiding the "snapshot" feature of the capture stress protocol. An excellent example of this type of study is work on greylag geese exploring correlations between fecal corticosteroids and both ontogenetic changes and social status (e.g., Frigerio et al. 2001). In many of these studies, the researchers previously used a capture stress protocol to assess plasma corticosteroid concentrations, but have intentionally moved to fecal analysis to take advantage of its more integrated nature and its minimal interference with natural behaviors.

Corticosteroids released into the blood have two ultimate fates—they either bind to a receptor and are eventually degraded by the target cell; or they are processed by the liver and eventually excreted. Processing by the liver is necessary because of the hydrophobic nature of steroids. The liver places polar side chains on the steroid backbone in order to form a conjugate (Brownie 1992). This makes the hormone inactive in that it can no longer enter a cell and bind to its intracellular receptor, and water soluble so that it can be excreted into the urine or feces. However, because corticosteroids are conjugated prior to excretion, very little of the corticosteroid in the feces is actually the native corticosteroid in the plasma (i.e., cortisol or corticosterone). It is actually the corticosteroid metabolites that are excreted. Consequently, we will refer to fecal corticosteroid metabolites (FGM) for the remainder of this section.

The beauty of the fecal steroid method is that you do not need to handle an animal to collect feces, and often do not even need the animal present. Verifying which animal goes with which fecal sample can be done in a number of ways. Animals can be observed through binoculars from a distance, defecation locations noted, and samples collected after the animals have moved away (e.g., Pride 2005; Franceschini et al. 2008). One innovative technique for finding feces in free-living animals is to use dogs (Wasser et al. 2004). By using the natural olfactory prowess of the canine nose, researchers can not only identify the scat of the target species, but also avoid the scat of non-target species. Individuals are then identified post-collection using genetic techniques (von der Ohe et al. 2004; Hunt et al. 2006). In fact, many trained dogs have sufficient skill at discriminating scat that they can identify individual animals, thereby skipping genetic identifications (Wasser et al. 2009). Dogs also provide the opportunity to collect feces as quickly as possible after defecation and under extreme habitat conditions such as in the open ocean (Hunt et al. 2006).

Once collected, the FGM are extracted from the feces and assayed, usually using a radioimmunoassay (RIA) for either corticosterone or cortisol. Several commercial RIA kits have been found to measure FGM concentrations in a number of species and appear to cross-react with a variety of metabolites (Wasser et al. 2000). However, species can differ dramatically in what kinds of metabolites are actually secreted, so a number of validations, both technical and biological, are required (Moestl et al. 2005; Palme 2005; Palme et al. 2005). Most of the non-field studies included in Table 6.2 were conducted in order to validate the method on that particular species.

B. Weaknesses of the Fecal Steroid Techniques

Collecting feces in order to assess the corticosteroid status, and thereby "stress," of an animal appears simple and elegant. After all, the steroids are just sitting in the waste ready to be picked up and measured without ever having to disturb the animal. However, the devil is in the details. Several excellent recent reviews (e.g., Millspaugh and Washburn 2004; Goymann 2005; Klasing 2005; Moestl et al. 2005; Palme 2005; Touma and Palme 2005; Sheriff et al. 2011) critically examine a number of complex and confounding technical and biological issues concerning FGM measurements of steroid metabolites in general and comparisons with blood levels (e.g., Figure 6.12) that we will summarize later in this chapter and in Figure 6.15. Successfully addressing many of these issues requires extensive validation work. The inescapable conclusion when taking all of these issues into account is that measuring FGM is anything but a simple technique.

Several aspects of sample collection and storage can dramatically alter FGM measurements (Millspaugh and Washburn 2004; Moestl et al. 2005). What is becoming clear is that each of the various steps of going from defecation to the RIA assay bench is fraught with danger. Problems begin with the sample collection itself. Although most studies to date using FGM measurements have been under captive conditions (e.g., Table 6.2), the ultimate goal of most researchers is to apply the technique to free-ranging animals. However, most wild animals do not defecate into controlled and regulated environments such as cages or clean paddocks. They do it in the woods, the savannah, the water, and so on. Unfortunately, environmental conditions can alter measured FGM concentrations, an effect that becomes a bigger problem the longer the samples remain uncollected after defecation. For example, simulated rainfall in the laboratory increased FGM concentrations compared to an aliquot of the same sample not exposed to simulated rainfall, an effect attributed to bacterial breakdown of metabolites not measured by the RIA antibody into metabolites that were recognized (Washburn and Millspaugh 2002). These results clearly indicate potential problems with samples collected under humid or wet conditions. Furthermore, if the authors are correct in the mechanism, the specific metabolites excreted in each species and the antibody used for the RIA could both affect the direction of the change: the bacteria could just as easily degrade the metabolites that the antibody recognizes into ones that the antibody does not. Other weather conditions have not been found to affect FGM concentrations (Washburn and Millspaugh 2002; Mashburn and Atkinson 2004), but the impact of the predominant environmental conditions on FGM concentrations would likely have to be assessed for each study.

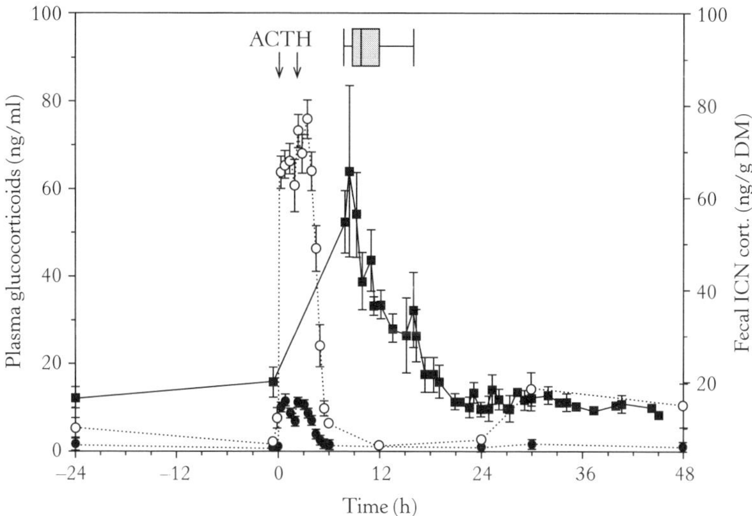

FIGURE 6.12: Time lag between exogenous ACTH injection and FGM excretion into the feces in non-pregnant, lactating dairy cattle. Open circles represent plasma cortisol and closed circles represent plasma corticosterone. Closed squares represent FGM concentrations. The lines and shaded box above the FGM peak represent the range, median, 25th, and 75th percentile values for the presence of nylon bags in the fecal samples.

Reprinted with permission from Morrow et al. (2002). Courtesy of Elsevier.

Large fecal mass can also be a problem for larger mammals. FGMs are not randomly distributed throughout the feces (e.g., Millspaugh and Washburn 2003). The solution to this problem is multiple subsampling or extensive mixing of the feces prior to sampling (e.g., Beehner and Whitten 2004). This is likely to be a problem with any fecal sample too large to collect the feces in its entirety.

Once collected, different short-term storage techniques for transporting the samples back to the lab can create different changes to FGM concentrations (Millspaugh and Washburn 2004). FGM concentrations can be altered when samples are stored in various preservatives, such as ethanol and acetic acid (Khan et al. 2002; Millspaugh et al. 2003), and the effects are not consistent. Some sort of preservative is often unavoidable due to import requirements to avoid infectious disease spread, but even untreated samples are subject to change. The currently accepted "best technique" is to quickly freeze untreated fecal samples for transport and storage (Hunt and Wasser 2003; Lynch et al. 2003; Moestl et al. 2005; Palme 2005). Unfortunately, the method of freezing seems to affect FGM concentrations, with concentrations frozen in liquid N_2 lower than with storage on ice alone (Tempel and Gutierrez 2004).

Long-term storage appears to be even more problematic. A detailed study by Hunt and Wasser (2003) on different preservation methods indicated that the FGM concentrations that are measured changed with every preservation and storage method except lyophilization (freeze drying), although the changes were damped when the samples were also frozen. Of special concern was that samples stored in ethanol had as much as a 300% increase in measured FGM concentrations (Hunt and Wasser 2003). On the other hand, freezing fresh samples can result in substantial nonlinear changes over time (Khan et al. 2002). Most studies have reported an increase in FGMs over time when fecal samples are stored frozen (Khan et al. 2002; Hunt and Wasser 2003), but others report that frozen samples are relatively stable (Beehner and Whitten 2004). In sum, each individual collection and storage technique adds its own pitfalls to FGM analyses. These problems are not insurmountable, but it is becoming clear that each step in the path from collection to assay must be validated.

Because corticosteroids are metabolized prior to excretion, there is very little measurable corticosterone or cortisol in the feces. Injections of radio-labeled corticosteroids indicate that the liver metabolizes the hormones in multiple ways, resulting in many excreted metabolites (Moestl et al. 2005). The best way to measure FGM concentrations, therefore, is to use a separation technique such as HPLC to identify the specific metabolites and their relative contributions (Touma and Palme 2005). However, this approach is very expensive and extraordinarily time-consuming to perform on more than a few animals. Consequently, most studies use an RIA or an ELISA to estimate FGMs. There are a number of antibodies that appear to adequately measure at least some metabolites and are able to detect changes due to ACTH injections (e.g., Wasser et al. 2000; Young et al. 2004; Moestl et al. 2005; Heistermann et al. 2006), but there is widespread acknowledgement that these antibodies do not measure all, or even most, of the excreted metabolites. The best features of these assays are that they are relatively inexpensive, easy to perform, and provide reasonable estimates of FGM concentrations. Unfortunately, it is clear that different species secrete different metabolite mixtures (e.g., Bahr et al. 2000; Young et al. 2004), possibly a result of different degradation enzymes (Vylitova et al. 1998). Consequently, a specific antibody may or may not be a good measure of FGMs for an individual species (e.g., Goymann et al. 1999). The result is that each species of interest requires its own validation experiments to determine the best, or at least an adequate, assay for detecting biologically relevant changes in FGM concentrations. In fact, many of the studies in Table 6.2 are reports whose sole purpose was to validate an assay system for the species of interest. Furthermore, an implicit assumption of many of these studies is that the FGM mixture does not change over time in an individual, or between sexes, life-history stages, diet, and so on (Goymann 2012). If the mixture did change, FGM measurements might change even though plasma corticosteroid concentrations remained the same (or vice versa). To our knowledge, this assumption has not been rigorously tested. However, there is potential for serious concern. Goymann (2005) measured fecal testosterone metabolites in stonechats and found equivalent concentrations in males and females, even though males have 12 times the plasma testosterone concentrations (Figure 6.13). He speculates that this is a result of other steroids forming metabolites that cross-react with the testosterone antibody. If this occurs with presumed FGMs as well, the reliability of FGM measurements would decline.

The equivalent testosterone concentrations in males and females found by Goymann highlight an important issue in FGM analyses. Corticosteroids exert their biological effects by binding to receptors, and they have access to these receptors via the plasma. As far as we know, there are no receptors for

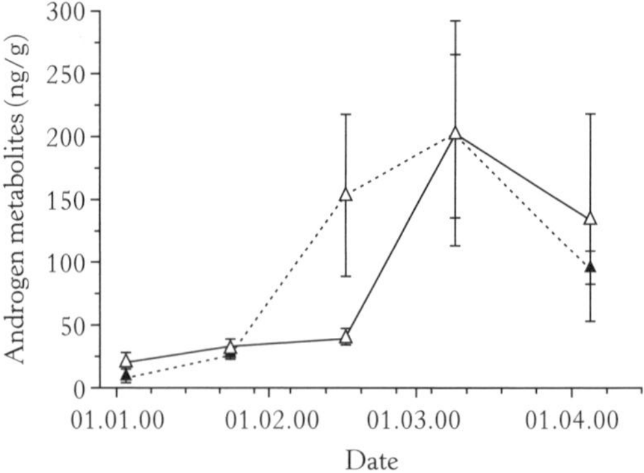

FIGURE 6.13: Seasonal testosterone metabolite patterns in male (closed triangles) and female (open triangles) European stonechats. In males, testosterone metabolite levels correspond very well both to validations using a GnRH challenge and blood plasma levels with a peak of 1.0 ng/ml testosterone in March. Female plasma levels of testosterone are much lower (0.08 ng./ml) at the same time, despite similar levels of testosterone metabolites in the females and males.

Reprinted with permission from Goymann (2005). Courtesy of Wiley.

corticosteroid metabolites. Therefore, measuring FGMs is only useful insofar as they reflect plasma concentrations of actual corticosterone (or cortisol). In order to ensure that what is measured truly reflects biologically relevant changes in FGMs, a number of other validation steps have been proposed. Although we will not go into them in detail here, they include verifying extraction techniques, determining recovery rates after extraction, assessing the accuracy and precision of the assay, and determining the cross-reactivity with other steroid metabolites (Moestl et al. 2005; Palme 2005). The above validation steps are primarily technical, but it is becoming increasing clear that biological validation is also vital (Goymann 2012). When measured concurrently, changes in plasma corticosteroid concentrations often do not match changes in FGM concentrations.

One ubiquitous feature of FGM analysis is the enormous variation in concentrations between different samples from the same individual. For example, when measured concurrently, the variability in fecal testosterone metabolites was found to be 2–5 times higher in feces than testosterone concentrations in plasma (Hirschenhauser et al. 2000). This variability between samples exists even in individuals serving as controls, where the plasma corticosteroid concentrations are presumed to not have changed.

There are many sources of this increased variability. Perhaps foremost is variation in the interval between defecations. If we assume a constant excretion rate into the lumen of the gut, then digesta that remain in the gastrointestinal tract for longer will naturally have higher FGM concentrations. In addition, since there is a delay in when the peak in plasma corticosteroids appears as FGMs (see later in this chapter), defecations closer or further away from the peak in excretion will naturally vary in FGM concentrations. Other potential sources include individual differences (some individuals show greater inter-sample variation than others (Scheiber et al. 2005), non-homogeneous distribution within a fecal sample (Millspaugh and Washburn 2003), varying contributions of urine contamination (e.g., Ludders et al. 2001; Washburn et al. 2003; Goymann 2005), and variation inherent in small fecal sample sizes (samples with very small fecal mass have increasing FGM measurements; Millspaugh and Washburn 2004).

The variability between samples wreaks havoc, of course, with analysis of variance (ANOVA) tests and makes it very difficult to discern statistically significant, biologically relevant differences. One way to compensate for this variability is to collect multiple samples corresponding to a treatment and to use their mean instead of individual samples in the analyses. Scheiber et al. (2005) directly tested how many samples would be required to counteract the inter-sample variability in greylag geese. They determined that at least three, and preferably four, equivalent samples provided a sufficiently good estimate of an individual's "endocrine profile" that can be used to discern significant differences between treatment groups.

Scheiber et al.'s results have two major implications. First, their data indicate that FGM analysis will work far better for stressors that maintain their intensity for a long period, probably needing to span a multitude of defecations. Chronic stressors, such as conspecific social interactions (e.g., Kotrschal et al. 1998; Creel 2001; Goymann and Wingfield 2004), weather conditions (e.g., Frigerio et al. 2004), and human-initiated habitat degradation (e.g., Creel et al. 2002; Arlettaz et al. 2007), would fit this criterion. In addition, natural long-term changes, such as daily rhythms (e.g., Cyr and Romero 2008) or puberty (e.g., Gesquiere et al. 2005), would provide useful targets for study. Scheiber et al.'s second implication, however, is that FGM analysis is a particularly poor technique for exploring responses to short-term acute stressors, especially in those species that have long periods between defecations. The inter-sample variability is likely to be too great to discern treatment effects. A potential solution is to perform each experiment multiple times and combine the fecal samples, but this is unlikely to be feasible for many field studies.

There can be substantial variability associated with different biological factors, such as diurnal changes, seasonal variation, specific life-history needs, sex, age, and reproductive status (Millspaugh and Washburn 2004). Each of these factors has been shown to influence both basal plasma corticosteroid concentrations, as well as how individuals respond to a stressor. It is reasonable to assume that these plasma changes will be reflected in FGM concentrations as well, thereby adding a further layer of complexity to interpreting FGM changes. Perhaps the most difficult problem with FGM analysis is that the measured concentrations are heavily dependent upon both the preferred food for a specific species (i.e., herbivores vs. frugivores vs. carnivores, etc.) and the specific diet of the individual at the time of measurement (Dantzer et al. 2011). For example, the amount of dietary fiber appears to influence FGM measurements (Wasser et al. 1993) and closely related species can digest fiber differently (Varo and Amat 2008). One of the key factors that determines the ultimate FGM concentrations is gut transport time, or the time it takes for the digesta to travel from the duodenum to the rectum.

In an elegant study, Morrow et al. (2002) showed that the peak of FGM excretion is tied to the gut transport time. They created a chronic fistula in the duodenum positioned close to the entry of the bile duct (the main route of steroid excretion into the digesta) in dairy cattle. They then inserted a nylon bag into the duodenum concurrent to an injection of exogenous ACTH. The peak in FGM excretion closely matched when the nylon bag was excreted (Figure 6.12). However, the gut transport time changed, as did the FGM peak, when the cattle altered their diet. Lactating cows in the spring consumed more food with greater water content, resulting in greater defecation rates and greater total fecal output, than non-lactating cows in the fall. This coincided with a shorter gut transport time in the spring, going from 16.6 hours in the fall (range 9.5–44.1 h) to 9.76 hours in the spring (range 7.6–15.96 h). There was a similar shift in the peak FGM excretion.

Unfortunately, Morrow et al. could not determine whether the gut transport time had an impact on total FGM concentrations because there was also a seasonal difference in the cows' sensitivity to ACTH. However, this is likely to be the case. Longer gut transport rates expose the digesta to a number of factors that can potentially alter the ultimate FGM concentrations, including circadian changes in plasma concentrations, a longer time for metabolites to be secreted into the digesta, longer exposure to degrading effects of gut bacteria, and so on (Hirschenhauser et al. 2005; Touma and Palme 2005). Differences in gut transport rates might be the mechanism underlying differences in FGM concentrations from the rainy and dry seasons (Chinnadurai et al. 2009). Furthermore, the analysis by Morrow et al. (2002) relied upon the cows' frequent defecation rate (Figure 6.12). It would be much more difficult to time sample collection to the peak in FGM excretion in species that defecate less frequently (Goymann et al. 2002).

Similar to the effects of diet at the individual level are the effects of diet at the species level. Nectarivores, carnivores, piscivores, insectivores, granivores, frugivores, herbivores, and omnivores all have different gut morphologies that can affect fecal retention times and degree of microbial activity (Klasing 2005). Diet can be especially problematic for omnivores that change diet frequently (von der Ohe et al. 2004). Furthermore, there is speculation that carnivores can also pass their prey's corticosteroids through their gut (von der Ohe and Servheen 2002), which would artificially elevate FGM concentrations. The problem of dietary preferences can become especially acute if a species relies upon a different diet at different times during the annual cycle. As a practical matter, it will be difficult to compare FGM concentrations from animals on different diets without extensive validation work.

Unfortunately, one of the unavoidable facts of FGM analyses is that most of the validation work must be done on captive animals (Millspaugh and Washburn 2004), even though the ultimate goal is usually to apply the technique to wild free-ranging animals. A number of studies, however, indicate that captive animals are not physiologically equivalent to free-living animals. Bringing wild animals into captivity changes HPA axis regulation, both on the order of weeks to months (e.g., Marra et al. 1995; Romero and Wingfield 1999; Washburn et al. 2003) and on the order of years to generations (e.g., Krass et al. 1979; Kunzl and Sachser 1999). Few studies have attempted to connect laboratory and field data when it comes to FGM analyses.

Furthermore, given that assessing the presence of chronic stress is the stated goal for most FGM studies, it is surprising that few validation studies have attempted to ascertain FGM dynamics in animals known to be chronically stressed. Most validation studies restrict their biological validation to an ACTH injection, thereby mimicking an acute stress response, and occasionally a validation study will apply an acute stressor itself. The resultant elevations in FGM concentrations are then assumed to reflect the expected increases due to chronic stressors. However, many studies from the biomedical literature indicate that chronic and acute stress responses are not equivalent. Consequently, the assumption that FGM responses to acute stressors "validate" FGM responses to chronic stressors may not be fully justified.

Cyr and Romero (2008) tested both these two points, and the resultant data are cause for concern. They subjected captive European starlings to chronic stress for 18 days. The plasma corticosterone concentrations in these birds underwent a biphasic response (Figure 6.14), with an increase in concentrations in the first few days followed by a decrease in concentrations as the regulation of the HPA axis changed (Rich and Romero 2005). However, as you can see in Figure 6.14, there was no resultant change in FGM concentrations throughout the chronic stress period. In other words, the chronic release of corticosterone into the plasma was not reflected in FGM concentrations, directly contradicting the assumption that most researchers make. However, when a similar chronic stress protocol was applied to starlings in the field, the predicted increase in FGM concentrations was detected (Cyr and Romero 2008). Other studies have also demonstrated a correlation between plasma corticosteroids and FGM concentrations (Sheriff et al. 2010), but many other studies have not. Clearly, both the impact of captivity on corticosteroid regulation and the difference between acute and chronic responses are underappreciated confounding factors in FGM studies.

Nonetheless, FGM analyses have great attraction. The samples are easy to collect, and the desirability of avoiding the handling of an animal for sample collection is often a driving factor in adopting FGM analysis. However, it is becoming clear that entering into an FGM study should not be taken lightly. This is not an easy technique, and the benefits often do not outweigh the disadvantages. In the end, FGM analysis is only useful if it accurately reflects plasma corticosteroid concentrations. After all, the goal is to understand biological impact of the steroids, and the biological

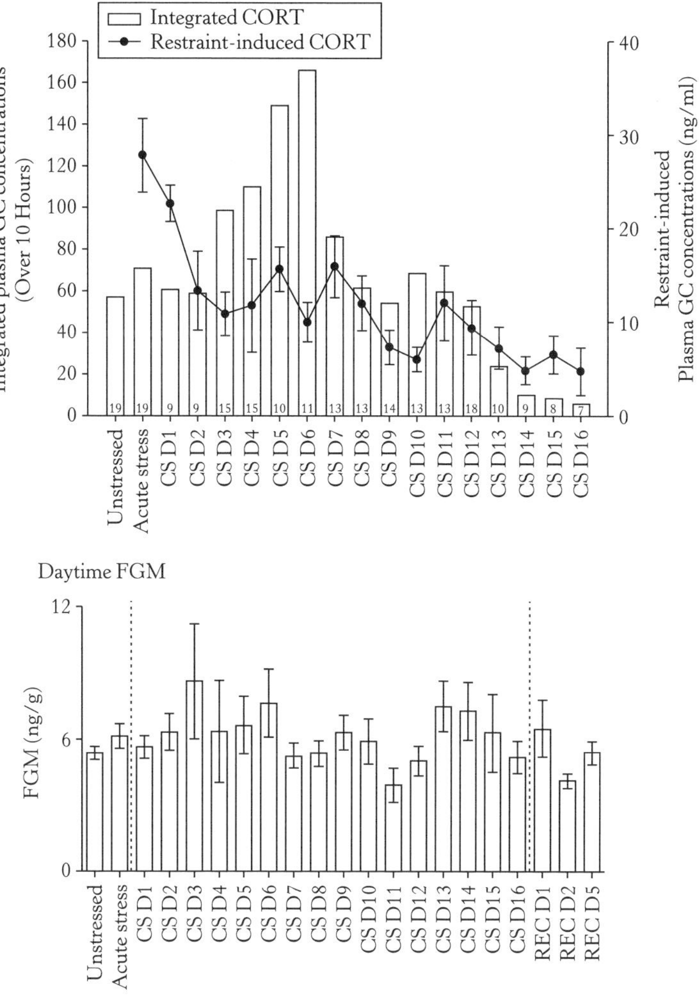

FIGURE 6.14: Top panel: plasma corticosterone. The white bars represent plasma corticosterone concentrations integrated over a 10-hour day period in unstressed, acutely stressed (30-minute restraint), and chronically stressed (CS) European starlings. Samples sizes are inside the bars. The black line represents the acute restraint-induced GC concentrations of acutely stressed and chronically stressed starlings. Bottom panel: fecal glucocorticoid metabolite (FGM) concentrations. Groups are the same as in top panel, and REC represents recovery or days after the completion of the chronic stress protocol. Dotted vertical lines denote the onset and completion of the chronic stress protocol. Note that the FGM concentrations do not match the plasma concentrations.

impact is through receptors that have access to plasma steroids. Without verifying a plasma-fecal connection, the data are difficult to interpret at best and potentially very misleading. A successful study will need to be as confident as possible that changes in FGM do reflect changes in plasma steroid concentrations (e.g., Sheriff et al. 2010).

The overwhelming message from the literature is that establishing the plasma-fecal link is time-consuming and expensive. Each step of the process needs independent validation because nearly every variation at each step has been shown to differentially alter the measured FGM output (Figure 6.15). In addition, because even closely related species process FGMs differently, there must be a customized process for each species of interest. The most common method of "validating" a fecal assay is to inject ACTH and verify that FGM concentrations increase. This method is useful for determining whether individuals in identical conditions have elevated plasma corticosteroid concentrations, but it is clearly insufficient

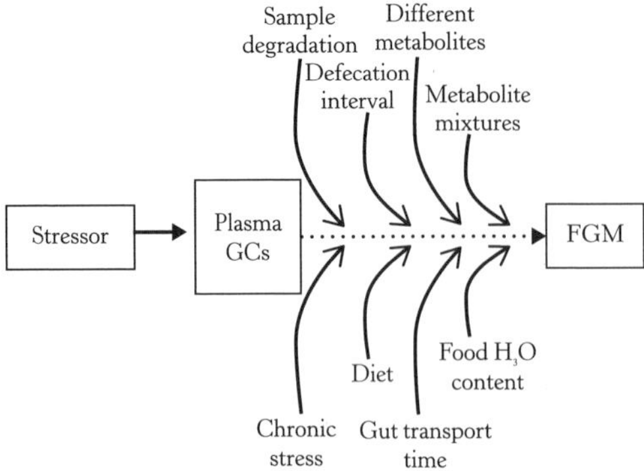

FIGURE 6.15: Summary of confounding variables that can alter fecal glucocorticoid metabolite (FGM) measurements even when plasma glucocorticoids (GCs) do not change.

validation by itself if the goal is to explore the other forms of variation discussed at the beginning of this chapter. Without extensive validation, there are simply too many unknowns at each step of the measurement process to be confident that the measured values for FGMs will form a solid foundation for exploring variability associated with different habitats, environments, and/or individual variation.

The combination of all the factors mentioned in this section indicates that FGM analysis should never be viewed as a quick method for assessing stress. When all the validation work is performed properly and the plasma-fecal link is strong, the results can be spectacular. But those results come at the end of a long and arduous process.

IV. URINE AND SALIVARY GLUCOCORTICOIDS

Corticosteroid clearance from the plasma does not only occur through the feces. In fact, based upon tracer studies of radio-labeled corticosteroids injected into the plasma, up to 80%–90% of corticosteroid metabolites are secreted in urine in several species (Bahr et al. 2000; Teskey-Gerstl et al. 2000; Ganswindt et al. 2003). In mice, however, more radio-labeled corticosteroids are secreted in the feces than in the urine, and the exact ratio depends upon the time of day (Touma et al. 2003). This suggests that at least some validation work is necessary in order to be confident that changes in urinary corticosteroids reflect changes in plasma.

Significant corticosteroids are also present in saliva. Measuring salivary cortisol is a common technique when studying humans (Lovas et al. 2006). However, this technique works best in animals trained to open their mouths to researchers (i.e., in captive situations). Salivary measurements are also likely to be much more useful in mammals—neither of us has had the courage to try to measure corticosteroids in the saliva of birds or reptiles.

Many of the difficulties in processing fecal samples are avoided when collecting urine or saliva. For example, urine and saliva have the distinct advantage that they contain the native steroid and not a metabolite. This meant that a study by Hiebert et al. (2000a) demonstrated that measuring corticosteroid metabolites from the cloacal fluid (urine) of hummingbirds did not require extraction. However, this study also highlights the sensitivity to assay conditions of measuring corticosteroid metabolites. After significant effort, Hiebert et al. successfully validated their assay for measuring corticosteroid metabolites in hummingbird urine. Soon after the paper was published, however, the last stocks of the specific antibody used in the assay were consumed. Apparently, the single animal used to produce the antibody had died several years before and the company had run out of previously stored supplies. Unfortunately, no other commercially available antibody has been able to duplicate the published results (S. Hiebert, personal communication), likely a result of few antibodies being sensitive enough to measure the extremely low amounts of steroids available in the urine of these tiny birds. Consequently, a promising technique was stillborn, and urinary corticosteroids from hummingbirds have not been reported since (but this may be changing; P. González-Gómez, personal communication).

The collection and analysis of urinary and salivary steroids are useful primarily in captive studies or in zoological settings. We are aware of only three studies in which urine samples have been successfully collected from free-living animals. Muller and Wrangham (2004) were able to collect urine opportunistically from free-ranging chimpanzees in Kibale National Park, Uganda. They were careful to collect urine in plastic bags on poles from individuals, not contaminated with feces. They also pipetted urine off vegetation (taking care to test whether vegetation compounds interfered with the assay). They found that urine cortisol levels correlated positively with male dominance rank and with rates of aggression among males. Conversely, urine cortisol correlated negatively with food availability (Muller and Wrangham 2004). Jaimez et al. (2011) also pipetted urine off leaves in a study in gray-cheeked mangabeys and found that animals in disturbed habitats had elevated urinary cortisol and disrupted diurnal patterns.

Dwarf mongooses engage in extensive scent marking. Creel et al. (1992) cleverly placed rubber pads where the mongooses liked to scent mark and successfully collected the resultant urine. This technique might be adapted for use in other species that urinate in predictable sites. Creel et al. also collected urine from mongooses during normal trapping, and although they found no differences between the urinary corticosteroids measured in free-ranging and trapped individuals, a lack of a difference would likely need to be verified for other species.

Urinary corticosteroids have also been measured in a few amphibian species (Narayan et al. 2010; Narayan et al. 2011a; Narayan et al. 2011b), but the most common measurement of urinary corticosteroids is in the tank water of fish (Scott and Ellis 2007), although these steroids may also be released across the gills. Except for fish, however, non-mammalian studies are still uncommon.

To our knowledge, salivary corticosteroids have only been measured once in free-ranging animals. Laboratory or captive-related studies have generally used swabs to collect saliva from a range of animals, including bottlenose dolphins (Pedernera-Romano et al. 2006), hamadryas baboons (Pearson et al. 2008), guinea pigs (Fenske 1996), Asian elephants (Dathe et al. 1992), and white-tailed deer (Millspaugh et al. 2002). Cross et al. (2004) trained marmosets to lick and chew a cotton-wool swab coated in banana, from which they could reliably extract saliva, and hence cortisol, for measurement. Similarly, Higham et al. (2010) used a swab baited with Tang drink crystals to entice free-living rhesus macaques (but habituated to human presence) to chew on a swab and thereby provide a saliva sample. Perhaps placing a similarly baited swab in the field where other species are known to congregate, or enticed to congregate (such as a salt lick for deer), would provide sufficient saliva for analysis, although it appears that the type of attractant can affect corticosteroid measurements (Dreschel and Granger 2009).

V. MONITORING HEART RATE AND CATECHOLAMINES

Most techniques for assessing either the presence/absence or the magnitude of a stress response in wild animals focus on the corticosteroid arm of the stress response. Very few studies attempt to measure the sympathetic response, even though for many stressors the fight-or-flight response is likely to be the primary mediator for immediate survival. In large part, this focus on corticosteroids is a direct result of the relative speeds of the two responses. Whereas there is a several-minute lag between stressor and corticosteroid release, the sympathetic nervous system is activated almost instantaneously. Consequently, it is very difficult to ascertain an animal's baseline (pre-stressor) sympathetic state, which is a vital component of determining both the presence and magnitude of a response to a stressor. Studies that have attempted to assess sympathetic activation have generally followed two different approaches.

The first approach has been to measure circulating plasma catecholamines, epinephrine (adrenalin) and norepinephrine (noradrenalin). Since the catecholamines are primary mediators of the fight-or-flight response (see Chapter 2), increases in plasma concentrations should indicate activation of sympathetic responses. Several studies have measured plasma epinephrine and norepinephrine in wild animals held in captivity. For example, catecholamines can change seasonally in birds (Chaudhuri and Maiti 1989), and increase in response to handling in American alligators (Lance and Elsey 1999a, 1999b) and exercise in toads (Romero et al. 2004). A few other studies have examined catecholamine concentrations in free-living animals. Catcholamines can vary depending upon life-history stage (Hamann et al. 2003) and have been shown to increase in response to capture in Kemp's ridley sea turtles (Hoopes et al. 2000) and a fish, the blue mao mao (Lowe and Wells 1996). However, the results can often be contradictory across studies. For example, female green turtles that successfully laid eggs had higher catecholamine concentrations than those who were unsuccessful (AlKindi et al. 2008), but in another study female green turtles that were disturbed and consequently abandoned egg laying showed no changes in catecholamines (Jessop and Hamann 2004). In a further example, catecholamines appeared to be elevated shortly after capture in Kemp's ridley sea turtles (Hoopes et al. 2000) but did not change from approximately 30 seconds to 10 minutes after capture in green sea turtles (Hamann et al. 2003).

The likely reason for the different results reported by different investigators is that the catecholamine response is so rapid. Catecholamines are released extremely rapidly (Sapolsky et al. 2000), and even the fastest reported collection of blood samples (Hamann et al. 2003) is far too slow to ascertain pre-stimulus concentrations. The only way to reliably ascertain plasma catecholamine concentrations would be to implant a chronic cannula into the vein, which is difficult in wild animals and impossible for free-living animals. It is illuminating that the majority of studies that have attempted to measure plasma catecholamines in free-living animals have used reptilian species. It is possible that heterothermic reptiles release catecholamines more slowly than homeotherms, especially when cold, so that very rapid collection of plasma samples can reflect pre-stressor concentrations, though to our knowledge this has not been verified. Until this work is done, plasma catecholamine concentrations are unlikely to provide much help in understanding the fight-or-flight response.

A related technique, so far used only in the laboratory, is to use the iris dilation reaction as an indirect measure of sympathetic activation (Carr and Zozzaro 2004). The diameter of the Texas toad iris is extremely sensitive to sympathetic activation, so that a stressor that stimulates a sympathetic response will quickly induce dilation of the iris. This assay might be adaptable to field conditions and, if so, could potentially provide a sensitive and non-invasive index of sympathetic responses, at least in some species.

One consequence of sympathetic activation is an increase in heart rate. This increase can be extraordinarily rapid and results from both direct sympathetic enervation and an increase in plasma catecholamines (see Chapter 2). Consequently, there have been a number of studies that have used increases in heart rate as an index of sympathetic activation. There have been three major techniques used to monitor heart rate changes in free-living animals.

The first has been to supply artificial eggs to incubating birds. When birds sit to incubate, these artificial eggs come in contact with a specialized, and often highly vascularized, brood patch that they use to transmit heat to the incubating eggs (Gill 1995). The eggs can then be equipped with either an infrared sensor that measures reflectance of the infrared beam as the blood pulses through the brood patch (e.g., Nimon et al. 1996) or a sensitive microphone that can pick up the sounds of pulsing blood (e.g., Ellenberg et al. 2006; Arnold et al. 2011). These artificial eggs have been very useful in measuring heart rate changes in response to actual or potential stressors.

Most of the focus to date has been on determining the impact of ecotourism. The impact of human disturbance on heart rate has been monitored in gentoo penguins (Nimon et al. 1995), Humboldt penguins (Ellenberg et al. 2006), royal penguins (Holmes et al. 2005), and northern giant petrels (De Villiers et al. 2006). Although the use of these artificial eggs has proven very useful in monitoring sympathetic activation, their use is clearly limited to incubating birds, thereby greatly restricting their general usefulness. In addition, there are several technical issues that have still to be addressed. For instance, the brood patch of incubating common eiders responds to a human approach with a decrease in temperature (Criscuolo et al. 2001), and it is unclear whether that change in temperature might affect the infrared signal.

The second major technique for measuring heart rate has been to use radio-transmitters either implanted into the animal or worn as a backpack. Implantable heart rate radio-transmitters have been used for decades for biomedical research and are commercially available (e.g., Data Sciences International). Not only are these commercial transmitters widely used in laboratory mammals, but they have also been used in birds, including chickens (Savory and Kostal 1997) and European starlings (Nephew et al. 2003). These transmitters are small (about 4 g—but weights are getting smaller) and reliable, but they have a very short range (< 40 cm) that limits their usefulness outside a laboratory. The transmitters that have been used in the field are large (25 g and up), which has limited their use to relatively large animals. Another disadvantage of transmitters is that the animal must remain within range to detect the signal—this range is several hundred meters for the current devices. If the animal goes out of range, any potential data are lost. Even given these constraints, radio-transmitters have been used to monitor heart rate in a number of species in field, or semi-field, conditions. Some examples are listed in Table 6.3. A search of the literature indicates that heart rate transmitters were used relatively frequently in field research for about a decade from the mid-1970s to the mid-1980s, with few studies thereafter until the last few years. Much of the resurgent interest in using heart rate transmitters is likely linked to new technologies that have decreased their weight and made transmitters available for a much wider number of species. Although these technological advances are just beginning, the next few years are likely to see a revitalization of these types of studies (Cooke et al. 2004).

TABLE 6.3: EXAMPLES OF SPECIES WHERE HEART RATE WAS MEASURED AS AN INDEX OF STRESS USING TRANSMITTERS FROM FREE-LIVING OR SEMI-FREE-LIVING INDIVIDUALS

Mammals	
Bottlenose dolphin (*Tursiops truncates*)	Miksis et al. (2001)
Roe deer (*Capreolus capreolus*)	Theil et al. (2004)
Red deer (*Cervus elaphus*)	Espmark and Langvatn (1985)
White-tailed deer (*Odocoileus oirginianus*)	Moen (1978)
Reindeer (Rangifer tarandus)	Nilsson et al. (2006)
Mountain sheep (*Ovis canidensis*)	Macarthur et al. (1982)
Woodchuck (*Marmota monax*)	Smith and Woodruff (1980)
Beaver (*Castor canadensis*)	Swain et al. (1988)
European badger (*Meles meles*)	Schutz et al. (2006)
European rabbit (*Oryctolagus cuniculus*)	Eiserman (1992)
American opossum (*Didelphis marsupialis*)	Gabrielsen and Smith (1985)
Birds	
Black duck (*Anas rubripes*)	Harms et al. (1997)
Willow ptarmigan (*Lagopus lagopus*)	Steen et al. (1988)
Svalbard ptarmigan (*Lagopus mutus*)	Gabrielsen et al. (1985)
Greylag goose (*Anser anser*)	Wascher et al. (2008)
Greater white-front goose (*Anser albifrons*)	Ely et al. (1999)
Tule greater white-front goose (*Anser albifrons elgasi*)	Ackerman et al. (2004)
Herring gull (*Larus argentatus*)	Kanwisher et al. (1978)
White-eyed vireo (*Vireo griseus*)	Bisson et al. (2009)
Black-capped vireo (*Vireo atricapilla*)	Bisson et al. (2011)
Prairie falcon (*Falco mexicanus*)	Ellis et al. (1991)
Reptiles	
Alligator (*Alligator mississippiensis*)	Smith et al. (1974)
Ornate box turtle (*Terrapene ornate*)	Smith and Decarvalho (1985)

There has been a plethora of studies in the past few decades using heart rate loggers in free-living animals. Loggers differ from transmitters in that they store the heart rate signal onboard the device for later download. This can provide a huge advantage if animals are not likely to remain within range of a transmitter and has especially been useful in studies of diving animals. However, this leads to the disadvantage of it being difficult to connect individual acute stressor events to the changes in heart rate recorded by the logger. It can be difficult to recreate a stress response and ascribe it to a specific acute event when that response occurred several days earlier and yet lasted only seconds. As a consequence, the majority of studies using heart rate loggers have been interested in energetic rather then stress questions. Given the strong correlations between heart rate and energy expenditures (see Chapter 4), long-term changes in heart rates related to different activities (such as resting, foraging, mating, etc.) provide an excellent index of relative energy consumptions associated with these activities. Comparatively few studies have used loggers to attempt to assess sympathetic activation in response to stressors (e.g., Weimerskirch et al. 2002). New technology, including smaller loggers with better internal clocks to synchronize with external stressors, have the potential to greatly increase the usefulness of loggers in studying sympathetic activation during stress in free-living animals.

There is one other technique that would seem ideal for studying the fight-or-flight response—measuring flight initiation distances (other terms used are "flushing distance" and "escape flight distance"). The idea is that the distance at which an animal chooses to flee, from either a predator or, under more controlled conditions, a human simulating a predator, should be a sensitive measurement of the fight-or-flight response. After all, "flight" is one of the key concepts in the fight-or-flight response. This technique has been used extensively by wildlife managers to assess the sensitivity of animals to human disturbance (reviewed by Tarlow and Blumstein 2007). Unfortunately, as discussed in Chapter 2, the term "fight-or-flight response" is only shorthand for the sympathetic arm of the stress response. It turns out that flight initiation distance is a poor indicator of sympathetic responses.

The problem is that the flight initiation distance depends upon a multitude of factors that are not associated with the stressor per se, such as time of day, angle of approach, starting distance, and so on (reviewed by Tarlow and Blumstein 2007). For example, birds in good condition show higher flight initiation distances than birds in poor condition (Beale and Monaghan 2004), the opposite of what might be predicted. In fact, anti-predator and anti-stressor (e.g., fleeing from storms) behavior can be so context dependent that it is difficult to make a priori predictions about how an animal should react (Wingfield and Ramenofsky 1997; Eilam 2005). The inability to make strong a priori predictions makes using flight initiation distances as a marker of the stress response problematic at best. Furthermore, flight initiation distances are not always good indices of predator exposure (Adams et al. 2006; Roedl et al. 2007) and they are poorly correlated with heart rate changes. For example, royal penguins elevate heart rate as a human approaches the nest even though they never flush off the nest (Holmes et al. 2005), and other species elevate their heart rate when humans are tens of meters away without overt behavioral responses (e.g., Gabrielsen et al. 1985; De Villiers et al. 2006; Ellenberg et al. 2006). Taken together, flight initiation distances can be useful for determining when a stressor might start to impact fitness, but it is unlikely to ever be useful as a tool for studying the stress response itself.

Sympathetic activation is clearly the most difficult aspect of the stress response to measure in free-living animals. The only technique that has shown any promise of success is measuring changes in heart rate as an index for the sympathetic response. However, the miniaturization of electronics, coupled with GPS (global positioning satellite) technology, has the potential to revolutionize this area and open up exciting new areas for research (Wikelski et al. 2007). Assuming these changes take place, however, what types of variability discussed at the beginning of this chapter are likely to be amenable for study? Studies of heart rate changes are likely to be applicable to all four levels of analysis. Although speculative at this time, animals might adjust both their basal heart rates and their heart rate responses to stressors when they colonize different habitats and when they are exposed to different environmental conditions, as well as showing facultative changes and individual differences. Our understanding of how, why, and when free-living animals use sympathetic activation in response to stressors is in its infancy and is ripe for further study.

VI. IMMUNOLOGY TECHNIQUES IN THE FIELD

Over the past 20 years there has been an explosive interest in how free-living animals apportion resources to maintain the immune system in the face of other life history demands. However, the literature has been plagued by different techniques used to assess how well the immune system is working—immunocompetence. Perhaps there is no single technique that can assess immune function across the board. Therefore it is critical to use a technique that most closely answers the question posed. There is considerable debate about this, and we review some techniques below.

A. Heterophil/Lymphocyte Ratios

One technique that is growing in popularity is to take a blood smear on a slide, count white blood cells, and determine the differential counts of various white blood cell types. There are several excellent reviews describing its use in poultry and free-living species (e.g., Maxwell 1993; Siegel 1995; Vleck 2001; Davis et al. 2008). Briefly, the two most prevalent white blood cell types in birds are heterophils and lymphocytes. Changes in the ratio of these two cell types are correlated with individual health and/or other indices of stress (Maxwell 1993; Siegel 1995). Specifically, there is considerable evidence that increases in heterophil/lymphocyte ratios are driven by increases in corticosteroids (Davis et al. 2008). In general, unhealthy animals show a marked increase in heterophils and a decrease in lymphocytes. Consequently, an increase in the heterophil/lymphocyte ratio can be a useful index for whether the animal has been exposed to a stressor.

Although heterophil/lymphocyte ratios can vary considerably between individuals (Vleck et al. 2000), the ratio appears to be consistent within an individual for at least several months, as long as the individual is not exposed to a stressor (Horak et al. 2002). In addition, heterophil/lymphocyte ratios do not appear to change quickly, with no significant change with one hour of handling (Davis 2005). Taken together, these data suggest that changes in heterophil/lymphocyte ratios will accurately reflect long-term (chronic) but not short-term (acute) changes in environmental stimuli. However, it is also clear that a consistent increase in heterophil/lymphocyte ratios only occurs with mild to moderate stressors—the relative proportions of white blood cell types differ significantly in response to severe stressors (Maxwell 1993). On the other hand, increases in heterophil/lymphocyte ratios have been correlated with higher mortality (Suorsa et al. 2004; Hylton et al. 2006; Kilgas et al. 2006b), suggesting that heterophil/lymphocyte ratios might provide a robust indicator of the overall health and potential fitness of an individual.

Perhaps because the technique was used primarily in human and agricultural studies, measuring heterophil/lymphocyte ratios has only recently been widely adopted for free-ranging species (Davis et al. 2008). In her 2001 review, Vleck (2001) commented on the paucity of studies in free-living birds. Since that review, there has been a surge of studies. Researchers have used heterophil/lymphocyte ratios to assess the "stress" associated with decreased food availability (Totzke et al. 1999; Pap and Markus 2003), differing habitat types (Suorsa et al. 2004; Kilgas et al. 2006a; Owen and Moore 2006) including urban habitats (Bonier et al. 2007a), pollution (Eeva et al. 2005; Schulz et al. 2006; Schulz et al. 2007), life-history trade-offs (Moreno et al. 2002; Ilmonen et al. 2003; Edler et al. 2004; Sanz et al. 2004; Friedl and Edler 2005; Garamszegi et al. 2006; Laiolo et al. 2007), parasite infestation (Shutler et al. 2004; Lobato et al. 2005; Boughton et al. 2006; Laiolo et al. 2007), translocations (Groombridge et al. 2004), overall health or body condition (Averbeck 1992; Hanauska-Brown et al. 2003; Alvarez et al. 2006; Hylton et al. 2006; Artacho et al. 2007; Pfaff et al. 2007), impact of field techniques (Kreger and Mench 1993; Morici et al. 1997; Newman et al. 2005; Schulz et al. 2005), and conspecific interactions (Lopez et al. 2005). In addition, a few studies have begun to focus on other vertebrates. Heterophil/lymphocyte ratios have now been measured in turtles (Work et al. 2001; Case et al. 2005; Xinran et al. 2007), snakes (Kreger and Mench 1993), lizards (Kreger and Mench 1993), and alligators (Morici et al. 1997). Clearly, this is a technique that is growing in popularity.

Although mammals do not have heterophils, the functional equivalent is neutrophils, yet measuring the neutrophil/lymphocyte ratio as an index of stress is not as prevalent in wild mammals and has primarily been used in animal husbandry settings. When it has been used, there appears to be a similar change as occurs in birds. Dairy cattle that have been dehorned, for example, demonstrated an increase in the neutrophil/lymphocyte ratio that paralleled an increase in cortisol (Doherty et al. 2007), as do pigs exposed to a transport stressor (McGlone et al. 1993). Similar correlations between elevated cortisol concentrations and increased neutrophil/lymphocyte ratios have been shown in several captive primates (Morrow-Tesch et al. 1993; Kim et al. 2005). In addition, blind mole rats show an increased neutrophil/lymphocyte ratio when encountering an unknown conspecific (Zuri et al. 1998). The increase in neutrophil/lymphocyte ratio appears to be secondary to an increase in cortisol in mammals (Rossdale et al. 1982; Widowski et al. 1989). Only a handful of studies have measured neutrophil/lymphocyte ratios in free-living mammals. They indicate that capture can increase the neutrophil/lymphocyte ratio (Presidente and Correa 1981; Hajduk et al. 1992; Weber et al. 2002) and that the neutrophil/lymphocyte ratio can vary seasonally (Bradley et al. 1988). Furthermore, the heterophil/lymphocyte ratio soon after handling in European rabbits was correlated with survival when the animals were in captivity (Calvete et al. 2005). These studies suggest that increases in neutrophil/lymphocyte ratios in mammals represent a similar response as increases in heterophil/lymphocyte ratios in birds. In all taxa studied to date, increases in the ratio appear to indicate that the animal is experiencing a significant sustained stressor.

In a review on using heterophil/lymphocyte ratios in birds, Vleck (2001) identified a number of drawbacks in using this technique to assess stress in free-living animals. First, the relative numbers of heterophils and lymphocytes can vary among closely related species, and even among different studies of the same species, making it imperative that a reference range for unstressed animals be available for each species of interest. Unfortunately, these baseline reference ranges are not often available, and determining them in unstressed free-living animals can be difficult. Second, a number of studies have indicated that the heterophil/lymphocyte ratio can vary as individuals age or enter different life-history stages (Vleck et al. 2000; Friedl and Edler 2005; Owen and Moore 2006;

Mortimer and Lill 2007). Third, selection experiments in domesticated birds (Siegel 1995) suggest that heterophil/lymphocyte ratios may vary significantly in a heritable manner, making it difficult to distinguish between individual variation and variation in response to environmental changes.

Another drawback is that it is not always clear how heterophil/lymphocyte ratios relate to circulating corticosteroids. Many studies have shown that changes in heterophil/lymphocyte ratios are closely linked to changes in plasma corticosteroid concentrations (e.g., Vleck et al. 2000; Newman et al. 2005; Boughton et al. 2006), and that corticosteroids may actually be driving the changes in heterophil/lymphocyte ratios (e.g., Rossdale et al. 1982; Widowski et al. 1989; Maxwell 1993; Morici et al. 1997), but many other studies have not shown this link (e.g., Collette et al. 2000; Ilmonen et al. 2003; Case et al. 2005; Newman et al. 2005; Bonier et al. 2007a; Mueller et al. 2011). Several studies also show that heterophil/lymphocyte ratios are not particularly sensitive to short-term acute stressors. The long-term stressors that do elicit an increase in heterophil/lymphocyte ratios are also known to increase corticosteroid concentrations, making the lack of correlation more troubling. Given that corticosteroids are often considered the *sina qua non* of a stress response, it is not clear how to reconcile these differences. Several researchers suggest that heterophil/lymphocyte ratios may provide a better long-term measure of stress than individual "snapshots" of corticosteroid concentrations (e.g., Maxwell 1993; Siegel 1995; Vleck 2001). They claim that increases in heterophil/lymphocyte ratios are less variable and more enduring than corticosteroid responses. However, the presumed superiority of heterophil/lymphocyte ratios mostly is in reference to single samples of corticosteroids rather than the modern capture stress protocol covered earlier in this chapter. It is not clear whether the heterophil/lymphocyte ratio would still be considered superior to the improved capture stress protocol.

There is also a potential problem in using an immune system measure as a generalized measure for stress. Infections can alter immune parameters in the absence of other stimuli, but the impact on heterophil/lymphocyte ratios is not consistent. There are reports of an increase (Ots et al. 2001; Sanz et al. 2004), a decrease (Bonier et al. 2007a), and no change (Boughton et al. 2006) in heterophil/lymphocyte ratios in infected individuals. Infections, of course, can be stressors, but if the goal of a study is to determine whether a different stressor is present (e.g., habitat degradation), different infection rates could be a serious confounding variable if heterophil/lymphocyte ratios were the only measure. This has been suggested as a mechanism to explain the differences in heterophil/lymphocyte ratios between free-living and captive animals (Ewenson et al. 2001).

It should also be of concern that the dynamics that create a consistent increase in heterophil/lymphocyte ratios break down during severe stressors (Maxwell 1993). If the relative severity of the stressor is suspected before the study, then this problem could potentially be avoided. However, if the severity is unknown, it may be very difficult to distinguish between a lack of any stressors and the presence of severe stressors. Finally, it is unclear how important this technique will be in different taxonomic classes. The original work on measuring heterophil/lymphocyte ratios was done in domesticated fowl, and very little work was been done on other taxa.

We identified four types of variation that we would like to be able to study in free-living animals. How well do measurements of heterophil/lymphocyte ratios help us in evaluating variability? The first type of variation was adaptations to specific environments. Measuring heterophil/lymphocyte ratios appears to be useful in this regard, especially in terms of short-term adaptations, that is, on a physiological time scale. Comparing adaptations on an evolutionary time scale is more problematic since heterophil/lymphocyte ratios are known to vary considerably between closely related species and appear to be able to be selected for (Siegel 1995).

The second type of variation was in response to environmental change. It appears that much more work is necessary before heterophil/lymphocyte ratios can provide much illumination on these questions. If heterophil/lymphocyte ratios vary seasonally and with different life-history stages, comparing across these stages will be very difficult. However, future work assessing how heterophil/lymphocyte ratios change over the yearly cycle and the life span of an individual has the potential to make measurements of heterophil/lymphocyte ratios much more valuable for these types of questions.

The third type of variation, facultative changes within a season or life-history stage, appears to be the best fit for using differences in heterophil/lymphocyte ratios. Studies at this level avoid the problem of heterophil/lymphocyte ratios changing over the year and allow comparisons of stress responses between different groups or populations. This is the level targeted by most of the extant studies.

Comparing individual differences, the fourth type of variation, is just beginning. Vital to answering questions at this level would be establishing heterophil/lymphocyte ratios in non-stressed individuals. Establishing these reference ranges is usually missing and will often be difficult to obtain without resorting to other methods (at which point many of the benefits of the technique are lost). However, this seems to be an area where significant progress can be made.

B. Inflammation Responses

A widespread technique, especially in mammals and birds, is to inject an antigen such as sheep red blood cells, or keyhole limpet hemocyanin, subcutaneously and to measure the degree of inflammation. In mammals the injection is typically in the pinna of the ear so that thickness of the swelling can be measured directly compared to controls. In birds typically the injection is in the wing web (between the humerus and the radius/ulna) and thickness is measured using a caliper. Although this technique provides a rather crude index of immune function, it appears to be effective. The problem, however, is in the interpretation. Virtually all papers using this technique regard a thicker swelling to indicate a better immune response than less swelling (reviewed in Martin et al. 2010). However, one could also argue that less swelling to the same amount of antigen could indicate a more vigorous and efficient immune system. This problem has not been resolved.

C. Sickness Behavior

As mentioned in Chapter 5, sickness behavior is thought to be adaptive in potentiating the immune response to infection by changing food intake and social behavior, and regulating fever (e.g., Hart 1988). One way to induce sickness behavior is by intravenous injection of lipopolysaccharide (LPS—essentially bacteria cell walls), which tricks the immune system into responding to an apparent infection, but without live pathogens. Typically, animals injected with LPS will show pronounced sickness behavior within an hour and the effect lasts for up to one to two days (e.g., Owen-Ashley et al. 2008). This is a technique that can be used in the field to determine seasonal and sex differences in response to LPS as well as condition, age, and many other variables (Ashley and Wingfield 2012). Field studies rarely measure sickness behavior per se but rather look at deficits in other behavior such as response of males to a simulated territorial intrusion (aggression) after LPS or control injection. The technique is attractive because a behavioral response is used rather than an indirect measure of a complex immune response.

D. Bacteria-Killing Capacity

Until techniques are developed to measure key cytokines in blood as a direct measure of the immune response, the previous techniques were the best we had until a novel assay was developed that involves taking fresh blood from the focal animal and dropping it onto petri dishes with cultures of bacteria (*Escherischia coli*). After a standard amount of time, the numbers of cultures killed by the immune cells in the blood give a measure of the potential immune response (Tieleman et al. 2005). This capacity can be compared across sexes, seasons, and so on. The power of this technique is that interpretation is straightforward—bacteria-killing capacity is a direct measure of the potential immune response. A drawback is preparing Petri dishes with live bacteria cultures and transporting them to remote field locations. Clearly, considerable prior logistical planning will be needed.

VII. CORTICOSTEROID MANIPULATION

Although not technically a method for measuring stress in wild animals, many studies have attempted to manipulate the corticosteroid portion of the stress response, either by adding corticosteroid via injections, implants, and so forth, or administering various blockers of synthesis, such as receptor agonists and antagonists. There have generally been three goals of these studies. One is to study the function of corticosteroids in order to understand basic corticosteroid physiology. The second is to mimic chronic elevations of corticosteroids that are presumed to occur during chronic stress. Third, corticosteroid implants are used to study ultimate evolutionary questions, such as asking what the impact would be on reproduction if corticosteroid concentrations were higher. All three goals have been targets of both laboratory and field studies.

Implants are created by either embedding corticosteroids in a wax, packing corticosteroids into silastic tubing, or placing corticosteroids in newly developed gel materials (French et al. 2007). All three approaches yield relatively slow release of the steroid over a number of days. Either the concentration of the steroid in the wax or the length of the silastic tubing can provide different doses. There has been some disagreement over the proper controls for implant studies. Some researchers advocate a cholesterol-packed implant in order to add a steroid-like substance that is roughly akin to using a vehicle control. Other researchers are concerned that cholesterol is a precursor to steroid synthesis and could be used to create steroids and thus is not a benign substance. These researchers advocate using a blank implant. Currently, most field studies use blank implants as controls.

Laboratory studies especially have taken advantage of implants. One of the most important techniques in endocrinology is the removal/replacement study. Adrenalectomy is the classic surgical technique for removing corticosteroids. Using primarily laboratory rodents, implants have traditionally provided the yin to adrenalectomy's yang. Adrenalectomy removed the endogenous source of the steroids, and implants containing different steroid concentrations helped recover function (e.g., Darlington et al. 1990a; Akana et al. 1992). Chemical adrenalectomy, especially using the drug mitotane (Breuner et al. 2000), has been also used to eliminate (or at least reduce) corticosteroid release, but so far few chemical adrenalectomy studies have been paired with implants in a removal/replacement study (Wingfield and Ramenofsky 1999). Implants have also been used in a number of field studies (e.g., Wingfield and Silverin 1986; Astheimer et al. 2000), although most of these investigations have been interested more in the elevation of corticosteroids rather than replacement.

Implants have a number of advantages for field studies. First, they allow the manipulation of the corticosteroid arm of the stress response. This opens a number of possibilities for experimental approaches and can move a study away from relying solely on correlative evidence. Furthermore, removing corticosteroids (i.e., adrenalectomy) is simply not a viable option in the field. Adrenalectomized animals die within a few weeks under stressor-free laboratory conditions (Darlington et al. 1990a; Darlington et al. 1990b) and would presumably perish even quicker in the wild. Chemical adrenalectomy via mitotane might be a viable option because it reduces rather than eliminates corticosteroid release (Breuner et al. 2000), but mitotane does not appear to work in all species (C. Breuner, personal communication) and, to our knowledge, has not yet been attempted in a field context.

There are also several major advantages related to the ease of use and the relative benign nature of implants. The typical subcutaneous implantation is an easy surgical manipulation, allowing wild animals to be quickly captured, implanted, and released. Implants are also relatively long lasting. Experiments can extend for several days at least. The combination of rapid recovery and long-lasting effects allows researchers to examine corticosteroid impact on natural behaviors after minimal disturbance to the animal's normal routine. In addition, implants have a limited life span. This restricts implant effects to a few days to weeks, resulting in little long-term harm to the animal. Furthermore, the animal does not need to be recaptured to remove the implant.

Finally, there are excellent advantages of implants for studies of evolutionary questions. Because there appears to be a trade-off between higher corticosteroid release to help counteract stressors and lower corticosteroid release to avoid deleterious exposures, a major unanswered question in corticosteroid physiology is why concentrations are what they are. Why aren't the concentrations higher? And if they were higher, what would the trade-offs be? These questions are difficult to answer by only studying endogenous concentrations. Natural release is likely finely balanced to minimize potential deleterious effects, following the ideas of Ketterson et al. (Ketterson et al. 1996; Ketterson and Nolan 1999; Ketterson et al. 2005; McGlothlin and Ketterson 2008) on phenotypic engineering. Consequently, supra-physiological concentrations are necessary to expose either compensatory adaptations or potential deleterious effects, and providing supra-physiological doses is one of the strengths of implants. Examples include breeding arctic birds that are insensitive to the behavior effects of corticosterone during the extremely short breeding season (Astheimer et al. 2000), and molting birds where exogenous corticosterone interferes with the normal replacement of feathers (Romero et al. 2005). These experiments are difficult to design (see caveats discussed later in this chapter), but implants can provide useful indirect evidence on the evolutionary constraints on the corticosteroid system.

There are a number of serious drawbacks that indicate that data from implant manipulations should be interpreted cautiously. Unfortunately, most implants only provide crude control over dose. There are a number of reasons for this problem. Wax implants have been finely titrated to provide consistent doses in rodents (e.g., Akana et al. 1992), but the types of wax, which determine how quickly the wax dissolves (thereby releasing the embedded steroids), have been chosen and optimized for mammalian body temperatures. Species with different body temperatures will dissolve the wax at varying rates, resulting in different doses. For example, birds with their higher body temperatures dissolve the wax too quickly (Müller et al. 2009), and reptiles with their lower body temperature would presumably dissolve the wax too slowly. One solution to this problem has been to use dermal patches that contain corticosteroids that can diffuse across the skin (Knapp and Moore 1997; Wada and Breuner 2008), thereby making external "implants." Other implants of unknown matrix (e.g., from Innovative Research) are useful to deliver relatively low physiological doses (e.g., Bonier et al. 2007b). Additionally, a steroid can be complexed in cyclodextrins that can be added at various doses to water, or in the case of hummingbirds, in nectar (Hiebert et al. 2000b). Controls are given cyclodextrins only. The cyclodextrins are dissolved by enzymatic action in the gut, thus releasing steroid that is taken up into the blood. The problem here is that the actual dose administered is dependent not only on the concentration in the water/nectar, but also on how much liquid the individual chooses to imbibe.

Silastic tubing implants avoid the problems associated with dissolving wax. However, they have many drawbacks of their own. First, corticosteroids do not diffuse easily through the tubing. To allow sufficient corticosteroid to diffuse into the animal, one end of the tubing is usually left open. However, this removes some of the control over dose and timing of release. In our experience, silastic implants can release corticosteroids anywhere from three days to several weeks. The shorter time frames provide a bolus of steroid that quickly reaches supra-physiological concentrations but rapidly dissipates. The longer time frames provide a lower bolus, but inconsistent durations. In neither case do the silastic implants provide a smooth release of steroid, which is typical of the wax implants. Furthermore, it is not uncommon to remove silastic implants after several weeks and find undissolved steroid remaining in the tubing. Measurements of plasma concentrations indicate that these implants failed to release the steroid. As a result of these problems, it is important to use plasma concentrations to verify and quantify both the amount of steroids released and the release duration for each implant study. When this is not possible for a particular study, interpretations should be made cautiously, especially if there are hyper-responders (supra-physiological dose?) or non-responders (failed implant?).

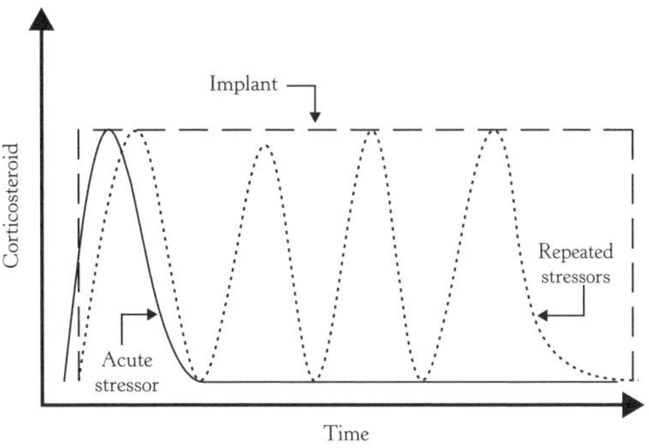

FIGURE 6.16: Theoretical schematic of how corticosteroid release from implants compares to endogenous release after either an acute stressor or repeated acute stressors (e.g., chronic exposure).

Even if the implants work as intended, they still provide a dose of corticosteroid that is very different in its dynamics from endogenous release. In response to a stressor, endogenous corticosteroid release increases, and then negative feedback begins to reduce further release (see Chapter 2). Implants, on the other hand, bypass negative feedback and produce a relatively constant elevated concentration of steroid (Figure 6.16). The body attempts to compensate for this abnormal elevation by decreasing synthesis, storage, and release of releasing factors (e.g., CRF and ACTH), changing CBG concentrations, and down-regulating corticosteroid receptors. The latter effect is especially problematic for interpreting implant studies. Implants are normally used to increase the physiological effects of corticosteroids, and yet the act of increasing corticosteroid concentrations over the lifetime of an implant will lead to fewer corticosteroid receptors and ultimately reduced corticosteroid impact. It is not always appreciated that implants create an animal with a very different physiology than non-manipulated controls. Corticosteroid concentrations are not simply elevated while everything else remains constant.

A. Circadian Disruption

The constant nature of corticosteroid release with implants also creates problems with normal circadian rhythms. Endogenous corticosteroids are released in a circadian rhythm, with the peak occurring at the beginning of the active phase (see Chapter 2). This rhythm is integral to normal energy regulation (Dallman et al. 1993; Dallman and Bhatnagar 2001). Implants disrupt this normal physiology. Implants provide relatively constant elevated concentrations of steroids, but it is unknown whether constant high corticosteroids or multiple high bursts on top of a normal circadian rhythm better reflect natural up-regulation of corticosteroid concentrations. There have been a number of attempts to avoid disrupting the underlying circadian rhythm. Corticosteroid injections provide a rapid bolus of steroid that is cleared quickly and more closely mimics a natural response to a stressor (Remage-Healey and Romero 2001), but this technique requires multiple and frequent handling of the animal to maintain elevated concentrations. Similarly, a recent technique paints exposed skin with a solution of corticosteroids dissolved in DMSO, an organic solvent that readily carries the steroid across the skin (Busch et al. 2008a; Busch et al. 2008b). This technique avoids the stress of an injection, but otherwise has the same advantages and drawbacks as multiple injections. Perhaps the most ingenious solution to this problem was pioneered by Breuner et al. (1998). They injected corticosterone into live mealworms and presented them to birds. When consumed by the birds, the mealworms release a bolus of corticosterone that mimicked the endogenous release in response to an acute stressor. This technique allows the researcher to elevate corticosteroids without the other physiological responses to a stressor and without disrupting the normal underlying circadian rhythm.

B. Mimicking Chronic Stress

Many studies use implants to mimic chronic stress. However, the endocrine profile for a chronically stressed free-living animal is not yet clear (Dickens and Romero 2013). Some studies suggest that chronic stress results in either long-term elevations of corticosteroids (e.g., Creel 2001) or in the inability to turn off the stress response (e.g., Sapolsky and Share 1994), but other studies suggest that chronic stress can result in lower corticosteroid concentrations and an attenuated response to acute stressors (e.g., Blanchard et al. 1995; Rich and Romero 2005; Cyr and Romero 2007). Furthermore, endogenous (via chronic stress) and exogenous (via implant) corticosteroids can have different physiological effects in the same experimental system (Romero et al. 2005; Strochlic and Romero 2008). The results from these disparate studies have not yet been reconciled, and doing so is the subject of current research. It is not beyond possibility that different species, different populations, and even different individuals will differ in whether they show elevated or attenuated corticosteroid responses. However, the implication is that implants may or may not act as good mimics for chronic stress. Until this issue is resolved, mimicking chronic stress with implants should be interpreted cautiously.

Despite the potential pitfalls and intricacies of interpretation, corticosteroid implants provide a useful technique in field endocrinologists' toolkit. When used correctly, they can provide experimental evidence to bolster correlative data. However, given the drawbacks presented earlier, the usefulness of implants is often limited. Of special concern are when implant studies are used as the exclusive, or even the main, evidence in support of a hypothesis. Implants are most likely to be useful in producing a supplementary line of evidence, but seem to be ill suited to addressing questions of individual variation. Given the stochastic nature of the corticosteroid release from some implants, this technique is not reliable for assessing individual variation. When used in the field, there will be no way to know whether individual differences result from natural individual variation in the physiological effects of corticosteroids, or from simple differences in dose.

VIII. EMERGING TECHNIQUES

In this section we will review some new and innovative techniques. Many of them are creative solutions for addressing problems in specific species, and may not be generalized to other taxa. Others have recently been proposed and may be widely applicable once sufficient validation work has been performed. They have been developed for various reasons to replace or supplement the collection of urine, feces, or saliva for glucocorticoid measurements described earlier.

A. Corticosteroids in Hair and Feathers

There has been extensive effort to measure steroid concentrations in hair. The original impetus was an attempt to detect illicit steroid use in human (e.g., Gambelunghe et al. 2007) and animal (e.g., Gratacos-Cubarsi et al. 2006) athletes. Glucocorticoids were not an initial target for these studies. Instead, the goal was to detect androgen usage and other drugs of abuse.

In 2006, Davenport et al. (2006) published the first paper analyzing cortisol in hair. They showed that the hair of captive rhesus macaques contained sufficient cortisol to be measured. After clipping the hair and washing it with a series of methanol extractions, cortisol was analyzed with a standard radioimmunoassay. The cortisol appears to be deposited during growth and was correlated with concurrent concentrations of salivary cortisol. However, once the growing hair leaves the follicle, cortisol embedded in that hair is no longer in equilibrium with the plasma. It thus appears that cortisol in mammalian hair forms a record of the individual's cortisol milieu at the time the hair was formed. Hair cortisol analysis has now been applied to humans (e.g., Kalra et al. 2007), dogs and cats (Accorsi et al. 2008), various primates (Fourie and Bernstein 2011), caribou (Ashley et al. 2011), and grizzly bears (Macbeth et al. 2010).

Recent work has extended this technique to measure corticosterone in feathers (Bortolotti et al. 2008; Bortolotti et al. 2009a; Bortolotti et al. 2009b; Harms et al. 2010; Mougeot et al. 2010; Fairhurst et al. 2011). Similar to hair, each feather reflects the hormonal milieu at the time of growth, although since feathers grow differently than hair, the calculations for feather corticosteroid levels may be different (Bortolotti 2010). In addition, even though native corticosterone appears to be deposited in feathers (Koren et al. 2012), at least some of the corticosterone is unconjugated (Bortolotti et al. 2008), and it is still unclear which kinds of assays will work best at detecting the corticosteroids (Lattin et al. 2011).

Given the newness of this technique, there are a number of technical and biological issues that still need to be addressed. Many of the validation steps necessary for applying a fecal analysis to a new species or collection regimen will also need to be worked out for corticosteroids in hair and feathers. For example, we will need to determine whether there are species differences in how efficiently the corticosteroids are incorporated, how natural species variability in plasma corticosteroid concentrations affect hair/feather concentrations, whether the speed of hair or feather growth alters subsequent corticosteroid deposition, whether there are any effects of changing diets, and how robust corticosteroids are to various storage and/or collection conditions (for example, if feathers or hair are picked up from the ground, will they still accurately reflect the original corticosteroid titers?), and so on.

Once these details are worked out, there will be tremendous potential with this technique. We can envision numerous projects, including ones in which hormonal titers can be ascertained without even seeing the animal. Examples might include collecting hair from barbed wire snags and collecting feathers from abandoned nests. We predict, however, that studies of corticosteroids in hair and feathers will end up with many similarities to fecal analyses. Both are non-invasive techniques that provide a more integrated picture of the plasma steroid milieu, and both analyses will likely be better suited to studying long-term stressors instead of short-term acute stressors. The biggest contrast is the time frame that is being integrated. With fecal analyses, plasma corticosteroids are being integrated over the period since the last defecation. With hair and feather analyses, the plasma corticosteroids are being integrated over a period of days to weeks—during the time when the hair or new feather was growing. Consequently, hair/feather analyses will be complementary to other techniques and will provide a window on a time frame not currently available except through repeated serial sampling using other techniques. We are very excited about the potential future of hair and feather analyses.

B. Corticosteroids in Whale Blow

Marine mammals have proved daunting species for measuring stress hormones. However, given the endangered status of many species, there has been tremendous interest in ascertaining whether these animals are responding to stressors, especially anthropogenic stressors (NRC 2005). Several attempts have been made to measure cortisol in various marine mammals, with varying success. Some marine mammal species, such as seals and sea lions, spend some time on land and can easily be accessed to collect blood samples (e.g., Sangalang and Freeman 1976; Bartsh et al. 1992; Engelhard et al. 2002). However, even in these cases, getting baseline measures of cortisol can be difficult, which one study only accomplished by shooting the animals (Sangalang and Freeman 1976). The earliest anyone else has reported being able to take a blood sample was 6 minutes after administering a light anesthetic (Engelhard et al. 2002), far too long to be confident that the measured concentrations represent a true baseline, as the authors readily admit. On the other hand, the cetaceans do not come to land, and so corticosteroids must be assessed in free-swimming animals. This generally entails lengthy capture methods in nets (Wright et al. 2007), and samples are rarely collected in under 30 minutes from the beginning of the capture process (e.g., Koopman et al. 1995; Ortiz and Worthy 2000). For those species whose feces float, fecal analysis provides an excellent alternative (Hunt et al. 2006). However, fecal and/or urine samples are not available for the majority of cetaceans.

An innovative technique to measure steroids non-invasively from free-swimming cetaceans was presented by Hogg et al. (2005) and was described in detail at a subsequent meeting (Hogg et al. 2006). Whale blow (i.e., the rapid exhalation from the blow hole when cetaceans break the ocean surface to breathe) contains significant amounts of mucus. This mucus can be captured by holding a nylon mesh, attached to a long pole held from the deck of a boat, inside the spray as the whale blows. The mucus exudate can then be extracted and analyzed for steroids. Although the validation work for cortisol has not yet been published, cortisol is in the blow in sufficient concentrations to be measured (C. Hogg, personal communication). Although clearly much more validation work is necessary, measuring cortisol in whale blow has the potential to be an excellent technique for evaluating cortisol responses in cetaceans.

C. Corticosteroids in Aquarium Water

It has always been problematic to sample aquatic animals such as fish and amphibians, especially in the field, because actually catching the animal, restraining it, and obtaining the sample can take considerable time and is particularly distressing to the animal. Imagine if you were captured and held underwater while a sample was collected—the reverse of what a fish will experience! It is important to point out that some field researchers have developed techniques to capture and sample fish underwater in the ocean or rivers (e.g., Godwin and Thomas 1993; Pottinger 1998), and this is an impressive field skill indeed. Nonetheless, for many fish, and perhaps amphibians too, the animals are so small that even if captured they are virtually impossible to bleed. A novel way of getting around this is to maintain the animals in aquaria in captivity, conduct manipulations (e.g., social interactions), and measure steroid concentrations in the aquarium water (Scott and Ellis 2007). Fish excrete steroids in urine and feces, and some may leak out through the gills. Samples of aquarium water can be extracted and measured for steroids. This innovative method has allowed some key investigations of stress and social interactions underlying hormones and behavior (e.g., Bender et al. 2006). A drawback is that steroids excreted must take time to equilibrate after a social interaction, and thus rapid changes may not be possible to determine.

D. Blood-Sucking Bugs

A few studies have recently been published using blood-sucking insects to collect plasma samples for steroid analysis. The technique has been applied to several species, including domestic rabbits (Voigt et al. 2004), three species of captive primates (Thomsen and Voigt 2006), and free-living common terns (Becker et al. 2006). The technique entails placing a hungry insect, usually *Dipetalogaster maximus* (Reduviidae, Heteroptera), in close proximity to the skin and protecting the insect with a wire mesh to keep the target animal from eating the bug, or placing it in a false egg in incubating birds. The bug then consumes a blood meal and, before the meal can be digested, the blood is removed and analyzed.

This technique has several advantages (Voigt et al. 2006). The proboscis of the insect is significantly smaller than a normal hypodermic needle, and the insect injects a local anesthetic as it feeds; consequently, the insect removes blood with less overall disturbance than does a human. The insect also uses a natural anticoagulant so that samples do not have to be treated to prevent clotting. The insects also do not appear to begin digestion for some time. At least in the rabbit, corticosteroid concentrations were stable for over 24 hours (Voigt et al. 2004). Finally, at least in some contexts, blood-sucking insects can be used in the field. Becker et al. (2006) hollowed out an egg, covered a small opening with wire mesh, and placed it under an incubating tern. The insect then fed and was collected several hours later.

Two major drawbacks, however, currently limit the usefulness of this technique. The first is that there is not yet a proven and strong link between plasma corticosteroid concentrations and what is measured in the bug's blood meal. This is a similar problem addressed recently for fecal measurements (see previous section in this chapter). To be really useful, the levels measured in the bugs must be an accurate reflection of what is in the plasma. The second major drawback relates to its potential generality for field studies. The technique requires two fundamental conditions—that the insect has access to the animal of interest and that the researcher has subsequent access to the insect. Satisfying these two conditions will be difficult for many species and for different times of the year. For example, although the bug technique worked well for incubating terns, it is unclear whether a similar success will be possible when birds are not incubating and thus are not sitting on eggs. In sum, we believe that this technique has the potential to make a significant contribution to the measurement of corticosteroids under certain field conditions, but that those contributions will be limited until a strong link between plasma and blood meal has been forged.

E. Telomere Shortening

Telomeres are repetitive DNA regions at the ends of every eukaryotic chromosome that do not appear to code for any genes. Because DNA synthetic enzymes cannot replicate the entire chromosome during cell division, the telomere region of each chromosome shortens by about 20–30 base pairs. Consequently, telomeres normally function as a cap on the chromosome that allows replication to occur without losing vital genetic information. Cells are thought to stop replicating when telomere length shortens beyond a critical length, so that telomere length can be used as a marker for cell age (i.e., the number of times it has been replicated) and, by extension, organism age and senescence (Monaghan and Haussmann 2006; Vleck et al. 2007).

Although allowing efficient DNA replication appears to be the primary role for telomeres, oxidative stress also shortens telomeres (Epel et al. 2004). Because oxidative stress at the cellular level is associated with environmental stressors, possibly mediated through corticosteroids, telomere shortening is thought to be a marker for an animal's exposure to stressors (Haussmann and Marchetto 2010). Evidence for this relationship is fairly well established in human medicine and it is starting to be applied in free-living species. For example, non-surviving alpine swifts displayed increased telomere shortening rates compared to those that survived (Bize et al. 2009); telomeres in wild house mice were significantly shortened in response to chronic psychological stress (Kotrschal et al. 2007); and telomere shortening rate predicted survival in free-living jackdaws (Salomons et al. 2009). It thus appears that telomeres may be good markers of cumulative stress exposure in wild animals (Haussmann and Marchetto 2010).

The use of telomeres as an index of stressor exposure in free-living populations is just beginning. The technique holds great promise for evaluating lifetime stress exposure and is therefore most likely to be useful for exploring variation in responses to environmental and habitat changes. Telomere shortening is likely to have limited use, however, for studying facultative stress responses (see the beginning of this chapter), and unless long-term longitudinal studies are undertaken (e.g., Salomons et al. 2009), it is not clear how useful telomeres will be in assessing individual differences.

IX. FLUCTUATING ASYMMETRY

Bilateral creatures are defined by the symmetry between the left and right sides of their bodies. During development, numerous molecular developmental mechanisms serve to ensure that growth proceeds as symmetrically as possible. Anything that disrupts those molecular mechanisms will create asymmetry between the two sides of the organism, although how this occurs is not well understood. The degree of asymmetry is thought to reflect the degree of underlying disruption in the developmental pathways. Asymmetry derived from this disruption is termed "fluctuating asymmetry" because which side becomes larger is random, not programmed (as opposed to directional asymmetry, such as the one hypertrophied claw in many fiddler crabs). Stress (although the term is loosely defined in these studies) is believed to be a major, if not the predominant, environmental cause of fluctuating asymmetry. A number of excellent reviews have evaluated the usefulness of fluctuating asymmetry for assessing the stress experienced by an animal during development (e.g., Bjorksten et al. 2000; Lens et al. 2002; Knierim et al. 2007).

Fluctuating asymmetry has a number of advantages for quantifying stress, not least of which is its ease of measurement (Lens et al. 2002). Theoretically, all that is required is the measurement of the same trait (e.g., tarsus length) from both sides of the body. This requires minimal equipment—often only a good pair of calipers—and rapid assessment of these traits can result in large sample sizes being collected rather easily. In addition, fluctuating asymmetry likely reflects long-term stress that would be difficult to detect using the other techniques described in this chapter.

Although there is great appeal in a simple and quick assessment of stress, there remain a number of significant drawbacks. Perhaps the worst drawback is that fluctuating asymmetry does not appear to reliably indicate developmental stress. Several reviews have evaluated the quality of the evidence that fluctuating asymmetry reflects the degree of stress during development and have concluded that the data are equivocal (e.g., Bjorksten et al. 2000; Lens et al. 2002; Knierim et al. 2007). Partially this is a result of few well-designed studies that explicitly study this link. All three reviews feel that measuring fluctuating asymmetry is still a promising technique and call for more work to resolve the inconsistencies.

However, even if fluctuating asymmetry were found to have a robust connection with stress, there are a number of other drawbacks that would decrease its usefulness. First, the asymmetry would result from stress during the period of development of the measured trait. This means that fluctuating asymmetry will be more useful for evaluating stress during development and will have limited utility for assessing stress during the majority of an animal's life. Consequently, fluctuating asymmetry will have limited use for studying facultative stress responses (see the beginning of this chapter). Likewise, it is not clear how useful fluctuating asymmetry will be in assessing individual differences. There appear to be sufficient stochastic processes during development that changes in symmetry in response to stress are difficult to detect at the individual level (Knierim et al. 2007). A stress signal is more likely to be detected at the population level. This means that, assuming a strong link can be forged between stress and fluctuating asymmetry, this technique will be most useful for exploring variation in responses to environmental and habitat changes.

X. PTILOCHRONOLOGY

Ptilochronology is the study of the growth of bird feathers, and specifically the formation of growth bars that reflect different protein deposition rates over a 24-hour cycle. The formation of these bars is sensitive to the nutritional status of the bird, which creates an obvious link to stressors that serve to reduce a bird's nutritional status. Grubb (2008) has written an excellent book that reviews ptilochronology and the connection to stress.

In many ways, ptilochronology is a technique related to fluctuating asymmetry. It focuses on developmental processes and so shares many of the advantages and drawbacks. Furthermore, ptilochonology is limited to studies on birds and to stressors that decrease the energy allocated to feather growth. However, it can be a very useful technique under these limited conditions.

XI. INTROCEREBROVENTRICULAR INJECTIONS IN THE FIELD

Behavior is obviously an important facet of any stress response and there are numerous techniques in animal behavior that can be applied to field studies of stress. Neural regulation of that behavior, however, has generally been restricted to the laboratory. Traditionally, suspected neuroactive peptides have been surgically injected directly into the brain, with subsequent monitoring of short-term behavioral changes. These studies implicitly assume that results can be generalized to freely behaving animals and that observed effects do not simply reflect laboratory conditions. Furthermore, results are assumed to reflect behavioral effects of endogenously released peptides in natural situations. Testing these assumptions outside the laboratory has been considered infeasible, if not impossible, due to difficulties in catching, observing, and administering short-acting peptides to wild animals.

We introduced a novel stereotaxic-like method for injecting substances into the lateral ventricles of small passerine birds (Romero and Wingfield 1997; Romero et al. 1998a). After capture, each bird is immediately anesthetized and placed on a Plexiglass surgical stage. A small hole is made in the skull, and hormones and neurotransmitters are injected directly into the lateral ventricle. Surgeries are completed within 6–10 minutes, and birds are released in 30–45 minutes. Behavioral effects of the hormones and neurotransmitters are then compared to treatment by a vehicle.

This technique has opened up a number of possibilities for studying the neurobiological mechanisms underlying natural behavioral responses. Rapid surgeries and a portable apparatus allow experiments without confounding variables from the laboratory. This permits studies of the regulation of ethologically relevant behaviors such as increased foraging during moderate storms (Astheimer et al. 1992) or abandonment of territories during severe storms (Wingfield et al. 1995b). Furthermore, there is no reason that the technique could not be extended to other vertebrate taxa.

However, there are several drawbacks to the technique. First, the required surgery can be disruptive to natural behavior. In the studies performed to date, only approximately two-thirds of the control birds resumed normal behavior, and even that was at a lower rate (Romero et al. 1998a). The technique is likely to be most useful when studying robust behavioral responses such as territorial defense. Second, few species, and no wild species, have stereotaxic brain atlases constructed for them. This makes accessing discrete brain regions very difficult. Although techniques have been introduced for injecting into other areas of the brain (Richardson and Boswell 1993), those techniques require far more involved surgery and would further decrease the chance of a bird showing natural behavior after the injection. Consequently, for all practical purposes, this technique will be

TABLE 6.4: SUMMARY OF TYPES OF VARIATION PROFITABLY ADDRESSED BY EACH TECHNIQUE FOR STUDYING STRESS IN FREE-LIVING ANIMALS

	Adaptations to Specific Habitats	Responses to Environmental Change	Facultative Changes	Individual Differences
Capture stress protocol	√	√	√	√
Fecal glucocorticoids	√	√	√	?
Urinary and salivary glucocorticoids	√	√	√	√
Monitoring heart rate	√	√	√	√
Heterophil/lyphocyte ratios	√	?	√	
Glucocorticoids in hair and feathers	√	√		√
Whale blow	√	√	√	√
Blood-sucking insects	?	?	?	?
Fluctuating asymmetry	√	√		
Ptilochronology	√	√		
Field introcerebroventricular injections	?	√		√

limited to global injections into the lateral ventricles. As an anecdote, one of us (JCW) recaptured one of the birds that received an injection into a cerebral ventricle four years after the event and on exactly the same territory! Although the technique may disturb the birds in the short term, long-term prospects appear to be normal.

XII. GLUCOCORTICOIDS IN EGG YOLK

Earlier work by Schwabl pioneered the measurement of steroid hormones deposited into egg yolk by the mother. These early studies were extensively validated and precipitated a broad front of subsequent work by many authors working on egg-laying vertebrates (Schwabl 1996). Measurement of steroid hormones in yolk, and their subsequent manipulation, provided valuable new insight into the effects of stress and maternal effects on development. Some of these studies focused on the extent to which stress in the environment, physical and social, affected a breeding female, resulting in the deposition of corticosteroids in yolk and/or albumin (e.g., Hayward and Wingfield 2004; Downing and Bryden 2008). Higher levels of corticosteroids in yolk are regarded a measurement of stress in breeding females, reflect circulating corticosteroids in the mother at the time of laying, and may influence the phenotype that develops (Hayward and Wingfield 2004; Hayward et al. 2005). However, there are still a number of technical difficulties that remain to be worked out in measuring corticosteroids in yolk, including determining how much corticosteroid is in the yolk (Rettenbacher et al. 2009).

Although much more work remains to be done in relation to stress and development, it must be pointed out here that severe stress would result in the cessation of laying and even abandonment of the nest (Chapters 4 and 5) and thus corticosteroids in yolk may represent high allostatic load for breeding females, but not sufficiently high corticosteroid levels to trigger a classic stress response. Implications for offspring developing from eggs with high corticosteroids remain to be clarified.

XIII. CONCLUSIONS

This chapter has presented some of the techniques that researchers have used to study stress in wild free-living animals. Table 6.4 summarizes these techniques, and predicts which of the four types of variation, presented at the beginning of this chapter, each technique would be best at addressing. One theme that should be apparent is that studying stress in field contexts is not easy. This probably should not be a surprise. After all, Selye formulated his General Adaptation Syndrome in part as a result of the difficulty of handling animals in a laboratory setting. The stress response is exquisitely sensitive to perceived or actual disturbances to an animal. Perhaps the biggest surprise should be that these stress responses can be studied in free-living animals at all.

REFERENCES

Accorsi, P. A., Carloni, E., Valsecchi, P., Viggiani, R., Garnberoni, M., Tarnanini, C., Seren, E., 2008. Cortisol determination in hair and faeces from domestic cats and dogs. *Gen Comp Endocrinol* 155, 398–402.

Ackerman, J. T., Takekawa, J. Y., Kruse, K. L., Orthmeyer, D. L., Yee, J. L., Ely, C. R., Ward, D. H., Bollinger, K. S., Mulcahy, D. M., 2004. Using radiotelemetry to monitor cardiac response of free-living tule greater white-fronted geese (*Anser albifrons elgasi*) to human disturbance. *Wilson Bull* 116, 146–151.

Adams, J. L., Camelio, K. W., Orique, M. J., Blumstein, D. T., 2006. Does information of predators influence general wariness? *Behav Ecol Sociobiol* 60, 742–747.

Adams, N. J., Cockrem, J. F., Taylor, G. A., Candy, E. J., Bridges, J., 2005. Corticosterone responses of grey-faced petrels (*Pterodroma macroptera gouldi*) are higher during incubation than during other breeding stages. *Physiol Biochem Zool* 78, 69–77.

Adams, N. J., Farnworth, M. J., Rickett, J., Parker, K. A., Cockrem, J. F., 2011. Behavioural and corticosterone responses to capture and confinement of wild blackbirds (*Turdus merula*). *Appl Anim Behav Sci* 134, 246–255.

Akana, S. F., Scribner, K. A., Bradbury, M. J., Strack, A. M., Walker, C. D., Dallman, M. F., 1992. Feedback sensitivity of the rat hypothalamo-pituitary-adrenal axis and its capacity to adjust to exogenous corticosterone. *Endocrinology* 131, 585–594.

AlKindi, A. Y. A., Al-Habsi, A. A., Mahmoud, I. Y., 2008. Changes in plasma levels of adrenaline, noradrenaline, glucose, lactate and CO2 in the green turtle, Chelonia mydas, during peak period of nesting. *Gen Comp Endocrinol* 155, 581–588.

Almedom, A. M., Teclemichael, T., Romero, L. M., Alemu, Z., 2005. Postnatal salivary cortisol and sense of coherence (SOC) in eritrean mothers. *Am J Human Biol* 17, 376–379.

Alvarez, F., Sanchez, C., Angulo, S., 2006. Relationships between tail-flicking, morphology, and body condition in Moorhens. *J Field Ornith* 77, 1–6.

Angelier, F., Moe, B., Weimerskirch, H., Chastel, O., 2007a. Age-specific reproductive success in a long-lived bird: Do older parents resist stress better? *J Anim Ecol* 76, 1181–1191.

Angelier, F., Shaffer, S. A., Weimerskirch, H., Chastel, O., 2006. Effect of age, breeding experience and senescence on corticosterone and prolactin levels in a long-lived seabird: The wandering albatross. *Gen Comp Endocrinol* 149, 1–9.

Angelier, F., Weimerskirch, H., Chastel, O., 2011. Capture and blood sampling do not affect foraging behaviour, breeding success and return rate of a large seabird: The black-browed albatross. *Polar Biol* 34, 353–361.

Angelier, F., Weimerskirch, H., Dano, S., Chastel, O., 2007b. Age, experience and reproductive performance in a long-lived bird: A hormonal perspective. *Behav Ecol Sociobiol* 61, 611–621.

Arlet, M. E., Grote, M. N., Molleman, F., Isbell, L. A., Carey, J. R., 2009. Reproductive tactics influence cortisol levels in individual male gray-cheeked mangabeys (Lophocebus albigena). Horm Behav 55, 210–216.

Arlettaz, R., Patthey, P., Baltic, M., Leu, T., Schaub, M., Palme, R., Jenni-Eiermann, S., 2007. Spreading free-riding snow sports represent a novel serious threat for wildlife. *Proc R Soc Lond B* 274, 1219–1224.

Armario, A., 2006. The hypothalamic-pituitary-adrenal axis: What can it tell us about stressors? *CNS Neurol Disord Drug Targ* 5, 485–501.

Arnold, J. M., Ordonez, R., Copeland, D. A., Nathan, R., Scornavacchi, J. M., Tyerman, D. J., Oswald, S. A., 2011. Simple and inexpensive devices to measure heart rates of incubating birds. *J Field Ornith* 82, 288–296.

Artacho, P., Soto-Gamboa, M., Verdugo, C., Nespolo, R. F., 2007. Using haematological parameters to infer the health and nutritional status of an endangered black-necked swan population. *Comp Biochem Physiol A* 147, 1060–1066.

Asa, C. S., Bauman, J. E., Coonan, T. J., Gray, M. M., 2007. Evidence for induced estrus or ovulation in a canid, the island fox (*Urocyon littoralis*). *J Mammal* 88, 436–440.

Aschauer, A., Hoffmann, I. E., Millesi, E., 2006. Endocrine profiles and reproductive output in European ground squirrels after unilateral ovariectomy. *Anim Repro Sci* 92, 392–400.

Ashley, N. T., Barboza, P. S., Macbeth, B. J., Janz, D. M., Cattet, M. R. L., Booth, R. K., Wasser, S. K., 2011. Glucocorticosteroid concentrations in feces and hair of captive caribou and reindeer following adrenocorticotropic hormone challenge. *Gen Comp Endocrinol* 172, 382–391.

Ashley, N. T., Wingfield, J. C., 2012. Sickness behavior in vertebrates. In: Demas, G. E., Nelson, R. J. (Eds.), *Ecoimmunology*. Oxford University Press, New York, pp. 45–91.

Astheimer, L. B., Buttemer, W. A., Wingfield, J. C., 1992. Interactions of corticosterone with feeding, activity and metabolism in passerine birds. *Ornis Scan* 23, 355–365.

Astheimer, L. B., Buttemer, W. A., Wingfield, J. C., 1995. Seasonal and acute changes in adrenocortical responsiveness in an arctic-breeding bird. *Horm Behav* 29, 442–457.

Astheimer, L. B., Buttemer, W. A., Wingfield, J. C., 2000. Corticosterone treatment has no effect on reproductive hormones or aggressive behavior in free-living male tree sparrows, *Spizella arborea*. *Horm Behav* 37, 31–39.

Averbeck, C., 1992. Haematology and blood chemistry of healthy and clinically abnormal great black-backed gulls larus-marinus and herring gulls *Larus-argentatus*. *Avian Path* 21, 215–223.

Bahr, N. I., Palme, R., Moehle, U., Hodges, J. K., Heistermann, M., 2000. Comparative aspects of the metabolism and excretion of cortisol in three individual nonhuman primates. *Gen Comp Endocrinol* 117, 427–438.

Bales, K. L., French, J. A., Hostetler, C. M., Dietz, J. M., 2005. Social and reproductive factors affecting cortisol levels in wild female golden lion tamarins (*Leontopithecus rosalia*). *Am J Primatol* 67, 25–35.

Barja, I., Silvan, G., Rosellini, S., Pineiro, A., Gonzalez-Gil, A., Camacho, L., Illera, J. C., 2007. Stress physiological responses to tourist pressure in a wild population of European pine marten. *J Steroid Biochem Mol Biol* 104, 136–142.

Barrett, G. M., Shimizu, K., Bardi, M., Asaba, S., Mori, A., 2002. Endocrine correlates of rank, reproduction, and female-directed aggression in male Japanese macaques (*Macaca fuscata*). *Horm Behav* 42, 85–96.

Bartsh, S. S., Johnston, S. D., Siniff, D. B., 1992. Territorial behavior and breeding frequency of male weddell seals (*Leptonychotes weddelli*) in relation to age, size, and concentrations of serum testosterone and cortisol. *Can J Zool* 70, 680–692.

Baylé, J. D., 1980. The adenohypophysiotropic mechanisms. In: Epple, A., Stetson, M.H. (Eds.), *Avian endocrinology*. Academic Press, New York, pp. 117–146.

Beale, C. M., Monaghan, P., 2004. Behavioural responses to human disturbance: A matter of choice? *Anim Behav* 68, 1065–1069.

Becker, P. H., Voigt, C. C., Arnold, J. M., Nagel, R., 2006. A non-invasive technique to bleed incubating birds without trapping: A blood-sucking bug in a hollow egg. *J Ornithol* 147, 115–118.

Beehner, J. C., McCann, C., 2008. Seasonal and altitudinal effects on glucocorticoid metabolites in a wild primate (*Theropithecus gelada*). *Physiol Behav* 95, 508–514.

Beehner, J. C., Whitten, P. L., 2004. Modifications of a field method for fecal steroid analysis in baboons. *Physiol Behav* 82, 269–277.

Belden, L. K., Moore, I. T., Mason, R. T., Wingfield, J. C., Blaustein, A. R., 2003. Survival, the hormonal stress response and UV-B avoidance in Cascades frog tadpoles (*Rana cascadae*) exposed to UV-B radiation. *Func Ecol* 17, 409–416.

Belden, L. K., Moore, I. T., Wingfield, J. C., Blaustein, A. R., 2005. Corticosterone and growth in Pacific treefrog (*Hyla regilla*) tadpoles. *Copeia* 424–430.

Bender, N., Heg, D., Hamilton, I. M., Bachar, Z., Taborsky, M., Oliveira, R. F., 2006. The relationship between social status, behaviour, growth and steroids in male helpers and breeders of a cooperatively breeding cichlid. *Horm Behav* 50, 173–182.

Benowitz-Fredericks, Z. M., Shultz, M. T., Kitaysky, A. S., 2008. Stress hormones suggest opposite trends of food availability for planktivorous and piscivorous seabirds in 2 years. *Deep Sea Res Part II Top Stud Oceanogr* 55, 1868–1876.

Bettinger, J. M., Tomasso, J. R., Isely, J. J., 2005. Hooking mortality and physiological responses of striped bass angled in freshwater and held in live-release tubes. *N Am J Fish Manag* 25, 1273–1280.

Bisson, I. A., Butler, L. K., Hayden, T. J., Kelley, P., Adelman, J. S., Romero, L. M., Wikelski, M. C., 2011. Energetic response to human disturbance in an endangered songbird. *Anim Conserv* 14, 484–491.

Bisson, I. A., Butler, L. K., Hayden, T. J., Romero, L. M., Wikelski, M. C., 2009. No energetic cost of anthropogenic disturbance in a songbird. *Proc R Soc Lond B* 276, 961–969.

Bize, P., Criscuolo, F., Metcalfe, N. B., Nasir, L., Monaghan, P., 2009. Telomere dynamics rather than age predict life expectancy in the wild. *Proc R Soc Lond B* 276, 1679–1683.

Bjorksten, T. A., Fowler, K., Pomiankowski, A., 2000. What does sexual trait FA tell us about stress? *Trends Ecol Evol* 15, 163–166.

Blanchard, D. C., Spencer, R. L., Weiss, S. M., Blanchard, R. J., McEwen, B., Sakai, R. R., 1995. Visible burrow system as a model of chronic social stress: Behavioral and neuroendocrine correlates. *Psychoneuroendocrinology* 20, 117–134.

Blas, J., Bortolotti, G. R., Tella, J. L., Baos, R., Marchant, T. A., 2007. Stress response during development predicts fitness in a wild, long lived vertebrate. *Proc Natl Acad Sci USA* 104, 8880–8884.

Blumstein, D. T., Patton, M. L., Saltzman, W., 2006. Faecal glucocorticoid metabolites and alarm calling in free-living yellow-bellied marmots. *Biol Lett* 2, 29–32.

Boinski, S., Swing, S. P., Gross, T. S., Davis, J. K., 1999. Environmental enrichment of brown capuchins (*Cebus apella*): Behavioral and plasma and fecal cortisol measures of effectiveness. *Am J Primatol* 48, 49–68.

Bókony, V., Lendvai, A. Z., Liker, A., Angelier, F., Wingfield, J. C., Chastel, O., 2009. Stress response and the value of reproduction: are birds prudent parents? *Am Nat* 173, 589–598.

Bonier, F., Martin, P. R., Sheldon, K. S., Jensen, J. P., Foltz, S. L., Wingfield, J. C., 2007a. Sex-specific consequences of life in the city. *Behav Ecol* 18, 121–129.

Bonier, F., Martin, P. R., Wingfield, J. C., 2007b. Maternal corticosteroids influence primary offspring sex ratio in a free-ranging passerine bird. *Behav Ecol* 18, 1045–1050.

Bonier, F., Quigley, H., Austad, S. N., 2004. A technique for non-invasively detecting stress response in cougars. *Wildlife Soc Bull* 32, 711–717.

Boonstra, R., McColl, C. J., 2000. Contrasting stress response of male Arctic ground squirrels and red squirrels. *J Exp Zool* 286, 390–404.

Boonstra, R., McColl, C. J., Karels, T. J., 2001. Reproduction at all costs: The adaptive stress response of male arctic ground squirrels. *Ecology (Washington DC)* 82, 1930–1946.

Boonstra, R., Singleton, G. R., 1993. Population declines in the snowshoe hare and the role of stress. *Gen Comp Endocrinol* 91, 126–143.

Bortolotti, G. R., 2010. Flaws and pitfalls in the chemical analysis of feathers: Bad news—good news for avian chemoecology and toxicology. *EcolApplic* 20, 1766–1774.

Bortolotti, G. R., Marchant, T., Blas, J., Cabezas, S., 2009a. Tracking stress: Localisation, deposition and stability of corticosterone in feathers. *J Exp Biol* 212, 1477–1482.

Bortolotti, G. R., Marchant, T. A., Blas, J., German, T., 2008. Corticosterone in feathers is a long-term, integrated measure of avian stress physiology. *Func Ecol* 22, 494–500.

Bortolotti, G. R., Mougeot, F., Martinez-Padilla, J., Webster, L. M. I., Piertney, S. B., 2009b. Physiological stress mediates the honesty of social signals. *Plos One* 4, e4983.

Bosson, C. O., Palme, R., Boonstra, R., 2009. Assessment of the stress response in Columbian ground squirrels: laboratory and field validation of an enzyme immunoassay for fecal cortisol metabolites. *Physiol Biochem Zool* 82, 291–301.

Boughton, R. K., Atwell, J. W., Schoech, S. J., 2006. An introduced generalist parasite, the sticktight flea (*Echidnophaga gallinacea*), and its pathology in the threatened Florida scrub-jay (*Aphelocoma coerulescens*). *J Parasitol* 92, 941–948.

Braasch, A., Palme, R., Hoppen, H. O., Becker, P. H., 2011. Body condition, hormonal correlates and consequences for survival in common tern chicks. *J Comp Physiol A* 197, 1009–1020.

Bradley, A. J., Kemper, C. M., Kitchener, D. J., Humphreys, W. F., How, R. A., Schmitt, L. H., 1988. Population ecology and physiology of the common rock rat *Zyzomys-argurus* Rodentia Muridae in tropical northwestern Australia. *J Mammal* 69, 749–764.

Brent, L. J. N., Semple, S., Dubuc, C., Heistermann, M., MacLarnon, A., 2011. Social capital and physiological stress levels in free-ranging adult female rhesus macaques. *Physiol Behav* 102, 76–83.

Breuner, C. W., Greenberg, A. L., Wingfield, J. C., 1998. Noninvasive corticosterone treatment rapidly increases activity in Gambel's white-crowned sparrows (*Zonotrichia leucophrys gambelii*). *Gen Comp Endocrinol* 111, 386–394.

Breuner, C. W., Jennings, D. H., Moore, M. C., Orchinik, M., 2000. Pharmacological adrenalectomy with mitotane. *Gen Comp Endocrinol* 120, 27–34.

Breuner, C. W., Lynn, S. E., Julian, G. E., Cornelius, J. M., Heidinger, B. J., Love, O. P., Sprague, R. S., Wada, H., Whitman, B. A., 2006. Plasma-binding globulins and acute stress response. *Horm Metab Res* 38, 260–268.

Breuner, C. W., Wingfield, J. C., Romero, L. M., 1999. Diel rhythms of basal and stress-induced corticosterone in a wild, seasonal vertebrate, Gambel's white-crowned sparrow. *J Exp Zool* 284, 334–342.

Brockman, D. K., Cobden, A. K., Whitten, P. L., 2009. Birth season glucocorticoids are related to the presence of infants in sifaka (*Propithecus verreauxi*). *Proc R Soc Lond B* 276, 1855–1863.

Brown, J. L., Bellem, A. C., Fouraker, M., Wildt, D. E., Roth, T. L., 2001. Comparative analysis of gonadal and adrenal activity in the black and white rhinoceros in North America by noninvasive endocrine monitoring. *Zoo Biology* 20, 463–486.

Brown, K. I., Nestor, K. E., 1973. Some physiological responses of turkeys selected for high and low adrenal response to cold stress. *Poult Sci* 52, 1948–1954.

Brown, M. B., Brown, C. R., 2009. Blood sampling reduces annual survival in cliff swallows (*Petrochelidon pyrrhonota*). *Auk* 126, 853–861.

Brownie, A. C., 1992. The metabolism of adrenal cortical steroids. In: James, V. H. T. (Ed.), *The adrenal gland*, 2nd Edition. Raven Press, New York, pp. 209–224.

Busch, D. S., Sperry, T. S., Peterson, E., Do, C. T., Wingfield, J. C., Boyd, E. H., 2008a. Impacts of frequent, acute pulses of corticosterone on condition and behavior of Gambel's white-crowned sparrow (*Zonotrichia leucophtys gambelii*). *Gen Comp Endocrinol* 158, 224–233.

Busch, D. S., Sperry, T. S., Wingfield, J. C., Boyd, E. H., 2008b. Effects of repeated, short-term, corticosterone administration on the hypothalamo-pituitary-adrenal axis of the white-crowned sparrow (*Zonotrichia leucophrys gambelii*). *Gen Comp Endocrinol* 158, 211–223.

Calisi, R. M., Bentley, G. E., 2009. Lab and field experiments: Are they the same animal? *Horm Behav* 56, 1–10.

Calvete, C., Angulo, E., Estrada, R., Moreno, S., Villafuerte, R., 2005. Quarantine length and survival of translocated European wild rabbits. *J Wildlife Manage* 69, 1063–1072.

Canoine, V., Hayden, T. J., Rowe, K., Goymann, W., 2002. The stress response of European stonechats depends on the type of stressor. *Behaviour* 139, 1303–1311.

Carere, C., Groothuis, T. G. G., Moestl, E., Daan, S., Koolhaas, J. M., 2003. Fecal corticosteroids in a territorial bird selected for different personalities: Daily rhythm and the response to social stress. *Horm Behav* 43, 540–548.

Carnegie, S. D., Fedigan, L. M., Ziegler, T. E., 2011. Social and environmental factors affecting fecal glucocorticoids in wild, female white-faced capuchins (*Cebus capucinus*). *Am J Primatol* 73, 861–869.

Carr, J. A., Zozzaro, P. E., 2004. The toad iris assay: a simple method for evaluating CRH action on the sympathetic nervous system. *Gen Comp Endocrinol* 135, 134–141.

Carragher, J. F., Rees, C. M., 1994. Primary and secondary stress responses in golden perch, *Macquaria-ambigua. Comp Biochem Physiol A* 107, 49–56.

Carroll, B., Feinberg, M., Greden, J., 1981. A specific laboratory test for the diagnosis of melancholia. *Arch Gen Psychiatry* 38, 15–23.

Case, B. C., Lewbart, G. A., Doerr, P. D., 2005. The physiological and behavioural impacts of and preference for an enriched environment in the eastern box turtle (*Terrapene carolina carolina*). *Appl Anim Behav Sci* 92, 353–365.

Cash, W. B., Holberton, R. L., Knight, S. S., 1997. Corticosterone secretion in response to capture and handling in free-living red-eared slider turtles. *Gen Comp Endocrinol* 108, 427–433.

Cavigelli, S. A., 1999. Behavioural patterns associated with faecal cortisol levels in free-ranging female ring-tailed lemurs, *Lemur catta. Anim Behav* 57, 935–944.

Chapman, C. A., Wasserman, M. D., Gillespie, T. R., Speirs, M. L., Lawes, M. J., Saj, T. L., Ziegler, T. E., 2006. Do food availability, parasitism, and stress have synergistic effects on red colobus populations living in forest fragments? *Am J Phys Anthropol* 131, 525–534.

Charbonnel, N., Chaval, Y., Berthier, K., Deter, J., Morand, S., Palme, R., Cosson, J. F., 2008. Stress and demographic decline: A potential effect mediated by impairment of reproduction and immune function in cyclic vole populations. *Physiol Biochem Zool* 81, 63–73.

Chastel, O., Lacroix, A., Weimerskirch, H., Gabrielsen, G. W., 2005. Modulation of prolactin but not corticosterone responses to stress in relation to parental effort in a long-lived bird. *Horm Behav* 47, 459–466.

Chaudhuri, S., Maiti, B. R., 1989. Changes in adrenal adrenaline and noradrenaline concentrations and blood glucose level during the seasonal gonadal cycle in the indian tree pie *Dendrocitta-vagabunda. J Yamashina Inst Ornithol* 21, 304–308.

Chelini, M. O. M., Otta, E., Yamakita, C., Palme, R., 2010. Sex differences in the excretion of fecal glucocorticoid metabolites in the Syrian hamster. *J Comp Physiol B* 180, 919–925.

Chinnadurai, S. K., Millspaugh, J. J., Matthews, W. S., Canter, K., Slotow, R., Washburn, B. E., Woods, R. J., 2009. Validation of fecal glucocorticoid metabolite assays for South African herbivores. *J Wildlife Manage* 73, 1014–1020.

Clark, T. D., Donaldson, M. R., Drenner, S. M., Hinch, S. G., Patterson, D. A., Hills, J., Ives, V., Carter, J. J., Cooke, S. J., Farrell, A. P., 2011. The efficacy of field techniques for obtaining and storing blood samples from fishes. *J Fish Biol* 79, 1322–1333.

Cleary, J. J., Pankhurst, N. W., Battaglene, S. C., 2000. The effect of capture and handling stress on plasma steroid levels and gonadal condition in wild and farmed snapper *Pagrus auratus* (Sparidae). *J World Aquacult Soc* 31, 558–569.

Clements, S. P., Hicks, B. J., Carragher, J. F., Dedual, M., 2002. The effect of a trapping procedure on the stress response of wild rainbow trout. *N Am J Fish Manage* 22, 907–916.

Coburn, S., Salman, M., Rhyan, J., Keefe, T., McCollum, M., 2010. Comparison of endocrine response to stress between captive-raised and wild-caught bighorn sheep. *J Wildlife Manage* 74, 532–538.

Cockrem, J. F., Potter, M. A., Candy, E. J., 2006. Corticosterone in relation to body mass in Adelie penguins (*Pygoscelis adeliae*) affected by unusual sea ice conditions at Ross Island, Antarctica. *Gen Comp Endocrinol* 149, 244–252.

Cockrem, J. F., Silverin, B., 2002. Variation within and between birds in corticosterone responses of great tits (*Parus major*). *Gen Comp Endocrinol* 125, 197–206.

Collette, J. C., Millam, J. R., Klasing, K. C., Wakenell, P. S., 2000. Neonatal handling of Amazon parrots alters the stress response and immune function. *Appl Anim Behav Sci* 66, 335–349.

Comendant, T., Sinervo, B., Svensson, E. I., Wingfield, J., 2003. Social competition, corticosterone and survival in female lizard morphs. *J Evolut Biol* 16, 948–955.

Cooke, S. J., Hinch, S. G., Wikelski, M., Andrews, R. D., Kuchel, L. J., Wolcott, T. G., Butler, P. J., 2004. Biotelemetry: A mechanistic approach to ecology. *Trends Ecol Evol* 19, 334–343.

Cornelius, J. M., Perfito, N., Zann, R., Breuner, C. W., Hahn, T. P., 2011. Physiological trade-offs in self-maintenance: Plumage molt and stress physiology in birds. *J Exp Biol* 214, 2768–2777.

Cree, A., Amey, A. P., Whittier, J. M., 2000. Lack of consistent hormonal responses to capture during the breeding season of the bearded dragon, *Pogona barbata. Comp Biochem Physiol* 126A, 275–285.

Creel, S., 2001. Social dominance and stress hormones. *Trends Ecol Evol* 16, 491–497.

Creel, S., Creel, N., Wildt, D. E., Monfort, S. L., 1992. Behavioural and endocrine mechanisms of reproductive suppression in Serengeti dwarf mongooses. *Anim Behav* 43, 231–245.

Creel, S., Creel, N. M., Monfort, S. L., 1996. Social stress and dominance. *Nature* 379, 212.

Creel, S., Creel, N. M., Monfort, S. L., 1997. Radiocollaring and stress hormones in african wild dogs. *Conserv Biol* 11, 544–548.

Creel, S., Fox, J. E., Hardy, A., Sands, J., Garrott, B., Peterson, R. O., 2002. Snowmobile activity and glucocorticoid stress responses in wolves and elk. *Conserv Biol* 16, 809–814.

Crino, O. L., Larkin, I., Phelps, S. M., 2010. Stress coping styles and singing behavior in the short-tailed singing mouse (*Scotinomys teguina*). *Horm Behav* 58, 334–340.

Criscuolo, F., Bertile, F., Durant, J. M., Raclot, T., Gabrielsen, G. W., Massemin, S., Chastel, O., 2006. Body mass and clutch size may modulate prolactin and corticosterone levels in eiders. *Physiol Biochem Zool* 79, 514–521.

Criscuolo, F., Gauthier-Clerc, M., Le Maho, Y., Gabrielsen, G. W., 2001. Brood patch temperature during provocation of incubating common eiders in Ny-Alesund, Svalbard. *Polar Res* 20, 115–118.

Crofoot, M., Mace, M., Azua, J., MacDonald, E., Czekala, N. M., 2003. Reproductive assessment of the great hornbill (*Buceros bicornis*) by fecal hormone analysis. *Zoo Biol* 22, 135–145.

Cross, N., Pines, M. K., Rogers, L. J., 2004. Saliva sampling to assess cortisol levels in unrestrained common marmosets and the effect of behavioral stress. *Am J Primatol* 62, 107–114.

Curley, J. P., Keverne, E. B., 2005. Genes, brains and mammalian social bonds. *Trends Ecol Evol* 20, 561–567.

Cyr, N. E., Romero, L. M., 2007. Chronic stress in free-living European starlings reduces corticosterone concentrations and reproductive success. *Gen Comp Endocrinol* 151, 82–89.

Cyr, N. E., Romero, L. M., 2008. Fecal glucocorticoid metabolites of experimentally stressed captive and free-living starlings: Implications for conservation research. *Gen Comp Endocrinol* 158, 20–28.

Dalerum, F., Creel, S., Hall, S. B., 2006. Behavioral and endocrine correlates of reproductive failure in social aggregations of captive wolverines (*Gulo gulo*). *J Zool* 269, 527–536.

Dallman, M. F., Bhatnagar, S., 2001. Chronic stress and energy balance: role of the hypothalamo-pituitary-adrenal axis. In: McEwen, B. S., Goodman, H. M. (Eds.), *Handbook of physiology*; Section 7: *The endocrine system*; Vol. IV: *Coping with the environment: Neural and endocrine mechanisms*. Oxford University Press, New York, pp. 179–210.

Dallman, M. F., Strack, A. M., Akana, S. F., Bradbury, M. J., Hanson, E. S., Scribner, K. A., Smith, M., 1993. Feast and famine: Critical role of glucocorticoids with insulin in daily energy flow. *Front Neuroendocrinol* 14, 303–347.

Dalmau, A., Ferret, A., Chacon, G., Manteca, X., 2007. Seasonal changes in fecal cortisol metabolites in Pyrenean chamois. *J Wildlife Manage* 71, 190–194.

Dantzer, B., McAdam, A. G., Palme, R., Boutin, S., Boonstra, R., 2011. How does diet affect fecal steroid hormone metabolite concentrations? An experimental examination in red squirrels. *Gen Comp Endocrinol* 174, 124–131.

Dantzer, B., McAdam, A. G., Palme, R., Fletcher, Q. E., Boutin, S., Humphries, M. M., Boonstra, R., 2010. Fecal cortisol metabolite levels in free-ranging North American red squirrels: Assay validation and the effects of reproductive condition. *Gen Comp Endocrinol* 167, 279–286.

Darlington, D. N., Chew, G., Ha, T., Keil, L. C., Dallman, M. F., 1990a. Corticosterone, but not glucose, treatment enables fasted adrenalectomized rats to survive moderate hemorrhage. *Endocrinology* 127, 766–772.

Darlington, D. N., Neves, R. B., Ha, T., Chew, G., Dallman, M. F., 1990b. Fed, but not fasted, adrenalectomized rats survive the stress of hemorrhage and hypovolemia. *Endocrinology* 127, 759–765.

Dathe, H. H., Kuckelkorn, B., Minnemann, D., 1992. Salivary cortisol assessment for stress detection in the Asian elephant *Elephas-maximus*: A pilot study. *Zoo Biology* 11, 285–289.

Dauphin-Villemant, C., Xavier, F., 1987. Nychthemeral variations of plasma corticosteroids in captive female *Lacerta vivipara* Jacquin: Influence of stress and reproductive state. *Gen Comp Endocrinol* 67, 292–302.

Davenport, M. D., Tiefenbacher, S., Lutz, C. K., Novak, M. A., Meyer, J. S., 2006. Analysis of endogenous cortisol concentrations in the hair of rhesus macaques. *Gen Comp Endocrinol* 147, 255.

Davidson, G. W., Thorarensen, H. T., Lokman, M., Davie, P. S., 1997. Stress of capture and captivity in kahawai *Arripis trutta* (Bloch and Schneider) (Perciformes: Arripidae). *Comp Biochem Physiol A* 118, 1405–1410.

Davis, A. K., 2005. Effect of handling time and repeated sampling on avian white blood cell counts. *J Field Ornith* 76, 334–338.

Davis, A. K., Maney, D. L., Maerz, J. C., 2008. The use of leukocyte profiles to measure stress in vertebrates: A review for ecologists. *Func Ecol* 22, 760–772.

Dawson, A., Howe, P. D., 1983. Plasma corticosterone in wild starlings (*Sturnus vulgaris*) immediately following capture and in relation to body weight during the annual cycle. *Gen Comp Endocrinol* 51, 303–308.

De Villiers, M., Bause, M., Giese, M., Fourie, A., 2006. Hardly hard-hearted: heart rate responses of incubating northern giant petrels (*Macronectes halli*) to human disturbance on sub-Antarctic Marion Island. *Polar Biol* 29, 717–720.

De Villiers, M. S., Van Jaarsveld, A. S., Meltzer, D. G. A., Richardson, P. R. K., 1997. Social dynamics and the cortisol response to immobilization stress of the African wild dog, *Lycaon pictus*. *Horm Behav* 31, 3–14.

Dehnhard, M., Clauss, M., Lechner-Doll, M., Meyer, H. H. D., Palme, R., 2001. Noninvasive monitoring of adrenocortical activity in roe deer (*Capreolus capreolus*) by measurement of fecal cortisol metabolites. *Gen Comp Endocrinol* 123, 111–120.

Dehnhard, M., Schreer, A., Krone, O., Jewgenow, K., Krause, M., Grossmann, R., 2003. Measurement of plasma corticosterone and fecal glucocorticoid metabolites in the chicken (*Gallus domesticus*), the great cormorant (*Phalacrocorax carbo*), and the goshawk (*Accipiter gentilis*). *Gen Comp Endocrinol* 131, 345–352.

Delehanty, B., Boonstra, R., 2009. Impact of live trapping on stress profiles of Richardson's ground squirrel (*Spermophilus richardsonii*). *Gen Comp Endocrinol* 160, 176–182.

Dembiec, D. P., Snider, R. J., Zanella, A. J., 2004. The effects of transport stress on tiger physiology and behavior. *Zoo Biol* 23, 335–346.

Denollet, J., 1998. Personality and coronary heart disease: The Type-D scale-16 (DS16). *Ann Behav Med* 20, 209–215.

Dickens, M. J., Delehanty, D. J., Romero, L. M., 2009. Stress and translocation: alterations in the stress physiology of translocated birds. *Proc R Soc Lond B* 276, 2051–2056.

Dickens, M. J., Romero, L. M., 2013. A consensus endocrine profile for a chronically stressed wild animal does not exist. *Gen Comp Endocrinol.* 191, 177–189.

Dittami, J., Katina, S., Mostl, E., Eriksson, J., Machatschke, I. H., Hohmann, G., 2008. Urinary androgens and cortisol metabolites in field-sampled bonobos (*Pan paniscus*). *Gen Comp Endocrinol* 155, 552–557.

Doherty, T. J., Kattesh, H. G., Adcock, R. J., Welborn, M. G., Saxton, A. M., Morrow, J. L., Dailey, J. W., 2007. Effects of a concentrated lidocaine solution on the acute phase stress response to dehorning in dairy calves. *J Dairy Sci* 90, 4232–4239.

Douglas, H. D., Kitaysky, A. S., Kitaiskaia, E. V., Maccormick, A., Kelly, A., 2009. Size of ornament is negatively correlated with baseline corticosterone in males of a socially monogamous colonial seabird. *J Comp Physiol B* 179, 297–304.

Downing, J. A., Bryden, W. L., 2008. Determination of corticosterone concentrations in egg albumen: A non-invasive indicator of stress in laying hens. *Physiol Behav* 95, 381–387.

Dreschel, N. A., Granger, D. A., 2009. Methods of collection for salivary cortisol measurement in dogs. *Horm Behav* 55, 163–168.

Dunlap, K. D., Schall, J. J., 1995. Hormonal alterations and reproductive inhibition in male fence lizards (*Sceloporus occidentalis*) infected with the malarial parasite *Plasmodium mexicanum*. *Physiol Zool* 68, 608–621.

Dunlap, K. D., Wingfield, J. C., 1995. External and internal influences on indices of physiological stress: I. Seasonal and population variation in adrenocortical secretion of free-living lizards, *Sceloporus occidentalis*. *J Exp Zool* 271, 36–46.

Ebensperger, L. A., Ramirez-Estrada, J., Leon, C., Castro, R. A., Tolhuysen, L. O., Sobrero, R., Quirici, V., Burger, J. R., Soto-Gamboa, M., Hayes, L. D., 2011. Sociality, glucocorticoids and direct fitness in the communally rearing rodent, *Octodon degus*. *Horm Behav* 60, 346–352.

Edler, R., Klump, G. M., Friedl, T. W. P., 2004. Do blood parasites affect reproductive performance in male red bishops (*Euplectes orix*)? A test of the Hamilton-Zuk hypothesis. *Ethol Ecol Evolution* 16, 315–328.

Eeva, T., Hasselquist, D., Langefors, A., Tummeleht, L., Nikinmaa, M., Ilmonen, P., 2005. Pollution related effects on immune function and stress in a free-living population of pied flycatcher *Ficedula hypoleuca*. *J Avian Biol* 36, 405–412.

Eilam, D., 2005. Die hard: A blend of freezing and fleeing as a dynamic defense—implications for the control of defensive behavior. *NeurosciBiobehav Rev* 29, 1181–1191.

Eiserman, K., 1992. Long-term heart rate responses to social stress in wild european rabbits: predominant effect of rank position. *Physiol Behav* 52, 33–36.

Ellenberg, U., Mattern, T., Seddon, P. J., Jorquera, G.L., 2006. Physiological and reproductive consequences of human disturbance in Humboldt penguins: The need for species-specific visitor management. *Biol Conserv* 133, 95–106.

Ellenberg, U., Setiawan, A. N., Cree, A., Houston, D. M., Seddon, P. J., 2007. Elevated hormonal stress response and reduced reproductive output in Yellow-eyed penguins exposed to unregulated tourism. *Gen Comp Endocrinol* 152, 54–63.

Ellis, D. H., Ellis, C. H., Mindell, D. P., 1991. Raptor responses to low-level jet aircraft and sonic-booms. *Environ Pollut* 74, 53–83.

Elsey, R. M., Lance, V. A., Joanen, T., McNease, L., 1991. Acute stress suppresses plasma estradiol levels in female alligators (*Alligator-mississippiensis*). *Comp Biochem Physiol A* 100, 649–651.

Ely, C. R., Ward, D. H., Bollinger, K. S., 1999. Behavioral correlates of heart rates of free-living greater white-fronted geese. *Condor* 101, 390–395.

Engelhard, G. H., Brasseur, S., Hall, A. J., Burton, H. R., Reijnders, P. J. H., 2002. Adrenocortical responsiveness in southern elephant seal mothers and pups during lactation and the effect of scientific handling. *J Comp Physiol B* 172, 315–328.

Epel, E. S., Blackburn, E. H., Lin, J., Dhabhar, F. S., Adler, N. E., Morrow, J. D., Cawthon, R. M., 2004. Accelerated telomere shortening in response to life stress. *Proc Natl Acad Sci USA* 101, 17312–17315.

Espmark, Y., Langvatn, R., 1985. Development and habituation of cardiac and behavioral-responses in young red deer calves (*Cervus-elaphus*) exposed to alarm stimuli. *J Mammal* 66, 702–711.

Evans, M. R., Roberts, M. L., Buchanan, K. L., Goldsmith, A. R., 2006. Heritability of corticosterone response and changes in life history traits during selection in the zebra finch. *J Evolut Biol* 19, 343–352.

Ewenson, E. L., Zann, R. A., Flannery, G. R., 2001. Body condition and immune response in wild zebra finches: Effects of capture, confinement and captive-rearing. *Naturwissenschaften* 88, 391–394.

Fairhurst, G. D., Frey, M. D., Reichert, J. F., Szelest, I., Kelly, D. M., Bortolotti, G. R., 2011. Does environmental enrichment reduce stress? An integrated measure of corticosterone from feathers provides a novel perspective. *Plos One* 6, e17663.

Fenske, M., 1996. Measurement of salivary cortisol in guinea pigs. *J Exper Animal Sci* 38, 13–19.

Fink, G.E.-i.-C., 2007. *Encyclopedia of stress*, 2nd Edition. Academic Press, Oxford.

Fletcher, Q. E., Boonstra, R., 2006. Impact of live trapping on the stress response of the meadow vole (*Microtus pennsylvanicus*). *J Zool (London)* 270, 473–478.

Foerster, S., Cords, M., Monfort, S. L., 2011. Social behavior, foraging strategies, and fecal glucocorticoids in female blue monkeys (*Cercopithecus mitis*): Potential fitness benefits of high rank in a forest guenon. *Am J Primatol* 73, 870–882.

Foley, C. A. H., Papageorge, S., Wasser, S. K., 2001. Noninvasive stress and reproductive measures of social and ecological pressures in free-ranging African elephants. *Conserv Biol* 15, 1134–1142.

Fourie, N. H., Bernstein, R. M., 2011. Hair cortisol levels track phylogenetic and age related differences in hypothalamic-pituitary-adrenal (HPA) axis activity in non-human primates. *Gen Comp Endocrinol* 174, 150–155.

Franceschini, C., Siutz, C., Palme, R., Millesi, E., 2007. Seasonal changes in cortisol and progesterone secretion in common hamsters. *Gen Comp Endocrinol* 152, 14–21.

Franceschini, M. D., Rubenstein, D. I., Low, B., Romero, L. M., 2008. Fecal glucocorticoid metabolites as an indicator of stress during translocation and acclimation in an endangered large mammal, the Grevy's zebra. *Anim Conserv* 11, 263–269.

French, S. S., McLemore, R., Vernon, B., Johnston, G. I. H., Moore, M. C., 2007. Corticosterone modulation of reproductive and immune systems trade-offs in female tree lizards: Long-term corticosterone manipulations via injectable gelling material. *J Exp Biol* 210, 2859–2865.

Friedl, T. W. P., Edler, R., 2005. Stress-dependent trade-off between immunological condition and reproductive performance in the polygynous red bishop (*Euplectes orix*). *Evolut Ecol* 19, 221–239.

Frigerio, D., Dittami, J., Mostl, E., Kotrschal, K., 2004. Excreted corticosterone metabolites co-vary with ambient temperature and air pressure in male greylag geese (*Anser anser*). *Gen Comp Endocrinol* 137, 29–36.

Frigerio, D., Moestl, E., Kotrschal, K., 2001. Excreted metabolites of gonadal steroid hormones and corticosterone in greylag geese (*Anser anser*) from hatching to fledging. *Gen Comp Endocrinol* 124, 246–255.

Frisch, A., Anderson, T., 2005. Physiological stress responses of two species of coral trout (*Plectropomus leopardus* and *Plectropomus maculatus*). *Comp Biochem Physiol A* 140, 317–327.

Frisch, A. J., Anderson, T. A., 2000. The response of coral trout (Plectropomus leopardus) to capture, handling and transport and shallow water stress. *Fish Physiol Biochem* 23, 23–34.

Funder, J. W., Pearce, P. T., Smith, R., Smith, A. I., 1988. Mineralocorticoid action: Target tissue-specificity is enzyme, not receptor, mediated. *Science* 242, 583–585.

Gabrielsen, G. W., Blix, A. S., Ursin, H., 1985. Orienting and freezing responses in incubating ptarmigan hens. *Physiol Behav* 34, 925–934.

Gabrielsen, G. W., Smith, E. N., 1985. Physiological responses associaed with feigned death in the American opossum. *Acta Physiol Scand* 123, 393–398.

Gallman, E. A., Isely, J. J., Tomasso, J. R., Smith, T. I. J., 1999. Short-term physiological responses of wild and hatchery-produced red drum during angling. *N Am J Fish Manage* 19, 833–836.

Gambelunghe, C., Sommavilla, M., Ferranti, C., Rossi, R., Aroni, K., Manes, N., Bacci, M., 2007. Analysis of anabolic steroids in hair by GC/MS/MS. *Biomed Chromat* 21, 369–375.

Ganswindt, A., Palme, R., Heistermann, M., Borragan, S., Hodges, J. K., 2003. Non-invasive assessment of adrenocortical function in the male African elephant (*Loxodonta africana*) and its relation to musth. *Gen Comp Endocrinol* 134, 156–166.

Garamszegi, L. Z., Merino, S., Toeroek, J., Eens, M., Martinez, J., 2006. Indicators of physiological stress and the elaboration of sexual traits in the collared flycatcher. *Behav Ecol* 17, 399–404.

Gerlinskaya, L. A., Zav'yalov, E. L., Evsikov, V. I., 2000. Variation of steroid hormones in the musk deer *Moschus moschiferus* (Moschidae, Artiodactyla) feces. *Zoologicheskii Zhurnal* 79, 608–614.

Gesquiere, L. R., Altmann, J., Khan, M. Z., Couret, J., Yu, J. C., Endres, C. S., Lynch, J. W., Ogola, P., Fox, E. A., Alberts, S. C., Wango, E. O., 2005. Coming of age: Steroid hormones of wild immature baboons (*Papio cynocephalus*). *Am J Primatol* 67, 83–100.

Gill, F. B., 1995. *Ornithology*. W. H. Freeman, New York.

Girard-Buttoz, C., Heistermann, M., Krummel, S., Engelhardt, A., 2009. Seasonal and social influences on fecal androgen and glucocorticoid excretion in wild male long-tailed macaques (*Macaca fascicularis*). *Physiol Behav* 98, 168–175.

Girling, J. E., Cree, A., 1995. Plasma corticosterone levels are not significantly related to reproductive stage in female common geckos (*Hoplodactylus maculatus*). *Gen Comp Endocrinol* 100, 273–281.

Gladbach, A., Gladbach, D. J., Koch, M., Kuchar, A., Mostl, E., Quillfeldt, P., 2011. Can faecal glucocorticoid metabolites be used to monitor body condition in wild upland geese *Chloephaga picta leucoptera*? *Behav Ecol Sociobiol* 65, 1491–1498.

Godwin, J. R., Thomas, P., 1993. Sex change and steroid profiles in the protandrous anemonefish *Amphiprion melanopus* (Pomacentridae, Teleostei). *Gen Comp Endocrinol* 91, 144–157.

Good, T., Khan, M. Z., Lynch, J. W., 2003. Biochemical and physiological validation of a corticosteroid radioimmunoassay for plasma and fecal samples in oldfield mice (*Peromyscus polionotus*). *Physiol Behav* 80, 405–411.

Goodson, J. L., 2005. The vertebrate social behavior network: Evolutionary themes and variations. *Horm Behav* 48, 11–22.

Goymann, W., 2005. Noninvasive monitoring of hormones in bird droppings: Physiological validation, sampling, extraction, sex differences, and the influence of diet on hormone metabolite levels. *Ann NY Acad Sci*, 1046, 35–53.

Goymann, W., 2012. On the use of non-invasive hormone research in uncontrolled, natural environments: the problem with sex, diet, metabolic rate and the individual. *Methods Ecol Evol* 3, 757–765.

Goymann, W., East, M. L., Wachter, B., Hoener, O. P., Moestl, E., Hofer, H., 2003. Social status does not predict corticosteroid levels in postdispersal male spotted hyenas. *Horm Behav* 43, 474–479.

Goymann, W., Moestl, E., Van't Hof, T., East, M. L., Hofer, H., 1999. Noninvasive fecal monitoring of glucocorticoids in spotted hyenas, *Crocuta crocuta*. *Gen Comp Endocrinol* 114, 340–348.

Goymann, W., Mostl, E., Gwinner, E., 2002. Corticosterone metabolites can be measured noninvasively in excreta of European stonechats (*Saxicola torquata rubicola*). *Auk* 119, 1167–1173.

Goymann, W., Trappschuh, M., Jensen, W., Schwabl, I., 2006. Low ambient temperature increases food intake and dropping production, leading to incorrect estimates of hormone metabolite concentrations in European stonechats. *Horm Behav* 49, 644–653.

Goymann, W., Wingfield, J. C., 2004. Allostatic load, social status and stress hormones: the costs of social status matter. *Anim Behav* 67, 591–602.

Graham, L. H., Brown, J. L., 1996. Cortisol metabolism in the domestic cat and implications for non-invasive monitoring of adrenocortical function in endangered felids. *Zoo Biol* 15, 71–82.

Grassman, M., Hess, D. L., 1992. Sex differences in adrenal function in the lizard *Cnemidophorus sexlineatus*: I. Seasonal variation in the field. *J Exp Zool* 264, 177–182.

Gratacos-Cubarsi, M., Castellari, M., Valero, A., Garcia-Regueiro, J. A., 2006. Hair analysis for veterinary drug monitoring in livestock production. *J Chromatog B* 834, 14–25.

Greenberg, N., Wingfield, J., 1987. Stress and reproduction: Reciprocal relationships. In: Norris, D. O., Jones, R. E. (Eds.), *Hormones and reproduction in fishes, amphibians, and reptiles*. Plenum Press, New York, pp. 461–503.

Gregory, L. F., Gross, T. S., Bolten, A. B., Bjorndal, K. A., Guillette, L. J., Jr., 1996. Plasma corticosterone concentrations associated with acute captivity stress in wild loggerhead sea turtles (*Caretta caretta*). *Gen Comp Endocrinol* 104, 312–320.

Gregory, L. F., Schmid, J. R., 2001. Stress responses and sexing of wild Kemp's ridley sea turtles (*Lepidochelys kempii*) in the Northeastern Gulf of Mexico. *Gen Comp Endocrinol* 124, 66–74.

Groombridge, J. J., Massey, J. G., Bruch, J. C., Malcolm, T. R., Brosius, C. N., Okada, M. M., Sparklin, B., 2004. Evaluating stress in a Hawaiian honeycreeper, *Paroreomyza montana*, following translocation. *J Field Ornith* 75, 183–187.

Gross, W. B., Siegel, P. B., 1985. Selective breeding of chickens for corticosterone response to social stress. *Poult Sci* 64, 2230–2233.

Grubb, T. C., 2008. *Ptilochronology: Feather time and the biology of birds*. Oxford University Press, New York.

Grutter, A. S., Pankhurst, N. W., 2000. The effects of capture, handling, confinement and ectoparasite load on plasma levels of cortisol, glucose and lactate in the coral reef fish Hemigymnus melapterus. *J Fish Biol* 57, 391–401.

Gulland, F. M. D., Haulena, M., Lowenstine, L. J., Munro, C., Graham, P. A., Bauman, J., Harvey, J., 1999. Adrenal function in wild and rehabilitated Pacific harbor seals (*Phoca vitulina richardii*) and in seals with phocine herpesvirus-associated adrenal necrosis. *Marine Mammal Sci* 15, 810–827.

Gutman, R., Dayan, T., Levy, O., Schubert, I., Kronfeld-Schor, N., 2011. The effect of the lunar cycle on fecal cortisol metabolite levels and foraging ecology of nocturnally and diurnally active spiny mice. *Plos One* 6, 9.

Haddy, J. A., Pankhurst, N. W., 2000. The efficacy of exogenous hormones in stimulating changes in plasma steroids and ovulation in wild black bream *Acanthopagrus butcheri* is improved by treatment at capture. *Aquaculture* 191, 351–366.

Hajduk, P., Copland, M. D., Schultz, D. A., 1992. Effects of capture on hematological values and plasma cortisol levels of free-range koalas *Phascolarctos-cinereus*. *J Wildlife Dis* 28, 502–506.

Hamann, M., Limpus, C. J., Whittier, J. M., 2003. Seasonal variation in plasma catecholamines and adipose tissue lipolysis in adult female green sea turtles (*Chelonia mydas*). *Gen Comp Endocrinol* 130, 308–316.

Hanauska-Brown, L. A., Dufty, A. M., Jr., Roloff, G. J., 2003. Blood chemistry, cytology, and body condition in adult northern goshawks (*Accipiter gentilis*). *J Raptor Res* 37, 299–306.

Handasyde, K. A., McDonald, I. R., Evans, B. K., 2003. Plasma glucocorticoid concentrations in free-ranging platypuses (*Ornithorhynchus anatinus*): Response to capture and patterns in relation to reproduction. *Comp Biochem Physiol A* 136A, 895–902.

Harms, C. A., Fleming, W. J., Stoskopf, M. K., 1997. A technique for dorsal subcutaneous implantation of heart rate biotelemetry transmitters in black ducks: Application in an aircraft noise response study. *Condor* 99, 231–237.

Harms, N. J., Fairhurst, G. D., Bortolotti, G. R., Smits, J. E. G., 2010. Variation in immune function, body condition, and feather corticosterone in nestling tree swallows (*Tachycineta bicolor*) on reclaimed wetlands in the Athabasca oil sands, Alberta, Canada. *Environ Pollut* 158, 841–848.

Harper, J. M., Austad, S. N., 2000. Fecal glucocorticoids: a noninvasive method of measuring adrenal activity in wild and captive rodents. *Physiol Biochem Zool* 73, 12–22.

Hart, B. L., 1988. Biological basis of the behavior of sick animals. *Neurosci Biobehav Rev* 12, 123–137.

Hartup, B. K., Olsen, G. H., Czekala, N. M., 2005. Fecal corticoid monitoring in whooping cranes (*Grus americana*) undergoing reintroduction. *Zoo Biol* 24, 15–28.

Harvey, S., Phillips, J. G., Rees, A., Hall, T. R., 1984. Stress and adrenal function. *J Exp Zool* 232, 633–645.

Hattingh, J., Pitts, N. I., Ganhao, M. F., 1988. Immediate response to repeated capture and handling of wild impala. *J Exp Zool* 248, 109–112.

Haussmann, M. F., Marchetto, N. M., 2010. Telomeres: Linking stress and survival, ecology and evolution. *Curr Zool* 56, 714–727.

Hayward, L. S., Satterlee, D. G., Wingfield, J. C., 2005. Japanese quail selected for high plasma corticosterone response deposit high levels of corticosterone in their eggs. *Physiol Biochem Zool* 78, 1026–1031.

Hayward, L. S., Wingfield, J. C., 2004. Maternal corticosterone is transferred to avian yolk and may alter offspring growth and adult phenotype. *Gen Comp Endocrinol* 135, 365–371.

Heath, J., 1997. Corticosterone levels during nest departure of juvenile American kestrels. *Condor* 99, 806–811.

Heidinger, B. J., Nisbet, I. C. T., Ketterson, E. D., 2006. Older parents are less responsive to a stressor in a long-lived seabird: A mechanism for increased reproductive performance with age? *Proc R Soc Lond B* 273, 2227–2231.

Heistermann, M., Palme, R., Ganswindt, A., 2006. Comparison of different enzyme-immunoassays for assessment of adrenocortical activity in primates based on fecal analysis. *Am J Primatol* 68, 257–273.

Hiebert, S. M., Ramenofsky, M., Salvante, K., Wingfield, J. C., Gass, C. L., 2000a. Noninvasive methods for measuring and manipulating corticosterone in hummingbirds. *Gen Comp Endocrinol* 120, 235–247.

Hiebert, S. M., Salvante, K. G., Ramenofsky, M., Wingfield, J. C., 2000b. Corticosterone and nocturnal torpor in the rufous hummingbird (*Selasphorus rufus*). *Gen Comp Endocrinol* 120, 220–234.

Higham, J. P., Vitale, A. B., Rivera, A. M., Ayala, J. E., Maestripieri, D., 2010. Measuring salivary analytes from free-ranging monkeys. *Physiol Behav* 101, 601–607.

Hirschenhauser, K., Kotrschal, K., Moestl, E., 2005. Synthesis of measuring steroid metabolites in goose feces. Ann NY Acad Sci, 1046, 138–153.

Hirschenhauser, K., Moestl, E., Peczely, P., Wallner, B., Dittami, J., Kotrschal, K., 2000. Seasonal relationships between plasma and fecal testosterone in response to GnRH in domestic ganders. *Gen Comp Endocrinol* 118, 262–272.

Hodgson, Z. G., Meddle, S. L., Roberts, M. L., Buchanan, K. L., Evans, M. R., Metzdorf, R., Gahr, M., Healy, S. D., 2007. Spatial ability is impaired and hippocampal mineralocorticoid receptor mRNA expression reduced in zebra finches (*Taeniopygia guttata*) selected for acute high corticosterone response to stress. *Proc R Soc Lond B* 274, 239–245.

Hogan, L. A., Johnston, S. D., Lisle, A. T., Keeley, T., Wong, P., Nicolson, V., Horsup, A. B., Janssen, T., Phillips, C. J. C., 2011. Behavioural and physiological responses of captive wombats (*Lasiorhinus latifrons*) to regular handling by humans. *Appl Anim Behav Sci* 134, 217–228.

Hogg, C., Rogers, T., Vickers, E. R., 2006. Reproductive hormones are unstable in some non-invasive samples. *J Exp Zool A: Comp Exp Biol* 305A, 133–133.

Hogg, C. J., Vickers, E. R., Rogers, T. L., 2005. Determination of testosterone in saliva and blow of bottlenose dolphins (*Tursiops truncatus*) using liquid chromatography-mass spectrometry. *J Chromatog B* 814, 339–346.

Holberton, R. L., Helmuth, B., Wingfield, J. C., 1996a. The corticosterone stress response in gentoo and king penguins during the non-fasting period. *Condor* 98, 850–854.

Holberton, R. L., Parrish, J. D., Wingfield, J. C., 1996b. Modulation of the adrenocortical stress response in neotropical migrants during autumn migration. *Auk* 113, 558–564.

Holberton, R. L., Wingfield, J. C., 2003. Modulating the corticosterone stress response: A mechanism for balancing individual risk and reproductive success in Arctic-breeding sparrows? *Auk* 120, 1140–1150.

Holmes, N., Giese, M., Kriwoken, L. K., 2005. Testing the minimum approach distance guidelines for incubating royal penguins *Eudyptes schlegeli*. *Biol Conserv* 126, 339–350.

Homan, R. N., Reed, J. M., Romero, L. M., 2003a. Corticosterone concentrations in free-living spotted salamanders (*Ambystoma maculatum*). *Gen Comp Endocrinol* 130, 165–171.

Homan, R. N., Regosin, J. V., Rodrigues, D. M., Reed, J. M., Windmiller, B. S., Romero, L. M., 2003b. Impacts of varying habitat quality on the physiological stress of spotted salamanders (*Ambystoma maculatum*). *Anim Conserv* 6, 11–18.

Hood, L. C., Boersma, P. D., Wingfield, J. C., 1998. The adrenocortical response to stress in incubating magellanic penguins (*Spheniscus magellanicus*). *Auk* 115, 76–84.

Hoopes, L. A., Landry, A. M., Stabenau, E. K., 2000. Physiological effects of capturing Kemp's ridley sea turtles, *Lepidochelys kempii*, in entanglement nets. *Can J Zool* 78, 1941–1947.

Hopkins, W. A., DuRant, S. E., 2011. Innate immunity and stress physiology of eastern hellbenders (*Cryptobranchus alleganiensis*) from two stream reaches with differing habitat quality. *Gen Comp Endocrinol* 174, 107–115.

Horak, P., Saks, L., Ots, I., Kollist, H., 2002. Repeatability of condition indices in captive greenfinches (*Carduelis chloris*). *Can J Zool* 80, 636–643.

Huber, S., Palme, R., Arnold, W., 2003. Effects of season, sex, and sample collection on concentrations of fecal cortisol metabolites in red deer (*Cervus elaphus*). *Gen Comp Endocrinol* 130, 48–54.

Hunt, K. E., Rolland, R. A., Kraus, S. D., Wasser, S. K., 2006. Analysis of fecal glucocorticoids in the North Atlantic right whale (*Eubalaena glacialis*). *Gen Comp Endocrinol* 148, 260–272.

Hunt, K. E., Wasser, S. K., 2003. Effect of long-term preservation methods on fecal glucocorticoid concentrations of grizzly bear and African elephant. *Physiol Biochem Zool* 76, 918–928.

Hylton, R. A., Frederick, P. C., de la Fuente, T. E., Spalding, M. G., 2006. Effects of nestling health on postfledging survival of wood storks. *Condor* 108, 97–106.

Ilmonen, P., Hasselquist, D., Langefors, A., Wiehn, J., 2003. Stress, immunocompetence and leukocyte profiles of pied flycatchers in relation to brood size manipulation. *Oecologia (Berlin)* 136, 148–154.

Jaimez, N. A., Bribiescas, R. G., Aronsen, G. P., Anestis, S., Watts, D., 2011. Urinary cortisol levels of grey cheeked mangabeys are higher in disturbed compared to undisturbed forest areas in Kibale National Park, Uganda. *Anim Conserv* 15, 240–247.

Jankowski, M. D., Wittwer, D. J., Heisey, D. M., Franson, J. C., Hofmeister, E. K., 2009. The adrenocortical response of greater sage grouse (*Centrocercus urophasianus*) to capture, ACTH injection, and confinement, as measured in fecal samples. *Physiol Biochem Zool* 82, 190–201.

Jenni-Eiermann, S., Glaus, E., Gruebler, M., Schwabl, H., Jenni, L., 2008. Glucocorticoid response to food availability in breeding barn swallows (*Hirundo rustica*). *Gen Comp Endocrinol* 155, 558–565.

Jessop, T. S., 2001. Modulation of the adrenocortical stress response in marine turtles (*Cheloniidae*): Evidence for a hormonal tactic maximizing maternal reproductive investment. *J Zool* 254, 57–65.

Jessop, T. S., Hamann, M., 2004. Hormonal and metabolic responses to nesting activities in the green turtle, *Chelonia mydas*. *J Exper Marine Biol Ecol* 308, 253–267.

Jessop, T. S., Tucker, A. D., Limpus, C. J., Whittier, J. M., 2003. Interactions between ecology, demography, capture stress, and profiles of corticosterone and glucose in a free-living population of Australian freshwater crocodiles. *Gen Comp Endocrinol* 132, 161–170.

Jimenez, G., Lemus, J. A., Melendez, L., Blanco, G., Laiolo, P., 2011. Dampened behavioral and physiological responses mediate birds' association with humans. *Biol Conserv* 144, 1702–1711.

Jones, M. A., Mason, G. J., Pillay, N., 2011. Correlates of birth origin effects on the development of stereotypic behaviour in striped mice, *Rhabdomys*. *Anim Behav* 82, 149–159.

Jones, R. B., Mills, A. D., Faure, J. M., Williams, J. B., 1994a. Restraint, fear, and distress in Japanese-quail genetically selected for long or short tonic immobility reactions. *Physiol Behav* 56, 529–534.

Jones, R. B., Satterlee, D. G., Ryder, F. H., 1994b. Fear of humans in Japanese quail selected for low or high adrenocortical response. *Physiol Behav* 56, 379–383.

Jones, S. M., Bell, K., 2004. Plasma corticosterone concentrations in males of the skink *Egernia whitii* during acute and chronic confinement, and over a diel period. *Comp Biochem Physiol* 137A, 105–113.

Jurke, M. H., Czekala, N. M., Lindburg, D. G., Millard, S. E., 1997. Fecal corticoid metabolite measurement in the cheetah (*Acinonyx jubatus*). *Zoo Biol* 16, 133–147.

Kalra, S., Einarson, A., Karaskov, T., VanUm, S., Koren, G., 2007. The relationship between stress and hair cortisol in healthy pregnant women. *Clin Invest Med* 30, E100–E104.

Kanwisher, J. W., Williams, T. C., Teal, J. M., Lawson, K. O., 1978. Radiotelemetry of heart rates from free-ranging gulls. *Auk* 95, 288–293.

Karsten, A. H., Turner, J. W., Jr., 2003. Fecal corticosterone assessment in the epaulette shark, *Hemiscyllium ocellatum*. *J Exp Zool* 299A, 188–196.

Ketterson, E. D., Nolan, V., Jr. 1999. Adaptation, exaptation, and constraint: A hormonal perspective. *Am Nat* 154, S4–S25.

Ketterson, E. D., Nolan, V., Cawthorn, M. J., Parker, P. G., Ziegenfus, C., 1996. Phenotypic engineering: Using hormones to explore the mechanistic and functional bases of phenotypic variation in nature. *Ibis* 138, 70–86.

Ketterson, E. D., Nolan, V., Sandell, M., 2005. Testosterone in females: Mediator of adaptive traits, constraint on sexual dimorphism, or both? *Am Nat* 166, S85–S98.

Khan, M. Z., Altmann, J., Isani, S. S., Yu, J., 2002. A matter of time: Evaluating the storage of fecal samples for steroid analysis. *Gen Comp Endocrinol* 128, 57–64.

Kilgas, P., Mand, R., Magi, M., Tilgar, V., 2006a. Hematological parameters in brood-rearing great tits in relation to habitat, multiple breeding and sex. *Comp Biochem Physiol A* 144, 224–231.

Kilgas, P., Tilgar, V., Mand, R., 2006b. Hematological health state indices predict local survival in a small passerine bird, the great tit (*Parus major*). *Physiol Biochem Zool* 79, 565–572.

Kim, C.-Y., Han, J. S., Suzuki, T., Han, S.-S., 2005. Indirect indicator of transport stress in hematological values in newly acquired cynomolgus monkeys. *J Med Primatol* 34, 188–192.

Kitaysky, A. S., Piatt, J. F., Wingfield, J. C., 2007. Stress hormones link food availability and population processes in seabirds. *Mar Ecol Prog Ser* 352, 245–258.

Kitaysky, A. S., Romano, M. D., Piatt, J. F., Wingfield, J. C., Kikuchi, M., 2005. The adrenocortical response of tufted puffin chicks to nutritional deficits. *Horm Behav* 47, 606–619.

Klasing, K. C., 2005. Potential impact of nutritional strategy on noninvasive measurements of hormones in birds. *Ann NY Acad Sci*, 1046, 5–16.

Klose, S. M., Smith, C. L., Denzel, A. J., Kalko, E. K. V., 2006. Reproduction elevates the corticosterone stress response in common fruit bats. *J Comp Physiol A* 192, 341–350.

Knapp, R., Moore, M. C., 1997. Male morphs in tree lizards have different testosterone responses to elevated levels of corticosterone. *Gen Comp Endocrinol* 107, 273–279.

Knierim, U., Van Dongen, S., Forkman, B., Tuyttens, F. A. M., Spinka, M., Campo, J. L., Weissengruber, G. E., 2007. Fluctuating asymmetry as an animal welfare indicator: A review of methodology and validity. *Physiol Behav* 92, 398–421.

Konjevic, D., Janicki, Z., Slavica, A., Severin, K., Krapinec, K., Bozic, F., Palme, R., 2011. Non-invasive monitoring of adrenocortical activity in free-ranging fallow deer (*Dama dama L.*). *Eur J Wildlife Res* 57, 77–81.

Koopman, H. N., Westgate, A. J., Read, A. J., Gaskin, D. E., 1995. Blood chemistry of wild harbor porpoises *Phocoena phocoena (L.)*. *Marine Mammal Sci* 11, 123–135.

Koren, L., Nakagawa, S., Burke, T., Soma, K. K., Wynne-Edwards, K. E., Geffen, E., 2012. Non-breeding feather concentrations of testosterone, corticosterone and cortisol are associated with subsequent survival in wild house sparrows. *Proc R Soc Lond B* 279, 1560–1566.

Kotrschal, A., Ilmonen, P., Penn, D. J., 2007. Stress impacts telomere dynamics. *Biol Lett* 3, 128–130.

Kotrschal, K., Hirschenhauser, K., Moestl, E., 1998. The relationship between social stress and dominance is seasonal in greylag geese. *Anim Behav* 55, 171–176.

Kralj-Fiser, S., Scheiber, I. B. R., Blejec, A., Moestl, E., Kotrschal, K., 2007. Individualities in a flock of free-roaming greylag geese: Behavioral and physiological consistency over time and across situations. *Horm Behav* 51, 239–248.

Krass, P. M., Bazhan, N. M., Reshetnikov, S. S., Trut, L. N., 1979. Adrenal reactivity to ACTH age changes in silver foxes inheriting different defensive behaviors. *Biol Bull Acad Sci USSR* 6, 306–310.

Kreger, M. D., Mench, J. A., 1993. Physiological and behavioral effects of handling and restraint in the ball python (*Python regius*) and the blue-tongued skink (*Tiliqua scincoides*). *Appl Anim Behav Sci* 38, 323–336.

Kunzl, C., Sachser, N., 1999. The behavioral endocrinology of domestication: a comparison between the domestic guinea pig (*Cavia aperea* f. *porcellus*) and its wild ancestor, the cavy (*Cavia aperea*). *Horm Behav* 35, 28–37.

Kuznetsov, V. A., Tchabovsky, A. V., Moshkin, M. P., 2006. Seasonal corticosterone dynamics in natural population of the speckled ground squirrel (*Spermophilus suslicus*). *Byulleten' Moskovskogo Obshchestva Ispytatelei Prirody Otdel Biologicheskii* 111, 68–70.

Laiolo, P., Serrano, D., Tella, J. L., Carrete, M., Lopez, G., Navarro, C., 2007. Distress calls reflect poxvirus infection in lesser short-toed lark *Calandrella rufescens*. *Behav Ecol* 18, 507–512.

Lance, V. A., Elsey, R. M., 1999a. Hormonal and metabolic responses of juvenile alligators to cold shock. *J Exp Zool* 283, 566–572.

Lance, V. A., Elsey, R. M., 1999b. Plasma catecholamines and plasma corticosterone following restraint stress in juvenile alligators. *J Exp Zool* 283, 559–565.

Landys-Ciannelli, M. M., Ramenofsky, M., Piersma, T., Jukema, J., Castricum Ringing, G., Wingfield, J. C., 2002. Baseline and stress-induced plasma corticosterone during long-distance migration in the bar-tailed godwit, *Limosa lapponica*. *Physiol Biochem Zool* 75, 101–110.

Lattin, C. R., Reed, J. M., DesRochers, D. W., Romero, L. M., 2011. Elevated corticosterone in feathers correlates with corticosterone-induced decreased feather quality: a validation study. *J Avian Biol* 42, 247–252.

Leary, C. J., Garcia, A. M., Knapp, R., 2006. Elevated corticosterone levels elicit non-calling mating tactics in male toads independently of changes in circulating androgens. *Horm Behav* 49, 425–432.

Leche, A., Busso, J. M., Navarro, J. L., Hansen, C., Marin, R. H., Martella, M. B., 2011. Non-invasive monitoring of adrenocortical activity in greater rhea (*Rhea americana*) by measuring fecal glucocorticoid metabolites. *J Ornithol* 152, 839–847.

Legagneux, P., Gauthier, G., Chastel, O., Picard, G., Bety, J., 2011. Do glucocorticoids in droppings reflect baseline level in birds captured in the wild? A case study in snow geese. *Gen Comp Endocrinol* 172, 440–445.

Lens, L., Van Dongen, S., Kark, S., Matthysen, E., 2002. Fluctuating asymmetry as an indicator of fitness: can we bridge the gap between studies? *Biol Rev* 77, 27–38.

Li, C., Jiang, Z., Tang, S., Zeng, Y., 2007. Influence of enclosure size and animal density on fecal cortisol concentration and aggression in Pere David's deer stags. *Gen Comp Endocrinol* 151, 202–209.

Lim, M. M., Young, L. J., 2006. Neuropeptidergic regulation of affiliative behavior and social bonding in animals. *Horm Behav* 50, 506–517.

Lindstrom, K. M., Hawley, D. M., Davis, A. K., Wikelski, M., 2005. Stress responses and disease in three wintering house finch (*Carpodacus mexicanus*) populations along a latitudinal gradient. *Gen Comp Endocrinol* 143, 231–239.

Linklater, W. L., MacDonald, E. A., Flamand, J. R. B., Czekala, N. M., 2010. Declining and low fecal corticoids are associated with distress, not acclimation to stress, during the translocation of African rhinoceros. *Anim Conserv* 13, 104–111.

Liu, J., Chen, Y., Guo, L., Gu, B., Liu, H., Hou, A., Liu, X., Sun, L., Liu, D., 2006. Stereotypic behavior and fecal cortisol level in captive giant pandas in relation to environmental enrichment. *Zoo Biol* 25, 445–459.

Lobato, E., Moreno, J., Merino, S., Sanz, J. J., Arriero, E., 2005. Haematological variables are good predictors of recruitment in nestling pied flycatchers (*Ficeduld hypoleuca*). *Ecoscience* 12, 27–34.

Long, J. A., Holberton, R. L., 2004. Corticosterone secretion, energetic condition, and a test of the migration modulation hypothesis in the hermit thrush (*Catharus guttatus*), a short-distance migrant. *Auk* 121, 1094–1102.

Lopez, G., Figuerola, J., Varo, N., Soriguer, R., 2005. White wagtails *Motacilla alba* showing extensive post-juvenile moult are more stressed. *Ardea* 93, 237–244.

Lovas, K., Thorsen, T. E., Husebye, E. S., 2006. Saliva cortisol measurement: Simple and reliable assessment of the glucocorticoid replacement therapy in Addison's disease. *J Endocrinol Invest* 29, 727–731.

Love, O. P., Shutt, L. J., Silfies, J. S., Bird, D. M., 2003. Repeated restraint and sampling results in reduced corticosterone levels in developing and adult captive American kestrels (*Falco sparverius*). *Physiol Biochem Zool* 76, 753–761.

Lowe, T. E., Wells, R. M. G., 1996. Primary and secondary stress responses to line capture in the blue mao mao. *J Fish Biol* 49, 287–300.

Lucas, J. R., Freeberg, T. M., Egbert, J., Schwabl, H., 2006. Fecal corticosterone, body mass, and caching rates of Carolina chickadees (*Poecile carolinensis*) from disturbed and undisturbed sites. *Horm Behav* 49, 634–643.

Ludders, J. W., Langenberg, J. A., Czekala, N. M., Erb, H. N., 2001. Fecal corticosterone reflects serum corticosterone in Florida sandhill cranes. *J Wildlife Dis* 37, 646–652.

Lutterschmidt, D. I., Mason, R. T., 2005. A serotonin receptor antagonist, but not melatonin, modulates hormonal responses to capture stress in two populations of garter snakes (*Thamnophis sirtalis parietalis* and *Thamnophis sirtalis concinnus*). *Gen Comp Endocrinol* 141, 259–270.

Lynch, J. W., Khan, M. Z., Altmann, J., Njahira, M. N., Rubenstein, N., 2003. Concentrations of four fecal steroids in wild baboons: Short-term storage conditions and consequences for data interpretation. *Gen Comp Endocrinol* 132, 264–271.

Lynch, J. W., Ziegler, T. E., Strier, K. B., 2002. Individual and seasonal variation in fecal testosterone and cortisol levels of wild male tufted capuchin monkeys, *Cebus apella nigritus*. *Horm Behav* 41, 275–287.

Lynn, S. E., Hunt, K. E., Wingfield, J. C., 2003. Ecological factors affecting the adrenocortical response, to stress in chestnut-collared and McCown's longspurs (*Calcarius ornatus, Calcarius mccownii*). *Physiol Biochem Zool* 76, 566–576.

Lynn, S. E., Porter, A. J., 2008. Trapping initiates stress response in breeding and non-breeding house sparrows Passer domesticus: Implications for using unmonitored traps in field studies. *J Avian Biol* 39, 87–94.

Lynn, S. E., Prince, L. E., Phillips, M. M., 2010. A single exposure to an acute stressor has lasting consequences for the hypothalamo-pituitary-adrenal response to stress in free-living birds. *Gen Comp Endocrinol* 165, 337–344.

Macarthur, R. A., Geist, V., Johnston, R. H., 1982. Cardiac and behavioral responses of mountain sheep to human disturbance. *J Wildlife Manage* 46, 351–358.

Macbeth, B. J., Cattet, M. R. L., Stenhouse, G. B., Gibeau, M. L., Janz, D. M., 2010. Hair cortisol concentration as a noninvasive measure of long-term stress in free-ranging grizzly bears (*Ursus arctos*): Considerations with implications for other wildlife. *Can J Zool* 88, 935–949.

Manzo, C., Zerani, M., Gobbetti, A., Maddalena Di Fiore, M., Angelini, F., 1994. Is corticosterone involved in the reproductive processes of the male lizard, *Podarcis sicula sicula*? *Horm Behav* 28, 117–129.

Marra, P. P., Holberton, R. L., 1998. Corticosterone levels as indicators of habitat quality: Effects of habitat segregation in a migratory bird during the non-breeding season. *Oecologia* 116, 284–292.

Marra, P. P., Lampe, K. T., Tedford, B. L., 1995. Plasma corticosterone levels in two species of *Zonotrichia* sparrows under captive and free-living conditions. *Wilson Bull* 107, 296–305.

Martin, L. B., Hopkins, W. A., Mydlarz, L. D., Rohr, J. R., 2010. The effects of anthropogenic global changes on immune functions and disease resistance. *Ann NY Acad Sci*, 1195, 129–148.

Martinez-Mota, R., Valdespino, C., Sanchez-Ramos, M. A., Serio-Silva, J. C., 2007. Effects of forest fragmentation on the physiological stress response of black howler monkeys. *Anim Conserv* 10, 374–379.

Mashburn, K. L., Atkinson, S., 2004. Evaluation of adrenal function in serum and feces of Steller sea lions (*Eumetopias jubatus*): Influences of molt, gender, sample storage, and age on glucocorticoid metabolism. *Gen Comp Endocrinol* 136, 371–381.

Mateo, J. M., Cavigelli, S. A., 2005. A validation of extraction methods for noninvasive sampling of glucocorticoids in free-living ground squirrels. *Physiol Biochem Zool* 78, 1069–1084.

Mathies, T., Felix, T. A., Lance, V. A., 2001. Effects of trapping and subsequent short-term confinement stress on plasma corticosterone in the brown treesnake (*Boiga irregularis*) on Guam. *Gen Comp Endocrinol* 124, 106–114.

Maxwell, M. H., 1993. Avian blood leucocyte responses to stress. *World Poultry Sci J* 49, 34–43.

Mayne, G. J., Martin, P. A., Bishop, C. A., Boermans, H. J., 2004. Stress and immune responses of nestling tree swallows (*Tachycineta bicolor*) and eastern bluebirds (*Sialia sialis*) exposed to nonpersistent pesticides and p,p,'- dichlorodiphenyldichloroethylene in apple orchards of southern Ontario, Canada.*Environ Toxicol Chem* 23, 2930–2940.

McGlone, J. J., Salak, J. L., Lumpkin, E. A., Nicholson, R. I., Gibson, M., Norman, R. L., 1993. Shipping stress and social status effects on pig performance, plasma cortisol, natural killer cell activity, and leukocyte numbers. *J Animal Sci* 71, 888–896.

McGlothlin, J. W., Ketterson, E. D., 2008. Hormone-mediated suites as adaptations and evolutionary constraints. *Phil Trans R Soc B* 363, 1611–1620.

McKenzie, S., Deane, E. M., 2005. Faecal corticosteroid levels as an indicator of well-being in the tammar wallaby, *Macropus eugenii*. *Comp Biochem Physiol A* 140, 81–87.

Meddle, S. L., Owen-Ashley, N. T., Richardson, M. I., Wingfield, J. C., 2003. Modulation of the hypothalamic-pituitary-adrenal axis of an Arctic-breeding polygynandrous songbird, the Smith's longspur, *Calcarius pictus*. *Proc R Soc Lond B* 270, 1849–1856.

Meka, J. M., McCormick, S. D., 2005. Physiological response of wild rainbow trout to angling: impact of angling duration, fish size, body condition, and temperature. *Fisheries Res (Amsterdam)* 72, 311–322.

Mellish, J. E., Hindle, A. G., Horning, M., 2010. A preliminary assessment of the impact of disturbance and handling on Weddell seals of McMurdo Sound, Antarctica. *Antarctic Sci* 22, 25–29.

Miksis, J. L., Grund, M. D., Nowacek, D. P., Solow, A. R., Connor, R. C., Tyack, P. L., 2001. Cardiac responses to acoustic playback experiments in the captive bottlenose dolphin (*Tursiops truncatus*). *J Comp Psychol* 115, 227–232.

Miller, M. W., Hobbs, N. T., Sousa, M. C., 1991. Detecting stress responses in Rocky Mountain bighorn sheep *Ovis-canadensis* reliability of cortisol concentrations in urine and feces. *Can J Zool* 69, 15–24.

Millspaugh, J. J., Washburn, B. E., 2003. Within-sample variation of fecal glucocorticoid measurements. *Gen Comp Endocrinol* 132, 21–26.

Millspaugh, J. J., Washburn, B. E., 2004. Use of fecal glucocorticoid metabolite measures in conservation biology research: Considerations for application and interpretation. *Gen Comp Endocrinol* 138, 189.

Millspaugh, J. J., Washburn, B. E., Milanick, M. A., Beringer, J., Hansen, L. P., Meyer, T. M., 2002. Non-invasive techniques for stress assessment in white-tailed deer. *Wildlife Soc Bull* 30, 899–907.

Millspaugh, J. J., Washburn, B. E., Milanick, M. A., Slotow, R., van Dyk, G., 2003. Effects of heat and chemical treatments on fecal glucocorticoid measurements: Implications for sample transport. *Wild Soc Bull* 31, 399–406.

Mizrahi, D. S., Holberton, R. L., Gauthreaux, S. A., Jr., 2001. Patterns of corticosterone secretion in migrating semipalmated sandpipers at a major spring stopover site. *Auk* 118, 79–91.

Moen, A.N., 1978. Seasonal changes in heart rates, activity, metabolism, and forage intake of white-tailed deer. *J Wildlife Manage* 42, 715–738.

Möstl, E., Rettenbacher, S., Palme, R., 2005. Measurement of corticosterone metabolites in birds' droppings: An analytical approach. *Ann NY Acad Sci*, 1046, 17–34

Monaghan, P., Haussmann, M. F., 2006. Do telomere dynamics link lifestyle and lifespan? *Trends Ecol Evol* 21, 47–53.

Monclus, R., Roedel, H. G., Palme, R., Von Holst, D., de Miguel, J., 2006. Non-invasive measurement of the physiological stress response of wild rabbits to the odour of a predator. *Chemoecology* 16, 25–29.

Moore, I. T., Lemaster, M. P., Mason, R. T., 2000. Behavioural and hormonal responses to capture stress in the male red-sided garter snake, *Thamnophis sirtalis parietalis*. *Anim Behav* 59, 529–534.

Moore, M. C., Thompson, C. W., Marler, C. A., 1991. Reciprocal changes in corticosterone and testosterone levels following acute and chronic handling stress in the tree lizard, *Urosaurus ornatus*. *Gen Compar Endocrinol* 81, 217–226.

Morato, R. G., Bueno, M. G., Malmheister, P., Verreschi, I. T. N., Barnabe, R. C., 2004. Changes in the fecal concentrations of cortisol and androgen metabolites in captive male Jaguars (*Panthera onca*) in response to stress. *Braz J Med Biol Res* 37, 1903–1907.

Morehead, D. T., 1998. Effect of capture, confinement and repeated sampling on plasma steroid concentrations and oocyte size in female striped trumpeter *Latris lineata* (Latrididae). *Mar Freshwater Res* 49, 373–377.

Moreno, J., Merino, S., Martinez, J., Sanz, J. J., Arriero, E., 2002. Heterophil/lymphocyte ratios and heat-shock protein levels are related to growth in nestling birds. *Ecoscience* 9, 434–439.

Morici, L. A., Elsey, R. M., Lance, V. A., 1997. Effect of long-term corticosterone implants on growth and immune function in juvenile alligators, *Alligator mississippiensis*. *J Exp Zool* 279, 156–162.

Morrow, C. J., Kolver, E. S., Verkerk, G. A., Matthews, L. R., 2002. Fecal glucocorticoid metabolites as a measure of adrenal activity in dairy cattle. *Gen Comp Endocrinol* 126, 229–241.

Morrow-Tesch, J. L., McGlone, J. J., Norman, R. L., 1993. Consequences of restraint stress on natural killer cell activity, behavior, and hormone levels in rhesus macaques (*Macaca mulatta*). *Psychoneuroendocrinology* 18, 383–395.

Mortimer, L., Lill, A., 2007. Activity-related variation in blood parameters associated with oxygen transport and chronic stress in little penguins. *Aust J Zool* 55, 249–256.

Mougeot, F., Martinez-Padilla, J., Bortolotti, G. R., Webster, L. M. I., Piertney, S. B., 2010. Physiological stress links parasites to carotenoid-based colour signals. *J Evol Biol* 23, 643–650.

Mueller, C., Jenni-Eiermann, S., Blondel, J., Perret, P., Caro, S. P., Lambrechts, M., Jenni, L., 2006. Effect of human presence and handling on circulating corticosterone levels in breeding blue tits (*Parus caeruleus*). *Gen Comp Endocrinol* 148, 163–171.

Mueller, C., Jenni-Eiermann, S., Jenni, L., 2011. Heterophils/Lymphocytes-ratio and circulating corticosterone do not indicate the same stress imposed on Eurasian kestrel nestlings. *Func Ecol* 25, 566–576.

Müller, C., Almasi, B., Roulin, A., Breuner, C. W., Jenni-Eiermann, S., Jenni, L., 2009. Effects of corticosterone pellets on baseline and stress-induced corticosterone and corticosteroid-binding-globulin. *Gen Comp Endocrinol* 160, 59–66.

Muller, M. N., Wrangham, R. W., 2004. Dominance, cortisol and stress in wild chimpanzees (*Pan troglodytes schweinfurthii*). *Behav Ecol Sociobiol* 55, 332–340.

Nakagawa, S., Moestl, E., Waas, J. R., 2003. Validation of an enzyme immunoassay to measure faecal glucocorticoid metabolites from Adelie penguins (*Pygoscelis adeliae*): A non-invasive tool for estimating stress? *Polar Biol* 26, 491–493.

Narayan, E., Molinia, F., Christi, K., Morley, C., Cockrem, J., 2010. Urinary corticosterone metabolite responses to capture, and annual patterns of urinary corticosterone in wild and captive endangered Fijian ground frogs (*Platymantis vitiana*). *Aust J Zool* 58, 189–197.

Narayan, E. J., Cockrem, J. F., Hero, J. M., 2011a. Urinary corticosterone metabolite responses to capture and captivity in the cane toad (*Rhinella marina*). *Gen Comp Endocrinol* 173, 371–377.

Narayan, E. J., Molinia, F. C., Kindermann, C., Cockrem, J. F., Hero, J. M., 2011b. Urinary corticosterone responses to capture and toe-clipping in the cane toad (*Rhinella marina*) indicate that toe-clipping is a stressor for amphibians. *Gen Comp Endocrinol* 174, 238–245.

Nephew, B.C., Kahn, S.A., Romero, L.M., 2003. Heart rate and behavior are regulated independently of corticosterone following diverse acute stressors. *Gen Comp Endocrinol* 133, 173–180.

Newell-Fugate, A., Kennedy-Stoskopf, S., Brown, J. L., Levine, J. F., Swanson, W. F., 2007. Seminal and endocrine characteristics of male Pallas' cats (*Otocolobus manul*) maintained under artificial lighting with simulated natural photoperiods. *Zoo Biol* 26, 187–199.

Newman, A. E. M., Pradhan, D. S., Soma, K. K., 2008. Dehydroepiandrosterone and corticosterone are regulated by season and acute stress in a wild songbird: Jugular versus brachial plasma. *Endocrinology* 149, 2537–2545.

Newman, S. H., Carter, H. R., Whitworth, D. L., Zinkl, J. G., 2005. Health assessments and stress response of Xantus's murrelets to capture, handling and radio-marking. Marine Ornithol 33, 147–154.

Nilsson, A., Ahman, B., Norberg, H., Redbo, I., Eloranta, E., Olsson, K., 2006. Activity and heart rate in semi-domesticated reindeer during adaptation to emergency feeding. *Physiol Behav* 88, 116–123.

Nimon, A. J., Schroter, R. C., Oxenham, R. K. C., 1996. Artificial eggs: Measuring heart rate and effects of disturbance in nesting penguins. *Physiol Behav* 60, 1019–1022.

Nimon, A. J., Schroter, R. C., Stonehouse, B., 1995. Heart-rate of disturbed penguins *Nature* 374, 415–415.

Noble, R. E., 2002. Diagnosis of stress. *Metab Clin Exp* 51, 37–39.

Norris, D. O., Donahue, S., Dores, R. M., Lee, J. K., Maldonado, T. A., Ruth, T., Woodling, J. D., 1999. Impaired adrenocortical response to stress by brown trout, *Salmo trutta*, living in metal-contaminated waters of the Eagle River, Colorado. *Gen Comp Endocrinol* 113, 1–8.

NRC, 2005. *Marine mammal populations and ocean noise: determining when noise causes biologically significant impacts.* U.S. National Research Council, Washington, DC, pp. 1–98.

Nunes, S., Pelz, K. M., Muecke, E. M., Holekamp, K. E., Zucker, I., 2006. Plasma glucocorticoid concentrations and body mass in ground squirrels: Seasonal variation and circannual organization. *Gen Comp Endocrinol* 146, 136–143.

O'Reilly, K. M., Wingfield, J. C., 2001. Ecological factors underlying the adrenocortical response to capture stress in arctic-breeding shorebirds. *Gen Comp Endocrinol* 124, 1–11.

Oates, J. E., Bradshaw, F. J., Bradshaw, S. D., Stead-Richardson, E. J., Philippe, D. L., 2007. Reproduction and embryonic diapause in a marsupial: Insights from captive female Honey possums, *Tarsipes rostratus* (Tarsipedidae). *Gen Comp Endocrinol* 150, 445–461.

Ortiz, R. M., Worthy, G. A. J., 2000. Effects of capture on adrenal steroid and vasopressin concentrations in free-ranging bottlenose dolphins (*Tursiops truncatus*). *Comp Biochem Physiol A* 125A, 317–324.

Ostner, J., Heistermann, M., Schulke, O., 2008. Dominance, aggression and physiological stress in wild male Assamese macaques (*Macaca assamensis*). *Horm Behav* 54, 613–619.

Ots, I., Kerimov, A. B., Ivankina, E. V., Ilyina, T. A., Horak, P., 2001. Immune challenge affects basal metabolic activity in wintering great tits. *Proc R Soc Lond B* 268, 1175–1181.

Ott, J. A., Mendonça, M. T., Guyer, C., Michener, W. K., 2000. Seasonal changes in sex and adrenal steroid hormones of gopher tortoises (*Gopherus polyphemus*). *Gen Comp Endocrinol* 117, 299–312.

Ouyang, J. Q., Hau, M., Bonier, F., 2011. Within seasons and among years: When are corticosterone levels repeatable? *Horm Behav* 60, 559–564.

Øverli, Ø., Pottinger, T. G., Carrick, T. R., Øverli, E., Winberg, S., 2002. Differences in behaviour between rainbow trout selected for high- and low-stress responsiveness. *J Exp Biol* 205, 391–395.

Owen, J. C., Moore, F. R., 2006. Seasonal differences in immunological condition of three species of thrushes. *Condor* 108, 389–398.

Owen-Ashley, N. T., Hasselquist, D., Raberg, L., Wingfield, J. C., 2008. Latitudinal variation of immune defense and sickness behavior in the white-crowned sparrow (*Zonotrichia leucophrys*). *Brain Behav Immun* 22, 614–625.

Palme, R., 2005. Measuring fecal steroids: Guidelines for practical application. Ann NY Acad Sci 1046, 75–80.

Palme, R., Fischer, P., Schildorfer, H., Ismail, M. N., 1996. Excretion of infused 14C-steroid hormones via faeces and urine in domestic livestock. *Anim Repro Sci* 43, 43–63.

Palme, R., Rettenbacher, S., Touma, C., El-Bahr, S. M., Moestl, E., 2005. Stress hormones in mammals and birds: Comparative aspects regarding metabolism, excretion, and noninvasive measurement in fecal samples. *Ann NY Acad Sci* 1046, 162–171.

Pankhurst, N. W., 2001. Stress inhibition of reproductive endocrine processes in a natural population of the spiny damselfish *Acanthochromis polyacanthus. Mar Freshwater Res* 52, 753–761.

Pap, P. L., Markus, R., 2003. Cost of reproduction, T-lymphocyte mediated immunocompetence and health status in female and nestling barn swallows *Hirundo rustica. J Avian Biol* 34, 428–434.

Pearson, B. L., Judge, P. G., Reeder, D. M., 2008. Effectiveness of saliva collection and enzyme-immunoassay for the quantification of cortisol in socially housed baboons. *Am J Primatol* 70, 1145–1151.

Pedernera-Romano, C., Valdez, R. A., Singh, S., Chiappa, X., Romano, M. C., Galindo, F., 2006. Salivary cortisol in captive dolphins (*Tursiops truncatus*): A non-invasive technique. *Anim Welfare* 15, 359–362.

Pedersen, S. S., Denollet, J., 2003. Type D personality, cardiac events, and impaired quality of life: A review. *Eur J Cardiovasc Prev Rehabil* 10, 241–248.

Peel, A.J., Vogelnest, L., Finnigan, M., Grossfeldt, L., O'Brien, J. K., 2005. Non-invasive fecal hormone analysis and behavioral observations for monitoring stress responses in captive western lowland gorillas (*Gorilla gorilla gorilla*). *Zoo Biol* 24, 431–445.

Pereira, R. J. G., Duarte, J. M. B., Negrao, J. A., 2006. Effects of environmental conditions, human activity, reproduction, antler cycle and grouping on fecal glucocorticoids of free-ranging Pampas deer stags (*Ozotoceros bezoarticus bezoarticus*). *Horm Behav* 49, 114–122.

Pereyra, M. E., Wingfield, J. C., 2003. Changes in plasma corticosterone and adrenocortical response to stress during the breeding cycle in high altitude flycatchers. *Gen Comp Endocrinol* 130, 222–231.

Perfito, N., Schirato, G., Brown, M., Wingfield, J. C., 2002. Response to acute stress in the Harlequin Duck (*Histrionicus histrionicus*) during the breeding season and moult: Relationships to gender, condition, and life-history stage. *Can J Zool* 80, 1334–1343.

Perfito, N., Zann, R. A., Bentley, G. E., Hau, M., 2007. Opportunism at work: Habitat predictability affects reproductive readiness in free-living zebra finches. *Func Ecol* 21, 291–301.

Perkins, D. E., Holberton, R. L., Boere, G. C., Galbraith, C. A., Stroud, D. A., 2006. Indicators of body condition, energy demand and breeding success in the ruddy turnstone Arenaria interpres, a species of concern. *Waterbirds around the world: A global overview of the conservation, management and research of the world's waterbird flyways.* International conference on waterbirds held in Edinburgh in April 2004, pp. 551–552.

Pfaff, J. A., Zanette, L., MacDougall-Shackleton, S. A., MacDougall-Shackleton, E. A., 2007. Song repertoire size varies with HVC volume and is indicative of male quality in song sparrows (*Melospiza melodia*). *Proc R Soc Lond B* 274, 2035–2040.

Place, N. J., Kenagy, G. J., 2000. Seasonal changes in plasma testosterone and glucocorticosteroids in free-living male yellow-pine chipmunks and the response to capture and handling. *J Comp Physiol B* 170, 245–251.

Ponzio, M. F., Monfort, S. L., Busso, J. M., Dabbene, V. G., Ruiz, R. D., Fiol De Cuneo, M., 2004. A non-invasive method for assessing adrenal activity in the Chinchilla (Chinchilla lanigera). *J Exp Zool* 301A, 218–227.

Poole, W. R., Nolan, D. T., Wevers, T., Dillane, M., Cotter, D., Tully, O., 2003. An ecophysiological comparison of wild and hatchery-raised Atlantic salmon (*Salmo salar L.*) smolts from the Burrishoole system, western Ireland. *Aquaculture* 222, 301–314.

Popp, L. G., Serafni, P. P., Reghelin, A. L. S., Spercoski, K. M., Roper, J. J., Morais, R. N., 2008. Annual pattern of fecal corticoid excretion in captive Red-tailed parrots (*Amazona brasiliensis*). *J Comp Physiol B* 178, 487–493.

Pottinger, T. G., 1998. Changes in blood cortisol, glucose and lactate in carp retained in anglers' keepnets. *J Fish Biol* 53, 728–742.

Presidente, P. J. A., Correa, J. J., 1981. Hematology plasma electrolytes and serum biochemical values of *Trichosurus-vulpecula* Marsupialia Phalangeridae. *Aust J Zool* 29, 507–518.

Pride, R. E., 2005. Optimal group size and seasonal stress in ring-tailed lemurs (*Lemur catta*). *Behav Ecol* 16, 550.

Quillfeldt, P., Möstl, E., 2003. Resource allocation in Wilson's storm-petrels Oceanites oceanicus determined by measurement of glucocorticoid excretion. *Acta Ethol* 5, 115–122.

Rangel-Negrin, A., Alfaro, J. L., Valdez, R. A., Romano, M. C., Serio-Silva, J. C., 2009. Stress in Yucatan spider monkeys: effects of environmental conditions on fecal cortisol levels in wild and captive populations. *Anim Conserv* 12, 496–502.

Redmond, L. J., Murphy, M. T., 2011. Multistate mark-recapture analysis reveals no effect of blood sampling on survival and recapture of Eastern kingbirds (*Tyrannus tyrannus*). *Auk* 128, 514–521.

Reeder, D. M., Kosteczko, N. S., Kunz, T. H., Widmaier, E. P., 2004. Changes in baseline and stress-induced glucocorticold levels during the active period in free-ranging male and female little brown myotis, *Myotis lucifugus* (Chiroptera: Vespertilionidae). *Gen Comp Endocrinol* 136, 260–269.

Rehbinder, C., Hau, J., 2006. Quantification of cortisol, cortisol immunoreactive metabolites, and immunoglobulin A in serum, saliva, urine, and feces for noninvasive assessment of stress in reindeer. *Can J Vet Res* 70, 151–154.

Remage-Healey, L., Romero, L. M., 2001. Corticosterone and insulin interact to regulate glucose and triglyceride levels during stress in a bird. *Am J Physiol* 281, R994–R1003.

Reneerkens, J., Morrison, R. I. G., Ramenofsky, M., Piersma, T., Wingfield, J. C., 2002. Baseline and stress-induced levels of corticosterone during different life cycle substages in a shorebird on the high arctic breeding grounds. *Physiol Biochem Zool* 75, 200–208.

Rettenbacher, S., Mostl, E., Groothuis, T. G. G., 2009. Gestagens and glucocorticoids in chicken eggs. *Gen Comp Endocrinol* 164, 125–129.

Rich, E. L., Romero, L. M., 2005. Exposure to chronic stress downregulates corticosterone responses to acute stressors. *Am J Physiol* 288, R1628–R1636.

Richardson, R. D., Boswell, T., 1993. A method for third ventricular cannulation of small passerine birds. *Physiol Behav* 53, 209–213.

Rittenhouse, C. D., Millspaugh, J. J., Washburn, B. E., Hubbard, M. W., 2005. Effects of radiotransmitters on fecal glucocorticoid metabolite levels of three-toed box turtles in captivity. *Wildlife Soc Bull* 33, 706–713.

Roedl, T., Berger, S., Romero, L. M., Wikelski, M., 2007. Tameness and stress physiology in a predator-naive island species confronted with novel predation threat. *Proc R Soc Lond B* 274, 577–582.

Rogovin, K., Randall, J. A., Kolosova, I., Moshkin, M., 2003. Social correlates of stress in adult males of the great gerbil, *Rhombomys opimus*, in years of high and low population densities. *Horm Behav* 43, 132–139.

Romero, L. M., 2001. Mechanisms underlying seasonal differences in the avian stress response. In: Dawson, A., Chaturvedi, C. M. (Eds.), *Avian endocrinology*. Narosa Publishing House, New Delhi, pp. 373–384.

Romero, L. M., 2002. Seasonal changes in plasma glucocorticoid concentrations in free-living vertebrates. *Gen Comp Endocrinol* 128, 1–24.

Romero, L. M., 2004. Physiological stress in ecology: Lessons from biomedical research. *Trends Ecol Evol* 19, 249–255.

Romero, L. M., Cyr, N. E., Romero, R. C., 2006a. Corticosterone responses change seasonally in free-living house sparrows (*Passer domesticus*). *Gen Comp Endocrinol* 149, 58–65.

Romero, L. M., Dean, S. C., Wingfield, J. C., 1998a. Neurally-active stress peptide inhibits territorial defense in wild birds. *Horm Behav* 34, 239–247.

Romero, L. M., Holt, D. W., Maples, M., Wingfield, J. C., 2006b. Corticosterone is not correlated with nest departure in snowy owl chicks (*Nyctea scandiaca*). *Gen Comp Endocrinol* 149, 119–123.

Romero, L. M., Holt, D. W., Petersen, J. L., 2009. Flushing effects and seasonal changes on corticosterone levels in adult long-eared owls *Asio otus*. *Ardea* 97, 603–608.

Romero, L. M., Meister, C. J., Cyr, N. E., Kenagy, G. J., Wingfield, J. C., 2008. Seasonal glucocorticoid responses to capture in wild free-living mammals. *Am J Physiol* 294, R614-R622.

Romero, L. M., Ramenofsky, M., Wingfield, J. C., 1997. Season and migration alters the corticosterone response to capture and handling in an arctic migrant, the white-crowned sparrow (*Zonotrichia leucophrys gambelii*). *Comp Biochem Physiol* 116C, 171–177.

Romero, L. M., Reed, J. M., 2005. Collecting baseline corticosterone samples in the field: is under three minutes good enough? *Comp Biochem Physiol Part A: Mol Integr Physiol* 140, 73–79.

Romero, L. M., Reed, J. M., 2008. Repeatability of baseline corticosterone concentrations. *Gen Comp Endocrinol* 156, 27–33.

Romero, L. M., Reed, J. M., Wingfield, J. C., 2000. Effects of weather on corticosterone responses in wild free-living passerine birds. *Gen Comp Endocrinol* 118, 113–122.

Romero, L. M., Romero, R. C., 2002. Corticosterone responses in wild birds: the importance of rapid initial sampling. *Condor* 104, 129–135.

Romero, L. M., Soma, K. K., Wingfield, J. C., 1998b. Changes in pituitary and adrenal sensitivities allow the snow bunting (*Plectrophenax nivalis*), an arctic-breeding song bird, to modulate corticosterone release seasonally. *J Comp Physiol B* 168, 353–358.

Romero, L. M., Soma, K. K., Wingfield, J. C., 1998c. Hypothalamic-pituitary-adrenal axis changes allow seasonal modulation of corticosterone in a bird. *Am J Physiol* 274, R1338–R1344.

Romero, L. M., Soma, K. K., Wingfield, J. C., 1998d. The hypothalamus and adrenal regulate modulation of corticosterone release in redpolls (*Carduelis flammea*—an arctic-breeding song bird). *Gen Comp Endocrinol* 109, 347–355.

Romero, L. M., Strochlic, D., Wingfield, J. C., 2005. Corticosterone inhibits feather growth: Potential mechanism explaining seasonal down regulation of corticosterone during molt. *Comp Biochem Physiol Part A: Mol Integr Physiol* 142, 65–73.

Romero, L. M., Wikelski, M., 2001. Corticosterone levels predict survival probabilities of Galápagos marine iguanas during El Niño events. *Proc Natl Acad Sci USA* 98, 7366–7370.

Romero, L. M., Wikelski, M., 2006. Diurnal and nocturnal differences in hypothalamic-pituitary-adrenal axis function in Galapagos marine iguanas. *Gen Comp Endocrinol* 145, 177–181.

Romero, L. M., Wingfield, J. C., 1997. A novel stereotaxic-like method for injecting into the lateral ventricles of small passerine birds. *Physiol Behav* 62, 1109–1112.

Romero, L. M., Wingfield, J. C., 1999. Alterations in hypothalamic-pituitary-adrenal function associated with captivity in Gambel's white-crowned sparrows (*Zonotrichia leucophrys gambelii*). *Comp Biochem Physiol* 122B, 13–20.

Romero, L. M., Wingfield, J. C., 2001. Regulation of the hypothalamic-pituitary-adrenal axis in free-living pigeons. *J Comp Physiol B* 171, 231–235.

Romero, S. M. B., Pereira, A. F., Garofalo, M. A. R., Hoffmann, A., 2004. Effects of exercise on plasma catecholamine levels in the toad, *Bufo paracnemis*: Role of the adrenals and neural control. *J Exp Zool A: Comp Exp Biol* 301A, 911–918.

Rossdale, P. D., Burguez, P. N., Cash, R. S. G., 1982. Changes in blood neutrophil lymphocyte ratio related to adreno cortical function in the horse. *Equine Vet J* 14, 203–298.

Rubenstein, D. R., 2007. Stress hormones and sociality: Integrating social and environmental stressors. *Proc R Soc Lond B* 274, 967–975.

Salomons, H. M., Mulder, G. A., van de Zande, L., Haussmann, M. F., Linskens, M. H. K., Verhulst, S., 2009. Telomere shortening and survival in free-living corvids. *Proc R Soc Lond B* 276, 3157–3165.

Sands, J., Creel, S., 2004. Social dominance, aggression and faecal glucocorticoid levels in a wild population of wolves, *Canis lupus*. *Anim Behav* 67, 387–396.

Sangalang, G. B., Freeman, H. C., 1976. Steroids in the plasma of the gray seal, *Halichoerus grypus*. *Gen Comp Endocrinol* 29, 419–422.

Sanz, J. J., Moreno, J., Merino, S., Tomas, G., 2004. A trade-off between two resource-demanding functions: Post-nuptial moult and immunity during reproduction in male pied flycatchers. *J Anim Ecol* 73, 441–447.

Sapolsky, R. M., 1982. The endocrine stress-response and social status in the wild baboon. *Horm Behav* 16, 279–287.

Sapolsky, R. M., 1987. Stress, social status, and reproductive physiology in free-living baboons. In: Crews, D. (Ed.) *Psychobiology of reproductive behavior: An evolutionary perspective.* Prentice-Hall, Englewood Cliffs, NJ, pp. 291–322.

Sapolsky, R. M., 1992. *Stress, the aging brain, and the mechanisms of neuron death.* MIT Press, Cambridge, MA.

Sapolsky, R. M., 2001. Physiological and pathophysiological implications of social stress in mammals. In: McEwen, B. S., Goodman, H. M. (Eds.), *Handbook of physiology*; Section 7: *The endocrine system*; Vol. IV: *Coping with the environment: Neural and endocrine mechanisms.* Oxford University Press, New York, pp. 517–532.

Sapolsky, R. M., Altmann, J., 1991. Incidence of hypercortisolism and dexamethasone resistance increases with age among wild baboons. *Biol Psych* 30, 1008–1016.

Sapolsky, R. M., Romero, L. M., Munck, A. U., 2000. How do glucocorticoids influence stress-responses? Integrating permissive, suppressive, stimulatory, and preparative actions. *Endocr Rev* 21, 55–89.

Sapolsky, R. M., Share, L. J., 1994. Rank-related differences in cardiovascular function among wild baboons: Role of sensitivity to glucocorticoids. *Am J Primatol* 32, 261–275.

Satterlee, D. G., Johnson, W. A., 1988. Selection of Japanese quail for contrasting blood corticosterone response to immobilization. *Poult Sci* 67, 25–32.

Satterlee, D. G., Jones, R. B., 1997. Ease of capture in Japanese quail of two lines divergently selected for adrenocortical response to immobilization. *Poult Sci* 76, 469–471.

Savory, C. J., Kostal, L., 1997. Application of a radiotelemetry system for chronic measurement of blood pressure, heart rate, EEG, and activity in the chicken. *Physiol Behav* 61, 963–969.

Scheiber, I. B. R., Kralj, S., Kotrschal, K., 2005. Sampling effort/frequency necessary to infer individual acute stress responses from fecal analysis in greylag geese (Anser anser). *Ann NY Acad Sci*, 1046, 154–167.

Scheibler, E., Weinandy, R., Gattermann, R., 2004. Social categories in families of Mongolian gerbils. *Physiol Behav* 81, 455–464.

Scheuerlein, A., Van't Hof, T. J., Gwinner, E., 2001. Predators as stressors? Physiological and reproductive consequences of predation risk in tropical stonechats (*Saxicola torquata axillaris*). *Proc R Soc Lond B* 268, 1575.

Schjolden, J., Stoskhus, A., Winberg, S., 2005. Does individual variation in stress responses and agonistic behavior reflect divergent stress coping strategies in juvenile rainbow trout? *Physiol Biochem Zool* 78, 715–723.

Schoech, S. J., Ketterson, E. D., Nolan, V., 1999. Exogenous testosterone and the adrenocortical response in dark-eyed juncos. *Auk* 116, 64–72.

Schulz, J. H., Gao, X., Millspaugh, J. J., Bermudez, A. J., 2007. Experimental lead pellet ingestion in mourning doves (*Zenaida macroura*). *Am Midl Nat* 158, 177–190.

Schulz, J. H., Millspaugh, J. J., Bermudez, A. J., Gao, X., Bonnot, T. W., Britt, L. G., Paine, M., 2006. Acute lead toxicosis in mourning doves. *J Wildlife Manage* 70, 413–421.

Schulz, J. H., Millspaugh, J. J., Washburn, B. E., Bermudez, A. J., Tomlinson, J. L., Mong, T. W., He, Z., 2005. Physiological effects of radiotransmitters on mourning doves. *Wildlife Society Bull* 33, 1092–1100.

Schutz, K. E., Agren, E., Amundin, M., Roken, B., Palme, R., Morner, T., 2006. Behavioral and physiological responses of trap-induced stress in European badgers. *J Wildlife Manage* 70, 884–891.

Schwabl, H., 1995. Individual variation of the acute adrenocortical response to stress in the white-throated sparrow. *Zoology* 99, 113–120.

Schwabl, H., 1996. Maternal testosterone in the avian egg enhances postnatal growth. *Comp Biochem Physiol A* 114, 271–276.

Schwabl, H., Ramenofsky, M., Schwabl-Benzinger, I., Farner, D. S., Wingfield, J. C., 1988. Social status, circulating levels of hormones, and competition for food in winter flocks of the white-throated sparrow. *Behaviour* 107, 107–121.

Scott, A. P., Ellis, T., 2007. Measurement of fish steroids in water: A review. *Gen Comp Endocrinol* 153, 392–400.

Selva, N., Cortes-Avizanda, A., Lemus, J. A., Blanco, G., Mueller, T., Heinrich, B., Donazar, J. A., 2011. Stress associated with group living in a long-lived bird. *Biol Lett* 7, 608–610.

Sheldon, L. D., Chin, E. H., Gill, S. A., Schmaltz, G., Newman, A. E. M., Soma, K. K., 2008. Effects of blood collection on wild birds: an update. *J Avian Biol* 39, 369–378.

Sher, L., 2005. Type D personality: The heart, stress, and cortisol. *QJM* 98, 323–329.

Sheriff, M. J., Bosson, C. O., Krebs, C. J., Boonstra, R., 2009. A non-invasive technique for analyzing fecal cortisol metabolites in snowshoe hares (*Lepus americanus*). *J Comp Physiol B* 179, 305–313.

Sheriff, M. J., Dantzer, B., Delehanty, B., Palme, R., Boonstra, R., 2011. Measuring stress in wildlife: techniques for quantifying glucocorticoids. *Oecologia* 166, 869–887.

Sheriff, M. J., Krebs, C. J., Boonstra, R., 2010. Assessing stress in animal populations: Do fecal and plasma glucocorticoids tell the same story? *Gen Comp Endocrinol* 166, 614–619.

Shutler, D., Mullie, A., Clark, R. G., 2004. Tree swallow reproductive investment, stress, and parasites. *Can J Zool* 82, 442–448.

Siegel, H. S., 1995. Stress, strains and resistance. *Brit Poultry Sci* 36, 3–22.

Silverin, B., 1997. The stress response and autumn dispersal behaviour in willow tits. *Anim Behav* 53, 451–459.

Silverin, B., 1998. Behavioural and hormonal responses of the pied flycatcher to environmental stressors. *Anim Behav* 55, 1411–1420.

Silverin, B., Arvidsson, B., Wingfield, J., 1997. The adrenocortical responses to stress in breeding Willow Warblers *Phylloscopus trochilus* in Sweden: Effects of latitude and gender. *Func Ecol* 11, 376–384.

Silverin, B., Wingfield, J. C., 1998. Adrenocortical responses to stress in breeding pied flycatchers *Ficedula hypoleuca*: Relation to latitude, sex and mating status. *J Avian Biol* 29, 228.

Sims, C. G., Holberton, R. L., 2000. Development of the corticosterone stress response in young northern mockingbirds (*Mimus polyglottos*). *Gen Comp Endocrinol* 119, 193–201.

Smith, E. N., Allison, R. D., Crowder, W. E., 1974. Bradycardia in a free ranging American alligator. *Copeia*, 1974, 770–772.

Smith, E. N., Decarvalho, M. C., 1985. Heart rate response to threat and diving in the ornate box turtle, *Terrapene-ornata*. *Physiol Zool* 58, 236–241.

Smith, E. N., Woodruff, R. A., 1980. Fear bradycardia in free-ranging woodchucks, *Marmota-monax*. *J Mammal* 61, 750–753.

Smith, G. T., Wingfield, J. C., Veit, R. R., 1994. Adrenocortical response to stress in the common diving petrel, *Pelecanoides urinatrix*. *Physiol Zool* 67, 526–537.

Sorato, E., Kotrschal, K., 2006. Hormonal and behavioural symmetries between the sexes in the Northern bald ibis. *Gen Comp Endocrinol* 146, 265–274.

Sousa, M. B. C., Ziegler, T. E., 1998. Diurnal variation on the excretion patterns of fecal steroids in common marmoset (*Callithrix jacchus*) females. *Am J Primatol* 46, 105–117.

Staley, A. M., Blanco, J. M., Dufty, A. M., Jr., Wildt, D. E., Monfort, S. L., 2007. Fecal steroid monitoring for assessing gonadal and adrenal activity in the golden eagle and peregrine falcon. *J Comp Physiol B* 177, 609–622.

Stead-Richardson, E., Bradshaw, D., Friend, T., Fletcher, T., 2010. Monitoring reproduction in the critically endangered marsupial, Gilbert's potoroo (*Potorous gilbertii*): Preliminary analysis of faecal oestradiol-17 beta, cortisol and progestagens. *Gen Comp Endocrinol* 165, 155–162.

Steen, J. B., Gabrielsen, G. W., Kanwisher, J. W., 1988. Physiological aspects of freezing behavior in willow ptarmigan hens. *Acta Physiol Scand* 134, 299–304.

Strier, K. B., Ziegler, T. E., Wittwer, D. J., 1999. Seasonal and social correlates of fecal testosterone and cortisol levels in wild male muriquis (*Brachyteles arachnoides*). *Horm Behav* 35, 125–134.

Strochlic, D. E., Romero, L. M., 2008. The effects of chronic psychological and physical stress on feather replacement in European starlings (*Sturnus vulgaris*). *Comp Biochem Physiol Part A: Mol Integr Physiol* 149, 68–79.

Suarez-Dominguez, E. A., Morales-Mavil, J. E., Chavira, R., Boeck, L., 2011. Effects of habitat perturbation on the daily activity pattern and physiological stress of the spiny tailed iguana (*Ctenosaura acanthura*). *Amphibia-Reptilia* 32, 315–322.

Suorsa, P., Helle, H., Koivunen, V., Huhta, E., Nikula, A., Hakkarainen, H., 2004. Effects of forest patch size on physiological stress and immunocompetence in an area-sensitive passerine, the Eurasian treecreeper (*Certhia familiaris*): An experiment. *Proc R Soc Lond B* 271, 435–440.

Superina, M., Carreno, N., Jahn, G. A., 2009. Characterization of seasonal reproduction patterns in female pichis *Zaedyus pichiy* (Xenarthra: Dasypodidae) estimated by fecal sex steroid metabolites and ovarian histology. *Anim Repro Sci* 116, 358–369.

Swain, U. G., Gilbert, F. F., Robinette, J. D., 1988. Heart rates in the captive, free-ranging beaver. *Comp Biochem Physiol A* 91, 431–435.

Tarlow, E. M., Blumstein, D. T., 2007. Evaluating methods to quantify anthropogenic stressors on wild animals. *Appl Anim Behav Sci* 102, 429–451.

Tempel, D. J., Gutierrez, R. J., 2003. Fecal corticosterone levels in California spotted owls exposed to low-intensity chainsaw sound. *Wildlife Soc Bull* 31, 698–702.

Tempel, D. J., Gutierrez, R. J., 2004. Factors related to fecal corticosterone levels in California spotted owls: Implications for assessing chronic stress. *Conserv Biol* 18, 538–547.

Teskey-Gerstl, A., Bamberg, E., Steineck, T., Palme, R., 2000. Excretion of corticosteroids in urine and faeces of hares (*Lepus europaeus*). *J Comp Physiol B* 170, 163–168.

Theil, P. K., Coutant, A. E., Olesen, C. R., 2004. Seasonal changes and activity-dependent variation in heart rate of roe deer. *J Mammal* 85, 245–253.

Thiel, D., Jenni-Eiermann, S., Palme, R., 2005. Measuring corticosterone metabolites in droppings of capercaillies (*Tetrao urogallus*). *Ann NY Acad Sci*, 1046, 96–108.

Thomsen, R., Voigt, C. C., 2006. Non-invasive blood sampling from primates using laboratory-bred blood-sucking bugs (*Dipetalogaster maximus*; Reduviidae, Heteroptera). *Primates* 47, 397–400.

Tieleman, B. I., Williams, J. B., Ricklefs, R. E., Klasing, K. C., 2005. Constitutive innate immunity is a component of the pace-of-life syndrome in tropical birds. *Proc R Soc Lond B* 272, 1715–1720.

Totzke, U., Fenske, M., Hueppop, O., Raabe, H., Schach, N., 1999. The influence of fasting on blood and plasma composition of herring gulls (*Larus argentatus*). *Physiol Biochem Zool* 72, 426–437.

Touma, C., Palme, R., 2005. Measuring fecal glucocorticoid metabolites in mammals and birds: The importance of validation. *Ann NY Acad Sci*, 1046, 54–74.

Touma, C., Sachser, N., Mostl, E., Palme, R., 2003. Effects of sex and time of day on metabolism and excretion of corticosterone in urine and feces of mice. *Gen Comp Endocrinol* 130, 267–278.

Turner, J. W., Jr., Nemeth, R., Rogers, C., 2003. Measurement of fecal glucocorticoids in parrotfishes to assess stress. *Gen Comp Endocrinol* 133, 341–352.

Tyrrell, C. L., Cree, A., 1998. Relationships between corticosterone concentration and season, time of day and confinement in a wild reptile (tuatara, *Sphenodon punctatus*). *Gen Comp Endocrinol* 110, 97–108.

Valverde, R. A., Owens, D. W., Mackenzie, D. S., Amoss, M. S., 1999. Basal and stress-induced corticosterone levels in olive ridley sea turtles (*Lepidochelys olivacea*) in relation to their mass nesting behavior. *J Exp Zool* 284, 652–662.

Van Jaarsveld, A. S., Skinner, J. D., 1992. Adrenocortical responsiveness to immobilization stress in spotted hyenas (*Crocuta crocuta*). *Comp Biochem Physiol A* 103, 73–79.

Varo, N., Amat, J. A., 2008. Differences in food assimilation between two coot species assessed with stable isotopes and particle size in faeces: Linking physiology and conservation. *Comp Biochem Physiol Part A: Mol Integr Physiol* 149, 217–223.

Vasconcellos, A. S., Chelini, M. O. M., Palme, R., Guimaraes, M., Oliveira, C. A., Ades, C., 2011. Comparison of two methods for glucocorticoid evaluation in maned wolves. *Pesqui Vet Bras* 31, 79–83.

Vera, F., Antenucci, C. D., Zenuto, R. R., 2011. Cortisol and corticosterone exhibit different seasonal variation and responses to acute stress and captivity in tuco-tucos (*Ctenomys talarum*). *Gen Comp Endocrinol* 170, 550–557.

Vleck, C. M., 2001. Comparison of corticosterone and heterophil to lymphocyte ratios as indicators of stress in free-living birds. In: Dawson, A., Chaturvedi, C. M. (Eds.), *Avian endocrinology*. Narosa Publishing House, New Delhi, pp. 401–411.

Vleck, C. M., Haussmann, M. F., Vleck, D., 2007. Avian senescence: Underlying mechanisms. *J Ornithol* 148, S611–S624.

Vleck, C. M., Vertalino, N., Vleck, D., Bucher, T. L., 2000. Stress, corticosterone, and heterophil to lymphocyte ratios in free-living Adelie penguins. *Condor* 102, 392–400.

Voigt, C. C., Fassbender, M., Dehnhard, M., Wibbelt, G., Jewgenow, K., Hofer, H., Schaub, G. A., 2004. Validation of a minimally invasive blood-sampling technique for the analysis of hormones in domestic rabbits, *Oryctolagus cuniculus* (Lagomorpha). *Gen Comp Endocrinol* 135, 100–107.

Voigt, C. C., Peschel, U., Wibbelt, G., Frolich, K., 2006. An alternative, less invasive blood sample collection technique for serologic studies utilizing triatomine bugs (Heteroptera; insecta). *J Wildlife Dis* 42, 466–469.

von der Ohe, C. G., Servheen, C., 2002. Measuring stress in mammals using fecal glucocorticoids: Opportunities and challenges. *Wildlife Soc Bull* 30, 1215–1225.

von der Ohe, C. G., Wasser, S. K., Hunt, K. E., Servheen, C., 2004. Factors associated with fecal glucocorticoids in Alaskan brown bears (*Ursus arctos horribilis*). *Physiol Biochem Zool* 77, 313–320.

Voss, M., Shutler, D., Werner, J., 2010. A hard look at blood sampling of birds. *Auk* 127, 704–708.

Vylitova, M., Miksik, I., Pacha, J., 1998. Metabolism of corticosterone in mammalian and avian intestine. *Gen Comp Endocrinol* 109, 315–324.

Wack, C. L., Fox, S. F., Hellgren, E. C., Lovern, M. B., 2008. Effects of sex, age, and season on plasma steroids in free-ranging Texas horned lizards (*Phrynosoma cornutum*). *Gen Comp Endocrinol* 155, 589–596.

Wada, H., Breuner, C. W., 2008. Transient elevation of corticosterone alters begging behavior and growth of white-crowned sparrow nestlings. *J Exp Biol* 211, 1696–1703.

Wada, H., Moore, I. T., Breuner, C. W., Wingfield, J. C., 2006. Stress responses in tropical sparrows: Comparing tropical and temperate Zonotrichia. *Physiol Biochem Zool* 79, 784–792.

Walker, C.-D., Anand, K. J. S., Plotsky, P. M., 2001. Development of the hypothalamic-pituitary-adrenal axis and the stress response. In: McEwen, B. S., Goodman, H. M. (Eds.), *Handbook of physiology*; Section 7: *The endocrine system*; Vol. IV: *Coping with the environment: Neural and endocrine mechanisms*. Oxford University Press, New York, pp. 237–270.

Wallner, B., Moestl, E., Dittami, J., Prossinger, H., 1999. Fecal glucocorticoids document stress in female barbary macaques (*Macaca sylvanus*). *Gen Comp Endocrinol* 113, 80–86.

Wascher, C. A. F., Amold, W., Kotrschal, K., 2008. Heart rate modulation by social contexts in greylag geese (*Anser anser*). *J Comp Psychol* 122, 100–107.

Washburn, B. E., Millspaugh, J. J., 2002. Effects of simulated environmental conditions on glucocorticoid metabolite measurements in white-tailed deer feces. *Gen Comp Endocrinol* 127, 217–222.

Washburn, B. E., Millspaugh, J. J., Schulz, J. H., Jones, S. B., Mong, T., 2003. Using fecal glucocorticoids for stress assessment in mourning doves. *Condor* 105, 696–706.

Wasser, S. K., Bevis, K., King, G., Hanson, E., 1997. Noninvasive physiological measures of disturbance in the northern spotted owl. *Conserv Biol* 11, 1019–1022.

Wasser, S. K., Davenport, B., Ramage, E. R., Hunt, K. E., Parker, M., Clarke, C., Stenhouse, G., 2004. Scat detection dogs in wildlife research and management: Application to grizzly and black bears in the Yellowhead Ecosystem, Alberta, Canada. *Can J Zool* 82, 475–492.

Wasser, S. K., Hunt, K. E., 2005. Noninvasive measures of reproductive function and disturbance in the barred owl, great horned owl, and northern spotted owl. *Ann NY Acad Sci*, 1046, 109–137.

Wasser, S. K., Hunt, K. E., Brown, J. L., Cooper, K., Crockett, C. M., Bechert, U., Millspaugh, J. J., Larson, S., Monfort, S. L., 2000. A generalized fecal glucocorticoid assay for use in a diverse array of nondomestic mammalian and avian species. *Gen Comp Endocrinol* 120, 260–275.

Wasser, S. K., Smith, H., Madden, L., Marks, N., Vynne, C., 2009. Scent-matching dogs determine number of unique individuals from scat. *J Wildlife Manage* 73, 1233–1240.

Wasser, S. K., Thomas, R., Nair, P. P., Guidry, C., Southers, J., Lucas, J., Wildt, D. E., Monfort, S. L., 1993. Effects of dietary fibre on faecal steroid measurements in baboons (*Papio cynocephalus cynocephalus*). *J Reprod Fertil* 97, 569–574.

Watson, S. L., McCoy, J. G., Stavisky, R. C., Greer, T. F., Hanbury, D., 2005. Cortisol response to relocation stress in Garnett's bushbaby (*Otolemur garnettii*). *Cont Topics Lab Animal Sci* 44, 22–24.

Weber, D. K., Danielson, K., Wright, S., Foley, J. E., 2002. Hematology and serum biochemistry values of dusky-footed wood rat (*Neotoma fuscipes*). *J Wildlife Dis* 38, 576–582.

Weimerskirch, H., Shaffer, S. A., Mabille, G., Martin, J., Boutard, O., Rouanet, J. L., 2002. Heart rate and energy expenditure of incubating wandering albatrosses: Basal levels, natural variation, and the effects of human disturbance. *J Exp Biol* 205, 475–483.

Weingrill, T., Gray, D. A., Barrett, L., Henzi, S. P., 2004. Fecal cortisol levels in free-ranging female chacma baboons: Relationship to dominance, reproductive state and environmental factors. *Horm Behav* 45, 259–269.

Wells, K. M. S., Washburn, B. E., Millspaugh, J. J., Ryan, M. R., Hubbard, M. W., 2003. Effects of radio-transmitters on fecal glucocorticoid levels in captive dickcissels. *Condor* 105, 805–810.

Whitten, P. L., Stavisky, R., Aureli, F., Russell, E., 1998. Response of fecal cortisol to stress in captive chimpanzees (*Pan troglodytes*). *Am J Primatol* 44, 57–69.

Widowski, T. M., Curtis, S. E., Graves, C. N., 1989. The neutrophil lymphocyte ratio in pigs fed cortisol. *Can J Animal Sci* 69, 501–504.

Wikelski, M., Kays, R. W., Kasdin, N. J., Thorup, K., Smith, J. A., Swenson, G. W., Jr., 2007. Going wild: What a global small-animal tracking system could do for experimental biologists. *J Exp Biol* 210, 181–186.

Williams, T. D., 2008. Individual variation in endocrine systems: moving beyond the "tyranny of the Golden Mean."*Phil Trans R Soc B* 363, 1687–1698.

Wilson, C. M., Holberton, R. L., 2004. Individual risk versus immediate reproductive success: A basis for latitudinal differences in the adrenocortical response to stress in yellow warblers (*Dendroica petechia*). *Auk* 121, 1238–1249.

Wingfield, J. C., 1988. Changes in reproductive function of free-living birds in direct response to environmental perturbations. In: Stetson, M. H. (Ed.) *Processing of environmental information in vertebrates*. Springer-Verlag, Berlin, pp. 121–148.

Wingfield, J. C., 1994. Modulation of the adrenocortical response to stress in birds. In: Davey, K. G., Peter, R. E., Tobe, S. S. (Eds.), *Perspectives in comparative endocrinology*. National Research Council of Canada, Ottawa, pp. 520–528.

Wingfield, J. C., DeViche, P., Sharbaugh, S., Astheimer, L. B., Holberton, R., Suydam, R., Hunt, K., 1994a. Seasonal changes of the adrenocortical responses to stress in redpolls, *Acanthis flammea*, in Alaska. *J Exp Zool* 270, 372–380.

Wingfield, J. C., Hunt, K., Breuner, C., Dunlap, K., Fowler, G. S., Freed, L., Lepson, J., 1997. Environmental stress, field endocrinology, and conservation biology. In: Clemmons, J. R., Buchholz, R. (Eds.), *Behavioral approaches to conservation in the wild*. Cambridge University Press, Cambridge, UK, pp. 95–131.

Wingfield, J. C., Kubokawa, K., Ishida, K., Ishii, S., Wada, M., 1995a. The adrenocortical response to stress in male bush warblers, *Cettia diphone*: A comparison of breeding populations in Honshu and Hokkaido, Japan. *Zool Sci* 12, 615–621.

Wingfield, J. C., O'Reilly, K. M., Astheimer, L. B., 1995b. Modulation of the adrenocortical responses to acute stress in Arctic birds: A possible ecological basis. *Am Zool* 35, 285–294.

Wingfield, J. C., Ramenofsky, M., 1997. Corticosterone and facultative dispersal in response to unpredictable events. *Ardea* 85, 155–166.

Wingfield, J. C., Ramenofsky, M., 1999. Hormones and the behavioral ecology of stress. In: P. H. M. Balm (Ed.), *Stress Physiology in Animals*, Sheffield Academic Press, Sheffield, U.K., pp. 1–51.

Wingfield, J. C., Ramos-Fernandez, G., Nunez-de la Mora, A., Drummond, H., 1999. The effects of an "El Nino" southern oscillation event on reproduction in male and female blue-footed boobies, *Sula nebouxii*. *Gen Comp Endocrinol* 114, 163–172.

Wingfield, J. C., Romero, L. M., 2001. Adrenocortical responses to stress and their modulation in free-living vertebrates. In: McEwen, B. S., Goodman, H. M. (Eds.), *Handbook of physiology*; Section 7: *The endocrine system*; Vol. IV: *Coping with the environment: Neural and endocrine me*chanisms. Oxford University Press, New York, pp. 211–234.

Wingfield, J. C., Silverin, B., 1986. Effects of corticosterone on territorial behavior of free-living male song sparrows *Melospiza melodia*. *Horm Behav* 20, 405–417.

Wingfield, J. C., Smith, J. P., Farner, D. S., 1982. Endocrine responses of white-crowned sparrows to environmental stress. *Condor* 84, 399–409.

Wingfield, J. C., Suydam, R., Hunt, K., 1994b. The adrenocortical responses to stress in snow buntings (*Plectrophenax nivalis*) and Lapland longspurs (*Calcarius lapponicus*) at Barrow, Alaska. *Comp Biochem Physiol* 108C, 299–306.

Wingfield, J. C., Vleck, C. M., Moore, M. C., 1992. Seasonal changes of the adrenocortical response to stress in birds of the Sonoran Desert. *J Exp Zool* 264, 419–428.

Woodruff, J. A., Lacey, E. A., Bentley, G., 2010. Contrasting fecal corticosterone metabolite levels in captive and free-living colonial tuco-tucos (*Ctenomys sociabilis*). *J Exper Zool A* 313A, 498–507.

Work, T. M., Rameyer, R. A., Balazs, G. H., Cray, C., Chang, S. P., 2001. Immune status of free-ranging green turtles with fibropapillomatosis from Hawaii. *J Wildlife Dis* 37, 574–581.

Wright, A. J., Aguilar Soto, N., Baldwin, A. L., Bateson, M., Beale, C. M., Clark, C., Deak, T., Edwards, E. F., Fernández, A., Godinho, A., Hatch, L., Kakuschke, A., Lusseau, D., Martineau, D., Romero, L. M., Weilgart, L., Wintle, B., Notarbartolo di Sciara, G., Martin, V., 2007. Do marine mammals experience stress related to anthropogenic noise? *Int J Comp Psychol* 20, 274–316.

Xinran, C., Cuijuan, N., Lijun, P., 2007. Effects of stocking density on growth and non-specific immune responses in juvenile soft-shelled turtle, *Pelodiscus sinensis*. *Aquaculture Res* 38, 1380–1386.

Young, K. M., Brown, J. L., Goodrowe, K. L., 2001. Characterization of reproductive cycles and adrenal activity in the black-footed ferret (*Mustela nigripes*) by fecal hormone analysis. *Zoo Biol* 20, 517–536.

Young, K. M., Walker, S. L., Lanthier, C., Waddell, W. T., Monfort, S. L., Brown, J. L., 2004. Noninvasive monitoring of adrenocortical activity in carnivores by fecal glucocorticold analyses. *Gen Comp Endocrinol* 137, 148–165.

Young, L. J., Wang, Z. X., 2004. The neurobiology of pair bonding. *Nature Neurosci* 7, 1048–1054.

Zav'yalov, E. L., Gerlinskaya, L. A., Evsikov, V. I., 2003. Estimation of stress level in the bank vole *Clethrionomys glareolus* (Rodentidae, Rodentia) by fecal corticosterone. *Zoologicheskii Zhurnal* 82, 508–513.

Zav'yalov, E. L., Gerlinskaya, L. A., Ovchinnikova, L. E., Evsikov, V. I., 2007. Stress and territorial structure of a local water vole (*Arvicola terrestris*) population. *Zoologicheskii Zhurnal* 86, 242–251.

Zerani, M., Amabili, F., Mosconi, G., Gobbetti, A., 1991. Effects of captivity stress on plasma steroid levels in the green frog, *Rana esculenta*, during the annual reproductive cycle. *Comp Biochem Physiol* 98A, 491–496.

Zuri, I., Gottreich, A., Terkel, J., 1998. Social stress in neighboring and encountering blind mole-rats (*Spalax ehrenbergi*). *Physiol Behav* 64, 611–620.

7

Responses to Natural Perturbations

Variation in Available Energy

I. INTRODUCTION

Natural perturbations of the environment involve numerous abiotic and biotic factors that interact to threaten homeostasis, food availability, and territory or home range integrity. Biotic factors include food available (Eg in Chapter 3), parasites, diseases, and social interactions. In this chapter we assess factors that have a direct relationship to changes in energy. Of course, many stressors have indirect impacts on energy. Examples include effects of weather that increase allostatic load and are potentially stressful, which we will discuss in Chapter 8, and other biotic factors, including social- and health-related issues, which we will discuss in Chapter 9. We acknowledge that there is considerable overlap with this Chapter and Chapters 8 and 9 because these types of perturbations interact at many levels. It is perhaps heuristic, however, to assemble the evidence from the literature on stressors that have a direct impact on energy as a first attempt to assess these complex interactions and to determine what future directions should then be pursued in field and laboratory experiments. The literature is indeed vast on these topics, and we have made no attempt to cover everything, but we have tried to provide good evidence for a very representative set that address the key points.

Perturbation factors can be classified into three types, as outlined by Wingfield (2013a, 2013b; see also Chapter 1 of this volume). Specific examples of *abiotic indirect labile perturbation factors* are listed in Table 7.1. As reviewed in Chapter 4, responses to indirect labile perturbation factors involve activation of the autonomic nervous system and secretions of the adrenal medulla such as epinephrine. As soon as the perturbation has passed, recovery is quick, and individuals return to their predictable daily routines of the normal life cycle. There have been very few field investigations on this group of perturbation factors, and they have been covered in Chapter 4 and will not be considered further here.

In contrast, *abiotic direct labile perturbation factors* are longer term, that is, hours to days (examples in Table 7.1; Wingfield 2013b). These potentially trigger allostatic responses resulting in an individual abandoning its normal life-history stage because of reduced or restricted access to biotic resources such as food, shelter, and so on. Hormonal responses to direct labile perturbation factors, reactive scope, typically involve the hypothalamo-pituitary-adrenal cortex (HPA) axis culminating in the release of glucocorticoids (e.g., Sapolsky et al. 2000; Wingfield 2003; Romero et al. 2009).

Third, *abiotic permanent perturbation factors* leading to adaptation or local extinction (examples in Table 7.1) involve changes in the environment and occur following major events such as changes

TABLE 7.1: TYPES OF ABIOTIC PERTURBATION FACTORS

Abiotic Indirect Labile Perturbation Factors	Abiotic Direct Labile Perturbation Factors	Abiotic Permanent Perturbation Factors
Sudden severe storm (e.g., tornado, thunderstorm, freezing rain and other ice conditions)	Prolonged storms or temporary climate change (e.g., El Niño Southern Oscillation Event)	Global climate change
Fire (localized)	Fire (on a large scale)	Human disturbance (urbanization, habitat degradation)
Flood from rain that fell many kilometers away and not in the local area (e.g., desert stream beds, arroyos, or wadis)	Heat and drought	Pollution (endocrine disruption)
Earthquakes, tsunamis, volcanic eruption	Cold	
Accident (e.g. run/crawl/fly/swim from a falling rock)	Hypoxia	
	Extremes of pH	
	Extremes of osmotic pressure	
	Trace element deficiency	
	High pressure	
	Intense solar radiation	

After Wingfield 2013a, 2013b.

in climate and direct disturbance of anthropogenic origin. Because these are permanent, or extremely long term (e.g., hundreds of years), organisms must undergo similarly permanent acclimation to the event, and many individuals may die, or reproductive success might be reduced to such an extent that extinction follows. However, some individuals are able to show sufficient acclimation/adaptation that will change many aspects of the life cycle but that allow them to survive. Selection for those individuals that can adapt may be intense, and eventually those phenotypes will persist (McEwen and Wingfield 2003; Wingfield 2003). Because permanent perturbation factors select for those individuals that adapt to new conditions, it is unlikely that there are permanent increases in activation of the HPA axis. These individuals adapt to new conditions and do not show the symptoms of chronic stress; they return to a different "normal" life cycle that now matches the new conditions. For example, freezing temperatures during the breeding season may be a powerful stressor for a species that is not accustomed to it, but once that species has adapted to conditions during an ice age, freezing temperatures are now normal. In many ways, this is what we mean when we say that a species has adapted—local conditions are no longer stressful. As far as we know, this point has not been investigated in free-living organisms following a permanent perturbation. Other aspects of this relating to human disturbance and conservation will be discussed in later chapters.

Labile perturbation factors that affect energy availability are many, but we will focus on more well-known examples here, mostly direct labile perturbation factors. They include habitat quality, climatic events such as El Niño Southern Oscillation events, famine, and hypoxia, especially during metabolically expensive life-history events such as migration and molt.

II. HABITAT QUALITY

The quality of the habitat in which organisms live involves many interacting factors of abiotic and biotic origin. Quality can involve the degree of shelter from weather, as well as predators, food availability, access to that food, and low incidence of disease and parasites. Each individual experiences its environment in a unique way and differently from its neighbor just meters away. Internal differences (such as parasite load and injuries, social status) and external differences (including microhabitat, presence of predators, etc.) all play a role. They interact, resulting in complex individual experiences of the local environment. This in turn determines how organisms respond by regulating physiology, morphology, and behavior (Wingfield et al. 2011). Given these individual experiences, it is probable, indeed frequent, that one individual may experience potentially stressful conditions, but its neighbor may not. For these reasons it is important to consider how the habitat is configured and how this relates to quality.

Configuration is defined as the way in which parts or elements of something are arranged to fit together (Wingfield et al. 2011). First, it is important to include internal state (e.g., parasites, energy reserves, injury, age, and so on), and to integrate this with external conditions in relation to territory/home range quality, weather and exposure, shelter, predators, population density, and social status to determine how challenging environmental conditions may be and thus the potential for Eo (Wingfield et al. 2011). The configuration of habitat that provides sufficient food (Eg) so that it can fuel seasonal routines (e.g., breeding, migration, molt, etc.) and shelter when the weather turns bad or when predators are nearby should be as favorable for fitness as possible. Trophic resources (Eg) must also be sufficient to cover the energetic costs of internal components such as parasites, injury, and social status (Ee + Ei). Some examples of the complex interactions of external and internal factors are listed in Table 7.2 (from Wingfield et al. 2011). It is also important to point out that prior experience of extreme events can, through learning, result in additional behavioral traits for dealing with perturbations in the future of that individual's life span.

TABLE 7.2: POTENTIAL COMPONENTS OF HABITAT CONFIGURATION

External	Internal
Territory/home range	Body condition
Location (central/peripheral)	Age
Food availability	Parasite load
Weather	Injury
Exposure to weather	Proactive/reactive coping style
Shelter	Social status
Population density	Pollutant load
Predator density/variety	Developmental experience
Human disturbance	Maternal (paternal) effects
Presence of mate (social status)	Ability to access food resources
Group size (social status)	
Heterospecific competition (non-predator)	
Invasive species	

From Wingfield et al. (2011), courtesy of Academica Sinica.

The assessment of these complex interactions, the interaction of abiotic and biotic factors, will require theoretical and biophysical approaches to come up with testable predictions under natural conditions. Porter et al. (2002) and Pörtner and Farrell (2008) present models for ecological predictions concerning distribution, energetic requirements, and predator-prey interactions. These are relevant for identifying potential conditions when Eo is likely to increase, especially at the individual level, and how components of the external, internal, and social environments might combine to increase allostatic load (Ee + Ei + Eo). There is also an important temporal component to habitat quality. Trophic resources (Eg) may be abundant for a limited but predictable period, or abundant for a limited but unpredictable period. This could have profound implications for allostatic load. On the other hand, Eg may never be particularly high, that is, trophic resources are dispersed and difficult to obtain, or high but concentrated in certain seasons or patchily distributed. Social status can be an important factor for allostatic load by limiting access to resources when available, whereas those individuals with higher social status are not so limited. However, Goymann and Wingfield (2004) have pointed out that high social status may also increase allostatic load in certain contexts.

A. Terrestrial Habitats

Circulating corticosteroid levels and the response to acute stress are related to many aspects of life histories and environmental conditions, including food supply and habitat (Ricklefs and Wikelski 2002). In some species, males and females may segregate into different habitats on their wintering grounds. In the American redstart on its non-breeding grounds in Jamaica, males tend to predominate in higher quality habitat such as mangroves, and females predominate in lower quality habitat such as dry scrub (Marra et al. 1993). A field study showed that, soon after migrant arrival in October, all redstarts in the female-dominated habitat had similar baseline levels of blood corticosterone to those in the male-dominated habitat. However, by spring, just prior to departure on vernal migration, baseline levels of corticosterone were much higher in redstarts in female-dominated habitat, regardless of age and sex (Figure 7.1; Marra and Holberton 1998). In autumn, birds in both habitats showed

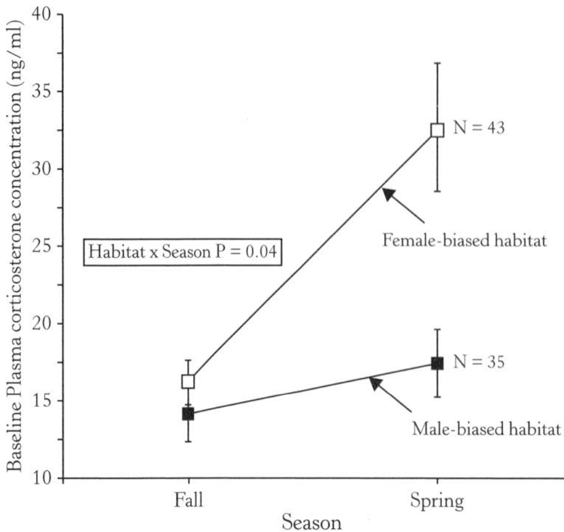

FIGURE 7.1: Plasma baseline levels (mean. 1 SE) of corticosterone in American redstarts at time of capture (baseline) in male- and female-biased habitat types in fall (October) and spring (late March/early April) on the non-breeding grounds in Jamaica, West Indies. Sexes combined due to non-significant effects of sex in ANOVA.

From Marra and Holberton (1998), with permission and courtesy of Springer-Verlag.

marked increases in circulating corticosterone following capture, handling, and restraint, whereas in spring only birds in the male-dominated habitat showed the same increase to acute stress (Figure 7.2; Marra and Holberton 1998). Birds from the female-dominated habitat showed no significant increase of corticosterone over baseline levels (Figure 7.2). Clearly redstarts (mostly females) in lower quality habitat undergo a decrease in body condition over winter compared with redstarts (mostly males) in better quality habitat. The implications for migration and reproduction remain unknown but could be important.

Habitat quality and geographical range of populations depend upon a variety of biotic and abiotic factors. The song wren in Panama is common in rain forest, but abundance declines markedly down a rainfall gradient southward toward the Pacific side of the isthmus. Song wrens inhabiting less preferred habitat in drier parts of their range had lower body condition and higher baseline levels of circulating corticosterone than birds in the wetter forest close to the Caribbean side of the isthmus (Figure 7.3; Busch et al. 2011). In Carolina chickadees, birds from a disturbed site (a recently logged forest) had higher fecal levels of corticosteroids than those sampled in undisturbed forest and in a residential area (Lucas et al. 2006). Body mass of chickadees in the disturbed site was lower than in the undisturbed site but higher than in birds sampled in the residential area. A laboratory experiment showed that with ad libitum food, all populations underwent the same seasonal changes in body weight and fecal corticosteroid levels, and caching rates were similar. The authors suggest that the different corticosteroid levels in birds from the disturbed area were not simply because of disturbance, but may be related to lower quality of habitat.

Field investigation into the "island syndrome," in which organisms face different

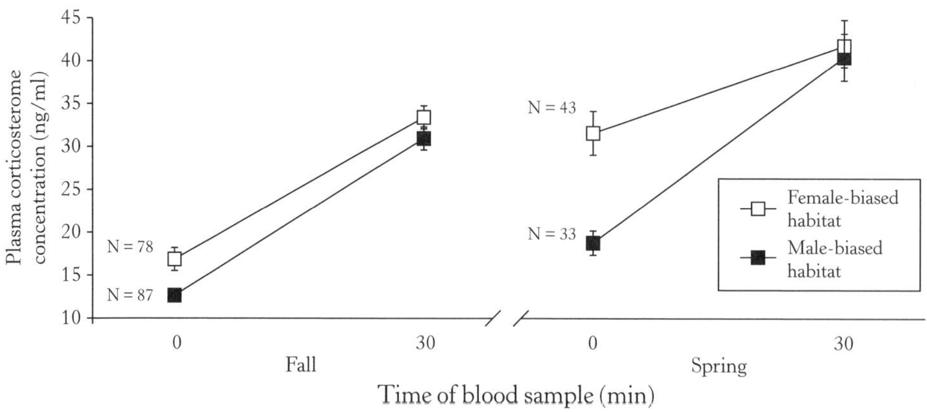

FIGURE 7.2: Profiles of corticosterone secretion at the time of capture (0) and 30 minutes after capture (30) in American redstarts in female- and male-dominated habitat types in fall (October) and spring (late March/early April) on the non-breeding grounds in Jamaica. Sexes and ages combined due to non-significant effects of both in ANOVA.

From Marra and Holberton (1998), with permission and courtesy of Springer-Verlag.

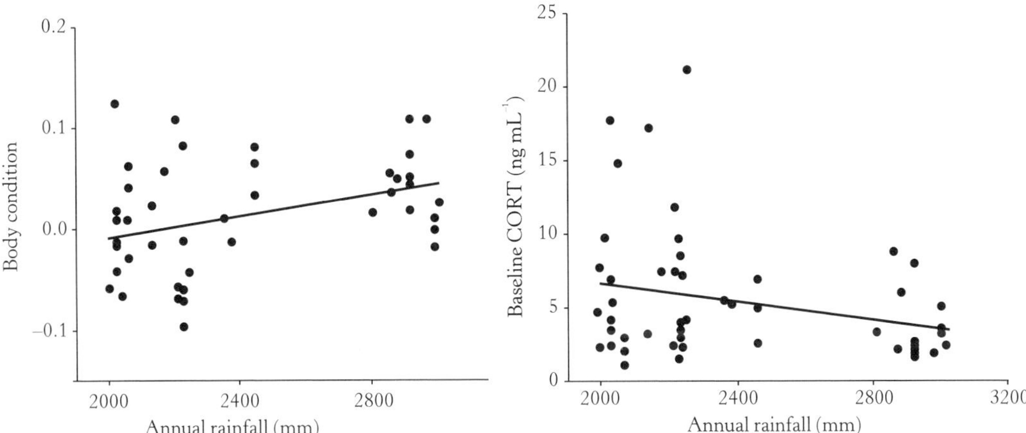

FIGURE 7.3: Significant linear regression relationships from best-fit path models of song wrens across their geographical range on the isthmus of Panama, an area characterized by a strong rainfall gradient.

From Busch et al. (2011), with permission, British Ecological Society.

ecological conditions than their conspecifics on the mainland, showed reduced species diversity, leading to fewer predators and lower interspecific competition in island ecosystems. Blondel (2000) looked at populations of blue tits in Corsica (in the Mediterranean) and in the European mainland in France. Two populations were studied at each site, one in summer green habitat (with high abundance of caterpillars in spring) and the other in evergreen habitat (with lower and later emergence of caterpillars; Muller et al. 2007). Baseline corticosterone levels were lower in island populations of blue tits (Figure 7.4) compared with mainland birds, indicating a possible effect of insular island syndrome. Baseline levels of corticosterone did not differ in blue tits between summer green and evergreen habitats on the island or mainland. Corticosterone levels after capture, handling, and restraint stress were higher in the evergreen population with less caterpillars to feed young than in the summer green site. This effect was more marked on the island population (Muller et al. 2007).

In free-living chicks of the Eurasian tree creeper, plasma levels of corticosterone were generally negatively related to body condition and survival (Figure 7.5; Suorsa et al. 2003) Furthermore, these authors found that corticosterone levels were higher in conditions of poor food supply. Forest fragmentation also was correlated with plasma corticosterone, with higher circulating levels in birds in smaller patches of forest (Suorsa et al. 2003). However, a low-quality diet does not appear to be equivalent to low food availability. A short period of poor food during the nestling phase of zebra finches decreased growth but did not elevate corticosterone titers (Honarmand et al. 2010).

There is often not a simple relationship, however, between forage availability and corticosteroid concentrations. In a review of field studies of chimpanzees and other primates, Seraphin et al. (2006) concluded that habitat quality, defined in terms of dietary plant availability and other characteristics, can influence urinary corticosteroid metabolites in complex ways. Studies in various reptile species are also not consistent. Field studies of brown tree snakes, an invasive species in Guam, show that multiple indices of body condition may be important to tease apart the complex relationships with corticosteroid secretion (Waye and Mason 2008). Animals with greater body condition (indicative of good populations of prey) had lower baseline corticosterone levels (Waye and Mason 2008). In contrast, there were no differences in plasma levels of corticosterone in free-ranging desert tortoises from two habitats of differing quality (Dickinson et al. 2002). In addition, the relationship between corticosteroids and habitat quality can often be more complex than simply with baseline levels. The Western fence lizard has a very broad distribution across arid and semi-arid areas of the western United States. A comparison of blood corticosterone levels in populations of fence lizards at three sites on the edge of their distribution with three populations at the center of their range revealed no consistent differences in baseline corticosterone. But, maximum plasma corticosterone after capture, handling, and restraint

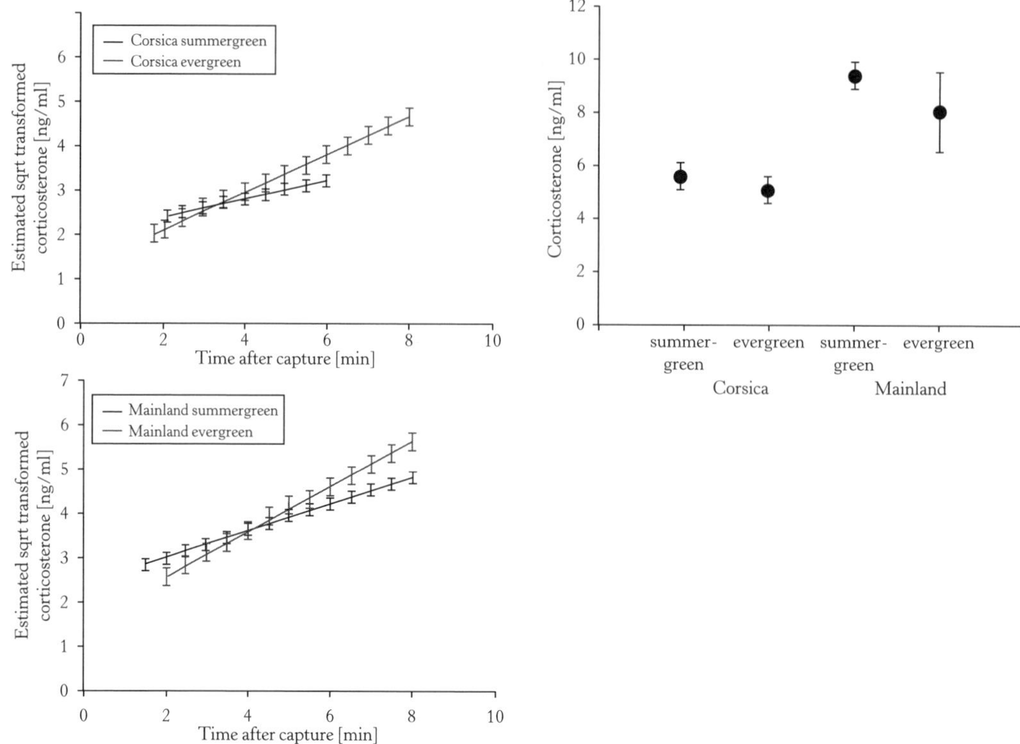

FIGURE 7.4: Baseline corticosterone levels of blue tits breeding in habitats of different quality on Corsica and mainland Southern France. Individuals on the Mediterranean island of Corsica had significantly lower levels than their conspecifics in southern France near Montpellier. There was no significant difference between individuals breeding in the summer green downy oak habitat and those breeding in the evergreen holm oak habitat.

From Muller et al. (2007), with permission and courtesy of Elsevier Press.

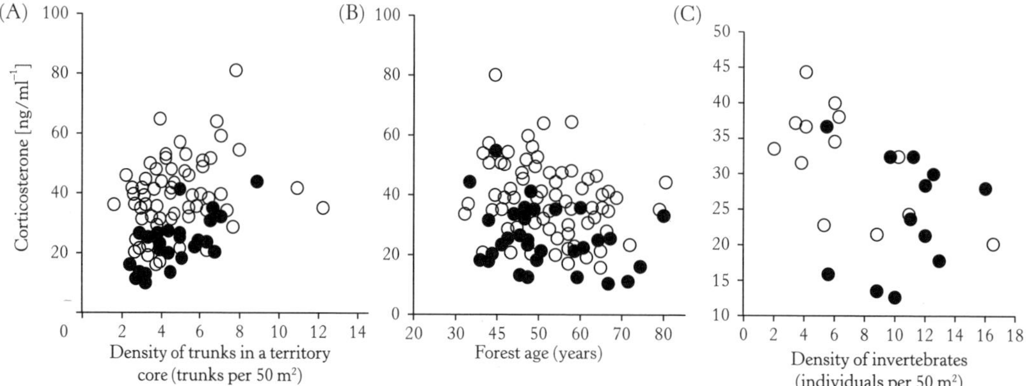

FIGURE 7.5: (A) Relationship between density of tree trunks (trunks per 50 m^2) at the territory core area and the corticosterone level in the heaviest chick of each brood in the Eurasian tree creeper. Corticosterone increased with greater forest density in both first broods (represented by open circles) and second broods (represented by filled circles). (B) Relationship between forest age at the territory core area and corticosterone level in the heaviest chick of each brood. Corticosterone decreased in older forests in both first and second broods. (C) Relationship between mean density of invertebrates on tree trunks and the mean corticosterone level in the brood (all nestlings sampled). Corticosterone decreased with increasing food availability in first broods but not second broods.

From Suorsa et al. (2003), with permission and courtesy of the Royal Society.

was higher in populations living at the margin of their normal range, particularly in those individuals with lowest body condition (Figure 7.6; Dunlap and Wingfield 1995). However, the difference in maximum corticosterone levels in lizards from marginal habitat remained in populations held in identical laboratory conditions, suggesting that body condition was not the only factor involved. These data are consistent with the hypothesis that lower quality habitat at the edge of a normal range is accompanied by higher activity of the adrenocortical response to acute stress. Wilson (1990) and Wilson and Wingfield (1992) concluded that seasonal and individual variation in basal corticosterone in side-blotched lizards was related more closely to intrinsic reproductive cycles (e.g., oogenic state) and ontogenetic changes (juveniles vs. adult) than seasonal or geographic differences in environmental quality. Males had higher corticosterone concentrations than females in the spring, but interpreting this finding is difficult because during the spring sampling period relatively few females had emerged from hibernation. It is thus impossible to determine whether this difference in basal corticosterone is due to an intrinsic sexual difference or whether it is related to emergence from hibernation (Dauphin-Villemant et al. 1987). The apparent lack of any consistent seasonal variation is possibly due to asynchronous breeding cycles among populations (Wilson 1990; Wilson and Wingfield 1992).

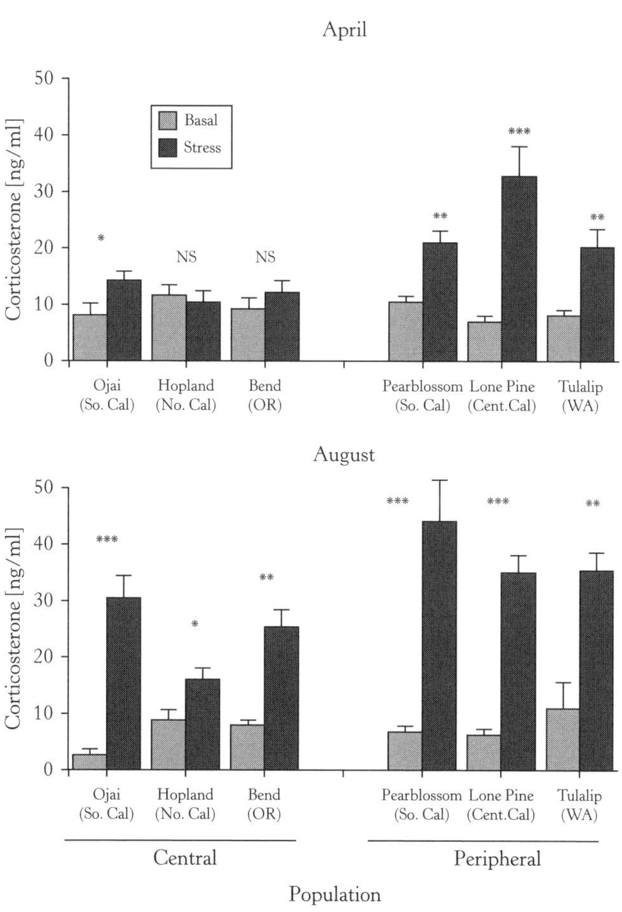

FIGURE 7.6: Plasma corticosterone concentration in six populations of western fence lizards during April and August. Blood was collected immediately after capture (within 1 min) for basal concentrations (filled bars) or 1 hour after capture for stress concentrations (hatched bars). Asterisks indicate significant differences between basal and stress values.

* $P < 0.05$; ** $P < 0.01$; *** $P < 0.001$; NS, not significant.

From Dunlap and Wingfield (1995), courtesy of Wiley Liss.

Interpreting habitat-related differences in corticosteroids can be difficult because many other factors may be involved. For example, in southern Sweden, pied flycatchers prefer to nest in deciduous forests rather than coniferous forests. Moreover, the density of breeding birds and reproductive success was highest in the deciduous forest. Simulated territorial intrusions (STI) to test the aggression of breeding birds in the two habitats showed that flycatchers were generally more aggressive in response to STI and had higher plasma levels of testosterone in the deciduous versus coniferous forests (Figure 7.7; Silverin 1998). However, circulating levels of corticosterone were also higher in the preferred habitat, deciduous forest, than in the suboptimal coniferous forest (Figure 7.8; Silverin 1998). This may have been because the density of birds was higher and there was more competition in the preferred habitat. These data are the opposite of what many others have found, and emphasize that many factors should be taken into consideration when determining adrenocortical responses to habitat quality (e.g., Bonier et al. 2009). Working with a breeding population of pied flycatchers in Wales (United Kingdom), Kern et al. (2005) found that plasma corticosterone levels increased during incubation and provisioning of nestlings in females and during the parental phase in males, suggesting an effect of substage of the nesting cycle that also must be taken into account. The increase in corticosterone, however, appears to be related to gluconeogenesis required to support parental activities (Kern et al. 2007).

If poor-quality habitat does result in increased corticosteroid levels, it could have a profound impact. Treatment of male barn owls with corticosterone to simulate a stress event resulted in decreased provisioning rates of chicks (Almasi et al. 2008). These data suggest that higher corticosteroid levels resulting from a poor-quality habitat could have repercussions on parental care. Similar results have been obtained for the effects of corticosterone treatment on territorial

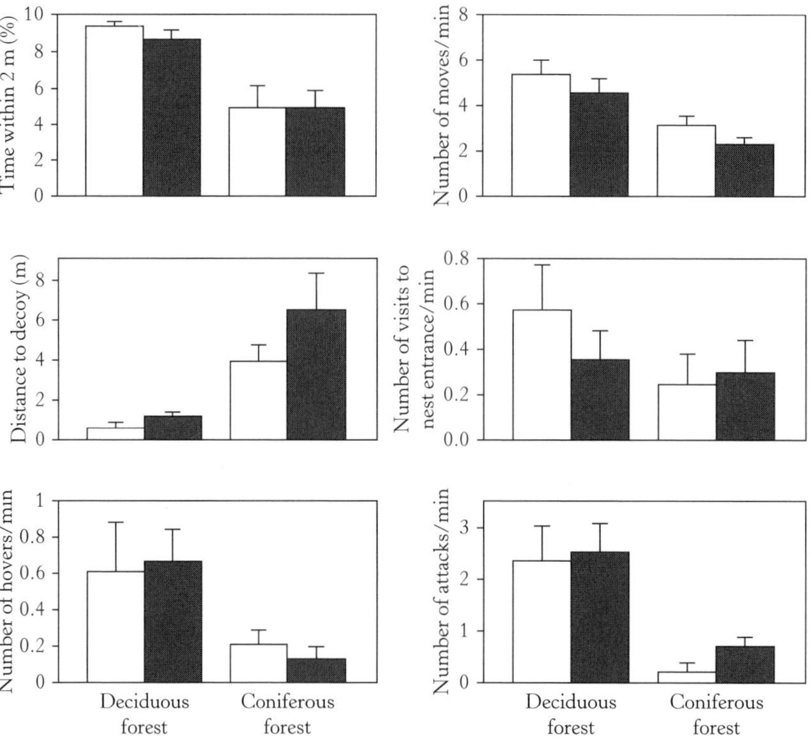

FIGURE 7.7: Behavior of free-living male pied flycatchers during a 10-minute exposure to a simulated territorial intrusion (a stuffed male pied flycatcher placed on the roof of the nestbox + flycatcher song from a tape recorder). The experiments were done before the nest-building periods of 1993 (open bars) and 1994 (solid bars) and in two breeding habitats (deciduous and coniferous forests).

From Silverin (1998), with permission and courtesy of Elsevier.

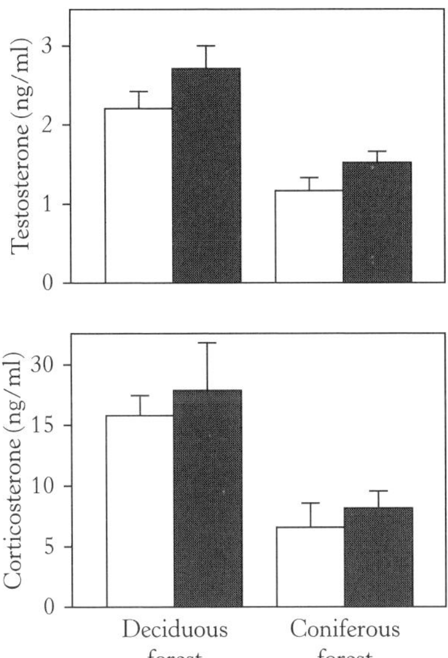

FIGURE 7.8: Circulating levels of testosterone and corticosterone in territorial, free-living, unmated, male pied flycatchers from two habitats in southwest Sweden. Blood samples were collected before the nest-building periods of 1995 (open bars) and 1996 (solid bars) in a deciduous and a coniferous forest. None of these males had been exposed to simulated territorial intrusions.

From Silverin (1998), with permission and courtesy of Elsevier.

aggression and parental care in pied flycatchers (Silverin 1986) and song sparrows (Wingfield and Silverin 1986). Experimental supplementation of food in free-living vertebrates is one way to increase habitat quality and often results in earlier onset of breeding (Figure 7.9; e.g., Boutin 1990; Schoech et al. 2007). Supplemental food also decreased baseline corticosterone levels in blood relative to controls in free-living song sparrows (Clinchy et al. 2004) and Florida scrub jays (Schoech et al. 2007) compared to birds on un-supplemented territories. Schoech et al. (2007) hypothesized that low circulating corticosterone in the early breeding season, at least in females, may provide information that environmental conditions are conducive to onset of nesting and egg-laying. Corticosterone's role, however, appears to be more complex. Small doses of corticosterone were experimentally administered to females noninvasively by offering mealworms injected with corticosterone three times a day. This treatment resulted in an acute increase in circulating corticosterone, well within the physiological range, compared with control females. Corticosterone treatment did not significantly advance clutch initiation dates more than supplemental feeding alone, suggesting that cues to initiate nesting involve other regulatory pathways (Figure 7.9; Schoech et al. 2007). On the other hand, treatment of corticosterone via subcutaneous Silastic implants in female zebra finches that elevated blood corticosterone levels to those seen in response to acute stress decreased plasma vitellogenin and decreased the proportion of treated females that initiated egg-laying compared to controls (Salvante and Williams 2003). Furthermore, in those females that did breed, egg-laying was delayed by corticosterone treatment (Salvante and Williams 2003) Clearly corticosterone, as well as ecological context, can influence breeding decisions, but the relationship, and likely the mechanisms, are complex.

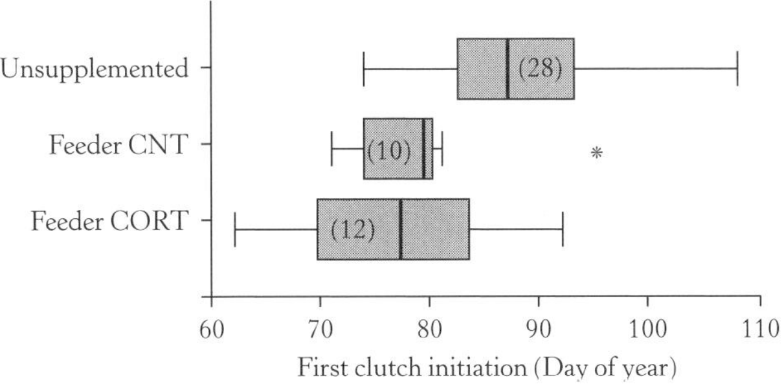

FIGURE 7.9: Dates of first clutch initiation for female Florida scrub jays in each treatment group. Boxes indicate the inter-quartile range with a vertical bar at the median. The data range and potential outliers are shown with whiskers and asterisks. Numbers in parenthesis are samples sizes (numbers of territories) for each group. The Feeder groups indicate groups that had supplemental food available via a feeder, and CORT indicates groups that were fed mealworms containing corticosterone (with CNT indicating the associated controls).

From Schoech et al. (2007), with permission and courtesy of Elsevier.

B. Marine Habitats

Habitat quality is difficult to assess in marine habitats. One example where this has been attempted is with oceanic seabirds that forage far out at sea. Field evidence continues to build supporting the general conclusion that baseline corticosteroids are an indicator of foraging conditions. High blood corticosteroid levels appear related to poor conditions (weather and food availability), and low corticosteroid levels appear related to good conditions. For example, plasma levels of corticosterone were explained by variation in foraging success and distance traveled in black-legged kittiwakes. Birds that were less successful had higher baseline corticosterone when returning to the breeding colony compared to levels just prior to leaving (Angelier et al. 2007a). Plasma corticosterone levels were also higher in breeding black-legged kittiwakes when food resources were scarce (Kitaysky et al. 1999b; Kitaysky et al. 2003; Buck et al. 2007). Similar results were found in free-living common murres, a piscivore, in the Bering Sea. Baseline corticosterone levels increased when foraging conditions were bad (Benowitz-Fredericks et al. 2008), especially during the chick substage of nesting during years when food availability (fish populations) was not coincident with nesting, compared to years in which the parental phase and maximum fish populations did coincide (Doody et al. 2008). Baseline corticosterone was also highest with projected feeding effort in Adelie penguins (Angelier et al. 2008). Finally, as penguins fast while incubating or attending young chicks, there appears to be a critical energy level in terms of stores, below which animals abandon eggs or young and return to the ocean to refeed (e.g., Groscolas et al. 2008). It is likely that the amount of energy stored and the time taken for the mate to refeed and return to relieve its mate are dependent upon the quality of the foraging area.

An increase in foraging effort in adults also seems to affect offspring. For example, chicks of black-legged kittiwakes near Kodiak Island, Alaska, had higher blood levels of corticosterone in years when foraging was poor (Brewer et al. 2008). However, corticosteroid levels in parents and offspring do not always match. A field study of breeding Wilson's storm-petrels in the Tres Hermanos (Three Brothers Hill) colony on King George Island (62°14'S, 58°40'W), South Shetland Islands in the maritime Antarctic, revealed that in a year when food availability was low, fecal corticosteroid metabolite levels of chicks were high during the period of starvation (Quillfeldt and Möstl 2003). Fecal corticosteroids were negatively correlated with body condition in chicks, whereas corticosteroids did not change in adults. These data suggest that in years of low food abundance, adults protect their own body condition by reducing the provisioning of chicks (Quillfeldt and Möstl 2003).

It is generally thought that as parental effort increases, due to decreasing quality of habitat and foraging, many long-lived species reduce their parental effort in favor of self-preservation. Harding et al. (2009) experimentally increased flight costs by clipping the flight feathers of little auks breeding in East Greenland, thereby simulating increased reproduction costs (increased allostatic load). Clipped little auks and their untreated mates both lost more body mass than unclipped controls and their partners, and also had higher plasma levels of baseline corticosterone (Figures 7.10 and 7.11). Furthermore, chicks of a clipped and untreated pair also fledged at a

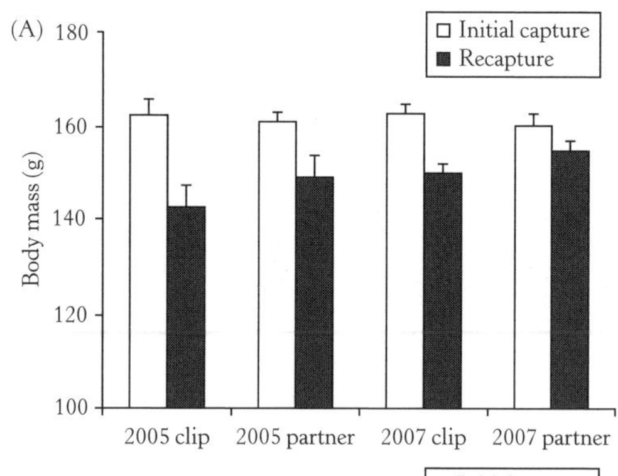

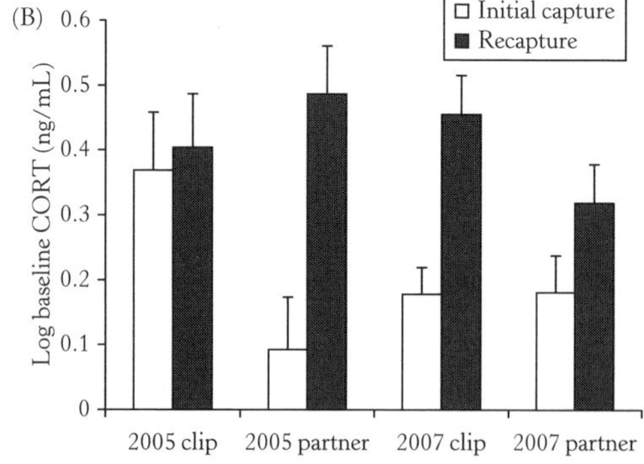

FIGURE 7.10: Values of (A) body mass in experimental little auks (clipped birds and partners to clipped birds) and (B) circulating baseline CORT levels (log-transformed) during the initial capture (before clipping) and recapture session.

From Harding et al. (2009), with permission and courtesy of the British Ecological Society.

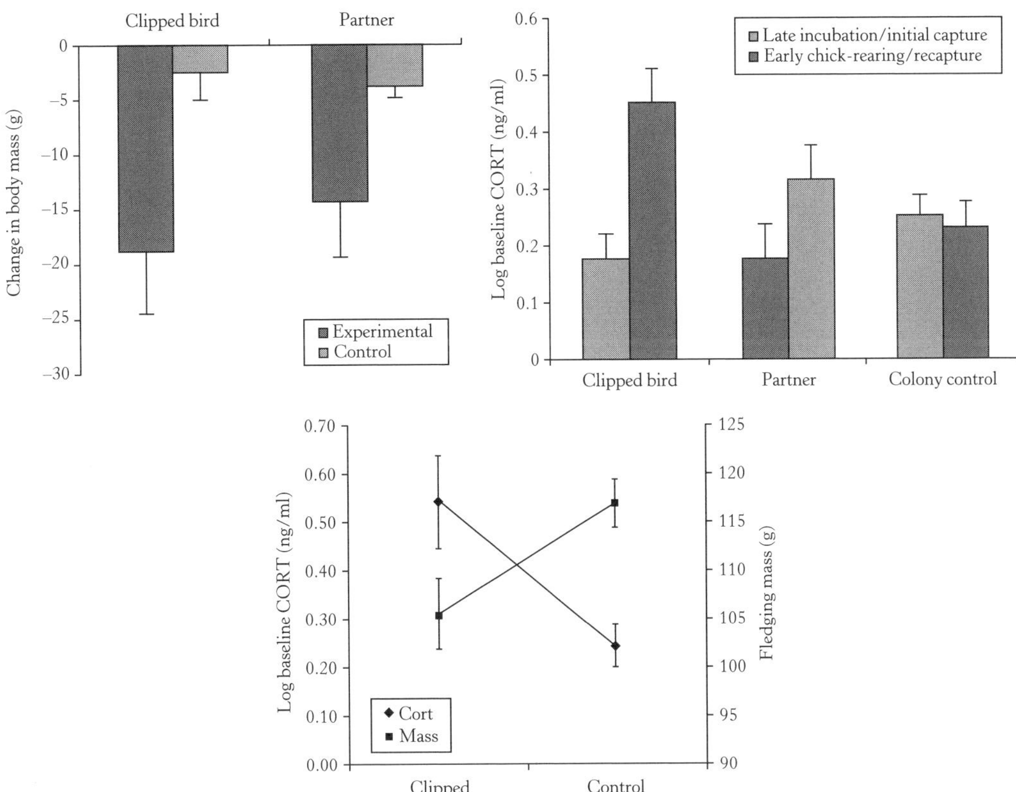

FIGURE 7.11: Top left caption. Changes in body mass of little auks, experimental and control adults. Top right caption. Corticosteroid (CORT) levels (log-transformed) in two capture groups: experimental pairs at initial capture and incubation colony control birds; and experimental pairs at recapture and chick-rearing colony birds. There was no significant difference in CORT levels in the three groups during the first capture. CORT levels in clipped birds were significantly higher than controls during the second capture session. Bottom caption. Chicks with a clipped parent had higher baseline CORT levels and fledged at a significantly lower body mass than chicks in the control group.

From (Harding et al. 2009). With permission and courtesy of the British Ecological Society.

lower body mass and had elevated plasma levels of corticosterone than did controls (Figure 7.11). Harding et al. (2009) conclude that the little auk, a fairly long-lived seabird, can increase foraging effort to some extent. On the other hand, increasing allostatic load by raising wing loading by adding 45 gram weights to Cory's shearwaters during incubation increased foraging time and a lower rate of mass gain while at sea, but resulted in no change in baseline corticosterone compared with controls (Navarro et al. 2008).

Although most work in this area has focused on avian species, other taxa appear to respond similarly. In a study of captive Steller's sea lions, food restriction, including quality of fish in the diet, resulted in an increase in plasma cortisol as body mass decreased. IGF-1 levels decreased, whereas no changes in thyroid hormones were seen (Figure 7.12; du Dot et al. 2009). Fecal corticosteroids in free-living populations of Steller's sea lions showed a negative correlation with changes in population size: those populations that were decreasing had higher corticosteroid levels (Kitaysky et al. 2007a). These population declines may be a result of loss of habitat quality in terms of fish available in the foraging grounds.

III. EL NIÑO SOUTHERN OSCILLATION EVENTS

The El Niño Southern Oscillation (ENSO; Trenberth 1997; Enfield 2001) is a major climatic event that prevails when a warm water layer originating from the Pacific Ocean overlays cold water of the Humboldt Current off the west coast of South America. The area affected by this layer of warm water varies tremendously and can be

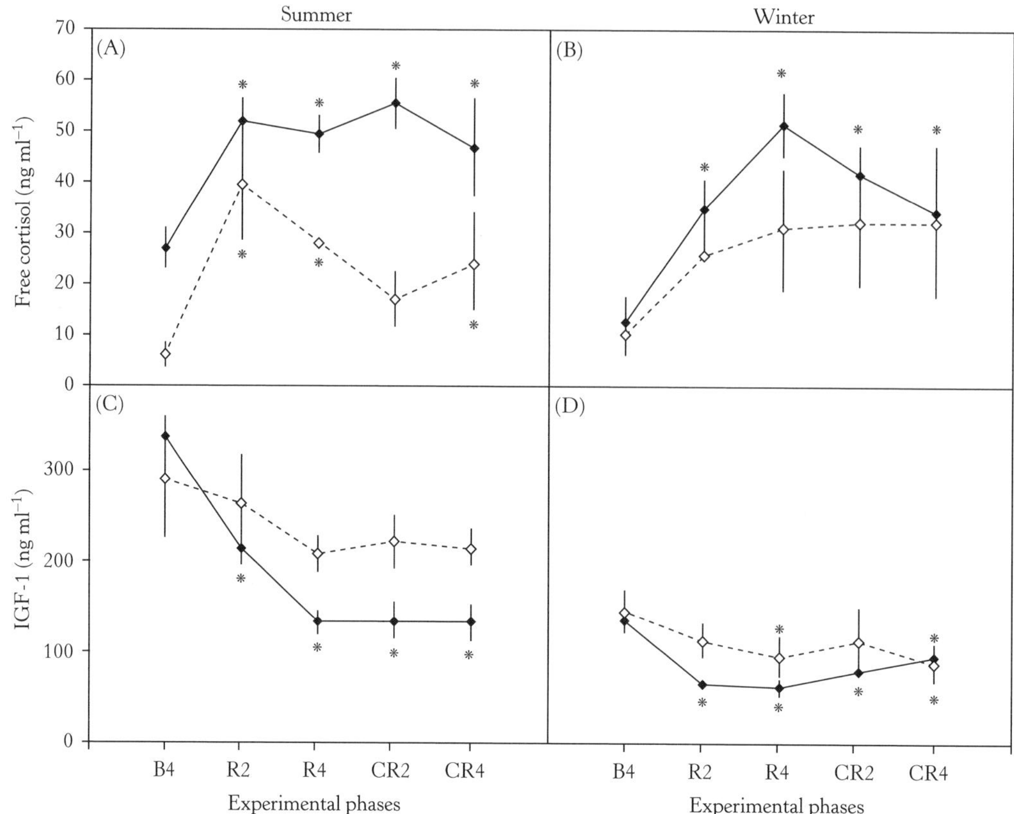

FIGURE 7.12: Mean ±SE serum concentration of free cortisol and IGF-1 in eight female Steller sea lions segregated by age class (filled diamonds: juveniles; and open diamonds: subadults) measured at the end of the baseline (B4), and after 2 and 4 weeks of restricted food intake (R2 and R4) and a controlled refeeding (CR2 and CR4) period. The two graphs on the left (A and C) represent the data collected during the summer 2005 experiment and the two graphs on the right (B and D) during the winter 2006 experiment. The asterisks indicate significant within-group differences compared to the respective B4 measurement.

From du Dot et al. (2009), with permission and courtesy of Elsevier.

as large as 5000 kilometers or more across the eastern Pacific Ocean. In these cases, an ENSO event can affect weather on oceans and landmasses globally (Ropelewski and Halpert 1987). This in turn can mean increases or decreases in food resources, depending upon whether drought or abundant rain conditions prevail. Seabirds worldwide are particularly vulnerable to ocean conditions during ENSO events in terms of food availability and the distance traveled to find that food from land-based breeding sites, as well as weather conditions that determine the energetic costs of flying under less than ideal conditions to forage. The opposite event is called La Niña, when colder water from the Humboldt Current prevails.

Extensive rainfall or droughts can result from ENSO events, and the former is followed by prodigious productivity of plant growth and arthropods. For example, land birds such as Galapagos finches can breed up to 15 consecutive months (Gibbs and Grant 1987) with individual reproductive capacity affected by an interaction of age and population density (Wilson et al. 2007). In contrast, warm water during an ENSO event has very low levels of nutrients, and primary marine productivity is reduced. Algal growth declines to virtually zero, the food chain collapses, fish stocks decline precipitously, and the sub-tidal zone of the Galapagos Islands becomes barren. Fishes and marine iguanas that depend on algal growth in this sub-tidal zone starve in large numbers during ENSO events (e.g., Laurie 1989; Wikelski and Trillmich 1997). Some seabird species that feed on fish and marine life close to shore also lose body condition and may fail to breed. A La Niña event results in nearly the opposite conditions. Sea temperatures are lower, accompanied by an upwelling of nutrients followed by rich algal blooms, increases of marine invertebrates, and increasing fish populations. Inshore feeding seabirds now have sufficient food to breed successfully. However, drought conditions prevail on land, with reduced primary productivity and a decline in arthropod numbers. Many land birds now have very restricted breeding seasons or may fail to nest successfully (e.g., Lack 1950; Grant and Grant 1980).

Variation in longer term climatic events such as ENSO that last several months, or even years, have raised a number of questions of whether baseline and maximum circulating levels of corticosteroids following acute stress are adjusted in response to these climatic events (e.g., Wingfield and Sapolsky 2003). Modulation of the adrenocortical responses to acute stress will be discussed in depth in Chapter 10, but some evidence will be introduced here, relevant to responses to perturbations of the environment. The brood value hypothesis (Bókony et al. 2009) predicts that adrenocortical responses to climatic conditions and acute stressors would be higher when conditions precluded successful reproduction. In other words, individuals faced with reduced reproductive success, and thus lower fitness value of that brood of young, would show a greater adrenocortical response to acute stress and thus greater probability of abandoning that breeding attempt. Brood value will also vary according to life span, with longer-lived organisms tending to show greater responsiveness to acute stress while breeding than shorter-lived organisms. This is because shorter-lived organisms will always have a higher brood value as a result of fewer possible breeding seasons. In seabirds, lower brood value potentially results during the ENSO year, and in land birds it would be during the La Niña year.

In Galapagos penguins and flightless cormorants, species dependent upon abundant fish for successful breeding, corticosterone levels were higher in the El Niño year compared to La Niña conditions. Offshore feeding seabirds, such as great frigate birds and red-footed boobies, showed no effects of ENSO on baseline or plasma levels of corticosterone (Wingfield et al., submitted), possibly because their pelagic food source was less affected by ENSO than in those foraging inshore. Terrestrial birds such as Galapagos finches, doves, and mockingbirds showed less dramatic differences in adrenocortical responses to acute stress with the ENSO event when trophic resources were good. Two small species (< 18 g) are an exception and had, contrary to predictions, increased baseline corticosterone and stress responses during ENSO conditions (Wingfield et al., submitted). It is possible that smaller species may be more susceptible to inclement weather during ENSO than larger species. These data point out that modulation of adrenocortical responses to stress with climatic conditions should address ecological conditions as well as body condition and breeding status.

A field investigation of another tropical Pacific seabird, nesting blue-footed boobies in a colony on Isla Isabel, off the Pacific coast of Sinaloa, Mexico, revealed zero reproductive success during the ENSO event of 1993. Approximately 20% of pairs in the colony attempted to breed and some hatched chicks. However, because during ENSO there was insufficient food to feed both adults and their chicks, all the latter died by day 18 of age, resulting in total loss of reproductive success (Figure 7.13; Wingfield et al. 1999). In contrast, when La Niña conditions prevailed in 1994, most pairs in the colony bred successfully. A comparison of both baseline plasma levels of corticosterone and the adrenocortical responses to capture, handling, and restraint in male and female blue-footed boobies on Isla Isabel were similar in the El Niño and La Niña years of 1993 and 1994 (Figure 7.13; Wingfield et al. 1999). Circulating testosterone levels were slightly lower in males and females during ENSO as expected, given that most birds did not initiate nesting. In blue-footed boobies and other seabirds, brood reduction is a typical response to adverse breeding conditions, and adults may cease to feed chicks if food supply is reduced and invest available food in self-preservation (see further discussion later in this chapter). However, although predictions of the brood value hypothesis were not supported in this study, a question can be raised of whether baseline and maximum corticosterone responses to acute stress during ENSO events may be adjusted prior to such events. Other field studies may shed light on this.

An ENSO's impact on reproduction is not restricted to birds. A study of Galapagos marine iguanas during ENSO conditions in 1998 and La Niña conditions in 1999 indicated that the widespread disappearance of intertidal algae during the ENSO resulted in substantial increases in corticosterone (Romero and Wikelski 2001). As a result of different currents surrounding the Galapagos archipelago, an ENSO has different impacts on the algal forage on different islands. Figure 7.14 shows that corticosterone

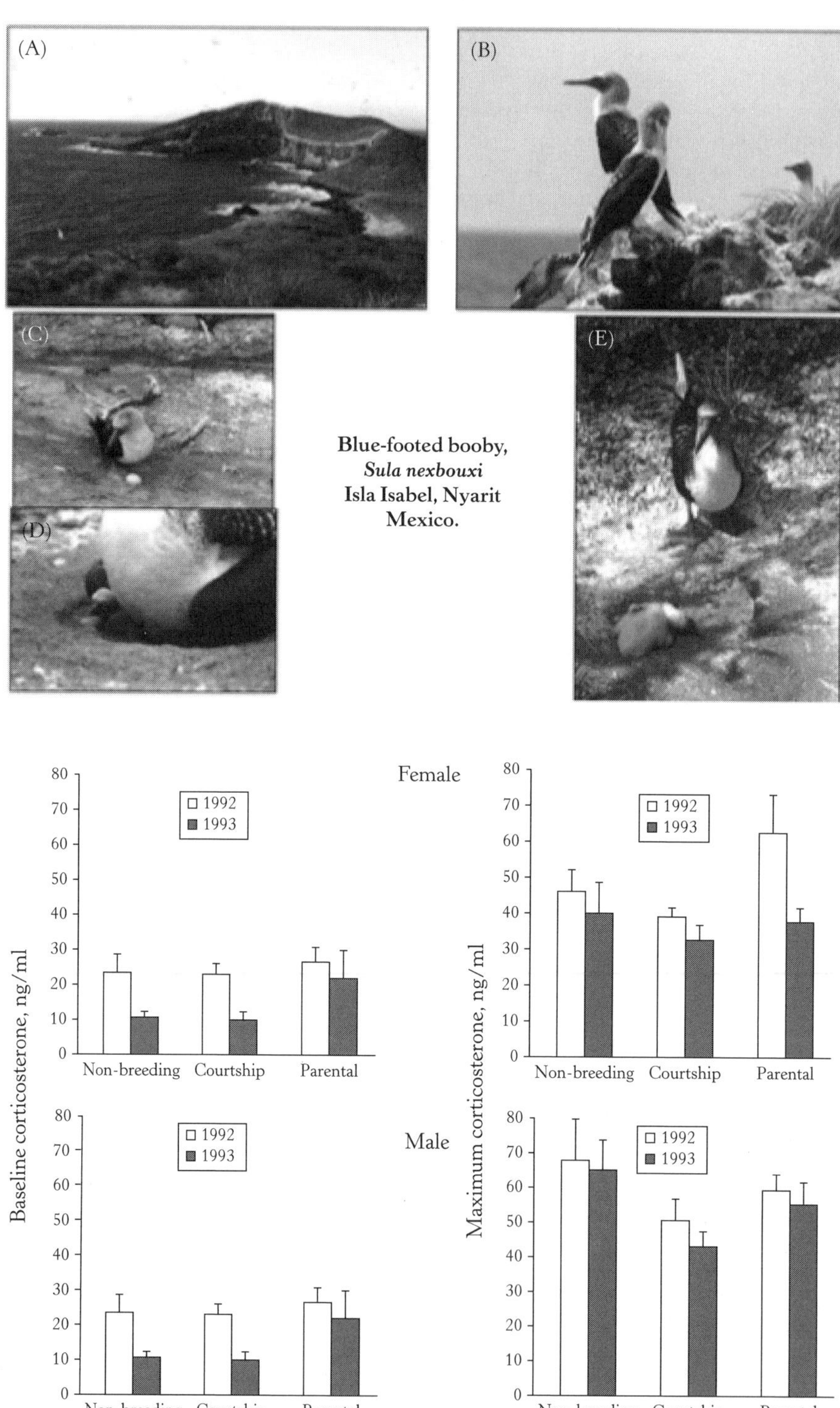

FIGURE 7.13: Seabirds worldwide can be affected by El Niño Southern Oscillation (ENSO) events as abundance of food and occurrence of inclement weather change dramatically. The blue-footed booby (panel B) breeds extensively on Isla Isabel (panel A) off the coast of Nyarit, Mexico. They lay one or two eggs (panel C), and chicks (panel D) are entirely dependent upon fish brought by the parents. In the ENSO event of 1993, very few blue-footed boobies attempted to breed; of those that did, the young died of starvation (panel D). Because adults chose a self-preservation strategy, corticosterone levels were not elevated (lower panel).

From Wingfield et al. (1999), courtesy of Elsevier. All photos by John C. Wingfield.

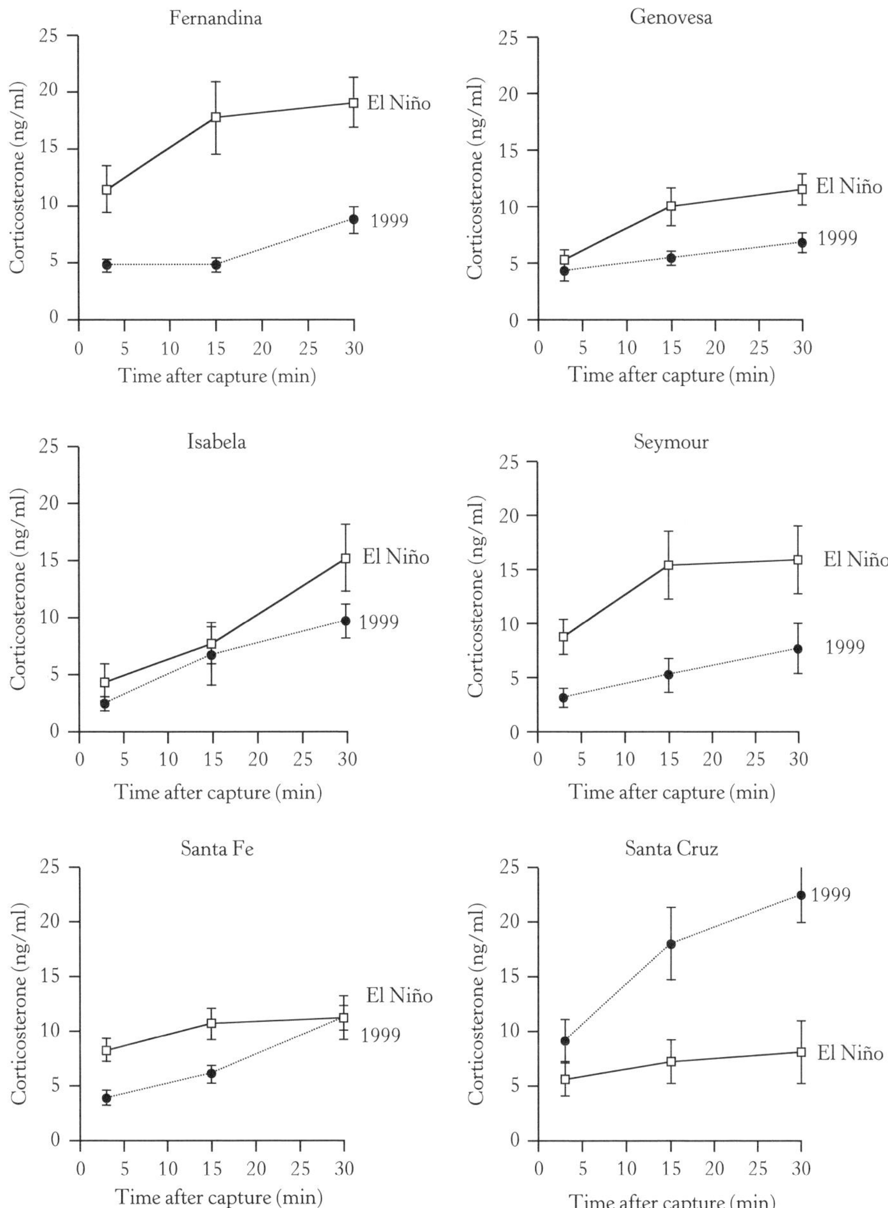

FIGURE 7.14: Corticosterone responses to the stress of capture and handling in marine iguanas captured on six different islands during La Niña conditions of 1999 and the El Niño of 1998.

Reprinted with permission from Romero and Wikelski (2001).

concentrations were elevated at five of the six island populations of marine iguanas, with the variation in the severity of the response matching the severity of algal die-off. The lone exception was Santa Cruz, where substantial runoff from the ENSO rains flushed nutrients into the bay near the study population so that algae was plentiful. The lack of such runoff during La Niña conditions meant that conditions were reversed for marine iguanas at Santa Cruz, which was reflected in their corticosterone concentrations (Figure 7.14). The corticosterone concentrations also closely matched the breeding success of the iguanas on those islands during those years: the higher the corticosterone, the lower the reproductive success.

ENSO events change sea surface temperatures and food distribution beyond the tropics, including throughout the Pacific and even globally. This in turn has dramatic effects in determining the distribution of many seabirds such as petrels (Procellariformes) and whether they breed or not that year (e.g., Warham 1996). In the common murre and the black-legged kittiwake, food abundance around breeding islands in the Gulf of Alaska can accurately predict corticosterone levels in breeding adults. Baseline plasma corticosterone was lower when food abundance was high (Kitaysky et al. 1999b; Buck et al. 2007; Kitaysky et al. 2007b; Kitaysky et al. 2010), consistent with the brood value hypothesis. This is in turn affects corticosterone titers of developing chicks, that is, baseline levels are lower when they are fed more. Ultimately, effects on reproductive success and survival can be profound (e.g., Kitaysky et al. 2003; Kitaysky et al. 2005).

It is also important to be careful to control for substages of breeding to tease apart potential ENSO effects. For example, stress responses in the black-legged kittiwakes described earlier were also higher during the incubation phase compared to other breeding substages. In grey-faced petrels there were no sex differences or changes with breeding substage in baseline corticosterone levels in blood, but there was a weak negative relationship of the adrenocortical response to capture stress (Adams et al. 2005). ENSO conditions can also delay the onset of breeding. For example, a weak ENSO in 2003 resulted in late breeding in rhinoceros auklets, whereas in 2004 (cooler waters, greater primary production, and more food in the northeastern Pacific Ocean) laying dates were earlier (Addison et al. 2008). Other environmental factors such as moonlight may affect the distribution and abundance of prey species, and when they are present, can in turn affect circulating levels of corticosterone such as in Nazca boobies breeding on the Galapagos Islands (Tarlow et al. 2003).

Angelier and Chastel (2009) suggest that the adrenocortical stress response during the parental phase of nesting can be modulated (baseline, degree of increase, and maximum levels of corticosteroids) in relation to ecological conditions and age. Additionally, the prolactin stress response (decrease in plasma levels) may be involved owing to its role in regulating parental behavior and thus parental investment. Interaction of corticosterone and prolactin effects could be very important in determining the degree of parental effort in relation to environmental perturbations both acute and chronic (e.g., ENSO events). Experimental elevation of circulating corticosterone in black-legged kittiwakes inhibited prolactin secretion compared to controls (Angelier et al. 2009a). In king penguins, abandonment of the egg or chick occurred primarily when parent fat reserves reached a critical low level. Sudden termination of reproductive effort was accompanied by higher baseline corticosterone and a decrease in plasma levels of prolactin (Groscolas et al. 2008). In the snow petrel of the Antarctic region, adrenocortical responses to acute stress were negatively correlated with body condition during incubation but not the prolactin response. Furthermore, unlike black-legged kittiwakes, injection of ACTH (to increase endogenous corticosterone) had no effect on circulating prolactin (Angelier et al. 2009b). Why these differences in adrenocortical and prolactin stress responses to acute perturbations exist remain unknown. Further investigations under natural conditions are needed to determine the ecological bases of variation, including responses to weather and food, as well as other factors including age and life span.

Foraging itself may play a role in adrenocortical function. Baseline plasma corticosterone levels were highest after arrival at the nest following a foraging trip in wandering albatrosses, but then declined proportional to the success of that foraging trip (i.e., how much food was provisioned to the chick; Angelier et al. 2007a). On the other hand, post-foraging corticosterone was lower in nesting Adélie penguins (McQueen et al. 1999; Angelier et al. 2008), indicating that success of the foraging trip (environmental conditions) and length of the trip required to replenish body condition could be important factors regulating adrenocortical function. However, Beaulieu et al. (2010) also found no correlation of baseline plasma corticosterone with length of foraging trips associated with the extent and rate of melt of sea ice. These data suggest that physical conditions affecting access to foraging areas may be less of a factor influencing adrenocortical function than actual food availability.

The role of corticosteroids and foraging success, however, is complex. Although black-legged kittiwakes breeding in poorer body condition because of decreased food availability had higher baseline plasma corticosterone, experimentally increased corticosterone by implants resulted in increased body condition (Kitaysky et al. 2003; Lanctot et al. 2003; Angelier et al. 2007b). These authors suggest that this effect is through corticosterone-induced increased foraging, but only if food availability is sufficiently high to result in higher food intake following increased foraging effort. In other words, decreased food availability elevates corticosterone, which in turn stimulates increased foraging, but that increased foraging only results in better body condition if the foraging is successful. In other field studies, breeding black-legged kittiwakes had a higher adrenocortical response and lower prolactin response to acute stress. In contrast, failed breeders showed the opposite responses (Chastel et al. 2005). Presumably, the easing of allostatic load once breeding fails makes an increase in corticosteroids less imperative. Clearly, breeding status is important, and in ENSO years, when food availability is reduced and less breeding occurs, the corticosterone and prolactin stress responses may also be lower. Seabirds at higher latitudes in the Northern and Southern Hemispheres provide fascinating comparisons to similar environmental conditions associated with ENSO events and may allow us to tease apart the effects of ecological and body conditions from phylogenetic differences.

The role that blood-binding proteins such as CBG may have in regulating free corticosterone (i.e., not bound to CBG) levels in blood (Breuner and Orchinik 2001; Breuner and Orchinik 2002) is also very important. CBG is thought to determine how much "free" hormone is available to enter target cells and bind to receptors. In pelagic seabirds such as black-legged kittiwakes, variation in baseline and maximum plasma corticosterone, as well as CBG-binding capacity of blood, varied from year to year and colony to colony, but the variation appeared to be associated with environmental cues such as local food supplies (Shultz and Kitaysky 2008). In the Laysan albatross, although circulating corticosterone levels rose during incubation fasts, and body condition declined, an increase in CBG may serve to protect the reproductive attempt by keeping free levels of corticosterone low (Sprague 2009). In tufted puffins, on the other hand, total and free levels of baseline and maximum corticosterone levels in plasma (after capture stress) were higher just prior to egg laying than during incubation. CBG-binding capacity in plasma was also positively correlated with body condition during the chick rearing phase, whereas free corticosterone baselines were negatively correlated (Williams et al. 2008). More studies of CBG-binding capacity throughout nesting will be needed to fully understand the complex dynamics of adrenocortical function and ecological conditions in oceanic seabirds.

Finally, there is growing evidence that weather events result in skews of sex ratios in some species. In some cases, females tend to rear more males in good years and more females in poorer years when ENSO events prevail. Assuming that females are "cheaper" to raise because they tend to be smaller than males suggests mechanisms affecting sex ratio, but there were no differences in baseline corticosterone titers (Addison et al. 2008). On the other hand, although there were no differences in chick responses to stress such as reduced food (Cameron-MacMillan et al. 2007; Addison et al. 2008), parent rhinoceros auklets and common murres may feed sons and daughters differentially according to environmental conditions such as ENSO.

IV. FAMINE VERSUS FEAST

Food abundance and access to that food (availability) owing to ecological conditions, weather, social status, and so on, are ubiquitous issues that have complex interrelationships with mediators of homeostasis and allostasis (reactive scope). We have focused thus far in this chapter on habitat quality in terrestrial and oceanic birds, but we must now address evidence from experimental laboratory investigations on available energy. Our understanding of the roles that catecholamines and corticosteroids play in metabolism (Chapter 5) was derived almost exclusively from laboratory studies, and primarily on laboratory rodents and humans. How closely do these mechanisms match what is observed in free-living species? Unfortunately, recent evidence suggests that corticosteroids might not regulate metabolism in free-living animals exactly as the laboratory data would suggest.

There have been hints through the years that corticosteroids did not always "work" as they were supposed to when it came to glucose regulation. Figure 7.15 is a good example. Although epinephrine elicited a robust increase in glucose concentrations in turkeys, corticosterone had no effect (Thurston et al. 1993). In fact, the difference between catecholamine and corticosteroid regulation of glucose concentrations during the immediate phase of the stress response has been highlighted by a number of studies. Rapid increases in blood glucose in wild-caught fish, for example, does not coincide with the profile of cortisol release (Frisch and Anderson 2000; Grutter and Pankhurst 2000), an effect also seen in the laboratory (Vijayan et al. 1994), nor do changes in glucose and cortisol correlate in fish selected for high and low cortisol concentrations (Trenzado et al. 2003). Notice how different these results are from the classic response discussed in Chapter 5, and specifically the data from Figure 5.2, where corticosteroids elicited a robust increase in blood

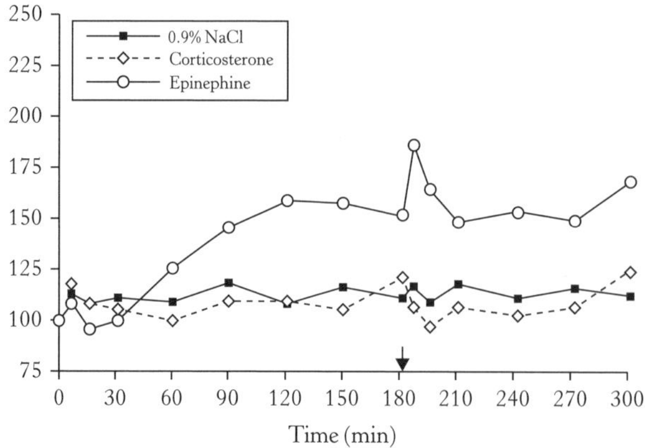

FIGURE 7.15: Plasma glucose concentrations expressed as the percent of pretreatment levels (T0) during continuous infusion of epinephrine and corticosterone in domestic turkeys. The arrow at 180 min represents a bolus injection of 3–20 times the infusion dose.

Reprinted with permission from Thurston et al. (1993). Courtesy of Elsevier.

glucose. Not only do the fish and turkey data support the general model of Figure 5.1, indicating that corticosteroids are not the primary regulator of glucose in the period directly after capture, they provide further evidence that corticosteroids are not the prime regulators of glucose concentrations.

What was the difference between the data presented in Figure 7.15 and Figure 5.2? Although there could be taxonomic differences between mammals and birds, the real difference might be subtler, and has far more interesting implications. All of the original studies, and almost all of the subsequent studies, have used fasted animals. This made a great deal of sense. After all, why would you study the impact of corticosteroids on glucose levels in fed animals? Dissecting the specific actions of corticosteroids from the confounding complexity of the hormonal milieu that manages the postprandial rise in glucose would be daunting. On the other hand, how realistic is it for corticosteroids to be secreted only when the animal is fasting? Stressors are unpredictable and can occur at any time, including when an animal has just fed.

There is building evidence that corticosteroids regulate glucose concentrations differently when glucose titers are elevated after animals have fed (e.g., Vijayan et al. 1993). For example, Figure 7.16 indicates that captive European starlings show a classic increase in glucose concentrations during the overnight fast, but not during the day when they are typically feeding (Remage-Healey and Romero 2000). Figure 7.17 indicates that this appears to be a direct consequence of feeding and does not simply reflect a diel difference in responses. There are two other key points from Figure 7.17. First, the peak in glucose in the fasted animals is approximately the same as the baseline glucose concentrations in the fed animals. This suggests that corticosteroids are unable to elevate glucose beyond postprandial concentrations. Second, the 30-minute increase in glucose is far faster than the 90–120 minute increase from Figure 5.2. This suggests that the rise in glucose is due primarily to catecholamines, not corticosteroids, as has also been shown for other species (e.g., Vijayan and Moon 1994). In fact, Figure 7.18 indicates that exogenous corticosteroids are unable to alter glucose concentrations in captive starlings during either the day or night (Remage-Healey and Romero 2001), suggesting that corticosteroids are completely ineffective at altering blood glucose concentrations within 2.5 hours. Corticosteroids are also ineffective at counteracting the effects of insulin (Remage-Healey and Romero 2001; Remage-Healey and Romero 2002). Furthermore, there is also evidence that the degree of fasting, and especially blood glucose concentrations, can in turn influence the corticosteroid response to a stressor (e.g. Kirschbaum et al. 1997; Gonzalez-Bono et al. 2002).

So what are we to make of these data? They do not fit easily into the dogma of corticosteroid actions described in Chapter 5. It seems that there are two potential answers: that corticosteroid function in birds is very different from that in mammals; or that corticosteroids regulate glucose concentrations very differently when there are already high glucose concentrations from a recent

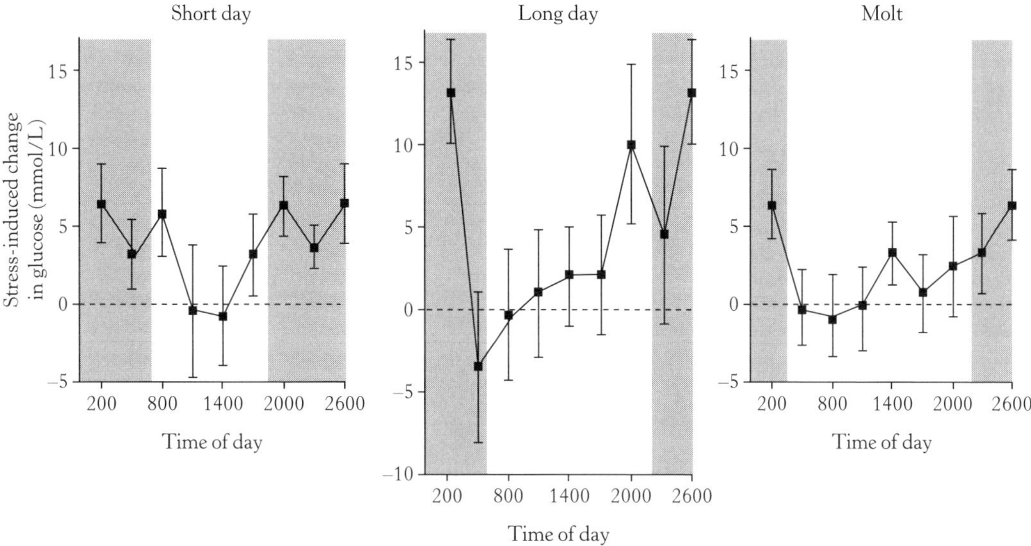

FIGURE 7.16: Glucose increases from baseline during a 30-minute restraint in captive European starlings. Birds were held on two different photoperiods, and on a long-day photoperiod while undergoing molt (the replacement of feathers). Dark bars represent periods when the lights were off.

Reprinted with permission from Remage-Healey and Romero (2000). Courtesy of Elsevier.

meal. Given the wide taxonomic conservation in many corticosteroid functions, we find it unlikely that birds are so completely different from mammals in how corticosteroids regulate glucose. In addition, other mammalian species show a similar lack of corticosteroid effects on glucose when in a fed state (e.g., Sernia and McDonald 1977; Yamada et al. 1993). Instead, these experiments may point out how little we currently know about how energy is regulated during stress. Anyone who has ever spent time watching most wild species is struck by how much time they devote to finding food. Most individuals are probably never completely fasting during their active period, but are also never completely sated. The classic figures in the physiology texts of glucose concentrations varying around several discrete meals during the day may have little relevance for an individual that is constantly foraging for small food items throughout the active period. What this type of energy intake means for how corticosteroids help regulate energy flow is completely unknown.

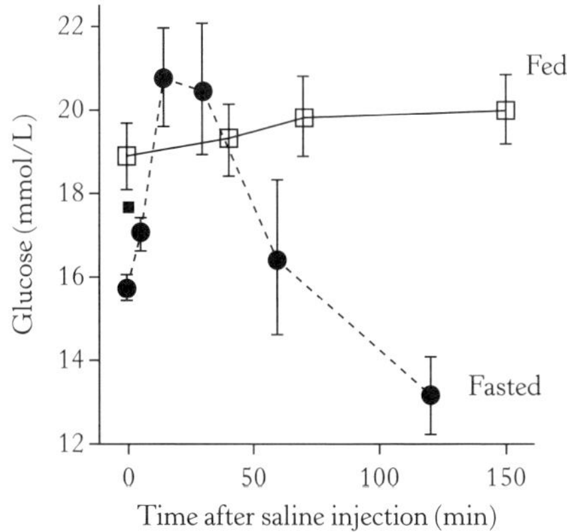

FIGURE 7.17: Glucose concentrations due to handling and restraint in ad libitum fed and overnight fasted captive European starlings. Both groups were tested in the morning approximately an hour after lights on (unpublished data from LMR).

One avenue that might be profitable is to examine differences in glucose regulation by corticosteroids in predators and herbivores. A rabbit that is grazing all day, or a bird that is constantly gleaning small insects from tree branches, has a very different meal schedule than the lion or eagle that consumes food in relatively large, yet irregular, batches. The responses to fasting are likely to be very different, as well as the functioning of corticosteroids. For example, carnivorous birds rely much more heavily on gluconeogenesis from amino acids than other bird species because the majority of their energy comes from the protein of their prey (Klasing 1998). The consequences of these differences remain largely unexplored. After all, most captive and domesticated species used in stress research are more similar to rabbits

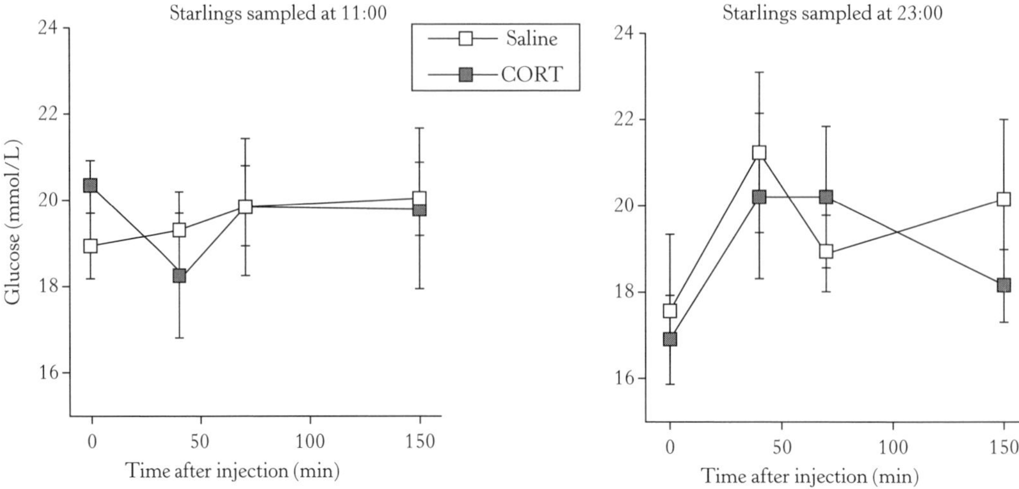

FIGURE 7.18: Glucose concentrations after exogenous corticosteroid (CORT) injections in captive European starlings after a morning feed (11:00) or during an overnight fast (23:00).

Reprinted with permission from Remage-Healey and Romero (2001). Courtesy of American Physiological Society.

than to lions. However, the comparative study of carnivores is likely to provide exciting insights into how corticosteroids regulate glucose concentrations during emergencies.

A. Starvation

The discussion in the previous section focused on short-term fasts, such as during the daily inactive period or over the course of a few hours. Longer fasts, lasting days, weeks, or even months, are likely to be important stressors for wild animals (see Chapter 1). The role of energy stores in helping animals survive these periods has been known for a long time. In an early example, Bumpus (1899) documented that the heaviest sparrows (and thus likely the fattest) were more likely to survive a severe storm. Many subsequent studies have expanded upon these initial observations and have gone further to show that poor body condition can correlate with elevated corticosteroid concentrations (reviewed in Wingfield et al. 1997). Clearly, the role of corticosteroids in metabolism likely plays a central role in helping wild animals survive these types of stressors. We should keep in mind, however, that periods of starvation are extreme events that require emergency responses—responses that are likely to be very different from responses required for normal everyday fasts. But at what point does fasting become severe enough to be called starvation? It should also be noted that starvation in response to reduced food availability is generally involuntary. However, some organisms also fast voluntarily, such as described earlier in seabirds that have long incubation bouts (up to 60 days or more) during which they are unable to feed (see further discussion later in this section). Mechanisms underlying responses to starvation must, therefore, take involuntary and voluntary processes into account.

There are generally considered to be three phases of starvation that are vital for survival (Phillips 1994): a short phase of rapid protein degradation; a longer phase in which protein degradation is slowed and calories are mainly derived from fat; and a final phase of rapid protein degradation, ultimately leading to death (Cahill 1976). Figure 7.19 summarizes these major changes. Phase I utilizes glucose metabolism, and especially glycogen breakdown, supplemented by

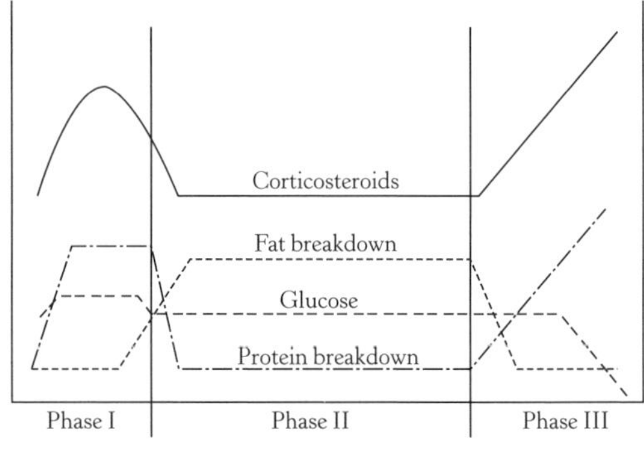

FIGURE 7.19: Schematic of corticosteroid and metabolic changes during the three phases of starvation.

the breakdown of easily mobilizable protein. Phase I ends when glucose and glycogen stores are exhausted. The short-term fasts discussed in the previous section take place exclusively within phase I. Phase II then shifts to fatty acid metabolism in an effort to save protein. The exhaustion of glucose and glycogen stores with the concomitant shift to gluconeogenesis also results in a decrease in overall glucose utilization during phase II (Cherel et al. 1988a). This is accompanied by increased glucagon concentrations (Totzke et al. 1999), altered glucagon function (Bernard et al. 2003), decreased insulin levels (Cahill 1976) and, at least in reptiles, a change in pancreatic B cell morphology (Godet et al. 1984). Fatty acid metabolism during phase II results in the production of ketone bodies used by tissues, especially the brain, in lieu of glucose (Owen et al. 1983). Finally, phase III relies upon breakdown of essential proteins for energy after fatty acids are depleted (Cahill 1976; Robin et al. 1987; Vleck and Vleck 2002). The shift from phase II to III is marked by a decrease in fatty acid oxidation (Cherel and Le Maho 1985; Bernard et al. 2002b), but the decrease in fatty acid concentrations does not appear to be the signal for the phase transition (Bernard et al. 2002a). In fact, the identification of the physiological trigger (such as thresholds in protein levels or fat stores, an increase in plasma ketones, etc.) for entering phase III, and thus increasing corticosteroid concentrations, is currently unknown.

The phase shifts, especially in relation to protein catabolism, appear to be regulated by corticosteroids (Dallman et al. 1993; Challet et al. 1995; Nasir et al. 1999). Corticosteroid concentrations generally increase during a short-term fast (phase I), although their response to further stressors is often blunted (Astheimer et al. 1992; Dallman et al. 1993; Dallman et al. 1999; Lynn et al. 2003). Phase II, however, is typified by low corticosteroid concentrations in most species studied to date, including penguins (e.g., Cherel and Le Maho 1985; Cherel et al. 1988c; Le Ninan et al. 1988; Hood et al. 1998; Groscolas and Robin 2001), common eiders (Bourgeon et al. 2006), and rainbow trout (Pottinger et al. 2003). There are some exceptions, however. Young northern elephant seals (Ortiz et al. 2001; Ortiz et al. 2003; Champagne et al. 2005) and lactating fur seals (Guinet et al. 2004) show a slow increase in corticosteroids over the fast, although in both species there are normal life-history events that create other substantial metabolic demands. Young northern elephant seals maintain growth throughout the post-weaning fast, suggesting that corticosteroids might be interacting with other metabolic hormones to increase growth. Female seals utilize a rare life-history strategy of lactating during the fast, so that the increase in corticosteroids may be related to maintaining protein mobilization for milk production (Guinet et al. 2004; Champagne et al. 2006; Houser et al. 2007). It is also important to re-emphasize that corticosteroid function during phase II of a prolonged voluntary fast, such as occurs in capital breeders (those species that fund reproduction through pre-accumulated reserves) like the seals, may be quite different from corticosteroid function during phase II of an involuntary fast, such as occurs when insufficient food is available. Although much of the work on phase II responses in wild animals has been done on capital breeders (e.g., the penguins, eiders, and seals cited earlier), the little work that has been done on involuntary fasts has supported the general model presented in Figure 7.19 (see following discussion).

In contrast, corticosteroids increase dramatically during the phase II–III transition (Cherel et al. 1988c; Le Ninan et al. 1988). The corticosteroids are thought to be the trigger for the shift to protein metabolism as well as changes in behavior. However, the interactions between corticosteroids and starvation are complex since caloric restriction can alter HPA function both peripherally, by remodeling adrenal steroidogenic tissue (e.g., Carsia and McIlroy 1998; McIlroy et al. 1999), and centrally, by disrupting normal diurnal variation and negative feedback (Fichter and Pirke 1986; McIlroy et al. 1999; Dallman et al. 2004).

There is an important distinction, however, between starvation and decreases in food availability. The corticosteroid responses to starvation are different from the responses to food restriction. A number of studies have maintained animals at a percentage of their free-feeding body weight. In general, those studies have shown an increase in corticosteroids (e.g., Freeman et al. 1981; Savory and Mann 1997; Lynn et al. 2003; Kitaysky et al. 2005; Perez-Rodriguez et al. 2006; Rosen and Kumagai 2008; Strochlic and Romero 2008). Many of these studies have used food restriction, or foods of lower caloric content, to model periods of limited or unpredictable food in the environment. In these cases, the elevated corticosteroids are interpreted to facilitate an increase in foraging behavior in adults (e.g., Pravosudov et al. 2001) and to increase begging behavior in young seabirds (e.g., Kitaysky et al.

1999a; Kitaysky et al. 1999b; Kitaysky et al. 2001a; Kitaysky et al. 2001b; Walker et al. 2005).

The length of time that phase II lasts is heavily dependent upon the individual. In humans, approximately 0.5 kilograms of body weight is lost per day during phase II, about one-quarter of which is lean tissue, with the rest being fat (Cahill 1976). Very obese humans can survive for over a year with essentially zero calorie intake (Stewart and Fleming 1973), although data from Irish hunger strikers suggest that an average human survives for approximately two months and loses 40% of his or her body weight (Elia 2000). However, medical problems become acute after losing approximately 18% of body weight, and loss of 30% of weight becomes life-threatening (Crosby et al. 2007). Furthermore, under-nutrition in humans may have lifelong effects. Birds have also been shown to lose a constant amount of weight during a fast (Ancel et al. 1998), but smaller birds may only have enough stored fat to fast for one day (Klasing 1998). Consequently, phase II duration, and ultimately survival, is tightly linked to the total fat stores maintained by the individual at the beginning of the fast. This is likely to be an important factor in survival at both the individual and species level. Within a species, the fattest individuals in a population of wild animals are likely to survive the longest. Between species, those species that have greater fat storage capacities are going to be more resistant to starvation conditions. Red-legged partridges, for example, appear to enter phase III after only 48 hours (Rodriguez et al. 2005), and some bird species may skip phase II altogether (Klasing 1998).

B. Voluntary Fasting

The ability to fast while breeding is also found in many large avian species such as geese. Nesting birds may fast for up to 2.5 months (Geleon 1981), showing almost complete anorexia (Mrosovsky and Sherry 1980), with three similar phases of fasting and protein sparing (Le Maho et al. 1981). Fasting can occur despite access to food (Portugal et al. 2007). Penguins breeding in Antarctic regions also show the three phases of starvation and are excellent models for what begins as a voluntary fast. The processes discovered in penguins appear to represent many species of animals that fast "voluntarily" during breeding, migration, or other predictable life-history stages. Because of the substantial amount of work that has been done on various penguins, we will focus the rest of this section on these species.

Many penguin species maintain an extended fast when incubating their eggs. During this fast, they show all three classic phases of starvation. When they enter phase III, however, they abandon their eggs and return to the sea to forage (e.g., Ancel et al. 1998; Vleck and Vleck 2002), thus ending their fast. Furthermore, after breeding, emperor and king penguins remain on land or ice for several weeks while completely replacing their plumage and without eating. Thus they are vulnerable to inclement weather and cold while drawing on endogenous reserves of fat and protein for energy and plumage production (Groscolas and Cherel 1992). Additionally, it should be noted that the insulating properties of their plumage are compromised while molting, and they must stay out of the ocean while not feeding, possibly leading to even greater vulnerability to storms (Adams and Brown 1990). During the molt they may lose up to 45% of body mass and 50% of body protein.

Field endocrine studies indicated that plasma T4 increased at the onset of molt, whereas T3 increased during molt and may be involved in energy expenditure while fasting (but see Jenni-Eiermann et al. 2002 for the opposite observations in red knots). Insulin levels did not change throughout molt in penguins or in the post-molt period when animals returned to the sea. Although corticosterone and glucagon levels remained stable throughout the period of molt and fasting, both hormones increased dramatically as the birds returned to the ocean (Groscolas and Cherel 1992).

In general, larger birds and mammals tend not to initiate periods of torpor during fasting (see Chapter 8). Instead they reduce locomotor activity and resting metabolic rates, and can show a slight decrease in core temperature (Cherel et al. 1988b), resulting in some energy savings. Additionally, huddling in severe weather can reduce energy expenditure in emperor penguins close to basal metabolic rate (Le Maho et al. 1976). Single emperor penguins that are unable to huddle in the severe cold of the Antarctic winter lose weight twice as rapidly during phase II than penguins that have an opportunity to huddle (Le Maho 1983). Reduced locomotor activity, coupled with huddling, further reduced energetic costs. For example, on average during severe weather, emperor penguins move less than 30 meters a day (Le Maho 1983). Similar reductions in locomotion and grouping behavior have been observed in high latitude rock ptarmigan in winter (Stokkan et al. 1986; Stokkan 1992). In king penguin chicks, huddling in winter results in savings of energy that can lengthen the voluntary winter fast up to 84 days, compared with only 44 days in summer (Barré 1984). However, huddling can be short and of variable duration among individuals (1–2 hours; Gilbert et al. 2006). Apparently this was not because of differential access to huddles, as individuals appear to have equal access. Energy savings in huddling penguins appears to be mostly through reduced metabolic rate (and activity) and avoidance of exposure to ambient temperatures for long periods (Gilbert et al. 2007). Interestingly, core temperatures of breeding male emperor penguins fasting on the ice in mid-winter were stable in incubating birds but may drop up to 1°C in birds that had lost an egg.

Phase II of fasting in emperor penguins was also accompanied by an almost nonexistent escape response to capture by the investigators. However, when phase III was reached, there was an 8–15-fold increase in spontaneous locomotor activity and a robust escape response during attempts at capture (Robin et al. 1998). This was related to increased plasma levels of corticosterone and uric acid, and a decrease in plasma beta-hydroxybutyrate. Robin et al. (1998) suggest these metabolic changes triggered a re-feeding signal and hence increased locomotor activity. These behavioral changes are in complete contrast to increased locomotor activity in captive white-crowned sparrows and dark-eyed juncos deprived of food (Ketterson and King 1977; Astheimer et al. 1992; Ramenofsky et al. 1992). These observations in songbirds have been suggested to be similar to phase III in larger avian species (Cherel et al. 1988b).

The rise in corticosteroids that coincides with entering phase III are believed to trigger egg abandonment (Groscolas and Robin 2001; Criscuolo et al. 2005; Cockrem et al. 2006). In king penguins, corticosterone levels increase and prolactin decreases in adults just prior to nest abandonment, when energy stores are depleted and birds are entering phase III of starvation (Groscolas et al. 2008). Such dramatic responses may avoid potential lethal effects of prolonged fasting in phase III. However, there is evidence that adult breeding king penguins may tolerate greater loss of body condition if they started breeding earlier and thus have a greater chance of fledging young that season (Groscolas et al. 2008).

Plasma levels of corticosterone were elevated during voluntary fasting when incubating compared to arrival from a feeding trip in Adélie penguins (McQueen et al. 1999; Vleck and Vleck 2002) and can be elevated further in phase III of fasting (just before they must leave for the ocean). However, in 2001 a large iceberg stopped the movement of pack ice in the Ross Sea, Antarctica, and the penguins weighed less than normal because they had to travel farther on ice to reach open sea to find food and then return. Corticosterone levels in blood were highest in departing birds compared to birds that were returning after a foraging trip, consistent with the self-preservation hypothesis (Cockrem et al. 2006). On the other hand, in an East Antarctica population of Adelie penguins, plasma levels of corticosterone did not differ between years of early versus later retreat of sea ice, possibly because access to open ocean is closer than other areas (Beaulieu et al. 2010). It thus appears that the degree of effort required to reach foraging areas can affect corticosteroid titers.

Some king penguin chicks also fast throughout the sub-Antarctic winter because the parents are unable to find sufficient food (Cherel and Le Maho 1985; Cherel et al. 1987). Additionally, king penguin chicks in phases I and II of fasting are accompanied by a 2–3-fold reduction in the magnitude of the adrenocortical response to capture stress (Corbel et al. 2010). Note that the fasting in penguin chicks is very different from fasting in penguin adults. The adults can always abandon their eggs and/or chicks and thus end the fast. Penguin chicks do not have this option. They are reliant upon their parents for food, and if the parents do not provide it, they cannot forage on their own. However, a lengthy post-hatch fast is a predictable life-history event for these chicks as they often wait for extended periods between feedings. As a result, penguin chicks can experience both a voluntary and an involuntary fast, which leads us to the next section.

C. Involuntary Fasting

One useful model for studying the impact of corticosteroids during starvation has been the Galápagos marine iguana. This species has adapted to conditions in the semi-arid Galápagos archipelago by relying exclusively on the rich marine algae growing in the intertidal and sub-tidal seas surrounding the islands (Wikelski and Trillmich 1994; Wikelski et al. 1997). Their reliance on a single food source appears to be a result of endosymbiotic bacteria in the gut that allows them to digest the marine algae, but not other plants (Mackie et al. 2004). Every few years, however, the Galápagos marine iguanas are subjected to El Niño–induced famine conditions. The algal forage that iguanas rely upon depends on this nutrient-rich upwelling, so that algae disappear during an ENSO. Figure 7.20 shows iguanas foraging during El Niño and non–El Niño conditions. The collapse of algal forage can result in widespread starvation, with the potential of iguana populations declining by 90% during severe ENSO events (Laurie 1989; Wikelski and Trillmich 1997).

Marine iguanas have several major advantages as a model for examining the role of glucocorticoids in surviving natural stressors. First, their reliance on one food source subjects them to

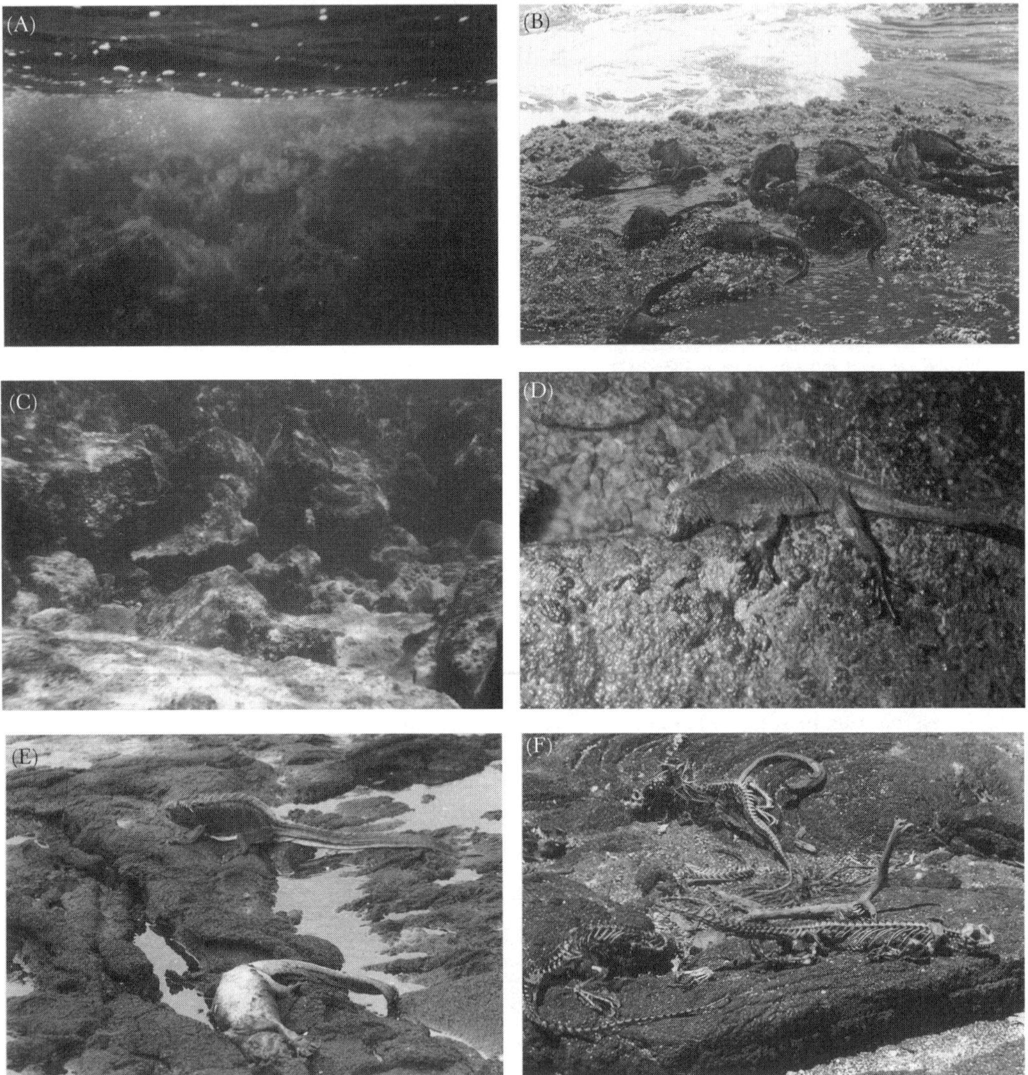

FIGURE 7.20: The Galápagos Islands under normal conditions and during an El Niño. (A) Underwater forage conditions during a normal year. (B) Marine iguanas foraging on the abundant subtidal algae during a normal year. (C) Underwater forage conditions during a severe El Niño (1997–1998). Water temperatures in the Galápagos Archipelago, normally 18°–23°C, remained elevated up to 32°C for nearly 18 months (Oberhuber et al. 1998). This led to a severe reduction in the algal forage and resulted in widespread starvation. (D) Marine iguana trying to forage during an El Niño. (E) Marine iguanas during the height of the 1997–1998 El Niño. Even though conditions were the same on each island, some individuals were surviving, whereas others had already died. (F) The aftermath of a severe El Niño—marine iguana carcasses on the beach approximately a year after the cessation of El Niño conditions.

All photos by LMR.

a fairly regular cycle of unintentional fasting, and potential starvation, every few years. This helps control for many of the difficulties in studying wild animal responses to stress under inherently unpredictable natural conditions. Second, these iguanas have essentially no natural predators on many of the islands (Kruuk and Snell 1981), leaving the ENSO-induced starvation as the major, and perhaps only, stressor in their lives. This is a powerful advantage since predation pressure can be a major confounding factor when studying stress under natural conditions. Third, even though these iguanas can live several decades, they are highly sedentary and rarely move from a several hundred meter area of coastline (Wikelski and Trillmich 1994). This allows us to return multiple times to monitor individual animals. Fourth, the Galápagos are famous for their tame animals, and the marine iguanas are no exception. They easily tolerate human approach and, because they are reptiles, are usually basking on warm rocks. This makes the iguanas easy to capture.

We exploited these advantages to examine the role of corticosteroids in marine iguanas undergoing starvation resulting from ENSO conditions. During 1997 and 1998, one of the longest and most severe ENSO events on record struck the Galápagos Islands. We captured marine iguanas, took blood samples, and assessed body condition within one week before widespread nutrient upwelling ended the 1998 ENSO conditions. Although algal forage did exist, it was sparse and heavily grazed. Many animals were in extremely poor condition, and carcasses were abundant. Surprisingly, however, some animals appeared to cope adequately (Figure 7.20E). We then repeated the study exactly one year after the El Niño event, when the algal forage had returned and surviving animals had recovered.

Figure 7.21 shows that El Niño conditions induced an intriguing biphasic response in corticosteroid concentrations (Romero and Wikelski 2001). There was no impact on corticosteroids for a wide range of body conditions. Even though all animals had experienced starvation conditions for 18 months, those individuals who were able to maintain body condition had corticosteroid concentrations indistinguishable from individuals of similar body condition when algae were plentiful. Only as body condition worsened and crossed a threshold did corticosteroid levels begin to increase. By itself, an enforced reduction in food availability appeared insufficient to stimulate corticosteroid release.

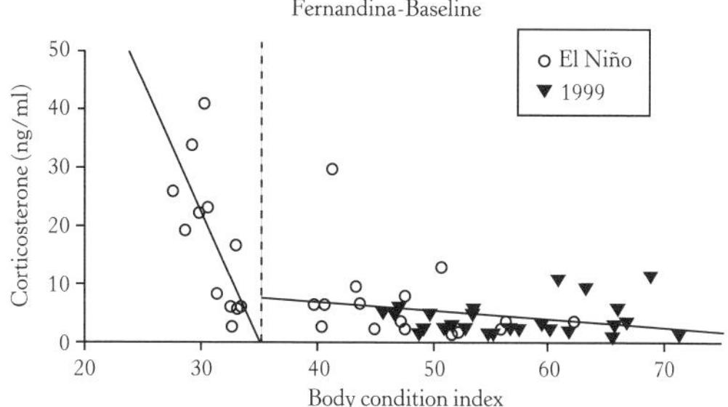

FIGURE 7.21: Relationship between body condition and corticosteroid concentrations in Galápagos marine iguanas. Data were collected from animals on Fernandina Island during the 1997–1998 El Niño and approximately one year after El Niño conditions had ended. Corticosteroid concentrations were determined in blood samples collected within 2 minutes of capture and the body condition index was a ratio of weight and length. Results were similar on other islands.

Reprinted with permission from Romero and Wikelski (2001).

A body condition index of 35 (Figure 7.21) was a consistent threshold on the three worst hit islands for switching to elevated corticosteroid levels (Romero and Wikelski 2001), despite island differences in the range of body sizes (Wikelski and Trillmich 1997). This raises an interesting question: What is occurring physiologically when body condition crosses this threshold? Because the body condition index is linked directly to body weight (after controlling for bone mass by taking the ratio with body length), the condition index is a rough indication of the energy stored as protein and fat. As a result, the threshold looks suspiciously like the transition from phase II to phase III of starvation. The surge in corticosteroids matches the increase in Figure 7.19, and other species also show distinct changes in physiology and behavior at a threshold of decreasing body mass (e.g., Cherel and Le Maho 1985; Ancel et al. 1998). In further support, just like other species that enter phase III, iguanas with a body condition index less than 35 are unlikely to survive.

What role does the corticosteroid surge play during phase II? The discussion in this section clearly suggests that the increase in corticosteroids served as a last-ditch effort to mobilize protein reserves for survival (i.e., the entrance to phase III). Increasing corticosteroids titers could prolong life by accessing these protein stores. If a single blood sample were taken during an animal's progression through the starvation period (a "snapshot"), the predicted relationship would look very much like the data in Figure 7.21, especially if animals were at asynchronous stages of the process. Furthermore, Figure 7.21 only contains data from surviving iguanas—those unable to mount a sufficient response may have already died. Consequently, these data match the penguin studies showing that an increase in corticosteroids, and thereby protein breakdown, occurs at nest abandonment and provides birds with the extra energy needed to return to sea to forage, preventing death from starvation (e.g., Cherel et al. 1988c; Groscolas and Robin 2001; Vleck and Vleck 2002). Given that ENSO conditions could end at any moment, delaying death by even a week or two might be all that is needed for the individual's survival.

There is, however, an alternative possibility. High corticosteroid titers could be the actual trigger for death. Increased corticosteroid release appears to be the mechanism that causes death in post-spawning salmonid species (Dickhoff 1989) and males from several species of Australian marsupials (e.g., Barnett 1973; Bradley et al. 1980; Bradley 1987). Consequently, corticosteroid release in marine iguanas could be the final step in tissue breakdown, with the process of dying only truly beginning when corticosteroids levels begin to rise. Which explanation is correct is not discernable from data collected to date. The bias of most researchers, based upon corticosteroids' survival benefits during acute stress, is that corticosteroids are aiding survival, but the data so far are mixed (Breuner et al. 2008). Whether corticosteroid secretion during phase III of starvation is a net positive or a net negative for survival is an important unanswered question in corticosteroid physiology.

Regardless of whether corticosteroids during phase III are beneficial or not, it appears that survival can be enhanced if the transition between phase II to phase III can be delayed. A recent study in marine iguanas measured four aspects of corticosteroid physiology in healthy iguanas prior to an El Niño (Romero and Wikelski 2010). Measures included baseline corticosterone, corticosterone titers after 30 minutes of restraint, the maximal corticosterone response assessed after an ACTH challenge, and the efficacy of negative feedback assessed with a dexamethasone (DEX) challenge (see Chapter 6). A few months later, a mild El Niño killed approximately one-third of the animals. Analysis of the data collected prior to the El Niño revealed that neither baseline, stress-induced, nor maximal responses predicted which iguanas would later succumb to starvation during the El Niño (Romero and Wikelski 2010). Efficacy of negative feedback, however, was predictive, with those iguanas showing the weakest negative feedback most likely to die (Figure 7.22). When combined with Figure 7.21, these data suggest that the ability to limit the duration of corticosteroid release (i.e. strong negative feedback) can delay an iguana entering phase III of starvation.

The importance of negative feedback makes sense in terms of reactive scope (Chapter 3). Figure 7.23 shows that natural variation in baseline, stress-induced, and maximal corticosterone are unlikely to alter an animal's reactive scope (Romero 2012). This is because each of these responses is rapid and will not contribute to long-term wear and tear. In contrast, a weak negative feedback will extend the time that corticosteroids are in the reactive homeostasis range, thus contributing to wear and tear. This increase in wear and tear will further add to the decrease in reactive scope (Figure 7.23) and will shorten the time before corticosteroids enter homeostatic overload. In other words, the weak negative feedback leads to a more rapid decrease in reactive scope, making the animal more vulnerable as the famine conditions continue.

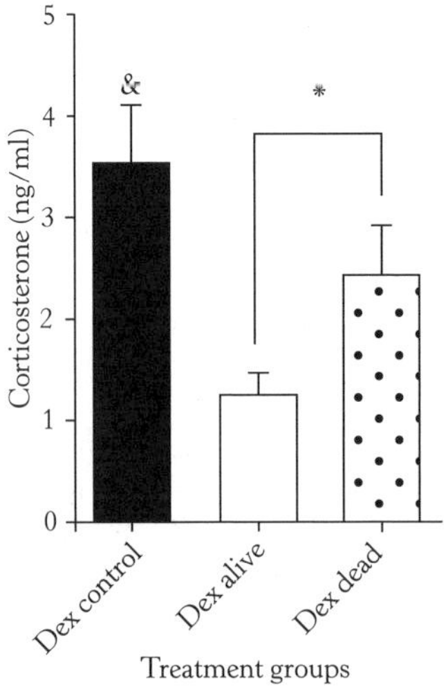

FIGURE 7.22: Comparison of corticosterone titers following dexamethasone (DEX) administration in marine iguanas captured prior to an El Niño. Assignment of individual iguanas to Alive or Dead categories was made subsequent to the El Niño. DEX injection tested the efficacy of negative feedback.

Reprinted with permission from Romero and Wikelski (2010). Courtesy of the Royal Society.

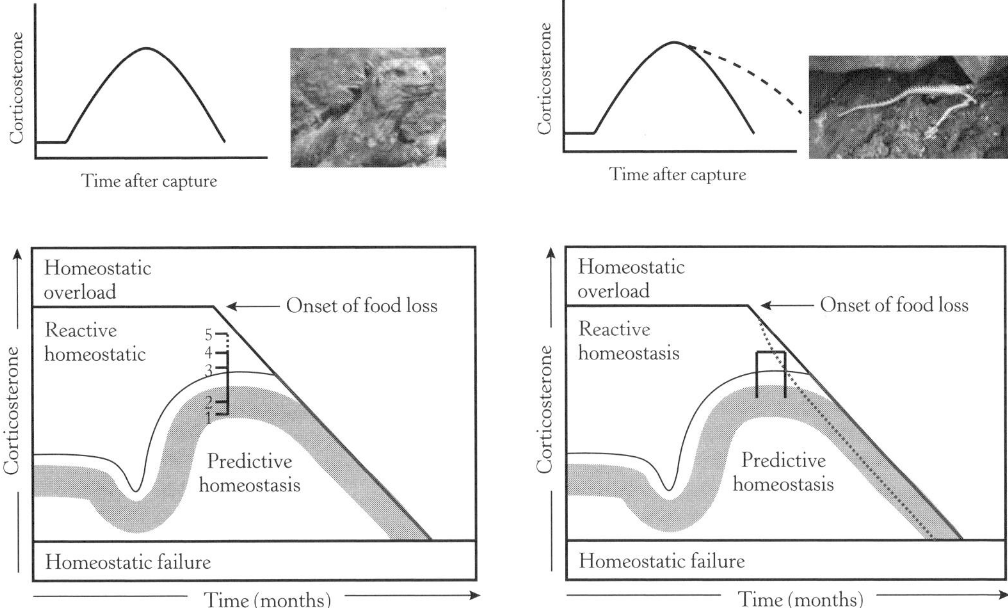

FIGURE 7.23: Interpreting the results of Figure 7.22 using the reactive scope model. Top left panel represents the corticosterone response with a strong negative feedback response in those iguanas most likely to survive. The dotted line in the top right panel represents the weak negative feedback response in those iguanas most likely to die. In the bottom panels, the onset of food loss results in wear and tear. This is modeled by a decrease in reactive scope beginning at the arrow. This is partially compensated for by a decrease in predictive homeostasis. The vertical line on the bottom left panel represents a normal acute corticosterone response in an animal with strong negative feedback. Numbers represent different levels of this response. Levels 1 and 2 are within the predictive homeostasis range and represent animals with different baseline titers of corticosterone. Levels 3 and 4 are within the reactive homeostasis range and represent animals with different responses to capture and handling. Level 5 represents the maximal corticosterone response after stimulation by ACTH. None of these different levels will alter the decrease in reactive scope, and none of these differences predicted individual iguana survival. The inverted U on the right side represents the longer sustained corticosterone response of an animal with weaker negative feedback. The longer response adds to wear and tear, thus resulting in an accelerated decrease in reactive scope, as represented by the dashed black line. The decrease in reactive scope would make these animals more likely to enter homeostatic overload earlier during the El Niño, and thus more likely to die.

Figure adapted from Romero (2012). Courtesy of Elsevier.

V. CACHING BEHAVIOR

Access to food supplies can be unpredictable, especially when weather conditions worsen and may increase secretions of glucocorticoids. Mountain chickadees of high elevation forests in western North America cope with limited and uncertain food supplies over the winter period by storing food in caches when food is plentiful in late summer and autumn. Corticosteroids appear to play an important role in this critical behavior.

In a captive experiment, mountain chickadees were maintained on a limited (food restricted) and unpredictable (time for access varied) food source for over 90 days (Pravosudov et al. 2001). Food-restricted birds had higher baseline plasma corticosterone levels than controls on ad libitum food. However, there were no differences in their adrenocortical responses to acute stress (capture, handling, and restraint). Females responded more quickly and reached higher levels of corticosterone during acute stress than males. The data are consistent with the hypothesis that free-living birds resident in a winter area and with unpredictable food supplies should have higher baseline plasma corticosterone for prolonged periods in order to stimulate feeding activity and fat storage (Pravosudov et al. 2001). This could have implications for long-term deleterious effects of high corticosterone unless these birds have alternate feeding strategies, such as access to food caches. The data are also consistent with the field evidence on weather effects in other species. In another study, mountain chickadees subjected to long-term (90 days) elevation (intermediate) of corticosterone with subcutaneous implants resulted in greater food consumption, higher food-caching activity, and greater efficiency of caching than controls (Pravosudov 2003, 2005). These authors also showed enhanced spatial memory performance compared to controls, an important attribute to being able to retrieve many hundreds of food items stored in various locations. Noninvasive corticosterone treatment, using ingestion of mealworms injected with corticosterone, elevated food retrieval from stored sites but had no effect on caching behavior compared with controls (Saldanha et al. 2000). The number of retrieved seeds eaten and storage sites visited also did not differ from controls, suggesting that corticosterone has effects on appetite and/or activity. Pravosudov (2005) concluded that moderate but chronic elevation of corticosterone may enhance performance in unpredictable environments by facilitating foraging, food caching, and cache retrieval.

Seasonal effects appear to be important for adrenocortical function and food caching/retrieval. Baseline and maximum plasma levels of corticosterone in mountain chickadees were the same on long and short days (Pravosudov et al. 2002). However, birds reached maximum plasma corticosterone levels in response to capture stress more rapidly (5–20 min) on long days than on short days with females responding faster than males (Pravosudov et al. 2002). While photoperiod does apparently affect the adrenocortical response to stress, data indicate that changes in baseline corticosterone levels and effects on spatial memory and foraging are regulated by other environmental factors. Subordinate birds cached less food, were less efficient in cache retrieval, and had reduced spatial memory ability compared with dominant birds (Pravosudov et al. 2003). This was unexpected and may suggest that juveniles may have lower survival during bad weather in winter or must migrate to more benign habitats at lower elevations. Curiously, dominant birds had higher maximum corticosterone levels (stress series) than subordinates, although the overall pattern of response was the same in both groups. Also curiously, subordinates did not have higher baseline corticosterone than dominants (Pravosudov et al. 2003).

VI. CORTICOSTEROIDS AND AVIAN MIGRATION

It is important to remember that not all periods of extensive energy use are emergencies. Many normal life-history events are energetically costly, the preeminent one being reproduction. One event that has garnered significant interest in terms of the role of corticosteroids is avian migration.

There are three major phases of the migratory process: development of the migratory state (zugdisposition), which includes premigratory fattening (hyperphagia); mature capability, which allows the initiation of migratory flight (zugunrhue or migratory restlessness) and the flight itself; and termination of the migratory life-history stage, in which hyperphagia subsides and birds lose weight (e.g., Ramenofsky and Wingfield 2006; Ramenofsky and Wingfield 2007) Corticosteroids make attractive candidates as an important regulator during all three of these stages. This makes sense on two levels. First, regulating the energetic requirements necessary to support the massive changes in energy storage, followed by rapid utilization, fits well with known corticosteroid functions discussed earlier in this chapter, especially at baseline concentrations. Second, high fat loads likely pose a trade-off between needing fuel for migration but decreasing speed and maneuverability needed to escape from predators (Witter and Cuthill 1993). Corticosteroids might be expected to play a role in that trade-off. Consequently, a number of studies have explored the role that corticosteroids play throughout migration.

A. Premigratory Fattening

Most of the work on corticosteroids and migration has focused on the premigratory hyperphagia period. Providing the fuel for migration requires an extensive period of hyperphagia that often lasts for several weeks (Blem 1990). Some bird species can accumulate fat at the rate of 10% of body weight per day, and some shore birds can double their weight in only two weeks of foraging (Klasing 1998). The fat is stored in numerous depots throughout the body, including subcutaneously, in visceral fat depots, in the liver, and even inside muscle (Berthold 1993; Jenni-Eiermann and Jenni 1996).

The role of corticosteroids in fat deposition and appetite makes it likely that they would play important roles in hyperphagia. Extensive evidence suggests that this is the case. Although the regulation of food intake is as complicated and multifaceted in birds as in mammals (Kuenzel 1994; Boswell et al. 1995; Boswell et al. 1997; Denbow 1999; Boswell 2005), both laboratory and field studies in birds parallel the mammalian literature in indicating the importance of corticosteroids as an indirect regulator of feeding behavior. For example, corticosteroid administration directly into the brain induces hyperphagia in captive ring doves (Koch et al. 2002). Interestingly, in the laboratory, corticosteroid implants may only increase foraging behavior when birds are in migratory condition (Gray et al. 1990) or are fasting (Astheimer et al. 1992). Ramenofsky et al. (1999) have shown that the natural increase in endogenous corticosteroids during migration is restricted to the day. Nighttime concentrations do not change, meaning that there is an alteration in the diel rhythm, not simply an overall increase throughout 24 hours. Similar data have been collected in other species (e.g., Schwabl et al. 1991). Since the species that have been studied do not forage at night, corticosteroid increases during the day would make sense if corticosteroids were regulating hyperphagia and lipid storage.

Corticosteroids also appear to regulate the metabolic shift that allows food to be preferentially stored as fat. Corticosteroid implants administered to dark-eyed juncos under laboratory conditions, for example, increased fat storage at the expense of flight muscle (Gray et al. 1990). Although such studies with exogenous corticosteroid administration should be interpreted with caution, parallel results have been obtained in the field. Corticosteroid concentrations are negatively correlated with fat stores in migratory garden warblers captured while refueling (Schwabl et al. 1991), and Figure 7.24 provides an example of corticosteroid concentrations also increasing in bar-tailed godwits during refueling (i.e., the birds become fatter and weigh more) at a migratory stopover site (Landys-Ciannelli et al. 2002).

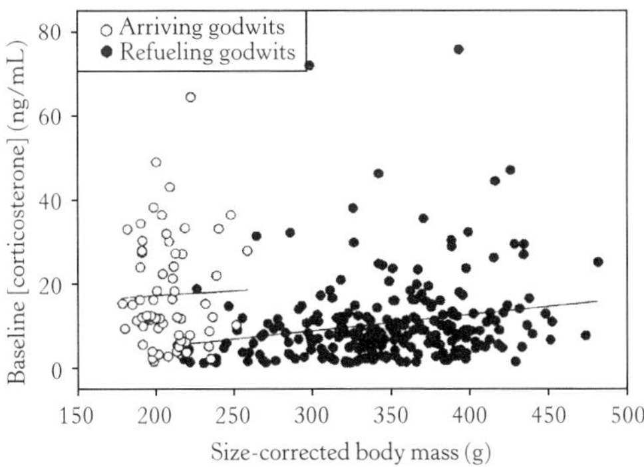

FIGURE 7.24: Baseline plasma corticosterone of bar-tailed godwits arriving at a refueling site on the Wadden Sea. Baseline levels are regressed against size-corrected body mass. Corticosterone was significantly higher in arriving godwits than in refueling birds. In refueling birds, corticosterone correlated positively with size-corrected body mass.

Reprinted with permission from Landys-Ciannelli et al. (2002). Courtesy of University of Chicago Press.

Note, however, that the correlation of corticosteroids and body mass in Figure 7.24 is primarily with baseline titers, suggesting that premigratory fattening is regulated via type I (MR) receptors. Interestingly, Landys et al. (2004a, 2004b) have shown that hyperphagia and fat storage are regulated by different receptors. Using a type II (GR) receptor blocker (RU486), they inferred that type II receptors help promote hyperphagia, but not fatty acid and triglyceride trafficking. The latter effect reinforces the conclusions drawn from the mammalian literature (e.g., Dallman et al. 2004) that normal energy trafficking is regulated by baseline concentrations of corticosteroids working through the MR receptors. Consequently, the change in energy flow during premigratory fattening is regulated mostly by modulating baseline corticosteroid concentrations and does not require stress-induced levels (Landys et al. 2006). The actions of corticosteroids during premigratory fattening are thus very different from their role during starvation as discussed in the previous section.

Gaining fat is not the only goal during the premigratory hyperphagic period. Avoiding getting eaten is also a high priority. Probably because high fat loads decrease flight performance, and thus make the animal more susceptible to predation (Witter and Cuthill 1993), the amount of fat accumulated can depend upon the presence, or perceived presence, of a predator (e.g., Lank et al. 2003; Cimprich and Moore 2006; Lind and Cresswell 2006; Nemeth and Moore 2007). The decrease in fat accumulation appears to result from a decrease in fuel deposition rate (Schmaljohann and Dierschke 2005), a process that clearly implicates corticosteroids. Although it is not yet known whether corticosteroids serve as mediators of the trade-off between fattening and predator avoidance, it is likely to be a fruitful area of research.

B. Initiation of Flight

The drive to initiate a bout of migratory flight is manifested in the laboratory as a general increase in activity and has been termed "migratory restlessness." Corticosteroids have been implicated as a trigger for this behavior because they are elevated in the laboratory in birds showing migratory restlessness (Lohmus et al. 2003). Furthermore, corticosteroids returned to normal when the behavior was disrupted (Schwabl et al. 1991). Figure 7.25 shows that corticosteroids increased just prior to the onset of migratory restlessness only in birds held on long-days, that is, those that were in migratory condition, and are coincident to the onset of activity typical of migratory restlessness (Landys et al. 2004c). Contrary to stimulation of feeding by corticosteroids, however, stimulation of migratory restlessness does not appear to be regulated by type II receptors (Landys et al. 2004b), indicating that these different behavioral changes are regulated by different receptor types. The trigger to begin a migratory flight might also be linked indirectly to corticosteroids because flight appears to be initiated when a threshold of fat is reached (Cochran and Wikelski 2005; Schaub et al. 2008). Consequently, the evidence that corticosteroids might also regulate the behavioral initiation of migratory flight is building, although there are few studies to date.

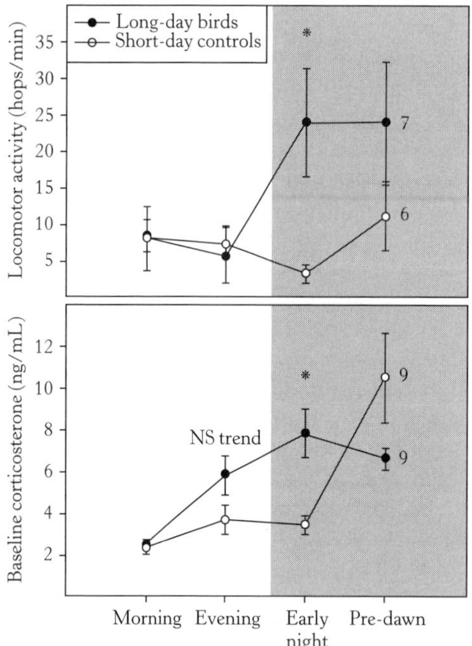

FIGURE 7.25: Average locomotor activity (top panel) and plasma corticosterone levels (bottom panel) of long-day birds and short-day controls. The shaded area denotes samples that were collected during the dark phase.

Reprinted with permission from Landys et al. (2004c). Courtesy of Elsevier.

C. Migratory Flight

Corticosteroids may also play a major role in helping fuel the migratory flight because the act of flying is a very costly behavior for birds (Blem 1990). This cost is magnified for the period of migration, especially for those species that migrate thousands of kilometers in one hop. The primary fuel for migration is fat, which appears to be derived both from liver stores and from mobilization of fat depots (Landys et al. 2005). Fat is then used directly by the muscles, rather than being converted to glucose (Jenni-Eiermann and Jenni 2001; McWilliams et al. 2004; Sweazea and Braun 2006). Protein is also important, but in a process reminiscent of phase III of starvation, appears to only become used after fat stores are largely depleted (Jenni and Jenni-Eiermann 1998; Schwilch et al. 2002; Landys et al. 2005). However, the degree of protein utilization also depends upon the species, with insectivores relying more heavily on protein to fuel migratory flight than omnivores (Gannes 2001). This suggests that, whatever role corticosteroids play in regulating energy trafficking during migratory flight, it is likely to show species differences.

The migratory flight itself can place enormous strain on an individual. In species with unlimited stopover sites, such as species that migrate over land, birds usually fly until the recently deposited fuel reserves are exhausted (Cochran and Wikelski 2005). These birds then land and spend a period of time refueling for the next hop. For species with limited refueling sites, such as shorebirds dependent upon distant mudflats, birds not only completely consume their lipid fuel reserves but also metabolize major parts of their muscles and intestines (Piersma and Gill 1998). Consequently, many ultra-long distance migrants mobilize substantial protein during the flight. For example, after a 5400-kilometer non-stop flight in great knots, a medium-sized shore bird, there were significant reductions in the mass of all measured organs except for brain and lungs (Battley et al. 2000).

Although measuring corticosteroids in the middle of a migratory flight is likely impossible, the dramatic mobilization of fat and protein required by such a Herculean effort as a 5400-kilometer flight is likely mediated, at least partially, by corticosteroids. There are a number of studies that provide circumstantial evidence that corticosteroids are elevated during the migratory flight. Figure 7.26 shows early data on racing pigeons indicating that a long flight back to the home roost resulted in elevated corticosteroid

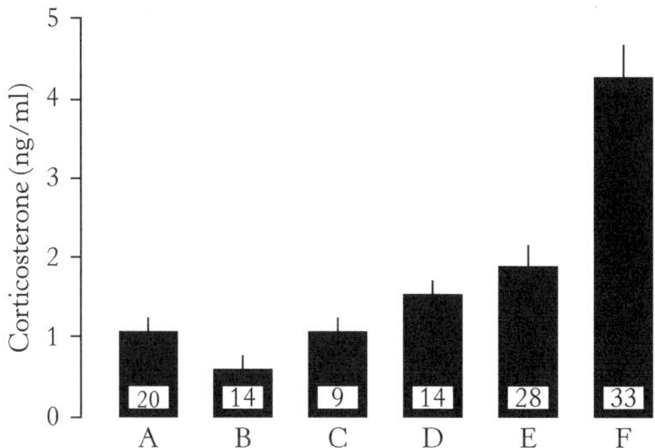

FIGURE 7.26: Concentrations of corticosterone in the plasma of experienced racing pigeons following short (< 100 m, Group E) or long-distance (> 180 km) flight (Group F), in comparison with non-exercised birds that were bled before the release of the exercised birds (Group A) or at the time of their return to the home loft (Group B) or after transportation to the release site (Group C) or after being carried 100 m back to the home loft (Group D).

Reprinted with permission from Haase et al. (1986). Courtesy of Elsevier.

concentrations (Haase et al. 1986). Although homing flights are not strictly migratory, the physiological processes are probably similar. Several other studies have found higher corticosteroid concentrations in long-distance migrant shorebirds that had recently arrived at either the breeding grounds (e.g., Reneerkens et al. 2002) or at refueling sites (Ramenofsky et al. 1995). Figure 7.24 shows an example of these types of data (Landys-Ciannelli et al. 2002). The godwits just arriving at the refueling site have, on average, higher corticosteroid concentrations than those in the process of refueling.

The corticosteroid concentrations from arriving godwits in Figure 7.24, however, are still below titers from godwits exposed to a stressor such as restraint. In general, the increase in concentrations associated with flight are still in the baseline range (Landys et al. 2006). A number of studies have examined whether the increase in baseline levels during migratory flight alters a subsequent corticosteroid response to stress. Several studies suggest that the response to stress is damped (e.g., Holberton 1999; Holberton and Dufty 2005) and that the damping is most pronounced in the leanest birds with the least fat reserves (Long and Holberton 2004). These studies led Holberton et al. (1996) to propose the Migration Modulation Hypothesis. This hypothesis posits that (1) corticosteroids will be elevated throughout the migratory period in order to facilitate hyperphagia and storage of fuel as fat, and (2) corticosteroid responses to stress will be suppressed in order to avoid protein catabolism in flight muscles. The evidence for this hypothesis is currently mixed. Although the foundation of the hypothesis was built on studies of small migrants, such as warblers, studies in other species have failed to find either sustained increases in corticosteroids (e.g., Figure 7.24) or damped stress responses during migration (e.g., Romero et al. 1997; Reneerkens et al. 2002; Nilsson and Sandell 2009).

Although much of this work on migration is just beginning, there is building evidence that corticosteroids play a major role in regulating the behavioral and physiological changes associated with migration. Migration, however, poses a different model for understanding corticosteroid metabolic functions than other events such as fasting or starvation. Migration is a normal life-history event in many species, and corticosteroids appear to exert their effects primarily at baseline concentrations. Migration is not an emergency life-history stage, so it is not surprising that corticosteroids function differently via different receptors. In the end, what we have learned about corticosteroid regulation of energy trafficking in free-living birds during migration is likely to be analogous to other non-emergency life-history stages, such as reproduction, but it would be inappropriate to extrapolate what we discover in migration studies to responses to stress. In other words, migration and the emergency life-history stage are very different.

Finally, there is an alternative hypothesis for why corticosteroids might be elevated during migration. It might be less a function of energy regulation, but instead migration might itself be a stressor. One inescapable feature of migration, especially long-distance migration, is the looming presence of the unknown just over the horizon. Migrants are faced with a massive amount of novelty as they fly through unfamiliar habitats and arrive at unfamiliar destinations. Novelty and uncertainty will be a factor for both juveniles, who are arriving at areas for the first time (Mettke-Hofmann and Greenberg 2005), and experienced adults, who might be encountering unanticipated changes in previously familiar habitats, such as late snow melt on breeding sites (Breuner and Hahn 2003; Wingfield et al. 2004) or predators that have taken up residence (Ramenofsky and Wingfield 2006). From Chapter 3 we know that novelty and uncertainty are potent stressors. It is possible that both the uncertainty itself and the anticipation of that uncertainty could result in elevated corticosteroid concentrations. There is circumstantial evidence that arriving at a new site after a migratory flight is stressful since heart rate spikes at this time (Cochran and Wikelski 2005), although the spike may also reflect changing from cruising to more active flying. Furthermore, in one captive study, the peak in corticosteroid concentrations was correlated to the period of stable mass just prior to a migratory flight, rather than the preceding hyperphagia period (Piersma et al. 2000). In another study, even though captive birds maintained a normal annual pattern of fattening coincident with the period of migration, corticosteroid concentrations strongly decreased with the length of time in captivity and were not correlated with hyperphagia (Piersma and Ramenofsky 1998). The authors interpreted this decrease to indicate that captive birds had learned that captive conditions were no longer stressful. Note, however, that we are suggesting that the uncertainty of the situation at arrival serves as the stressor, not the physical activity itself. As far as we know, this hypothesis remains untested.

VII. MOLT

The growth of certain tissues in adults, rather than growth during development, is one model of how corticosteroids can have a profound impact on growth in wild species. One focus has been on the avian molt, the seasonal replacement of flight and body feathers by birds in the late summer and early autumn. Since feathers are routinely abraded and broken, it is important for birds to periodically replace their feathers, although how often depends upon the size of the species. Figure 7.27 illustrates how worn plumage can become during the routine wear and tear of an annual cycle. Note that other vertebrates also show types of molt (Figure 7.28), although the effects of glucocorticoids in molt in many vertebrates remains unclear (Silverin and Wingfield 2010).

A. Disrupting the Avian Molt

The majority of avian species down-regulate corticosteroid release, both baseline and stress-induced, during molt (reviewed by Romero 2002). There is building evidence that birds down-regulate corticosteroid release during molt in order to avoid the protein catabolic activity of corticosteroids from directly inhibiting the protein deposition necessary to produce feathers.

Undamaged feathers are critical for birds for a number of reasons. First, replacing worn feathers is important for efficient energy usage during flight. Old feathers provide significantly less power at each wing beat than new feathers (Swaddle and Witter 1997; Swaddle et al. 1999; Williams and Swaddle 2003) and both empirical and modeling studies suggest that birds with lost or broken feathers have reduced aerodynamic efficiency (Tucker 1991; Chai 1997; Hedenström and Sunada 1999; Swaddle et al. 1999; Williams and Swaddle 2003). Decreased efficiency can clearly lead to an increased need for energy consumption (Dawson et al. 2000), which likely explains why many species spend less time flying during molt (Ginn and Mellville 1983; Jenni and Winkler 1994). Second, good-quality feathers are important for thermoregulation. Lower quality feathers can result in lower overwinter survival due to thermoregulatory energy expenditure (Nilsson and Svensson 1996). The increased energy expenditure on thermoregulation also apparently led to reduced reproductive success the following year (Nilsson and Svensson 1996). Third, good-quality feathers can be a key component in mate selection (e.g., Fitzpatrick 1998; Ferns and Lang 2003). One indicator of feather quality, wider growth bars, have been correlated with reproductive success (e.g., Takaki et al. 2001) and might be an indirect indicator of territory quality (Witter and Lee 1995). Finally, and perhaps most important in the context of stress, intact feathers are vital for optimal predator escape. Both feather gaps in the wing and decreased power from old feathers can increase the susceptibility to predation by decreasing aerial maneuverability (Hedenström and Sunada 1999) and reducing the takeoff angle a bird can achieve when surprised by a predator (Swaddle and Witter 1997). In fact, experimentally creating feather gaps can lead directly to increased predation (Slagsvold and Dale 1996).

Given these important roles that feathers play, feather production must be tightly regulated so that the end result of a successful molt is a complete set of structurally sound feathers. However, the costs associated with feather loss and subsequent regrowth are impressive. Feathers are composed of 95% protein, particularly the amino acids cysteine and methionine (Murphy and King 1992), and account for as much as 40% of the dry weight of an individual (Ginn and Mellville 1983). Protein production is not restricted to the feathers, however. The entire body is rebuilt, including changes in integument, bone restructuring, increases in total blood volume, changes in water

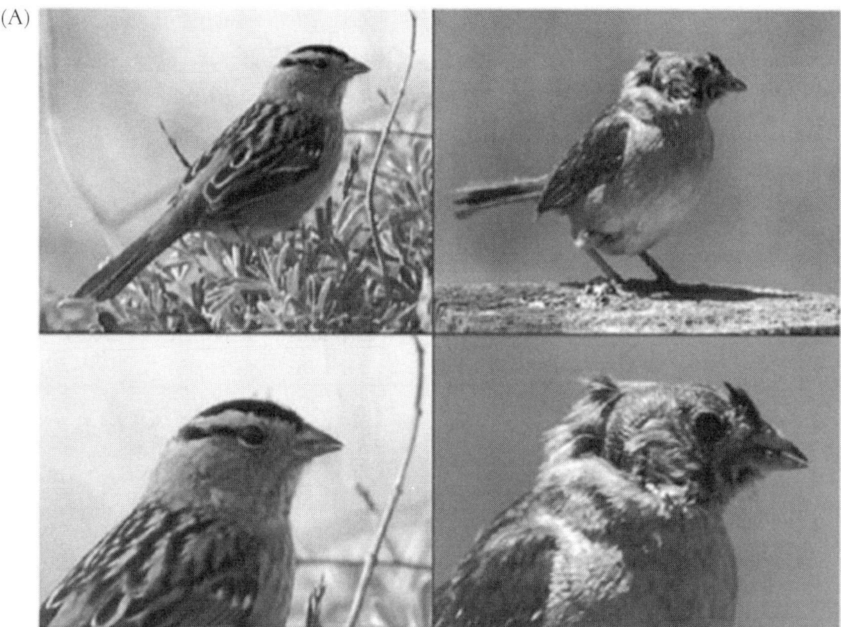

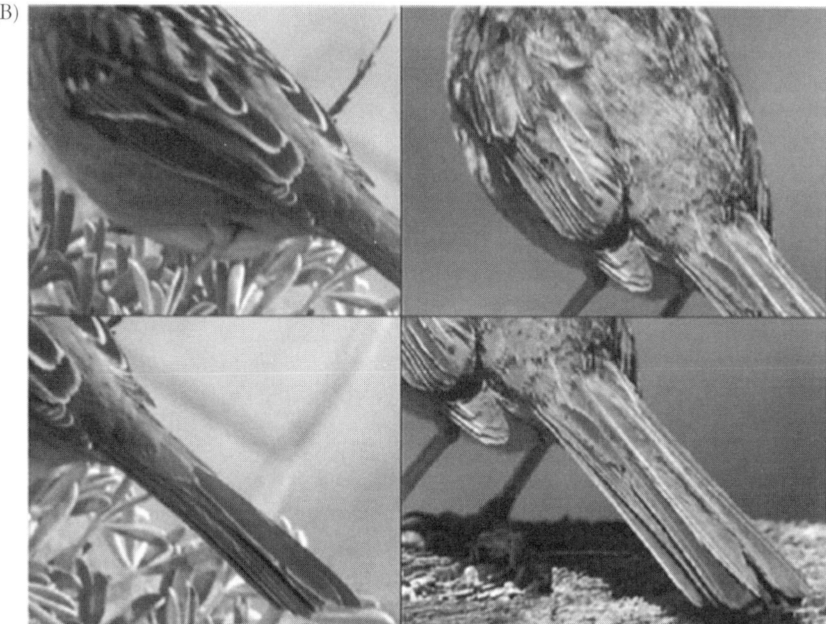

FIGURE 7.27: (A) Why molt? Nuttall's white-crowned sparrows on the left-hand side have fresh breeding plumage, while those on the right have extremely worn plumage at the end of the breeding season in July. Some feathers (e.g., on the head, right panels) may have been lost while fighting. Note also the faded coloration of feathers in the right-hand panels.

Photos by J. C. Wingfield, taken on the Pacific coast of central California.

(B) Close up of fresh plumage (left-hand panels) and worn plumage (right-hand panels) in Nuttall's white-crowned sparrows. Note the extreme wear on the right-hand panels and the dramatic fading of color. This worn plumage is completely replaced by molt.

Photos by J. C. Wingfield. Reprinted with permission from Wingfield and Silverin (2000). Courtesy of Elsevier.

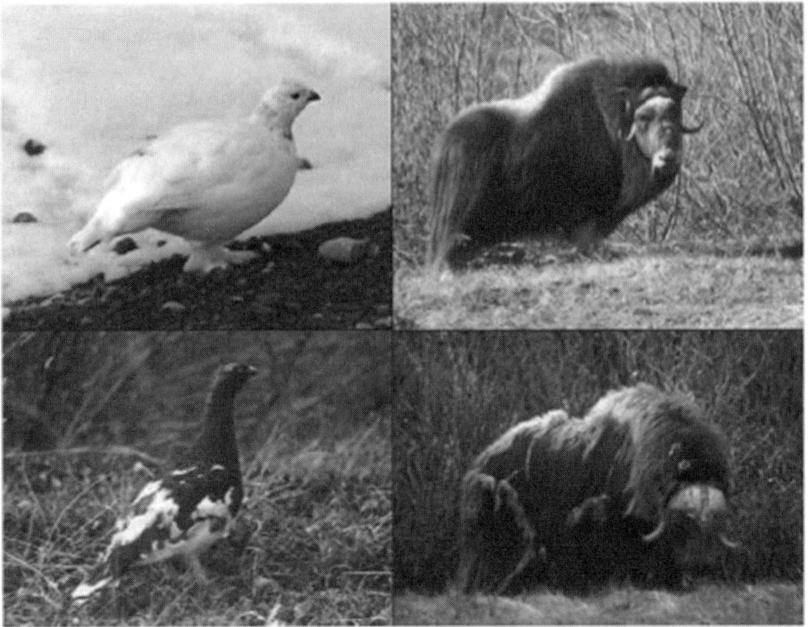

FIGURE 7.28: Examples of seasonal changes in pelage. Seasonal changes in plumage coloration in willow ptarmigan on the North Slope of Alaska. Top left panel shows typical all-white winter plumage, cryptic in snow but also highly insulated against the Arctic winter weather. Lower left panel shows summer plumage, more cryptic in the absence of snow. The top right panel shows a musk ox on the North Slope of Alaska in full winter pelage with long outer guard hairs and thick insulating hair beneath. Lower right panel shows a musk ox in spring, shedding large chunks of insulating hair. This will be replaced the following autumn.

Photos by J. C. Wingfield. Reprinted with permission from Wingfield and Silverin (2000). Courtesy of Elsevier.

turnover, and growth of flight muscles (Jenni and Winkler 1994). As a consequence, there is about 25% turnover of the total protein in the bird (Klasing 1998). Most birds lose weight during molt (Cherel et al. 1994; Hedenstrom 2003), but alter the muscle to body weight ratio thought to improve flight performance during molt (Chai 1997; Lind and Jakobsson 2001; Hedenstrom 2003). Interestingly, however, feather proteins are more costly to synthesize than are muscle proteins (Lindstrom et al. 1993). Accomplishing all this tissue growth and remodeling can result in increased basal metabolic rates of 9%–111% depending upon the species (Murphy and King 1992; Lindstrom et al. 1993; Klaassen 1995; Murphy 1996; Murphy et al. 1998).

The massive protein production during molt may be incompatible with the actions of corticosteroids because corticosteroids can inhibit protein synthesis and stimulate gluconeogenesis via protein catabolism. If so, this would explain why so many species down-regulate corticosteroid release during molt. In order to replace worn feathers and to survive the immediate feather replacement period, a delicate metabolic balance must exist. Unforeseen metabolic demands during the molt, such as those created by physical and psychological stressors, could disrupt this balance and negatively impact both immediate and future survival. The suppression of plasma corticosteroid release would allow for normal amino acid deposition at the site of feather synthesis and a normal rate of feather growth, and would prevent decreased fitness resulting from elevated corticosteroids.

The role of corticosteroids in shifting metabolism from protein production to protein catabolism suggests that elevated concentrations would disrupt normal feather growth. Recent evidence suggests that corticosteroids do interfere with molt. Figure 7.29 shows that exogenous corticosteroids inhibit feather growth rates by as much as 1 millimeter per feather per day (Romero et al. 2005). There appears to be an optimal molt duration, dependent upon species. Compressing molt into a shorter time can decrease feather quality, overwinter survival, and reproductive success (Nilsson and Svensson 1996; Dawson et al. 2000; Hall 2000; Serra 2001; Dawson 2004), but lengthening the duration of molt can result in more time

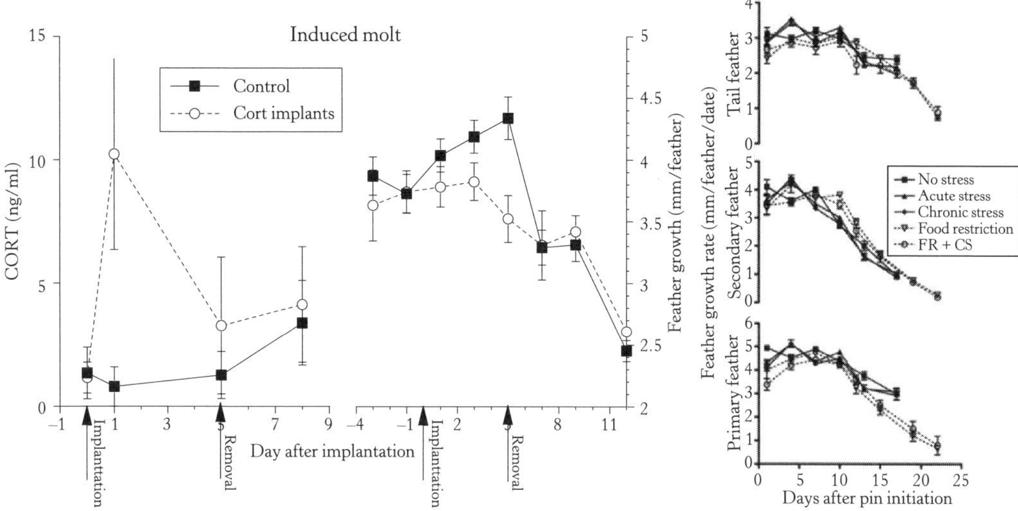

FIGURE 7.29: Left panel: Corticosterone implants (open symbols) decrease the growth rates of feathers in captive European starlings compared to controls (closed symbols). Feather growth rates were determined by measuring primary, secondary, and tail feathers throughout the replacement period.

Reprinted with permission from Romero et al. (2005). Courtesy of Elsevier.

Right panel: Natural stressors had no impact on feather growth rates.

Reprinted with permission from Strochlic and Romero (2008). Courtesy of Elsevier.

spent in a state of increased susceptibility (Borras et al. 2004). Consequently, the slower growth rate induced by corticosteroids could be very costly.

Furthermore, exogenous corticosteroids can significantly degrade feather quality (DesRochers et al. 2009; Manniste and Horak 2011). In general, feathers were lighter and weaker, consistent with the hypothesis that high concentrations of corticosteroids inhibit protein availability for feather production. Fault bars, or bands of decreased protein content in the growing feather, are also a commonly reported effect of stress on feather development (Witter and Lee 1995; Carbonell and Telleria 1999; Bortolotti et al. 2002; Jovani and Blas 2004). Decreases in feather quality could have significant implications for individual survival. Lighter feathers could increase the rate of feather abrasion (Dawson et al. 2000), and weaker feathers could break and create gaps in the wings (affecting wing surface area and wing loading; Jovani and Blas 2004), both of which would lead to a decrease in flight performance. Elevated corticosterone in the feathers has also been correlated with a degraded ornamentation used in social signaling (Bortolotti et al. 2009).

These data suggest that a physiological trade-off is taking place in molting birds. On one hand, elevated corticosteroids are important in regulating energy flow during emergencies. Down-regulation of corticosteroid release may thus compromise the ability to respond to and/or recover from a stressor. On the other hand, elevated corticosteroids appear to have profound impacts on growing feathers. Down-regulation of corticosteroids during molt may be necessary to ensure a successful molt. The ultimate amount of corticosteroids released during molt may be a compromise between these two opposing physiological sequelae.

If elevated corticosteroids were so devastating to a successful molt, then birds should avoid damaging concentrations at all costs. Two lines of evidence suggest that this appears to be the case. First, in contrast to exogenous corticosteroids, Figure 7.29 indicates that endogenous corticosteroid release induced by both acute and chronic stressors fails to inhibit feather growth rates (Strochlic and Romero 2008). The HPA axis appears to be finely tuned to prevent corticosteroid concentrations from ever reaching concentrations that inhibit feather growth or degrade feather quality (Remage-Healey and Romero 2002). Exogenous corticosteroids short-circuited this balance, thereby exposing the underlying mechanistic reason for the down-regulation of corticosteroids during molt. Second, although different species utilize different mechanisms (e.g., reduced pituitary sensitivity to CRF/AVT, reduced adrenal sensitivity to ACTH, etc.) to down-regulate corticosteroid release during molt (Romero 2001), the end result is the same—lowered corticosteroid concentrations. Apparently, the end result is so important that the exact physiological mechanism used to reduce corticosteroid release is relatively unimportant (and may suggest multiple evolutionary origins). The conclusion we can draw from these data is that a complete set of feathers appears to be more important for a bird's survival than the ability of corticosteroids to respond maximally to a stressor.

In summary, elevated corticosteroids inhibit aspects of growth in adult birds, although the mechanism does not appear to be through the growth hormone or IGF axes. Furthermore, the potential to disrupt molt appears to have exposed a physiological trade-off in corticosteroid function that ties directly into evolutionary processes. It is not clear, however, whether this can be generalized to other taxa. Some mammalian species, for example, also undergo a seasonal molt (replacement of hair), but at least in seals, this is accompanied by elevated rather than reduced corticosteroid concentrations in some species (Ashwellerickson et al. 1986), but not in others (Boily 1996).

VIII. CONCLUSION

We have focused this chapter on environmental stressors that directly impact energy utilization. As we discussed in the introduction, the stressors presented in this chapter are only a small subset of the stressors that we could have covered. However, from this subset we can identify a few common themes. First is that the role of catecholamines in energy regulation in free-living animals has barely been studied. This is a wide-open area, and yet with the introduction of small radio-transmitters that can monitor heart rate (Chapter 6) and the data from laboratory studies, this is likely to be an interesting avenue of investigation in the future. Second is that the role of the corticosteroids is quite complex. This should not be surprising. Biomedicine has struggled for decades to understand the role of corticosteroids in energy regulation in humans and laboratory species. The inclusion of differences in energy regulation in non-traditional study species, as well as environmental variability, can be daunting for these studies. However, one theme that does arise is that emergency regulation of energy appears to be mainly regulated by type II (GR) receptors, and non-emergency regulation appears to be mainly regulated by type I (MR) receptors. It is encouraging that this division also matches the biomedical evidence. It suggests that much of the information from the biomedical literature will be broadly applicable to field studies, and that the differences will likely be very illuminating.

REFERENCES

Adams, N. J., Brown, C. R., 1990. Energetics of molt in penguins. In: Davis, L. S., Darby, J. T. (Eds.), *Penguin biology*, Academic Press, San Diego, pp. 297–315.

Adams, N. J., Cockrem, J. F., Taylor, G. A., Candy, E. J., Bridges, J., 2005. Corticosterone responses of grey-faced petrels (*Pterodroma macroptera gouldi*) are higher during incubation than during other breeding stages. *Physiol Biochem Zool* 78, 69–77.

Addison, B., Kitaysky, A. S., Hipfner, J. M., 2008. Sex allocation in a monomorphic seabird with a single-egg clutch: Test of the environment, mate quality, and female condition hypotheses. *Behav Ecol Sociobiol* 63, 135–141.

Almasi, B., Roulin, A., Jenni-Eiermann, S., Jenni, L., 2008. Parental investment and its sensitivity to corticosterone is linked to melanin-based coloration in barn owls. *Horm Behav* 54, 217–223.

Ancel, A., Fetter, L., Groscolas, R., 1998. Changes in egg and body temperature indicate triggering of egg desertion at a body mass threshold in fasting incubating blue petrels (*Halobaena caerulea*). *J Comp Physiol B* 168, 533–539.

Angelier, F., Bost, C. A., Giraudeau, M., Bouteloup, G., Dano, S., Chastel, O., 2008. Corticosterone and foraging behavior in a diving seabird: The Adelie penguin, *Pygoscelis adeliae*. *Gen Comp Endocrinol* 156, 134–144.

Angelier, F., Chastel, O., 2009. Stress, prolactin and parental investment in birds: A review. *Gen Comp Endocrinol* 163, 142–148.

Angelier, F., Clement-Chastel, C., Gabrielsen, G.W., Chastel, O., 2007a. Corticosterone and time-activity Black-legged budget: An experiment with kittiwakes. *Horm Behav* 52, 482–491.

Angelier, F., Clement-Chastel, C., Welcker, J., Gabrielsen, G. W., Chastel, O., 2009a. How does corticosterone affect parental behaviour and reproductive success? A study of prolactin in black-legged kittiwakes. *Func Ecol* 23, 784–793.

Angelier, F., Moe, B., Blanc, S., Chastel, O., 2009b. What factors drive prolactin and corticosterone responses to stress in a long-lived bird species (snow petrel *Pagodroma nivea*)? *Physiol Biochem Zool* 82, 590–602.

Angelier, F., Shaffer, S. A., Weimerskirch, H., Trouve, C., Chastel, O., 2007b. Corticosterone and foraging behavior in a pelagic seabird. *Physiol Biochem Zool* 80, 283–292.

Ashwellerickson, S., Fay, F. H., Elsner, R., 1986. Metabolic and hormonal correlates of molting and regeneration of pelage in Alaskanharbor and spotted seals (*Phoca vitulina* and *Phoca largha*). *Can J Zool* 64, 1086–1094.

Astheimer, L. B., Buttemer, W. A., Wingfield, J. C., 1992. Interactions of corticosterone with feeding, activity and metabolism in passerine birds. *Ornis Scan* 23, 355–365.

Barnett, J. L., 1973. A stress response in *Antechinus stuartii* (MacLeay). *Aust J Zool* 21, 501–513.

Barré, H., 1984. Metabolic and insulative changes in winter—and summer-acclimatized King Penguin chicks. *J Compar Physiol B* 154, 317–324.

Battley, P. F., Piersma, T., Dietz, M. W., Tang, S. X., Dekinga, A., Hulsman, K., 2000. Empirical evidence for differential organ reductions during trans-oceanic bird flight. *Proc R Soc Lond B* 267, 191–195.

Beaulieu, M., Dervaux, A., Thierry, A. M., Lazin, D., Le Maho, Y., Ropert-Coudert, Y., Spee, M., Raclot, T., Ancel, A., 2010. When sea-ice clock is ahead of Adelie penguins' clock. *Func Ecol* 24, 93–102.

Benowitz-Fredericks, Z. M., Shultz, M. T., Kitaysky, A. S., 2008. Stress hormones suggest opposite trends of food availability for planktivorous and piscivorous seabirds in 2 years. *Deep-Sea Res II-Top Stud Oceanogr* 55, 1868–1876.

Bernard, S. F., Fayolle, C., Robin, J. P., Groscolas, R., 2002a. Glycerol and NEFA kinetics in long-term fasting king penguins: phase II versus phase III. *J Exp Biol* 205, 2745–2754.

Bernard, S. F., Mioskowski, E., Groscolas, R., 2002b. Blockade of fatty acid oxidation mimics phase II-phase III transition in a fasting bird, the king penguin. *Am J Physiol* 283, R144–R152.

Bernard, S. F., Thil, M. A., Groscolas, R., 2003. Lipolytic and metabolic response to glucagon in fasting king penguins: phase II vs. phase III. *Am J Physiol* 284, R444-R454.

Berthold, P., 1993. *Bird migration: A general survey.* Oxford University Press, New York.

Blem, C. R., 1990. Avian energy storage. In: Power, D. (Ed.) *Current ornithology.* Plenum, New York, pp. 59–113.

Blondel, J., 2000. Evolution and ecology of birds on islands: Trends and prospects. *Vie Milieu* 50, 205–220.

Boily, P., 1996. Metabolic and hormonal changes during the molt of captive gray seals (*Halichoerus grypus*). *Am J Physiol* 270, R1051–R1058.

Bókony, V., Lendvai, A. Z., Liker, A., Angelier, F., Wingfield, J. C., Chastel, O., 2009. Stress response and the value of reproduction: are birds prudent parents? *Am Nat* 173, 589–598.

Bonier, F., Martin, P. R., Moore, I. T., Wingfield, J. C., 2009. Do baseline glucocorticoids predict fitness? *Trends Ecol Evol* 24, 634–642.

Borras, A., Cabrera, T., Cabrera, J., Senar, J. C., 2004. Interlocality variation in speed of moult in the Citril finch (*Serinus citrinella*). *Ibis* 146, 14–17.

Bortolotti, G. R., Dawson, R. D., Murza, G. L., 2002. Stress during feather development predicts fitness potential. *J Anim Ecol* 71, 333–342.

Bortolotti, G. R., Mougeot, F., Martinez-Padilla, J., Webster, L. M. I., Piertney, S. B., 2009. Physiological stress mediates the honesty of social signals. *Plos One* 4, e4983.

Boswell, T., 2005. Regulation of energy balance in birds by the neuroendocrine hypothalamus. *J Poultry Sci* 42, 161–181.

Boswell, T., Lehman, T. L., Ramenofsky, M., 1997. Effects of plasma glucose manipulations on food intake in white-crowned sparrows. *Comp Biochem Physiol A* 118, 721–726.

Boswell, T., Richardson, R. D., Seeley, R. J., Ramenofsky, M., Wingfield, J. C., Friedman, M. I., Woods, S. C., 1995. Regulation of food intake by metabolic fuels in white-crowned sparrows. *Am J Physiol* 38, R1462–R1468.

Bourgeon, S., Martinez, J., Criscuolo, F., Le Maho, Y., Raclot, T., 2006. Fasting-induced changes of immunological and stress indicators in breeding female eiders. *Gen Comp Endocrinol* 147, 336–342.

Boutin, S., 1990. Food supplementation experiments with terrestrial vertebrates: Patterns, problems, and the future. *Can J Zool* 68, 203–220.

Bradley, A. J., 1987. Stress and mortality in the red-tailed phasogale, *Phasogale calura* (Marsupalia: Dasyuridae). *Gen Comp Endocrinol* 67, 85–100.

Bradley, A. J., McDonald, I. R., Lee, A. K., 1980. Stress and mortality in a small marsupial (*Antechinus stuartii*, Macleay). *Gen Comp Endocrinol* 40, 188–200.

Breuner, C. W., Hahn, T. P., 2003. Integrating stress physiology, environmental change, and behavior in free-living sparrows. *Horm Behav* 43, 115–123.

Breuner, C. W., Orchinik, M., 2001. Seasonal regulation of membrane and intracellular corticosteroid receptors in the house sparrow brain. *J Neuroendocrinol* 13, 412–420.

Breuner, C. W., Orchinik, M., 2002. Beyond carrier proteins: Plasma binding proteins as mediators of corticosteroid action in vertebrates. *J Endocrinol* 175, 99–112.

Breuner, C. W., Patterson, S. H., Hahn, T. P., 2008. In search of relationships between the acute adrenocortical response and fitness. *Gen Comp Endocrinol* 157, 288–295.

Brewer, J. H., O'Reilly, K. M., Kildaw, S. D., Buck, C. L., 2008. Interannual variation in the adrenal responsiveness of black-legged kittiwake chicks (*Rissa tridactyla*). *Gen Comp Endocrinol* 156, 361–368.

Buck, C. L., O'Reilly, K. A., Kildaw, S. D., 2007. Interannual variability of black-legged kittiwake productivity is reflected in baseline plasma corticosterone. *Gen Comp Endocrinol* 150, 430–436.

Bumpus, H., 1899. The elimination of the unfit as illustrated by the introduced sparrow, *Passer domesticus*. *Mar Biol Lab, Biol Lect* (Woods Hole, 1898), 209–228.

Busch, D. S., Robinson, W. D., Robinson, T. R., Wingfield, J. C., 2011. Influence of proximity to a geographical range limit on the physiology of a tropical bird. *J Anim Ecol* 80, 640–649.

Cahill, G. F. J., 1976. Starvation in man. *Clin Endocrinol Metab* 5, 397–415.

Cameron-MacMillan, M. L., Walsh, C. J., Wilhelm, S. I., Storey, A. E., 2007. Male chicks are more costly to rear than females in a monogamous seabird, the common murre. *Behav Ecol* 18, 81–85.

Carbonell, R., Telleria, J. L., 1999. Feather traits and ptilochronology as indicators of stress in Iberian blackcaps *Sylvia atricapilla*. *Bird Study* 46, 243–248.

Carsia, R. V., McIlroy, P. J., 1998. Dietary protein restriction stress in the domestic turkey (*Meleagris gallopavo*) induces hypofunction and remodeling of adrenal steroidogenic tissue. *Gen Comp Endocrinol* 109, 140–153.

Chai, P., 1997. Hummingbird hovering energetics during moult of primary flight feathers. *J Exp Biol* 200, 1527–1536.

Challet, E., le Maho, Y., Robin, J. P., Malan, A., Cherel, Y., 1995. Involvement of corticosterone in the fasting-induced rise in protein utilization and locomotor activity. *Pharmacol BiochemBehav* 50, 405–412.

Champagne, C. D., Houser, D. S., Crocker, D. E., 2005. Glucose production and substrate cycle activity in a fasting adapted animal, the northern elephant seal. *J Exp Biol* 208, 859–868.

Champagne, C. D., Houser, D. S., Crocker, D. E., 2006. Glucose metabolism during lactation in a fasting animal, the northern elephant seal. *Am J Physiol* 291, R1129–R1137.

Chastel, O., Lacroix, A., Weimerskirch, H., Gabrielsen, G. W., 2005. Modulation of prolactin but not corticosterone responses to stress in relation to parental effort in a long-lived bird. *Horm Behav* 47, 459–466.

Cherel, Y., Burnol, A. F., Leturque, A., Lemaho, Y., 1988a. Invivo glucose utilization in rat tissues during the 3 phases of starvation. *Metab Clin Exp* 37, 1033–1039.

Cherel, Y., Charrassin, J. B., Challet, E., 1994. Energy and protein requirements for molt in the king penguin Aptenodytes patagonicus. *Am J Physiol* 266, R1182–1188.

Cherel, Y., Le Maho, Y., 1985. Five months of fasting in king penguin chicks: Body mass loss and fuel metabolism. *Am J Physiol* 18, R387–R392.

Cherel, Y., Robin, J. P., Lemaho, Y., 1988b. Physiology and biochemistry of long-term fasting in birds. *Can J Zool* 66, 159–166.

Cherel, Y., Robin, J. P., Walch, O., Karmann, H., Netchitailo, P., Le Maho, Y., 1988c. Fasting in king penguin. I. Hormonal and metabolic changes during breeding. *Am J Physiol* 254, R170–177.

Cherel, Y., Stahl, J.C., Lemaho, Y., 1987. Ecology and physiology of fasting in king penguin chicks. *Auk* 104, 254–262.

Cimprich, D. A., Moore, F. R., 2006. Fat affects predator-avoidance behavior in gray catbirds (*Dumetella carolinensis*) during migratory stopover. *Auk* 123, 1069–1076.

Clinchy, M., Zanette, L., Boonstra, R., Wingfield, J. C., Smith, J. N. M., 2004. Balancing food and predator pressure induces chronic stress in songbirds. *Proc R Soc Lond B* 271, 2473–2479.

Cochran, W. W., Wikelski, M., 2005. Individual migratory tactics of new world *Catharus* thrushes: Current knowledge and future tracking options from space. In: Greenberg, R., Marra, P. P. (Eds.), *Birds of two worlds: The ecology and evolution of migration*. Johns Hopkins University Press, Baltimore, MD, pp. 274–289.

Cockrem, J. F., Potter, M. A., Candy, E. J., 2006. Corticosterone in relation to body mass in Adelie penguins (*Pygoscelis adeliae*) affected by unusual sea ice conditions at Ross Island, Antarctica. *Gen Comp Endocrinol* 149, 244–252.

Corbel, H., Geiger, S., Groscolas, R., 2010. Preparing to fledge: the adrenocortical and metabolic responses to stress in king penguin chicks. *Func Ecol.* 24, 82–92.

Criscuolo, F., Chastel, O., Bertile, F., Gabrielsen, G.W., Le Maho, Y., Raclot, T., 2005. Corticosterone alone does not trigger a short term behavioural shift in incubating female common eiders Somateria mollissima, but does modify long term reproductive success. *J Avian Biol* 36, 306–312.

Crosby, S. S., Apovian, C. M., Grodin, M. A., 2007. Hunger strikes, force-feeding, and physicians' responsibilities. *JAMA* 298, 563–566.

Dallman, M. F., Akana, S. F., Bhatnagar, S., Bell, M. E., Choi, S., Chu, A., Horsley, C., Levin, N., Meijer, O., Soriano, L. R., Strack, A.M., Viau, V., 1999. Starvation: Early signals, sensors, and sequelae. *Endocrinology* 140, 4015–4023.

Dallman, M. F., la Fleur, S. E., Pecoraro, N. C., Gomez, F., Houshyar, H., Akana, S. F., 2004. Minireview: Glucocorticoids—food intake, abdominal obesity, and wealthy nations in 2004. *Endocrinology* 145, 2633–2638.

Dallman, M. F., Strack, A. M., Akana, S. F., Bradbury, M. J., Hanson, E. S., Scribner, K. A., Smith, M., 1993. Feast and famine: Critical role of glucocorticoids with insulin in daily energy flow. *Front Neuroendocrinol* 14, 303–347.

Dauphin-Villemant, C., Leboulenger, F., Vaudry, H., Xavier, F., 1987. Interrenal activity in a female lizard, *Lacerta vivipara*: Annual variations of plasma corticosteroids and responsiveness of interrenal tissue to ACTH. *Gen Comp Endocrinol* 66, 31.

Dawson, A., 2004. The effects of delaying the start of moult on the duration of moult, primary feather growth rates and feather mass in common starlings *Sturnus vulgaris*. *Ibis* 146, 493–500.

Dawson, A., Hinsley, S. A., Ferns, P. N., Bonser, R. H. C., Eccleston, L., 2000. Rate of moult affects feather quality: A mechanism linking current reproductive effort to future survival. *Proc R Soc Lond B* 267, 2093–2098.

Denbow, D. M., 1999. Food intake regulation in birds. *J Exp Zool* 283, 333–338.

DesRochers, D. W., Reed, J. M., Awerman, J., Kluge, J., Wilkinson, J., van Griethuijsen, L. I., Aman, J., Romero, L. M., 2009. Exogenous and endogenous corticosterone alter feather quality. *Comp Biochem Physiol A Mol Integr Physiol* 152, 46–52.

Dickhoff, W. W., 1989. Salmonids and annual fishes: Death after sex. In: *Development, maturation, and senescence of neuroendocrine systems: A comparative approach*. Academic Press, New York, pp. 253–266.

Dickinson, V. M., Jarchow, J. L., Trueblood, M. H., 2002. Hematology and plasma biochemistry reference range values for free-ranging desert tortoises in Arizona. *J Wildlife Dis* 38, 143–153.

Doody, L. M., Wilhelm, S. I., McKay, D. W., Walsh, C. J., Storey, A. E., 2008. The effects of variable foraging conditions on common murre (*Uria aalge*) corticosterone concentrations and parental provisioning. *Horm Behav* 53, 140–148.

du Dot, T. J., Rosen, D. A. S., Richmond, J. P., Kitaysky, A. S., Zinn, S. A., Trites, A. W., 2009. Changes in glucocorticoids, IGF-I and thyroid hormones as indicators of nutritional stress and subsequent refeeding in Steller sea lions (*Eumetopias jubatus*). *Comp Biochem Physiol A* 152, 524–534.

Dunlap, K. D., Wingfield, J. C., 1995. External and internal influences on indices of physiological stress: I. Seasonal and population variation in adrenocortical secretion of free-living lizards, *Sceloporus occidentalis*. *J Exp Zool* 271, 36–46.

Elia, M., 2000. Hunger disease. *Clin Nutrition* 19, 379–386.

Enfield, D. B., 2001. Evolution and historical perspective of the 1997–1998 El Nino-Southern Oscillation event. *Bull Marine Sci* 69, 7–25.

Ferns, P. N., Lang, A., 2003. The value of immaculate mates: Relationships between plumage quality and breeding success in shelducks. *Ethology* 109, 521–532.

Fichter, M. M., Pirke, K. M., 1986. Effect of experimental and pathological weight loss upon the hypothalamo-pituitary-adrenal axis. *Psychoneuroendocrinology* 11, 295–305.

Fitzpatrick, S., 1998. Birds' tails as signaling devices: Markings, shape, length, and feather quality. *Am Nat* 151, 157–173.

Freeman, B. M., Manning, A. C. C., Flack, I. H., 1981. The effects of restricted feeding on the adrenal-cortical activity in the immature domestic fowl. *Brit Poultry Sci* 22, 295–303.

Frisch, A. J., Anderson, T. A., 2000. The response of coral trout (Plectropomus leopardus) to capture, handling and transport and shallow water stress. *Fish Physiol Biochem* 23, 23–34.

Gannes, L. Z., 2001. Comparative fuel use of migrating passerines: Effects of fat stores, migration distance, and diet. *Auk* 118, 665–677.

Geleon, A., 1981. Modifications du comportement au cours du cycle annuel de l'oie landaise. *Can J Zool* 63, 2810–2816.

Gibbs, H. L., Grant, P. R., 1987. Ecological consequences of an exceptionally strong El Nino event on Darwin's finches. *Ecology* 68, 1735–1746.

Gilbert, C., Le Maho, Y., Perret, M., Ancel, A., 2007. Body temperature changes induced by huddling in breeding male emperor penguins. *Am J Physiol* 292, R176-R185.

Gilbert, C., Robertson, G., Le Maho, Y., Naito, Y., Ancel, A., 2006. Huddling behavior in emperor penguins: Dynamics of huddling. *Physiol Behav* 88, 479–488.

Ginn, H. B., Mellville, D. S., 1983. *Moult in birds: BTO guide 19*. British Trust for Ornithology, Tring, UK.

Godet, R., Mattei, X., Dupe-Godet, M., 1984. Alterations of endocrine pancreas B cells in a sahelian reptile (*Varanus exanthematicus*) during starvation. *J Morphol* 180, 173–180.

Gonzalez-Bono, E., Rohleder, N., Hellhammer, D. H., Salvador, A., Kirschbaum, C., 2002. Glucose but not protein or fat load amplifies the cortisol response to psychosocial stress. *Horm Behav* 41, 328–333.

Goymann, W., Wingfield, J. C., 2004. Allostatic load, social status and stress hormones: the costs of social status matter. *Anim Behav* 67, 591–602.

Grant, P. R., Grant, B. R., 1980. The breeding and feeding characteristics of Darwin's finches on Isla Genovesa, Galapagos. *Ecol Monogr* 50, 381–410.

Gray, J. M., Yarian, D., Ramenofsky, M., 1990. Corticosterone, foraging behavior, and metabolism in dark-eyed juncos, *Junco hyemalis*. *Gen Comp Endocrinol* 79, 375–384.

Groscolas, R., Cherel, Y., 1992. How to molt while fasting in the cold: The metabolic and hormonal adaptations of emperor and king penguins. *Ornis Scan* 23, 328–334.

Groscolas, R., Lacroix, A., Robin, J. P., 2008. Spontaneous egg or chick abandonment in energy-depleted king penguins: A role for corticosterone and prolactin? *Horm Behav* 53, 51–60.

Groscolas, R., Robin, J. P., 2001. Long-term fasting and re-feeding in penguins. *Comp Biochem Physiol A Mol Integr Physiol* 128, 645–655.

Grutter, A. S., Pankhurst, N. W., 2000. The effects of capture, handling, confinement and ectoparasite load on plasma levels of cortisol, glucose and lactate in the coral reef fish Hemigymnus melapterus. *J Fish Biol* 57, 391–401.

Guinet, C., Servera, N., Mangin, S., Georges, J. Y., Lacroix, A., 2004. Change in plasma cortisol and metabolites during the attendance period ashore in fasting lactating subantarctic fur seals. *Comp Biochem Physiol A* 137, 523–531.

Haase, E., Rees, A., Harvey, S., 1986. Flight stimulates adrenocortical activity in pigeons (*Columba livia*). *Gen Comp Endocrinol* 61, 424–427.

Hall, K. S. S., 2000. Lesser whitethroats under time-constraint moult more rapidly and grow shorter wing feathers. *J Avian Biol* 31, 583–587.

Harding, A. M. A., Kitaysky, A. S., Hall, M. E., Welcker, J., Karnovsky, N. J., Talbot, S. L., Hamer, K. C., Gremillet, D., 2009. Flexibility in the parental effort of an Arctic-breeding seabird. *Func Ecol* 23, 348–358.

Hedenstrom, A., 2003. Flying with holey wings. *J Avian Biol* 34, 324–327.

Hedenström, A., Sunada, S., 1999. On the aerodynamics of moult gaps in birds. *J Exp Biol* 202, 67–76.

Holberton, R. L., 1999. Changes in patterns of corticosterone secretion concurrent with migratory fattening in a neotropical migratory bird. *Gen Comp Endocrinol* 116, 49–58.

Holberton, R. L., Dufty, A. M., Jr., 2005. Hormones and variation in life history strategies of migratory and nonmigratory birds. In: Greenberg, R., Marra, P. P. (Eds.), *Birds of two worlds: The ecology and evolution of migration*. Johns Hopkins University Press, Baltimore, MD, pp. 290–302.

Holberton, R. L., Parrish, J. D., Wingfield, J. C., 1996. Modulation of the adrenocortical stress response in neotropical migrants during autumn migration. *Auk* 113, 558–564.

Honarmand, M., Goymann, W., Naguib, M., 2010. Stressful dieting: Nutritional conditions but not compensatory growth elevate corticosterone levels in zebra finch nestlings and fledglings. *Plos One* 5, e12930.

Hood, L. C., Boersma, P. D., Wingfield, J. C., 1998. The adrenocortical response to stress in incubating magellanic penguins (*Spheniscus magellanicus*). *Auk* 115, 76–84.

Houser, D. S., Champagne, C. D., Crocker, D. E., 2007. Lipolysis and glycerol gluconeogenesis in simultaneously fasting and lactating northern elephant seals. *Am J Physiol* 293, R2376–R2381.

Jenni, L., Jenni-Eiermann, S., 1998. Fuel supply and metabolic constraints in migrating birds. *J Avian Biol* 29, 521–528.

Jenni, L., Winkler, R., 1994. *Moult and ageing of European passerines*. Academic Press, London.

Jenni-Eiermann, S., Jenni, L., 1996. Metabolic differences between the postbreeding, moulting and migratory periods in feeding and fasting passerine birds. *Func Ecol* 10, 62–72.

Jenni-Eiermann, S., Jenni, L., 2001. Postexercise ketosis in night-migrating passerine birds. *Physiol Biochem Zool* 74, 90–101.

Jenni-Eiermann, S., Jenni, L., Piersma, T., 2002. Temporal uncoupling of thyroid hormones in red knots: T3 peaks in cold weather, T4 during moult. *Journal Ornithol* 143, 331–340.

Jovani, R., Blas, J., 2004. Adaptive allocation of stress-induced deformities on bird feathers. *J Evolut Biol* 17, 294–301.

Kern, M., Bacon, W., Long, D., Cowie, R. J., 2005. Blood metabolite and corticosterone levels in breeding adult pied flycatchers. *Condor* 107, 665–677.

Kern, M. D., Bacon, W., Long, D., Cowie, R. J., 2007. Blood metabolite levels in normal and handicapped pied flycatchers rearing broods of different sizes. *Comp Biochem Physiol A* 147, 70–76.

Ketterson, E. D., King, J. R., 1977. Metabolic and behavioral-responses to fasting in white-crowned sparrow (Zonotrichia-Leucophrys-Gambelii). *Physiol Zool* 50, 115–129.

Kirschbaum, C., Bono, E. G., Rohleder, N., Gessner, C., Pirke, K. M., Salvador, A., Hellhammer, D. H., 1997. Effects of fasting and glucose load on free cortisol responses to stress and nicotine. *J Clin Endocrinol Metabol* 82, 1101–1105.

Kitaysky, A., Rosen, D. A. S., Trites, A. W., 2007a. *Endocrine response of Steller sea lions to nutritional stress*. Final Report to the Marine Mammal Research Consortium. University of Alaska, Fairbanks.

Kitaysky, A. S., Kitaiskaia, E. V., Piatt, J. F., Wingfield, J. C., 2003. Benefits and costs of increased levels of corticosterone in seabird chicks. *Horm Behav* 43, 140–149.

Kitaysky, A. S., Kitaiskaia, E. V., Wingfield, J. C., Piatt, J. F., 2001a. Dietary restriction causes chronic elevation of corticosterone and enhances stress response in red-legged kittiwake chicks. *J Comp Physiol B* 171, 701.

Kitaysky, A. S., Piatt, J. F., Hatch, S. A., Kitaiskaia, E. V., Benowitz-Fredericks, Z. M., Shultz, M. T., Wingfield, J. C., 2010. Food availability and population processes: severity of nutritional stress during reproduction predicts survival of long-lived seabirds. *Func Ecol* 24, 625–637.

Kitaysky, A. S., Piatt, J. F., Wingfield, J. C., 2007b. Stress hormones link food availability and population processes in seabirds. *Mar Ecol-Prog Ser* 352, 245–258.

Kitaysky, A. S., Piatt, J. F., Wingfield, J. C., Romano, M., 1999a. The adrenocortical stress-response of black-legged kittiwake chicks in relation to dietary restrictions. *J Comp Physiol B* 169, 303–310.

Kitaysky, A. S., Romano, M. D., Piatt, J. F., Wingfield, J. C., Kikuchi, M., 2005. The adrenocortical response of tufted puffin chicks to nutritional deficits. *Horm Behav* 47, 606–619.

Kitaysky, A. S., Wingfield, J. C., Piatt, J. F., 1999b. Dynamics of food availability, body condition and physiological stress response in breeding black-legged kittiwakes. *Func Ecol* 13, 577–584.

Kitaysky, A. S., Wingfield, J. C., Piatt, J. F., 2001b. Corticosterone facilitates begging and affects resource allocation in the black-legged kittiwake. *Behav Ecol* 12, 619.

Klaassen, M., 1995. Moult and basal metabolic costs in males of two subspecies of stonechats: The European *Saxicola torquata rubicula* and the East African *S t axillaris*. *Oecologia* 104, 424–432.

Klasing, K. C., 1998. *Comparative avian nutrition*. CAB International, New York.

Koch, K. A., Wingfield, J. C., Buntin, J. D., 2002. Glucocorticoids and parental hyperphagia in ring doves (*Streptopelia risoria*). *Horm Behav* 41, 9–21.

Kruuk, H., Snell, H., 1981. Prey selection by feral dogs from a population of marine iguanas (*Amblyrhynchus cristatus*). *J Appled Ecology* 18, 197–204.

Kuenzel, W. J., 1994. Central neuroanatomical systems involved in the regulation of food intake in birds and mammals. *J Nutrition* 124, S1355–S1370.

Lack, D., 1950. Breeding seasons in the Galapagos. *Ibis* 92, 268–278.

Lanctot, R. B., Hatch, S. A., Gill, V. A., Eens, M., 2003. Are corticosterone levels a good indicator of food availability and reproductive performance in a kittiwake colony? *Horm Behav* 43, 489–502.

Landys, M. M., Piersma, T., Guglielmo, C. G., Jukema, J., Ramenofsky, M., Wingfield, J.C., 2005. Metabolic profile of long-distance migratory flight and stopover in a shorebird. *Proc R Soc Lond B* 272, 295–302.

Landys, M. M., Piersma, T., Ramenofsky, M., Wingfield, J. C., 2004a. Role of the low-affinity glucocorticoid receptor in the regulation of behavior and energy metabolism in the migratory red knot Calidris canutus islandica. *Physiol Biochem Zool* 77, 658–668.

Landys, M. M., Ramenofsky, M., Guglielmo, C. G., Wingfield, J. C., 2004b. The low-affinity glucocorticoid receptor regulates feeding and lipid breakdown in the migratory Gambel's white-crowned sparrow *Zonotrichia leucophrys gambelii*. *J Exp Biol* 207, 143–154.

Landys, M. M., Ramenofsky, M., Wingfield, J. C., 2006. Actions of glucocorticoids at a seasonal baseline as compared to stress-related levels in the regulation of periodic life processes. *Gen Comp Endocrinol* 148, 132–149.

Landys, M. M., Wingfield, J. C., Ramenofsky, M., 2004c. Plasma corticosterone increases during migratory restlessness in the captive white-crowned sparrow *Zonotrichia leucophrys gambelli*. *Horm Behav* 46, 574–581.

Landys-Ciannelli, M. M., Ramenofsky, M., Piersma, T., Jukema, J., Wingfield, J. C., 2002. Baseline and stress-induced plasma corticosterone during long-distance migration in the bar-tailed godwit, *Limosa lapponica*. *Physiol Biochem Zool* 75, 101–110.

Lank, D. B., Butler, R. W., Ireland, J., Ydenberg, R. C., 2003. Effects of predation danger on migration strategies of sandpipers. *Oikos* 103, 303–319.

Laurie, W. A., 1989. Effects of the 1982–1983 El Nino-Southern Oscillation event on marine iguana (*Amblyrhynchus cristatus*, Bell, 1825) populations in the Galapagos islands. In: Glynn, P. (Ed.) *Global ecological consequences of the 1982–1983 El Nino-Southern Oscillation*. Elsevier, New York, pp. 121–141.

Le Maho, Y., 1983. Metabolic adaptations to long-term fasting in antarctic penguins and domestic geese. *J Thermal Biol* 8, 91–96.

Le Maho, Y., Delclitte, P., Chatonnet, J., 1976. Thermoregulation in fasting emperor penguins under natural conditions. *Am J Physiol* 231, 913–922.

Le Maho, Y., Vankha, H. V., Koubi, H., Dewasmes, G., Girard, J., Ferre, P., Cagnard, M., 1981. Body-composition, energy-expenditure, and plasma metabolites in long-term fasting geese. *Am J Physiol* 241, E342–E354.

Le Ninan, F., Cherel, Y., Sardet, C., Le Maho, Y., 1988. Plasma hormone levels in relation to lipid and protein metabolism during prolonged fasting in king penguin chicks. *Gen Compar Endocrinol* 71, 331–337.

Lind, J., Cresswell, W., 2006. Anti-predation behaviour during bird migration; the benefit of studying multiple behavioural dimensions. *J Ornithol* 147, 310–316.

Lind, J., Jakobsson, S., 2001. Body building and concurrent mass loss: Flight adaptations in tree sparrows. *Proc R Soc Lond B* 268, 1915–1919.

Lindstrom, A., Visser, G. H., Daan, S., 1993. The energetic cost of feather synthesis is proportional to basal metabolic rate. *Physiol Zool* 66, 490–510.

Lohmus, M., Sandberg, R., Holberton, R. L., Moore, F. R., 2003. Corticosterone levels in relation to migratory readiness in red-eyed vireos (*Vireo olivaceus*). *Behav Ecol Sociobiol* 54, 233–239.

Long, J. A., Holberton, R. L., 2004. Corticosterone secretion, energetic condition, and a test of the migration modulation hypothesis in the hermit thrush (*Catharus guttatus*), a short-distance migrant. *Auk* 121, 1094–1102.

Lucas, J. R., Freeberg, T. M., Egbert, J., Schwabl, H., 2006. Fecal corticosterone, body mass, and caching rates of Carolina chickadees (*Poecile carolinensis*) from disturbed and undisturbed sites. *Horm Behav* 49, 634–643.

Lynn, S. E., Breuner, C. W., Wingfield, J. C., 2003. Short-term fasting affects locomotor activity, corticosterone, and corticosterone binding globulin in a migratory songbird. *Horm Behav* 43, 150–157.

Mackie, R. I., Rycyk, M., Ruemmler, R. L., Aminov, R. I., Wikelski, M., 2004. Biochemical and microbiological evidence for fermentative digestion in free-living land iguanas (*Conolophus pallidus*) and marine iguanas (*Amblyrhynchus cristatus*) on the Galapagos archipelago. *Physiol Biochem Zool* 77, 127–138.

Manniste, M., Horak, P., 2011. Effects of immune activation and glucocorticoid administration on feather growth in greenfinches. *J Exper Zool A* 315A, 527–535.

Marra, P. P., Holberton, R. L., 1998. Corticosterone levels as indicators of habitat quality: effects of habitat segregation in a migratory bird during the non-breeding season. *Oecologia* 116, 284–292.

Marra, P. P., Sherry, T. W., Holmes, R. T., 1993. Territorial exclusion by a long-distance migrant warbler in Jamaica: A removal experiment with American redstarts (*Setophaga ruticilla*). *Auk* 110, 565–572.

McEwen, B. S., Wingfield, J. C., 2003. The concept of allostasis in biology and biomedicine. *Horm Behav* 43, 2–15.

McIlroy, P., Kocsis, J. F., Weber, H., Carsia, R., 1999. Dietary protein restriction stress in the domestic fowl (*Gallus gallus domesticus*) alters adrenocorticostropin-transmembranous signaling and corticosterone negative feedback in adrenal steroidogenic cells. *Gen Comp Endocrinol* 113, 255–266.

McQueen, S. M., Davis, L. S., Young, G., 1999. Sex steroid and corticosterone levels of Adelie penguins (*Pygoscelis adeliae*) during courtship and incubation. *Gen Comp Endocrinol* 114, 11–18.

McWilliams, S. R., Guglielmo, C., Pierce, B., Klaassen, M., 2004. Flying, fasting, and feeding in birds during migration: A nutritional and physiological ecology perspective. *J Avian Biol* 35, 377–393.

Mettke-Hofmann, C., Greenberg, R., 2005. Behavioral and cognitive adaptations to long-distance migration. In: Greenberg, R., Marra, P. P. (Eds.), *Birds of two worlds: The ecology and evolution of migration*. Johns Hopkins University Press, Baltimore, MD, pp. 114–123.

Mrosovsky, N., Sherry, D. F., 1980. Animal anorexias. *Science* 207, 837–842.

Muller, C., Jenni-Eiermann, S., Blondel, J., Perret, P., Caro, S. P., Lambrechts, M. M., Jenni, L., 2007. Circulating corticosterone levels in breeding blue tits Parus caeruleus differ between island and mainland populations and between habitats. *Gen Comp Endocrinol* 154, 128–136.

Murphy, M. E., 1996. Energetics and nutrition of molt. In: Carey, C. (Ed.), *Avian energetics and nutritional ecology*. Chapman and Hall, New York, pp. 158–198.

Murphy, M. E., King, J. R., 1992. Energy and nutrient use during moult by white-crowned sparrows *Zonotrichia leucophrys gambelii*. *Ornis Scan* 23, 304–313.

Murphy, M. T., Cornell, K. L., Murphy, K. L., 1998. Winter bird communities on San Salvador, Bahamas. *J Field Ornith* 69, 402–414.

Nasir, A., Moudgal, R. P., Singh, N.B., 1999. Involvement of corticosterone in food intake, food passage time and *in vivo* uptake of nutrients in the chicken (*Gallus domesticus*). *Brit Poultry Sci* 40, 517–522.

Navarro, J., Gonzalez-Solis, J., Viscor, G., Chastel, O., 2008. Ecophysiological response to an experimental increase of wing loading in a pelagic seabird. *J Exper Marine Biol Ecol* 358, 14–19.

Nemeth, Z., Moore, F. R., 2007. Unfamiliar stopover sites and the value of social information during migration. *J Ornithol* 148, S369–S376.

Nilsson, A. L. K., Sandell, M. I., 2009. Stress hormone dynamics: An adaptation to migration? *Biol Lett* 5, 480–483.

Nilsson, J. A., Svensson, E., 1996. The cost of reproduction: A new link between current reproductive effort and future reproductive success. *Proc R Soc Lond B* 263, 711–714.

Oberhuber, J. M., Roeckner, E., Christoph, M., Esch, M., Latif, M., 1998. Predicting the 97 el-nino event with a global climate model. *Geophys Res Let* 25, 2273–2276.

Ortiz, R. M., Houser, D. S., Wade, C. E., Ortiz, C. L., 2003. Hormonal changes associated with the transition between nursing and natural fasting in northern elephant seals (*Mirounga angustirostris*). *Gen Comp Endocrinol* 130, 78–83.

Ortiz, R. M., Wade, C. E., Ortiz, C. L., 2001. Effects of prolonged fasting on plasma cortisol and TH in postweaned northern elephant seal pups. *Am J Physiol* 280, R790-R795.

Owen, O. E., Caprio, S., Reichard, G. A., Jr., Boden, G., Owen, R. S., 1983. Ketosis of starvation: A revisit and new perspectives. *Clin Endocrinol Metab* 12, 359–379.

Perez-Rodriguez, L., Blas, J., Vinuela, J., Marchant, T. A., Bortolotti, G. R., 2006. Condition and androgen levels: are condition-dependent and testosterone-mediated traits two sides of the same coin? *Anim Behav* 72, 97–103.

Phillips, W. J., 1994. Starvation and survival: some military considerations. *Military Med* 159, 513–516.

Piersma, T., Gill, R. E., 1998. Guts don't fly: Small digestive organs in obese bar-tailed godwits. *Auk* 115, 196–203.

Piersma, T., Ramenofsky, M., 1998. Long-term decreases of corticosterone in captive migrant shorebirds that maintain seasonal mass and moult cycles. *J Avian Biol* 29, 97–104.

Piersma, T., Reneerkens, J., Ramenofsky, M., 2000. Baseline corticosterone peaks in shorebirds with maximal energy stores for migration: A general preparatory mechanism for rapid behavioral and metabolic transitions? *Gen Comp Endocrinol* 120, 118–126.

Porter, W. P., Sabo, J. L., Tracy, C. R., Reichman, O. J., Ramankutty, N., 2002. Physiology on a landscape scale: Plant-animal interactions. *Integ Comp Biol* 42, 431–453.

Pörtner, H. O., Farrell, A. P., 2008. Ecology: Physiology and climate change. *Science* 322, 690–692.

Portugal, S. J., Green, J. A., Butler, P. J., 2007. Annual changes in body mass and resting metabolism in captive barnacle geese (*Branta leucopsis*): The importance of wing moult. *J Exp Biol* 210, 1391–1397.

Pottinger, T. G., Rand-Weaver, M., Sumpter, J. P., 2003. Overwinter fasting and re-feeding in rainbow trout: plasma growth hormone and cortisol levels in relation to energy mobilisation. *Comp Biochem Physiol B* 136, 403–417.

Pravosudov, V. V., 2003. Long-term moderate elevation of corticosterone facilitates avian food-caching behaviour and enhances spatial memory. *Proc R Soc Lond B* 270, 2599–2604.

Pravosudov, V. V., 2005. Corticosterone and memory in birds. In: Dawson, A., Sharp, J. P. (Eds.), *Functional avian endocrinology*, Narosa Press, New Delhi, pp. 271–284.

Pravosudov, V. V., Kitaysky, A. S., Saldanha, C. J., Wingfield, J. C., Clayton, N. S., 2002. The effect of photoperiod on adrenocortical stress response in mountain chickadees (*Poecile gambeli*). *Gen Comp Endocrinol* 126, 242–248.

Pravosudov, V. V., Kitaysky, A. S., Wingfield, J. C., Clayton, N. S., 2001. Long-term unpredictable foraging conditions and physiological stress response in mountain chickadees (*Poecile gambeli*). *Gen Comp Endocrinol* 123, 324–331.

Pravosudov, V. V., Mendoza, S. P., Clayton, N. S., 2003. The relationship between dominance, corticosterone, memory, and food caching in mountain chickadees (*Poecile gambeli*). *Horm Behav* 44, 93–102.

Quillfeldt, P., Möstl, E., 2003. Resource allocation in Wilson's storm-petrels Oceanites oceanicus determined by measurement of glucocorticoid excretion. *Acta Ethol* 5, 115–122.

Ramenofsky, M., Gray, J. M., Johnson, R. B., 1992. Behavioral and physiological adjustments of birds living in winter flocks. *Ornis Scan* 23, 371–380.

Ramenofsky, M., Piersma, T., Jukema, J., 1995. Plasma corticosterone in bar-tailed godwits at a major stop-over site during spring migration. *Condor* 97, 580–585.

Ramenofsky, M., Savard, R., Greenwood, M. R. C., 1999. Seasonal and diel transitions in physiology and behavior in the migratory dark-eyed junco. *Comp Biochem Physiol A Mol Integr Physiol* 122, 385–397.

Ramenofsky, M., Wingfield, J. C., 2006. Behavioral and physiological conflicts in migrants: the transition between migration and breeding. *J Ornithol* 147, 135–145.

Ramenofsky, M., Wingfield, J. C., 2007. Regulation of migration. *Bioscience* 57, 135–143.

Remage-Healey, L., Romero, L. M., 2000. Daily and seasonal variation in response to stress in captive starlings (*Sturnus vulgaris*): Glucose. *Gen Comp Endocrinol* 119, 60–68.

Remage-Healey, L., Romero, L. M., 2001. Corticosterone and insulin interact to regulate glucose and triglyceride levels during stress in a bird. *Am J Physiol* 281, R994-R1003.

Remage-Healey, L., Romero, L. M., 2002. Corticosterone and insulin interact to regulate plasma glucose but not lipid concentrations in molting starlings. *Gen Comp Endocrinol* 129, 88–94.

Reneerkens, J., Morrison, R. I. G., Ramenofsky, M., Piersma, T., Wingfield, J. C., 2002. Baseline and stress-induced levels of corticosterone during different life cycle substages in a shorebird on the high arctic breeding grounds. *Physiol Biochem Zool* 75, 200–208.

Ricklefs, R. E., Wikelski, M., 2002. The physiology/life-history nexus. *Trends Ecol Evolu* 17, 462–468.

Robin, J. P., Boucontet, L., Chillet, P., Groscolas, R., 1998. Behavioral changes in fasting emperor penguins: Evidence for a "refeeding signal" linked to a metabolic shift. *Am J Physiol* 274, R746–R753.

Robin, J. P., Cherel, Y., Girard, H., Geloen, A., LeMaho, Y., 1987. Uric acid and urea in relation to protein catabolism in long-term fasting geese. *J Comp Physiol B* 157, 491–499.

Rodriguez, P., Tortosa, F. S., Villafuerte, R., 2005. The effects of fasting and refeeding on biochemical parameters in the red-legged partridge (*Alectoris rufa*). *Comp Biochem Physiol A* 140, 157–164.

Romero, L. M., 2001. Mechanisms underlying seasonal differences in the avian stress response. In: Dawson, A., Chaturvedi, C. M. (Eds.), *Avian endocrinology*. Narosa Publishing House, New Delhi, pp. 373–384.

Romero, L. M., 2002. Seasonal changes in plasma glucocorticoid concentrations in free-living vertebrates. *Gen Comp Endocrinol* 128, 1–24.

Romero, L. M., 2012. Using the reactive scope model to understand why stress physiology predicts survival during starvation in Galapagos marine iguanas. *Gen Comp Endocrinol* 176, 296–299.

Romero, L. M., Dickens, M. J., Cyr, N. E., 2009. The reactive scope model: A new model integrating homeostasis, allostasis, and stress. *Horm Behav* 55, 375–389.

Romero, L. M., Ramenofsky, M., Wingfield, J. C., 1997. Season and migration alters the corticosterone response to capture and handling in an arctic migrant, the white-crowned sparrow

(*Zonotrichia leucophrys gambelii*). *Comp Biochem Physiol* 116C, 171–177.

Romero, L. M., Strochlic, D., Wingfield, J. C., 2005. Corticosterone inhibits feather growth: potential mechanism explaining seasonal down regulation of corticosterone during molt. *Comp Biochem Physiol A Mol Integr Physiol* 142, 65–73.

Romero, L. M., Wikelski, M., 2001. Corticosterone levels predict survival probabilities of Galápagos marine iguanas during El Niño events. *Proc Natl Acad Sci USA* 98, 7366–7370.

Romero, L. M., Wikelski, M., 2010. Stress physiology as a predictor of survival in Galapagos marine iguanas. *Proc R Soc Lond B* 277, 3157–3162.

Ropelewski, C. F., Halpert, M. S., 1987. Global and regional scale precipitation patterns associated with the El Niño/Southern Oscillation. *Monthly Weather Rev* 115, 1606–1626.

Rosen, D. A. S., Kumagai, S., 2008. Hormone changes indicate that winter is a critical period for food shortages in Steller sea lions. *J Comp Physiol B* 178, 573–583.

Saldanha, C. J., Schlinger, B. A., Clayton, N. S., 2000. Rapid effects of corticosterone on cache recovery in mountain chickadees (*Parus gambeli*). *Horm Behav* 37, 109–115.

Salvante, K. G., Williams, T. D., 2003. Effects of corticosterone on the proportion of breeding females, reproductive output and yolk precursor levels. *Gen Comp Endocrinol* 130, 205–214.

Sapolsky, R. M., Romero, L. M., Munck, A. U., 2000. How do glucocorticoids influence stress-responses? Integrating permissive, suppressive, stimulatory, and preparative actions. *Endocr Rev* 21, 55–89.

Savory, C. J., Mann, J. S., 1997. Is there a role for corticosterone in expression of abnormal behaviour in restricted-fed fowls? *Physiol Behav* 62, 7–13.

Schaub, M., Jenni, L., Bairlein, F., 2008. Fuel stores, fuel accumulation, and the decision to depart from a migration stopover site. *Behav Ecol* 19, 657–666.

Schmaljohann, H., Dierschke, V., 2005. Optimal bird migration and predation risk: A field experiment with northern wheatears Oenanthe oenanthe. *J Anim Ecol* 74, 131–138.

Schoech, S. J., Bowman, R., Bridge, E. S., Morgan, G. M., Rensel, M. A., Wilcoxen, T. E., Boughton, R. K., 2007. Corticosterone administration does not affect timing of breeding in Florida scrub-jays (*Aphelocoma coerulescens*). *Horm Behav* 52, 191–196.

Schwabl, H., Bairlein, F., Gwinner, E., 1991. Basal and stress-induced corticosterone levels of garden warblers Sylvia-borin during migration. *J Compar Physiol* 161B, 576–580.

Schwilch, R., Grattarola, A., Spina, F., Jenni, L., 2002. Protein loss during long-distance migratory flight in passerine birds: adaptation and constraint. *J Exp Biol* 205, 687–695.

Seraphin, S. B., Whitten, P. L., Reynolds, V., 2006. The interaction of hormones with ecological factors in male Budongo forest chimpanzees. In: Newton-Fisher, N. E., Notman, H., Paterson, J. D., Reynolds, V. (Eds.), *Primates of Western Uganda*. Springer, New York, pp. 93–104.

Sernia, C., McDonald, I. R., 1977. Metabolic effects of cortisol, corticosterone and adrenocorticotropin in a prototherian mammal *Tachyglossus aculeatus* (Shaw). *J Endocrinol* 75, 261–269.

Serra, L., 2001. Duration of primary moult affects primary quality in grey plovers *Pluvialis squatarola*. *J Avian Biol* 32, 377–380.

Shultz, M. T., Kitaysky, A. S., 2008. Spatial and temporal dynamics of corticosterone and corticosterone binding globulin are driven by environmental heterogeneity. *Gen Comp Endocrinol* 155, 717–728.

Silverin, B., 1986. Corticosterone-binding proteins and behavioral effects of high plasma levels of corticosterone during the breeding period in the pied flycatcher. *Gen Comp Endocrinol* 64, 67–74.

Silverin, B., 1998. Territorial behavioural and hormones of pied flycatchers in optimal and suboptimal habitats. *Anim Behav* 56, 811.

Silverin, B., Wingfield, J. C., 2010. Wintering strategies. In: Breed, M., Moore, J. (Eds.), *Encyclopedia of animal behavior*, Elsevier Press, London, pp. 597–605.

Slagsvold, T., Dale, S., 1996. Disappearance of female pied flycatchers in relation to breeding stage and experimentally induced molt. *Ecology* 77, 461–471.

Sprague, R. S., 2009. *Glucocorticoid physiology and behavior during life history transitions in Laysan albatross* (Phoebastria immutabilis). Ph.D. Thesis, University of Montana, Missoula, p. 89

Stewart, W. K., Fleming, L. W., 1973. Features of a successful therapeutic fast of 382 days duration. *Postgraduate Med J* 49, 203–209.

Stokkan, K. A., 1992. Energetics and adaptations to cold in ptarmigan in winter. *Ornis Scan* 23, 366–370.

Stokkan, K. A., Sharp, P. J., Unander, S., 1986. The annual breeding cycle of the high-arctic Svalbard ptarmigan (*Lagopus mutus hyperboreus*). *Gen Comp Endocrinol* 61, 446–451.

Strochlic, D. E., Romero, L. M., 2008. The effects of chronic psychological and physical stress on feather replacement in European starlings (*Sturnus vulgaris*). *Comp Biochem Physiol A Mol Integr Physiol* 149, 68–79.

Suorsa, P., Huhta, E., Nikula, A., Nikinmaa, M., Jäntti, A., Helle, H., Hakkarainen, H., 2003. Forest management is associated with physiological stress in an old-growth forest passerine. *Proc R Soc Lond B* 270, 963–969.

Swaddle, J. P., Williams, E. V., Rayner, J. M. V., 1999. The effect of simulated flight feather moult on escape take-off performance in starlings. *J Avian Biol* 30, 351–358.

Swaddle, J. P., Witter, M. S., 1997. The effects of molt on the flight performance, body mass, and behavior of European starlings (*Sturnus vulgaris*): An experimental approach. *Can J Zool* 75, 1135–1146.

Sweazea, K. L., Braun, E. J., 2006. Oleic acid uptake by in vitro English sparrow skeletal muscle. *J Exp Zool A Comp Exp Biol* 305A, 268–276.

Takaki, Y., Eguchi, K., Nagata, H., 2001. The growth bars on tail feathers in the male Styan's grasshopper warbler may indicate quality. *J Avian Biol* 32, 319–325.

Tarlow, E. M., Hau, M., Anderson, D. J., Wikelski, M., 2003. Diel changes in plasma melatonin and corticosterone concentrations in tropical Nazca boobies (*Sula granti*) in relation to moon phase and age. *Gen Comp Endocrinol* 133, 297–304.

Thurston, R. J., Bryant, C. C., Korn, N., 1993. The effects of corticosterone and catecholamine infusion on plasma glucose levels in chicken (Gallus domesticus) and turkey (*Melagris gallapavo*) *Comp Biochem Physiol C* 106, 59–62.

Totzke, U., Hubinger, A., Korthaus, G., Bairlein, F., 1999. Fasting increases the plasma glucagon response in the migratory garden warbler (*Sylvia borin*). *Gen Comp Endocrinol* 115, 116–121.

Trenberth, K. E., 1997. The definition of El Nino. *Bull Am Meteorol Soc* 78, 2771–2777.

Trenzado, C. E., Carrick, T. R., Pottinger, T. G., 2003. Divergence of endocrine and metabolic responses to stress in two rainbow trout lines selected for differing cortisol responsiveness to stress. *Gen Comp Endocrinol* 133, 332–340.

Tucker, V. A., 1991. The effect of molting on the gliding performance of a Harris hawk (*Parabuteo unicinctus*). *Auk* 108, 108–113.

Vijayan, M. M., Maule, A. G., Schreck, C. B., Moon, T. W., 1993. Hormonal control of hepatic glycogen metabolism in food-deprived continuously swimming coho salmon (*Oncorhynchus kisutch*). *Can J Fish Aquat Sci* 50, 1676–1682.

Vijayan, M. M., Moon, T. W., 1994. The stress response and the plasma disappearance of corticosteroid and glucose in a marine teleost, the sea raven. *Can J Zool* 72, 379–386.

Vijayan, M. M., Reddy, P. K., Leatherland, J. F., Moon, T. W., 1994. The effects of cortisol on hepatocyte metabolism in rainbow trout: mA study using the steroid analog RU486. *Gen Comp Endocrinol* 96, 75–84.

Vleck, C. M., Vleck, D., 2002. Physiological condition and reproductive consequences in Adelie penguins. *Integ Comp Biol* 42, 76–83.

Walker, B. G., Wingfield, J. C., Boersma, P. D., 2005. Age and food deprivation affects expression of the glucocorticosteroid stress response in Magellanic penguin (Spheniscus magellanicus) chicks. *Physiol Biochem Zool* 78, 78–89.

Warham, J., 1996. *The behavior, population biology and physiology of the petrels.* Academic Press, New York.

Waye, H. L., Mason, R. T., 2008. A combination of body condition measurements is more informative than conventional condition indices: Temporal variation in body condition and corticosterone in brown tree snakes (*Boiga irregularis*). *Gen Comp Endocrinol* 155, 607–612.

Wikelski, M., Carrillo, V., Trillmich, F., 1997. Energy limits to body size in a grazing reptile, the Galapagos marine iguana. *Ecology* 78, 2204–2217.

Wikelski, M., Trillmich, F., 1994. Foraging strategies of the Galapagos marine iguana (*Amblyrhynchus cristatus*): Adapting behavioral rules to ontogenetic size change. *Behaviour* 128, 255–279.

Wikelski, M., Trillmich, F., 1997. Body size and sexual size dimorphism in marine iguanas fluctuate as a result of opposing natural and sexual selection: An island comparison. *Evolution* 51, 922–936.

Williams, C. T., Kitaysky, A. S., Kettle, A. B., Buck, C. L., 2008. Corticosterone levels of tufted puffins vary with breeding stage, body condition index, and reproductive performance. *Gen Comp Endocrinol* 158, 29–35.

Williams, E. V., Swaddle, J. P., 2003. Moult, flight performance and wingbeat kinematics during take-off in European starlings *Sturnus vulgaris. J Avian Biol* 34, 371–378.

Wilson, B. S., 1990. *Latitudinal variation in the ecology of a lizard: Seasonal differences in mortality and physiology.* Ph.D. Thesis, University of Washington, Seattle,

Wilson, B. S., Wingfield, J. C., 1992. Correlation between female reproductive condition and plasma-corticosterone in the lizard Uta-Stansburiana. *Copeia* 1992, 691–697.

Wilson, S., Norris, D. R., Wilson, A. G., Arcese, P., 2007. Breeding experience and population density affect the ability of a songbird to respond to future climate variation. *Proc R Soc Lond B* 274, 2539–2545.

Wingfield, J. C., 2003. Control of behavioural strategies for capricious environments. *Anim Behav* 66, 807–815.

Wingfield, J. C., 2013a. The comparative biology of environmental stress: Behavioural endocrinology and variation in ability to cope with novel, changing environments. *Anim Behav* 85, 1127–1133.

Wingfield, J. C., 2013b. Ecological processes and the ecology of stress: The impacts of abiotic environmental factors. *Func Ecol* 27, 37–44.

Wingfield, J. C., Hunt, K., Breuner, C., Dunlap, K., Fowler, G. S., Freed, L., Lepson, J., 1997. Environmental stress, field endocrinology, and conservation biology. In: Clemmons, J. R., Buchholz, R. (Eds.), *Behavioral approaches to conservation in the wild*. Cambridge University Press, Cambridge, UK, pp. 95–131.

Wingfield, J. C., Kelley, J. P., Angelier, F., 2011. What are extreme environmental conditions and how do organisms cope with them? *Curr Zool* 57, 363–374.

Wingfield, J. C., Owen-Ashley, N., Benowitz-Fredericks, Z. M., Lynn, S., Hahn, T. P., Wada, H., Breuner, C., Meddle, S., Romero, L. M., 2004. Arctic spring: The arrival biology of migrant birds. *Acta Zool Sinica* 50, 948–960.

Wingfield, J. C., Ramos-Fernandez, G., Nunez-de la Mora, A., Drummond, H., 1999. The effects of an "El Nino" southern oscillation event on reproduction in male and female blue-footed boobies, *Sula nebouxii*. *Gen Comp Endocrinol* 114, 163–172.

Wingfield, J. C., Sapolsky, R. M., 2003. Reproduction and resistance to stress: When and how. *J Neuroendocrinol* 15, 711.

Wingfield, J. C., Silverin, B., 1986. Effects of corticosterone on territorial behavior of free-living male song sparrows *Melospiza melodia*. *Horm Behav* 20, 405–417.

Witter, M. S., Cuthill, I. C., 1993. The ecological costs of avian fat storage. *Phil Trans R Soc London B* 340, 73–92.

Witter, M. S., Lee, S. J., 1995. Habitat structure, stress and plumage development. *Proc R Soc Lond B* 261, 303–308.

Yamada, F., Inoue, S., Saitoh, T., Tanaka, K., Satoh, S., Takamura, Y., 1993. Glucoregulatory hormones in the immmobilization stress-induced increase of plasma glucose in fasted and fed rats. *Endocrinology* 132, 2199–2205.

8

Responses to Natural Perturbations

Tempests—Weather and Climate Events

I've lived in a good climate, and it bores the hell out of me.
I like weather rather than climate.

JOHN STEINBECK, *Travels with Charlie (1962)*

I. INTRODUCTION

Perhaps the most ubiquitous labile perturbation factors are related to weather events. They can be very brief (e.g., thunderstorms and tornadoes), more prolonged (e.g., hurricanes, cold snaps, and heat waves), or very long term (e.g., El Niño Southern Oscillation events [ENSO] and the alternate condition, La Niña, which can last for weeks to months). It is highly likely that all organisms must cope with a weather event at some time in their life cycles. In this chapter we will review the various weather scenarios and behavioral responses that vertebrates show, and then go on to summarize hormonal responses that regulate coping strategies for weather (emergency life-history stage). Although behavioral responses to weather are diverse, the mediators of the coping mechanisms within the emergency life-history stage may be much more conserved (Wingfield and Ramenofsky 2011).

There are numerous accounts of the catastrophic effects of weather throughout history. In one example, Gilbert White, an eighteenth-century naturalist living in Selbourne, southern England, documents one particularly severe weather event (White 1860). He writes that in 1771 a Dr. Johnson wrote to him describing a spring season that was so severe in the Island of Skye, Scotland, that it is remembered by the name of "black spring." To quote "the snow, which seldom lies at all, covered the ground for eight weeks; many cattle died, and those that survived were extremely emaciate." White goes on to describe the local weather in the south; "never were so many barren cows known as in the spring following that dreadful period. Whole dairies missed being in calf together. At the end of March, the face of the earth was naked to a surprising degree: wheat hardly to be seen, and no signs of any grass; turnips all gone, and sheep in a starving way; all provisions rising in price. Farmers cannot sow for want of rain" (White 1860). Such extreme events are probably rare at any one locality, but weather events of lesser magnitude that nonetheless can potentially disrupt the predictable life cycle are much more frequent (Elkins 1983; Wingfield and Ramenofsky 2011). Furthermore, there is growing evidence that one of the corollaries of global climate change is that the frequency, duration and intensity of severe weather events is increasing worldwide (e.g., Meehl 2000; Meehl et al. 2000; Munich Rev 2002; Wingfield et al. 2011). Implications for sustainability across a broad front are profound (Parmesan et al. 2000; Rosenzweig et al. 2001), with predictions of accompanying increases in mortality (Deschenes and Moretti 2009).

Migrant birds may be particularly vulnerable to weather events because they arrive on their breeding grounds in spring as early as possible to claim the best territories and begin breeding as soon as conditions allow. However, spring migration and arrival are influenced strongly by weather (see section F), with weather at arrival most critical because weather en route usually has no relevance to that on the breeding grounds (Newton 1973). In non-migrants, winter weather may have a great impact on survival, especially if it is unusually severe with prolonged periods of sub-freezing temperatures, heavy snow, and so forth. Generally, if birds are able to access their food supply, then survival will be higher despite severe conditions (Perrins 1979). Nonetheless, spring weather can be particularly devastating because late snowfall may result in total loss of broods of young. Cool weather and heavy rains during the nestling and post-fledging periods may result in chick mortality because caterpillars are less active and harder to find (Perrins 1979). Conversely, hotter weather can result in more rapid growth of caterpillars and earlier pupation, leading also to reduced food after fledging and consequent chick mortality. If these effects of weather are linked with changes in other perturbations, such as the number of predators, then survival can be affected even more.

Given the general effects of weather summarized briefly in the preceding paragraph, it is clear that these perturbations lend themselves to allostatic load modeling and reactive scope (Chapter 3). It is also important to point out that there are probably two distinct processes that animals must cope with—weather versus climate—as suggested by the quote from Steinbeck at the start of this chapter. Weather reflects the day-to-day conditions, complete with predicted and unpredicted events of local and regional atmospheric conditions. Climate, on the other hand, represents the averages of local weather conditions for each day, collected over many years (Kruckeberg 1991). In Seattle, Washington, for example, summers are referred to as cool, but some days in July and August can be extremely hot (in excess of 35°C). Likewise, winters are referred to as mild and wet, but every few years deep snow and temperatures well below freezing occur for prolonged periods of weeks. To quote Kruckeberg (1991), "weather is for day-to-day living, climate is for charts, textbooks and patient observers."

Wind extremes can be devastating, knocking down trees over large areas and even changing local ecological conditions and communities of organisms. Such weather events can have profound consequences as a result. Quoting Kruckeberg (1991) again, "the so-called Law of the mean is important for accounting for the perpetuation of long-term trends. But the law of the extreme often marks the end of a trend and initiation of a new one." He notes also that micro-climates deviate dramatically from "weather station" data and are essential for plants and animals to persist during periods of weather and other extremes (Kruckeberg 1991). These factors must be considered very carefully to fully understand why some animals are able to cope with a capricious environment and others cannot. Individual differences in seemingly identical conditions (e.g., Williams 2008) may then be explained.

Investigating the effects of inclement weather on animals in their natural habitat is difficult because these perturbations are by nature unpredictable, at least in the long term. For these reasons, any field study on the effects of weather has to be opportunistic and requires fieldwork under trying conditions. Once the weather turns bad, the logical tendency is to find shelter and abandon the field research being conducted until the perturbation passes. However, a few resolute biologists have withstood the urge to go indoors as inclement weather threatens. They discovered a novel suite of behavioral and physiological traits by which organisms cope with weather (Gessaman and Worthen 1982; Elkins 1983; Wingfield and Ramenofsky 1999; Wingfield and Romero 2001; Wingfield and Ramenofsky 2011). These coping mechanisms, across all vertebrate taxa, provide the flexibility to deal with increasingly capricious environments in which global climate change and human disturbance in general provide additional challenges (e.g., Travis 2003). It is important to bear in mind that although organisms prepare for predictable changes of climate (e.g., seasons), they must also be able to respond in a facultative way to unpredictable weather conditions, often on short notice (Wingfield and Jacobs 1999; Jacobs and Wingfield 2000; Wingfield 2008).

II. BEHAVIORAL AND GLUCOCORTICOID RESPONSES TO WEATHER AND CLIMATE EVENTS

The frameworks provided by the concepts of allostasis, reactive scope, and physiological state levels (Chapter 3) allow interpretation of the effects of rising intensity of storms or other climatic events (e.g., drought, floods, heat, etc.) to increase allostatic load. An increase of Eo (energy required to obtain food under trying conditions), often simultaneously with decreasing Eg (food available in the environment), can result in allostatic overload type 1. If Eo is integrated with other contributors to allostatic load, such as reproductive effort, then an increase of Eo precipitated by weather can result in breeding failure, followed by elevated secretion of the mediators of allostasis. Over the past 30 years, field investigations have collected data on weather events indicating that common underlying themes are present across vertebrates, with implications for understanding the responses of individuals and populations to global change in general.

A. Weather and the Breeding Season

Breeding seasons of vertebrates in general incur considerable energetic costs that make them particularly vulnerable to inclement weather events. For example, for one Arctic-breeding seabird, the thick-billed murre, even though ice conditions at breeding sites vary tremendously from year to year, the birds initiate egg laying within a narrow time span (Gaston and Nettleship 1981; Gaston et al. 2005). The researchers note that internal rhythms/photoperiod regulate gonadal development, but initiation of egg development leading to laying is dependent upon local factors. These local weather factors will affect egg size. In addition, both wind speed and sea conditions affect the feeding success of marine birds that catch fish and thus how much they feed their young. In general, these authors found no correlation of chick feeding rate and wind in thick-billed murres until wind speeds exceeded 50 kilometers per hour. Only under extreme wind conditions was there a deleterious effect on chick feeding rates (Gaston et al. 2005). In some years, unusual heat results in a greater populations of mosquitoes, and the combination of high temperature and loss of blood from mosquitoes results in failure of incubation and higher mortality (Gaston et al. 2002). It is possible that ongoing climate change in the Arctic could result in more frequent heat and insect events such as this.

Inclement weather also affected hunting success in breeding American kestrels, which resulted in kestrel nestlings that were smaller and lighter at fledging than those raised during good weather (Dawson and Bortolotti 2000). High rainfall and lower environmental temperature were correlated with similar trends in breeding black kites (Hiraldo et al. 1990) by significantly decreasing the frequency of prey capture attempts and thus less food for nestlings (Sergio 2003). Conversely, higher temperatures increased foraging success in black kites. A negative relationship between weather over the year and body condition of female black kites prior to laying could have been mediated through the ability of males to hunt successfully and provision their mates (Sergio 2003). Cold wet weather from February to April reduced the numbers of breeding European sparrow hawks (Newton and Marquiss 1986). When the weather was warm and dry during the same period, egg laying occurred earlier, clutch sizes were larger, and breeding success greater than in cold and wet conditions (Newton and Marquiss 1986).

In addition to affecting time of breeding and numbers of eggs, weather can have behavioral effects that can have an enormous impact on reproductive success. Brooding time of chicks by females in a Scottish population of hen harriers was longer in cold weather. Provisioning rates of male harriers were negatively related to temperature and rainfall, and lower provisioning rates were accompanied by greater chick mortality rates (Redpath et al. 2002). The opposite effect was observed in a Spanish population of harriers: fledging rates were negatively related to summer high temperatures (Redpath et al. 2002), suggesting that effects of temperature, and precipitation, on breeding success may be evident at different latitudes, but the mechanisms involved may be opposite depending upon location and weather extremes. Many other examples of how inclement weather may reduce reproductive success and even disrupt breeding have been reviewed by Wingfield and Ramenofsky (2011).

Behavioral responses to weather can have an important role in resilience to climate change (Sergio 2003). Breeding seasons of many vertebrate species in mid-latitudes are occurring earlier, probably as a result of global warming effects (e.g., Saether et al. 2000). The physiological responses to weather, particularly hormonal, can mediate many of the behavioral responses described in Chapters 3 through 5. It is important now to give examples from investigations of free-living vertebrates that show changes in physiological mediators of stress in response to labile perturbation factors.

Allostatic load is expected to rise steadily as breeding progresses and particularly when feeding young (Figure 8.1). These costs are represented by the line Ey, the added energy required to produce young and raise them to independence, above those of Ee and Ei combined. In many ways Ey has parallels to Eo, but Ey is always part of the predictable life cycle. We can assume that the cost of Ey must remain below Eg, but as Ey increases, then vulnerability to storms and other labile perturbation factors (Eo) becomes greater, with the potential for allostatic overload type 1 (Figure 8.1 upper panel). The outcome is similar if a decrease in Eg is modeled (Figure 8.1 lower panel; see also Wingfield 2004). The reactive scope model (Chapter 3) would predict rising levels of the mediators of allostasis, leading to homeostatic overload and high levels of glucocorticoids.

In male white-crowned sparrows, baseline corticosterone levels increase during nesting and decline thereafter as predicted from Figure 8.1 (Wingfield et al. 1983; Wingfield and Ramenofsky 2011). A severe and prolonged storm in May 1980 forced breeding pairs to abandon their nests and territories despite the presence of nestlings. Circulating levels of corticosterone were greatly elevated during the storm compared to those of males sampled in a year with no storm (Wingfield and Farner 1978; Wingfield et al. 1983; Figure 8.2). When the period of severe storms had abated and birds were re-nesting, plasma levels of corticosterone were normal for that time of year (Figure 8.2). Subcutaneous fat stores were virtually depleted during the storm, but returned to normal afterward when re-nesting. Note that male white-crowned sparrows had normal levels of luteinizing hormone and testosterone during the storm (Figure 8.3). These data suggest that high levels of corticosterone accompanying homeostatic overload act directly to suppress expression of reproductive behavior, rather than indirectly through decreased secretion of sex steroids.

Subsequent investigations of inclement weather disrupting breeding seasons have not always been consistent with the predictions noted earlier (Wingfield 1984). The allostasis/reactive scope concepts provide frameworks to understand this (Figure 8.1). The additional energy needed to incubate eggs and feed young to fledging and independence will rise steadily. Fledging should occur while Eg is still sufficient to fuel increasing allostatic load (Figure 8.1, top panel).

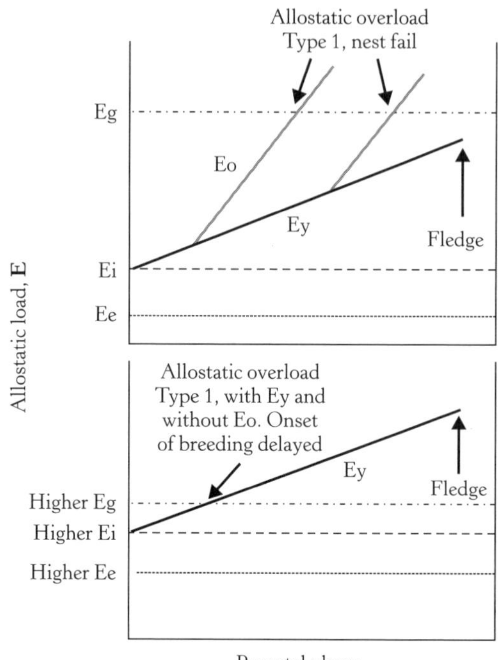

FIGURE 8.1: Ey, the extra energy and nutrients required to incubate eggs, then raise young to fledging and independence, increases steadily as the season progresses. Fledging occurs while Eg is still sufficient to fuel increasing allostatic load (top panel). A further perturbation, Eo, will increase allostatic load even faster (grey lines), and when it exceeds Eg (allostatic overload type 1) the nest and young will be abandoned. However, a perturbation would take longer to reach allostatic overload early in the parental phase (left-hand Eo) than an identical perturbation later (right-hand Eo). Timing of the parental phase is thus critical to ensure that Eg is sufficient to permit the growth and fledging of offspring. Storms during the parental phase can be particularly disruptive to breeding because Eo increases may exceed Eg quickly. Conditions early in the breeding season are usually more severe than later in spring and summer (such as lower Eg in early spring and higher Ee + Ei as a result of lower temperature and more energy needed to forage). Then Ey, the extra energy and nutrients required to raise young to fledging, will increase allostatic load immediately even without further Eo (lower panel). In this scenario, delayed onset of breeding (until Eg increases and Ee + Ei decrease) will occur but not necessarily because of allostatic overload type 1, but because local conditions are not conducive to the onset of breeding. On the other hand, if breeding does commence, then these individuals would be more susceptible to storms early in the season. Thus corticosteroids may or may not be involved at this time.

From Wingfield and Ramenofsky (2011), courtesy of Elsevier Press.

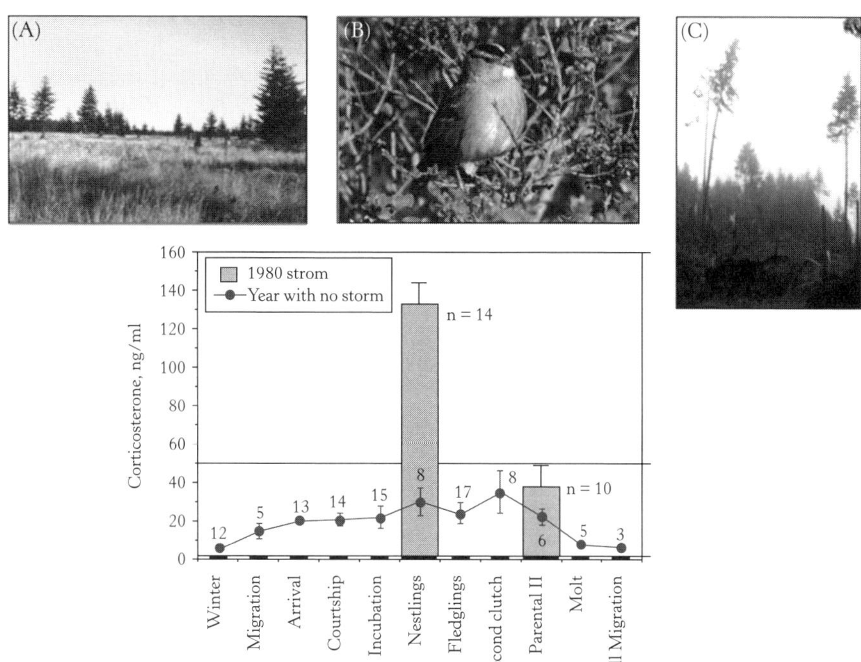

FIGURE 8.2: The Puget Sound sub-species of white-crowned sparrow (B) nests on or near the ground in open areas near forest edge (A). In May 1980 there were periods of inclement weather resulting in blow-downs of trees (C) near breeding habitat. Breeding sparrows abandoned breeding territories and even formed small flocks during this period. Corticosterone levels in free-living birds were greatly elevated over those in birds captured in 1979 when there were no severe storms (bar and line graph). Note that during the second parental phase (after the storms had passed), plasma levels of corticosterone had decreased and were identical to those at the same time in 1979.

From Wingfield et al. (1983), courtesy of Allen Press, the American Ornithologists' Union and Wingfield and Ramenofsky (2011), courtesy of Elsevier Press.

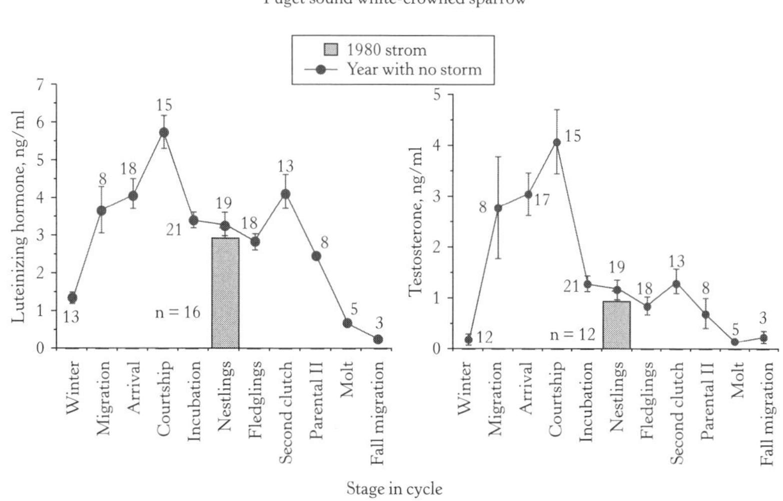

FIGURE 8.3: Plasma levels of luteinizing hormone (LH) and testosterone show typical cycles during the breeding season for socially monogamous birds such as the Puget Sound white-crowned sparrow (black lines). LH levels tend to peak at each sexual phase for each brood and are lower during the parental phases. Testosterone levels peak early in the season when establishing territories and remain lower thereafter. During the severe storms of 1980 (see Figure 8.5), plasma levels of LH and testosterone were identical to those of 1979 (no severe storms).

From Wingfield and Farner (1978); Wingfield et al. (1983), courtesy of Allen Press and the American Ornithologists' Union.

A labile perturbation factor will elevate Eo (grey lines), and when it exceeds Eg the individual is in allostatic overload type 1. As mediators of allostasis increase further, the nest and young will be abandoned. However, looking at Figure 8.1, rising Eo resulting from a perturbation would take longer to reach allostatic overload early in the parental phase (left-hand Eo in Figure 8.1) than an identical perturbation later in the breeding season (right hand Eo, Figure 8.1). Clearly, the timing of a perturbation during the parental phase is critical. Inclement weather later in the parental phase can be particularly disruptive to breeding because Eo will exceed Eg more rapidly. Conversely, early in the breeding season, environmental conditions are more severe, including lower Eg and greater Ee + Ei as a result of, for example, lower temperature and more energy needed to forage. Because Ey would elevate allostatic load immediately, even without further Eo (lower panel of Figure 8.1), then delayed onset of breeding will occur until Eg increases and Ee + Ei decrease, but not necessarily because of allostatic overload type 1. Rather, local conditions are not conducive to onset of breeding, egg-laying is delayed, and we can predict that glucocorticoids may not be involved. On the other hand, if breeding is initiated early, then individuals would be more susceptible to storms early in the season because Eo would rise quickly and Eg is still low. In this scenario Ey is already close to Eg, and any perturbation that adds Eo would result in allostatic overload type 1, elevating glucocorticoids and interrupting the nesting attempt (Wingfield and Ramenofsky 2011). The following field examples of storms and reproduction provide some support for these hypotheses.

Responses of free-living song sparrows to severe storms before and after onset of breeding are consistent with the scenarios suggested in Figure 8.1. A late snowstorm (200–300 mm) on April 6, 1982, in the Dutchess County region of New York State was followed by freezing temperatures for six days. In 1981 temperatures were above freezing throughout this period. In early April, gonadal recrudescence is occurring (Figure 8.4), but in 1982, song sparrows sampled during and after the snowstorm had significantly lower plasma levels of LH and testosterone in males and females compared with the same time in 1981 when there was no storm (Figure 8.4; Wingfield 1985a; Wingfield 1985b). Ovarian follicle diameter was smaller during the storm in 1982 (Fig. 8.4), consistent with the prediction that gonadal development should be slower in severe weather. However, there were no differences in plasma corticosterone levels between April 1981 and 1982, and subcutaneous fat score and body weight were inconsistent (Figure 8.5; Wingfield 1985a; Wingfield 1985b). These observations match the predictions of Figure 8.1. A storm early in the breeding season may result in phenological conditions that regulate reproductive development and onset of breeding, but the increased allostatic load from the storm this early in the breeding season was not sufficient to induce overload type 1 (Figure 8.1). Laboratory experiments show that low temperature decreased the rate of photoperiodically induced gonadal development, whereas high temperatures increased recrudescence (e.g., Wingfield et al. 1997; Perfito et al. 2006; Silverin et al. 2009). Moreover, plasma corticosterone levels were not affected as long as food availability remained sufficient (Wingfield et al. 1997).

According to Figure 8.1, inclement weather late in the breeding season, when parental and allostatic load is already high, may be potentially disruptive, as illustrated in white-crowned sparrows by Wingfield et al. (Figure 8.2; Wingfield et al. 1983). Eastern song sparrows in Dutchess County, New York State, endured periods of heavy rain for 10 days in May and June 1982 that resulted in severe flooding compared with 1981. Environmental temperatures were similar between years (Wingfield 1985a; Wingfield 1985b; Wingfield and Ramenofsky 2011). Song sparrows abandoned nests and moved to higher ground during the floods then returned to their territories later in June when the rain eased and the floods receded. Re-nesting followed soon after return (Wingfield 1985b; Wingfield 1985a). Similar to Figure 8.3, there were no differences in plasma levels of reproductive hormones in either male or female song sparrows in 1981 and during the inclement weather in 1982 (Figure 8.6). In 1982, males had higher circulating corticosterone levels during the rainy period than during the same time in 1981 (Figure 8.7). This is consistent with the predictions from Figure 8.1. Storms may be more disruptive to breeding during the parental phase when Ey is increasing rapidly, so that an additional perturbation Eo adds to Ey, resulting in allostatic overload type 1. On the other hand, females showed no increase in plasma corticosterone concentrations during the storm period of 1982. Gender differences in baseline plasma levels of glucocorticoids, as well as stressed levels (measured after 30–60 mins of capture, handling, and restraint stress; see Chapters 3 and 6), are widespread in the literature and may represent sexual differences in parental investment (e.g., Wingfield et al. 1995; Bókony et al. 2009).

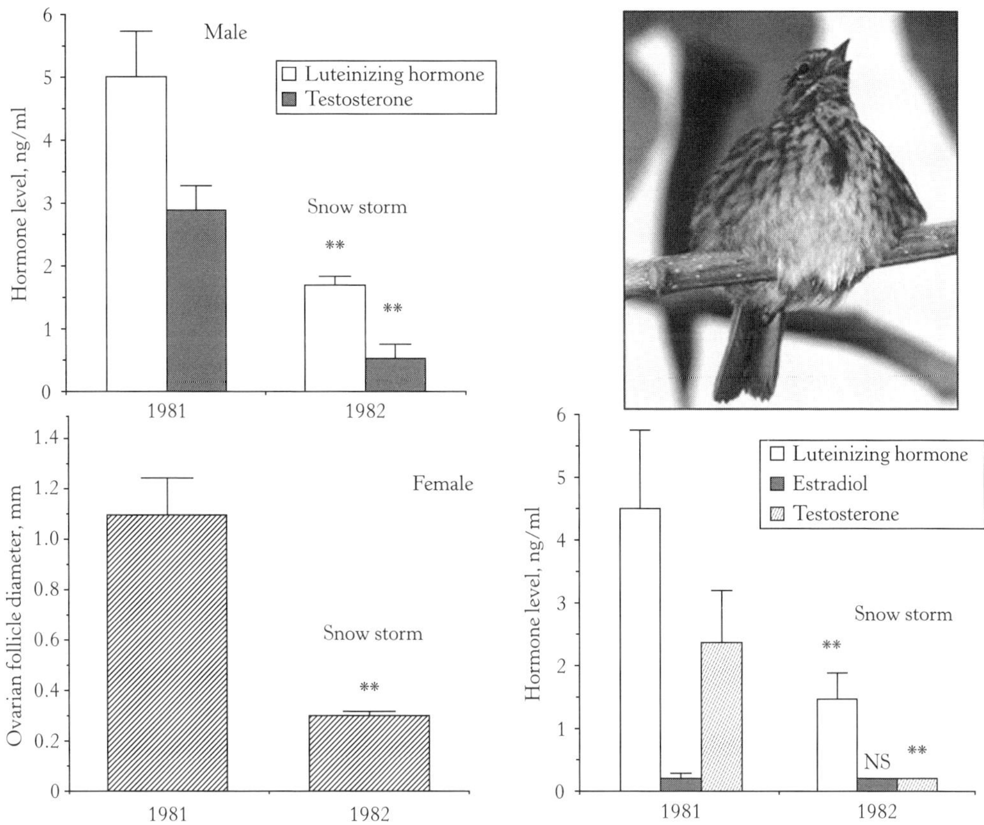

FIGURE 8.4: Effects of a spring snowstorm in 1982 on gonadal development and plasma levels of luteinizing hormone (LH), testosterone, and estradiol in male and female song sparrows. Comparisons are made with the same time in 1981 when weather was much warmer with no snow cover. In males both LH and testosterone levels were significantly lower during the snowstorm in 1982 compared to males in 1981. Similarly in females, plasma levels of LH and testosterone, but not estradiol, were also lower during the snowstorm in 1982 compared with 1981. Furthermore, the diameter of ovarian follicles were significantly less in 1982.

From Wingfield (1985a, 1985b). Courtesy of Wiley. Photo by J. C. Wingfield.

Effects of weather on adrenocortical function are now well known. Table 8.1 summarizes baseline and stressed plasma levels of corticosterone (from capture, handling and restraint) in Arctic birds sampled at Barrow, Alaska, on the Arctic Ocean coast during the later part of the breeding season and in relation to inclement weather. In these cases there were no gender differences (unlike early in the season) and no correlations with weather, including temperature and precipitation (Romero et al. 2000). As an adaptation to breeding in severe environments, it is possible that these birds have become resistant to inclement weather because the nesting season is so short at high latitudes. A delay in onset of nesting and slowed parental care are not options. The more significant effects of inclement weather on baseline and stressed plasma corticosterone levels that occur in Arctic birds during the post-breeding molt, a different life-history stage that follows the breeding season, are consistent with this hypothesis (Table 8.1; Romero et al. 2000).

The allostasis/reactive scope models allow us to make predictions about when inclement weather can delay onset of breeding or disrupt reproductive function (Figure 8.1). However, potential mechanisms are probably complex, and much more field investigation is needed on free-living populations in ecological contexts. Song sparrows in western Washington State breed in low, coastal habitats as well as at high elevations in the Cascade Mountains. Cool spring weather at higher elevation sites in May 1988 was accompanied by elevated corticosterone levels versus sparrows sampled at the same time at lower elevation sites (Figure 8.8; Wingfield and

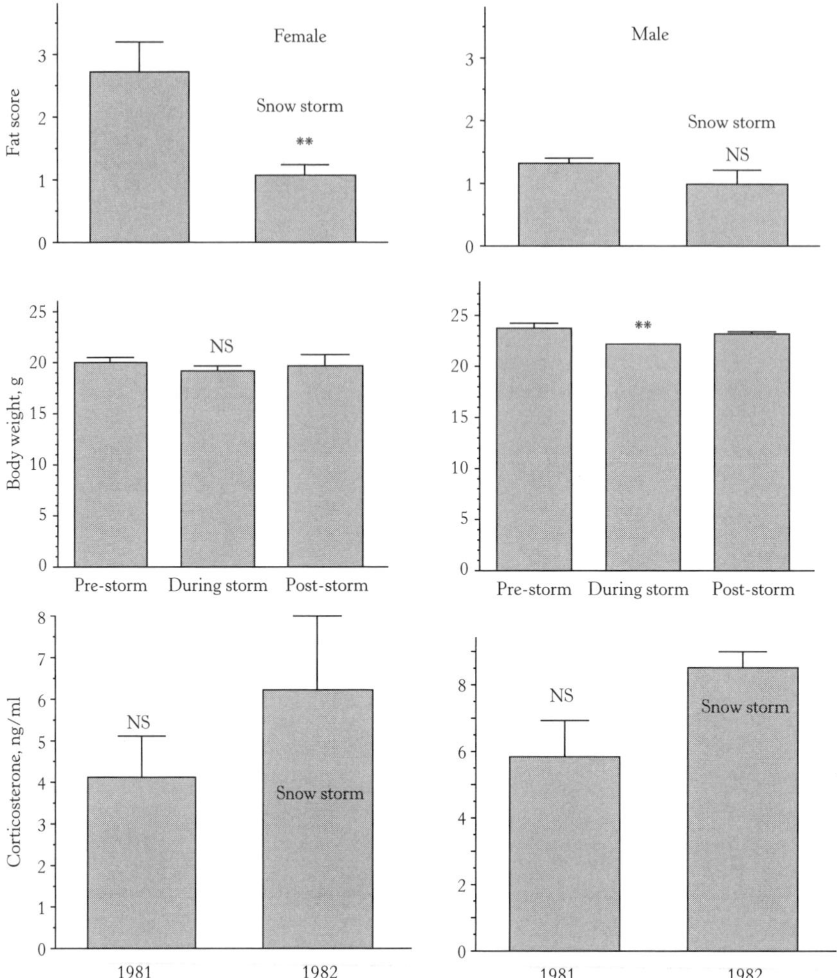

FIGURE 8.5: Effects of a spring snowstorm in 1982 on subcutaneous fat score (top panel), body weight (middle panel), and plasma levels of corticosterone in female and male song sparrows in Dutchess County, New York. Comparisons are made with the same time (early April) in 1981 when the weather was warmer with no snow cover. Fat score was lower during the snowstorm in females but not males compared with the same time in 1981. Although females showed no changes in body weight before, during, and after the storm in 1982, males had significantly lower weight during the storm. Comparing baseline plasma levels of corticosterone during the snowstorm in 1982 versus fine weather at the same time in 1981 revealed no significant differences.

From Wingfield (1985a, 1985b). Courtesy of Wiley.

Ramenofsky 2011). During incubation in dusky flycatchers breeding at an alpine site in the Sierra Nevada of California (Pereyra and Wingfield 2003), baseline levels of corticosterone increased dramatically in relation to longer periods of precipitation. Those birds experiencing 4–5 days of precipitation had higher corticosterone levels than those experiencing less precipitation. In contrast, harlequin ducks breeding along rivers in the Olympic Mountains of western Washington State showed an increase in baseline and stress-induced plasma corticosterone as the breeding season progressed. High river flow following extended periods of precipitation had no effect, but both baseline and stress-induced corticosterone levels were negatively correlated with body condition in females (Perfito et al. 2002). Interestingly, this species has precocial young, and adult females play a mostly escort role in caring for young, which may mean that Ey is shallower (Figure 8.1) than for a songbird raising altricial young.

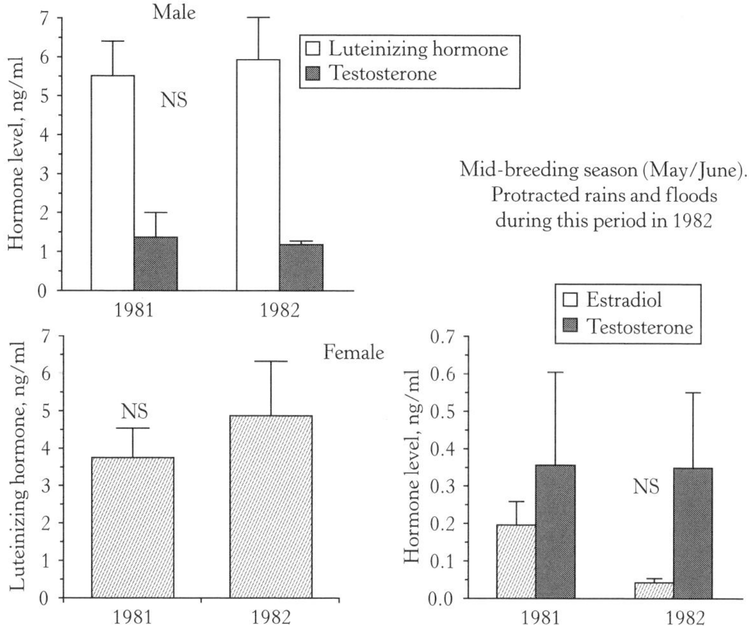

FIGURE 8.6: Effects of a protracted period of rains and subsequent floods on plasma levels of luteinizing hormone (LH), testosterone, and estradiol in male and female song sparrows in Dutchess County, New York, in 1982. Comparisons are made with song sparrows sampled at the same time of year and location, and similar reproductive status in 1981 (when there were no protracted periods of rain or floods). In contrast to the effects of a snowstorm earlier in the breeding season, there were no significant differences in any reproductive hormone plasma levels between years.

From Wingfield (1985a, 1985b). Courtesy of Wiley.

Seasonal and abrupt changes in weather have been shown to affect physiology and behavior in all major groups of vertebrates, including humans. A seasonal study of plasma total and free corticosteroids and urinary corticosteroids in young men from the Khabarovsk region of eastern Russia showed an increase in plasma levels of corticosteroids during winter, but an increase in excreted corticosteroids in summer. Elevated levels of biologically active (free) corticosteroids were found in response to bad weather at all seasons (Uchakina 1977). The extreme continental climate in Turkmenistan (central Asia) has hot dry summers and cold winters. Plasma levels of 17-hydroxy-corticosteroids of humans in this region were slightly higher in summer than winter, although urinary concentrations did not change (Sultanov et al. 2001). However, this study did find that the occupation of individuals also had an effect possibly confounding seasonal changes. Heavy labor and emotional tension, coupled with summer heat, tended to increase blood cortisol levels (Sultanov et al. 2001).

Distance runners are affected by weather, especially by high humidity and heat that tend to decrease performance (Suping et al. 1992). However, there is also a tendency for urinary 17-hydroxycorticosteroids to increase more after training in winter than in hotter and more humid conditions of summer—the opposite of performance (Suping et al. 1992). Sample size was limited and thus more research is needed to determine the association of corticosteroids and distance running under severe conditions in humans. Additional evidence suggests that high temperature and humidity have significant effects to reduce performance in distance runners (Vihma 2010). Moreover, weak associations of mood and weather with reduced sunshine were the strongest factors resulting in "lower" mood, perhaps affecting many activities (Persinger 1975).

Female baboons of Amboseli, Kenya, showed increases in fecal glucocorticoid levels during a prolonged dry season when food and water became scarce. However, this increase did not disrupt breeding, suggesting that the increases in corticosteroids were with baseline variation

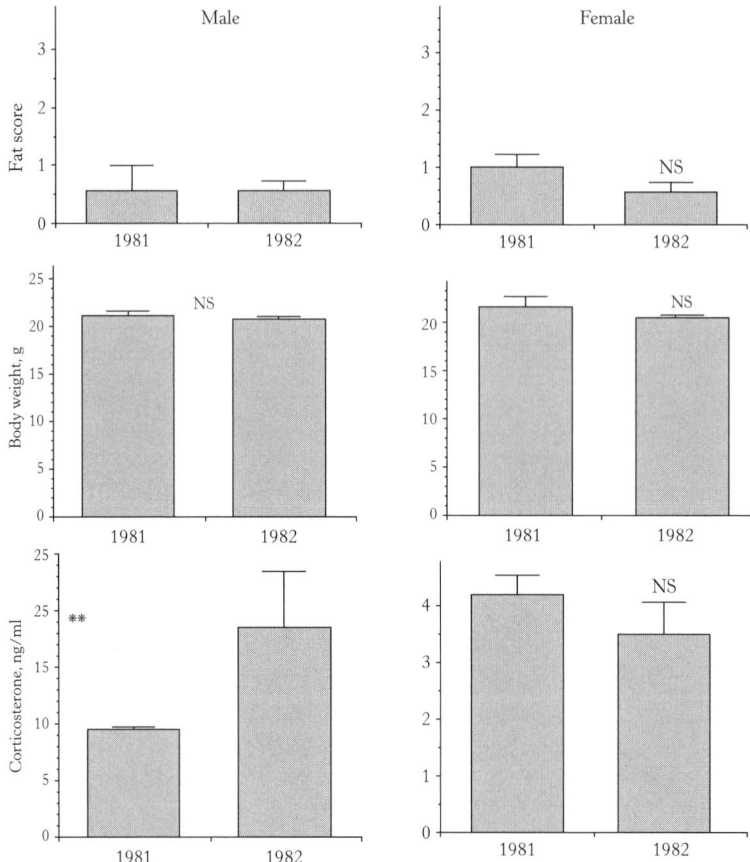

FIGURE 8.7: Effects of a protracted period of rains and subsequent floods on subcutaneous fat score (top panel), body weight (middle panel), and plasma levels of corticosterone in male and female song sparrows in Dutchess County, New York, in 1982. Comparisons are made with song sparrows sampled at the same time of year and location, and similar reproductive status in 1981 (when there were no protracted periods of rain or floods). There were no significant differences in fat score and body mass between years in either males for females. However, plasma levels of corticosterone were significantly higher in males during the rains and floods of 1982. Females showed no differences in circulating corticosterone.

From Wingfield (1985a, 1985b). Courtesy of Wiley.

TABLE 8.1: CORTICOSTERONE LEVELS IN RELATION TO WEATHER AT BARROW

	Breeding		Molt	
	Baseline	Stress	Baseline	Stress
Lapland longspur	No	Yes 37%–39%	Yes 47%–53%	Yes 41%–73%
Snow bunting	No	No	Yes 19%	Yes 25%–30%
Common redpoll adult	No	No	Yes 35%–59%	Yes 36%–60%
Juvenile			Yes 44%–88%	Yes 48%–58%

Correlations of baseline (i.e., blood levels sampled within 3 minutes of capture) and stress levels (after 30–60 minutes of capture, handling, and restraint stress) with weather in arctic breeding birds: snow buntings, Lapland longspurs, and common redpolls. The "yes/no" indicates whether corticosterone was correlated with weather conditions, and if correlation did exist, the percentage indicates the amount of variability explained by the weather conditions (i.e., the r^2).

Reprinted with permission from Romero et al. (2000). Courtesy of Elsevier.

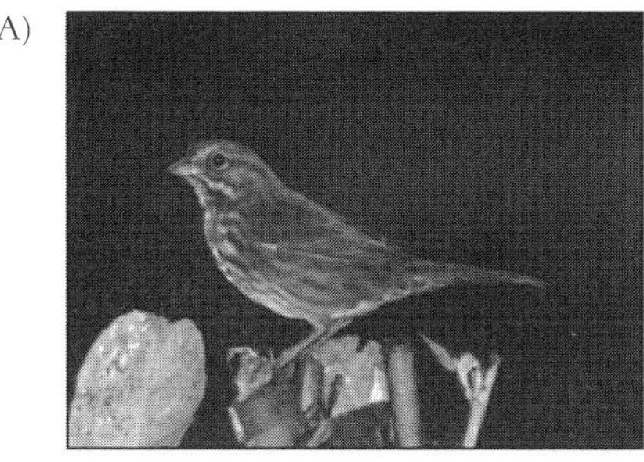

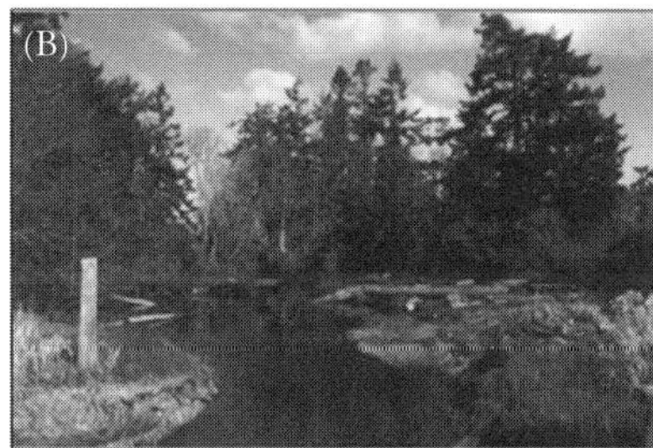

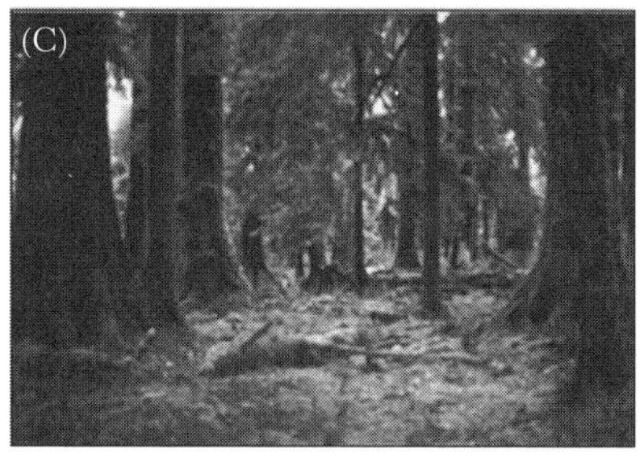

FIGURE 8.8: Effects of cool spring weather and elevation on plasma levels of corticosterone in male song sparrows (panel A) during the early breeding season in western Washington State in 1987 and 1988. Panel B shows typical low elevation habitat (0–10 meters) close to water in the Puget Sound region. Panel C shows higher elevation habitat (500–1000 meters) near the Pack Forest Experimental Station near Mt. Rainier. Cold spring temperatures in 1988 were accompanied by higher corticosterone levels versus 1987 at the higher elevation sites. Corticosterone levels were lower at the same time at the low elevation sites on Whidbey Island in Puget Sound.

All photos by J. C. Wingfield. From Wingfield and Ramenofsky (2011), courtesy of Elsevier Press.

and not into homeostatic overload range when breeding would be interrupted (Gesquiere et al. 2008). Behavioral adjustments are also critically important during inclement weather. During an exceptionally cold January, pronghorn antelopes of southern Alberta and northern Montana began moving south (Bruns 1977). These animals are efficient at pawing away snow to get at forage, but the harder and deeper the snow, the more they must work to get at food (i.e., higher allostatic load). Pronghorn routinely use microhabitats with reduced wind speed and shallower, softer snow to rest and sleep. In the most severe winds, when wind chills were extreme, they oriented the anterior parts of the body downwind and even curved the head along the body to reduce exposed surface area (Bruns 1977). Investigations of glucorticosteroid dynamics and action during these periods are needed to explore possible adaptive responses to severe weather conditions.

B. Heat, Drought, and Deserts

Periods of extreme heat, often accompanied by drought, are frequent at lower latitudes, particularly in deserts, although such conditions can also occasionally be found in other regions during unusually hot, dry weather. These conditions can be disruptive to the life cycle, particularly breeding seasons. Species that are adapted to xeric conditions adjust their life cycles around brief and usually unpredictable rainy seasons (e.g., Miller 1963; Williams and Tieleman 2001; Tieleman 2002; Tieleman et al. 2002; Perfito et al. 2006; Perfito et al. 2007).

Animals adjust to changing conditions of desert environments by integrating behavior and physiology to both reduce exposure to the most severe conditions and use food as a source of water (e.g., Bartholomew 1964; Schmidt-Nielsen 1965). For example, small birds cease activity during the hottest part of the day and retire to refugia where exposure to heat is less (Bartholomew

1964; Wolf 2000). Verdins can lower metabolic rate by as much as 50% in microhabitats sheltered from wind and solar radiation, but such a strategy has the disadvantage of decreasing cooling by evaporative water loss fourfold (Wolf and Walsberg 1996). In the Sonoran Desert of North America, both verdins and black tailed gnatcatchers frequently occupy thermal refugia such as knot holes and clefts in the bark of trees (Wolf et al. 1996). Other structures, including nests, can also be used to shelter from extreme heat (e.g., Ricklefs and Hainsworth 1968; reviewed in Wingfield and Ramenofsky 2011). If no shelter from solar radiation is available, behavioral traits including fluffed back and crown feathers to allow circulation of air, as opposed to trapping it for insulation in cold environments. Panting, exposing the edges of limbs, wetting of plumage, and so on, all contribute to the dissipation of heat (e.g., Calder and King 1994; Gill 1995; Wingfield and Ramenofsky 2011).

Mechanisms by which life cycles are regulated in arid and semi-arid regions remain unclear, but care should be taken to separate mechanisms involved where organisms can predict the timing of hot, dry seasons and prepare from mechanisms when responding to unpredicted hot and dry weather. When periods of hot and dry weather can be predicted (seasonality), two hypotheses explain environmental control of life-history stages (e.g., reproductive function based on the allostatic load models of Figure 8.1). Rain and subsequent associated cues, such as green grass and food supply, provide local predictive information to regulate gonadal maturation and onset of nesting (Vleck and Priedkalns 1985; Perfito et al. 2008). In this scenario, wet conditions stimulate whereas dry conditions inhibit breeding (Vleck and Priedkalns 1985; Perfito et al. 2008). From Figure 8.1 we can predict that as Ey increases during incubation and raising young, perturbations such as extreme droughts and heat could act as direct labile perturbation factors leading to disruption of the life cycle (elevation of Eo in addition to Ey, Figure 8.1) with potential activation of an emergency life-history stage (see Wingfield and Ramenofsky 2011 for further details).

A hormonal mechanism by which the dry season, or drought, may inhibit reproductive function in birds was proposed by Cain and Lien (1985). Water restriction of bobwhite quail resulted in elevated levels of corticosterone, and treatment of quail with doses of corticosterone that mimicked circulating levels generated by the stress of water restriction resulted in decreased weights of testes, ovaries, and oviducts, accompanied by reductions of sperm and egg production. Inhibition of reproduction by drought could thus be mediated through stress-induced corticosteroid secretion to inhibit reproductive function (Cain and Lien 1985). In support of the hypothesis, Sapolsky (1987) reported that plasma levels of testosterone were lower during a severe drought in East Africa in adult male olive baboons. However, other studies suggest that corticosteroids are not involved in delaying reproduction during droughts. In free-living populations of the white-browed sparrow weaver in the Luangwa valley of Zambia (Wingfield et al. 1991), a prolonged dry season was accompanied by widespread failure to initiate breeding during the period when nests are usually initiated in August–December 1987 (Wingfield and Ramenofsky 2011, and for review). Breeding began in full when rains started in January and February. In male and female white-browed sparrow weavers there were no differences in body weight and fat between drought and normal years (Wingfield et al. 1991). Plasma levels of corticosterone showed a slight increase during breeding, but there were no effects of drought on plasma levels of corticosterone in either sex (Wingfield and Ramenofsky 2011). Much more field and laboratory investigation is needed to understand the hormonal correlates and mechanisms underlying adjustments of breeding in relation to drought and extreme heat.

Delay of breeding in relation to drought could be due to other factors associated with resources for breeding. The contributions of Ey and Eo will be key, and it is likely that many species adapted for life in arid and semi-arid habitats are not stressed by dry conditions per se and allostatic load may not be high (see also Tieleman 2002; Tieleman et al. 2002 for discussion). Cain and Lien's (1985) mechanism for drought inhibition of breeding because of stress would be restricted to exceptionally severe and prolonged droughts, or to those species that are not adapted to semi-arid environments. In other words, Eo could increase, rapidly raising allostatic load and potential overload (Figure 8.1). Including social factors in the responses to rainfall is also important, as shown in the cooperatively breeding superb starling. Baseline and maximal stress-induced corticosterone levels change in different ways during dry and wet seasons, depending upon status (Rubenstein 2007). Subordinate starlings had higher circulating baseline and stress-induced corticosterone in drier years, whereas non-breeders or breeders showed no such relationships.

In zebra finches from arid regions of the Australian continent, water restriction for 11 weeks resulted in a decrease in LH levels compared to controls (Perfito et al. 2006). Access to *ad libitum* water was followed by a rise in LH, but no differences in immunoreative-gonadotropin-releasing hormone-I (ir-GnRH-1) or ir-GnRH-II in the hypothalamus. These data support the prediction that environmental conditions conducive to onset of nesting can stimulate release of GnRH and LH, rather than poor conditions eliciting a delay to accommodate full reproductive development. There was no evidence that elevated corticosteroids were associated with inhibition of breeding. Rather, cues associated with conditions permissive to nesting stimulated breeding or perhaps released an inhibition (Perfito et al. 2007; Perfito et al. 2008). These data are consistent with the effects of water on a semi-aquatic population of song sparrows in western Washington State (Wingfield et al. 2012). Populations of song sparrows closer to water tend to be denser than those further away from streams, lakes, and bogs. In an unusually dry spring, males were still territorial, but responded less strongly to a simulated territorial intrusion (Wingfield et al. 2012). In a captive study, males and females that had access to open water baths showed greater photoperiodically induced gonadal growth than controls with no access to open water (all had access to drinking water through a glass tube). Body weights and fat scores were not affected by treatment, suggesting that periodic drought may not be stressful per se, but inhibits reproductive function by as yet unknown mechanisms (see Wingfield and Ramenofsky 2011 for further discussion).

Many birds of the Sonoran Desert breed during periods of restricted water availability compared with species breeding in suburban and riparian habitats. Acute stress of capture, handling, and restraint (see Chapters 3 and 6) showed that desert birds such as black-throated sparrow, cactus wren, and curve-billed thrasher suppressed their adrenocortical responses to stress during the breeding season in summer compared to the much cooler winter. Inca dove and Abert's towhee, species of more mesic habitats, in contrast, did not modulate the adrenocortical response to acute stress (Wingfield et al. 1992). Baseline corticosterone levels did not differ between seasons. In the summer of 1990 there was a period of extreme heat in which temperatures reached 44°C and greater (50°C!), and Inca doves and Abert's towhees showed no change in baseline corticosterone level except for a slight elevation in male towhees but below those following capture stress (Figure 8.9). However, in black-throated sparrows sampled in open desert during the period of extreme heat, baseline corticosterone levels had increased to those generated by capture stress (Figure 8.9; Wingfield et al. 1992). These authors suggested that birds in suburban and riparian habitats (more mesic with extensive shade plants and access to water) were able to withstand the heat better than black-throated sparrows in open desert.

Effects of drought and extreme heat are also major concerns in many vertebrate taxa. Camels were able to withstand many days to weeks of dehydration, even under extreme heat conditions of deserts. Experimental dehydration of camels up to 11 days with complete denial of water resulted in an increase in plasma sodium levels in both spring (cooler) and summer conditions, but the increase was greatest in the latter. Plasma renin activity was enhanced mostly during dehydration in summer and returned to control values after rehydration. Plasma aldosterone increased slightly during dehydration, but increased dramatically after rehydration. Curiously, plasma levels of cortisol did not change (Finberg et al. 1978). These data are consistent with the renin-angiotensin-aldosterone system regulating salt and water balance during a heat and dehydration event, but cortisol does not seem to be directly involved, and the animals were not stressed in the classic sense, despite what would be extreme conditions to most terrestrial vertebrates.

Heat can also be a major stressor for fish. For example, salmon swimming upstream may have to cope with changes in temperature as they enter smaller and smaller streams that are more susceptible to changes in temperature. In one study, juvenile Chinook salmon elevated cortisol concentrations when faced with a moderate increase in temperature similar to those experienced in groundwater-fed tributary streams but a decrease in cortisol, interpreted as chronic stress, when faced with a stronger increase in temperature similar to those experienced in side-channel streams (Quigley and Hinch 2006).

In many arid regions exemplified by northwestern India, animals such as sheep have to walk long distances to find sufficient forage, under often severe conditions of aridity and heat. Ewes of a hardy arid region strain, Malpura, were experimentally subjected to a 14-kilometer walk compared with controls from 09.00 to 15.00 hours (a period of high ambient heat). They were not allowed to eat or drink during this period (Sejian et al. 2012). Plasma levels of cortisol

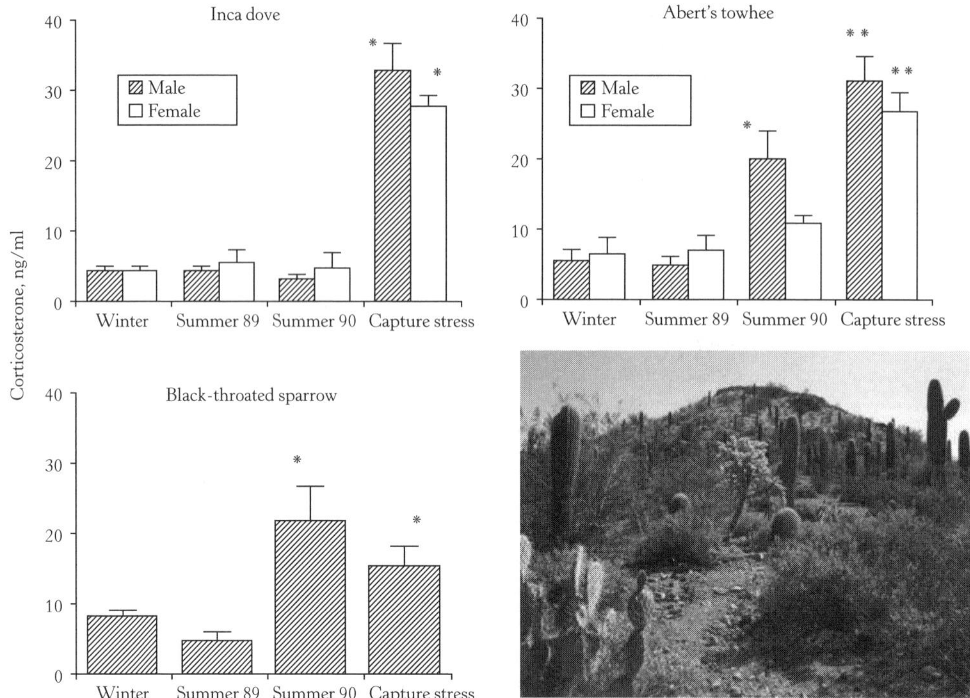

FIGURE 8.9: Plasma levels of corticosterone in relation to season, ambient temperature, and capture stress in the Inca dove, Abert's towhee, and black-throated sparrow. All birds were sampled on breeding grounds in mesic (Inca dove and Abert's towhee) versus xeric (black-throated sparrow) habitat in the Sonoran Zone of southeastern Arizona. The lower right-hand panel shows typical Sonoran Desert. There were no differences in baseline corticosterone levels from winter to summer in any species. During a period of extreme heat in summer 1990, birds in mesic habitat of suburbs and riparian habitat showed little change in baseline corticosterone versus levels reached during exposure to capture, handling, and restraint stress (top panels). However, black-throated sparrows breeding in the desert habitat showed marked increase in baseline corticosterone levels during the extreme heat of June 1990. Because these levels were similar to those induced by capture stress, it suggests that the extreme heat may have been stressful.

From Wingfield et al. (1992). Courtesy of Wiley. Photo by J. C. Wingfield.

increased two-fold in the walking group, whereas there was no change in reproductive hormones, estradiol and progesterone (Sejian et al. 2012). Conversely, plasma T3 and T 4 decreased. These data are consistent with the hypothesis that individuals that are adapted to severe weather may show increases in corticosteroids but not to levels that are potentially in the stress range (level C, reactive homeostasis, Chapter 3). Malpura ewes subjected to experimental heat stress (40°C for 6 hours a day) showed a much larger increase in plasma cortisol compared to controls, and much higher than walking stress. Again, thyroid hormones decreased (Sejian et al. 2010). Restricted nutrition (30% of daily intake) had a marginal effect on cortisol, but a combination of heat stress and reduced feed resulted in much higher cortisol, suggesting a truly stressful situation (level C. reactive homeostasis).

In great gerbils living in arid regions of Uzbekistan, fecal corticosteroid levels correlated positively with prior number of days with temperatures > 30°C (Rogovin et al. 2008). Fecal corticosteroids were also associated with population density and food availability, but generally were not associated with disappearance of males (mortality) from the population. Only in one year of the study did fecal corticosteroids correlate positively with disappearance, a year when population density was highest (Rogovin et al. 2008). This is another example of elevated levels of corticosteroids during the heat of summer, but only in the hottest years and then not necessarily associated with assumed mortality.

Many terrestrial reptiles such as lizards thermoregulate behaviorally. They choose to position themselves in shade versus open ground or in exposed parts of trees versus on the shaded side (e.g., Adolph 1990). Similarly, they can use the same strategies to thermoregulate seasonally and in response to sudden changes in weather. European sand lizards near the northern edge of their range in Sweden have earlier lay dates in warmer springs when there are more opportunities for basking in the sun (Olsson and Shine 1997). Similarly, in Australian blue-tongued skinks, individuals are much more active on sunny hot days (Koenig et al. 2002). Reptiles likely use behavioral thermoregulation to avoid the potential for heat stress in deserts or extreme heat events.

Nests of the Australian subalpine skink can be vulnerable to variations in ambient temperature. Warmer than usual temperatures tended to increase hatching success, advance hatching dates, and increase offspring size and locomotor performance. These effects were more dramatic if the variation in temperature occurred earlier in the incubation period (Shine and Elphick 2001). Several species of terrestrial reptiles have the ability to channel rainwater to the mouth via capillary action through interscalar spaces. Arching the body can accentuate this effect so that some lizards can harvest drinking water even in light rainfall (e.g., Sherbrooke 1990). These traits allow individuals to acclimate to potentially stressful conditions.

Female green turtles, as other marine turtles, are vulnerable to heat stress when coming on land to dig nests and lay eggs. Laying females exposed to heat stress on an island off northeastern Australia showed a significant increase in plasma corticosterone but much less magnitude of a change than in non-breeding (ocean ranging) females. These data suggest that female green turtles modulate their adrenocortical response to environmental stressors during laying (Jessop et al. 2000) and potentially avoid interruption of reproductive function under potentially severe conditions. However, effects of global warming may be key here, increasing the potential for more pronounced responses to heat events while on land.

Predicted rises in global temperatures, including those of oceans and fresh water, will have potentially deleterious effects on fish and other aquatic organisms. In the Antarctic fish *Pagothenia nborchgrevinki*, plasma cortisol levels increased after temperature increased from near 0°C to 5°C and 8°C (Ryan 1995), a relatively small rise but perhaps an extreme event for polar species. Warm water species will be able to move to higher latitudes (Sharma et al. 2007), but cold water species may have more and more restricted ranges. In the future, fish in tropical and subtropical shallower waters such as estuaries, mangroves, and lagoons will face some of the most severe environmental conditions (Blaber 2002). Heat shock proteins (HSPs) play an important role in the cellular response to heat stress, and other perturbations, as in other vertebrates (Basu et al. 2002). But their regulation by the endocrine system remains much less well known. Heat shock proteins increase in response to a variety of stressors including heat, pathogen exposure, cold shock, and environmental contaminants (Iwama et al. 1998). On the other hand, HSP 70 levels in several tissues of stream-living fishes showed seasonal changes and tended to be lowest in winter and higher in spring and autumn, with a second low in summer (Fader et al. 1994). The authors recommend caution when interpreting baseline HSP 70 levels as indicators of stress. Cortisol administration by intraperitoneal injection into tilapia and rainbow trout had no effect on gill and liver expression of HSP 70 in the absence of heat stress (Basu et al. 2001). However, cortisol treatment post–heat stress, suppressed HSP 70 expression by over 30%. Interrelationships of HSP expression and glucocorticoids during responses to environmental stress remain enigmatic, and more experimental research is needed across all vertebrates.

Temperature stress and corticosteroids are known to inhibit growth in fish (Mommsen et al. 1999). In sunshine bass, plasma IGF-1 levels were higher at 25°C and 30°C than at the range 4–20°C. A 15-minute period of confinement stress also decreased IGF-1 as did low temperature. However, treatment with cortisol did not affect IGF-1, suggesting that temperature stressors decrease IGF-1 independently of cortisol (Davis and Peterson 2006). Gilthead sea bream, like many temperate zone fish, will move to warmer waters in winter. If they are unable to do so, or are exposed to unusually cold temperatures, then they can develop "winter syndrome," which includes lethargy, characteristic sideways and backward swimming, and reduced reaction to external stimuli. Frequently the immune system is less active, resulting in more infections (e.g., Gallardo et al. 2003). Winter syndrome also is accompanied by an increase in plasma cortisol (Tort et al. 1998).

In walleye, confinement stress of young fish, stocking procedures, and transport to lakes resulted in marked increases in cortisol but these were back to baseline in 24 hours post-transport

(Parsons and Reed 2001). There was no effect on over-winter survival, but handling stress, and presumably higher cortisol, resulted in fish taking much longer to seek cover when released, resulting in elevated predation risk (Barton and Haukenes 1999). Arctic char show winter emaciation because they fast for 9–10 months a year. In the summer months they migrate to seawater and feed, resulting in dramatic increases in body weight and fat (Jorgensen et al. 1997). Fish acclimated to a specific water temperature or range of temperatures show marked physiological and behavioral responses if water temperature is rapidly decreased—cold shock. Such decreases in water temperature may also occur if a fish moves along a natural thermocline or in response to storms, seiches (sudden change in water level in a lake or inland sea), and so on. In some cases, death may occur (Donaldson et al. 2008). Behavioral effects include uncoordinated swimming and respiration rates accompanied by increases in plasma cortisol levels (Donaldson et al. 2008). However, Carruth et al. (2002) point out that variables such as maturational state may complicate the relationship of plasma cortisol to environmental stress.

C. Amphibians, Weather, and Facultative Metamorphosis

Amphibians have been subjected to widespread environmental stress, disease, and human disturbance, and this group is one of the most threatened globally. Over-winter survival of boreal toads in Colorado was positively correlated with minimum daily winter air temperature, that is, reduced survival at lower temperatures (Scherer et al. 2008). During the active season in summer, a combination of high temperatures and xeric conditions may reduce the amount of energy stores that toads can accumulate for winter hibernation, thus reducing the likelihood of survival (Scherer et al. 2008). Similarly, in a Romanian population of frogs, warmer spring temperatures and rainfall advance emergence and spawning (Hartel 2008). Thus global warming could have significant effects on these amphibians. On the other hand, decreases in rainfall and higher summer temperatures over several years do not appear to be responsible for catastrophic declines of rainforest frog populations in the montane regions of Queensland, Australia (Laurance 1996). Other factors such as disease may be responsible and could be exacerbated by weather variables. Measurements of urinary corticosteroid metabolites in captive and free-living Fijian ground frogs showed increases in corticosteroids following capture and handling, and captive animals had generally lower levels and did not show the same magnitude of seasonal changes as animals under natural conditions (Narayan et al. 2010). This suggests that amphibians, as other vertebrates, show similar responses to environment.

Some variants of the "take it or leave it" strategies include facultative developmental changes. In western spadefoot toads, premature drying of ponds results in facultative metamorphosis. This can be accelerated experimentally by lowering water levels in tanks in captive conditions (Denver 1998) and was accompanied by precocious increases in tadpoles of the whole body contents of thyroid hormones, triodothyronine and thyroxine, as well as corticosterone. Injections of CRF activated both thyroid hormone and corticosterone secretion, which in turn precipitated facultative metamorphosis (Denver 1997). Crowding, limited resources, and predation, as well as habitat desiccation, may also trigger this response (reviewed in Denver 1997; Hayes 1997). Similarly, crowding, as well as other stressors, increased corticosterone levels and precipitated premature metamorphosis in the boreal toad. This in turn allowed the animals to leave the pond in a physiological state more suited to a terrestrial life (Hayes 1997) (see Chapter 11 for further discussion).

D. Cold

Weather with lower temperatures can be challenging for ectothermic and endothermic vertebrates alike. Small birds are particularly vulnerable, and those species that do not migrate to escape the cold of winter at higher latitudes and altitudes tend to use micro-habitats and/or employ physiological mechanisms such as torpor to endure periods of low temperature. Reinertsen (1983), in a review of the physiological and behavioral adaptations for small birds surviving the night in arctic and subarctic regions, described how thermoregulatory responses to cold include seeking microclimates such as a cavity in a tree, a well-insulated nest, snow caves, and so on. Although some species do not seek shelter, even seemingly ineffective components of the immediate environment, such as branches of trees, may offer some protection. Huddling is common in some birds and mammals during cold weather, but bear in mind that animals also huddle for many reasons, including protection from predators and for social reasons. Nonetheless, in small mammals and birds huddling provides energetic advantages when ambient temperatures decline below the thermo-neutral zone and can be particularly effective if huddling occurs in a shelter and/or accompanied by hypothermia (Vickery and Millar 1984). For example, a small songbird, the bushtit, can undergo slight hypothermia at colder temperatures, but also will huddle in tight groups, especially during the night. This can reduce metabolism by about 20% compared to isolated birds, thereby conserving energy when cold weather reduces food supply (Chaplin 1982). Similar observations in black-tailed gnatcatchers showed that roosting may occur communally in the co-opted domed nest of a verdin. This small songbird normally does not flock, but 15–16 birds were observed roosting in this nest (Walsberg 1990). Temperature inside the nest was elevated over the outside ambient temperature. The sociable weaver constructs a massive communal nest with separate nest cavities occupied by an individual pair and young. In the winter, the nests are used as roost sites, with the advantage of social roosting reducing heat loss and costs of enduring cold winter nights (White et al. 1975). Many more anecdotal observations of microhabitat use, as well as detailed ecophysiological studies of birds in cold weather, have been reviewed by Wingfield and Ramenofsky (2011).

Small songbirds enduring the arctic winter have similar lower critical temperatures, as do mid-latitude and tropical species (Steen 1958). They must, therefore, increase metabolic rate to maintain body temperature, and some can reduce body temperature at night or during the worst weather (Steen 1958). Many fluff out their plumage to trap air and reduce heat loss, allowing them to survive low temperatures at night at 50%–70% of daytime metabolism (Steen 1958). Retraction of extremities, and the placement of the head (with bare eyes and bill as potential sources of heat loss) under a wing or beneath feathers on the back, are other ways of reducing heat loss (e.g., Reinertsen 1983; Calder and King 1994; reviewed in Wingfield and Ramenofsky 2011). Andreev (1999) reviews the diversity of ways in which birds wintering in extreme cold utilize energy sources. Some, such as willow ptarmigan, use widespread but low energy sources like willow shrubs (*Salix* sp). Others may store food items individually or segregate by sex into different habitats (e.g., Andreev 1991b). In all cases, wintering birds tend to minimize energy utilization as described earlier, including restricting themselves to short foraging times under extremely low ambient temperatures (Andreev 1999). Using the allostatic load model, this would mean minimizing heat loss, Ee, and decreasing Ei (Figure 8.1).

To summarize Andreev (Andreev 1991a, 1991b, 1999), territorial aggression and dominance-subordinance relations in extreme cold tend to be reduced. Furthermore, social behavior can minimize foraging time by reducing the risk of predation, another factor that is highly important when coping with severe weather and disruption of normal life-history stages. Collectively, these are additional components of the facultative behavioral and physiological responses to labile perturbation factors. Energy reserves during episodes of extreme cold are also critical, and use of these stores ideally should be minimized (Andreev 1999). In contrast, in summer no such minimization of energy use occurs as birds begin breeding. The offspring of high arctic and alpine tundra species must grow quickly under unstable weather conditions, restricted food resources, and unpredictably fluctuating food supplies. Clearly, Eg (food available in the environment), Ee, and Ei must be monitored closely (Figure 8.1) to keep allostatic load at a minimum (Wingfield and Ramenofsky 2011).

A comparison of southern and northern populations of pied flycatchers in Finland revealed that northern birds lay smaller clutches and have greater fat reserves than southern populations (Eeva et al. 2002). This potentially increased fledging success when the weather turned cold and rainy. Despite smaller clutch size in northern populations, reproductive success may be enhanced in poor weather (Eeva et al. 2002). This is also consistent with the stringency hypothesis (Wilson 1975; Ettinger and King 1980) in which some populations produce fewer offspring than they might be able to raise in a breeding season with fair weather. However, if inclement conditions occur, then a smaller investment in reproduction would be offset by greater reproductive success. Additionally, the development of homeothermy in nestling songbirds is accompanied by huddling behavior to reduce heat loss, especially when ambient temperatures decrease (Marsh 1980).

In a completely different type of habitat, beaches, estuaries, mud flats, and so on, shorebirds must forage harder to find food when temperature drops and prey such as worms and bivalves move deeper into substrate (Evans 1976). Although many shorebirds deposit fat in winter, during periods of inclement weather when food is harder to obtain and not sufficient for daily energetic needs (lower Eg and higher Eo in Figure 8.1), they must draw upon their reserves of fat and, in many cases, protein reserves from muscles as well (Davidson and Evans 1982). In two common European shorebirds in Scotland, redshanks and oystercatchers, mortality increased dramatically during severe weather in January and February 1979. Analysis of salvaged carcasses revealed that virtually all fat deposits and protein reserves from pectoralis muscles had been depleted. In another sudden period of exceptionally low temperatures in January 1982, redshanks and oystercatchers were able to mobilize fat stores quickly, but apparently they were unable to mobilize protein fast enough and many died (Davidson and Evans 1982).

Regulation of fat deposits in relation to potential inclement seasons (winter) has been less well studied, but in birds of the north temperate zone the mechanism appears to involve photoperiod (e.g., King and Farner 1966; Calder and King 1994). Fat deposits of yellow buntings at a roost in England during winter were correlated with the expected mean temperature for that time of year and not with actual temperatures experienced. This is consistent with the hypothesis that winter fattening is regulated by the annual change in photoperiod (Evans 1969).

Behavioral responses to weather events play a vital role in ameliorating potential stressful consequences that supplement deposition of energy stores in fat. In many ways, such behavioral responses are analogous to those pointed out for desert animals (Bartholomew 1964; Schmidt-Nielsen 1965). Grouse and other species burrow into snow to withstand extreme cold (Formozov 1946; Korhonen 1980, 1981; Pruitt 2005). Temperatures in burrows can be 20°–30°C higher than outside the burrow. Moreover, CO_2 did not appear to accumulate to any deleterious extent (Korhonen 1980). In some species such as white-tailed ptarmigan and rock ptarmigan, sometimes several birds dig winter roosts in snow banks, and may huddle as well to conserve energy. These roosts can also serve as refugia during snow and wind storms, with birds remaining in the burrows for most of the day if needed (Braun et al. 1983; Holder and Montgomerie 1993). Willow ptarmigan can spend up to 80% of the day in snow burrows, which allows them to survive extreme cold (Stokkan 1992; Hannon et al. 1998). Ptarmigan in the high arctic island of Svalbard (77°–80°N) maintain as much as 30% of body mass as stored fat that is used as a buffer against extreme cold and severe storms. Additionally, during storms, reduced activity decreases daily energy budgets, enhancing the ability to withstand severe weather (Stokkan et al. 1986; Stokkan 1992).

It is well known that even small songbirds can be active and survive during the winter at high latitudes. Redpolls and Siberian tits burrow in snow and use tree holes to insulate them from extreme cold and wind chill in the winter of northern latitudes (Sulkava 1969; Novikov 1972). These authors showed that both types of holes warmed to constant temperature within 30 minutes of occupancy by the birds. Curiously, Siberian tits preferred tree holes despite the temperature in snow burrows always being warmer. It is possible that closed snow burrows accumulated CO_2, forcing birds to leave within an hour to avoid asphyxiation. Snow adhering to tree braches, especially conifers (called qali) may force songbirds that forage in trees to wind-exposed areas where qali is blown off (Korhonen 1980, 1981; Pruitt 2005). In contrast, others can shelter under the accumulations of qali on trees to reduce heat loss.

How such facultative behavior is regulated remains to be determined, but there is evidence that thyroid hormones, rather than corticosteroids, may be involved in increased thermoregulatory capacity in winter in American goldfinches (Dawson et al. 1992). In support of this finding, it has been shown in captive red knots that T3 levels were elevated in winter when temperatures were low, whereas plasma T4 was highest during the annual molt and subsequent gain in weight (Jenni-Eiermann et al. 2002).

The behavioral patterns of mammals and birds at high latitudes can be highly influenced by patterns of snow cover. Obstructions to prevailing winds can result in snow-free areas to leeward that are crucial for birds and mammals to find food, for example seeds (Pruitt 2005). At mid-latitude continental regions, large land birds such as great bustards show facultative migration away from severe weather conditions in winter. Deep snow appears to be a trigger of this facultative migration, rather than low environmental temperature, possibly because access to food is greatly reduced (i.e., decreased Eg in Figure 8.1). However, this migration can occur even when food is available, suggesting that additional factors may also be important (Streich et al. 2006).

Insectivorous songbird species, such as American pipits and perhaps other species in alpine areas, use arthropod food sources from the alpine vegetation (Hendricks 1987). There is also an aeolian source of arthropods—the fallout on snow fields (see Edwards and Banko 1976; Edwards 1987) that can be used as a temporary source of food during bad weather when arthropods on vegetation are less active and difficult to find.

Although more is currently known about responses to cold in free-living avian species, several examples suggest that these responses are not unique to birds. The Florida manatee is a marine mammal at the northern edge of the species range in the southeastern United States. In this region it can be exposed to cold waters during winter, resulting in a degenerative condition known as cold stress syndrome. All ages (except neonates) and sexes are affected by chronic exposure to cold water, resulting in emaciation, fat store depletion, lymphoid depletion, epidermal hyperplasia, pustular dermatitis, enterocolitis, and myocardial degeneration (Bossart et al. 2003). These multifactor symptoms could be reversed by moving the animals into warmer water. Racoon dogs in Hokkaido, Japan, winter in dens and sometimes communally. These behaviors, as well as reduced body temperatures by 2°–3°C, helped ameliorate the decrease in body weight over winter by 33%–35% (Kitao et al. 2009).

There are few studies of hormonal correlates of cold in free-living animals. In free-ranging Gelada baboons in Ethiopia, high altitude and low environmental temperatures were correlated with high corticosteroid metabolites in fecal samples (Beehner and McCann 2008). In contrast, weather conditions had no effects on fecal corticosterone metabolite levels in adult blue tits or pied flycatchers. However, in nestlings of both species, fecal corticosterone metabolite levels increased with decreasing temperature. This effect was not found in blue tit nestlings in a colder year, suggesting that sensitivity to ambient temperature may change from one year to the next (Lobato et al. 2008).

Recent laboratory evidence suggests, however, that acute exposure to cold can act as a stressor. Captive European starlings were exposed to a 30-minute decrease in ambient temperature of approximately 3°C using a portable air conditioner. The minor decrease in air temperature resulted in corticosterone release and a sustained increase in heart rate consistent with a fight-or-flight response (de Bruijn and Romero 2011). A rapid 3°C drop in air temperature mimics a fast-moving cold front, but whether free-living starlings react to such a stimulus in a manner similar to captive birds is currently unknown. Furthermore, hormonal responses to cold exposure might be highly species-specific. For example, juvenile American alligators have a range extending further north than any other crocodilian and, as expected, are more frequently exposed to cold weather. Immersion of juveniles into ice water resulted in complete immobility within 5 minutes that could be reversed by warming in tepid water (Lance and Elsey 1999). Although there were large increases in catecholamines in blood up to 1 hour post-treatment, plasma levels of corticosterone showed a much more modest rise. Exposure to acute cold conditions was less stressful than acute handling and restraint (Lance and Elsey 1999).

E. Heterothermy

Many animals can adjust their body temperature up or down in relation to environmental conditions and the need to conserve energy. Such heterothermy is widespread in birds and mammals that can reduce their body temperatures to varying degrees, especially at night and in relation to cold weather. Nocturnal hypothermia is an important mechanism to reduce energetic costs of long winter nights or unexpected cooler temperatures at other times of year. Reinertsen (1983) defines hypothermia as a body temperature 1°–8°C below normal (normothermia for a resting animal), whereas torpor involves a much greater reduction of body temperature with concomitant reductions in metabolic rate and heart rate and virtually no response to external stimuli (see also Geiser 2010). Hibernation, on the other hand, is defined by Reinertsen (1983) as a prolonged state of torpor throughout a long winter of 6 months or more. Torpor frequently is facultative and only overnight, followed by activity during the day. The ability to decrease metabolic rate and enter a hypothermic state is essential for some mammals and birds to endure severe environmental conditions. It is important to note that evidence indicates that a decrease in metabolic rate is regulated first, which then results in lower body temperature, not the other way around (Storey 2001). Here we will focus on heterothermy in response to perturbations of the environment, particularly weather, and not hibernation, which, when it occurs, is a component of the predictable life cycle.

Hypothermic responses are widespread in birds ranging in weight from 3 grams to 6500 grams. The minimum body temperatures reached vary continuously from 4°–38°C (normothermia in birds is about 40°C). There has been much debate about the physiology of heterothermy.

McKechnie and Lovegrove (2002) pointed out that torpor differs from hypothermia when resting, although the distinction between them is unclear. Assumption of a hypothermic state can be triggered by a combination of ecological and physiological factors, including in response to unpredicted temperature declines and other weather variables. To define precisely and then study heterothermy in mammals and birds, it is important to determine the normothermic body temperature first for each individual. Torpor can then be defined as a body temperature below that level (Barclay et al. 2001). Heterothermy may have evolved in relation to body size because small animals easily lose heat, or diet because food is often less available in the cold. Phylogenetic position appears to be less likely (Geiser 1998). Further, endothermy and torpor apparently evolved independently in birds and mammals.

An insectivorous bird, the poorwill, is able to endure a wide range of ambient temperature because it can enter torpor as well as tolerate high daytime temperatures. In winter, torpor periods can continue for several days. This state resembles hibernation shown in other vertebrates (Csada and Brigham 1992), but it is not hibernation in the true sense (Wang and Wolowyk 1988). The lowest body temperature recorded for any bird was in a torpid poorwill (5°C). Reproductively active birds may even enter torpor when nesting during inclement weather (Kissner and Brigham 1993). In poorwills, torpor occurs most frequently on both a daily and a facultative basis, especially in spring when cold and wet conditions are more prevalent (see also Ligon 1970). Torpor in birds and mammals can be seasonal (as in hibernation and estivation), or aseasonal and facultative (nocturnal hypothermia, daily torpor). Depending on the duration and degree of torpor, energy savings of 10%–88% may be achieved (Wang and Wolowyk 1988).

Torpor also appears to be widespread in tropical birds. For example, in the freckled nightjar of South Africa, the extent and duration of torpor were pronounced during the winter months, when flying insects are less common and weather is more likely to be bad (McKechnie et al. 2007). Because Caprimulgids such as whip-poor-wills forage at night and particularly when there is moonlight, dark cloudy weather could decrease foraging success. On the other hand, common nighthawks forage more during the day and would be less affected by weather, except for cold decreasing the numbers of flying insects. Additionally, owlet-nightjars and tawny frogmouths of Australia tended to enter torpor during the coldest months of the year (Brigham et al. 2000; Kortner et al. 2001).

As described earlier, many small birds and mammals survive extreme cold in winter at high latitude. Black-capped chickadees, songbirds weighing around 10–12 grams, are resident in central Alaska and survive extreme low temperatures in winter compared with populations at lower latitudes in western Washington State. Exposure of captive chickadees to –30°C showed an increase in fat stores, but standard metabolic rate did not vary with treatment or season. Birds went into nocturnal hypothermia down to 33.9°C ± 1.3°C from 41°C (Sharbaugh 2001). In contrast, Grossman and West (1977) found no nocturnal hypothermia in this population, whereas in Scandinavia, a closely related species, the willow tit, did enter nocturnal hypothermia in a subarctic (63°N) habitat (Reinertsen and Haftorn 1983). Plasma levels of corticosterone, both basal and after 30 minutes of capture, handling, and restraint, were higher in central Alaska populations of black-capped chickadees and boreal chickadees compared with a population of black-capped chickadees and chestnut-backed chickadees sampled in mid-winter in western Washington State (Wingfield, unpublished data).

Other examples include the Puerto Rican tody, a small (5–7g) non-passerine bird with an unusually low body temperature (36.7°C ± 1.2°C) compared to other small birds (40°–41°C). Todies were able to show heterothermy (27.9°–42.9°C) between ambient temperatures of 15°–40°C (Merola-Zwartjes and Ligon 2000) and body temperatures dropped up to 11°C during cold nights in the breeding season. Curiously, this phenomenon was restricted to females only. Torpor was not recorded in males (Merola-Zwartjes and Ligon 2000). Torpor is widespread in hummingbirds, although in the rufous hummingbird, frequency of torpor bouts varied with season (Hiebert 1993). Bouts of torpor were highest in autumn compared with spring and summer, reflecting different energetic requirements related to migration, breeding, and molt. Nonetheless, torpor can be used at any time, providing maximum flexibility of activity in relation to weather conditions.

There is some evidence that entrance into torpor can be regulated by corticosteroids. Corticosterone levels were elevated (in cloacal fluid) in the evening prior to a torpor bout in rufous hummingbirds during migration, and when sugar concentration of nectar was experimentally lowered. Torpor use also increased with increasing corticosterone (Hiebert et al. 2000a;

Hiebert et al. 2000b). In contrast, torpor bouts were less frequent and there was no correlation with corticosterone levels in cloacal fluid during molt. Experimental administration of corticosterone in artificial nectar (Hiebert et al. 2000a; Hiebert et al. 2000b) reduced food intake and increased use of torpor (Hiebert et al. 2004). Although much more research is needed to tease apart the fascinating mechanisms underlying use of torpor in birds, in mammals a hormone derived from adipose tissue, leptin, is associated with the induction of torpor (Gavrilova et al. 1999; see also Nelson 2004), and perhaps ghrelin as well (Gluck et al. 2006).

F. Snow, Ice, and Ground Feeding

Wintering at mid- to high latitudes can be difficult because snow and ice cover food resources. Some birds and mammals migrate to avoid snow and ice, and some mammals hibernate (Pielou 1994). For those that remain active despite extensive snow cover during the winter months, larger species can easily dig to find covered food, and small rodents can be active underneath snow, whereas for small passerines access to food can involve much more energetically expensive digging. At mid-latitudes, ground-feeding birds can abandon winter home ranges and migrate facultatively when snow and ice conditions become too severe (Wingfield and Ramenofsky 1997, 2011). These irruptive migrations (also called facultative dispersal) may extend from a few hundred meters to thousands of kilometers (see Chapter 9). Other strategies include seeking refugia to provide shelter and trophic resources sufficient to survive the rest of the winter. Many utilize "feeders" at human habitations, enabling them to remain in wintering areas where they could not have survived normally.

Songbirds such as dark-eyed juncos and white-throated sparrows feed almost exclusively on the ground, despite snow depths up to 40 centimeters (Wingfield and Ramenofsky 1997). They prefer to forage in open forest and along the vegetated edges of fields and glades, and males and females appear to forage at different times to minimize competition (Ramenofsky et al. 1992). These birds foraged in micro-habitats when snow depth exceeded 1–2 centimeters, including in bare patches of ground found beneath the conifer canopy and under scrub vegetation, where depth of snow was much less than in open forest or fields. Many birds and mammals depend on these micro-habitats for feeding in winter (e.g., Formozov 1946; Pruitt 1970). Snow caught on canopy vegetation forms "snow shadows" where berries, and even arthropods, can be easily found by small birds and mammals (Formozov 1946; Wingfield and Ramenofsky 1997). An inland Inuit term, *qamaniq* (Pruitt 1970, 1978, 2005), has been used to describe open or shallow depressions in snow cover beneath vegetation and has been adopted elsewhere, as in Wingfield and Ramenofsky (1997, 2011; Figure 8.10).

Temperature measurements in the wintering ranges of dark-eyed juncos and white-throated sparrows revealed that the *qamaniq* was 7°–10°C warmer than all other locations (Wingfield and Ramenofsky 1997, 2011). On sunny but otherwise cold winter days, temperature can rise to 18°C in qamaniq despite ambient air temperature outside of –2°C. *Qamaniq* and other micro-habitats are also potential refuges during winter storms by reducing exposure to wind and providing insulation from cold. However, under conditions of high winds, snow can be blown into the *qamaniq* and qali falls from surrounding vegetation, thereby increasing snow depth further (Formozov 1946; Wingfield and Ramenofsky 1997). Clearly, energetic demands of digging for food when the *qamaniq* is filled (Ee + Ei + Eo, Figure 8.1) at some point will exceed the energy likely to be gained from food (Eg, Figure 8.1). Allostatic overload type 1 could then trigger irruptive migration to alternate refugia and sources of food. Wingfield and Ramenofsky (1997) showed that after a severe storm in the mid-Hudson Valley of New York State that filled up the *qamaniq* with deep snow (snow depth greater than 5 cm, i.e., no longer providing a refuge with food), both white-throated sparrows and dark-eyed juncos began facultative movements looking for food. Although many may have moved only a few hundred meters to feeders in local homeowner's gardens, others are known to move several hundred kilometers south if no local refuges were available (Wingfield and Ramenofsky 1997, 2011). Furthermore, Rogers et al. (1993) showed that dark-eyed juncos wintering in Tennessee had elevated plasma levels of corticosterone during a snowstorm and they had begun moving away from their home range. Corticosterone levels in blood were lower in samples collected before or after the storm (Figure 8.10).

Severe weather in the central Great Plains of North America can have serious consequences for ground-feeding birds during the non-breeding season, and field studies have revealed similar results to those presented in the preceding paragraphs. Harris's sparrows wintering in flocks

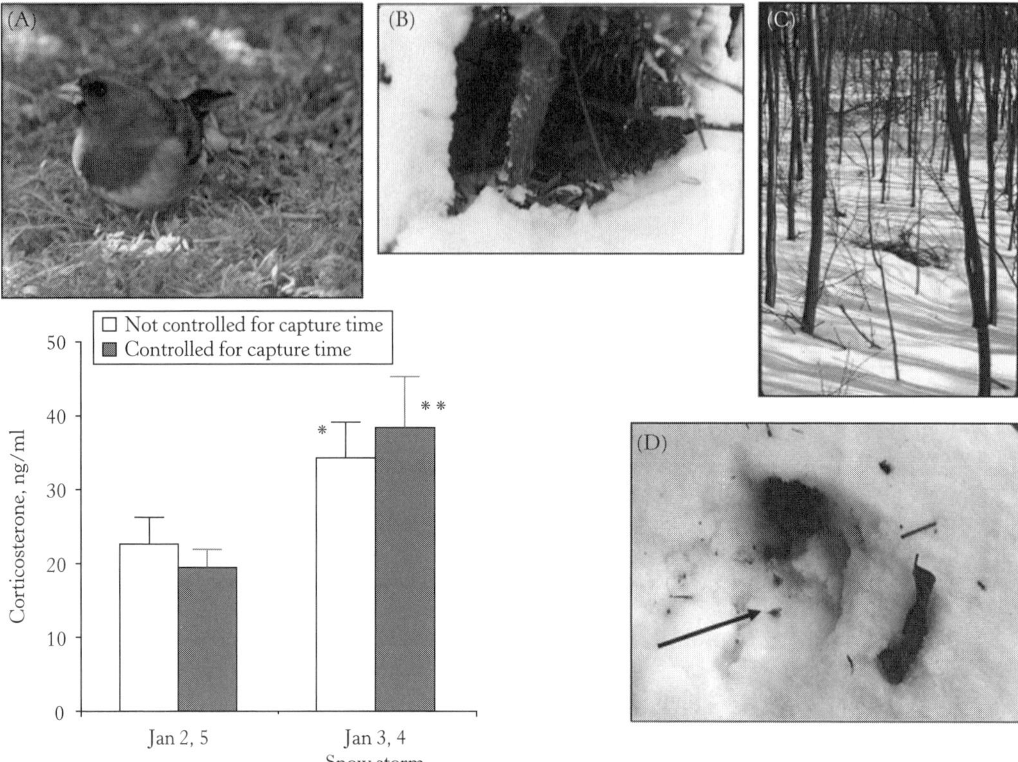

FIGURE 8.10: Ground-feeding birds utilize features of snow cover that allow them to obtain food in otherwise severe conditions. They find food in *qamaniq* (snow-free areas under vegetation—panel B) compared with panel C, where snow depth is deeper. Panel D shows seeds uncovered in shallow snow cover in *qamaniq*. Plasma levels of corticosterone in dark-eyed juncos (panel A) were sampled before, during, and after a snowstorm (lower left panel) that triggered an emergency life-history stage (abandonment of home range). Note that plasma corticosterone levels are significantly higher regardless of whether data are controlled for capture time (see Chapter 6).

From Rogers et al. (1993), with permission of the American Ornithologists' Union; Wingfield and Ramenofsky (1997), with permission of Ardea; Silverin and Wingfield (2010), with permission of Elsevier.

All photos by J. C. Wingfield.

that feed almost exclusively on the ground have a rigid dominance hierarchy, with dominant birds having more black feathering around the face and upper breast than subordinate birds (Figure 8.11). During a snowstorm, competition for food increases, but dominant birds have greater access to food than subordinates (i.e., social status affects Eg; see Goymann and Wingfield 2004). As expected, subordinate birds tended to have greater circulating levels of corticosterone than dominants. This could be because subordinates are being forced to the periphery of the flock, leading to foraging in potentially less productive patches, with a consequent increase in allostatic load (Figure 8.11; Rohwer and Wingfield 1981). In this example, Harris's sparrows chose to "ride out" the storm (the "take it" strategy of Wingfield and Ramenofsky 1997).

In another field study example, European blackbirds wintering in southern Germany typically revert to feeding on berries and fruit when other foods are covered by snowfall. Then competition for limited fruit increased, resulting in subordinate first-year birds of both sexes being forced to migrate south. By showing facultative migration, these birds avoided conflict with dominant adults. First-year European blackbirds of both sexes had elevated plasma levels of corticosterone compared to adults (Figure 8.12, Schwabl et al. 1985) consistent with predictions of Figure 8.1. In this example, the home range was abandoned, but individuals only moved as far as they needed to find alternate shelter and food.

These field studies of effects of severe weather events in wintering birds suggest that mechanisms underlying weather-induced allostatic overload

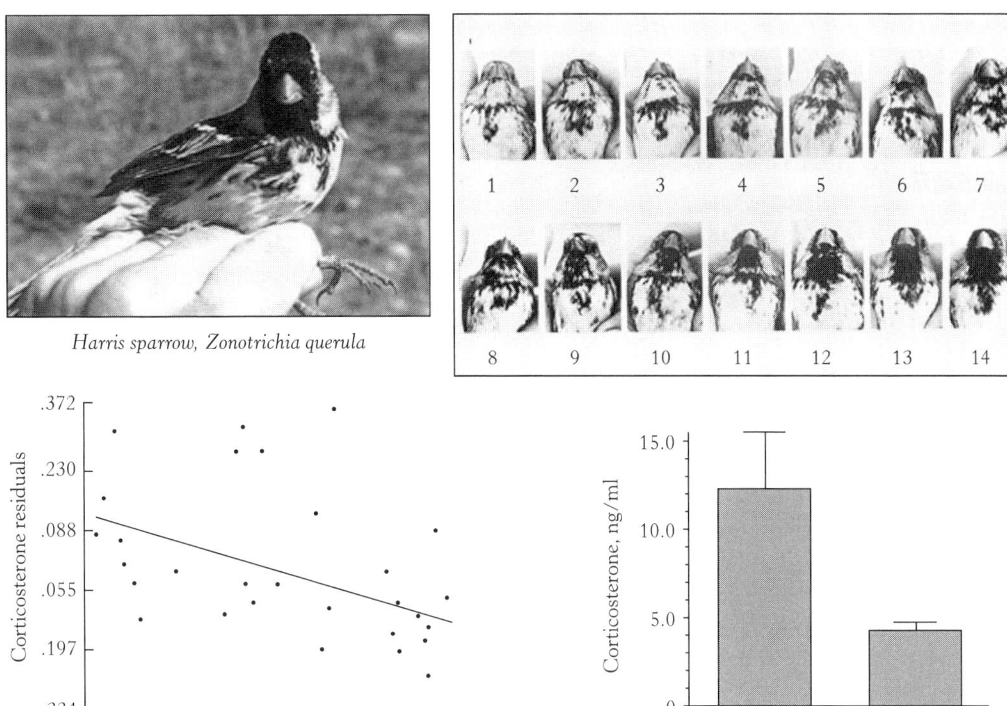

FIGURE 8.11: Harris's sparrows (upper left panel) winter in ground-feeding flocks in the central Great Plains of the United States. These flocks have rigid dominance hierarchies delineated by the amount of black feathering around the face and upper breast (upper right panel, number 1 is the most subordinate and number 14 the most dominant). During severe weather (snow), overall plasma levels of corticosterone were higher than in less severe winter weather (lower right panel), and dominants tended to have lower baseline levels of corticosterone than subordinates (lower left panel).

From Rohwer and Wingfield (1981), courtesy of Springer-Verlag.
Photo in upper left panel by John C. Wingfield.

type 1 may be similar across species despite differences in irruptive-type behavior. Extremes of weather in summer as well as winter may have deleterious effects. In central Honshu, Japan, great tit food supply was not affected by snow cover, but their home ranges increased and they tended to join mixed species flocks. Further, sites of foraging changed from the ground to the upper parts of trees (Nakamura and Shindo 2001). Coal tits foraging in winter in the Pyrenees of northern Spain used the inner parts of trees, including the trunks, when snow cover was heavy. They also used less energetic movements, such as hopping rather than flight foraging techniques (Brotons 1997). Note also that hatch dates of white-tailed ptarmigan were later in years when snow was deeper, but there was no relation to brood size (Clarke and Johnson 1992). Overall breeding success was negatively correlated with snow depth, probably related to nest site location, cover, and food availability in deep snow years.

For mammals winter conditions also frequently result in food sources being covered by snow and ice. Snow surfaces may become crusted and difficult to penetrate. Ice cover from freezing of rain onto terrestrial surfaces can be particularly devastating. Increasing freeze-thaw cycles in arctic regions result in more ice crust, which in turn excludes many terrestrial animals from their food (Callaghan et al. 2004). Smaller mammals such as voles that live beneath the snow layer may fare better, but exposure of the ground and subsequent ice cover could affect these animals as well. Moreover, more unusual weather episodes, such as freezing rain in arctic regions, affect native peoples in terms of mobility on the winter surface and the abundance of animal food such as caribou (Berkes and Jolly 2002).

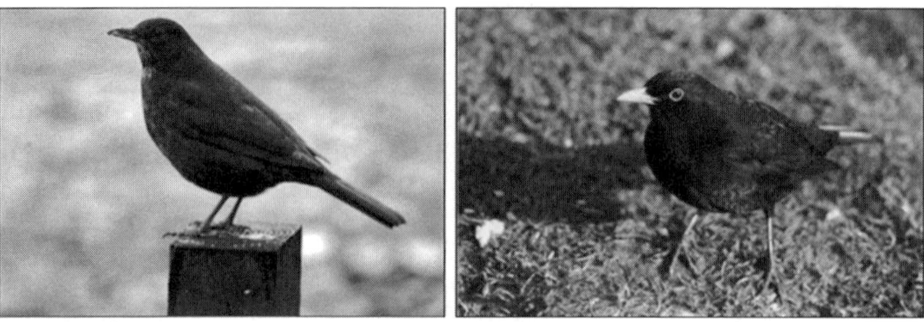

European blackbird, *Turdus merula*

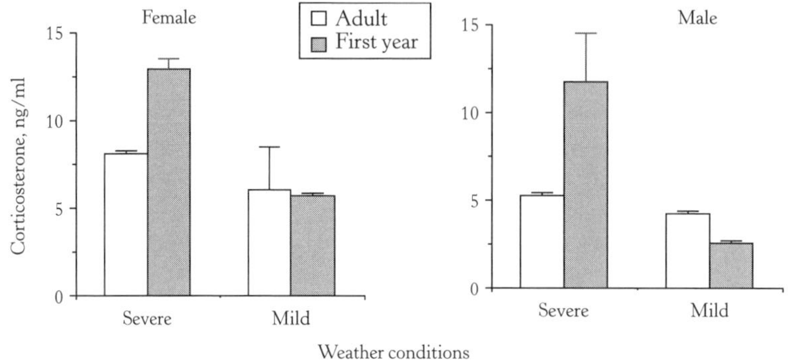

FIGURE 8.12: European blackbirds (female upper left panel, male upper right panel) wintering in southern Germany sometimes must endure severe weather, including snow that covers food resources. Competition for food following snow increases allostatic load to an extent that the less dominant juveniles of both sexes abandon home ranges and migrate further south to less severe conditions. These juveniles have higher baseline levels of corticosterone than adults that do not leave.

From Schwabl et al. (1985). Photos by John C. Wingfield.

Coyotes in Yellowstone National Park, Wyoming, reduce time spent hunting as snow depth and hardness of the snow surface increase, and temperatures decrease (Gese et al. 1996). Freezing rain can cover all terrestrial surfaces with ice, sometimes 1 centimeter or more thick, and the resultant ice crust can prevent many animals from foraging. Freezing rain is widespread throughout mid- to high latitudes and occurs when warm moist air releases rain and drizzle onto surfaces that are still well below freezing (Cortinas et al. 2004). Often, ice coating from freezing rain lasts only a few hours, but if these conditions persist, as in arctic regions, then there can be dramatic effects on wildlife. Caribou and reindeer populations are declining across the Holarctic region, possibly as a result of increased frequency of weather extremes, including ice that reduces access to food (Vors and Boyce 2009). These animals have to dig strenuously or even may show facultative migrations to avoid such extreme conditions. Wild reindeer in Norway showed no behavioral responses to weather in summer.

Norwegian reindeer calves show greater mortality after severe winters when they were in utero. Females may have been stressed by winter weather, resulting in smaller young in poorer condition (Weladji and Holand 2003). In a semi-domesticated herd of reindeer in Finnish Lapland, icing conditions that made access to forage difficult occurred about every seven years, resulting in decreased reproductive rate (calves per female) by almost 50%. Delayed snow melt also decreased reproductive rate (Helle and Kojola 2008). Global warming is resulting in more extremes of weather, including unseasonal freezing rain, deeper snow, and so on (Vors and Boyce 2009; Wingfield et al. 2011). For example, a catastrophic die-off of caribou on Peary Island, high arctic Canada, was associated with severe winter snow and ice conditions (Miller and Gunn 2003). Too much summer heat can also be a problem, because increased snow melt will increase insect densities, which can inhibit normal foraging behavior in reindeer (Hagemoen and Reimers 2002). Furthermore, reindeer foraging efficiency appears to decrease with increasing snow hardness. Their ability to paw through hard snow and form "craters" that allow access to forage beneath can be decreased fourfold with a threefold increase in hardness (Collins and Smith 1991). This suggests clearly that allostatic load increases sharply with snow hardness. Experimental studies of metabolic rate in black-tailed deer showed that these animals were more susceptible to precipitation and colder temperatures during summer than in winter (Parker 1988).

In semi-captive red deer near Vienna, Austria, fecal levels of cortisol metabolites peaked in the winter months, December and January. Furthermore, peak cortisol metabolites coincided with minimum temperatures and snow cover (Huber et al. 2003). Authors interpreted this as high corticosteroids helping the deer adapt to the coldest winter months.

G. Arrival of Migrant Birds in Arctic and Alpine Habitats

The majority of birds breeding in the Arctic migrate and spend the winter well below the Arctic Circle (Pielou 1994; Piersma 1994). In spring they must arrive on the tundra breeding grounds as early as possible to establish a breeding territory and initiate nesting (Hahn et al. 1995; O'Reilly and Wingfield 1995). Arrival in the Arctic in early spring can be challenging because of the unpredictable spring weather (Hahn et al. 1995; O'Reilly and Wingfield 1995). Timing of the annual spring snow melt can vary by as much as a month in arctic and alpine habitats, profoundly influencing when birds can settle and begin breeding. Severe storms and accompanying snow can occur at any time. On the other hand, ground temperatures can vary from below freezing to 45°C or more in direct sun, resulting in a complex and diverse array of local environmental conditions (see also Wingfield et al. 2004). The onset of breeding in alpine zones also generally occurs after snow melt and higher temperatures, but here also late storms can delay breeding in some years and reduce the possibility for re-nesting if the first clutch is lost (Martin and Wiebe 2004). In years when conditions result in late onset of breeding, reproductive success tends to be reduced. Because global warming may result in greater variation in extremes of weather events, alpine and arctic breeding species may be even more vulnerable to inclement weather during breeding (Martin and Wiebe 2004).

The problems facing arctic and alpine breeding birds at arrival in spring include the following (after Wingfield et al. 2004):

1. Migrant birds arrive in spring when conditions are still severe compared with wintering grounds far to the south.
2. Food supply early in the season is unpredictable.
3. The breeding season in arctic and alpine regions is brief, and individuals must initiate nesting immediately, despite severe conditions.
4. Even when nesting has begun, they must "resist" acute stressors such as inclement weather throughout the breeding season.

Arrival dates of many migrants to arctic and alpine breeding grounds tend to be consistent from year to year. However, arctic and alpine snow cover in spring on arrival of migrants can vary from complete in one year to patchy or none in another. Note that migrants cannot predict snow cover conditions until they arrive on the breeding grounds—snow cover on the migrating route provides no predictive help. For example, the snow cover south of the Brooks Range of Alaska in 2002 was 100% when songbirds were migrating, while at the same time snow cover north of the Brooks Range was 0%. However, after arrival in the breeding area there is a high possibility that snowstorms can occur at any time, requiring individuals to seek out microhabitats to shelter (Wingfield et al. 2004).

Depth of snow cover varies dramatically from year to year and in turn determines which areas melt out first and where migrant birds will be able to settle, at least during the early stages of the arrival period (Hahn et al. 1995). Snow depth along ridges scoured free of snow by winds may be only a few centimeters, whereas in valleys snow pack can be drifted to several meters deep in spots, especially in areas with taller vegetation. As spring progresses, the increasing angle of the sun's height above the horizon increases incident radiation (insolation), which can melt snow very rapidly. Darker surfaces of the first ground patches to become snow free absorb more radiant energy, resulting in higher temperatures (as much as 30°–60°C) at ground level compared with the open air (frequently below freezing at this time of year; Wingfield et al. 2004). When insolation is reduced by cloud cover, blocked by a mountain, or a low sun angle late in the day, then temperatures drop rapidly to below freezing (Wingfield et al. 2004). These daily cycles of temperature at ground level can fluctuate widely, but when the ground becomes snow-free it provides microhabitat for migrant birds. Of additional benefit is the observation that accumulation of new snow on these bare patches during late spring storms is greatly reduced compared to existing snow pack (Hahn et al. 1995).

Another environmental challenge facing migrant birds in arctic and alpine habitats is high wind speed that, in conjunction with low temperature, can result in extreme wind chill. Foraging behavior and locomotor movement among patches of food can be restricted, leading to reduced food intake and even potential competition for isolated patches of food. This would clearly increase allostatic load (Figure 8.1). Microhabitats (climates) are important at this time. Wind speed can be greatly attenuated close to the ground in vegetation (by over 90% in most habitats). Thus, despite apparently severe environmental conditions (measured at 1 meter above the ground, for example), local patches of ground that emerge from snow cover are much warmer than air temperature. These local patches provide shelter because of almost complete wind speed attenuation, resulting in greatly reduced wind chill (see Richardson et al. 2003; Martin and Wiebe 2004; Wingfield et al. 2004 for a comparison of arctic and alpine regions). This means that migrant songbirds arriving in arctic and alpine habitats only risk exposure to severe weather conditions when they move from one microhabitat to another over snow-covered areas. That said, some late spring snowstorms can be so severe that wind-blown snow can overwhelm microhabitats. These types of storms may force songbirds into shrinking areas with shelter, and eventually the birds may have to retreat south or to lower elevations (Breuner and Hahn 2003; Wingfield et al. 2004).

Unpredictability of conditions in arctic and alpine habitats during spring arrival of migrants (Figure 8.13) can also occur during the nesting season, and the potential for environmental stress and increased circulating levels of corticosteroids is high (Richardson et al. 2003; Martin and Wiebe 2004). Inclement weather, especially snowfall, in early spring can result in temporary abandonment of territories in mountain white-crowned sparrows breeding in alpine meadows of the Sierra Nevada mountains of California (Figures 8.13 and 8.14; Breuner and Hahn 2003; Hahn et al. 2004). Radio-tagged birds were shown to retreat down the mountain to refugia in more temperate zones when weather worsened, although there was variation in terms of individuals, gender, and so on (Figures 8.13 and 8.14; Hahn et al. 2004). Birds then returned when the inclement weather passed. Experimental implants of corticosterone into males in early spring delayed return to their alpine territories following an abandonment event compared with controls. Curiously, treatment with corticosterone had no effect on abandonment of the territory in fair weather, but did increase activity around the territory (Breuner and Hahn 2003). The adrenocortical response to stress was inversely related to body condition, suggesting that birds in poorer condition are more likely to move down the mountain to refugia during bad weather (Breuner and Hahn 2003).

Severe snowstorms with high winds and below freezing temperatures can occur at any time in the breeding season in the arctic and alpine habitats (Richardson et al. 2003; Martin and Wiebe 2004; Wingfield et al. 2004). Such storms have the potential to disrupt the breeding season, even resulting in complete reproductive failure. In a field study of Lapland longspurs on the North Slope of Alaska, a snowstorm lasting three days covered nests while females were incubating eggs (Figure 8.15; Astheimer et al. 1995). Females excavated holes in the snow, covering their nests so they could leave temporarily to find food while also being attentive to the nest. Because snow cover and low environmental temperatures during the storm decreased efficiency of feeding, females used stored fat to allow them to continue incubating while feeding less. After three days of the storm, fat stores were depleted and females abandoned their nests, forming wide-ranging foraging flocks with males. Adrenocortical responses to capture, handling, and restraint were greatly increased in both males and females compared to birds sampled before the storm (Figure 8.15; Astheimer et al. 1995). Female Lapland longspurs were able to tolerate allostatic overload type 1 for a few days using fat stores (see also Goymann and Wingfield 2004; Wingfield 2004) to substitute for reduced Eg (Figure 8.1). However, energetic requirements during such a severe and prolonged storm exceeded the ability of fat stores to substitute for Eg. Increasing levels of corticosterone resulting from allostatic overload type 1 eventually resulted in an emergency life-history stage and termination of nesting (Astheimer et al. 1995).

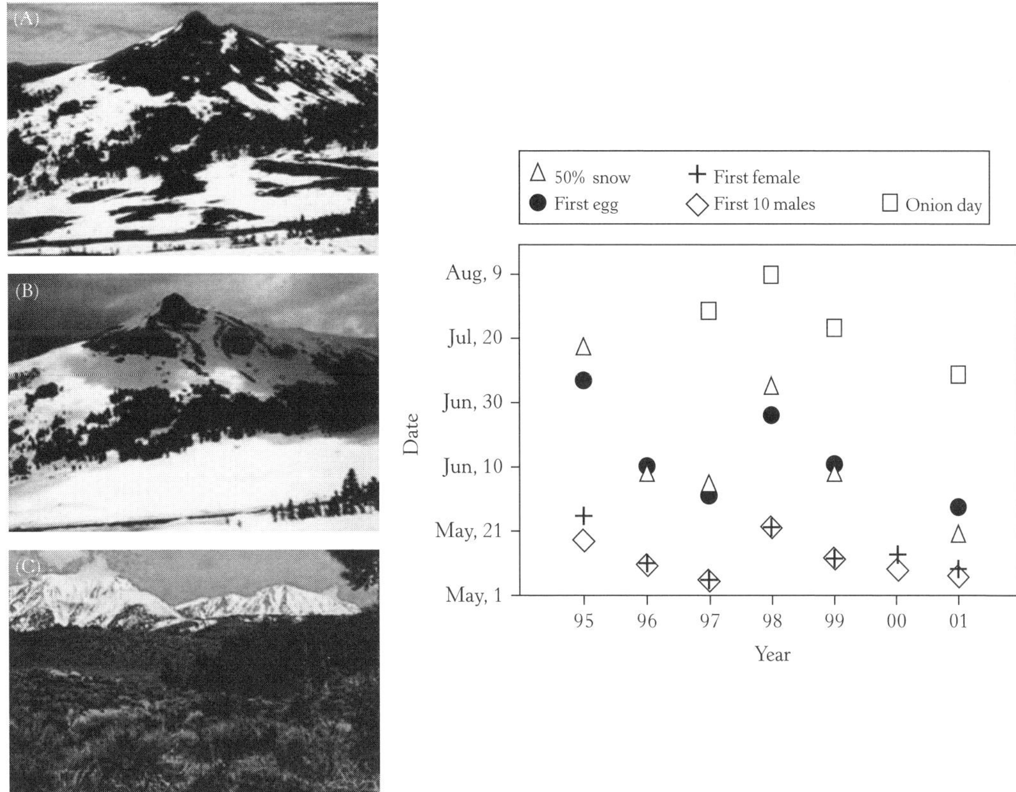

FIGURE 8.13: Left-hand panel: (A) Photograph of the main study area at Tioga Pass (3,000 m elevation) taken on June 1, 1997, a relatively light snow year. Note snow-free patches, which include subalpine willows and scrub pines; the first egg of the season was laid on that day. Snow melt was proceeding rapidly, and 50% snow cover was reached four days after the photograph was taken (June 5). (B) Same view of Tioga Pass as in A, on June 7, 1998, a heavy snow year. Note that subalpine willow and scrub-pine nesting sites are still almost entirely covered with snow remaining from winter. The strip of snow-free area across the bottom of the photograph is highway 120 (plowed). The first egg was not laid until June 26—more than three weeks later than in 1997, and 50% snow cover was not reached until July 6, a full month later than in 1997. (C) Low-elevation refuge habitat at the base of the eastern slope of the Sierra, a few kilometers east of Tioga Pass (2,200 m elevation), photographed on June 6, 1995, a very heavy snow year. Note that deciduous trees, such as quaking aspen (*Populus tremuloides*), are already in full leaf; snow cover at Tioga Pass was still 100% when the photograph was taken, and 50% snow cover was not reached until July 18. Site shown was used repeatedly by one female mountain white-crowned sparrow during snowstorms in spring 1995.

Right-hand panel: Relationship between two parameters indicative of environmental phenology ("onion day" and "date of 50% snow cover") and both arrival schedule and initiation of egg laying in Tioga Pass mountain white-crowned sparrows in seven years. Not all data are available for all years. Arrival schedule is plotted as date when tenth male was caught or when first female was caught (confidence in first female arrival is greater than for first male, owing to some males already being present when trapping began in some years). Egg-laying dates plotted represent date of first egg in the earliest nest on the main study area. Date of 50% snow cover is based on biweekly estimates of percentage of snow cover on the main study area, made consistently from the same elevated viewing point on the western slope above the main study area. Onion day represents the day when large patches of wild onions (*Allium* sp.) on the main study area are first judged to be in full bloom.

From Hahn et al. (2004) with permission and courtesy of the American Ornithologists' Union.

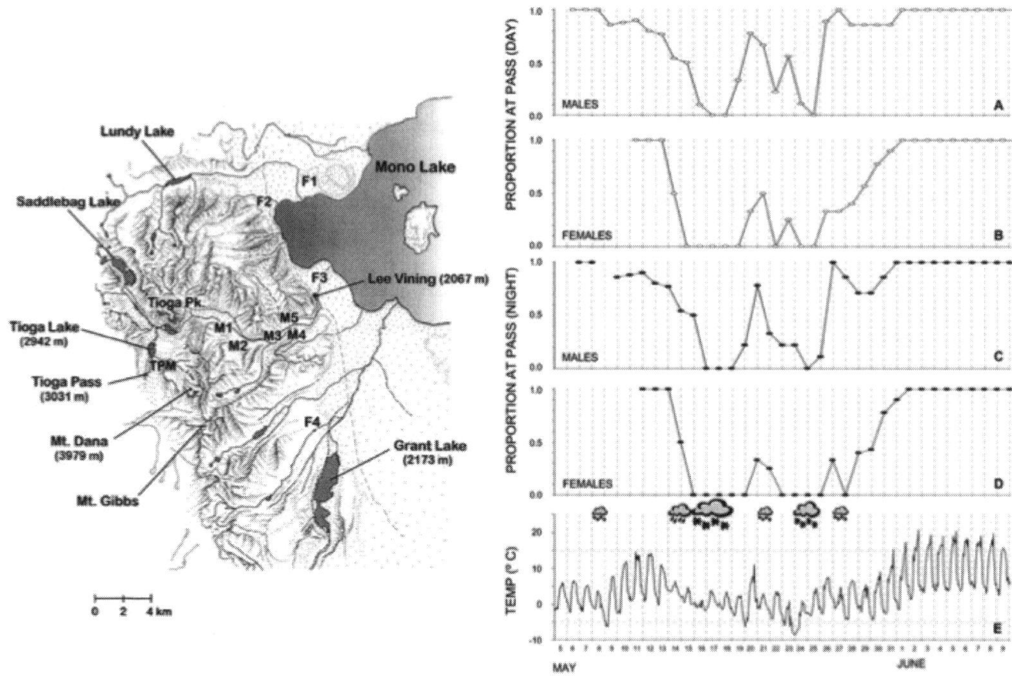

FIGURE 8.14: Left-hand panel: Map of low-elevation refugia positions in 1995, the year of the study with the heaviest residual winter snowpack. Females are indicated by F1–F4, and males by M1–M5. Sites plotted are those used repeatedly by each individual.

(TPM = Tioga Pass Meadow).

Right-hand panel: Prevalence of radiotagged mountain white-crowned sparrows at Tioga Pass during May and early June 1996, as functions of ambient temperature and weather at Tioga Pass. Top two panels (A and B: open circles) plot proportions of males and females at Tioga Pass during the day; next two panels (C and D: opaque circles) plot proportions spending the night there. Bottom panel (E) plots ambient temperature measured hourly in a cluster of pines in the middle of the study area. Rain and snow clouds indicate periods of adverse weather, overall size of clouds reflects general severity of storms, and widths of clouds span dates of precipitation. Numbers of radio-marked males were 1 on May 6, 4 on May 7, and 7–13 on all remaining dates plotted. Numbers of radio-marked females were 1 on May 11–12, 2 on May 13–19, and 3–10 on all remaining dates plotted.

From Hahn et al. (2004), with permission and courtesy of the American Ornithologists' Union.

H. Wind and Rain

Extremes of temperature and precipitation can have profound influences on the behavior and physiology of free-living birds (Wingfield and Ramenofsky 2011). If these conditions are combined with high wind, conditions can be severely exacerbated. High winds are frequently deleterious for foraging in many birds (Figure 8.16). The osprey feeds almost entirely on fish that it catches from the air over rivers, lakes, and coastal regions (Machmer and Ydenberg 1990). In Figure 8.16, we have modified a figure from Machmer and Ydenberg (1990) along the lines of allostatic load. The energy to be gained (in kJ, Eg) from the average size of fish captured can be estimated. The authors were also able to estimate wind speed on different days, and from this calculated the energy needed to fly out and catch fish (a measure of allostatic load, Ee + Ei + Eo, Figures 8.1 and 8.16). At high wind speeds, the energy expended in catching a fish exceeds that to be gained from the average fish capture, and the osprey enters allostatic overload type 1. At this point we would predict that the osprey would cease foraging and wait until conditions improved.

The opposite may be true for seabirds that rely on wind for dynamic soaring to forage successfully. Indeed some oceanic species may be unable to fly in calm conditions. There is a considerable literature on the effects of wind, frequently in combination with rain, but few studies have been conducted on mechanisms of coping in this type of weather (reviewed in Wingfield and Ramenofsky 2011).

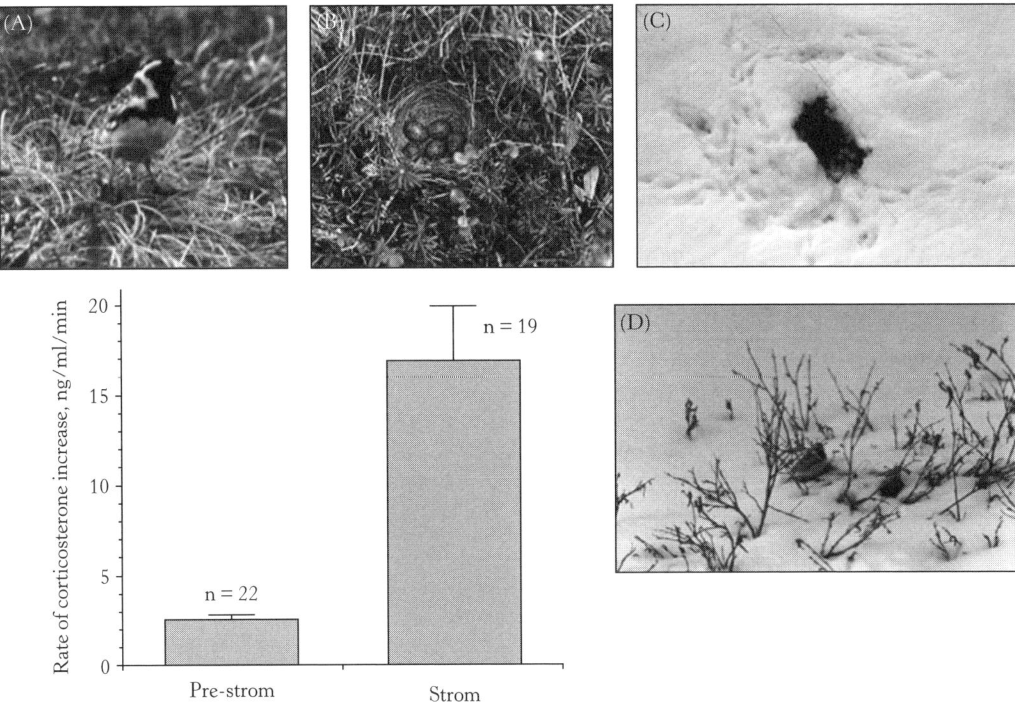

FIGURE 8.15: Lapland longspurs (panel A) breed throughout Arctic tundra regions. They nest on the ground (panel B), but when severe snowstorms occur, nests are frequently buried and females excavate holes through which they can leave to forage and then return to incubate (panel C). However, if snow cover persists for more than 3 days, the combination of high allostatic load of feeding in snow cover while also trying to incubate coupled with low Eg results in eventual abandonment of the nest and foraging over a wide area (panel D). At this time the adrenocortical response to capture stress was greatly enhanced in birds after abandonment of the nest (storm) compared to incubating birds before the storm (lower left panel).

From Astheimer et al. (1995) courtesy of Elsevier. Photos by Lee B. Astheimer, Bill Buttemer, and John C. Wingfield.

As has been reviewed for animals in extreme heat or cold, white-crowned and golden-crowned sparrows foraging in winter flocks in western Oregon favored microhabitats when possible (DeWoskin 1980). Increasing wind speed and decreasing temperature and solar radiation combined to elevate metabolic rate by as much as 20% in exposed, open flat field areas compared with more sheltered hedge rows. Sparrows often faced into the wind, when foraging activities allowed, favoring "streamlining and reduced resistance" (DeWoskin 1980). Other field investigations reveal how low temperature and high wind velocity affect the foraging behavior of forest birds in winter. Allostatic load tends to increase with wind speed, especially higher in trees near the canopy. In more severe conditions, birds may be forced to forage in less productive parts of the tree, such as near the trunk or in lower shrubs. Violent movements of higher and smaller branches in wind prohibit foraging in canopy-feeding birds (Grubb 1975; see also Wingfield and Ramenofsky 2011 for review). Furthermore, wind speed tends to be highest at the upper storey of the canopy and attenuated markedly at lower levels. These data suggest that in high winds, the lower storey of trees has less violent branch and twig movements and wind chill is also less. However, foraging conditions may be less rich, meaning that although allostatic load is reduced, Eg is lower (Wingfield and Ramenofsky 2011).

Canopy-feeding songbirds, and bark-feeding downy woodpeckers and white-breasted nuthatches, moved away from the windward edge of woodlots as wind speeds increased and temperatures declined (Dolby and Grubb 1999). Similar results were obtained in canopy-feeding songbirds foraging in wind and rain in western Washington State and in southern beech forests of New Zealand (Wingfield and Ramenofsky 2011). Furthermore, house sparrows frequented feeders with the most shelter, or reduced

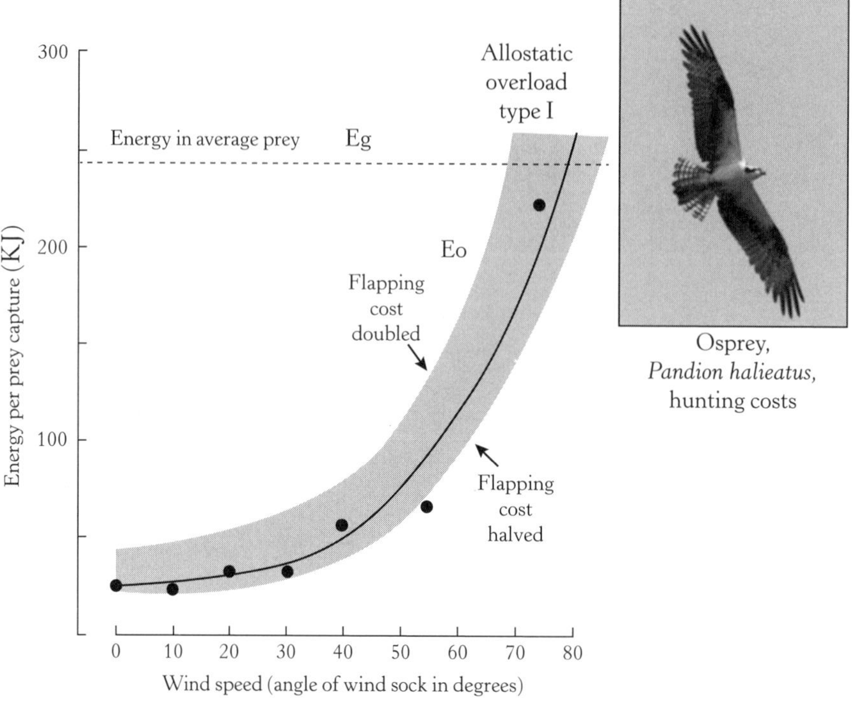

FIGURE 8.16: Osprey hunting energetics in relation to wind speed. The horizontal line shows the energy value of an average prey item (242 kJ). The data points in the figure show the estimates of energy needed to capture a prey item in each wind speed category, and the smooth function is a polynomial fitted to these points. The upper and lower boundaries of the shaded region show the effects of doubling and halving, respectively, the estimate of flapping power. The detrimental effects of weather increase sharply at wind speeds above 6.2 m/s, so that above about 7 m/s, the male's cost of capturing a fish exceeds the energetic gain.

From Machmer and Ydenberg (1990), Courtesy of NRC Press.

energetic cost, due to wind and cold (Grubb and Greenwald 1982).

Wind and temperature are important factors affecting the foraging of shorebirds on very exposed mud flats (Evans 1976). Wind tends to blow birds over, thereby increasing energetic demands for prey searching and capture. In black-bellied plovers, foraging efficiency and prey capture rates decreased and heat losses tended to be greater. Additionally, wind disturbs the surface of water, making it more difficult to locate prey (Evans 1976), or wind may dry exposed substrate, thus driving worms and bivalves deeper or back into water. Interactions of wind and tide can also reduce feeding efficiency. Wind and tide can exacerbate wave action dramatically and disturb the substrate, making feeding more difficult (Evans 1976), and resulting in individuals being forced to feed at the tide line, where competition with others becomes greater (Evans 1976). In general, inclement weather is accompanied by greatly increased energetic costs (allostatic load) for birds and other animals feeding in very exposed and flat environments.

On the other hand, there may often be an optimum wind speed. Low wind speeds may be deleterious for fishing success of common terns and Sandwich terns in shallow coastal seas (Dunn 1973). Calm, low wind speed conditions reduced fishing success probably because the terns had to work harder to hover and locate fish. Conversely, very windy conditions with waves obscured visual location of fish (Dunn 1973). On the other hand, increasing wind speed had no effect on foraging success or the rates of hovering and percentage of successful dives in the fish-eating osprey. However, a combination of cloudy weather and wind-induced rippling of the water surface reduced capture rates possibly because of reduced visibility of fish underwater (Grubb 1977). In contrast, Machmer and Ydenberg (Grubb 1977, 1990) found that wind speed and water surface conditions were the most important factors reducing foraging success of ospreys. All these factors tend to increase allostatic load (Figure 8.16).

Other examples in diverse habitats further illustrate how the allostatic load framework provides a potential common pathway for triggering an emergency life-history stage in response to weather events. Pelagic seabirds thrive in severe weather typical of many mid- and high-latitude oceans. Calm conditions may render some of the larger albatrosses unable to fly. Thus, pleasant calm weather is a labile perturbation factor for oceanic birds! Nonetheless, extremely severe gales can have debilitative effects on foraging seabirds (e.g., Elkins 1983), and seabird "wrecks" occur in which hundreds to thousands of individuals may be blown inland or wash up on beaches in a moribund state. The common diving petrel of the Southern Ocean may be an exception because under extreme weather conditions it can retreat to islands for shelter. They generally remain on oceanic waters within flying distance of their breeding grounds and will come to land during winter (Richdale 1945). They tend to be sighted closer to the islands on the windiest days and almost not sighted at all on less windy days. In June 1991 a severe storm near the South Georgia archipelago, with high winds, low temperatures, snow, and near zero visibility, reduced feeding efficiency (Veit et al. 1991), potentially accompanied by increased Eo (Figures 8.1 and 8.16). Body mass of common diving petrels captured during the storm was lower than those captured during calm weather. Moreover, plasma levels of corticosterone were higher during the storm when birds were observed moving toward nearby islands such as Annekov—a breeding locality and where burrows presumably provide shelter (Figure 8.17; Smith et al. 1994). These responses to severe weather conditions are remarkably similar to those of ground-feeding passerines in snow described earlier, and furthermore the responses of corticosterone secretion appear identical.

Aerial insectivorous species such as barn swallows are especially vulnerable to inclement weather, especially when breeding. Plasma

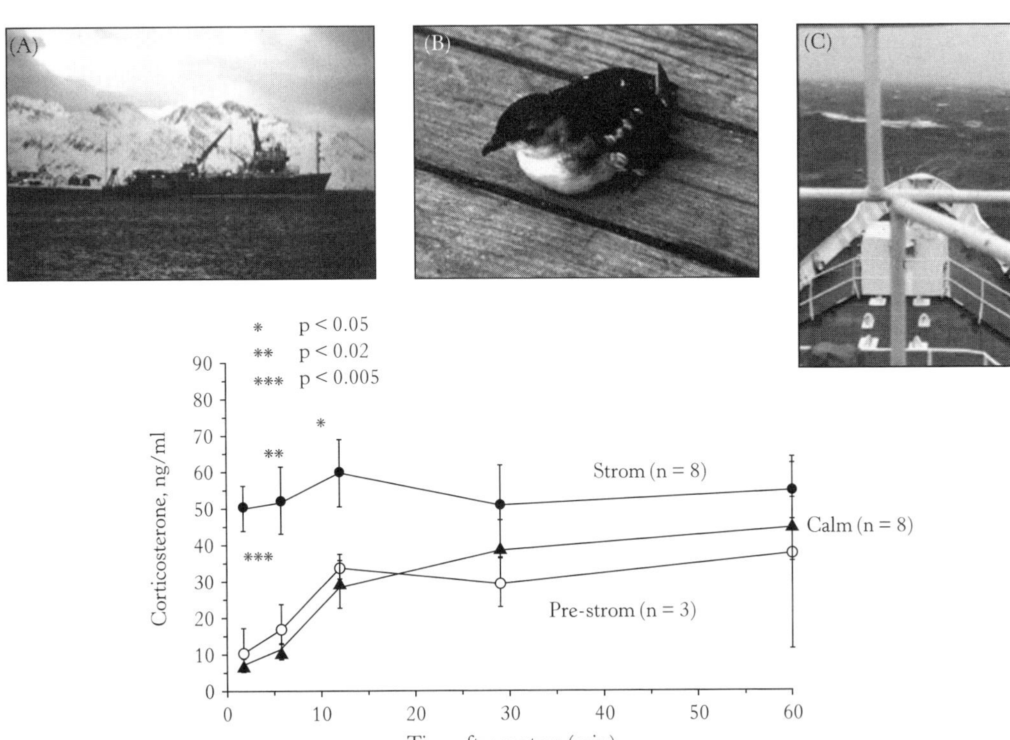

FIGURE 8.17: Plasma levels of corticosterone in common diving petrels (panel B) during calm weather (panel A), and just prior to and during (panel C) a severe storm off the South Georgia Islands. Bars are means and vertical lines the standard errors (lower panel).

Drawn from data in Smith et al. (1994), courtesy of University of Chicago Press.

Photos by Professor Troy Smith with permission.

corticosterone levels of free-living parents feeding young increased as mean daytime air temperature declined. Availability of flying insects declined, thus decreasing Eg (Jenni-Eiermann et al. 2008). The body condition of parent swallows deteriorated, and low temperature had a negative effect on the weights of nestlings (Jenni-Eiermann et al. 2008). Similar results were found during inclement weather in colonies of breeding cliff swallows; when flying insect numbers declined precipitously, corticosterone levels increased (Figure 8.18; Raouf et al. 2006). This effect was magnified in swallow colonies that were infested with blood-sucking parasites compared to colonies that had been experimentally fumigated to eliminate these parasites (Raouf et al. 2006). However, swallows with either very high or very low corticosterone levels in blood also had lower annual survival rates than birds with intermediate levels (Brown et al. 2005a). Furthermore, those with higher circulating concentrations of corticosterone that did survive tended to switch to other colonies when they returned the following year (Brown et al. 2005b).

I. Coping with a River in Spate

The effects of high water flows (spates) on fishes in rivers and streams can be dramatic, and there is an increasing interest in the impacts of such events for conservation and management purposes. Some spate events are natural, and others are anthropogenic. High flow rates can be a result of storms with copious rainfall as well as from release of water from upstream dams. Curiously, the effects of spates on other riverine vertebrates such as amphibians, stream specialist birds, and mammals are much less well known. The responses of fish to high water flow rates is highly variable, probably due to complex habitat configuration in rivers and streams, as well as because of highly variable ways in which investigators collect data and analyze them (Murchie et al. 2008).

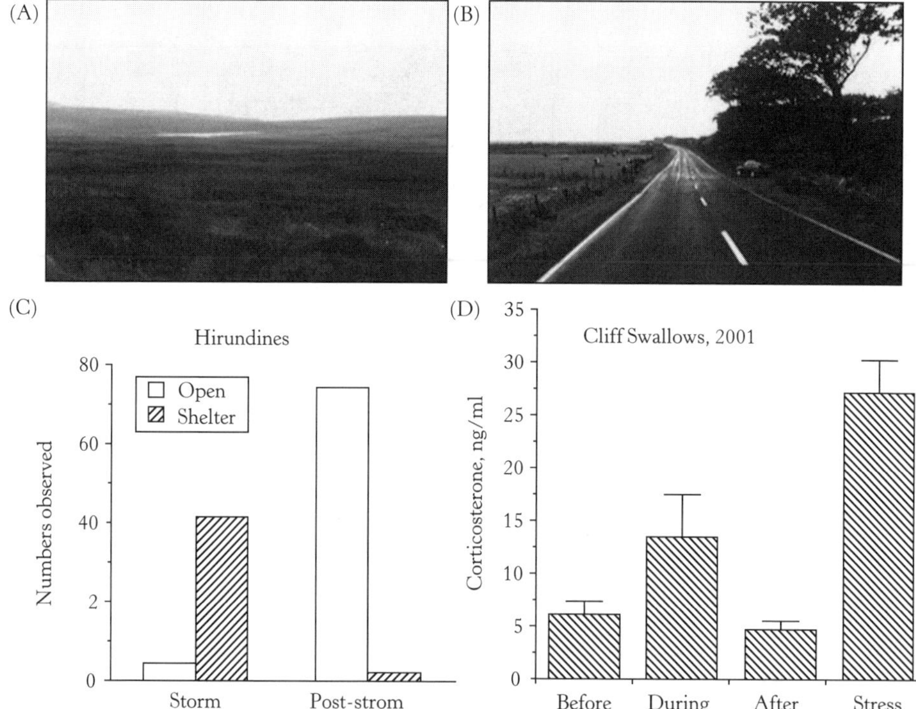

FIGURE 8.18: Swallows (Hirundines) feed exclusively on flying insects. Panel A shows a swath of Scottish moorland that many Hirundines use to catch flying midges and other insects. When inclement weather prevails, flying insect numbers drop to almost zero in such exposed areas and Hirundines are forced to congregate in sheltered areas on the lee side of copses (panel B) and similar shelter. Sometimes 50+ birds may be competing for flying insects in a sheltered area only 100 x 50 meters (panel C). In panel D, plasma levels of corticosterone were higher in cliff swallows during inclement weather, but not as high as in response to the acute stress of capture, handling, and restraint.

From Raouf et al. (2006); Wingfield and Ramenofsky (2011), with permission, courtesy of Elsevier Press. Photos by J. C. Wingfield.

Juvenile white sturgeons are potentially vulnerable to high water flow rates in rivers. Experiments on captive fish showed that increased water flow, and thus swimming speed to counteract flow, elevated oxygen consumption (Geist et al. 2005). However, electromyograms and radio tracking showed that free-living juvenile sturgeons sought shelter areas such as eddies to reduce swimming speed and thus energy expenditure (Geist et al. 2005). These data suggest that behavioral responses to high water flow rates are important coping mechanisms.

Male lake trout were fitted with radio-transmitters in a mountain river in Switzerland. The fish continued their upstream migration despite a spate in which flow rates increased from below 20 to over 90 m^3/S^{-1} (Monet and Soares 2001). However, not all species continue migrating in the face of high flow rates. In a similar radio-transmitter study of rainbow trout, individuals in the Tongariro River of New Zealand moved upstream regardless of minor changes in flow rate. However, a large flood resulted in downstream displacement. Once flow rates declined in the river, fish resumed their upstream migrations (Dedual and Jowett 1999). Similarly, in a stream in Southeast Alaska, both dollyvardens and cutthroat trout tend to move upstream in spring through summer. However, that movement can be blunted by high stream flow rates (Bryant et al. 2009).

Benthic algae form an important food base for many animals living in rivers, especially fish. Diatom communities in the benthos appear to be well adapted to storms, especially in gravel beds of temperate zone streams (Stevenson 1990). Storms can actually result in positive effects on algal communities, and only in the most severe, stream-bed-scouring storms are these communities affected adversely. On the other hand, increasing frequency and intensity of spate events tends to introduce greater variability in lotic ecosystems (Biggs et al. 2005) that could have important implications for food available for fish and for coping with those spates. Atlantic salmon juveniles in New Brunswick, Canada, are exposed to severe spates every two years or so. Curiously, feeding rates did not appear to be affected by a severe spate, probably because they were using sheltered areas. However, growth rates did decline during and after spates (Arndt et al. 2002). Truly massive floods, often accompanied by a debris flow of trees displaced from banks and large rocks, can have catastrophic effects on stream and rivers beds. Scouring can be extremely extensive, sometimes completely changing the stream characteristics (Roghair et al. 2002). Such a major flood in a river in Virginia in June 1995 completely depleted a population of brook trout compared to other areas of the river where the spate was less severe and the debris flow was decreased. The latter part of the river also had reduced densities of fish, but they were not eliminated. By 1998 the river had been re-colonized (Roghair et al. 2002).

Radio-tagged giant kokopu, a New Zealand fish, were followed before, during, and after spates. Some fish remained in their home range, some moved downstream and then returned after the spate, whereas yet others moved and then remained where they had settled (David and Closs 2002). During the height of a spate, fish tended to seek out refuges where water flow was greatly reduced by piles of debris or eddies formed by undercut banks. Fish moved to other areas of the stream, mostly at night, but otherwise stayed in low water velocity habitats until the spate subsided (Figure 8.19; David and Closs 2002).

Complex habitat configuration in rivers is important for fish to cope with fall and winter conditions such as floods. Radio-tagged cutthroat trout in rivers and streams with areas of large woody debris moved less than those with open channels. In the absence of woody debris, trout preferred areas with boulders and other shelter/eddy areas. During flood conditions, fish avoided open channels and congregated just downstream of woody debris piles and boulders (Harvey et al. 1999). A stream system in Poland is subject to occasional severe flooding after water release from a dam. Fish sheltered behind woody debris and boulder piles during high flows (Godlewska et al. 2003). They also found that both zoo- and phytoplankton populations declined markedly, requiring up to two weeks to recover (Godlewska et al. 2003). These data suggest that not only must fish find shelters during high water flows, but it may be a number of days before food levels return to normal for the time of year. This raises new significance for recovery mechanisms.

Radio-telemeters in chub in the upper Rhone Valley indicated that sheltering habitat such as clusters of boulders and woody debris are important for coping with intermittent floods caused by water release from a hydroelectric dam upstream (Allouche et al. 1999). In contrast, a population of cyprinid fish, the barbell, in British rivers showed less movement related to water flow compared to other species (Lucas and Batley 1996).

Native fishes in Arizona streams subject to severe seasonal flooding showed behavioral

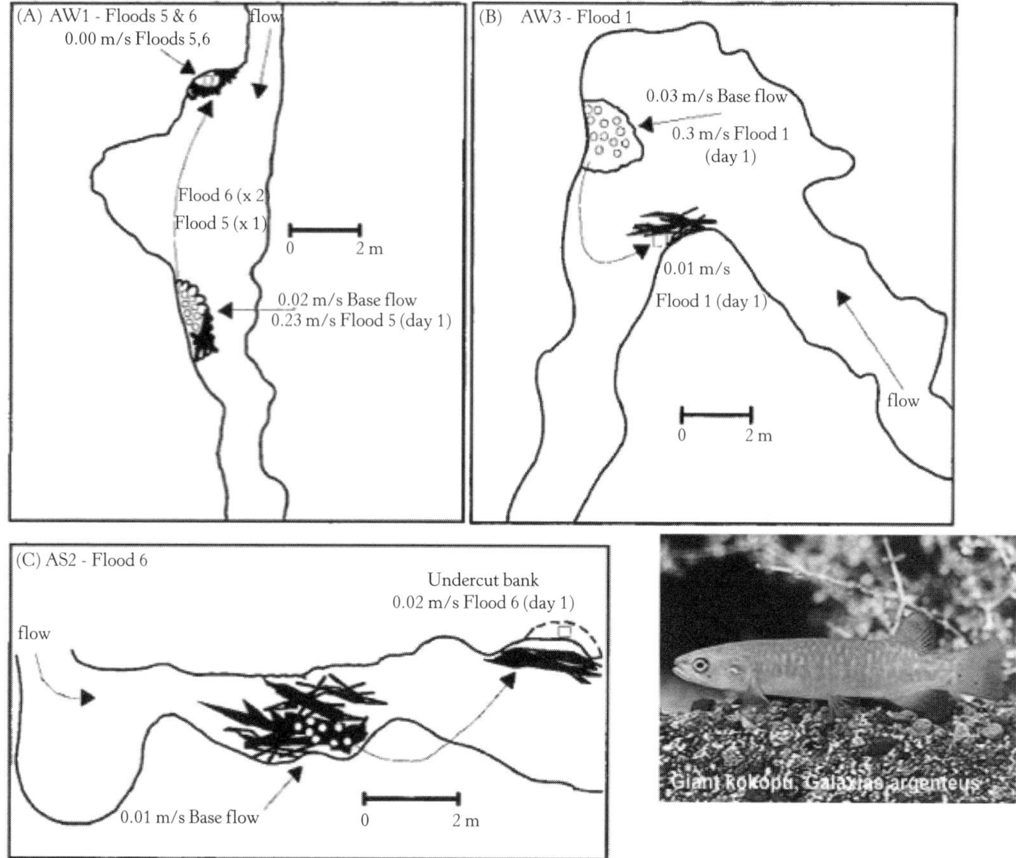

FIGURE 8.19: Micro-moves made by (A) fish AW1, (B) fish AW3, and (C) fish AS2, during various floods. Flow and movement of fish from their regular cover position (circles) to the refuge location (squares) are indicated. Fish AW1 used the refuge location two times (3 2) in flood 6 and one time (3 1) in flood 5.

From David and Closs (2002). Photo courtesy of the Department of Conservation, Government of New Zealand. Figure courtesy of The American Fisheries Society.

responses that facilitate coping with high water flow rates (Ward et al. 2003). In captive studies in which water flow rates were experimentally increased, suckers use mouth suction on the substrate to maintain position and relieve strong swimming activity, whereas speckled dace used pectoral fins as a prop to withstand high flow rates. In both cases these behavioral responses helped reduce active swimming in high flow rates, thus reducing energetic costs. These behaviors also allowed them to withstand higher water flow rates than introduced species (Ward et al. 2003). Such behaviors may be widespread in other species that regularly cope with floods.

Hurricane Iniki devastated much of the Island of Kaua'i in 1992. Streams were exposed to severe flash floods, and native fish such as *Eleotris sandwichensis* and *Stenogobius hawaiiensis* were absent in some streams. Another species, *Sicypterus stimpsoni*, was concentrated into downstream areas where aggression and reduced food availability resulted in decreased condition and absence of courtship behavior (Fitzsimons and Nishimoto 1995).

Investigations of hormonal responses of fish to spates are very sparse, and much more information is needed. River sediments suspended in water can result from spates, or from erosion and other factors. Experiments in which increasing sediment in water was used to simulate river conditions resulted in increases in whole body cortisol levels in whitetail shiners and spotfin chub from Appalachian rivers (Sutherland et al. 2008). So, not only flow rates, debris movement, and decreased food accompany floods, but turbidity can also be stressful. Following present-day land use practices, many river drainages experience spates of greater frequency and intensity. In general the diversity of fish species and biotic resources to sustain them were lower in streams that received higher frequencies of spate events (Helms et al. 2009).

Other potential stressors can also be associated with spates. Brown trout frequently form dominance hierarchies, particularly in stable environments such as fish tanks. However, when flow rate was experimentally increased to simulate a spate, the dominance hierarchies broke down and dominant fish failed to show continued higher growth rates than subordinates (Sloman et al. 2002). There were no differences in cortisol plasma levels between fish exposed to high flow rates versus controls, despite a change in hierarchies and reduced growth rates. In a final example, guppies in Trinidad that are heavily parasitized by worms show dramatically reduced recapture rates, but heavy rains in the wet season somehow decreased parasite load (van Oosterhout et al. 2007). Clearly many aspects of a spate could act as stressors, and further work is needed to determine whether stress mediators are involved in successful coping with these conditions.

III. CONCLUSIONS

The evidence is clear that weather has profound influences on behavior and that facultative physiological and endocrine mechanisms have evolved to cope with this type of environmental perturbation. It is also clear that many other factors, such as territory or home range quality, access to shelter and food, social status, body condition, parasite infection and injuries, all contribute to allostatic load, the daily expenditure required to go about daily and seasonal routines (Figure 8.1). Human disturbance through exploitation of natural resources, urbanization, pollution, and global climate change is an additional source of extreme environmental modification, and it is not surprising that many organisms are struggling to cope. The concept of allostasis, allostatic load, and allostatic overload provides a framework to understand how individuals must endure daily and seasonal routines, along with added wear and tear from unpredictable events, throughout their life cycles. The reactive scope model will allow us to predict how mediators of coping strategies should respond. So many factors can contribute to how an individual may respond to an identical event that no one individual experiences the environment in exactly the same way as another, and we must understand coping mechanisms at the individual level. Responses to weather are no exception.

A. Coping Mechanisms for Weather versus Climate

It is critically important to distinguish between climate, the ambient conditions averaged over many years, from current weather to which an individual is exposed (see also chapter 1). The latter requires facultative responses during and immediately after the event. The former is part of the predictable life cycle involving changing seasons. These, too, are changing as global climate change progresses, but that is a topic for a later chapter. Organisms time life-history stages, such as breeding, to occur at optimal times for reproductive success. Only when weather events push environmental variables beyond the climatic norm for a particular time of year are allostatic overload and stress likely. Increases in corticosteroid secretion occur in parallel, resulting in activation of the emergency life-history stage and appropriate coping strategies. Climatic events that change the timing of life-history stages such as breeding and migration act within the norms of seasonality in relation to phenology without necessarily any corticosteroid-related stress effects. As climate changes, there will be selection for those individuals that can adjust the timing of life-history stages to changing phenology. Others may not be able to do so.

Weather events are short-lived (hours to days), after which the normal life-history stage can be resumed quickly. Evidence is gathering that the intensity and duration of the weather event are proportional to allostatic load. As the frequency and intensity of weather events rise, then the potential for allostatic overload type 1 looms greater. Coping strategies allow individuals to survive short-lived perturbations in the best condition possible, but what will happen if these events occur more and more regularly?

It is becoming clear that elevated circulating levels of corticosteroids in response to unpredictable and potentially deleterious environmental events such as inclement weather are a common feature in diverse ecological contexts and in several taxa studied to date. Furthermore, increased circulating levels of corticosteroids in organisms responding to these labile perturbation factors are independent of season and habitat, although the degree to which the adrenocortical responses to stress are activated (reactive scope) does change. Opportunistic field observations, coupled with experimental evidence for the actions of corticosteroids in many physiological and behavioral changes associated with responses to the unpredictable, suggest common mechanisms across vertebrates. However, because the number of species studied is limited, and the spectrum of habitats and unpredictable events for which samples are available is still rather small, we should be cautious in generalizing too far.

REFERENCES

Adolph, S. C., 1990. Influence of behavioral thermoregulation on microhabitat use by 2 sceloporus lizards. *Ecology 71*, 315–327.

Allouche, S., Thevenet, A., Gaudin, P., 1999. Habitat use by chub (*Leuciscus cephalus L.* 1766) in a large river, the French Upper Rhone, as determined by radiotelemetry. *Archiv Fur Hydrobiologie 145*, 219–236.

Andreev, A. V., 1991a. Winter adaptations in the willow ptarmigan. *Arctic 44*, 106–114.

Andreev, A. V., 1991b. Winter habitat segregation in the sexually dimorphic black-billed Capercaillie Tetrao urogalloides. *Ornis Scan 22*, 287–291.

Andreev, A. V., 1999. Energetics and survival of birds in extreme environments. *Ostrich 70*, 13–22.

Arndt, S. K. A., Cunjak, R. A., Benfey, T. J., 2002. Effect of summer floods and spatial-temporal scale on growth and feeding of juvenile Atlantic salmon in two New Brunswick streams. *Trans Ame Fish Soc 131*, 607–622.

Astheimer, L. B., Buttemer, W. A., Wingfield, J. C., 1995. Seasonal and acute changes in adrenocortical responsiveness in an arctic-breeding bird. *Horm Behav 29*, 442–457.

Barclay, R. M. R., Lausen, C. L., Hollis, L., 2001. What's hot and what's not: Defining torpor in free-ranging birds and mammals. *Can J Zool 79*, 1885–1890.

Bartholomew, G. A., 1964. The roles of physiology and behavior in the maintenance of homeostasis in the desert environment. In: *Homeostasis and Feedback Mechanisms*, 18th Symp. Soc. Exp. Biol., Cambridge University Press, Cambridge, UK, pp. 7–29.

Barton, B. A., Haukenes, A. H., 1999. *Physiological stress and behavioral responses of juvenile walleye associated with handling and transport during stocking operations in South Dakota.* Completion Rep. 00–01. South Dakota Dept. Game, Fish and Parks, Pierre, S. D.

Basu, N., Nakano, T., Grau, E. G., Iwama, G. K., 2001. The effects of cortisol on heat shock protein 70 levels in two fish species. *Gen Comp Endocrinol 124*, 97–105.

Basu, N., Todgham, A. E., Ackerman, P. A., Bibeau, M. R., Nakano, K., Schulte, P. M., Iwama, G. K., 2002. Heat shock protein genes and their functional significance in fish. *Gene 295*, 173–183.

Beehner, J. C., McCann, C., 2008. Seasonal and altitudinal effects on glucocorticoid metabolites in a wild primate (*Theropithecus gelada*). *Physiol Behav 95*, 508–514.

Berkes, F., Jolly, D., 2002. Adapting to climate change: Social-ecological resilience in a Canadian Western Arctic community. *Conserv Ecol 5*, 18.

Biggs, B. J. F., Nikora, V. I., Snelder, T. H., 2005. Linking scales of flow variability to lotic ecosystem structure and function. *River Res Appl 21*, 283–298.

Blaber, S. J. M., 2002. 'Fish in hot water': the challenges facing fish and fisheries research in tropical estuaries. *J Fish Biol 61*, 1–20.

Bókony, V., Lendvai, A. Z., Liker, A., Angelier, F., Wingfield, J. C., Chastel, O., 2009. Stress response and the value of reproduction: are birds prudent parents? *Am Nat 173*, 589–598.

Bossart, G. D., Meisner, R. A., Rommel, S. A., Ghim, S.-J., Jensen, A. B., 2003. Pathological features of the Florida manatee cold stress syndrome. *Aquat Mamm 29*, 9–17.

Braun, C. E., Martin, K., Robb, L. A., 1983. White-tailed ptarmigan (Lagopus leucurus). No. 68. In: Poole, A., Gill, F. (Eds.), *The birds of North America*. Academy of Natural Sciences, Philadephia; American Ornithologists' Union, Washington, DC.

Breuner, C. W., Hahn, T. P., 2003. Integrating stress physiology, environmental change, and behavior in free-living sparrows. *Horm Behav 43*, 115–123.

Brigham, R. H., Kortner, G., Maddocks, T. A., Geiser, F., 2000. Seasonal use of torpor by free-ranging Australian owlet-nightjars (*Aegotheles cristatus*). *Physiol Biochem Zool 73*, 613–620.

Brotons, L., 1997. Changes in foraging behaviour of the Coal Tit Parus ater due to snow cover. *Ardea 85*, 249–257.

Brown, C. R., Brown, M. B., Raouf, S. A., Smith, L. C., Wingfield, J. C., 2005a. Effects of endogenous steroid hormone levels on annual survival in Cliff Swallows. *Ecology (Washington DC) 86*, 1034–1046.

Brown, C. R., Brown, M. B., Raouf, S. A., Smith, L. C., Wingfield, J. C., 2005b. Steroid hormone levels are related to choice of colony size in Cliff Swallows. *Ecology 86*, 2904–2915.

Bruns, E. H., 1977. Winter behavior of pronghorns in relation to habitat. *J Wildlife Manage 41*, 560–571.

Bryant, M. D., Lukey, M. D., McDonell, J. P., Gubernick, R. A., Aho, R. S., 2009. Seasonal movement of dolly varden and cutthroat trout with respect to stream discharge in a second-order stream in southeast Alaska. *N Am J Fish Manage 29*, 1728–1742.

Cain, J. R., Lien, R. J., 1985. A model for drought inhibition of bobwhite quail (*Colinus-Virginianus*) reproductive systems. *Comp Biochem Physiol A 82*, 925–930.

Calder, W. A., King, J. R., 1994. Thermal and caloric relations of birds. In: Farner, D. S., King, J. R. (Eds.), *Avian biology*, vol. *3*. Academic Press, New York, pp. 259–413.

Callaghan, T. V., Bjorn, L. O., Chernov, Y., Chapin, T., Christensen, T. R., Huntley, B., Ims, R. A., Johansson, M., Jolly, D., Jonasson, S., Matveyeva, N., Panikov, N., Oechel, W., Shaver, G., Elster, J., Jonsdottir, I. S., Laine, K., Taulavuori, K., Taulavuori, E., Zockler, C., 2004. Responses to projected changes in climate and UV-B at the species level. *Ambio 33*, 418–435.

Carruth, L. L., Jones, R. E., Norris, D. O., 2002. Cortisol and pacific salmon: A new look at the role of stress hormones in olfaction and home-stream migration. *Integ Comp Biol 42*, 574–581.

Chaplin, S. B., 1982. The energetic significance of huddling behavior in common bushtits (*Psaltriparus minimus*). *Auk 99*, 424–430.

Clarke, J. A., Johnson, R. E., 1992. The influence of spring snow depth on white-tailed ptarmigan breeding success in the Sierra-Nevada. *Condor 94*, 622–627.

Collins, W. B., Smith, T. S., 1991. Effects of wind-hardened snow on foraging by reindeer (Rangifer tarandus). *Arctic 44*, 217–222.

Cortinas, J. V., Bernstein, B. C., Robbins, C. C., Strapp, J. W., 2004. An analysis of freezing rain, freezing drizzle, and ice pellets across the United States and Canada: 1976–90. *Weather Forecast 19*, 377–390.

Csada, R. D., Brigham, R. M., 1992. Common poorwill, *Phalaenoptilus nuttalli*. No. 32. In: Poole, A., Gill, F. (Eds.), *The birds of North America*. Academy of Natural Sciences, Philadelphia; American Ornithologists' Union, Washington, DC.

David, B. O., Closs, G. P., 2002. Behavior of a stream-dwelling fish before, during, and after high-discharge events. *Trans Am Fish Soc 131*, 762–771.

Davidson, N. C., Evans, P. R., 1982. Mortality of redshanks and oystercatchers from starvation during severe weather. *Bird Study 29*, 183–188.

Davis, K. B., Peterson, B. C., 2006. The effect of temperature, stress, and cortisol on plasma IGF-I and IGFBPs in sunshine bass. *Gen Comp Endocrinol 149*, 219–225.

Dawson, R. D., Bortolotti, G. R., 2000. Reproductive success of American Kestrels: The role of prey abundance and weather. *Condor 102*, 814–822.

Dawson, W. R., Carey, C., Vanthof, T. J., 1992. Metabolic aspects of shivering thermogenesis in passerines during winter. *Ornis Scan 23*, 381–387.

de Bruijn, R., Romero, L. M., 2011. Behavioral and physiological responses of wild-caught European starlings (*Sturnus vulgaris*) to a minor, rapid change in ambient temperature. *Comp Biochem Physiol A 160*, 260–266.

Dedual, M., Jowett, I. G., 1999. Movement of rainbow trout (*Oncorhynchus mykiss*) during the spawning migration in the Tongariro River, New Zealand. *N Z J Marine Fresh Res 33*, 107–117.

Denver, R. J., 1997. Proximate mechanisms of phenotypic plasticity in amphibian metamorphosis. *Am Zool 37*, 172–184.

Denver, R. J., 1998. Hormonal correlates of environmentally induced metamorphosis in the Western spadefoot toad, *Scaphiopus hammondii*. *Gen Comp Endocrinol 110*, 326–336.

Deschenes, O., Moretti, E., 2009. Extreme weather events, mortality, and migration. *Rev Econ Stat 91*, 659–681.

DeWoskin, R., 1980. Heat exchange influence on foraging behavior of Zonotrichia flocks. *Ecology 61*, 30–36.

Dolby, A. S., Grubb, T. C., 1999. Effects of winter weather on horizontal vertical use of isolated forest fragments by bark-foraging birds. *Condor 101*, 408–412.

Donaldson, M. R., Cooke, S. J., Patterson, D. A., Macdonald, J. S., 2008. Cold shock and fish. *J Fish Biol 73*, 1491–1530.

Dunn, E. K., 1973. Changes in fishing ability of terns associated with windspeed and sea surface conditions. *Nature 244*, 520–521.

Edwards, J. S., 1987. Arthropods of alpine aeolian ecosystems. *Ann Rev Entomol 32*, 163–179.

Edwards, J. S., Banko, P. C., 1976. Arthropod fallout and nutrient transport: A quantitative study of Alaskan snowpatches. *Arctic Alpine Res 8*, 237–245.

Eeva, T., Lehikoinen, E., Ronka, M., Lummaa, V., Currie, D., 2002. Different responses to cold weather in two pied flycatcher populations. *Ecography 25*, 705–713.

Elkins, N., 1983. *Weather and bird behavior*. Poyser Press, Calton, UK.

Ettinger, A. O., King, J. R., 1980. Time and energy budgets of the willow flycatcher (*Empidonax traillii*) during the breeding season. *Auk 97*, 533–546.

Evans, P. R., 1969. Winter fat deposition and overnight survival of yellow buntings (*Emberiza citrinella L.*). *J Anim Ecol 38*, 415–423.

Evans, P. R., 1976. Energy balance and optimal foraging strategies in shorebirds: some implications for their distributions and movements in the non-breeding season. *Ardea 64*, 117–139.

Fader, S. C., Yu, Z. M., Spotila, J. R., 1994. Seasonal-variation in heat-shock proteins (Hsp70) in stream fish under natural conditions. *J Thermal Biol 19*, 335–341.

Finberg, J. P., Yagil, R., Berlyne, G. M., 1978. Response of the renin-aldosterone system in the camel to acute dehydration. *J Appl Physiol 44*, 926–930.

Fitzsimons, J. M., Nishimoto, R. T., 1995. Use of fish behavior in assessing the effects of Hurricane

Iniki on the Hawaiian island of Kaua'i. *Environ Biol Fish 43*, 39–50.

Formozov, A. N., 1946. Snow cover as an integral factor of the environment and its importance in the ecology of mammals and birds. *New Series, Zoology 5*: 1–152, Moscow Soc. Natur. English translation, Occ. Papers No. 1 (1963). Boreal Institute, University of Alberta, Edmonton.

Gallardo, M. A., Sala-Rabanal, M., Ibarz, A., Padros, F., Blasco, J., Fernandez-Borras, J., Sanchez, J., 2003. Functional alterations associated with "winter syndrome" in gilthead sea bream (*Sparus aurata*). *Aquaculture 223*, 15–27.

Gaston, A. J., Gilchrist, H. G., Hipfner, J. M., 2005. Climate change, ice conditions and reproduction in an Arctic nesting marine bird: Brunnich's guillemot (*Uria lomvia L.*). *J Anim Ecol 74*, 832–841.

Gaston, A. J., Hipfner, J. M., Campbell, D., 2002. Heat and mosquitoes cause breeding failures and adult mortality in an Arctic-nesting seabird. *Ibis 144*, 185–191.

Gaston, A. J., Nettleship, D. N., 1981. *The thick-billed murres of Prince Leopold Island.* Canadian Wildlife Service, Monograph Series 6. Canadian Wildlife Service, Ottawa, p. 350.

Gavrilova, O., Leon, L. R., Marcus-Samuels, B., Mason, M. M., Castle, A. L., Refetoff, S., Vinson, C., Reitman, M. L., 1999. Torpor in mice is induced by both leptin-dependent and -independent mechanisms. *Proc Natl Acad Sci USA 96*, 14623–14628.

Geiser, F., 1998. Evolution of daily torpor and hibernation in birds and mammals: Importance of body size. *Clini Exper Pharmacol Physiol 25*, 736–739.

Geiser, F., 2010. Hibernation, daily torpor and aestivation in mammals and birds: behavioral aspects. In: Breed, M., Moore, J. (Eds.), *Encyclopedia of animal Bbehavior.* Elsevier, New York, pp. 77–83.

Geist, D. R., Brown, R. S., Cullinan, V., Brink, S. R., Lepla, K., Bates, P., Chandler, J. A., 2005. Movement, swimming speed, and oxygen consumption of juvenile white sturgeon in response to changing flow, water temperature, and light level in the Snake River, Idaho. *Trans Am Fish Soc 134*, 803–816.

Gese, E. M., Ruff, R. L., Crabtree, R. L., 1996. Foraging ecology of coyotes (Canis latrans): The influence of extrinsic factors and a dominance hierarchy. *Can J Zool 74*, 769–783.

Gesquiere, L. R., Khan, M., Shek, L., Wango, T. L., Wango, E. O., Alberts, S. C., Altmann, J., 2008. Coping with a challenging environment: Effects of seasonal variability and reproductive status on glucocorticoid concentrations of female baboons (*Papio cynocephalus*). *Horm Behav 54*, 410–416.

Gessaman, J. A., Worthen, G. L., 1982. *The effect of weather on avian mortality.* Utah State University Printing Services, Logan, Utah.

Gill, F. B., 1995. *Ornithology.* W. H. Freeman, New York.

Gluck, E. F., Stephens, N., Swoap, S. J., 2006. Peripheral ghrelin deepens torpor bouts in mice through the arcuate nucleus neuropeptide Y signaling pathway. *Am J Physiol 291*, R1303–R1309.

Godlewska, M., Mazurkiewicz-Boron, G., Pociecha, A., Wilk-Wozniak, E., Jelonek, M., 2003. Effects of flood on the functioning of the Dobczyce reservoir ecosystem. *Hydrobiologia 504*, 305–313.

Goymann, W., Wingfield, J. C., 2004. Allostatic load, social status and stress hormones: The costs of social status matter. *Anim Behav 67*, 591–602.

Grossman, A. F., West, G. C., 1977. Metabolic-rate and temperature regulation of winter acclimatized black-capped chickadees *Parus-Atricapillus* of interior Alaska. *Ornis Scan 8*, 127–138.

Grubb, T. C., 1975. Weather-dependent foraging behavior of some birds wintering in a deciduous woodland. *Condor 77*, 175–182.

Grubb, T. C., 1977. Weather-dependent foraging in ospreys. *Auk 94*, 146–149.

Grubb, T. C., Greenwald, L., 1982. Sparrows and a brushpile: Foraging responses to different combinations of predation risk and energy-cost. *Anim Behav 30*, 637–640.

Hagemoen, R. I. M., Reimers, E., 2002. Reindeer summer activity pattern in relation to weather and insect harassment. *J Anim Ecol 71*, 883–892.

Hahn, T. P., Sockman, K. W., Breuner, C. W., Morton, M. L., 2004. Facultative altitudinal movements by mountain white-crowned sparrows (*Zonotrichia leucophrys oriantha*) in the Sierra Nevada. *Auk 121*, 1269–1281

Hahn, T. P., Wingfield, J. C., Mullen, R., Deviche, P. J., 1995. Endocrine bases of spatial and temporal opportunism in arctic-breeding birds. *Am Zool 35*, 259–273.

Hannon, S. J., Eason, P. K., Martin, K., 1998. Willow ptarmigan (*Lagopus lagopus*). No. 369. In: Poole, A., Gill, F. (Eds.), *The birds of North America.* Academy of Natural Sciences, Philadelphia; American Ornithologists' Union, Washington DC.

Hartel, T., 2008. Weather conditions, breeding date and population fluctuation in Rana dalmatina from central Romania. *Herpetol J 18*, 40–44.

Harvey, B. C., Nakamoto, R. J., White, J. L., 1999. Influence of large woody debris and a bankfull flood on movement of adult resident coastal cutthroat trout (Oncorhynchus clarki) during fall and winter. *Can J Fish Aquat Sci 56*, 2161–2166.

Hayes, T. B., 1997. Steroids as potential modulators of thyroid hormone activity in anuran metamorphosis. *Am Zool 37*, 185–194.

Helle, T., Kojola, I., 2008. Demographics in an alpine reindeer herd: Effects of density and winter weather. *Ecography 31*, 221–230.

Helms, B. S., Schoonover, J. E., Feminella, J. W., 2009. Assessing influences of hydrology, physicochemistry, and habitat on stream fish assemblages across a changing landscape. *J Ame Water Res Assoc 45*, 157–169.

Hendricks, P., 1987. Habitat use by nesting water pipits (*Anthus-Spinoletta*): A test of the snowfield hypothesis. *Arctic Alpine Res 19*, 313–320.

Hiebert, S., 1993. Seasonal-changes in body-mass and use of torpor in a migratory hummingbird. *Auk 110*, 787–797.

Hiebert, S. M., Ramenofsky, M., Salvante, K., Wingfield, J. C., Gass, C. L., 2000a. Noninvasive methods for measuring and manipulating corticosterone in hummingbirds. *Gen Comp Endocrinol 120*, 235–247.

Hiebert, S. M., Salvante, K. G., Ramenofsky, M., Wingfield, J. C., 2000b. Corticosterone and nocturnal torpor in the rufous hummingbird (*Selasphorus rufus*). *Gen Comp Endocrinol 120*, 220–234.

Hiebert, S. M., Wingfield, J. C., Ramenofsky, M., L., D., Gräfin zu Elz, A., 2004. Sex differences in the response of torpor to exogenous corticosterone during the onset of the migratory season in rufous hummingbirds. In: Barnes, B. M., Carey, H. V. (Eds.), *Life in the cold: Evolution, mechanisms, adaptation and application*. Twelfth International Hibernation Symposium, Institute of Arctic Biology, University of Alaska, Fairbanks, pp. 221–230.

Hiraldo, F., Veiga, J. P., Manez, M., 1990. Growth of nestling black kites *Milvus-Migrans*: Effects of hatching order, weather and season. *J Zool 222*, 197–214.

Holder, K., Montgomerie, R., 1993. Rock ptarmigan (*Lagopus mutus*). No. 51. In: Poole, A., Gill, F. (Eds.), *The birds of North America*. Academy of Natural Sciences, Philadelphia; American Ornithologists' Union, Washington, DC.

Huber, S., Palme, R., Arnold, W., 2003. Effects of season, sex, and sample collection on concentrations of fecal cortisol metabolites in red deer (*Cervus elaphus*). *Gen Comp Endocrinol 130*, 48–54.

Iwama, G. K., Thomas, P. T., Forsyth, R. H. B., Vijayan, M. M., 1998. Heat shock protein expression in fish. *Rev Fish Biol Fisheries 8*, 35–56.

Jacobs, J. D., Wingfield, J.C., 2000. Endocrine control of life-cycle stages: A constraint on response to the environment? *Condor 102*, 35–51.

Jenni-Eiermann, S., Glaus, E., Gruebler, M., Schwabl, H., Jenni, L., 2008. Glucocorticoid response to food availability in breeding barn swallows (*Hirundo rustica*). *Gen Comp Endocrinol 155*, 558–565.

Jenni-Eiermann, S., Jenni, L., Piersma, T., 2002. Temporal uncoupling of thyroid hormones in Red Knots: T3 peaks in cold weather, T4 during moult. *J Ornithologie 143*, 331–340.

Jessop, T. S., Hamann, M., Read, M. A., Limpus, C. J., 2000. Evidence for a hormonal tactic maximizing green turtle reproduction in response to a pervasive ecological stressor. *Gen Comp Endocrinol 118*, 407–417.

Jorgensen, E. H., Johansen, S. J. S., Jobling, M., 1997. Seasonal patterns of growth, lipid deposition and lipid depletion in anadromous Arctic charr. *J Fish Biol 51*, 312–326.

King, J. R., Farner, D. S., 1966. The adaptive role of winter fattening in the white-crowned sparrow with comments on its regulation. *Am Nat 100*, 403–418.

Kissner, K. J., Brigham, R. M., 1993. Evidence for the use of torpor by incubating and brooding common poorwills *Phalaenoptilus-Nuttallii. Ornis Scan 24*, 333–334.

Kitao, N., Fukui, D., Hashimoto, M., Osborne, P. G., 2009. Overwintering strategy of wild free-ranging and enclosure-housed Japanese raccoon dogs (*Nyctereutes procyonoides albus*). *Int J Biometeorol 53*, 159–165.

Koenig, J., Shine, R., Shea, G., 2002. The dangers of life in the city: Patterns of activity, injury and mortality in suburban lizards (*Tiliqua scincoides*). *J Herp 36*, 62–68.

Korhonen, K., 1980. Microclimate in the snow burrows of willow grouse (*Lagopus, Lagopus*). *Ann Zool Fenn 17*, 5–9.

Korhonen, K., 1981. Temperature in the nocturnal shelters of the redpoll (*Acanthis-Flammea L*) and the Siberian tit (*Parus-Cinctus Budd*) in winter. *Ann Zool Fenn 18*, 165–167.

Kortner, G., Brigham, R. M., Geiser, F., 2001. Torpor in free-ranging tawny frogmouths (*Podargus strigoides*). *Physiol Biochem Zool 74*, 789–797.

Kruckeberg, A. R., 1991. *The natural history of Puget Sound Country*. University of Washington Press, Seattle.

Lance, V. A., Elsey, R. M., 1999. Hormonal and metabolic responses of juvenile alligators to cold shock. *J Exp Zool 283*, 566–572.

Laurance, W. F., 1996. Catastrophic declines of Australian rainforest frogs: Is unusual weather responsible? *Biol Conserv 77*, 203–212.

Ligon, J. D., 1970. Still more responses of poor-will to low temperatures. *Condor 72*, 496.

Lobato, E., Merino, S., Moreno, J., Morales, J., Tomas, G., la Puente, J. M. D., Osorno, J. L., Kuchar, A., Mostl, E., 2008. Corticosterone metabolites in blue tit and pied flycatcher droppings: Effects of brood size, ectoparasites and temperature. *Horm Behav 53*, 295–305.

Lucas, M. C., Batley, E., 1996. Seasonal movements and behaviour of adult barbel Barbus barbus, a riverine cyprinid fish: Implications for river management. *J Appl Ecol 33*, 1345–1358.

Machmer, M. M., Ydenberg, R. C., 1990. Weather and osprey foraging energetics. *Can J Zool 68*, 40–43.

Marsh, R. L., 1980. Development of temperature regulation in nestling tree swallows. *Condor 82*, 461–463.

Martin, K., Wiebe, K.L., 2004. Coping mechanisms of alpine and arctic breeding birds: Extreme weather and limitations to reproductive resilience. *Integ Comp Biol 44*, 177–185.

McKechnie, A. E., Ashdown, R. A. M., Christian, M. B., Brigham, R. M., 2007. Torpor in an African caprimulgid, the freckled nightjar *Caprimuigus tristigma*. *J Avian Biol 38*, 261–266.

McKechnie, A. E., Lovegrove, B. G., 2002. Avian facultative hypothermic responses: A review. *Condor 104*, 705–724.

Meehl, G. A., 2000. An introduction to trends in extreme weather and climate events: Observations, socioeconomic impacts, terrestrial ecological impacts, and model projections. *Bull Am Meteorol Soc 81*, 413–416.

Meehl, G. A., Zwiers, F., Evans, J., Knutson, T., Mearns, L., Whetton, P., 2000. Trends in extreme weather and climate events: Issues related to modeling extremes in projections of future climate change. *Bull Am Meteorol Soc 81*, 427–436.

Merola-Zwartjes, M., Ligon, J. D., 2000. Ecological energetics of the Puerto Rican Tody: Heterothermy, torpor, and intra-island variation. *Ecology 81*, 990–1003.

Miller, A. H., 1963. Desert adaptations in birds. In: Sibley, C. G. (Ed.) *Proceedings of the 13th International Ornithological Congress American Ornithologists' Union*. Baton Rouge, pp. 666–674.

Miller, F. L., Gunn, A., 2003. Catastrophic die-off of Peary caribou on the western Queen Elizabeth Islands, Canadian High Arctic. *Arctic 56*, 381–390.

Mommsen, T. P., Vijayan, M. M., Moon, T. W., 1999. Cortisol in teleosts: dynamics, mechanisms of action, and metabolic regulation. *Rev Fish Biol Fisheries 9*, 211–268.

Monet, G., Soares, I., 2001. Tracking 48 and 150 MHZ radio-tagged male lake trout during their spawning migration in a mountain regulated river. *J Mt Ecol 6*, 7–19.

Munich Rev, 2002. *Topics: An annual review of natural catastrophes*. Munich Reinsurance Company Publications, Munich.

Murchie, K. J., Hair, K. P. E., Pullen, C. E., Redpath, T. D., Stephens, H. R., Cooke, S. J., 2008. Fish response to modified flow regimes in regulated rivers: Research methods, effects and opportunities. *River Res Appl 24*, 197–217.

Nakamura, M., Shindo, N., 2001. Effects of snow cover on the social and foraging behavior of the great tit Parus major. *Ecol Res 16*, 301–308.

Narayan, E., Molinia, F., Christi, K., Morley, C., Cockrem, J., 2010. Urinary corticosterone metabolite responses to capture, and annual patterns of urinary corticosterone in wild and captive endangered Fijian ground frogs (*Platymantis vitiana*). *Aust J Zool 58*, 189–197.

Nelson, R. J., 2004. Leptin: The "skinny" on torpor. *Am J Physiol 287*, R6–R7.

Newton, I., 1973. *Finches*. Taplinger Publishing, New York.

Newton, I., Marquiss, M., 1986. Population regulation in sparrowhawks. *J Anim Ecol 55*, 463–480.

Novikov, G. A., 1972. The use of under-snow refuges among small birds of the sparrow family. *Aquilo Ser Zool 13*, 95–97.

O'Reilly, K. M., Wingfield, J. C., 1995. Spring and autumn migration in arctic shorebirds: Same distance, different strategies. *Am Zool 35*, 222–233.

Olsson, M., Shine, R., 1997. The seasonal timing of oviposition in sand lizards (Lacerta agilis): Why early clutches are better. *J Evol Biol 10*, 369–381.

Parker, K. L., 1988. Effects of heat, cold, and rain on coastal black-tailed deer. *Can J Zool 66*, 2475–2483.

Parmesan, C., Root, T. L., Willig, M. R., 2000. Impacts of extreme weather and climate on terrestrial biota. *Bull Am Meteorol Soc 81*, 443–450.

Parsons, B. G., Reed, J. R., 2001. *Methods to reduce stress and improve over-winter survival of stocked walleye fingerlings*. Inv. Rep. 492. Minn. Dept. Nat. Resour., p. 14.

Pereyra, M. E., Wingfield, J. C., 2003. Changes in plasma corticosterone and adrenocortical response to stress during the breeding cycle in high altitude flycatchers. *Gen Comp Endocrinol 130*, 222–231.

Perfito, N., Bentley, G., Hau, M., 2006. Tonic activation of brain GnRH immunoreactivity despite reduction of peripheral reproductive parameters in opportunistically breeding zebra finches. *Brain Behav Evol 67*, 123–134.

Perfito, N., Kwong, J. M. Y., Bentley, G. E., Hau, M., 2008. Cue hierarchies and testicular development: Is food a more potent stimulus than day length in an opportunistic breeder (*Taeniopygia g. guttata*)? *Horm Behav 53*, 567–572.

Perfito, N., Schirato, G., Brown, M., Wingfield, J. C., 2002. Response to acute stress in the Harlequin duck (*Histrionicus histrionicus*) during the breeding season and moult: Relationships to gender, condition, and life-history stage. *Can J Zool 80*, 1334–1343.

Perfito, N., Zann, R. A., Bentley, G. E., Hau, M., 2007. Opportunism at work: habitat predictability affects reproductive readiness in free-living zebra finches. *Func Ecol 21*, 291–301.

Perrins, C. M., 1979. *British tits*. Collins, London.

Persinger, M. A., 1975. Lag responses in mood reports to changes in the weather matrix. *Int J Biometeorol 19*, 108–114.

Pielou, E. C., 1994. *A naturalist's guide to the Arctic*. University of Chicago Press, Chicago.

Piersma, T., 1994. *Close to the edge: Energetic bottlenecks and the evolution of migratory pathways in knots*. Ph.D. Thesis, Rijksuniversiteit Groningen. Published by Uitgeverij Het Open Boek, Texel, Netherlands, p. 366.

Pruitt, W. O. J., 1970. Some ecological aspects of snow. In: *Ecology of the subarctic regions*. United Nations Educational, Scientific and Cultural Organization, Paris, pp. 83–99.

Pruitt, W. O. J., 1978. *Boreal ecology*. Edward Arnold, London.

Pruitt, W. O. J., 2005. Why and how to study a snowcover. *Can Field Natl 119*, 118–128.

Quigley, J. T., Hinch, S. G., 2006. Effects of rapid experimental temperature increases on acute physiological stress and behaviour of stream dwelling juvenile chinook salmon. *J Thermal Biol 31*, 429–441.

Ramenofsky, M., Gray, J. M., Johnson, R. B., 1992. Behavioral and physiological adjustments of birds living in winter flocks. *Ornis Scan 23*, 371–380.

Raouf, S. A., Smith, L. C., Brown, M. B., Wingfield, J. C., Brown, C. R., 2006. Glucocorticoid hormone levels increase with group size and parasite load in cliff swallows. *Anim Behav 71*, 39–48.

Redpath, S. M., Arroyo, B. E., Etheridge, B., Leckie, F., Bouwman, K., Thirgood, S. J., 2002. Temperature and hen harrier productivity: from local mechanisms to geographical patterns. *Ecography 25*, 533–540.

Reinertsen, R. E., 1983. Nocturnal hypothermia and its energetic significance for small birds living in the Arctic and subarctic regions: A review. *Polar Res 1*, 269–284.

Reinertsen, R. E., Haftorn, S., 1983. Nocturnal hypothermia and metabolism in the willow tit *Parus-Montanus* at 63-degrees-N. *J Compar Physiol 151*, 109–118.

Richardson, M. I., Moore, I. T., Soma, K. K., Fu-Min, L., Wingfield, J. C., 2003. How similar are high latitude and high altitude habitats? A review and a preliminary study of the adrenocortical response to stress in birds of the Qinghai-Tibetan plateau. *Acta Zool Sin 49*, 1–19.

Richdale, L. E., 1945. Supplementary notes on the diving petrel. *Trans R Soc N Z 75*, 42–53.

Ricklefs, R. E., Hainsworth, F. R., 1968. Temperature dependent behavior of cactus wren. *Ecology 49*, 227–233.

Rogers, C. M., Ramenofsky, M., Ketterson, E. D., Nolan, V., Jr., Wingfield, J. C., 1993. Plasma corticosterone, adrenal mass, winter weather, and season in nonbreeding populations of dark-eyed juncos (*Junco hyemalis hyemalis*). *Auk 110*, 279–285.

Roghair, C. N., Dolloff, C. A., Underwood, M. K., 2002. Response of a brook trout population and instream habitat to a catastrophic flood and debris flow. *Trans Am Fish Soc 131*, 718–730.

Rogovin, K. A., Randall, J. A., Kolosova, I. E., Moshkin, M. P., 2008. Long-term dynamics of fecal corticosterone in male great gerbils (*Rhombomys opimus Licht.*) Effects of environment and social demography. *Physiol Biochem Zool 81*, 612–626.

Rohwer, S., Wingfield, J. C., 1981. A field-study of social-dominance, plasma-levels of luteinizing-hormone and steroid-hormones in wintering Harris sparrows. *Zeitschrift Tierpsychol J Comp Ethol 57*, 173–183.

Romero, L. M., Reed, J. M., Wingfield, J. C., 2000. Effects of weather on corticosterone responses in wild free-living passerine birds. *Gen Comp Endocrinol 118*, 113–122.

Rosenzweig, C., Iglesias, A., Yang, X. B., Epstein, P. R., Chivian, E., 2001. Climate change and extreme weather events: Implications for food production, plant diseases, and pests. *Global Change Human Health 2*, 90–104.

Rubenstein, D. R., 2007. Stress hormones and sociality: integrating social and environmental stressors. *Proc R Soc Lond B 274*, 967–975.

Ryan, S. N., 1995. The effect of chronic heat-stress on cortisol-levels in the Antarctic fish *Pagothenia-Borchgrevinki*. *Experientia 51*, 768–774.

Saether, B. E., Tufto, J., Engen, S., Jerstad, K., Rostad, O. W., Skatan, J. E., 2000. Population dynamical consequences of climate change for a small temperate songbird. *Science 287*, 854–856.

Sapolsky, R. M., 1987. Stress, social status, and reproductive physiology in free-living baboons. In: Crews, D. (Ed.) *Psychobiology of reproductive behavior: An evolutionary perspective*. Prentice-Hall, Englewood Cliffs, NJ, pp. 291–322.

Scherer, R. D., Muths, E., Lambert, B. A., 2008. Effects of weather on survival in populations of boreal toads in Colorado. *J Herp 42*, 508–517.

Schmidt-Nielsen, K., 1965. *Desert animals: Physiological problems of heat and water*. Oxford University Press, New York.

Schwabl, H., Wingfield, J. C., Farner, D. S., 1985. Influence of winter on endocrine state and behavior in European blackbirds (*Turdus-Merula*). *Zeitschrift Tierpsychol J Comp Ethol 68*, 244–252.

Sejian, V., Maurya, V. P., Naqvi, S. M. K., 2010. Adaptive capability as indicated by endocrine and biochemical responses of Malpura ewes subjected to combined stresses (thermal and nutritional) in a semi-arid tropical environment. *Int J Biometeorol 54*, 653–661.

Sejian, V., Maurya, V. P., Naqvi, S. M. K., 2012. Effect of walking stress on growth, physiological adaptability and endocrine responses in Malpura ewes in a semi-arid tropical environment. *Int J Biometeorol 56*, 243–252.

Sergio, F., 2003. From individual behaviour to population pattern: Weather-dependent foraging and breeding performance in black kites. *Anim Behav* 66, 1109–1117.

Sharbaugh, S. M., 2001. Seasonal acclimatization to extreme climatic conditions by black-capped chickadees (*Poecile atricapilla*) in interior Alaska (64 degrees N). *Physiol Biochem Zool 74*, 568–575.

Sharma, S., Jackson, D. A., Minns, C. K., Shuter, B. J., 2007. Will northern fish populations be in hot water because of climate change? *Global Change Biology 13*, 2052–2064.

Sherbrooke, W. C., 1990. Rain-harvesting in the lizard, *Phrynosoma-Cornutum*: Behavior and integumental morphology. *J Herp 24*, 302–308.

Shine, R., Elphick, M. J., 2001. The effect of short-term weather fluctuations on temperatures inside lizard nests, and on the phenotypic traits of hatchling lizards. *Biol J Linnean Soc 72*, 555–565.

Silverin, B., Gwinner, E., Van't Hof, T. J., Schwabl, I., Fusani, L., Hau, M., Helm, B., 2009. Persistent diel melatonin rhythmicity during the Arctic summer in free-living willow warblers. *Horm Behav 56*, 163–168.

Silverin, B., Wingfield, J. C., 2010. Wintering strategies. In: Breed, M., Moore, J. (Eds.), *Encyclopedia of animal behavior*. Elsevier Press, London, pp. 597–605.

Sloman, K. A., Wilson, L., Freel, J. A., Taylor, A. C., Metcalfe, N. B., Gilmour, K. M., 2002. The effects of increased flow rates on linear dominance hierarchies and physiological function in brown trout, *Salmo trutta*. *Can J Zool 80*, 1221–1227.

Smith, G. T., Wingfield, J. C., Veit, R. R., 1994. Adrenocortical response to stress in the common diving petrel, *Pelecanoides urinatrix*. *Physiol Zool 67*, 526–537.

Steen, J., 1958. Climatic adaptation in some small northern birds. *Ecology 39*, 625–629.

Steinbeck, J., 1962. *Travels with Charlie*. Viking Press, New York.

Stevenson, R. J., 1990. Benthic algal community dynamics in a stream during and after a spate. *J N Am Benthol Soc 9*, 277–288.

Stokkan, K. A., 1992. Energetics and adaptations to cold in ptarmigan in winter. *Ornis Scan 23*, 366–370.

Stokkan, K. A., Sharp, P. J., Unander, S., 1986. The annual breeding cycle of the high-arctic Svalbard ptarmigan (*Lagopus mutus hyperboreus*). *Gen Comp Endocrinol 61*, 446–451.

Storey, K.B., 2001. Turning down the fires of life: metabolic regulation of hibernation and estivation. In: Storey, K.B. (Ed.) Molecular Mechanisms of Metabolic Arrest, BIOS Sci. Publ., Oxford, pp. 1–21

Streich, W. J., Litzbarski, H., Ludwig, B., Ludwig, S., 2006. What triggers facultative winter migration of Great Bustard (*Otis tarda*) in Central Europe? *Eur J Wildlife Res 52*, 48–53.

Sulkava, S., 1969. On small birds spending the night in the snow. *Aquilo Ser Zool 7*, 33–37.

Sultanov, F. F., Klochkova, G. M., Mezidova, K. A., Ron'zhina, S. V., 2001. The effects of arid region conditions on the hormonal status of humans. (Translated from *Fiziologiya Cheloveka 27*, 74–85). *Human Physiol 27*, 65–67.

Suping, Z., Guanglin, M., Yanwen, W., Ji, L., 1992. Study of the relationships between weather conditions and the marathon race, and of meteortopic effects on distance runners. *Int J Biometeorol 36*, 63–68.

Sutherland, A. B., Maki, J., Vaughan, V., 2008. Effects of suspended sediment on whole-body cortisol stress response of two southern Appalachian minnows, *Erimonax monachus* and *Cyprinella galactura*. *Copeia* 2008, 234–244.

Tieleman, B. I., 2002. Avian adaptation along an aridity gradient. Ph.D. Thesis, University of Groningen, The Netherlands.

Tieleman, B. I., Williams, J. B., Buschur, M. E., 2002. Physiological adjustments to arid and mesic environments in larks (Alaudidae). *Physiol Biochem Zool 75*, 305–313.

Tort, L., Rotllant, J., Rovira, L., 1998. Immunological suppression in gilthead sea bream *Sparus aurata* of the North-West Mediterranean at low temperatures. *Comp Biochem Physiol A 120*, 175–179.

Travis, J. M. J., 2003. Climate change and habitat destruction: A deadly anthropogenic cocktail. *Proc R Soc Lond B 270*, 467–473.

Uchakina, R. V., 1977. Seasonal changes of corticosteroid content in practically healthy young persons under conditions of monsoon climate of Khabarovsk (in Russian, English abstract). *Probl Endokrinol (Moskva) 23*, 52–57.

van Oosterhout, C., Mohammed, R. S., Hansen, H., Archard, G. A., McMullan, M., Weese, D. J., Cable, J., 2007. Selection by parasites in spate conditions in wild Trinidadian guppies (*Poecilia reticulata*). *Int J Parasitol 37*, 805–812.

Veit, R. R., Kareivad, P. M., Doak, D. F., Engh, A., Heppell, S. F., Hollon, M., Jordan, C. E., Morgan, R. A., Morris, W. F., Nevitt, G. A., Smith, G. T., 1991. Foraging interactions between pelagic seabirds and Antarctic krill at South Georgia during winter 1991. *Antarctic J US 28*, 183–185.

Vickery, W. L., Millar, J. S., 1984. The energetics of huddling by endotherms. *Oikos 43*, 88–93.

Vihma, T., 2010. Effects of weather on the performance of marathon runners. *Int J Biometeorol 54*, 297–306.

Vleck, C. M., Priedkalns, J., 1985. Reproduction in zebra finches: Hormone levels and effect of dehydration. *Condor 87*, 37–46.

Vors, L. S., Boyce, M. S., 2009. Global declines of caribou and reindeer. *Global Change Biology 15*, 2626–2633.

Walsberg, G. E., 1990. Communal roosting in a very small bird: Consequences for the thermal and respiratory gas environments. *Condor 92*, 795–798.

Wang, L. C. H., Wolowyk, M. W., 1988. Torpor in mammals and birds. *Can J Zool 66*, 133–137.

Ward, D. L., Schultz, A. A., Matson, P. G., 2003. Differences in swimming ability and behavior in response to high water velocities among native and nonnative fishes. *Environ Biol Fish 68*, 87–92.

Weladji, R. B., Holand, O., 2003. Global climate change and reindeer: Effects of winter weather on the autumn weight and growth of calves. *Oecologia 136*, 317–323.

White, F. N., Bartholomew, G. A., Howell, T. R., 1975. Thermal significance of nest of sociable weaver *Philetairus-Socius*: Winter observations. *Ibis 117*, 171.

White, G., 1860. *The natural history of Selborne*. Gresham Books, London.

Williams, J. B., Tieleman, B. I., 2001. Physiological ecology and behavior of desert birds. In: Nolan, V., Thompson, C.F. (Eds.), *Current ornithology*, vol. *16*. Plenum Press, New York, pp. 299–353.

Williams, T. D., 2008. Individual variation in endocrine systems: Moving beyond the "tyranny of the Golden Mean." *Phil Trans R Soc B 363*, 1687–1698.

Wilson, E. O., 1975. *Sociobiology*. Belknapp Press, Cambridge, MA.

Wingfield, J. C., 1984. Influence of weather on reproduction. *J Exp Zool 232*, 589–594.

Wingfield, J. C., 1985a. Influences of weather on reproductive function in female Song sparrows, *Melospiza melodia. J Zool, Lond 205*, 545–558.

Wingfield, J. C., 1985b. Influences of weather on reproductive function in male Song sparrows, *Melospiza melodia. J Zool, Lond 205*, 525–544.

Wingfield, J. C., 2004. Allostatic load and life cycles: implications for neuroendocrine mechanisms. In: Schulkin, J. (Ed.), *Allostasis, homeostasis and the costs of physiological adaptation*, Cambridge University Press, Cambridge, pp. 302–342.

Wingfield, J. C., 2008. Comparative endocrinology, environment and global change. *Gen Comp Endocrinol 157*, 207–216.

Wingfield, J. C., Farner, D. S., 1978. The endocrinology of a naturally breeding population of the white-crowned sparrow (*Zonotrichia leucophrys pugetensis*). *Physiol Zoolog 51*, 188–205.

Wingfield, J. C., Hahn, T. P., Wada, M., Schoech, S. J., 1997. Effects of day length and temperature on gonadal development, body mass, and fat depots in white-crowned sparrows, *Zonotrichia leucophrys pugetensis. Gen Comp Endocrinol 107*, 44–62.

Wingfield, J. C., Hegner, R. E., Lewis, D. M., 1991. Circulating levels of luteinizing-hormone and steroid-hormones in relation to social-status in the cooperatively breeding white-browed sparrow weaver, *Plocepasser-Mahali. J Zool 225*, 43–58.

Wingfield, J. C., Helm, J., Sullivan, K., Meddle, S. L., 2012. The presence of water influences reproductive function in a semi-aquatic sparrow, the song sparrow (*Melospiza melodia morphna*). *Gen Comp Endocrinol. 178*, 485–493.

Wingfield, J. C., Jacobs, J. D., 1999. The interplay of innate and experiential factors regulating the life history cycle of birds. In: Adams, N., Slotow, R. (Eds.), *Proceedings of the 22nd International Ornithological Congress*, Birdlife South Africa, Johannesburg, pp. 2417–2443.

Wingfield, J. C., Kelley, J. P., Angelier, F., Chastel, O., Lei, F. M., Lynn, S. E., Miner, B., Davis, J. E., Li, D. M., Wang, G., 2011. Organism-environment interactions in a changing world: a mechanistic approach. *J Ornithol 152*, 279–288.

Wingfield, J. C., Moore, M. C., Farner, D. S., 1983. Endocrine responses to inclement weather in naturally breeding populations of white-crowned sparrows (*Zonotrichia leucophrys pugetensis*). *Auk 100*, 56–62.

Wingfield, J. C., O'Reilly, K. M., Astheimer, L. B., 1995. Modulation of the adrenocortical responses to acute stress in Arctic birds: A possible ecological basis. *Am Zool 35*, 285–294.

Wingfield, J. C., Owen-Ashley, N., Benowitz-Fredericks, Z. M., Lynn, S., Hahn, T. P., Wada, H., Breuner, C., Meddle, S., Romero, L. M., 2004. Arctic spring: The arrival biology of migrant birds. *Acta Zool Sinica 50*, 948–960.

Wingfield, J. C., Ramenofsky, M., 1997. Corticosterone and facultative dispersal in response to unpredictable events. *Ardea 85*, 155–166.

Wingfield, J. C., Ramenofsky, M., 1999. Hormones and the behavioral ecology of stress. In: Balm, P. H. M. (Ed.), *Stress Physiology in Animals*, Sheffield Academic Press, Sheffield, U.K., pp. 1–51.

Wingfield, J. C., Ramenofsky, M., 2011. Hormone-behavior interrelationships of birds in response to weather. In: Brockmann, H. J., Snowdon, C. T., Roper, T. J. (Eds.), *Advances in the study of behavior*, vol. *43*. Academic Press, New York, pp. 93–188.

Wingfield, J. C., Romero, L. M., 2001. Adrenocortical responses to stress and their modulation in free-living vertebrates. In: McEwen, B. S., Goodman, H. M. (Eds.), *Handbook of physiology*; Section 7: *The endocrine system*; Vol. IV: *Coping with the environment: Neural and endocrine mechanisms*. Oxford University Press, New York, pp. 211–234.

Wingfield, J. C., Vleck, C. M., Moore, M. C., 1992. Seasonal changes of the adrenocortical response to stress in birds of the Sonoran Desert. *J Exp Zool 264*, 419–428.

Wolf, B. O., 2000. Global warming and avian occupancy of hot deserts: a physiological and behavioral perspective. *Rev Chil Hist Nat 73*, 1–13.

Wolf, B. O., Walsberg, G. E., 1996. Thermal effects of radiation and wind on a small bird and implications for microsite selection. *Ecology 77*, 2228–2236.

Wolf, B. O., Wooden, K. M., Walsberg, G. E., 1996. The use of thermal refugia by two small desert birds. *Condor 98*, 424–428.

9

Responses to Natural Perturbations

Poxes, Predators, and Personalities

I. INTRODUCTION

Self-preservation is a daily, if not minute-by-minute, preoccupation of all organisms. Risk of infection, predation, and social pressures can change suddenly and dramatically. How individuals cope with these potential stressors will have a major impact on their ultimate survival. Differences in both internal physiology and external environmental features can be decisive. For example, habitat configuration may be critical in evading predation. Survival depends upon nearby refuges providing places to hide from predators, or alternatively, open landscape so that predators can be detected early and risk reduced. Similarly, the possibility of infection from the environment, including from social interactions, is another constant threat. Parasite load, while not necessarily affecting immediate health directly, can increase the energetic costs of daily and seasonal routines that increase allostatic load (Ee + Ei; see Chapter 3). If infection and/or disease does occur, then sickness behavior becomes part of the emergency life-history stage (ELHS) that allows the animal's immune system to eliminate or at least control disease. However, this comes at a cost that will increase allostatic load (Eo, Chapter 3).

In contrast to these environmental features, internal variation in physiology and behavior can also affect survival. For example, conspecific social interactions and status can have profound effects on predation risk as well as potential for infection and parasite load. Personality can influence how individuals cope with other perturbations of the environment as well. Proactive and reactive coping styles (e.g., Koolhaas et al. 1999) have been proposed as major coping styles for many animals, vertebrate and invertebrate. Behaviors associated with different developmental stages can also put animals at risk. Dispersal, for example, is a period of vulnerability in which individuals move away from familiar home ranges such as the natal territory. There is also risk during post-breeding exploration of potentially new areas for future reproduction. Additionally, unpredictable events, such as habitat destruction or modification, or occurrence of predators or invasive species, may necessitate immediate evacuation of an area, that is, facultative dispersal. Although these types of dispersal may seem to create an unacceptable level of risk, failure to respond will likely result in greatly increased allostatic load and reduced fitness.

Here we address environmental perturbations associated with self-preservation, such as immunocompetence and coping with infection (e.g., sickness behavior), risk of predation, social interactions (particularly how personalities can influence vulnerability to other perturbations), and the uncertainty of dispersal either by young individuals from their natal areas to facultative movements induced by perturbations of the environment. Evidence is building that stress mediators play major roles in helping animals survive these types of perturbations.

II. COPING WITH INFECTION

We summarized the actions of corticosteroids and other mediators in reactive scope on immune system function in Chapter 5. Over the past several decades, the rapidly growing field of ecological immunology has yielded important insights for understanding the impact that parasites and disease have upon host populations, life histories, and sexual selection (Ashley and Wingfield 2011; Nelson and Demas 2011). Moreover, because anti-parasite defenses of hosts are energetically costly to develop and maintain, there will be competition for resources with other life-history stages such as reproduction, migration, molt, and so on, as well as with overall growth and development of particular sexual ornaments (Sheldon and Verhulst 1996; Lochmiller and Deerenberg 2000; Norris and Evans 2000; Zuk and Stoehr 2002; Schmid-Hempel and Ebert 2003). Competition among life-history stages for resources also has survival costs, particularly those associated with immune system activation and function (Moret and Schmid-Hempel 2000; Hanssen et al. 2004; Eraud et al. 2009). Advances in this rapidly emerging field have been made to develop techniques and assays that quantify immunological performance, or "immunocompetence," in naturalistic settings, although conceptual challenges of how to link measures of immunocompetence to susceptibility to infection and fitness remain to be clarified (Adamo 2004; Viney et al. 2005). Nonetheless, ecologists and evolutionary biologists are exploring host-parasite interactions in relation to multidirectional communication among the immune, nervous, and endocrine systems (e.g., Demas 2004; Nelson and Demas 2011). These interrelationships regulate how host immunocompetence is synchronized with homeostatic mechanisms. How immune-endocrine-behavior relations predict susceptibility to infection within life-history and evolutionary contexts remain, however, major questions, especially regarding plasticity according to energy demands and life-history stage of the host (Zuk 1996; Ricklefs and Wikelski 2002; Demas 2004; Owen-Ashley and Wingfield 2007; Adelman and Martin 2009).

Before going on to explore mechanisms underlying the interrelationships of life histories, immunocompetence, ecology, and evolution, it is important to consider how they fit into the concept of perturbations of the environment and stress responses.

A. Injury, Disability, Parasite Load, and Disease

Recognition of infection or injury triggers the release of cytokines, which activates a suite of physiological and behavioral responses that include sickness behavior, fever, acute phase protein (APP) production from the liver, and activation of the hypothalamo-pituitary-adrenal (HPA) axis and subsequent release of corticosteroids (Figure 5.16; see also Chapters 3 and 5; e.g., Ashley and Wingfield 2011; Nelson and Demas 2011). These hormones will initially stimulate immune function, but later provide negative feedback at multiple levels to the overall circuit. Dotted and continuous lines in Figure 5.16 represent inhibitory and stimulatory actions, respectively.

The relationship between the emergency life-history stage (ELHS) and sickness behavior is presented in Figure 9.1. There are four major substages that may be expressed in varying combinations according to context and circumstances. They include the fight-or-flight response, proactive/reactive coping styles, facultative behavioral and physiological responses, and sickness behavior. Each of these substages can be initiated by labile perturbation factors (LPFs) in the environment that disrupt the normal life cycle (Figure 9.1). Sickness behavior and immune responses in general are critical components of the stress response (see Chapter 3; Sapolsky et al. 2000; Nelson and Demas 2011).

Using the allostasis model we can insert a line, Ep, which represents the additional energy required to fuel increasing ecto- and/or endo-parasite infections (Figure 9.2). As long as Ep remains below Eg, then the parasite load can be tolerated, assuming that no other pathological effects occur. However, such an individual is susceptible to further perturbations of the environment (Eo, in red, Figure 9.2). Note that as the parasite load (Ep) increases, then the same perturbation (Eo) will exceed Eg and trigger an

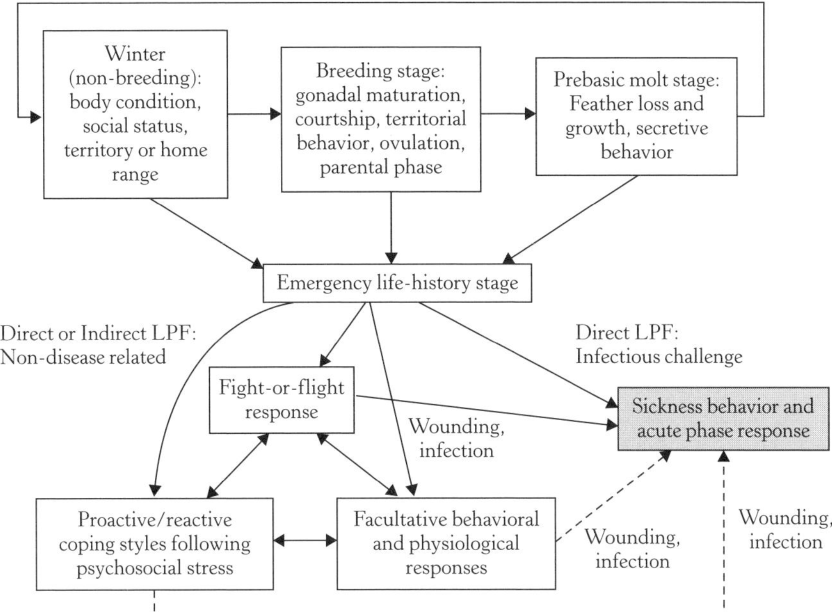

FIGURE 9.1: The emergency life-history stage (ELHS) and sickness behavior (modified from Wingfield 2003). There are four major sub-stages that may be expressed in varying combinations according to context and circumstances. LPFs are labile perturbations factors in the environment that disrupt the normal life cycle.

After Ashley and Wingfield (2011), courtesy of Oxford University Press.

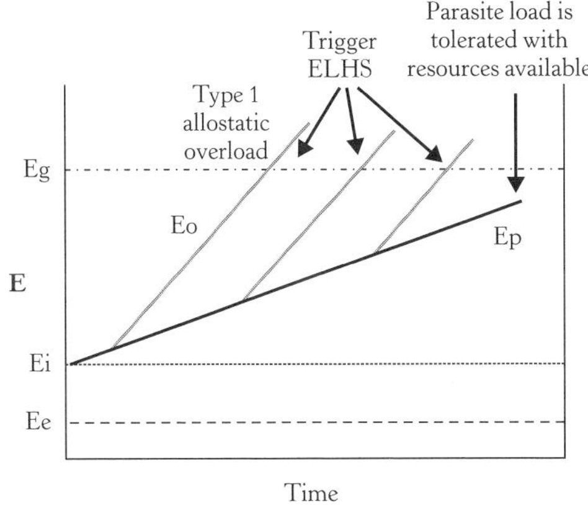

FIGURE 9.2: Representation of infections using the allostasis model. Ep represents the additional energy required to fuel increasing parasite infections and Eo represents further perturbations of the environment. Note that as Ep increases, the same Eo will exceed Eg and trigger an emergency life-history stage (ELHS) more quickly.

After Ashley and Wingfield (2011), courtesy of Oxford University Press.

ELHS more quickly. Increasing infection will also limit how much energy can be allocated to other life-history stages such as breeding (Figure 9.2).

Type 2 allostatic overload is initiated when there is sufficient or even excess energy available (Chapter 3), but the effects of social dysfunction, presence of predators, infection and/or injury, and other long-term changes in the environment increase Ee and Ei permanently, but not sufficiently to exceed Eg (Figure 9.3; Ashley and Wingfield 2011). There are many examples of this pathophysiological response in human societies and animals in captivity, and the long-term consequences can be debilitating, even though food supply is still sufficient to fuel such overload. Type 2 allostatic overload also makes an individual more susceptible to perturbations of the environment and thus allostatic overload type 1 (Ashley and Wingfield 2011). Allostatic overload type 2 may be long term (such as in cases of infection or injury) and can only be mitigated through learning and changes in social behavior and structure (McEwen and Wingfield 2003a). Allostatic overload type 2 may be a frequent consequence of infection and injury, as illustrated in Figure 9.3 (Ashley and Wingfield 2011). An individual infected with ecto- and/or endo-parasites will incur an increased allostatic load (Ep in left-hand panel, Figure 9.3). If it is assumed that this infection reaches a stable point, then the increased allostatic load becomes

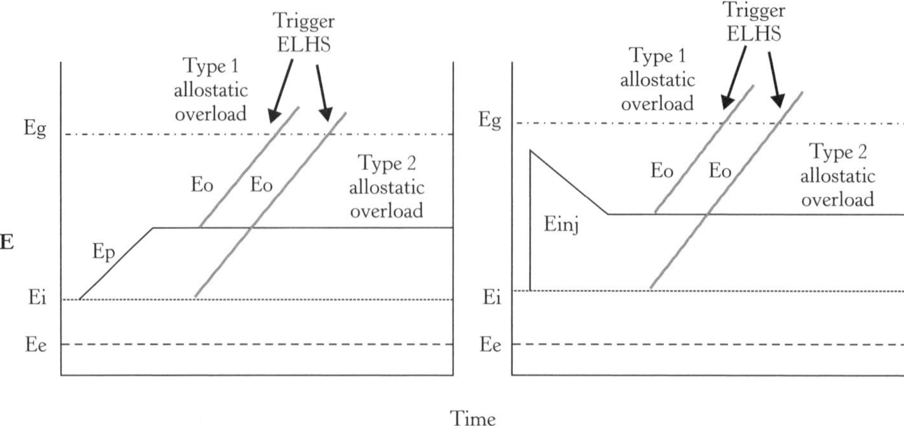

FIGURE 9.3: Relationship between infection (left panel) or injury (right panel) with allostatic overload type 2. Ep represents increased allostatic load due to infection, Einj represents increased allostatic load due to injury, Eo represents a further perturbation, and ELHS represents an emergency life-history stage.

After Ashley and Wingfield (2011), courtesy of Oxford University Press.

long term, consistent with allostatic overload type 2. Note that Eg has not been exceeded, but mediators of allostasis, such as corticosteroids and cytokines, may be high. In another example (right-hand panel, Figure 9.3), an injury may suddenly increase allostatic load (Einj), which then declines as the injury heals. If the injury does not completely heal or impairs daily routines, the allostatic load may become permanent, consistent with allostatic overload type 2. In both panels a further perturbation (Eo in red) will exceed Eg and trigger an ELHS more quickly in the individual with allostatic overload type 2 (Figure 9.3). In either case, allostatic overload type 2 will also limit how much energy can be allocated to other life-history stages such as breeding.

B. Sickness Behavior

The immune-neuroendocrine system function triggered by the acute phase response (APR) can be modulated, resulting in characteristic behavior, "sickness behavior," that occurs during the onset of infection (Hart 1988). Sickness behavior is a syndrome of behavioral traits (Figure 5.16) including anorexia (reduced appetite), adipsia (blunted thirst), reduced activity, soporific behavior, increased slow-wave sleep, anhedonia (inability to experience pleasure), hyperalgesia (reduced threshold to perception of pain), general withdrawal from social activities (e.g., territorial aggression, parental care, sexual behavior), reduced exploratory behavior, decreased libido, malaise, less grooming behavior, and, in some cases, impairment of learning and memory (Hart 1988; Kent et al. 1992; Dantzer et al. 1993; Exton 1997; Dantzer et al. 1998; Dunn and Swiergiel 1998; Maier and Watkins 1999; Kavaliers et al. 2000; Langhans 2000; Dantzer 2001; Konsman et al. 2002; Tizard 2008). In endothermic vertebrates, sickness behavior is frequently accompanied by shivering to increase heat production and ultimately fever (a rise in the thermoregulatory set-point). On the other hand, ectothermic vertebrates cannot regulate their body temperature directly and must seek warmer microhabitats. They may also adopt behavioral postures, such as a curled body position or a puffed out integument, to reduce heat loss (Hart 1988). In sum, such traits generally reduce the energy required to maintain a fever. Taken together, fever, sickness behavior, inflammation, hormonal changes, reduced intestinal motility, and regulated acute phase proteins (APPs) comprise the generalized APR in vertebrates (Andus et al. 1991; Baumann and Gauldie 1994).

The emerging field of Darwinian (evolutionary) medicine suggested that symptoms of disease are manifestations of infectious agents as well as host defenses (Ewald 1980; Williams and Nesse 1991). For example, fever in an ectothermic animal, the desert iguana, has been shown to have adaptive value (Kluger et al. 1975). After experimental infection with bacteria, desert iguanas can elevate body temperature by moving to warmer microhabitats and thus "induce" fever. Survival was enhanced, compared with infected iguanas kept in cool conditions (Vaughn et al.

1974; Kluger et al. 1975). Experimental investigations of endothermic vertebrates (e.g. infection of New Zealand white rabbits with bacteria) demonstrated that when treated with antipyretics survival was significantly less than controls that were allowed to develop fever normally (Kluger and Vaughn 1978). These data point to two benefits for mechanisms that allow individuals to combat infection:

1. Enhancement of innate and specific immunological defenses through temperature-dependent and independent mechanisms (Kluger 1991).
2. Inhibition of pathogenic bacteria and viruses exhibiting optimum growth at temperatures near or below the normal body temperature of hosts (Kluger 1979).

It should be borne in mind that fever can have negative effects upon fitness by elevating energy requirements and subsequent homeostatic disruption. However, the cost-benefit of fever outweighs the potential for morbidity and mortality (Kluger et al. 1998).

Hart (1988) argued that sickness behavior is an adaptive response that redirects energy to fever and immune defense and away from energy-expensive life-history traits such as foraging, reproduction, migration, growth, and social interactions. These concepts clearly point to sickness behavior and fever being important components of the ELHS (Ashley and Wingfield, 2011). Reduced activity would mitigate energy consumption by decreased convective heat loss accompanying movement and exposure to the elements, as well as reduced risk of predation.

In Chapter 3 we summarized the roles of primary mediators of allostasis: catecholamines, cytokines, and corticosteroids. They orchestrate behavioral and physiological alterations in response to changing environments and LPFs. Temporal patterns and combinations of these primary mediators (allostatic state or reactive scope) also vary according to the type of perturbation and potential for stress including infection (Romero et al. 2009). If food and/or energy reserves (e.g., fat stores) are sufficient to fuel homeostatic processes in the face of a perturbation, then these states can be sustained for periods of time, avoiding activation of an ELHS following allostatic overload (McEwen and Wingfield 2003a; Wingfield 2005a). It is generally agreed that the immune-neuroendocrine mechanisms of sickness behavior, and its modulation, can be incorporated into the framework of life-history theory and allostasis under natural conditions (Figures 9.2 and 9.3; Ashley and Wingfield 2011).

How do individuals cope with infection, and what are the proximate factors involved in modulation of sickness behavior (Hasselquist 2007; Owen-Ashley and Wingfield 2007; Adelman and Martin 2009; French et al. 2009)? The immune-neuroendocrine cascade of cytokines, peptides, and glucocorticoids is triggered when infectious agents and/or tissue damage are detected by circulating macrophages and dendritic cells (Figure 5.16). Phagocytic cells expressing toll-like receptors (TLR) can bind conserved pathogen-associated molecular patterns (PAMPs) on the outer surface of microbes. Release of alarmins from destroyed cells (Tizard 2008) provide further signals of infection or tissue damage. When activated, macrophages destroy infectious agents as well as express pro-inflammatory cytokines, such as interleukin 1-beta (IL-1β), IL-6, and tumor necrosis factor-alpha (TNF-μ). Autocrine and/or paracrine actions of these cytokines regulate a cascade of cytokine release to recruit other immune cells to the site of infection or injury. They also signal the brain and liver through the endocrine and neural pathways of the cascade, including the HPA axis (see also Chapter 5 and Figure 5.16). Central actions of cytokines include triggering metabolic and hormonal changes, underlying fever, sickness behavior, activation of the HPA axis, and inhibition of other systems associated with reproduction, metabolism and growth, and so on, as well as inhibiting prostaglandins such as PGE2 (Besedovsky et al. 1986; Rivier 1990; Rivier and Vale 1990; Turnbull and Rivier 1995; Kondo et al. 1997; Soto et al. 1998). Corticosteroids enhance immunological function in the short term (Dhabhar 2002), and then provide negative feedback to the immune-neuroendocrine cascade to inhibit an over-reactive immune response (Munck et al. 1984; Besedovsky et al. 1986; Besedovsky and DelRey 1996).

Comparative studies of modulation of immunocompetence in vertebrates, especially under natural conditions, provide convincing evidence that responses to infection disrupt the temporal sequence and duration of life-history stages (e.g., Nelson and Demas 2011). For example, the inhibitory effects of APR activation on the hypothalamic-pituitary-gonadal (HPG) axis are widespread, leading to lower reproductive success (Besedovsky and DelRey 1996). Sex differences are also apparent, with sexual activity being suppressed in female but not in male rats following

LPS or IL-1 treatment (Yirmiya et al. 1995; Avitsur and Yirmiya 1999). Experimental LPS administration also decreased territorial aggression and singing in reproductively mature male Gambel's white-crowned sparrows and song sparrows during the non-breeding, winter season (Owen-Ashley et al. 2006; Owen-Ashley and Wingfield 2006b). Furthermore, in female house sparrows, parental behavior was inhibited after LPS treatment compared with controls, and some females abandoned the nest completely (Bonneaud et al. 2003).

Considering sickness behavior as a component of the ELHS allows predictions of how an individual will respond to other perturbations of the environment. Sickness behavior has an energetic cost associated with it that increases allostatic load. Potentially allostatic overload type 1 explains why life-history stages such as reproduction may be suspended, or even deactivated, to allow energy reallocation to expressing sickness behavior and the APR. Note that these effects can be modulated according to the degree of reproductive investment, body condition, and so on. For example, the APR might be attenuated near the end of a successful breeding attempt. Following recovery from infection and/or injury, return to the normal life-history stage for that time of year will occur (Ashley and Wingfield, 2011).

Activation of sickness behavior and the APR can result in type 1 allostatic overload, but these can vary depending upon circumstances relating to Eg. It is important to bear in mind that a component of sickness behavior, reduction of food intake (anorexia), occurs despite Eg being unaffected. However, energetic demands of activating fever and other components of the APR are greatly elevated, resulting in an energetic crisis. This can be offset to varying degrees by regulating activity and other components of sickness behavior. Nonetheless, negative energy balance, accompanied by increased glucocorticoid levels, is an end result and threatens allostatic overload type 1. Therefore, we must adjust our energy models in order to compare sickness behavior responses in the context of classic type 1 allostatic overload (Figure 9.4; Ashley and Wingfield 2011). A major component of sickness behavior is that food intake may decline to zero, even though available energy (Eg) is unchanged (Figure 9.4B). The line Ef (energy from food intake) is thus independent of Eg (Figure 9.4A and we can remove it from Figure 9.4B). Here Eg is considered to be sufficient and will accommodate any increase in Ef. In an anorexic state, Ef is less than Ee (Figure 9.4B), and endogenous energy reserves (Er) must be drawn upon (Figure 9.4C and D; Ashley and Wingfield 2011). Eo, the additional energy needed for finding food during an LPF, must be substituted with the additional energy needed to produce an APR (Eapr) to fight infection (Figure 9.4C and D; Ashley and Wingfield 2011).

Energy reserves (Er) such as proteins, carbohydrates, and some lipids are available to fuel the APR and other immunological functions. Er will decline in an anorexic state, accompanied by loss of body weight. As Eapr increases, Er decreases, and the point at which Er intersects Ee + Ei represents the depletion of energy available to activate and maintain the APR—a form of allostatic overload type 2 (Figure 9.4C and D). It is predicted that re-feeding should occur at this point (increased Ef), or the individual will die. Considering an individual with high energy stores (Figure 9.4C), it is predicted that a stronger APR of longer duration will be possible compared to an individual with low energy reserves (Figure 9.4D). A foundation for explaining how sickness behavior is primarily modulated by energy limitation results from this framework, allowing the generation of specific hypotheses that can be experimentally tested. Because both high Er and low Er decline until reaching Ee + Ei, then a threshold minimum body weight should be strictly defended (Ashley and Wingfield 2011). This has been revealed in experimental studies (Bilbo et al. 2002; Owen-Ashley et al. 2006; Owen-Ashley and Wingfield 2006b; Owen-Ashley et al. 2008a; Buehler et al. 2009a). Further reduction in Er below Ee + Ei typically does not occur during an acute infection, because energy will be required to forage and search for food once the individual has recovered (Ashley and Wingfield 2011).

Remember that Eg has been sufficient throughout (Figure 9.4A) and regaining lost body weight is achievable once foraging behavior resumes. In some cases, chronic, debilitating disease induces cachexia and muscle wastage, and loss of body weight is not reversed, resulting in elevated potential for death. Energetic costs of the APR and the duration of potential type 1 allostatic overload depend on the amount of energy reserves (Er) regulating allostasis, even though Er might vary with seasonal fluctuations in food availability (Chapter 3; McEwen and Wingfield 2003a; Romero et al. 2009). Once again, the framework energy models provide a mechanism for generating predictions about how environmental conditions, social status, and disease and/or injury interact to regulate allostatic load and reactive scope, and how and when individuals are vulnerable to type 1 allostatic overload.

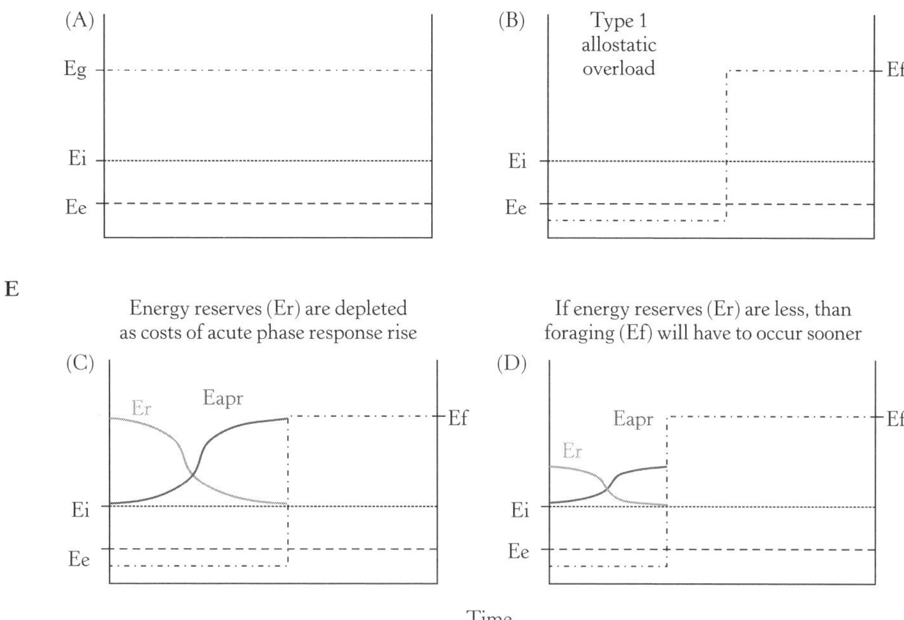

FIGURE 9.4: The concept of allostasis allows the modeling of sickness behavior using allostatic load as a metric of energetic costs (panel A) to mount an immune response. During activation of the acute phase response following infection and/or injury, anorexia is frequently a result. Thus, we remove Eg from panels B, C, and D, although it should be borne in mind that food (Eg) is probably always available. In panel B, we introduce a new term Ef (energy gained from food intake). Thus anorexia (very low Ef) results in immediate type 1 allostatic overload (Panel B). At this point, energy reserves (Er) must be tapped (red line in panel C) to fuel the rising energetic costs of mounting an APR (blue line in panel C). Once Er is depleted (intersection with Ee + Ei), then Ef must increase (panel C). If an individual has less Er, then the ability to mount an APR will be lessened and of shorter duration (panel D). Thus Ef will have to increase earlier. This model provides a basic framework to make predictions about how individuals should respond to infection and wounding depending upon circumstances and energy reserves.

After Ashley and Wingfield (2011), courtesy of Oxford University Press.

Next we will summarize possible mechanisms by which organisms modulate the expression of APRs and sickness behavior depending upon the fitness value of the activities to be sacrificed (such as breeding, migrating; Owen-Ashley and Wingfield 2007; Adelman and Martin 2009). As reviewed previously, the costs of sickness behavior and APRs mean fewer opportunities to breed and care for young, and so forth. In lactating mice, injections of LPS decreased nest-building behavior and increased time to retrieve pups, as expected. However, the LPS-induced decline in reproductive/parental behavior was not observed in controls when the ambient temperature was decreased to 6°C (Aubert et al. 1997), probably because at lower temperatures survival of pups is compromised in the absence of maternal care. In female rats, IL-1 reduced sexual behavior, again as expected, but had no effect on mating behavior in males. Curiously the suppressive effects of IL-1 on locomotor activity were similar in both sexes (Yirmiya et al. 1995). The authors suggest that male rats should maintain mating, even when sick, to increase fitness returns. No immediate fitness benefits would be gained in females owing to the high energetic costs of pregnancy and lactation and thus they should suppress sexual behavior, delay conception, and thereby decrease the chance of spontaneous abortion or other detriments of reproductive function (Avitsur and Yirmiya 1999).

Experimentally increased clutch size in free-living house sparrows elevates allostatic load of incubation and feeding young. Treatment of breeding females with LPS resulted in a small decline in feeding rates of nestlings compared with nests with fewer young. Presumably, fitness probabilities are increased with more young, resulting in modulation of the APR and sickness behavior (Owen-Ashley 2004). Injection of LPS during the winter (non-breeding season) in male song sparrows reduced territorial aggression and resulted in anorexia. However, injection of LPS into breeding males in the spring resulted in little or no response in territoriality (Owen-Ashley and Wingfield 2006b). This may be because a decrease in territorial aggression in response to LPS treatment in spring may result in lower reproductive success so that modulation of the expression of sickness behavior is beneficial (Ashley and Wingfield 2011). Indeed, expression of sickness behavior may depend upon a residual reproductive value (Adelman and Martin 2009), defined as the number of potential reproductive opportunities remaining in the individual's life span. Individuals with a high residual reproductive value are predicted to increase fitness by delaying reproduction, whereas those with a low residual reproductive value are predicted to decrease fitness when reproduction is delayed (Cluttonbrock 1984). Therefore when residual reproductive value is low, a reduced adrenocortical response to acute stress will also occur to enable successful breeding and to maximize fitness (Bókony et al. 2009). Modulation of sickness behavior in several contexts should also occur (for reviews, see Nelson and Demas 1996; Ashley and Wingfield 2011).

Migratory species may be able to avoid the impact of seasonal energy deficits by wintering in warmer areas that have more food and other resources, although risk of parasite infection is often greater at lower than higher latitudes (Piersma 1997). As a result, there will be seasonal differences in how resources will be allocated to fuel immunological defenses, and they will compete with functions of life-history stages over the annual cycle. Immunocompetence clearly varies seasonally, with examples in rodents showing blunted immune function in winter when food is limited and thermogenesis is higher (Nelson and Demas 1996; Nelson et al. 2002; Nelson 2004). The reverse, with enhanced components of immune function during winter, is also found, perhaps to mitigate energy deficits of winter (the winter immunoenhancement hypothesis, Nelson and Demas 1996).

On the other hand, experiments on immunocomptence in birds and other vertebrates have revealed equivocal results (Hasselquist 2007). Adaptive immune function is elevated on short-day (winter) conditions in some investigations (Bentley et al. 1998; Zuk and Johnsen 1998; Lozano and Lank 2003; Martin et al. 2004; Greenman et al. 2005), but in others enhanced immunocompetence occurs during the spring and summer breeding season (Hasselquist et al. 1999; Moller et al. 2003). Yet other investigations have shown no seasonal modulation of immune function at all (Gonzalez et al. 1999; Moore and Siopes 2000; Owen-Ashley et al. 2008a). Such variation in results may be because of seasonal fluctuations in energy stores (Er as well as Eg) (Demas and Nelson 2003; Demas 2004). For example, species that increase body fat (Er) during winter show immunoenhancement, whereas those that decrease fat (Er) show reduced immune function (Demas 2004) and appear to be independent of seasonal regulation by gonadal steroids and melatonin (Bentley et al. 1998; Wen et al. 2007; Prendergast et al. 2008). Experimental reduction of body fat (Er) in rodent species held on long days resulted in lower humoral immune function (Demas et al. 2003), indicating that the link between energy availability and immune function is important for seasonal changes in the expression of sickness behavior.

Siberian hamsters attenuate LPS-induced sickness behaviors on short days (Bilbo et al. 2002). In contrast, free-living male song sparrows show reduced sickness behavior responses to LPS in the early breeding season (i.e., on long days) compared to winter (on short days), as measured by a percentage of reduction in body weight compared with saline (SAL)-injected controls (Owen-Ashley and Wingfield 2006b). If male song sparrows were injected with LPS or saline, and were released back to their territories in both the non-breeding (January) or early breeding (April) seasons (these birds are territorial in both the breeding and non-breeding seasons), territorial aggressive behavior was decreased in LPS-treated males during the non-breeding season, but not in the spring (Owen-Ashley and Wingfield 2006b). LPS-treated males also were anorexic, and body weight declined in the winter, but not in the spring, suggesting modulation of the sickness behavior response in breeding males (Owen-Ashley and Wingfield 2006b).

Hyperphagia and preparatory activities leading to spring migration also modulate expression of sickness behavior (Figure 9.5C). A long-distance migrant that breeds in the Arctic, Gambel's white-crowned sparrow, shows hyperphagia and increases fat stores to a greater extent than conspecific Puget Sound white-crowned sparrows that migrate shorter distances (Wingfield et al. 1996; Wingfield et al. 1997). As predicted, when exposed to long day lengths to trigger development of the vernal migration life-history stage, Puget Sound white-crowned sparrows mount a greater sickness behavior response compared with Gambel's white-crowned sparrow (Owen-Ashley et al. 2008a). In constrast, anorexic responses to LPS, as measured by a percentage decrease in body weight, did not significantly differ between subspecies on winter-like short days. This is consistent with both subspecies having similar body weights in winter (Figure 9.5C). Curiously, female white-crowned sparrows showed no change in response to LPS with day length (Owen-Ashley et al. 2006), suggesting that additional factors, unknown at present, are involved in modulation of sickness behavior.

Free-living male song sparrows show opposing patterns of seasonal fat accumulation compared to captive white-crowned sparrows (compare Figure 9.5B and C). Non-migratory male song sparrows were heavier, with larger fat stores, during the winter than in spring, whereas Gambel's white-crowned sparrows exposed to long days developed extensive fat stores prior to migration (Wingfield et al. 1996). Thus there may be many, sometimes conflicting and sometimes synergistic, reasons that seasonal modulation of sickness behavior varies among species and in captive and free-living animals (Owen-Ashley and Wingfield 2007).

In the red knot, a long-distance migratory shore bird, predictable food shortages are experienced when tidal surges make food unavailable on mud flats twice a day (van Gils et al. 2006). However, when predictable tidal movements are coupled with unpredictable adverse weather, food availability may drop dramatically and knots endure bouts of fasting for several days (Zwarts et al. 1996; Vezina et al. 2009), resulting in substantial loss of body weight. If captive red knots were experimentally deprived of food for 18 hours per day, they failed to respond to LPS treatment by showing sickness behavior compared to controls (Buehler et al. 2009a). In contrast, birds allowed 22 hours of food access per day and treated with LPS showed marked anorexia relative to controls injected with saline (Buehler et al. 2009a). It is important to note that the dependence of expression of the APR on energy reserves is not limited to endotherms. When juvenile green iguanas are challenged with LPS injection, they tend to select warmer temperatures to behaviorally regulate body temperature. Iguanas can also show behavioral hypothermia (selection of colder temperatures) if energy reserves are not sufficient to sustain metabolism associated with higher temperatures and behavioral fever (Deen and Hutchison 2001).

Sickness behaviors can be modulated by social stimuli (Avitsur et al. 1997; Avitsur and Yirmiya 1999; Konsman et al. 2002). For example, the presence of a sexually receptive female has been shown to suppress sickness behavior in male rats (Aubert 1999; Avitsur and Yirmiya 1999), but not in male mice (Weil et al. 2006) or male white-crowned sparrows (Owen-Ashley 2004). Moreover, in male mice exposure to a receptive female actually resulted in an increase in hypothalamic IL-1 and TNF-α gene expression and a heightened anhedonic response compared to isolated males. Social status in dominance hierarchies also influences the expression of sickness behavior in male mice. Dominant mice have reduced activity and aggressive behavior after LPS treatment, but subordinate males were more active, showing defensive behaviors as well as social exploratory behavior (Cohn and de Sa-Rocha 2006). The authors suggest that dominant males were able to allocate resources to sickness behavior, while subordinate males could not and were forced to display defensive behaviors when housed with dominant males. It remains to be clarified whether modulation of sickness behaviors occurs in social hierarchal systems of wild vertebrates.

Absence of social contact can have a profound impact upon the activation of the APR and sickness behavior. Deprivation of parental care increased LPS-induced sickness behavior responses in pigs and impaired suckling behavior (Tuchscherer et al. 2006). Similar results were seen in mouse pups separated from their mothers (Avitsur and Sheridan 2009). This in turn suggests that early postnatal social environment can influence how individuals cope with disease in adulthood. Similarly, in adults caring for young, the presence or absence of offspring can influence the expression of sickness behavior (Aubert et al. 1997; Bonneaud et al. 2003), although further studies are needed to confirm this.

C. Proximate Mechanisms Regulating the Modulation of Sickness Behavior

Different arms of the vertebrate immune system (innate and adaptive immunity) interact in complex ways to orchestrate the APR, and these processes are connected with the suite of neuroendocrine and immune system hormones. Many of these hormones are potent immunoregulatory molecules involved in immune function. Energy reserves and allostasis are critical (Figure 9.4), and anorexia is a central component of sickness behavior, thus negating Eg as a factor. Energetic costs of an APR are high, and without Eg individuals must rely upon Er (e.g., fat, protein, and carbohydrate stores) (Figure 9.4; Ashley and Wingfield 2011). Er and body weight decline to a minimum threshold (Figure 9.4), following which individuals should resume feeding. If body weight declines below this minimum set-point, then

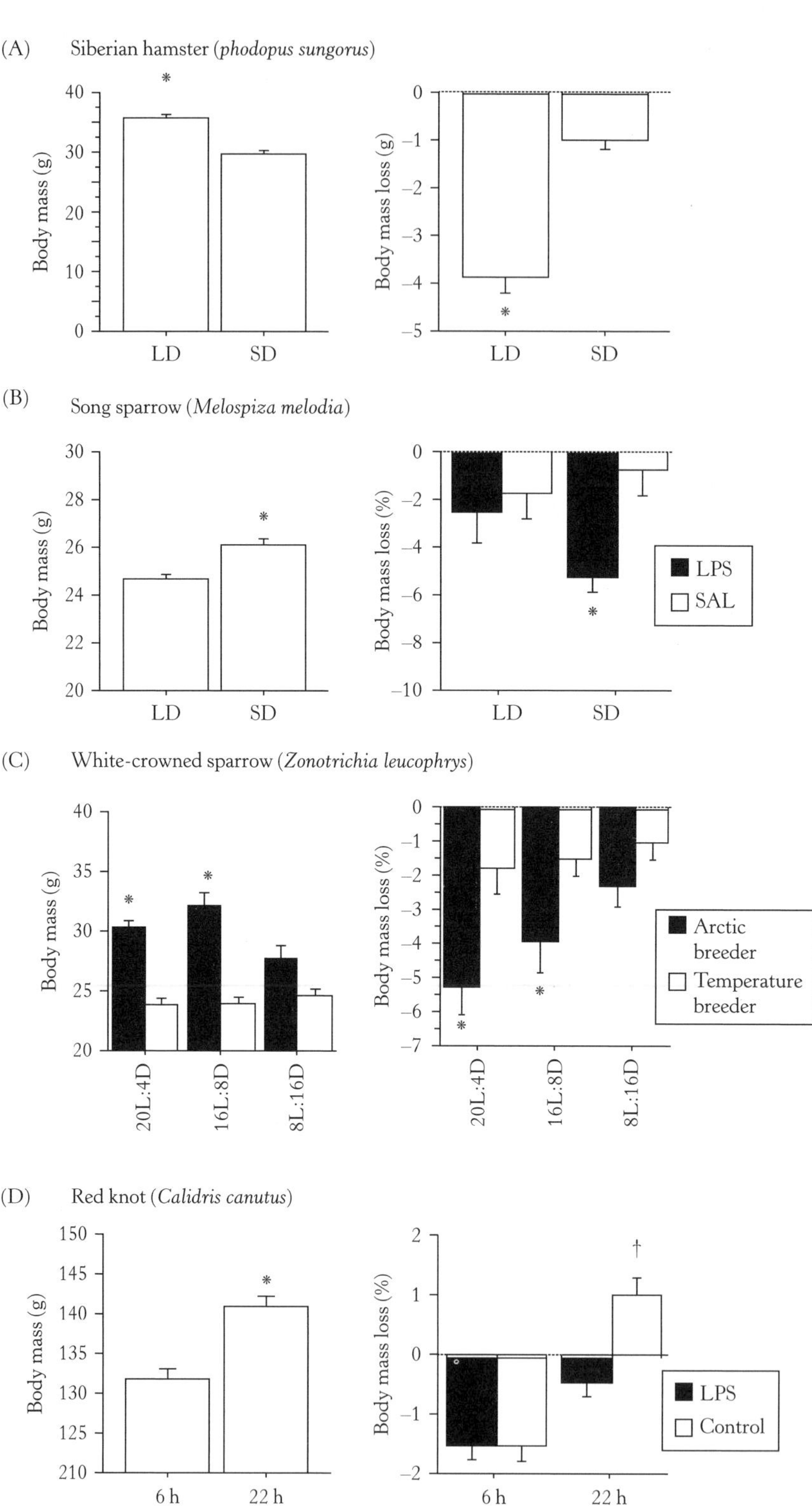

FIGURE 9.5: (Continued)

cachexia sets in, resulting in morbidity and mortality (Plata-Salaman 1996). Owen-Ashley and Wingfield (2007) termed this the "energy limitation hypothesis."

The role of hormones in the regulation of immune function is extremely complex, including corticosteroids, cytokines, prolactin, thyroid hormones, sex steroids, leptin, ghrelin, and melatonin (for review, see Ashley and Wingfield 2011). Here we will focus on the overwhelming evidence that corticosteroids regulate most, if not all, aspects of immunological function (Munck et al. 1984; Besedovsky and DelRey 1996; McEwen et al. 1997; Dhabhar 2002). Corticosteroids are essential to provide negative feedback to the APR and to prevent an overactive immune response (Besedovsky et al. 1986; Bateman et al. 1989; Baumann and Gauldie 1994). At the onset of infection or when exposed to acute stress, IL-1 and other cytokines stimulate the HPA axis to release corticosteroids, which then have an enhancing effect upon immunological function through early mobilization of immune cells and their redistribution (Dhabhar and McEwen 1999; Dhabhar 2002). This is in contrast to the better-known suppressive actions of corticosteroids in chronic stress situations. Such up-regulation may be adaptive, allowing animals to prepare for potential infection challenges such as wounding (Figure 9.1; Ashley and Wingfield 2011). Energy reserves and hormones, such as corticosteroids, play a role in regulating this response, but more experimental studies that manipulate energy levels, nutrition, and hormone levels are certainly needed.

III. PREDATION

The daily routine of finding food and so forth (Ee + Ei) can be markedly hampered by the presence of predators. This requires that an individual spend more time hiding rather than foraging, or proceeding with caution. The implications for Eo (more energy expended in finding food when predators are present) and Eg (food availability is effectively reduced because access to it is limited by the presence of predators) can be profound (see Chapter 6; McEwen and Wingfield 2003a). Furthermore, stress responses by potential prey could alter ecosystem functioning and energy available at other trophic levels (Hawlena and Schmitz 2010). For example, when red foxes, a major predator of birds and small mammals, declined in Sweden, grouse and other ground-dwelling animals increased, but their populations crashed when foxes recovered

FIGURE 9.5: A selection of studies that demonstrate the energy limitation hypothesis in regulating variation of sickness behavior in different life-history contexts. (A) Captive male Siberian hamsters lose body mass on short days and attenuate LPS-induced sickness responses as measured by a change in body mass 48 hours post-injection compared to long days. Note that pre-injection body mass is lower in short-day males compared to long-day subjects.

Modified from Bilbo et al. (2002). Courtesy of the Royal Society.

(B) Free-living male song sparrows exhibit an opposing seasonal pattern that involves suppression of sickness behavior during the breeding season (long days). Males injected with LPS (black bars) lost body mass 25 hours later during the winter (short days) compared to saline (SAL)-injected controls (white bars) in the same season. Males in the spring when defending breeding territories did not lose body mass compared to controls, suggesting insensitivity to LPS or an inability to mount a sickness response. These results are consistent with wintering sparrows being significantly heavier than breeding birds.

Modified from Owen-Ashley and Wingfield (2006a).

(C) Differences in sickness behavior responses (as measured by a 24-hour percentage change in body mass) in two subspecies of white-crowned sparrows that have different migratory strategies. The arctic-breeding subspecies (black bars) is a long-distance migrant and accumulates more body mass (g) and fat stores (not shown) upon vernal exposure to long days (16L:8D or 20L:4D) than the temperate-breeding subspecies (white bars). These changes in body mass parallel the magnitude of anorexic responses to LPS. Saline-injected controls are not shown in this figure.

Modified from Owen-Ashley et al. (2008b).

(D) Red knots given restricted access to food (6 hours of food access) fail to respond to LPS challenge compared to birds given 22 hours of food access as measured by a 24-hour percentage change in body mass. Restricted access to food decreased body mass (g), which is consistent with birds failing to mount a response.

Adapted from (Buehler et al. 2009b; Vézina et al. 2009).

Asterisk denotes a significant pair-wise difference. Dagger denotes a significant interaction in the overall ANOVA model, but no significant pair-wise difference.

After Ashley and Wingfield (2011), courtesy of Oxford University Press.

(Marcstrom et al. 1988). Foxes may drive three- to five-year cycles in voles as well, but a certain degree of unpredictability can result, and cycles can get out of synchrony if other sources of mortality, such as disease, deplete vole numbers. However, experimental removal of predators did not affect the vole cycle, suggesting that there is some degree of independence of predation that increases unpredictability even more (Lindstrom et al. 1994). Predator exclusions also result in increased reproductive success.

If populations of voles or other small mammal prey crash, then abundant predators may switch to other prey such as birds (e.g., Newton 1998). In northern Sweden islands, predator removal (red foxes and martens) resulted in increased reproductive success of capercaillie and black grouse. Breeding numbers increased the following year. When predators were not removed, grouse numbers were inversely correlated with vole abundance—that is, predators turned more to preying on grouse when voles were sparse (Marcstrom et al. 1988). Moreover, in the Arctic the brief breeding season means that migrant birds cannot delay the onset of breeding, and thus re-nesting following loss of a nest to a predator is rare (Wingfield et al. 2004). As a result, they cannot wait for predators to leave, or their numbers to change, as some avian species do in the tropics (Morton 1971).

It is not surprising that predator risk can increase circulating levels of corticosteroids (e.g., Sheriff et al. 2009). In fact, there may be a strong relationship between food availability and predator pressure, which Boonstra et al. (1998) and Clinchy et al. (2004) call the chronic stress hypothesis. This may also be an example of allostatic overload type 2 (see Chapter 3), in which chronic high levels of corticosteroids have deleterious but sub-lethal effects (e.g., McEwen and Wingfield 2003a). Clinchy et al. (2004) compared total plasma corticosterone levels in free-living populations of song sparrows in southwestern British Columbia, Canada. They used populations on islands as a low predator site and mainland populations as high predation risk sites. Food was then supplemented, or not, and the synergistic effects of food and predation risk was related to circulating corticosterone levels. Male sparrows at sites without food supplementation and high predation risk had the highest plasma levels of corticosterone compared with food-supplemented birds at sites with low predator risk (Clinchy et al. 2004). Sparrows at other sites had intermediate levels. Furthermore, this effect appeared to be greater in males than in females (Figure 9.6).

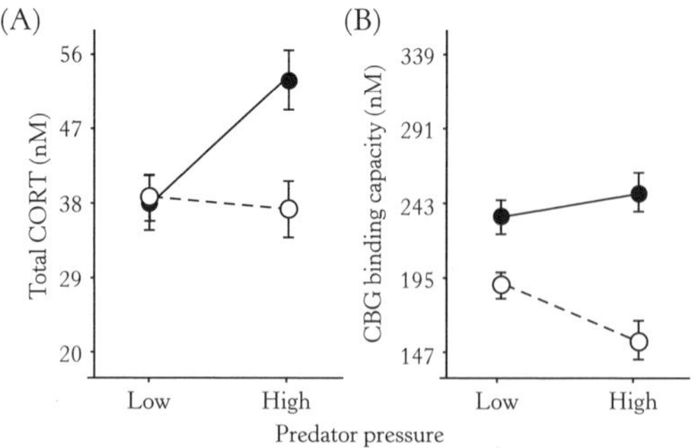

FIGURE 9.6: Plasma total corticosterone (CORT) concentrations (A) and corticosteroid binding globulin (CBG) binding capacities (B) in parental male (closed circles connected by solid line) and female (open circles connected by dashed line) song sparrows on day 6 of the chick rearing period, at low—and high predator pressure locations.

From Clinchy et al., (2004), courtesy of the Royal Society, London.

Clinchy et al. (2004) also measured CBG binding capacity in plasma, which allowed them to calculate a free corticosterone index, which revealed that unbound corticosterone levels were higher in both sexes at the high predation risk sites (Figures 9.6 and 9.7). Nonetheless, adrenocortical responses of males were still higher than in females at the high predation sites, including when mothers and fathers were feeding young at the same nest on the same day (Figure 9.8).

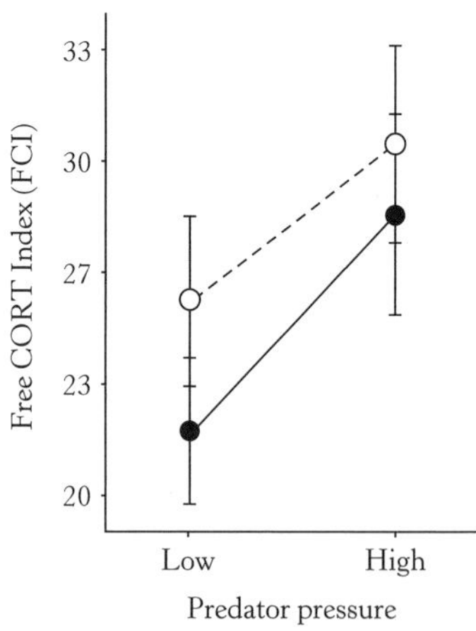

FIGURE 9.7: Free corticosterone (CORT) index (FCI) values in parental males (closed circles connected by solid line) and females (open circles connected by dashed line) on day 6 of the chick-rearing period, at low and high predator pressure locations.

From Clinchy et al. (2004), courtesy of the Royal Society, London.

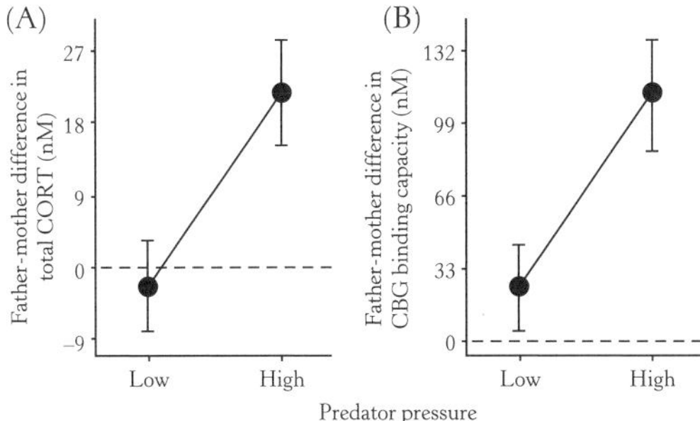

FIGURE 9.8: Difference in plasma total corticosterone (CORT) concentration (A) and corticosteroid binding globulin (CBG) binding capacity (B) between the father and mother caught at the same nest on the same day caring for day 6 chicks, at low and high predator pressure locations. Panels illustrate the value for the father minus the value for the mother. The horizontal dashed lines indicate no difference between the father and mother.

From Clinchy et al. (2004), courtesy of the Royal Society, London.

High predation risk may have long-term effects on survival and reproduction through chronic, sub-lethal stress. An example is the well-known predator-prey interrelationship of the snowshoe hare and the Canadian lynx (Figure 9.9; Krebs et al. 1995; Boonstra et al. 1998). The snowshoe hares in the Canadian boreal forest go through 10-year population cycles. Plasma levels of free cortisol in field-sampled (Yukon) hares were highest during a population decline and low in the 1990s (Figure 9.10; Boonstra et al. 1998). Additionally, CBG binding capacity was lowest, there was reduced testosterone, and a greater over-winter weight loss occurred during the population decline. The authors present evidence that these declines and high cortisol were a result of increased predation risk, not high population density or poor nutrition. Indeed, increased condition, improved reproductive function, and lower adrenocortical responses did not occur until predation risk subsided (Figure 9.11). Furthermore, although experimental enclosures prevented lynx

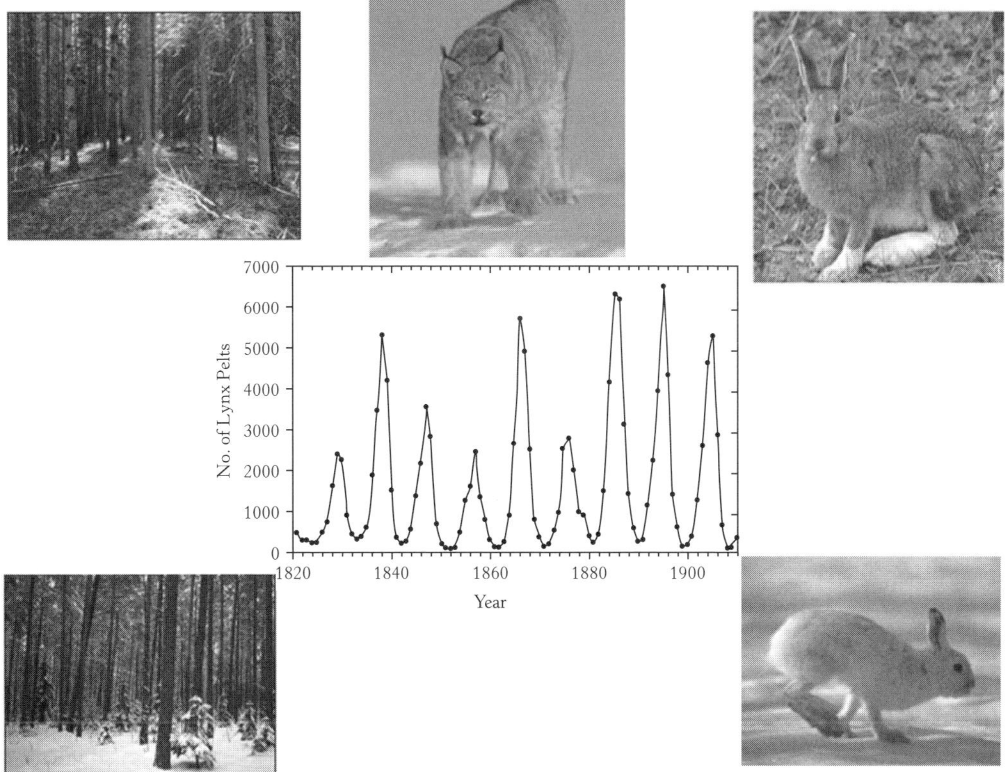

FIGURE 9.9: Boreal forests, snowshoe hares, and the Canadian lynx. The center panel shows cycles in lynx pelts traded through the Hudson's Bay Trading Company in the 1800s. Numbers cycle with great regularity dependent upon similar population cycles in the snowshoe hare.

From Krebs et al. (1995), courtesy of Science and Boonstra et al. (1998), courtesy of the Ecological Society of America.

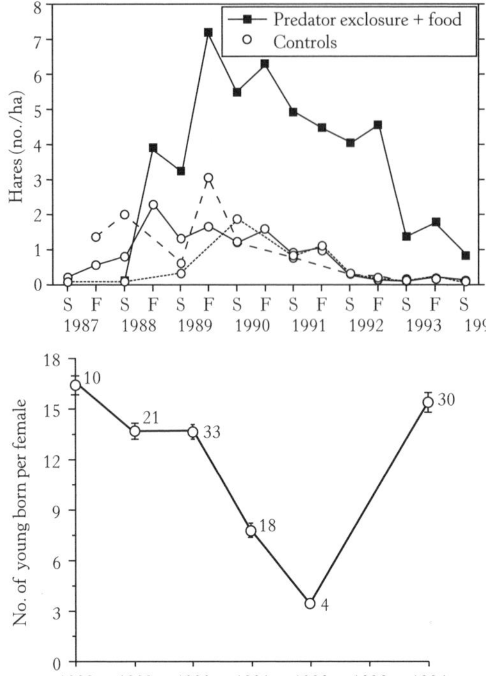

FIGURE 9.10: Top: Spring (S) and fall (F) densities of snowshoe hares in the southern Yukon on three control grids and on one Predator Exclosure + Food grid. The fence for the latter grid was built in 1988. Bottom: Total reproduction of live young per female snowshoe hare per year over the summer breeding season. Sample sizes are indicated beside each point.

From Boonstra et al. (1998), with permission and courtesy of the Ecological Society of America.

from killing snowshoe hares and led to increased hare density (Figure 9.10), the enclosures had no impact on adrenocortical function (Figure 9.11; Boonstra et al. 1998).

Predator threat can also increase plasma levels of corticosteroids in wild female show-shoe hares. Sheriff et al. (2009) hypothesize that corticosteroid-mediated effects on reproduction may also act to "program" their offspring to be timid (risk averse) when predator populations are high and risk of predation is greatest (Sheriff et al. 2009; Sheriff et al. 2010). A captive study of European hares showed that three short periods of arousal by human presence, probably interpreted as predation attempts by the hares, resulted in an increase in fecal corticosteroid concentrations (Teskey-Gerstl et al. 2000). Additionally, European rabbits exposed to the odor of a major predator, the red fox, increased their vigilance rates, but there were no differences in baseline plasma levels of corticosteroids or the responsiveness to ACTH challenge (Monclus et al. 2006b), although there was a difference in fecal corticosteroid metabolites (Monclus et al. 2006a). There was a similar lack of response to predator odor in meadow voles (Fletcher and Boonstra 2006). In general, corticosteroid responses by mammalian species to predator odors are not consistent (Apfelbach et al. 2005). In free-living yellow-bellied marmots, fecal concentrations of corticosteroid metabolites were positively correlated with predator pressure and alarm calls, and had both direct and indirect effects on the dispersal of pups (Blumstein et al. 2006; Monclus et al. 2011; see also discussion later in this chapter).

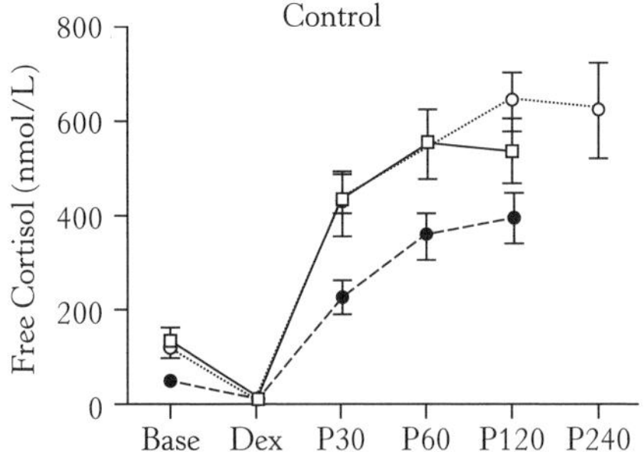

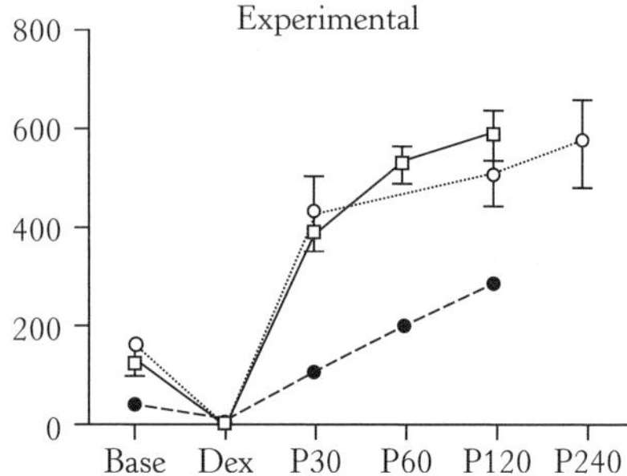

FIGURE 9.11: Responses over time in plasma concentrations of free cortisol in snowshoe hares from control (unmanipulated) and experimental (predator excluded; see Figure 9.10) grids. Data from two years of population decline (squares = 1991, diamonds = 1992) and one year of a population low (closed circles = 1994). Base levels indicate initial values, Dex indicates values 2 hours after the dexamethasone injection, and P30, P60, P120, and P240 indicate values 30, 60, 120, and 240 minutes after the adrenocorticotropic hormone (ACTH) injection.

From Boonstra et al. (1998), with permission and courtesy of the Ecological Society of America.

In a detailed study of the effects of laboratory rats (predators) on laboratory strains of mice (prey), Beekman (2004) showed that all mice exposed to the presence of a rat showed marked behavioral responses such as predator avoidance and coping behavior. This was accompanied by increases in plasma levels of ACTH and corticosterone, although there was variation in the magnitude of the response among strains of mice tested (Figure 9.12). Dialysis samples from regions of the brain of control and exposed mice also revealed increases in serotonin and norepinephrine as well as other neuroendocrine metabolites. Additionally, free corticosterone levels in brain dialysates showed significant increases during exposure to the rat, but the response was greatest in a subset of mice (Figure 9.13; Beekman 2004). Different laboratory experiments of mice exposed to cats also induced significant learning and memory deficiencies (El Hage et al. 2006), and in general predatory attacks can have lasting effects on brain function (Adamec et al. 2006).

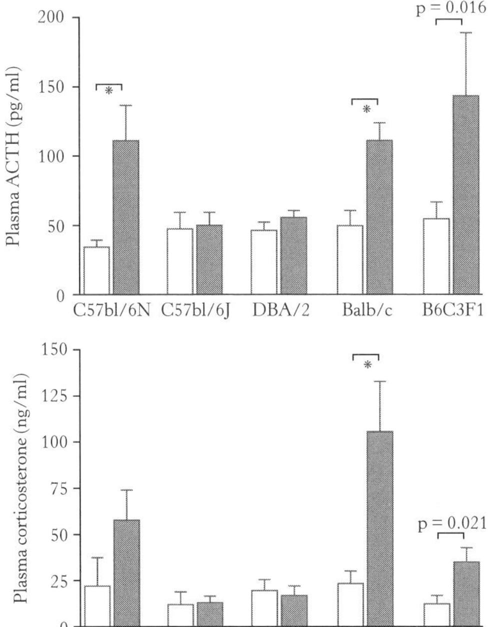

FIGURE 9.12: Average plasma levels of ACTH (top panel) and corticosterone (bottom panel) for five strains of mice under control conditions (open bars) or after half an hour of rat exposure (closed bars). Asterisks indicate a significant difference between control and exposed conditions.

From Beekman (2004), with permission.

A captive study of bank voles showed that when the experimental group was exposed to a major predator, the weasel, there was a decrease in foraging rate and hoarding of food for the winter (Ylonen et al. 2006). Fecal levels of corticosteroid metabolites were not different between the experimental group and the controls. Many rodents, such as Gunther's vole, respond to predator presence with reduced activity and foraging. Experimental playback of recorded calls of a major predator, the tawny owl, resulted in voles decreasing activity and foraging compared to controls exposed to the sound of a human voice. Some voles responded with hyperactive fleeing behavior (Eilam et al. 1999). Another rodent, the spiny mouse, showed no behavioral responses to owl calls, possible because this species lives in rock piles and is relatively protected from aerial predation, whereas voles live in exposed open fields. Curiously, exposure to owl calls resulted in an increase in plasma corticosteroid levels compared to controls in both species (Eilam et al. 1999).

In free-living pied flycatchers, nesting males will attack potential predators, both of themselves and of the nest. However, corticosterone-implanted males never attacked experimentally simulated predators such as great spotted woodpeckers, a nest predator, and a weasel, a predator of the adults (Silverin 1998). Exposure to the woodpecker elicited strong attack responses but no change in corticosterone levels compared to unmanipulated controls. Exposure to a weasel resulted in higher corticosterone and fewer attacks (Silverin 1998). Similarly, simulating predator presence at the nest in several free-living bird species elicited robust behavioral responses but no change in corticosteroid levels (Mueller et al. 2006; Butler et al. 2009). These are further examples of how behavioral responses to predators and adrenocortical responses are not necessarily linked. Indeed, if intense predator pressure meant serious risk of predation, then it may be preferable to not respond behaviorally and to show a corticosterone response.

A field study of free-living great tits in southern Sweden showed that when exposed to a stuffed and moving predator, Tengmalm's owl, birds responded with alarm calls and movements away. There was no increase in plasma levels of corticosterone 30 to 50 minutes after exposure. However, in a captive experiment, great tits showed more intense escape behavior when exposed to the stuffed owl. Plasma levels of corticosterone also increased markedly (Figure 9.14; Cockrem and Silverin 2002). When

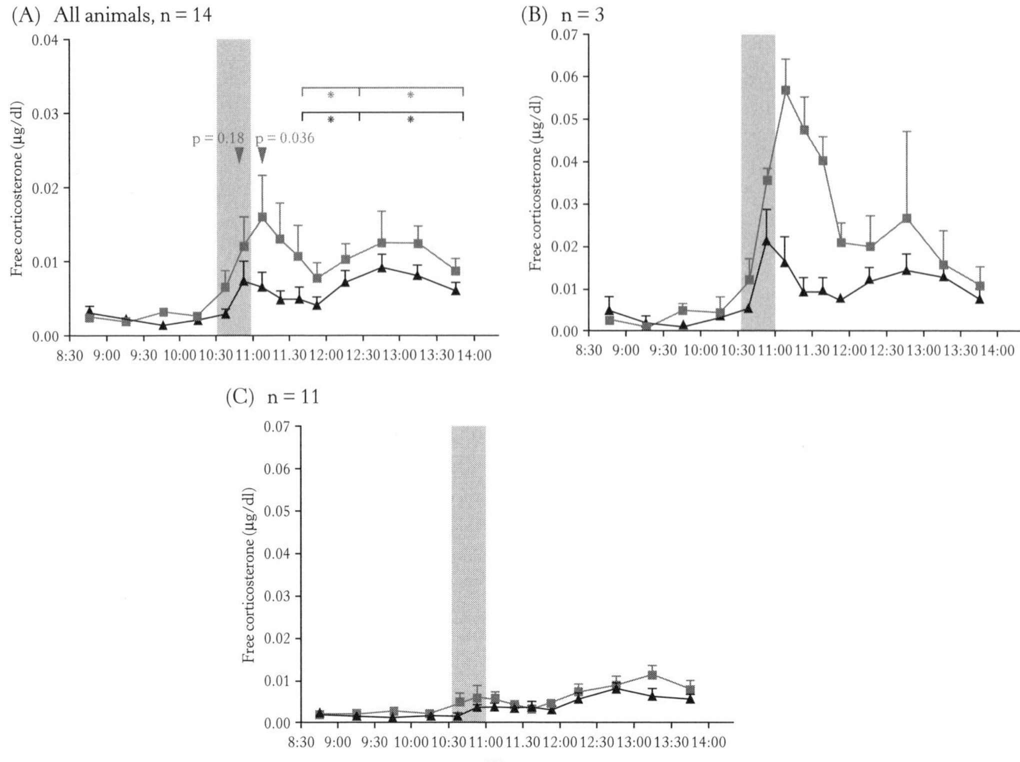

FIGURE 9.13: Average free corticosterone from dialysates of the brain. Time curves for all C57bl/6N mice of which the dialysate was analyzed (panel A) on day 1 (grey squares) and day 2 (black triangles) of rat exposure, as well as for 3 animals (panel B) of which the levels of free corticosterone clearly deviated from the other 11 animals (panel C). Note differences in Y-axis scaling. Shaded area signifies the time frame during which the rat was present. Only the figure in panel A was analyzed statistically.

Asterisks indicate a significant deviation from baseline level.

From Beekman (2004), with permission.

exposed to control stimuli—a non-predator, the brambling, or a slowly moving box—great tits did show some behavioral responses, but there was no effect on plasma levels of corticosterone (Figure 9.14; Cockrem and Silverin 2002). These authors suggest that the captive birds show a much more intense response to the predator than free-living birds because they were only able to flee to the edges of the flight aviary and thus were at greater risk of predation.

Free-living stonechats nesting in Kenya were less likely to initiate a second brood and showed greater inter-brood intervals if their territory was close to a songbird predator, the fiscal shrike (Scheuerlein et al. 2001). Males on territories close to shrikes had higher baseline levels of corticosterone and lower body condition than males on territories with no shrikes nearby, whereas females showed no differences (Scheuerlein et al. 2001). Captive European stonechats showed varying degrees of adrenocortical responses to stress depending upon the type of stressor. Exposure of captive birds to a predator, the tawny owl, elicited the strongest response (Figure 9.15; Canoine et al. 2002).

Offspring also respond to predators. This can be indirectly, through alarm calls of their parents, or directly through predator vocalizations. Although chicks of the American kestrel can respond behaviorally to experimental playback of recorded adult alarm calls, there were no effects on plasma corticosterone levels compared with controls (Dufty and Crandall 2005). Similarly, parental alarm calls played to chicks of white-crowned sparrows failed to elicit a corticosteroid response, even though handling induced a robust increase (Rivers et al. 2011). In contrast, when chicks of common blackbirds were exposed to playbacks of predator calls, they decreased corticosteroid concentrations (Ibanez-Alamo

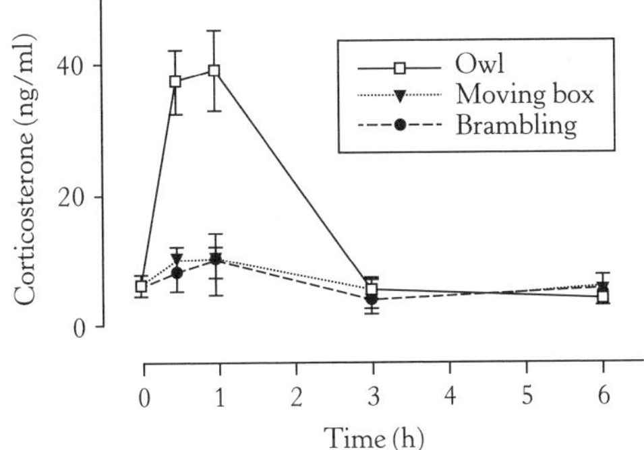

FIGURE 9.14: Plasma corticosterone levels in groups of great tits exposed to stimuli for 30 minutes and sampled at 30 minutes or exposed to stimuli for 60 minutes and sampled at 60 minutes or later after the start of the stimulus. Corticosterone levels measured in undisturbed birds in the aviary were taken as 0 h levels for all three stimuli.

From Cockrem and Silverin (2002), with permission and courtesy of Elsevier.

et al. 2011). The ultimate response by chicks likely depends upon the species, the type of predator, how the chicks detect the predator, and so on. Little work has been done on corticosteroid responses to predators in young animals, but the impacts on development and the ultimate fitness

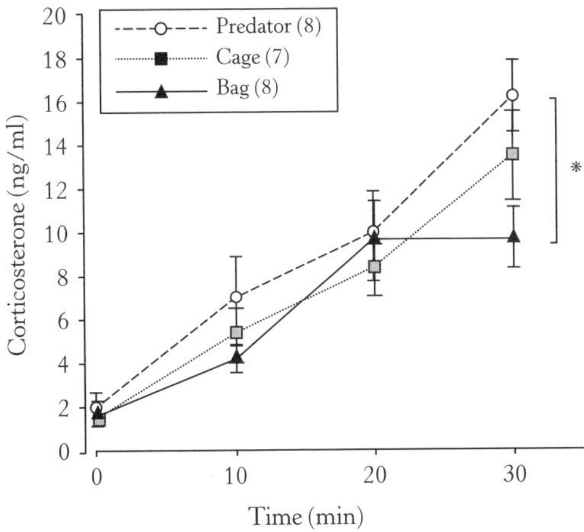

FIGURE 9.15: Stress-responses of stonechats exposed to a predator, kept in a cage or kept in a cloth bag. The increase in corticosterone levels (slope between baseline and 30 minutes) was significantly higher in the predator group than in the bag group. Also, corticosterone levels after 30 minutes were significantly higher in the predator than in the bag group.

From Canoine et al. (2002), with permission and courtesy of Brill, Leiden.

of the animal might be profound (Scheuerlein and Gwinner 2006).

Free-living elk in Montana and Wyoming change their behavior in response to predators such as wolves. These changes include altered patterns of aggregation and habitat selection, increased vigilance, and foraging patterns. Measurements of fecal progesterone concentrations revealed lower levels in females under greater predation risk, and this was associated with production of fewer calves (Figure 9.16; Creel et al. 2009). However, fecal corticosteroid metabolite levels were not related to wolf/elk ratios or to population density, suggesting that changes in foraging patterns in response to predation risk may be a more important determinant of progesterone and calf production (Creel et al. 2007).

Many vertebrate animals living on isolated islands and without predation risk show varying degrees of "tameness," especially when confronted with humans. Rödl et al. (2007) showed that marine iguanas on various Galápagos Islands were tamer when approached by a human on islands where predation risk was low (naïve animals) compared with islands where predators (e.g., dogs and cats) had been introduced for over 100 years (Figure 9.17). Furthermore, iguanas that were chased, captured, restrained, and held showed no adrenocortical response if naïve, but animals from islands with predators did respond. These data suggest that although the adrenocortical stress response can be greatly reduced in the absence of predators, it is restored if predators reappear (Figure 9.17; Roedl et al. 2007). However, island species may have a limit in the degree to which they can recover a normal response. Even though the Galápagos marine iguanas learned that humans could be predators (by catching and handling them), remote injections of epinephrine (via blow-gun darting) failed to initiate and only marginally augmented a flight-or-flight response (Vitousek et al. 2010). This suggests that the evolutionary development of "tameness" is accompanied by permanent changes in stress physiology, with these data suggesting a decrease in epinephrine receptors.

Individuals of the tree lizard have color morphs that vary in their responses to a major predator such as the collared lizard. The orange throated morph is more wary, initiates fleeing behavior at longer distances, and hides for longer periods in the presence of the predator compared with orange-blue and mottled morphs (Thaker et al. 2009b). Male tree lizards of all morphs showed an increase in corticosterone levels in

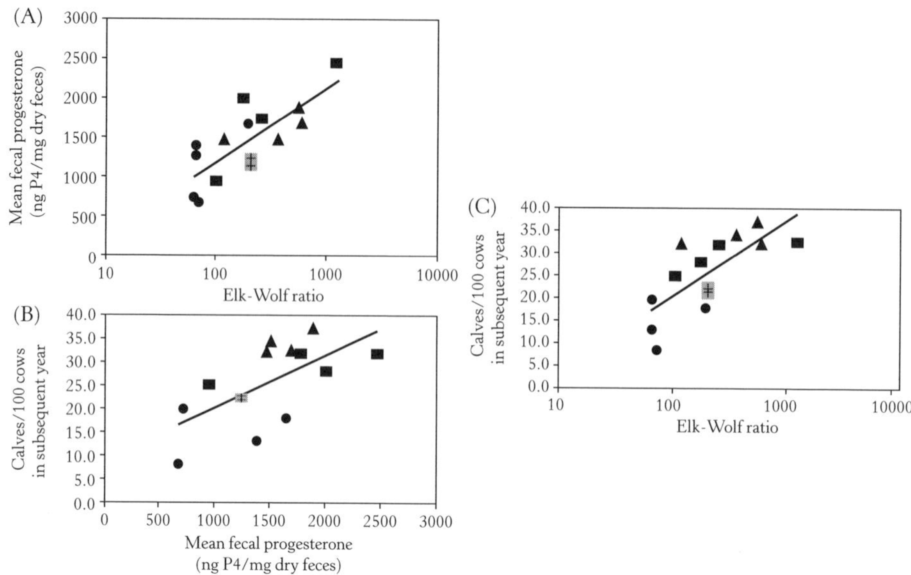

FIGURE 9.16: (A) Regression of elk mean fecal progesterone concentrations on predation pressure, measured by elk-wolf ratios, for five elk populations, 2002–2006. (B) Regression of calf-cow ratios in the subsequent year on mean fecal progesterone concentrations. (C) Regression of calf-cow ratios in the subsequent year on predation pressure.

Data point shapes denote different elk winter ranges.

From Creel et al. (2009), with permission, courtesy of the AAAS.

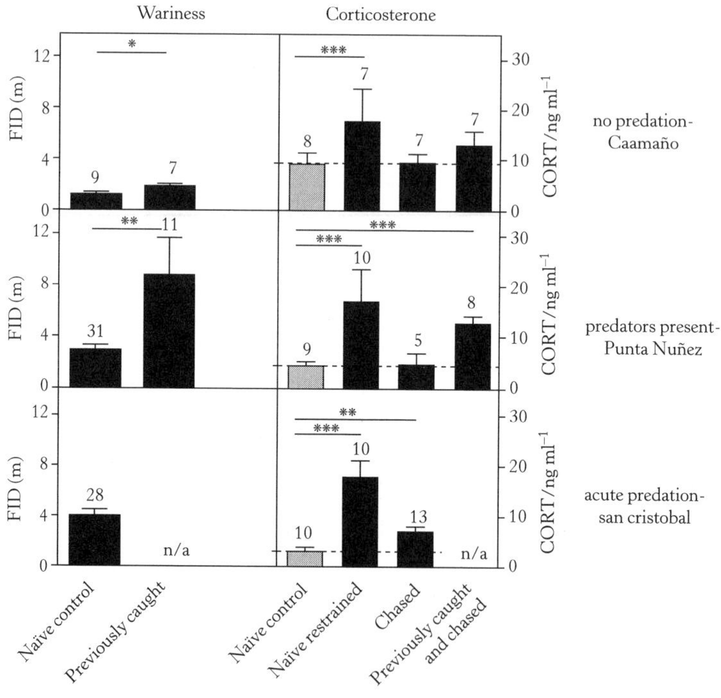

FIGURE 9.17: Wariness (as measured by flight initiation distance, FID—the distance at which an iguana begins to flee an approaching human) and corticosterone (CORT) concentrations at three sites differing in intensity of predation risk. Blood samples from naïve control animals were collected on an average 2 minutes after capture (i.e., CORT baselines), from naïve restrained animals 30 minutes after capture (i.e., CORT response to restraint in a bag). Chased and previously caught and chased animals were subjected to 15 minutes of experimental harassment prior to capture. In contrast to naïve chased individuals, the latter group had been caught and handled once, three to four weeks before. Dashed lines mark CORT baseline levels (average of the naïve control group).

From Rödl et al. (2007). Courtesy of the Royal Society, London.

blood after a single exposure to the approaching predator (Figure 9.18). Furthermore, the plasma corticosterone level post-encounter correlated strongly with the intensity of predator avoidance behavior displayed (Figure 9.19; Thaker et al. 2009b). In a semi-captive study (open enclosures), male tree lizards of different morphs were treated with non-invasive dermal patches to elevate plasma levels of corticosterone. Corticosterone treatment enhanced responses to the exposure to a caged collared lizard in male tree lizards of all morphs compared with controls. This included a quicker response, hiding for longer, and enhanced displays to the predator (Figure 9.20; Thaker et al. 2009a). However, orange morphs were still more wary following corticosterone treatment, suggesting that morph effects persist even when corticosterone levels are elevated. Blocking corticosteroid release prevents these behaviors, further supporting the regulatory role of corticosteroids in the anti-predator behaviors (Thaker et al. 2010).

Juvenile coho salmon are vulnerable to predation by lingcod and display typical wariness and

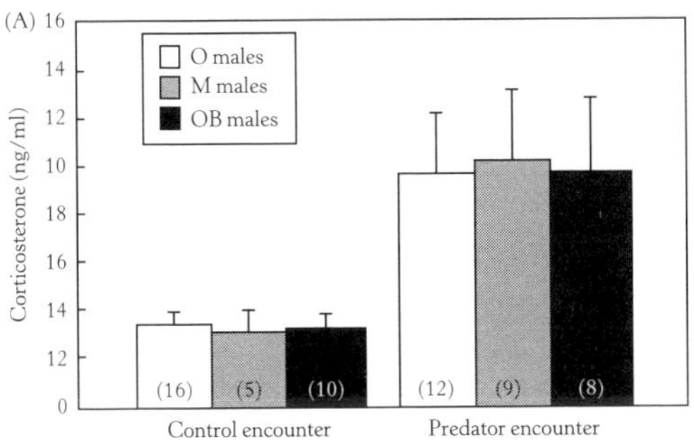

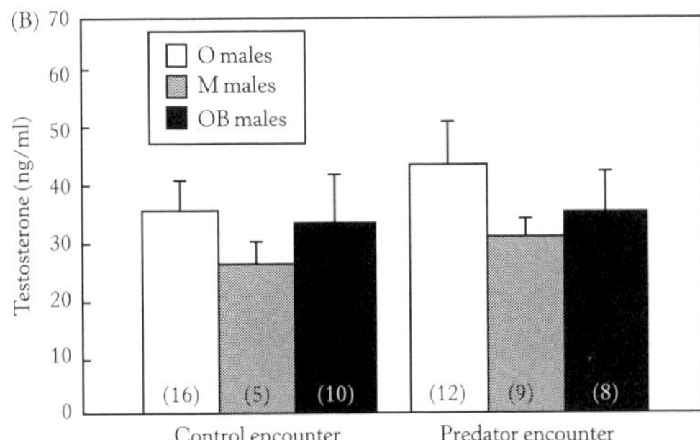

FIGURE 9.18: Plasma levels of corticosterone (A) and testosterone (B) in free-ranging male tree lizard morphs (distinguished by color of the dewlap: O = orange, M = mottled, and OB = orange-blue) after exposure to a control (stick) or predator (collared lizard). Sample sizes are reported within each bar.

From Thaker et al. (2009b), with permission and courtesy of Elsevier.

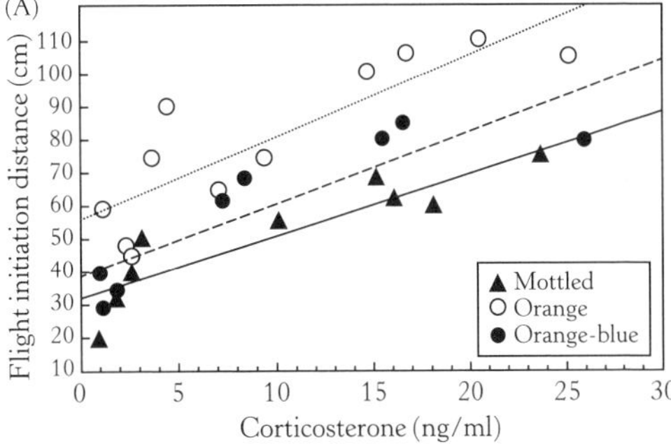

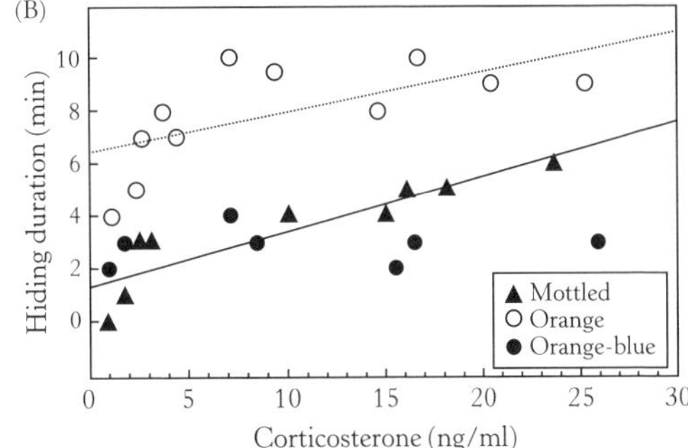

FIGURE 9.19: Correlations between plasma corticosterone levels after a predator encounter and flight initiation distance (A) and hiding duration (B) for free-ranging orange (open circles, dotted line), mottled (closed triangles, solid line) and orange-blue (closed circles, dashed line) males. Significant correlations are shown as regression lines. Males exposed to a control encounter are not shown.

From Thaker et al. (2009b), with permission and courtesy of Elsevier.

predation avoidance behavior in the presence of the predator. If juvenile cohos were stressed by capture and handling out of water for 1 minute, cortisol levels in blood increased markedly and remained high for at least 240 minutes. If a subgroup of these stressed fish were then exposed to predation by lingcod, predator avoidance was initially decreased but returned to levels of controls within 90 minutes, despite continuing high cortisol levels (Olla et al. 1992). These data are another example of behavioral responses to predators changing independently of corticosteroid levels in blood. When wintering European carp were subjected to exposure to a predator, the river otter, increased responses to stress, including metabolism and cortisol, were observed. On the other hand, juvenile winter flounder increased corticosteroid levels when exposed to some predators and not others (Breves and Specker 2005).

In contrast, some studies indicate a close connection between predator presence, corticosteroid

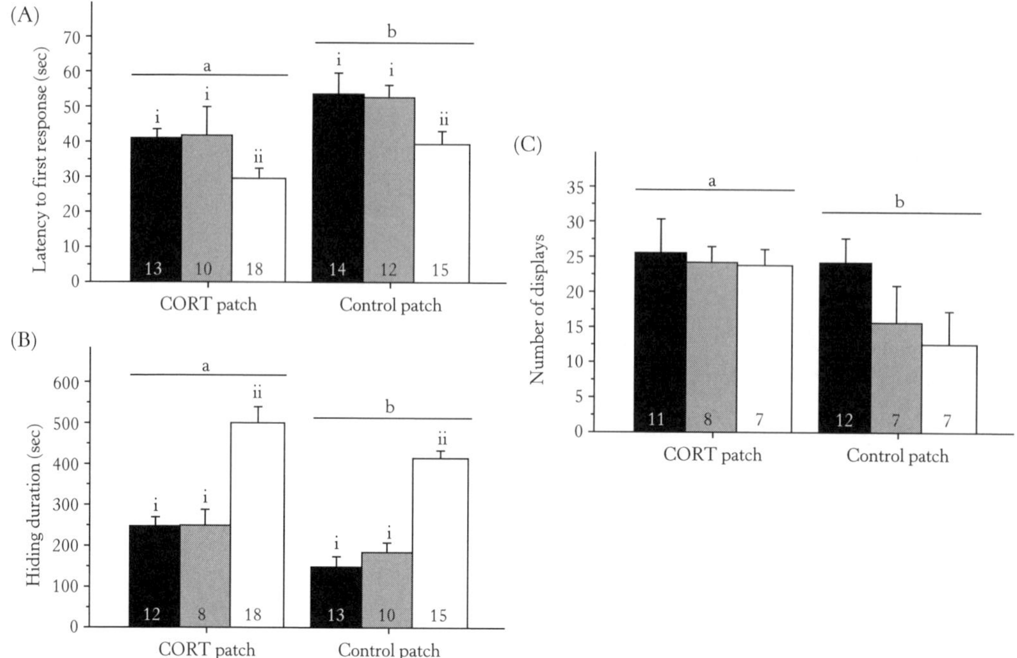

FIGURE 9.20: Antipredator responses of orange-blue (black bars), mottled (gray bars), and orange (white bars) male tree lizard morphs with a corticosterone dermal patch (CORT patch) or a control patch during a 20-minute predator exposure. Letters denote significant differences between endocrine treatment groups in their (A) latency to first respond, regardless of the behavioral tactic, (B) hiding duration for those who hid, and (C) number of displays for those who displayed toward the predator. Roman numerals denote significant differences between the male morphs irrespective of the endocrine treatment group. Sample sizes are denoted within each bar.

From Thaker et al. (2009a), with permission and courtesy of Elsevier.

release, and changes in behavior. Gulf toadfish belong to a group of fish that use vocalizations, via a sexually dimorphic vocal organ, to attract mates. When free-living gulf toadfish are exposed to sonar clicks of foraging bottlenose dolphins, they rapidly increase corticosteroid levels and suppress calling behavior (Remage-Healey et al. 2006). This response appears to be a direct non-genomic effect of corticosteroids inhibiting the function of central pattern generators that regulate vocal behavior (Remage-Healey and Bass 2004, 2006a, 2006b). However, the impact of corticosteroids on predator-avoidance behavior can depend upon the type of predator. Exogenous corticosteroids applied to eastern fence lizards normally elicited hiding behavior, likely effective at decreasing predation from native snakes and birds (Trompeter and Langkilde 2011). But when exogenous corticosteroids were applied to lizards from sites invaded by fire ants, they increased movement away from the ground, a behavior likely more effective at decreasing fire ant predation (Trompeter and Langkilde 2011).

It is well known that many wild animals respond to the presence of humans as they would to any predator (e.g., Frid and Dill 2002; Mueller et al. 2006; Carter et al. 2008). Indeed it is the perception of humans as predators that is central to the efficacy of the stress series described in Chapter 6 in which the capture, handling, and restraint of wild vertebrates almost invariably results in an acute increase in corticosteroid secretion. Free-living blue tits frequently give alarm calls and hesitate to enter nest boxes when humans approach the nest area. However, the degree of arousal to the presence of humans was not related to baseline levels of corticosterone. Nonetheless, all birds showed marked increases in circulating corticosterone following capture and handling (Mueller et al. 2006). The authors review other publications of this kind and conclude that behavioral responses to the presence of predators and the adrenocortical responses are independent, with corticosterone responses occurring only in the most life-threatening situations.

Predator presence can also lead to an inhibition of corticosteroid release. Female loggerhead turtles nesting on island beaches of the Great Barrier Reef, Australia, are exposed to attack from tiger sharks. Injuries from these attacks range from superficial lacerations to severe, potentially lethal, trauma to the body. Despite such predation risk, and sometimes major injury, female turtles will continue to emerge on the beaches and lay eggs (Jessop et al. 2004). Females tend to show significant reduction in their sensitivity of the adrenocortical response to capture, handling, and restraint, and turtles with injuries showed identical responses to uninjured turtles (Jessop et al. 2004). The authors suggest that the reduced sensitivity to acute stress may be part of the mechanisms that allow injured females to continue nesting despite the potentially lethal consequences of those injuries. Similarly, tadpoles of western spadefoot toads initiate a behaviorally quiescent state, accompanied by a decrease in whole-body corticosteroids, when exposed to predators (Fraker 2008). Interestingly, this response appears to be triggered by a pheromone from other tadpoles (Fraker 2008).

Overall it appears that the effects of predators on adrenocortical function in vertebrates appear to be mixed at best. One thing that is becoming clear is that only under conditions of immediate predation risk is there a stronger potential of a corticosteroid response. There are likely differences across species owing to the type of predator as well. Much further work is needed to understand the underlying mechanisms of behavioral and physiological responses to predator risk and whether this presents an example of allostatic overload type 2.

IV. SOCIAL PRESSURES

The spectrum of environmental perturbation factors ranges from the physical to the social, and organisms must cope with all of these throughout the life cycle. Facultative responses in social systems and the hormone-behavior mechanisms underlying them have been well investigated in laboratory animals, but such complex systems remain poorly understood in natural settings. In this section we will focus primarily on studies in naturalistic settings in an attempt to identify common themes across vertebrates and to identify gaps where additional work is needed, rather than provide an exhaustive overview of a burgeoning literature.

There are several physiological and behavioral strategies that animals responding to perturbations (such as infection, predators, and social pressures in the field) can adopt to redirect them away from the normal life-history stages (e.g., breeding, migrating) into survival mode. As summarized in Chapter 3, these components of the emergency life-history stage allow the individual to respond to a perturbation and avoid chronic stress (Wingfield and Ramenofsky 1999; Wingfield and Romero 2001; Wingfield 2004). The complexities of social behavioral systems and their control (for an excellent synthesis, see Adkins-Regan 2005) present a challenge, especially in relation to the emergency life-history stage. The expression of aggression can occur in so many contexts, hormonal control mechanisms are complex and sometimes contradictory (Wingfield 2005b). For example, anti-predator aggression (or against a dominant conspecific) is well known in many vertebrates (e.g., Sapolsky et al. 1997), but aggression may also be expressed in other contexts in response to perturbations, especially in relation to food shortages, competition for shelter, and so on. Bearing in mind such complexity and the general lack of a framework, we attempt to summarize what is known about responses to social pressures and the competition that may follow.

A. Allostasis and Hormone-Behavior Interactions: Some Context

The concept of allostasis, maintaining stability through change, and the reactive scope of mediators once again can provide a framework to investigate the complex influences of social interactions and coping mechanisms (Chapter 3; McEwen 2000; McEwen and Wingfield 2003a). A schematic representation of allostatic load (solid lines) and corticosteroid secretion (gray shading) is given in Figure 9.21 to provide context from Chapter 3. As a reminder, Ee = existence energy (resting metabolism); Ei = energy required to obtain food and process it under ideal conditions; Eo = additional energy required to obtain food and process it under non-ideal conditions; Eg = energy to be gained from the environment. In panel (A) of Figure 9.21, allostatic load and corticosteroid concentrations increase as the energy requirements of the organism (Eo) increase. In panel (B), allostatic overload type 1 occurs when Eo exceeds the amount of available energy in the environment (Eg), and corticosteroids trigger an emergency life-history stage (ELHS). The ELHS suppresses other life-history stages, resulting in a net decrease in allostatic load and corticosteroid concentrations below Eg. The animal

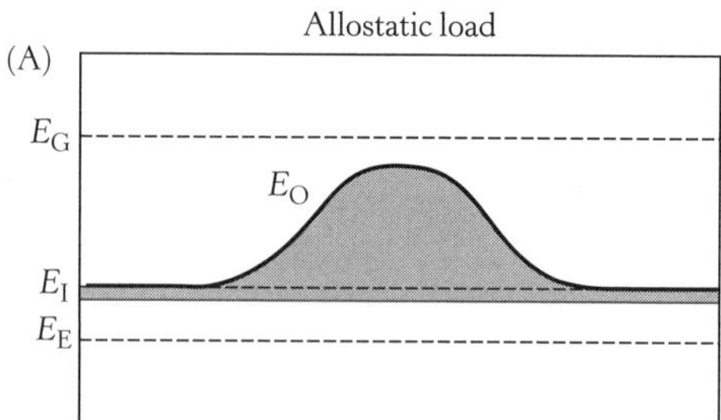

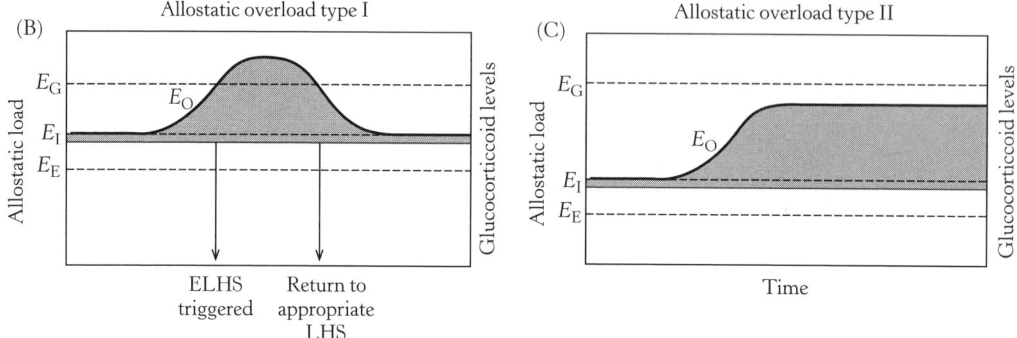

FIGURE 9.21: Schematic representation of allostatic load (solid lines) and corticosteroid secretion (gray shading). (A) Allostatic load. (B) Allostatic overload type 1. (C) Allostatic overload type 2.

Ee = existence energy (resting metabolism), Ei = energy required to obtain food and process it under ideal conditions, Eo = additional energy required to obtain food and process it under nonideal conditions, Eg = energy to be gained from the environment. Modified after McEwen and Wingfield (2003a).

From Goymann and Wingfield (2004), courtesy of Elsevier.

can now survive the perturbation in positive energy balance. In panel (C), allostatic overload type 2: owing to permanent perturbations such as social conflict, Eo increases and remains high. Corticosteroid concentrations increase and remain high, but since Eo does not exceed Eg, no ELHS is triggered (McEwen and Wingfield 2003a; Goymann and Wingfield 2004; Wingfield 2004).

Body condition is a major factor (Figure 9.22) that could influence allostatic load and overload when individuals trigger an ELHS in response to a labile perturbation factor (LPF). In birds, fat score is used as one measure of body condition on a scale of 0 (no fat) to large bulging fat bodies under the skin of the furculum and abdomen (5 in Figure 9.23; see Wingfield and Farner 1978). When Eo forces an individual into negative energy balance, if it is able to mobilize fat, then this will effectively increase Eg (Figure 9.22). The fat score is used to represent the degree by which Eg can be enhanced by utilizing endogenous reserves. If the individual has no fat (score 0), then the individual will be unable to supplement Eg. As fat score increases, then Eg can be increased to a maximum of 5 (Figure 9.22). Thus allostatic load (Ee + Ei + Eo) must be greater for fatter individuals to trigger an ELHS. In the upper panel (A), the LPF is brief and Eo increases above Eg, but only the leanest individuals must trigger an ELHS. Those with the highest fat scores are able to weather the LPF. In the lower panel (B), the LPF is more intense and lasts longer. Eo increases so that all individuals, the leanest and the fattest, must trigger an ELHS, but at different times after the onset of the LPF (i.e., individuals with highest fat scores are able to weather the LPF for longer). In both scenarios, as the LPF passes and Eo declines, allostatic load decreases below Eg and the original life-history stage can be resumed (Wingfield 2004).

A different way to model the effects of body condition on allostatic load and overload, leading to when an ELHS is triggered, is to decrease Eg. Many weather events act as labile perturbation factors to decrease available food (Figure 9.23). In the upper panel (A), the LPF is brief, but Eg still drops below Ee + Ei. However, if individuals

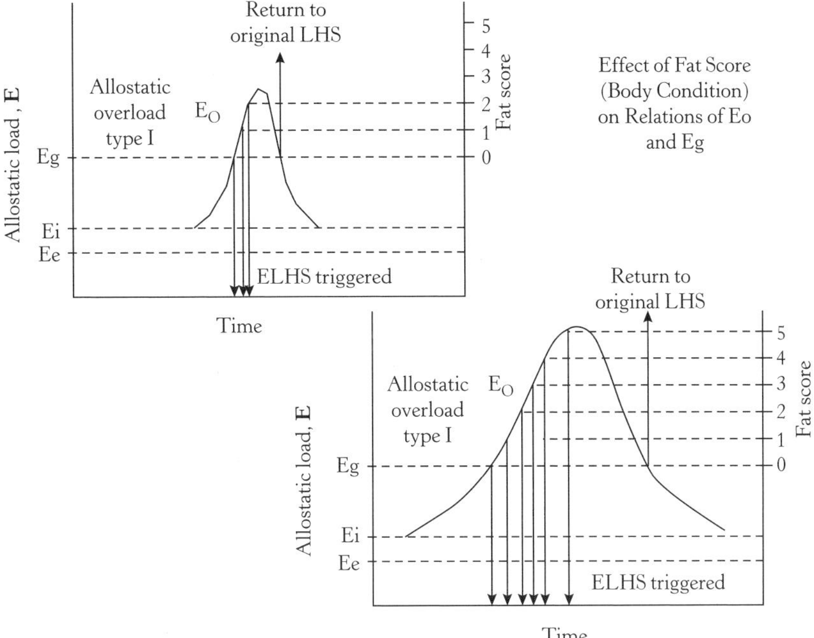

FIGURE 9.22: Body condition is a major factor that could influence when individuals trigger an ELHS in response to a labile perturbation factor (LPF). The fat score is used to represent the degree by which Eg can be increased with stored energy. Allostatic load (Ee + Ei + Eo) must be greater for fatter individuals to trigger an ELHS. The upper panel represents a brief LPF where only the leanest individuals must trigger an ELHS. The bottom panel represents a more intense LPF where all individuals, the leanest and the fattest, must trigger an ELHS.

From Wingfield (2004), courtesy of Cambridge University Press.

are able to mobilize fat, then those with greater fat scores can remain in their life-history stage (LHS) for longer, and only those with no fat (score 0) or a score of 1 trigger an ELHS. In the bottom panel (B), the LPF is more intense and lasts longer. In this case, Eg drops below even Ee, and all individuals except those with the highest fat score (5) must trigger an ELHS. When Eg increases again after the LPF passes, then the original, or an appropriate, life-history stage can be resumed. Note again that as Eg decreases, the leanest individuals trigger the ELHS first (Wingfield 2004). With this primer in mind, we can go on to discuss social interactions.

B. Competition in the Face of Food Shortages

Few environmental situations induce such intense aggression as a shortage of food. However, control of aggression under such circumstances has received scant attention, at least on a comparative scale. In tropical breeding blue-footed boobies, competition between siblings in a nest resulted in elevated corticosterone in the subordinate (Ramos-Fernandez et al. 2000), but food shortage in general had little effect on adults (Wingfield et al. 1999), suggesting that food was, perhaps, sufficient for the adults but not for feeding both chicks as well. Whether or not corticosterone facilitates aggression over food in this species remains to be determined. It is possible that maternal effects may be important in some species in which young compete with their siblings, or even kill them, in response to food shortage. In breeding cattle egrets, dominant siblings hatched from eggs with higher plasma levels of testosterone in yolk (Schwabl et al. 1997) and neonatal siblicidal spotted hyenas have elevated levels of androgens that stem from maternal precursor hormones (Glickman et al. 1992; Licht et al. 1992; Licht et al. 1998). Furthermore, in canaries, chicks hatching from eggs with higher testosterone concentrations in yolk grew faster, presumably by being more competitive in begging for food from the parents (Schwabl 1993; Schwabl et al. 1997). Mechanisms underlying the effects of corticosterone and testosterone on aggression over food remain to be determined. Begging behavior is influenced profoundly by developmental factors and environment with complex neural and

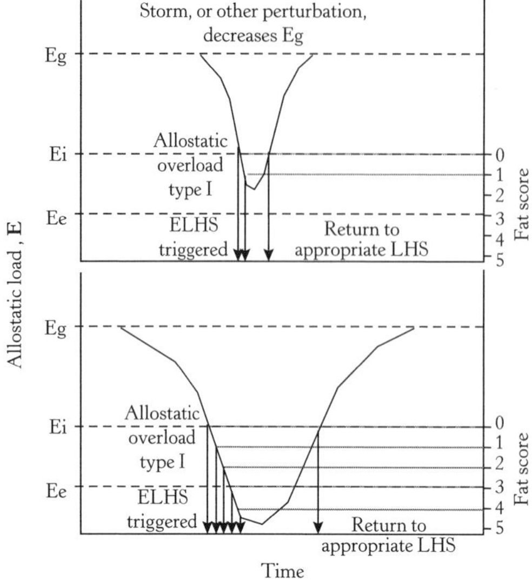

FIGURE 9.23: Using a decrease in Eg to model effects of body condition on when an ELHS is triggered. Upper panel shows a brief LPF where Eg drops below Ee + Ei. Individuals with greater fat scores can remain in their life-history stage (LHS) and only those with little fat (score 0–1) trigger an ELHS. Bottom panel shows a more-intense and longer-lasting LPF where Eg drops below even Ee, and all individuals except the fattest must trigger an ELHS.

From Wingfield (2004), courtesy of Cambridge University Press.

hormonal controls (Schwabl and Lipar 2002), and glucocorticoids can be included in the spectrum of regulatory mechanisms.

Socioecological theory predicts that competition for food is associated with linear dominance hierarchies with reproductive and other advantages for high-ranking individuals. A field study of female blue monkeys in Kenya showed that high-ranking females with priority of access to choice food items had lower fecal levels of glucocorticoids (Foerster et al. 2011). Dominant female ring-tailed lemurs had the highest fecal corticoid levels but also initiated more agonistic encounters in relation to competition and not reproductive status per se (Cavigelli et al. 2003). In free-living olive baboons sampled in Kenya, presumably dominant males with greater copulation success were able to increase testosterone levels in blood and show greater cortisol elevations following competition stress (Sapolsky 1982). In general there are rapid changes in testosterone and corticosteroids during competition among individuals, but the ways in which secretion of these steroids hormones are affected vary widely with species and contexts. Competition for food is one context. Wobber et al. (2010) conducted studies of bonobos and chimpanzees that differ markedly in their food-sharing behavior. Hierarchies are more rigid in chimpanzees, whereas bonobos show more flexibility and share food more readily. Male bonobos underwent a decrease in salivary cortisol in a situation of sharing food, whereas chimpanzees showed no change in cortisol but a decrease in testosterone. In a different situation in which competition for food was likely (with a dominant individual), then cortisol levels tended to rise in bonobos, whereas testosterone levels increased in chimpanzees (Wobber et al. 2010). The authors suggest that bonobos and chimpanzees differ in their perceptions of the situation as either a stressor or a dominance contest, and these perceptions may influence the hormonal responses in complex ways.

Many species of shore birds, such as red knots, forage for mollusks on open mud flats at low tide. Depending upon numbers of birds in a flock and other factors such as weather, competition for food can vary markedly. In captive knots, food was provided in varying quantities at unpredictable times of day to mimic the vagaries of tides and weather (Reneerkens et al. 2002). Interactions among birds over competition for food were positively associated with higher plasma levels of corticosterone (Figure 9.24), consistent with a role for corticosteroids regulating aggression over access to resources.

Serum levels of cortisol in male Brandt's voles were higher in males winning in experimentally staged food competitions (Li et al. 2007). This potential role of corticosteroids in competition for food may explain at least partially why in some investigations dominant animals have higher blood or fecal levels of corticosteroids. In the Eurasian water vole, free-living males had higher corticosteroid levels in situations of high competition for food and mates (Zavjalov et al. 2012). Corticosterone has a regulatory role in the prenatal control of juvenile dispersal in lizards and may have a role in reducing competition, including for food, between mother and offspring (De Fraipont et al. 2000). In this case, offspring exposed to higher maternal corticosterone were less likely to disperse. In another scenario, it has been hypothesized that competition among tadpoles increases the production of corticosteroids, and this may suppress growth and development (Glennemeier and Denver 2002). Whole-body corticosterone levels in leopard frog tadpoles raised in different densities and

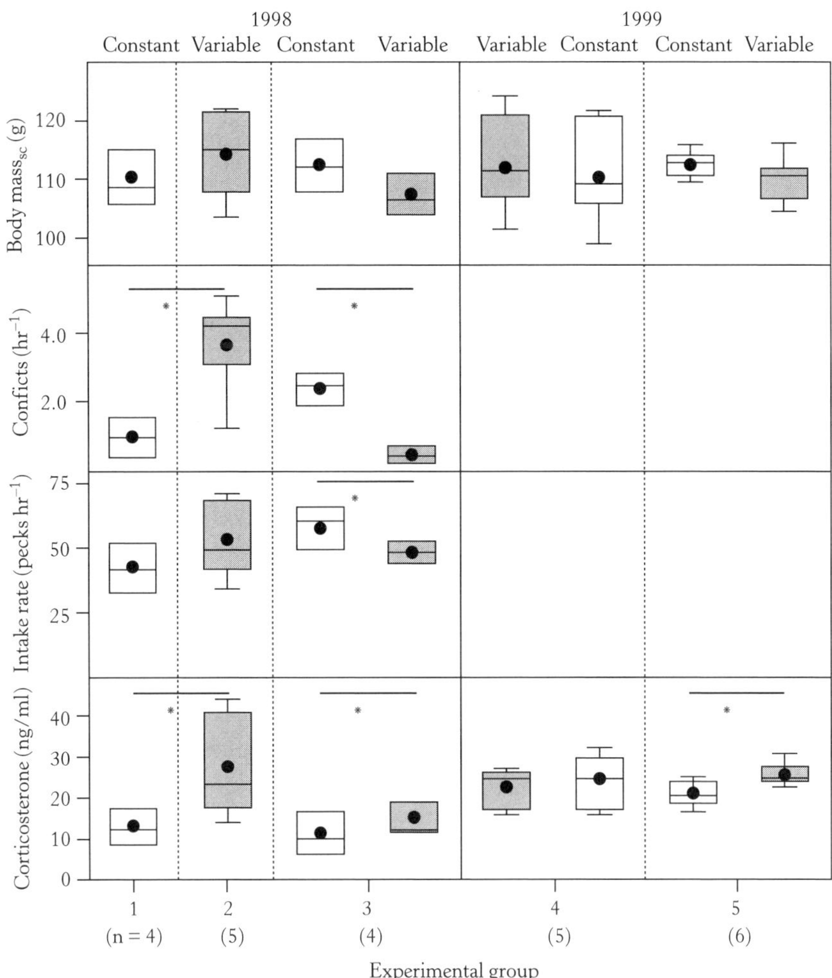

FIGURE 9.24: Summary of treatment differences in size corrected body mass, conflicts, food intake, and circulating corticosterone concentration during constant (unshaded boxes) and variable (shaded boxes) feeding schedules in five experimental groups. The boxes enclose the 50% of the values and the vertical lines show the range of individual averages. Note that there are no vertical lines indicating the range when sample size equals or is less than four, but that the boxes enclose the full range in those cases. The dividing lines within the boxes indicate the median, and the black dots indicate the averages. The number of individual birds studied in each group is given in parentheses on the *x* axis. A horizontal line with asterisk marks statistically significant differences.

From Reneerkens et al. (2002), courtesy of Wily Liss Inc.

at three different levels of food availability were higher at greater densities with more competition for food. This was accompanied by suppression of growth. Treatment of tadpoles with metyrapone (to reduce synthesis of corticosterone) reversed the negative effects on growth but had no effect on development rate (Glennemeier and Denver 2002).

In a pelagic seabird, the black-legged kittiwake breeding in the Bering Sea and Alaska coast, plasma levels of corticosterone increase in relation to shortage of food (fish) in both adults and chicks (Kitaysky et al. 1999). The release of corticosterone in black-legged kittiwake chicks triggers a behavioral cascade: first an increase in begging of chicks accompanied by aggression toward nest mates, followed by an increase in food provisioning of those chicks by parents (Kitaysky et al. 2001; Kitaysky et al. 2003). Thus hormonally induced begging behavior and aggression over access to food triggers compensatory behavior in adults to ameliorate potential stress and detriments later in life (Kitaysky et al. 2003) (see Chapter 5 for more details).

C. Social Status, Aggression, and Perturbations of the Environment

Cooperation and social support provide many advantages when living in social groups, but social conflict and competition may introduce disadvantages. Social conflicts elevate allostatic load, followed by increased levels of corticosteroids and often decreased health (Sapolsky 2005; DeVries et al. 2007). Individuals in groups experience different levels of allostatic load according to status, which in turn may predict relative corticosteroid levels of dominant and subordinate individuals. It has been quite rightly pointed out that there may actually be no obvious energetic costs of dominance/subordinance status per se (Walsberg 2003), especially in stable hierarchies. However, shortages of food or competition for shelter in the face of perturbations can result in situations that increase allostatic load, for example in finding enough food, in relation to social status (McEwen and Wingfield 2003b). It is also possible that although social status per se may not incur greater allostatic load, access to Eg can be affected, with subordinate animals deferring to dominants when food is patchy. In this case, Eg is essentially decreased for subordinates, leading to greater susceptibility to additional LPFs.

An analysis of the available data from free-ranging mammals and birds using phylogenetic independent contrasts of allostatic load and relative levels of corticosteroids revealed that relative allostatic load of social status predicted whether dominant or subordinate members of a social unit express higher or lower levels of corticosteroids (Goymann and Wingfield 2004). If the allostatic load of dominance rank (the sum of acquisition and maintenance) is higher than the allostatic load of being subordinate, then dominants are significantly more likely to have elevated levels of corticosteroids. Conversely, if allostatic load of social status is greatest in subordinates, then they are significantly more likely to express higher levels of corticosteroids (Goymann and Wingfield 2004). Social status and differences in allostatic load and corticosteroid concentrations are presented in Figure 9.25. The panels on the left represent a situation in which Ee and Ei are low, and those on the right represent a situation in which Ee and Ei are elevated, for example, because of breeding activities. A similar outcome could be imagined if Ee and Ei remained low, as on the left, but Eg decreased. In (a) social status had little impact on allostatic load (or the same impact on members of all social ranks), and there were no differences in allostatic load and glucocorticoid concentrations between dominants and subordinates. In (b) allostatic load fell more heavily on subordinates and, as a consequence, corticosteroid concentrations were higher in subordinates than in dominants. An ELHS is, therefore, more likely to be triggered in subordinates. In (c) allostatic load and, as a consequence, glucocorticoid concentrations were higher in dominants than in subordinates, and an ELHS is more likely to be triggered in dominants than in subordinates (Goymann and Wingfield 2004). Figure 9.26 then shows the relationships between relative allostatic load and relative glucocorticoid (GC) concentrations of dominants: as the allostatic load increases, so do the corticosteroid levels (Goymann and Wingfield 2004).

An alternative way to describe how social status may effect Eo is shown in Figure 9.27 (Wingfield 2004). Because dominance status often determines access to many resources including food (Eg), the degree by which Eo increases will be proportional to social status. The most dominant individuals will experience less of an increase in Eo because they have easier access to Eg. Subordinates, on the other hand, will have much less access to Eg, thus incurring a higher increase in Eo and allostatic load. In the left-hand panel (A) of Figure 9.27, Eg is high and thus only the most subordinate individuals will accrue an allostatic load that exceeds Eg. More dominant animals with greater access to Eg will be able to weather the LPF without Ee + Ei + Eo exceeding Eg. In the right-hand panel (B), Eg is lower, and coupled with Eo it can be seen that even dominants may eventually have an allostatic load that exceeds Eg, thus triggering an ELHS. Note that in both scenarios, the subordinates will trigger an ELHS before more dominant individuals, even when Eg is low.

Perhaps the best-known work on the impact on social status on corticosteroid release in free-living animals has been done on baboons (summarized by Sapolsky 2001, 2005). For example, hierarchy instability, such as when new aggressive males join the troop, leads to elevated corticosteroid concentrations (e.g., Bergman et al. 2005; Engh et al. 2006b). The overwhelming impression one gets from this work is that baboons are very good at stressing each other. In their case, social living creates multiple challenges. Work indicating how their corticosteroids respond to those challenges forms the foundation for models presented in Figures 9.25 and 9.27. However, conspecific interactions in other species also elicit corticosteroid

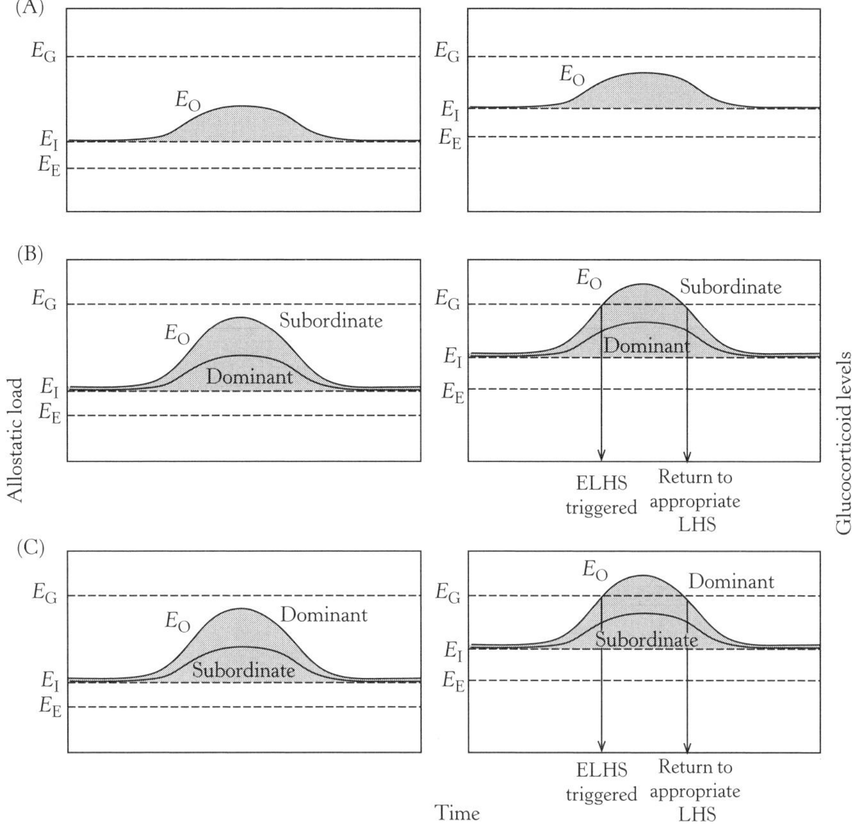

FIGURE 9.25: Social status impacts on allostatic load (solid lines) and glucocorticoid concentrations (gray shading). Ee and Ei are low in left panels and high in right panels. (A) Little impact of social status on allostatic load and no differences between dominants and subordinates. (B) Allostatic load falls more heavily on subordinates. (C) Allostatic load is higher in dominants.

From Goymann and Wingfield (2004), courtesy of Elsevier.

release. For example, calling behavior in free-living Gulf toadfish results in elevated corticosteroids (Remage-Healey and Bass 2005), and increased corticosteroid release in response to social stress in hermit thrushes appears to induce solitary non-territorial behavior, known as floaters, rather than flocking in the winter (Brown and Long 2007). On the other hand, group living can have benefits. For example, social support in free-living greylag geese can result in attenuated corticosteroid release (Scheiber et al. 2009), and enforcing social isolation in a social species can elevate corticosteroids (Apfelbeck and Raess 2008).

One other important social relationship in many species is the pair bond. Although to our knowledge there has not been any assessment of whether corticosteroids are associated with normal pair bond formation, forced pair formation with unattractive partners in female Gouldian finches resulted in elevated corticosteroids (Griffith et al. 2011). On the other hand, breaking a pair bond appears to be a strong stressor. Zebra finches form lifelong monogamous pairs. Figure 9.28A shows that corticosterone is elevated 24 hours after a pair is separated (Remage-Healey et al. 2003). When the pair is reunited, corticosterone titers return to pre-separation levels. Whether the separated animals were housed singly (Figure 9.28A) or with other same-sex birds (Figure 9.28B) made no difference—the separation itself appeared to be highly stressful. A similar response was demonstrated in free-living black-legged kittiwakes, where natural changing of pairs resulted in elevated baseline corticosterone (Angelier et al. 2007), and in free-ranging female chacma baboons, where loss of a close relative to predation resulted in elevated fecal corticosteroids (Engh et al. 2006a).

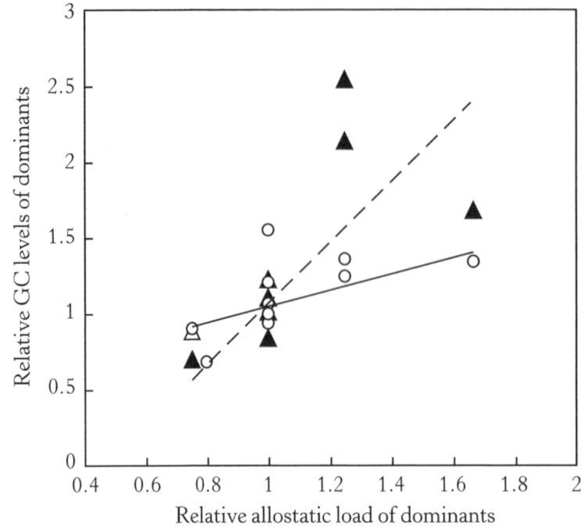

FIGURE 9.26: Relation between relative allostatic load and relative glucocorticoid (GC) concentrations of dominants, as derived from phylogenetic independent contrasts for females (triangles) and males (circles).

From Goymann and Wingfield (2004), courtesy of Elsevier.

D. Personalities and Coping Styles

Proactive and reactive coping styles allow vertebrates to deal with psychosocial stress among conspecifics. Coping styles have been classified in various ways, but a review by Koolhaas et al. (1999) has been useful as a framework that suggests a grouping that is applicable to vertebrates in general. The proactive coping style is an active response to a social challenge involving aggression, whereas the reactive coping style is characterized by behavioral immobility and low aggression (Koolhaas et al. 1999). This framework

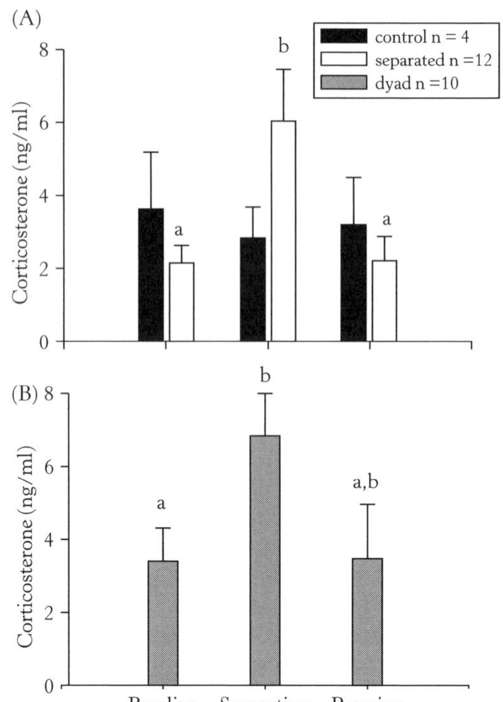

FIGURE 9.28: Plasma corticosterone responses to mate separation and reunion under different housing conditions. Corticosterone was elevated in pairs that were acoustically and visually separated and returned to baseline upon reunion (A, separated). When separated individuals were kept in same-sex dyads during separation, corticosterone was elevated and returned to baseline upon pair mate reunion (B, dyad).

Reprinted with permission from Remage-Healey et al. (2003).

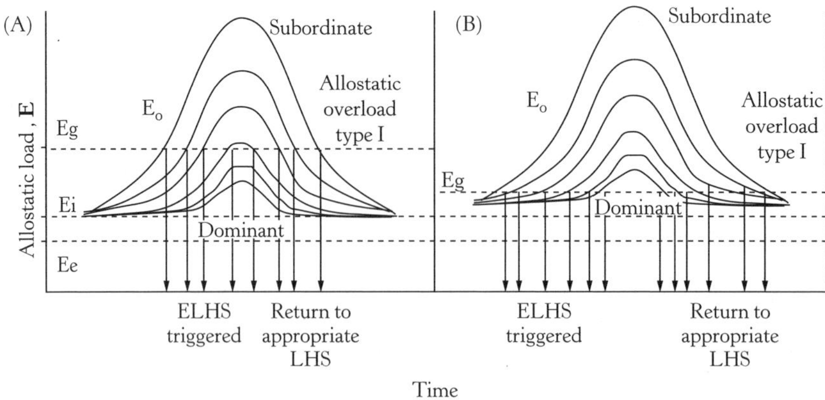

FIGURE 9.27: Impact of social status on potential to trigger an ELHS. The degree by which Eo increases will be proportional to social status. In the left-hand panel (A), Eg is high and thus only the most subordinate individuals will accrue an allostatic load that exceeds Eg. In the right-hand panel (B), Eg is lower so that even dominants may eventually have an allostatic load that exceeds Eg.

From Wingfield (2004), courtesy of Cambridge University Press.

has been very useful in assessing coping styles in a wide variety of organisms from invertebrates to vertebrates and has provided an assessment of possible common mechanisms involved. It should also be pointed out that these coping styles are not always clear-cut, and within a population there can be a continuum from reactive on one extreme to proactive at the other, with many intermediate scenarios. Furthermore, although some individuals develop coping styles as a result of genetic control, or through epigenetic mechanisms such as maternal effects during development (see Chapter 5), there is also evidence that individuals may switch strategies throughout the life cycle as circumstances allow and new opportunities arise. In this section, we review some examples in an attempt to point out where further research is needed.

Emerging theory suggests that individuals should invest more in parental care as the value of a brood increases. This in turn could influence the development of coping styles. At a mechanistic level this would include changing sensitivity to acute stressors to avoid abandonment of the brood. Brood value is related to parental care, and modulation of the adrenocortical response to an acute stress has two hypotheses: the brood value hypothesis (large broods have high fitness potential) and the workload hypothesis (allostatic load; large broods are energetically demanding for parents).

In an experiment on house sparrows, Lendvai and Chastel (2008) experimentally removed males (for 48 hours) from free-living pairs feeding young. Female house sparrows increased their feeding rates (workload) but were unable to fully compensate, resulting in decreased condition of the nestlings (decreased brood value) compared with controls that had both mates feeding young. After the 48-hour experimental period, females feeding young alone had a greater adrenocortical response to a standardized stressor (capture handling and restraint) than females feeding young with their mates (Lendvai and Chastel 2008). This is consistent with the brood value hypothesis (Bókony et al. 2009). The results are also consistent with the findings of Hegner and Wingfield (1987) in which free-living male house sparrows implanted with testosterone fed young less than controls. Female mates were unable to fully compensate for this detriment in parental behavior, and fledging success declined significantly. These data could also be interpreted in relation to personalities, but environmental and social factors here can change from one brood to the next, resulting in a change in apparent personality and coping style.

It is also important to point out here that there is growing evidence that adverse effects of stress can be ameliorated by social allies in mammals and in birds (Frigerio et al. 2001; Frigerio et al. 2003; Scheiber et al. 2009), further complicating the expression of personalities among individuals. Stöwe et al. (2008) studied corticosterone excretion patterns of hand-raised ravens at three developmental stages: chicks in the nest; post-fledging; and when independent of their parents. Corticosterone metabolites in feces were higher during the nestling phase than either post-fledging or when independent. How this may relate to social interactions when older deserves further study, but post-fledging birds with higher corticosteroid metabolite levels stayed closer to conspecifics and groomed them for longer than birds with lower levels. In another example, barn owl males have varying sizes of melanin spots on the ventral apterium, with larger spotted males showing less parental provisioning than males with no or smaller spots, consistent with apparent personality traits (Almasi et al. 2008). Corticosterone implants into free-living and breeding males resulted in a marked decline in provisioning rates in males with smaller spots versus controls. Corticosterone treatment in males with larger spots was much less effective on provisioning rates, and these birds seemed more resistant to the effects of corticosterone. It is possible that large spots signal resistance to acute stress. Reduced provisioning resulted in a decrease in nestling growth rates but not reproductive success (Almasi et al. 2008). Moderately elevated corticosterone may thus trigger behavioral responses that maximize lifetime reproductive success.

E. Population Density

It is well known that high-density living, especially in captive animals such as in agriculture and aquaculture settings, tends to result in poor growth rates, lower body condition, and reduced reproductive performance. Furthermore, transmission of disease and mortality from aggression in crowded situations can also reduce fitness. The early work of Christian (e.g., Christian et al. 1965) showed that many paradigms of crowding increased adrenocortical activity in mice and resulted in chronic stress symptoms. These results have been frequently extrapolated to wild animals, but few have actually documented the effects of high density under truly natural conditions. Because the experiments reviewed in Christian et al. (1965) frequently involved extreme crowding, whether or not such results are relevant for animals under natural conditions has been questioned (e.g., Chitty 1996). Nonetheless, high-density living is common for raising agricultural animals and for fish in aquaculture. Thus, crowding stress has important implications for farming, but may also be important in nature, especially in relation to the effects of invasive species, habitat degradation, and fragmentation, when more animals have less space in which to live. Although the direct causes of high mortality under natural conditions of crowding probably include poor nutrition, aggression, and transmission of disease, corticosteroids can indirectly exacerbate these problems.

Brown lemmings captured in the field under conditions of high density and just on emergence from snow in June showed adrenal hypertrophy consistent with hyper-adrenocortical function and accompanied by high basal levels of adrenal steroids and high content of pituitary ACTH (Andrews and Strohbehn 1971). These effects were much less pronounced in females, especially those that were pregnant. Furthermore, males revealed greater rates of mortality, with signs of chronic stress indicated by adrenal hyperfunction, cardiac hypertrophy, and renal disease (Andrews and Strohbehn 1971). The authors conclude that social environment changes in relation to population size can have marked effects on adrenal function and survival in addition to physical environment effects.

High-density living, or crowding stress, tends to reduce growth rates in many fish. Long-term crowding stress in captive brown trout increased plasma cortisol levels for at least 25 days compared to controls held at lower density. However, after 39 days of high-density treatment, plasma cortisol levels were the same as in fish held at low density. Cortisol levels in blood of both groups were even lower after 119 days, and there were no differences in interrenal histology (Pickering and Stewart 1984). The authors conclude that although crowding may increase cortisol and reduce growth rate initially, after an acclimation period fish adjust to high-density living. Crowding captive zebra fish at high density (40 fish/liter) for three hours (acute stress) or for five days (chronic stress) versus controls held at densities of 0.25 fish/liter) resulted in fourfold increases in whole-body concentrations of cortisol (Ramsay et al. 2006). This response to crowding was reduced in fish held at high density and given food, but was heightened in fish that were held at high density and food restricted. Indeed, there was no increase in cortisol concentrations in fed fish held at high density, suggesting an interaction of crowding and feeding (Ramsay et al. 2006). Similarly in sub-adult striped bass, brief confinement and crowding stress increased plasma levels of cortisol (MacFarsane 1984). High stocking density of captive gilthead seabream, an important Mediterranean food fish, increased plasma cortisol levels and resulted in many symptoms of chronic stress, including decreased immune function, compared to controls held at lower density (Montero et al. 1999). The tropical fishes, blue gouramis, were held either in bisexual pairs or as groups of eight. Grouping tended to increase the size of interrenal cell nuclei consistent with hyper-adrenocortical function, but there were no effects on testicular function (Pollak and Christian 1977). In females, interrenal hypertrophy was not apparent, but ovaries remained in an immature state and body weight was less than fish held in pairs.

Much more work, especially in the field, is needed to understand how population density may influence allostatic load in general and the reactive scope of mediators of stress. Effects of further perturbations of the environment might be extreme in some cases.

V. DISPERSAL

Animals undergo several forms of movements during their life cycles. Some of these are very predictable, for example, post-development dispersal and migrations between breeding and wintering areas. Some species are also partial migrants, where within a population a single individual is either consistently migratory or sedentary from year to year—called obligate partial migration, irrespective of environmental conditions (Wingfield and Silverin 2002, 2009). Obligate partial migration may be regulated by endogenous controls, but in other species individuals may switch between migratory or sedentary traits. When an individual shifts from being sedentary to migratory, it is called facultative partial migration or irruptive migration, depending on the prevailing environmental conditions at the time (Wingfield and Silverin 2002, 2009). What determines whether an individual will migrate or not includes competition for resources, establishment of a winter or non-breeding group, age and dominance relationships, or date of birth in relation to time of year, such as early in the breeding season or late (Schwabl and Silverin 1990). Partial migrations are usually short distance and rarely more than a few hundred kilometers. On the other hand, some facultative (irruptive) migrations are the result of changes in food availability in their original breeding, or wintering, areas and can involve movements over thousands of kilometers. During these irruptive episodes, animals can move in enormous numbers, usually on an unpredictable schedule. In birds, typically facultative, irruptive, species are predators, for example the snowy owl, but also include seed-eating birds such as crossbills and nutcrackers (Wingfield and Silverin 2002, 2009).

The many known types of movements are extremely complex, and there is debate as to what types of movements represent dispersal. Moreover, experiments designed to explore hormone mechanisms tend to be contradictory (Ramenofsky 1990; Schwabl and Silverin 1990; Wingfield et al. 1990; Ramenofsky and Wingfield 2007), but a role for corticosteroids in the dispersal of mammals, birds, and reptiles appears to be more consistent (reviewed in Wada et al. 2008). Wingfield and Silverin (2002, 2009) outlined possible life-history stages that include some form of movement that could be construed as dispersal as follows:

1. Juvenile dispersal is an ontogenetic life-history stage that will occur once in an individual's life cycle. Thus the hormone mechanisms involved may be entirely distinct from those regulating other types of movements.
2. Regular autumnal, or post-breeding, migration life-history stage of the entire population, the mirror image of vernal, or pre-breeding, migration.
3. Programmed partial migration in which certain individuals always show an autumnal migration life-history stage (and, therefore, vernal migration also), and others never migrate. Presumably those that do migrate have control mechanisms similar to those in 2.
4. Facultative migration, or irruptive movements that occur in response to unpredictable perturbations of the environment. This type of movement should be included in the emergency life-history stage and may have a completely different endocrine basis.

Given these categories of movements of animals, we can explore what is known about endocrine mechanisms. Much more information is needed, but the diversity of strategies within very closely related species offers many exciting models for future experiments. Here we will focus on postnatal dispersal and facultative movements—that is, those most likely to be precipitated by perturbations of the environment (see Chapter 7 for the role of corticosteroids in migration).

A. Juveniles

Post-juvenile, or postnatal, dispersal is probably ubiquitous among animals. Dispersal of offspring and of adults is a fundamental process of the life cycle with many ecological consequences relating to population dynamics, growth, and adaptation (Cote et al. 2010). It is a major developmental transition in many species and is often used to prospect for future breeding sites. Successfully identifying good breeding sites can have dramatic consequences for future reproductive success (Betts et al. 2008). However, there may be major energetic costs, risks of predation, and so on, to the disperser, but suites of morphological, physiological, and behavior specializations may have evolved to reduce those costs. These traits may also be markedly affected by personality (Figure 9.29; Cote et al. 2010). Behavioral traits such as boldness and aggressiveness (proactive) versus reactive types may vary, dependent upon maternal effects and environmental conditions (see section earlier in this chapter). The mechanisms underlying these dispersal traits and prospecting behavior remain largely unknown, but some field investigations suggest possible productive avenues for further research. Furthermore, because these dispersal events have been correlated with potentially stressful conditions, such as low food availability (Korpimaki and Lagerstrom 1988) or low social status (Ellsworth and Belthoff 1999), corticosteroid titers are an attractive possibility. Corticosteroids have profound regulatory effects on many developmental processes (see Chapters 5 and 11), such as ontogeny of organs prior to birth, parturition/hatching events in mammals and birds, metamorphosis-type events in fish and amphibians, and dispersal behavior in many tetrapod vertebrates (Wada 2008). Environmental influences during development, including maternal effects, can affect corticosteroid secretions and in turn phenotype. These complex mechanisms may be very important for organisms to cope with global climate change

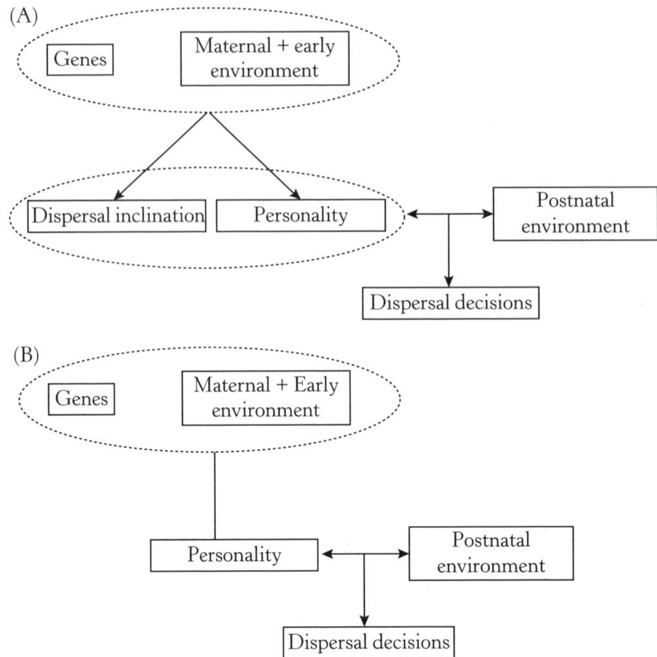

FIGURE 9.29: Two suggested ontogenetic pathways linking dispersal behavior and personality traits in varying environmental conditions. (A) The correlation between personality and dispersal inclination is coordinated by a shared gene-environment interaction, but the actual dispersal decisions that any given individual makes are influenced by its postnatal environment. (B) The set of personality traits is determined by gene-environment interactions during offspring development, and then dispersal decisions depend on the interaction between environmental conditions and personality traits.

From Cote et al. (2010), with permission and courtesy of the Royal Society, London.

from physiology and behavior of adaptation including postnatal dispersal (reviewed in Wada 2008; Meylan et al. 2012).

Seasonal and energetic constraints are usually a much greater challenge for young animals born later in the breeding season. In common hamsters, pups begin to disperse soon after weaning. Fecal levels of corticosteroid metabolites in juveniles late in the breeding season were higher during onset of dispersal than in juveniles born earlier in the year (Figure 9.30; Siutz and Millesi 2012). Furthermore, young animals immigrating to new areas later in the dispersal process also had higher fecal corticosteroid metabolite levels (Figure 9.31; Siutz and Millesi 2012). The authors suggest that because common hamsters go into hibernation in October, late-born juveniles have less time to prepare, resulting in greater energetic demands, exposure to predators, and so forth. In other words, allostatic load may be much higher for late-born individuals. Similarly, in free-living yellow-bellied marmots, fecal concentrations of corticosteroid metabolites were positively correlated with predator pressure and had both direct and indirect effects on dispersal of pups (Monclus et al. 2011). Age was also involved. Older females with high levels of corticosteroid metabolites in feces tended to have fewer pups, and the sex ratio was biased toward females. Sons from these litters also tended to disperse farther than sons of older marmot females with lower fecal levels of corticosteroids (Monclus et al. 2011). Male-biased and larger litters were found in younger mothers with lower fecal corticosteroid levels. These data suggest that age-related effects could allow marmot mothers to adjust the potential fitness of their offspring according to fluctuating environmental conditions.

A field study of the communally breeding and semi-fossorial rodent, the degu, revealed that fecal levels of corticosteroids showed no relationship to group sizes of juveniles at dispersal. Thus the mechanisms for competition and dispersal in this group of animals remain unknown (Quirici et al. 2011). In free-living degus, direct fitness decreases with group size, but the latter was not related to fecal levels of corticosteroids in females.

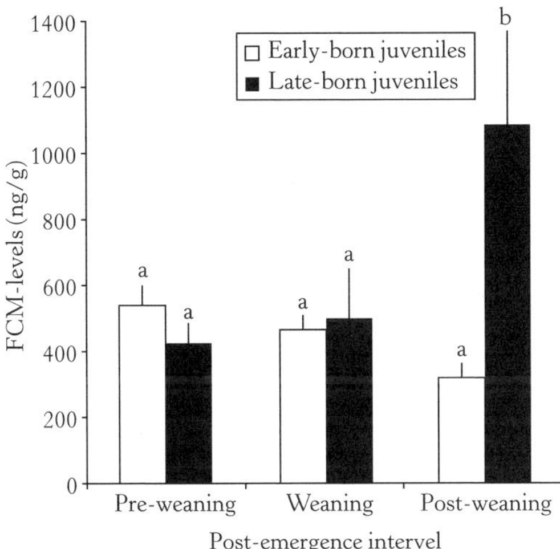

FIGURE 9.30: Fecal corticosteroid metabolite (FCM) concentrations in early- and late-born juvenile common hamsters during the pre-weaning, weaning, and post-weaning period. Early-born individuals emerged from the natal burrow between June 1 and July 7, late-born juveniles between July 29 and September 20. Groups with the same letter do not differ significantly.

From Siutz and Millesi (2012), with permission and courtesy of Elsevier Press.

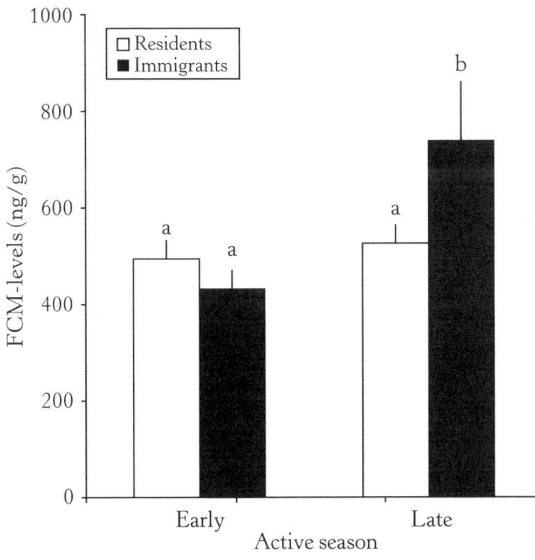

FIGURE 9.31: Fecal corticosteroid metabolite (FCM) levels in resident (born in the study area) and immigrated juvenile hamsters. Individuals that immigrated early (before July 26) and late in the season (after August 17) are compared. Groups with the same letter do not differ significantly.

From Siutz and Millesi (2012), with permission and courtesy of Elsevier Press.

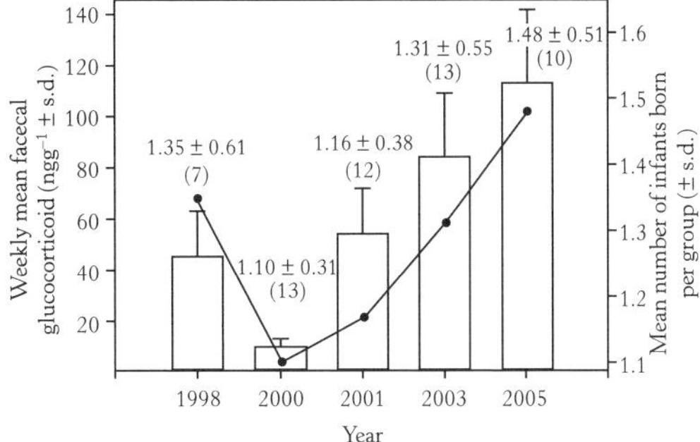

FIGURE 9.32: Annual variation of weekly mean fecal corticosteroid concentrations in focal males is strongly linked to the presence of infants. Annual changes in male weekly mean fecal corticosteroids parallel annual changes in mean number of infants born per group. Values in parentheses indicate number of groups sampled.

From Brockman et al. (2009), with permission and courtesy of the Royal Society, London.

However, fecal corticosteroid levels did increase with number of offspring produced and survival of young to at least first reproductive age in two out of the three years of study (Ebensperger et al. 2011). The authors conclude that their data support the corticosteroid adaptation hypothesis in which reproductive effort is the major influence on corticosteroid secretion.

In free-living white-faced capuchins in Costa Rica, fecal corticosteroid metabolite levels were highest in females during the dry season compared with the rainy season. Furthermore, excreted corticosteroids were also higher in pregnant females than in lactating individuals or in other reproductive states (Carnegie et al. 2011). In addition to these seasonal and reproductive events, females also showed higher corticosteroids when social instability among dominant males was prevalent, possibly leading to increased infanticide activity (Carnegie et al. 2011). In the plural breeding lemur, the sifaka, fecal corticosteroid metabolite levels increased in males coincident with a dispersal event in which younger subordinate males were evicted by dominant adult males (Brockman et al. 2009). Fecal corticosteroids were highest during the period when infants were present and were not related to age, dominance status, social stability, and so on (Figure 9.32; Brockman et al. 2009).

Cease et al. (2007) posit that in free-living male red-sided garter snakes, seasonal modulation of the HPA axis is linked in a temporal sense to dispersal post-breeding. Baseline plasma levels of corticosterone were higher in courting males than in those dispersing to feeding grounds up to 20 kilometers distant. Furthermore, courting males show no increase in corticosterone to the acute stress of capture and handling, whereas dispersing males do show a response (Cease et al. 2007). These authors suggest that changing dynamics of the HPA axis may play an important role in the transition from breeding to dispersal and feeding during the life cycle of these snakes.

Young sea turtles dig their way out of nests and disperse into the ocean, moving quickly into offshore areas. In hatchling green sea turtles, plasma corticosterone levels increased significantly while they were digging upward through sand and peaked between three and five hours after swimming activity had begun (Hamann et al. 2007). Lactate levels indicating anaerobic activity also increased in the hatchling turtles while digging. The changes in corticosterone are consistent with marked increases in metabolic activity associated with this intensive and rapid post-hatching dispersal.

Perhaps the strongest support that corticosteroids may be the internal trigger for juvenile dispersal comes from studies of willow tits (Silverin et al. 1989; Silverin 1997). Not only do migrating juveniles have higher corticosteroid titers than do territorial juveniles (Silverin et al. 1989), but corticosteroid implants had a biphasic response depending upon how likely the juveniles were to disperse. During the period when juveniles often disperse from their natal territories, corticosteroid implants augmented the percentage of young birds that left. In contrast, later in the autumn, when willow tits had already established winter flocks, corticosteroid implants did not alter juvenile movement (Silverin 1997). Even though data are available for only a small number of species, what data are available thus indicate that corticosteroids play a major role in juvenile dispersal.

However, hormones other than corticosteroids are also likely involved in dispersal. For example, young eels (glass eels) in Europe migrate upstream into estuaries and disperse in freshwater drainages. Eels treated with T4 in captive conditions showed increased locomotor activity versus controls. Moreover, treatment with thiourea, which blocks synthesis of T4, decreased locomotor activity, consistent with the hypothesis that thyroid hormones may also play an important role on migration and dispersal (Edeline et al. 2005).

The dispersal of young animals is frequently dependent upon condition and also maternal phenotype. How processes leading up to dispersal are integrated remain largely unknown. However, clues are starting to become available. In lizards, Vercken et al. (2007) show that maternal circulating levels of corticosterone interact with phenotype. They found that the timing and duration of exposure to high plasma corticosterone affect juvenile phenotype. Early exposure to high corticosterone resulted in reduced body size and condition in juveniles, but this could be reversible. However, duration of the exposure to high concentrations of maternal corticosterone affects juvenile dispersal in a sex-specific manner. Vercken et al. (2007) found that in female-dominated clutches, longer exposure to corticosterone promoted philopatry, whereas shorter duration enhanced dispersal. These data clearly show that environmental influences during development, including maternal effects, can affect corticosteroid secretions and in turn dispersal phenotype. Once more, we see how complex mechanisms organizing important events in the life cycle may be critical for coping with global climate change—from physiology and behavior of adaptation, to postnatal dispersal (reviewed in Wada 2008; Meylan et al. 2012).

B. Adults

"Programmed" partial migration may also be very widespread in vertebrates, although the natural history is not well known, and regulatory mechanisms are even less well known. Many years ago, Lack (1954) suggested that reproductive hormones such as testosterone might suppress the migratory urge, thus avoiding premature departure from the breeding grounds if breeding is delayed. This also seems to be true for regular migrants, particularly females (Runfeldt and Wingfield 1985; Schwabl and Silverin 1990). Although seasonal changes in testosterone levels of free-living birds have been published for many species (Hirschenhauser et al. 2003), only two partially migratory species have been investigated so far: the European blackbird (Schwabl et al. 1984) and the willow tit (Silverin et al. 1986). European blackbirds showed no autumnal surge in testosterone plasma levels, that is, separate from the breeding season (Schwabl et al. 1984). In contrast, about 30% of juvenile female and male willow tits had a brief peak in circulating testosterone in autumn (Silverin et al. 1986). Curiously, adult willow tits showed no elevation of testosterone levels at that time. Furthermore, high testosterone levels in blood were also found in some juveniles along the autumn migration route. On the other hand, field experiments in which birds were given subcutaneous implants of testosterone revealed that elevated testosterone levels during autumn did not affect the sedentary behavior of individuals that do not migrate (Silverin et al. 1989). Results from these two partially migratory species indicate that testosterone may not be involved in the regulation or initiation of partial migration, but could, in some way, be a result of it.

The example for the willow tit differs from that postulated for dispersal of non-territorial and sedentary birds. The latter may disperse from their natal areas in the absence of parental aggression and even when there is plenty of food. The timing of dispersal in these latter examples has been related to body condition and/or social status. This appears to be what is happening in the non-territorial marsh tit (Nilsson and Smith 1985), where birds in good condition disperse earlier than those in bad condition.

C. Facultative

Because facultative migrations are difficult to predict, we are restricted to opportunistic studies. We are unaware of any studies that have been lucky enough to assess the physiological mechanisms underlying these movements. Given that many irruptive movements are associated with low food availability, corticosteroids are an attractive possible mechanism. Social factors may also be important, and much more is known about this aspect.

Migratory as well as resident birds in winter may gather in large flocks, where they compete for resources such as food, shelter, future mating partners, and so on. Resident birds that have formed flocks may then hold winter territories. These winter territories are often not necessarily those in which breeding may occur the following spring. Migratory birds may hold foraging territories on their migratory route for brief periods and may also establish territories on their winter grounds. Within wintering flocks, whether territorial or not, there is usually a strict social hierarchy. Social challenges may have a profound influence on an individual's chances of surviving the winter to breed the following spring. To increase winter survival, especially in relation to perturbations such as severe storms, and to gain access to breeding resources in spring, it is important for many resident birds to maintain, or even enhance, their social status in a winter group. However, it is likely that this is associated with costs of aggressive interactions with other birds in the group, resulting in reduced access to food, increased predation pressure, and greater exposure to weather (see Chapter 8). In turn, this will increase energetic demand (allostatic load) and, as a result, elevated plasma levels of corticosterone (McEwen and Wingfield 2003a; Goymann and Wingfield 2004).

Variation in social ranks may normally be associated with differences in allostatic load, leading to the assumption that sub-dominant individuals have higher basal plasma levels of corticosteroids than dominant individuals (von Holst 1998; Goymann and Wingfield 2004). Recent studies indicate that, at least in some avian species, allostatic load in fact may be higher in the dominant birds. For example, in wintering mallard and pintail flocks, dominant males showed a stronger corticosterone acute stress response than subordinate males (Poisbleau et al. 2005). On the other hand, there were no differences in baseline levels of corticosterone between dominant and sub-dominant males of these two species, indicating that low-ranked males are normally not more stressed than the high-ranked males.

Birds may also show variation of basal corticosterone levels depending upon the size of the flock. Willow tits form flocks in autumn and then together they defend a winter territory. These flocks consist of four to six individuals, two adults from the breeding pair on that territory that now forms the borders of the winter territory, and two to four unrelated juveniles. It is essential that juveniles become a member of a flock and join an adult pair to survive the winter. Only a fraction of the juveniles in the area succeed in becoming established in a winter group, and they must defend positions in the flock and prevent other juveniles from joining. This often results in aggression, at least early in the autumn when flocks are first established. Juveniles almost exclusively defend the borders of the winter territory and, probably because of prior residency, adults rarely participate in territory defense, nor do they have to fight to be a flock member. Furthermore, the juveniles are forced by the adults to forage in the more open upper parts of the canopies, exposing them to predators and to weather (Ekman 1989). Thus, juvenile willow tits are more vulnerable to both physical and psychological threats than adults, possibly accompanied by higher allostatic load. As predicted, juveniles in these winter flocks had higher basal levels of corticosterone than adults (Silverin et al. 1984). On the other hand, in flocks with only three members (for example two adults and one juvenile), allostatic load might be greater for adults as well because all had high basal corticosterone levels. Similar results have been found in social flocks of greylag geese. Members of small flocks (three to four members) had higher excreted corticosterone metabolites in their feces than members of larger groups (Scheiber et al. 2005).

VI. CONCLUDING REMARKS

This chapter and the preceding two chapters have reviewed a vast literature on the ways by which perturbations of the environment, from tempests to pestilences, trigger facultative and presumably adaptive behavioral and physiological responses. Most of these kinds of investigations have been conducted at least partially in the field, and therefore represent facultative responses under naturalistic conditions. Nonetheless, the sheer diversity and complexity of these responses and their relationships to age, gender, social status, and so on, present an almost daunting prospect for the future to tease apart common mechanisms and underlying themes that explain how life on Earth copes with a frequently capricious environment. It is now abundantly clear that some form of theoretical approach, including modeling and predictive frameworks, will be needed to fully understand the diversity of mechanisms by which animals cope and to form more realistic hypotheses from which predictions can be tested. The allostasis, allostatic load, and overload framework (McEwen and Wingfield 2003a) and the reactive scope of the mediators of allostasis (Romero et al. 2009) are heuristic and potentially very useful approaches to provide such a framework. In Chapter 3 we tried to tie these two complementary approaches together and hope that this will be the beginning of a more theoretical approach. The following chapters will address the future and many of the issues of our time, such as global climate change, habitat destruction and urbanization, spread of invasive species and disease, and pollution. How and why do animals, including ourselves, modulate physiological and behavioral response to natural perturbations and human-induced rapid environmental change? How does flexibility in reactive scope contribute to individual robustness and resilience in the face of global change and major upheavals of the "Anthropocene" era? These major issues will ultimately reveal to us how to approach sustainability of natural resources and how we harvest them, perhaps mitigate loss of biodiversity, and adjust our own actions in how we affect our home—planet Earth.

REFERENCES

Adamec, R. E., Blundell, J., Burton, P., 2006. Relationship of the predatory attack experience to neural plasticity, pCREB expression and neuroendocrine response. *Neurosci Biobehav Rev* 30, 356–375.

Adamo, S. A., 2004. How should behavioural ecologists interpret measurements of immunity? *Anim Behav* 68, 1443–1449.

Adelman, J. S., Martin, L. B., 2009. Vertebrate sickness behaviors: Adaptive and integrated neuroendocrine immune responses. *Integ Comp Biol* 49, 202–214.

Adkins-Regan, E., 2005. *Hormones and animal social behavior.* Monographs in Behavior and Ecology. Princeton University Press, Princeton, NJ.

Almasi, B., Roulin, A., Jenni-Eiermann, S., Jenni, L., 2008. Parental investment and its sensitivity to corticosterone is linked to melanin-based coloration in barn owls. *Horm Behav* 54, 217–223.

Andrews, R. V., Strohbehn, R., 1971. Endocrine adjustments in a wild lemming population during the 1969 summer season. *Comp Biochem Physiol A Comp Physiol* 38, 183–201.

Andus, T., Bauer, J., Gerok, W., 1991. Effects of cytokines on the liver. *Hepatology* 13, 364–375.

Angelier, F., Moe, B., Clement-Chastel, C., Bech, C., Chastel, O., 2007. Corticosterone levels in relation to change of mate in black-legged kittiwakes. *Condor* 109, 668–674.

Apfelbach, R., Blanchard, C. D., Blanchard, R. J., Hayes, R. A., McGregor, I. S., 2005. The effects of predator odors in mammalian prey species: A review of field and laboratory studies. *Neurosci Biobehav Rev* 29, 1123–1144.

Apfelbeck, B., Raess, M., 2008. Behavioural and hormonal effects of social isolation and neophobia in a gregarious bird species, the European starling (*Sturnus vulgaris*). *Horm Behav* 54, 435–441.

Ashley, N., Wingfield, J. C., 2011. Allostasis, life history modulation and hormonal regulation. In: R.J., Nelson., G., Demas (Eds.), *Sickness behavior in vertebrates.* Oxford University Press, London, pp. 45–91

Aubert, A., 1999. Sickness and behaviour in animals: A motivational perspective. *Neurosci Biobehav Rev* 23, 1029–1036.

Aubert, A., Goodall, G., Dantzer, R., Gheusi, G., 1997. Differential effects of lipopolysaccharide on pup retrieving and nest building in lactating mice. *Brain Behav Immun* 11, 107–118.

Avitsur, R., Cohen, E., Yirmiya, R., 1997. Effects of interleukin-1 on sexual attractivity in a model of sickness behavior. *Physiol Behav* 63, 25–30.

Avitsur, R., Sheridan, J. F., 2009. Neonatal stress modulates sickness behavior. *Brain Behav Immun* 23, 977–985.

Avitsur, R., Yirmiya, R., 1999. The immunobiology of sexual behavior: Gender differences in the suppression of sexual activity during illness. *Pharmacol Biochem Behav* 64, 787–796.

Bateman, A., Singh, A., Kral, T., Solomon, S., 1989. The immune-hypothalamic-pituitary-adrenal axis. *Endocr Rev* 10, 92–112.

Baumann, H., Gauldie, J., 1994. The acute phase response. *Immunol Today* 15, 74–80.

Beekman, M., 2004. *Behavioral, neurochemical and neuroendocrine effects of predator stress in mice.* Ph.D. Thesis, Ludwig Maximilians University, Munich, Germany,

Bentley, G. E., Demas, G. E., Nelson, R. J., Ball, G. F., 1998. Melatonin, immunity and cost of reproductive state in male European starlings. *Proc R Soc Lond B* 265, 1191–1195.

Bergman, T. J., Beehner, J. C., Cheney, D. L., Seyfarth, R. M., Whitten, P. L., 2005. Correlates of stress in free-ranging male chacma baboons, *Papio hamadryas ursinus. Anim Behav* 70, 703–713.

Besedovsky, H., Delrey, A., Sorkin, E., Dinarello, C.A., 1986. Immunoregulatory feedback between interleukin-1 and glucocorticoid hormones. *Science* 233, 652–654.

Besedovsky, H. O., DelRey, A., 1996. Immune-neuro-endocrine interactions: Facts and hypotheses. *Endocr Rev* 17, 64–102.

Betts, M.G., Hadley, A. S., Rodenhouse, N., Nocera, J. J., 2008. Social information trumps vegetation structure in breeding-site selection by a migrant songbird. *Proc R Soc Lond B* 275, 2257–2263.

Bilbo, S. D., Drazen, D. L., Quan, N., He, L. L., Nelson, R. J., 2002. Short day lengths attenuate the symptoms of infection in Siberian hamsters. *Proc R Soc Lond B* 269, 447–454.

Blumstein, D. T., Patton, M. L., Saltzman, W., 2006. Faecal glucocorticoid metabolites and alarm calling in free-living yellow-bellied marmots. *Biol Lett* 2, 29–32.

Bókony, V., Lendvai, A. Z., Liker, A., Angelier, F., Wingfield, J. C., Chastel, O., 2009. Stress response and the value of reproduction: Are birds prudent parents? *Am Nat* 173, 589–598.

Bonneaud, C., Mazuc, J., Gonzalez, G., Haussy, C., Chastel, O., Faivre, B., Sorci, G., 2003. Assessing the cost of mounting an immune response. *Am Nat* 161, 367–379.

Boonstra, R., Hik, D., Singleton, G. P., Tinnikov, A., 1998. The impact of predator-induced stress on the snowshore hare cycle. *Ecol Monogr* 68, 371–394.

Breves, J. P., Specker, J. L., 2005. Cortisol stress response of juvenile winter flounder (*Pseudopleuronectes americanus, Walbaum*) to predators. *J Exper Marine Biol Ecol* 325, 1–7.

Brockman, D. K., Cobden, A. K., Whitten, P. L., 2009. Birth season glucocorticoids are related to the presence of infants in sifaka (*Propithecus verreauxi*). *Proc R Soc Lond B* 276, 1855–1863.

Brown, D. R., Long, J. A., 2007. What is a winter floater? Causes, consequences, and implications for habitat selection. *Condor* 109, 548–565.

Buehler, D. M., Encinas-Viso, F., Petit, M., Vezina, F., Tieleman, B. I., Piersma, T., 2009a. Limited access to food and physiological trade-offs in a long-distance migrant shorebird. II. Constitutive immune function and the acute-phase response. *Physiol Biochem Zool* 82, 561–571.

Buehler, D. M., Encinas-Viso, F., Petit, M., Vèzina, F., Tieleman, B. I., Piersma, T., 2009b. Limited access to food and physiological trade-offs in a long distance migrant shorebird. II. Constitutive immune function and the acute-phase response. *Physiol Biochem Zool* 82, 561–571.

Butler, L. K., Bisson, I. A., Hayden, T. J., Wikelski, M., Romero, L. M., 2009. Adrenocortical responses to offspring-directed threats in two open-nesting birds. *Gen Comp Endocrinol* 162, 313–318.

Canoine, V., Hayden, T. J., Rowe, K., Goymann, W., 2002. The stress response of European stonechats depends on the type of stressor. *Behaviour* 139, 1303–1311.

Carnegie, S. D., Fedigan, L. M., Ziegler, T. E., 2011. Social and environmental factors affecting fecal glucocorticoids in wild, female white-faced capuchins (*Cebus capucinus*). *Am J Primatol* 73, 861–869.

Carter, J., Lyons, N. J., Cole, H. L., Goldsmith, A. R., 2008. Subtle cues of predation risk: starlings respond to a predator's direction of eye-gaze. *Proc R Soc Lond B* 275, 1709–1715.

Cavigelli, S. A., Dubovick, T., Levash, W., Jolly, A., Pitts, A., 2003. Female dominance status and fecal corticoids in a cooperative breeder with low reproductive skew: Ring-tailed lemurs (*Lemur catta*). *Horm Behav* 43, 166–179.

Cease, A. J., Lutterschmidt, D. I., Mason, R. T., 2007. Corticosterone and the transition from courtship behavior to dispersal in male red-sided garter snakes (*Thamnophis sirtalis parietalis*). *Gen Comp Endocrinol* 150, 124–131.

Chitty, D., 1996. *Do lemmings commit suicide? Beautiful hypotheses and ugly facts.* Oxford University Press, New York.

Christian, J. J., LLoyd, J. A., Davis, D. E., 1965. The role of endocrines in the self-regulation of mammalian populations. *Rec Prog Horm Res* 21, 501–578.

Clinchy, M., Zanette, L., Boonstra, R., Wingfield, J. C., Smith, J. N. M., 2004. Balancing food and predator pressure induces chronic stress in songbirds. *Proc R Soc Lond B* 271, 2473–2479.

Cluttonbrock, T. H., 1984. Reproductive effort and terminal investment in iteroparous animals. *Am Nat* 123, 212–229.

Cockrem, J. F., Silverin, B., 2002. Sight of a predator can stimulate a corticosterone response in the great tit (*Parus major*). *Gen Comp Endocrinol* 125, 248.

Cohn, D. W. H., de Sa-Rocha, L. C., 2006. Differential effects of lipopolysaccharide in the social behavior of dominant and submissive mice. *Physiol Behav* 87, 932–937.

Cote, J., Clobert, J., Brodin, T., Fogarty, S., Sih, A., 2010. Personality-dependent dispersal: characterization, ontogeny and consequences for spatially structured populations. *Phil Trans R Soc B* 365, 4065–4076.

Creel, S., Christianson, D., Liley, S., Winnie, J. A., Jr., 2007. Predation risk affects reproductive physiology and demography of elk. *Science (Washington DC)* 315, 960.

Creel, S., Winnie, J. A., Christianson, D., 2009. Glucocorticoid stress hormones and the effect of predation risk on elk reproduction. *Proc Natl Acad Sci USA* 106, 12388–12393.

Dantzer, R., 2001. Cytokine-induced sickness behavior: Where do we stand? *Brain Behav Immun* 15, 7–24.

Dantzer, R., Bluthé, R., Kent, S., Goodall, G., 1993. Behavioral effects of cytokines: an insight into mechanisms of sickness behavior. In: Desouza, E. G. (Ed.), *Neurobiology of cytokines.* Academic Press, San Diego,

Dantzer, R., Bluthe, R. M., Laye, S., Bret-Dibat, J. L., Parnet, P., Kelley, K. W., 1998. *Ann NY Acad Sci*, 840, 586–590.

De Fraipont, M., Clobert, J., John, H., Alder, S., 2000. Increased pre-natal maternal corticosterone promotes philopatry of offspring in common lizards *Lacerta vivipara. J Anim Ecol* 69, 404–413.

Deen, C. M., Hutchison, V. H., 2001. Effects of lipopolysaccharide and acclimation temperature on induced behavioral fever in juvenile Iguana iguana. *J Thermal Biol* 26, 55–63.

Demas, G. E., 2004. The energetics of immunity: A neuroendocrine link between energy balance and immune function. *Horm Behav* 45, 173–180.

Demas, G. E., Drazen, D. L., Nelson, R. J., 2003. Reductions in total body fat decrease humoral immunity. *Proc R Soc Lond B* 270, 905–911.

Demas, G. E., Nelson, R. J., 2003. Lack of immunological responsiveness to photoperiod in a tropical rodent, *Peromyscus aztecus hylocetes. J Comp Physiol B* 173, 171–176.

DeVries, A. C., Craft, T. K. S., Glasper, E. R., Neigh, G. N., Alexander, J. K., 2007. 2006 Curt P. Richter Award winner: Social influences on stress responses and health. *Psychoneuroendocrinology* 32, 587–603.

Dhabhar, F. S., 2002. A hassle a day may keep the doctor away: Stress and the augmentation of immune function. *Integ Comp Biol* 42, 556–564.

Dhabhar, F. S., McEwen, B. S., 1999. Enhancing versus suppressive effects of stress hormones on skin immune function. *Proc Natl Acad Sci USA* 96, 1059–1064.

Dufty, A. M., Crandall, M. B., 2005. Corticosterone secretion in response to adult alarm calls in American Kestrels. *J Field Ornith* 76, 319–325.

Dunn, A. J., Swiergiel, A. H., 1998. The role of cytokines in infection-related behavior. *Ann NY Acad Sci*, 840, 577–585.

Ebensperger, L. A., Ramirez-Estrada, J., Leon, C., Castro, R. A., Tolhuysen, L. O., Sobrero, R., Quirici, V., Burger, J. R., Soto-Gamboa, M., Hayes, L. D., 2011. Sociality, glucocorticoids and direct fitness in the communally rearing rodent, *Octodon degus. Horm Behav* 60, 346–352.

Edeline, E., Bardonnet, A., Bolliet, V., Dufour, S., Pierre, E., 2005. Endocrine control of Anguilla anguilla glass eel dispersal: Effect of thyroid hormones on locomotor activity and rheotactic behavior. *Horm Behav* 48, 53–63.

Eilam, D., Dayan, T., Ben-Eliyahu, S., Schulman, I., Shefer, G., Hendrie, C.A., 1999. Differential behavioural and hormonal responses of voles and spiny mice to owl calls. *Anim Behav* 58, 1085–1093.

Ekman, J., 1989. Ecology of non-breeding social-systems of parus. *Wilson Bull* 101, 263–288.

El Hage, W., Griebel, G., Belzung, C., 2006. Long-term impaired memory following predatory stress in mice. *Physiol Behav* 87, 45–50.

Ellsworth, E. A., Belthoff, J. R., 1999. Effects of social status on the dispersal behaviour of juvenile western screech-owls. *Anim Behav* 57, 883–892.

Engh, A. L., Beehner, J. C., Bergman, T. J., Whitten, P. L., Hoffmeier, R. R., Seyfarth, R. M., Cheney, D. L., 2006a. Behavioural and hormonal responses to predation in female chacma baboons (*Papio hamadryas ursinus*). *Proc R Soc Lond B* 273, 707–712.

Engh, A. L., Beehner, J. C., Bergman, T. J., Whitten, P. L., Hoffmeier, R. R., Seyfarth, R. M., Cheney, D. L., 2006b. Female hierarchy instability, male immigration and infanticide increase glucocorticoid levels in female chacma baboons. *Anim Behav* 71, 1227.

Eraud, C., Jacquet, A., Faivre, B., 2009. Survival cost of an early immune soliciting in nature. *Evolution* 63, 1036–1043.

Ewald, P. W., 1980. Evolutionary biology and the treatment of signs and symptoms of infectious disease. *J Theor Biol* 86, 169–176.

Exton, M. S., 1997. Infection-induced anorexia: Active host defence strategy. *Appetite* 29, 369–383.

Fletcher, Q. E., Boonstra, R., 2006. Do captive male meadow voles experience acute stress in response to weasel odour? *Can J Zool* 84, 583–588.

Foerster, S., Cords, M., Monfort, S. L., 2011. Social behavior, foraging strategies, and fecal glucocorticoids in female blue monkeys (*Cercopithecus mitis*): Potential fitness benefits of high rank in a forest guenon. *Am J Primatol* 73, 870–882.

Fraker, M. E., 2008. The dynamics of predation risk assessment: responses of anuran larvae to chemical cues of predators. *J Anim Ecol* 77, 638–645.

French, S. S., Moore, M. C., Demas, G. E., 2009. Ecological immunology: The organism in context. *Integ Comp Biol* 49, 246–253.

Frid, A., Dill, L., 2002. Human-caused disturbance stimuli as a form of predation risk. *Conserv Ecol* 6, 11.

Frigerio, D., Moestl, E., Kotrschal, K., 2001. Excreted metabolites of gonadal steroid hormones and corticosterone in greylag geese (*Anser anser*) from hatching to fledging. *Gen Comp Endocrinol* 124, 246–255.

Frigerio, D., Weiss, B., Dittami, J., Kotrschal, K., 2003. Social allies modulate corticosterone excretion and increase success in agonistic interactions in juvenile hand-raised graylag geese (*Anser anser*). *Can J Zool* 81, 1746–1754.

Glennemeier, K. A., Denver, R. J., 2002. Role for corticoids in mediating the response of Rana pipiens tadpoles to intraspecific competition. *J Exp Zool* 292, 32–40.

Glickman, S. E., Frank, L. G., Pavgi, S., Licht, P., 1992. Hormonal correlates of 'masculinization' in female spotted hyaenas (*Crocuta crocuta*). 1. Infancy to sexual maturity. *J Reprod Fertil* 95, 451–462.

Gonzalez, G., Sorci, G., de Lope, F., 1999. Seasonal variation in the relationship between cellular immune response and badge size in male house sparrows (*Passer domesticus*). *Behav Ecol Sociobiol* 46, 117–122.

Goymann, W., Wingfield, J. C., 2004. Allostatic load, social status and stress hormones: the costs of social status matter. *Anim Behav* 67, 591–602.

Greenman, C. G., Martin, L. B., Hau, M., 2005. Reproductive state, but not testosterone, reduces immune function in male house sparrows (*Passer domesticus*). *Physiol Biochem Zool* 78, 60–68.

Griffith, S. C., Pryke, S. R., Buttemer, W. A., 2011. Constrained mate choice in social monogamy and the stress of having an unattractive partner. *Proc R Soc Lond B* 278, 2798–2805.

Hamann, M., Jessop, T. S., Schauble, C. S., 2007. Fuel use and corticosterone dynamics in hatchling green sea turtles (*Chelonia mydas*) during natal dispersal. *J Exper Marine Biol Ecol* 353, 13–21.

Hanssen, S. A., Hasselquist, D., Folstad, I., Erikstad, K. E., 2004. Costs of immunity: immune responsiveness reduces survival in a vertebrate. *Proc R Soc Lond B* 271, 925–930.

Hart, B. L., 1988. Biological basis of the behavior of sick animals. *Neuroscie Biobehav Rev* 12, 123–137.

Hasselquist, D., 2007. Comparative immunoecology in birds: Hypotheses and tests. *J Ornithol* 148, S571-S582.

Hasselquist, D., Marsh, J. A., Sherman, P. W., Wingfield, J. C., 1999. Is avian humoral immunocompetence suppressed by testosterone? *Behav Ecol Sociobiol* 45, 167–175.

Hawlena, D., Schmitz, O. J., 2010. Physiological stress as a fundamental mechanism linking predation to ecosystem functioning. *Am Nat* 176, 537–556.

Hegner, R. E., Wingfield, J. C., 1987. Effects of experimental manipulation of testosterone levels on parental investment and breeding success in male house sparrows. *Auk* 104, 462–469.

Hirschenhauser, K., Winkler, H., Oliveira, R. F., 2003. Comparative analysis of male androgen responsiveness to social environment in birds: The effects of mating system and paternal incubation. *Horm Behav* 43, 508–519.

Ibanez-Alamo, J. D., Chastel, O., Soler, M., 2011. Hormonal response of nestlings to predator calls. *Gen Comp Endocrinol* 171, 232–236.

Jessop, T., Sumner, J., Lance, V., Limpus, C., 2004. Reproduction in shark-attacked sea turtles is supported by stress-reduction mechanisms. *Proc R Soc Lond B* 271, S91-S94.

Kavaliers, M., Colwell, D. D., Choleris, E., 2000. Parasites and behaviour: An ethopharmacological perspective. *Parasitol Today* 16, 464–468.

Kent, S., Bluthe, R. M., Kelley, K. W., Dantzer, R., 1992. Sickness behavior as a new target for drug development. *Trends Pharmacol Sci* 13, 24–28.

Kitaysky, A. S., Kitaiskaia, E. V., Piatt, J. F., Wingfield, J. C., 2003. Benefits and costs of increased levels of corticosterone in seabird chicks. *Horm Behav* 43, 140–149.

Kitaysky, A. S., Wingfield, J. C., Piatt, J. F., 1999. Dynamics of food availability, body condition and physiological stress response in breeding Black-legged Kittiwakes. *Func Ecol* 13, 577–584.

Kitaysky, A. S., Wingfield, J. C., Piatt, J. F., 2001. Corticosterone facilitates begging and affects resource allocation in the black-legged kittiwake. *Behav Ecol* 12, 619.

Kluger, M. J., 1979. *Fever: Its biology, evolution, and function*. Princeton University Press, Princeton, NJ.

Kluger, M. J., 1991. Fever: Role of pyrogens and cryogens. *Physiol Rev* 71, 93–127.

Kluger, M. J., Kozak, W., Conn, C. A., Leon, L. R., Soszynski, D., 1998. Role of fever in disease. *Ann NY Acad Sci*, 856, 224–233.

Kluger, M. J., Ringler, D. H., Anver, M. R., 1975. Fever and survival. *Science* 188, 166–168.

Kluger, M. J., Vaughn, L. K., 1978. Fever and survival in rabbits infected with *Pasteurella multocida*. *J Physiol* 282, 243–251.

Kondo, K., Harbuz, M. S., Levy, A., Lightman, S. L., 1997. Inhibition of the hypothalamic-pituitary-thyroid axis in response to lipopolysaccharide is independent of changes in circulating corticosteroids. *Neuroimmunomodulation* 4, 188–194.

Konsman, J. P., Parnet, P., Dantzer, R., 2002. Cytokine-induced sickness behaviour: mechanisms and implications. *Trends Neurosci* 25, 154–159.

Koolhaas, J. M., Korte, S. M., De Boer, S. F., Van Der Vegt, B. J., Van Reenen, C. G., Hopster, H., De Jong, I. C., Ruis, M. A. W., Blokhuis, H. J., 1999. Coping styles in animals: Current status in behavior and stress-physiology. *Neurosci Biobehav Rev* 23, 925–935.

Korpimaki, E., Lagerstrom, M., 1988. Survival and natal dispersal of fledglings of Tengmalm's owl in relation to fluctuating food conditions and hatching date. *J Anim Ecol* 57, 433–441.

Krebs, C. J., Boutin, S., Boonstra, R., Sinclair, A. R., Smith, J. N., Dale, M. R., Martin, K., Turkington, R., 1995. Impact of food and predation on the snowshoe hare cycle. *Science* 269, 1112–1115.

Lack, D., 1954. *The natural regulation of animal numbers*. Oxford University Press, London.

Langhans, W., 2000. Anorexia of infection: Current prospects. *Nutrition* 16, 996–1005.

Lendvai, A. Z., Chastel, O., 2008. Experimental mate-removal increases the stress response of female house sparrows: The effects of offspring value? *Horm Behav* 53, 395–401.

Li, F. H., Zhong, W. Q., Wang, Z. X., Wang, D. H., 2007. Rank in a food competition test and humoral immune functions in male Brandt's voles (*Lasiopodomys brandtii*). *Physiol Behav* 90, 490–495.

Licht, P., Frank, L. G., Pavgi, S., Yalcinkaya, T. M., Siiteri, P. K., Glickman, S. E., 1992. Hormonal correlates of 'masculinization' in female spotted hyaenas (*Crocuta crocuta*). 2. Maternal and fetal steroids. *J Reprod Fertil* 95, 463–474.

Licht, P., Hayes, T., Tsai, P., Cunha, G., Kim, H., Golbus, M., Hayward, S., Martin, M. C., Jaffe, R. B., Glickman, S. E., 1998. Androgens and masculinization of genitalia in the spotted hyaena (*Crocuta crocuta*). 1. Urogenital morphology and placental androgen production during fetal life. *J Reprod Fertil* 113, 105–116.

Lindstrom, E. R., Andren, H., Angelstam, P., Cederlund, G., Hornfeldt, B., Jaderberg, L., Lemnell, P. A., Martinsson, B., Skold, K., Swenson, J. E., 1994. Disease reveals the predator: Sarcoptic mange, red fox predation, and prey populations. *Ecology* 75, 1042–1049.

Lochmiller, R. L., Deerenberg, C., 2000. Trade-offs in evolutionary immunology: just what is the cost of immunity? *Oikos* 88, 87–98.

Lozano, G. A., Lank, D. B., 2003. Seasonal trade-offs in cell-mediated immunosenescence in ruffs (*Philomachus pugnax*). *Proc R Soc Lond B* 270, 1203–1208.

MacFarsane, R. B., 1984. Determination of corticosteroids in fish plasma by high performance liquid chromatography: Evaluation of the method using striped bass (Morone saxatalis). *Can J Fishe Aquat Sci* 41, 1280–1286.

Maier, S. F., Watkins, L. R., 1999. Bidirectional communication between the brain and the immune system: implications for behaviour. *Anim Behav* 57, 741–751.

Marcstrom, V., Kenward, R.E., Engren, E., 1988. The impact of predation on boreal tetraonids during vole cycles: An experimental study. *J Animal Ecol* 57, 859.

Martin, L. B., Pless, M., Svoboda, J., Wikelski, M., 2004. Immune activity in temperate and tropical house sparrows: A common-garden experiment. *Ecology* 85, 2323–2331.

McEwen, B. S., 2000. Allostasis and allostatic load: Implications for neuropsychopharmacology. *Neuropsychopharmacology* 22, 108–124.

McEwen, B. S., Biron, C. A., Brunson, K. W., Bulloch, K., Chambers, W. H., Dhabhar, F. S., Goldfarb, R. H., Kitson, R. P., Miller, A. H., Spencer, R. L., Weiss, J. M., 1997. The role of adrenocorticoids as modulators of immune function in health and disease: Neural, endocrine and immune interactions. *Brain Res Rev* 23, 79–133.

McEwen, B. S., Wingfield, J. C., 2003a. The concept of allostasis in biology and biomedicine. *Horm Behav* 43, 2–15.

McEwen, B. S., Wingfield, J. C., 2003b. Response to commentaries on the concept of allostasis. *Horm Behav* 43, 28–30.

Meylan, S., Miles, D. B., Clobert, J., 2012. Hormonally mediated maternal effects, individual strategy and global change. *Phil Trans R Soc B* 367, 1647–1664.

Moller, A. P., Erritzoe, J., Saino, N., 2003. Seasonal changes in immune response and parasite impact on hosts. *Am Nat* 161, 657–671.

Monclus, R., Roedel, H. G., Palme, R., Von Holst, D., de Miguel, J., 2006a. Non-invasive measurement of the physiological stress response of wild rabbits to the odour of a predator. *Chemoecology* 16, 25–29.

Monclus, R., Roedel, H. G., von Holst, D., 2006b. Fox odour increases vigilance in european rabbits: A study under semi-natural conditions. *Ethology* 112, 1186–1193.

Monclus, R., Tiulim, J., Blumstein, D. T., 2011. Older mothers follow conservative strategies under predator pressure: The adaptive role of maternal glucocorticoids in yellow-bellied marmots. *Horm Behav* 60, 660–665.

Montero, D., Izquierdo, M. S., Tort, L., Robaina, L., Vergara, J. M., 1999. High stocking density produces crowding stress altering some physiological and biochemical parameters in gilthead seabream, *Sparus aurata*, juveniles. *Fish Physiol Biochem* 20, 53–60.

Moore, C. B., Siopes, T. D., 2000. Effects of lighting conditions and melatonin supplementation on the cellular and humoral immune responses in Japanese quail *Coturnix coturnix japonica*. *Gen Comp Endocrinol* 119, 95–104.

Moret, Y., Schmid-Hempel, P., 2000. Survival for immunity: The price of immune system activation for bumblebee workers. *Science* 290, 1166–1168.

Morton, E. S., 1971. Nest predation affecting the breeding season of the clay-colored robin, a tropical song bird. *Science* 171, 920–921.

Mueller, C., Jenni-Eiermann, S., Blondel, J., Perret, P., Caro, S. P., Lambrechts, M., Jenni, L., 2006. Effect of human presence and handling on circulating corticosterone levels in breeding blue tits (*Parus caeruleus*). *Gen Comp Endocrinol* 148, 163–171.

Munck, A., Guyre, P. M., Holbrook, N.J., 1984. Physiological functions of glucocorticoids in stress and their relation to pharmacological actions. *Endocr Rev* 5, 25–44.

Nelson, R. J., 2004. Seasonal immune function and sickness responses. *Trends Immunol* 25, 187–192.

Nelson, R. J., Demas, G., 2011. *Sickness behavior in vertebrates*. Oxford University Press, London.

Nelson, R. J., Demas, G. E., 1996. Seasonal changes in immune function. *Q Rev Biol* 71, 511–548.

Nelson, R. J., Demas, G. E., Klein, S. L., Kriegsfeld, L. J., 2002. *Seasonal patterns of stress, immune function, and disease*. Cambridge University Press, Cambridge.

Newton, I., 1998. *Population limitation in birds*. Academic Press, Boston.

Nilsson, J. A., Smith, H. G., 1985. Early fledgling mortality and the timing of juvenile dispersal in the marsh tit *Parus palustris*. *Ornis Scan* 16, 293–298.

Norris, K., Evans, M. R., 2000. Ecological immunology: Life history trade-offs and immune defense in birds. *Behav Ecol* 11, 19–26.

Olla, B. L., Davis, M. W., Schreck, C. B., 1992. Comparison of predator avoidance capabilities with corticosteroid levels induced by stress in juvenile coho salmon *Trans Am Fish Soc* 121, 544–547.

Owen-Ashley, N. T., 2004. *Environmental regulation of immune-endocrine phenomena in songbirds*. Department of Zoology, University of Washington, Seattle.

Owen-Ashley, N. T., Hasselquist, D., Raberg, L., Wingfield, J. C., 2008a. Latitudinal variation of immune defense and sickness behavior in the white-crowned sparrow (*Zonotrichia leucophrys*). *Brain Behav Immun* 22, 614–625.

Owen-Ashley, N. T., Hasselquist, D., Råberg, L., Wingfield, J. C., 2008b. Latitudinal variation of immune defense and sickness behavior in the white-crowned sparrow (*Zonotrichia leucophrys*). *Brain Behav Immun* 22, 614–625.

Owen-Ashley, N. T., Turner, M., Hahn, T. P., Wingfield, J. C., 2006. Hormonal, behavioral, and thermoregulatory responses to bacterial lipopolysaccharide in captive and free-living white-crowned sparrows (*Zonotrichia leucophrys gambelii*). *Horm Behav* 49, 15–29.

Owen-Ashley, N. T., Wingfield, J. C., 2006a. Seasonal modulation of sickness behavior in free-living northwestern song sparrows (*Melospiza melodia morphna*). *J Exp Biol* 209, 3062–3070.

Owen-Ashley, N. T., Wingfield, J. C., 2006b. Seasonal modulation of sickness behavior in free-living northwestern song sparrows (*Melospiza melodia morphna*). *J Exp Biol* 209, 3062–3070.

Owen-Ashley, N. T., Wingfield, J. C., 2007. Acute phase responses of passerine birds: characterization and seasonal variation. *J Ornithol* 148, S583–S591.

Pickering, A. D., Stewart, A., 1984. Acclimation of the interrenal tissue of the brown trout, Salmo trutta L., to chronic crowding stress. *J Fish Biol* 24, 731–740.

Piersma, T., 1997. Do global patterns of habitat use and migration strategics co-evolve with relative investments in immunocompetence due to spatial variation in parasite pressure? *Oikos* 80, 623–631.

Plata-Salaman, C. R., 1996. Anorexia during acute and chronic disease. *Nutrition* 12, 69–78.

Poisbleau, M., Fritz, H., Guillon, N., Chastel, O., 2005. Linear social dominance hierarchy and corticosterone responses in male mallards and pintails. *Horm Behav* 47, 485–492.

Pollak, E. I., Christian, J. J., 1977. Social activation of the interrenal gland in the blue gourami, *Trichogaster trichopterus* (*Pisces, Belontiidae*). *Behav Biol* 19, 217–227.

Prendergast, B. J., Baillie, S. R., Dhabhar, F. S., 2008. Gonadal hormone-dependent and—independent regulation of immune function by photoperiod in Siberian hamsters. *Am J Physiol* 294, R384–R392.

Quirici, V., Faugeron, S., Hayes, L. D., Ebensperger, L. A., 2011. The influence of group size on natal dispersal in the communally rearing and semifossorial rodent, *Octodon degus*. *Behav Ecol Sociobiol* 65, 787–798.

Ramenofsky, M., 1990. Fat storage and fat metabolism in relation to migration. In: Gwinner, E. (Ed.), *Bird migration: Physiology and ecophysiology*. Springer-Verlag, Berlin, pp. 214–231.

Ramenofsky, M., Wingfield, J. C., 2007. Regulation of migration. *Bioscience* 57, 135–143.

Ramos-Fernandez, G., Nunez-de la Mora, A., Wingfield, J. C., Drummond, H., 2000. Endocrine correlates of dominance in chicks of the blue-footed booby (*Sula nebouxii*): Testing the challenge hypothesis. *Ethol Ecol Evolution* 12, 27–34.

Ramsay, J. M., Feist, G. W., Varga, Z. M., Westerfield, M., Kent, M. L., Schreck, C. B., 2006. Whole-body cortisol is an indicator of crowding stress in adult zebrafish, *Danio rerio*. *Aquaculture* 258, 565–574.

Remage-Healey, L., Adkins-Regan, E., Romero, L. M., 2003. Behavioral and adrenocortical responses to mate separation and reunion in the zebra finch. *Horm Behav* 43, 108–114.

Remage-Healey, L., Bass, A. H., 2004. Rapid, hierarchical modulation of vocal patterning by steroid hormones. *J Neurosci* 24, 5892–5900.

Remage-Healey, L., Bass, A. H., 2005. Rapid elevations in both steroid hormones and vocal signaling during playback challenge: A field experiment in Gulf toadfish. *Horm Behav* 47, 297–305.

Remage-Healey, L., Bass, A. H., 2006a. From social behavior to neural circuitry: Steroid hormones rapidly modulate advertisement calling via a vocal pattern generator. *Horm Behav* 50, 432–441.

Remage-Healey, L., Bass, A. H., 2006b. A rapid neuromodulatory role for steroid hormones in the control of reproductive behavior. *Brain Res* 1126, 27–35.

Remage-Healey, L., Nowacek, D. P., Bass, A. H., 2006. Dolphin foraging sounds suppress calling and elevate stress hormone levels in a prey species, the Gulf toadfish. *J Exp Biol* 209, 4444–4451.

Reneerkens, J., Piersma, T., Ramenofsky, M., 2002. An experimental test of the relationship between temporal variability of feeding opportunities and baseline levels of corticosterone in a shorebird. *J Exp Zool* 293, 81–88.

Ricklefs, R. E., Wikelski, M., 2002. The physiology/life-history nexus. *Trends Ecol Evol* 17, 462–468.

Rivers, J. W., Martin, L. B., Liebl, A. L., Betts, M. G., 2011. Parental alarm calls of the white-crowned sparrow fail to stimulate corticosterone production in nest-bound offspring. *Ethology* 117, 374–384.

Rivier, C., 1990. Role of endotoxin and interleukin-1 in modulating ACTH, LH and sex steroid secretion. *Adv Exper Med Biol* 274, 295–301.

Rivier, C., Vale, W., 1990. Cytokines act within the brain to inhibit luteinizing hormone secretion and ovulation in the rat. *Endocrinology* 127, 849–856.

Roedl, T., Berger, S., Romero, L. M., Wikelski, M., 2007. Tameness and stress physiology in a predator-naive island species confronted with novel predation threat. *Proc R Soc Lond B* 274, 577–582.

Romero, L. M., Dickens, M. J., Cyr, N. E., 2009. The reactive scope model—a new model integrating homeostasis, allostasis, and stress. *Horm Behav* 55, 375–389.

Runfeldt, S., Wingfield, J. C., 1985. Experimentally prolonged sexual-activity in female sparrows delays termination of reproductive activity in their untreated mates. *Anim Behav* 33, 403–410.

Sapolsky, R. M., 1982. The endocrine stress-response and social status in the wild baboon. *Horm Behav* 16, 279–287.

Sapolsky, R. M., 2001. Physiological and pathophysiological implications of social stress in mammals. In: McEwen, B. S., Goodman, H. M. (Eds.), *Handbook of physiology*; Section 7: *The endocrine system*; Vol. IV: *Coping with the environment: Neural and endocrine mechanisms*. Oxford University Press, New York, pp. 517–532.

Sapolsky, R. M., 2005. The influence of social hierarchy on primate health. *Science* 308, 648–652.

Sapolsky, R. M., Alberts, S. C., Altmann, J., 1997. Hypercortisolism associated with social subordinance or social isolation among wild baboons. *Arch Gen Psychiatry* 54, 1137–1143.

Sapolsky, R. M., Romero, L. M., Munck, A. U., 2000. How do glucocorticoids influence stress-responses? Integrating permissive, suppressive, stimulatory, and preparative actions. *Endocr Rev* 21, 55–89.

Scheiber, I. B. R., Kotrschal, K., Weiss, B. M., 2009. Benefits of family reunions: Social support in secondary greylag goose families. *Horm Behav* 55, 133–138.

Scheiber, I. B. R., Weiss, B. M., Frigerio, D., Kotrschal, K., 2005. Active and passive social support in families of greylag geese (*Anser anser*). *Behaviour* 142, 1535–1557.

Scheuerlein, A., Gwinner, E., 2006. Reduced nestling growth of East African Stonechats Saxicola torquata axillaris in the presence of a predator. *Ibis* 148, 468–476.

Scheuerlein, A., Van't Hof, T. J., Gwinner, E., 2001. Predators as stressors? Physiological and reproductive consequences of predation risk in tropical stonechats (Saxicola torquata axillaris). *Proc R Soc Lond B* 268, 1575.

Schmid-Hempel, P., Ebert, D., 2003. On the evolutionary ecology of specific immune defence. *Trends Ecol Evol* 18, 27–32.

Schwabl, H., 1993. Yolk is a source of maternal testosterone for developing birds. *Proc Natl Acad Sci USA* 90, 11446–11450.

Schwabl, H., Lipar, J., 2002. Hormonal regulation of begging behavior. In: Wright, J., Leonard, M. L. (Eds.), *The evolution of begging*. Kluwer Academic Publishers, Netherlands, pp. 221–244.

Schwabl, H., Mock, D. W., Gieg, J. A., 1997. A hormonal mechanism for parental favouritism. *Nature* 386, 231–231.

Schwabl, H., Silverin, B., 1990. Control of partial migration and autumnal behavior. In: Gwinner, E. (Ed.), *Bird migration*, Springer-Verlag, Berlin, Heidelberg, pp. 144–155.

Schwabl, H., Wingfield, J. C., Farner, D. S., 1984. Endocrine correlates of autumnal behavior in sedentary and migratory individuals of a partially migratory population of the European blackbird (*Turdus-Merula*). *Auk* 101, 499–507.

Sheldon, B. C., Verhulst, S., 1996. Ecological immunology: Costly parasite defences and trade-offs in evolutionary ecology. *Trends Ecol Evol* 11, 317–321.

Sheriff, M. J., Krebs, C. J., Boonstra, R., 2009. The sensitive hare: Sublethal effects of predator stress on reproduction in snowshoe hares. *J Anim Ecol* 78, 1249–1258.

Sheriff, M. J., Krebs, C. J., Boonstra, R., 2010. The ghosts of predators past: Population cycles and the role of maternal programming under fluctuating predation risk. *Ecology* 91, 2983–2994.

Silverin, B., 1997. The stress response and autumn dispersal behaviour in willow tits. *Anim Behav* 53, 451–459.

Silverin, B., 1998. Behavioural and hormonal responses of the pied flycatcher to environmental stressors. *Anim Behav* 55, 1411–1420.

Silverin, B., Viebke, P. A., Westin, J., 1984. Plasma levels of luteinizing hormone and steroid hormones in free-living winter groups of willow tits (*Parus montanus*). *Horm Behav* 18, 367–379.

Silverin, B., Viebke, P. A., Westin, J., 1986. Seasonal-changes in plasma-levels of LH and gonadal-steroids in free-living willow tits *Parus-Montanus*. *Ornis Scan* 17, 230–236.

Silverin, B., Viebke, P. A., Westin, J., 1989. Hormonal correlates of migration and territorial behavior in juvenile willow tits during autumn. *Gen Comp Endocrinol* 75, 148.

Siutz, C., Millesi, E., 2012. Effects of birth date and natal dispersal on faecal glucocorticoid concentrations in juvenile Common hamsters. *Gen Comp Endocrinol* 178, 323–329.

Soto, L., Martin, A. I., Millan, S., Vara, E., Lopez-Calderon, A., 1998. Effects of endotoxin lipopolysaccharide administration on the somatotropic axis. *J Endocrinol* 159, 239–246.

Stöwe, M., Bugnyar, T., Schloegl, C., Heinrich, B., Kotrschal, K., Möstl, E., 2008. Corticosterone excretion patterns and affiliative behavior over development in ravens (*Corvus corax*). *Horm Behav* 53, 208–216.

Teskey-Gerstl, A., Bamberg, E., Steineck, T., Palme, R., 2000. Excretion of corticosteroids in urine and faeces of hares (*Lepus europaeus*). *J Comp Physiol B* 170, 163–168.

Thaker, M., Lima, S. L., Hews, D. K., 2009a. Acute corticosterone elevation enhances antipredator behaviors in male tree lizard morphs. *Horm Behav* 56, 51–57.

Thaker, M., Lima, S.L., Hews, D.K., 2009b. Alternative antipredator tactics in tree lizard morphs: Hormonal and behavioural responses to a predator encounter. *Anim Behav* 77, 395–401.

Thaker, M., Vanak, A. T., Lima, S. L., Hews, D. K., 2010. Stress and aversive learning in a wild vertebrate: The role of corticosterone in mediating escape from a novel stressor. *Am Nat* 175, 50–60.

Tizard, I., 2008. Sickness behavior, its mechanisms and significance. *Animal Health Res Rev* 9, 87–99.

Trompeter, W. P., Langkilde, T., 2011. Invader danger: Lizards faced with novel predators exhibit an altered behavioral response to stress. *Horm Behav* 60, 152–158.

Tuchscherer, M., Kanitz, E., Puppe, B., Tuchscherer, A., 2006. Early social isolation alters behavioral and physiological responses to an endotoxin challenge in piglets. *Horm Behav* 50, 753–761.

Turnbull, A. V., Rivier, C., 1995. Regulation of the HPA axis by cytokines. *Brain Behav Immun* 9, 253–275.

van Gils, J. A., Spaans, B., Dekinga, A., Piersma, T., 2006. Foraging in a tidally structured environment by red knots (*Calidris canutus*): Ideal, but not free. *Ecology* 87, 1189–1202.

Vaughn, L. K., Bernheim, H. A., Kluger, M. J., 1974. Fever in the lizard *Dipsosaurus dorsalis*. *Nature* 252, 473–474.

Vercken, E., de Fraipont, M., Dufty, A. M. Jr, Clobert, J., 2007. Mother's timing and duration of corticosterone exposure modulate offspring size and natal dispersal in the common lizard (*Lacerta vivipara*). *Horm Behav* 51, 379–386.

Vézina, F., Petit, M., Buehler, D. M., Dekinga, A., Piersma, T., 2009. Limited access to food and physiological trade-offs in a long-distance migrant shorebird. I. Energy metabolism, behavior, and body-mass regulation. *Physiol Biochem Zool* 82, 549–560.

Vézina, F., Petit, M., Buehler, D. M., Dekinga, A., Piersma, T., 2009. Limited access to food and physiological trade-offs in a long-distance migrant shorebirds. I. Energy metabolism, behavior, and body-mass regulation. *Physiol Biochem Zool* 82, 549–560.

Viney, M. E., Riley, E. M., Buchanan, K. L., 2005. Optimal immune responses: Immunocompetence revisited. *Trends Ecol Evol* 20, 665–669.

Vitousek, M. N., Romero, L. M., Tarlow, E., Cyr, N. E., Wikelski, M., 2010. Island tameness: An altered cardiovascular stress response in Galapagos marine iguanas. *Physiol Behav* 99, 544–548.

von Holst, D., 1998. The concept of stress and its relevance for animal behavior. In: Moller, A. P., Milinski, M., Slater, P. J. B. (Eds.), *Stress and behavior*, Academic Press, New York, vol. 27. pp. 1–131.

Wada, H., 2008. Glucocorticoids: Mediators of vertebrate ontogenetic transitions. *Gen Comp Endocrinol* 156, 441–453.

Wada, H., Salvante, K. G., Stables, C., Wagner, E., Williams, T. D., Breuner, C. W., 2008. Adrenocortical responses in zebra finches (*Taeniopygia guttata*): Individual variation, repeatability, and relationship to phenotypic quality. *Horm Behav* 53, 472–480.

Walsberg, G. E., 2003. How useful is energy balance as a overall index of stress in animals? *Horm Behav* 43, 16–17.

Weil, Z. M., Bowers, S. L., Pyter, L. M., Nelson, R. J., 2006. Social interactions alter proinflammatory cytokine gene expression and behavior following endotoxin administration. *Brain Behav Immun* 20, 72–79.

Wen, J. C., Dhabhar, F. S., Prendergast, B. J., 2007. Pineal-dependent and—independent effects of photoperiod on immune function in Siberian hamsters (*Phodopus sungorus*). *Horm Behav* 51, 31–39.

Williams, G. C., Nesse, R. M., 1991. The dawn of Darwinian medicine. *Q Rev Biol* 66, 1–22.

Wingfield, J. C., 2003. Control of behavioural strategies for capricious environments. *Anim Behav* 66, 807–815.

Wingfield, J. C. (2004). Allostatic load and life cycles: implications for neuroendocrine mechanisms. In: Schulkin J. (Ed.), *Allostasis, homeostasis and the costs of physiological adaptation*, Cambridge University Press, Cambridge, pp. 302–342.

Wingfield, J. C., 2005a. The concept of allostasis: Coping with a capricious environment. *J Mammal* 86, 248–254.

Wingfield, J. C., 2005b. Modulation of the adrenocortical response to acute stress in breeding birds. In: Dawson, A., Sharp, P. J. (Eds.), *Functional avian endocrinology*. Narosa Publishing House, New Delhi, India, pp. 225–240.

Wingfield, J. C., 2006. Communicative behaviors, hormone-behavior interactions, and reproduction in vertebrates. In: Neil, J. D. (Ed.), *Physiology of reproduction*. Academic Press, New York, pp. 1995–2040.

Wingfield, J. C., Farner, D. S., 1978. The endocrinology of a naturally breeding population of the white-crowned sparrow (*Zonotrichia leucophrys pugetensis*). *Physiol Zool* 51, 188–205.

Wingfield, J. C., Hahn, T. P., Wada, M., Astheimer, L. B., Schoech, S., 1996. Interrelationship of day length and temperature on the control of gonadal development, body mass, and fat score in white-crowned sparrows, *Zonotrichia leucophrys gambelii*. *Gen Comp Endocrinol* 101, 242–255.

Wingfield, J. C., Hahn, T. P., Wada, M., Schoech, S. J., 1997. Effects of day length and temperature on gonadal development, body mass, and fat depots in white-crowned sparrows, *Zonotrichia leucophrys pugetensis*. *Gen Comp Endocrinol* 107, 44–62.

Wingfield, J. C., Owen-Ashley, N. T., Benowitz-Fredericks, Z. M., Lynn, S. E., Hahn, T. P., Wada, H., Breuner, C. M., Meddle, S. L., Romero, L. M., 2004. Arctic spring: The arrival biology of migrant birds. *Acta Zool Sinica* 50, 948–960.

Wingfield, J.C., and Ramenofsky, M. (1999). Hormones and the behavioral ecology of stress. In: Balm, P.H.M. (Ed.), *Stress Physiology in Animals*, Sheffield Academic Press, Sheffield, U.K., pp. 1–51.

Wingfield, J. C., Ramos-Fernandez, G., Nunez-de la Mora, A., Drummond, H., 1999. The effects of an "El Nino" southern oscillation event on reproduction in male and female blue-footed boobies, *Sula nebouxii*. *Gen Comp Endocrinol* 114, 163–172.

Wingfield, J. C., Romero, L. M., 2001. Adrenocortical responses to stress and their modulation in free-living vertebrates. In: McEwen, B. S., Goodman, H. M. (Eds.), *Handbook of physiology*; Section 7: *The endocrine system*; Vol. IV: *Coping with the environment: Neural and endocrine mechanisms*. Oxford University Press, New York, pp. 211–234

Wingfield, J. C., Schwabl, H., Mattocks, P. W. Jr., 1990. Endocrine mechanisms of migration. In: Gwinner, E. (Ed.), *Bird migration: Physiology and eco-physiology*. Springer-Verlag, New York, pp. 232–256.

Wingfield, J. C., Silverin, B., 2002. Ecophysiological studies of hormone–behavior relations in birds. In: Pfaff, D. W., Arnold, A. P., Etgen, A. M., Fahrbach, S. E., Rubin, R. T. (Eds.), *Hormones, brain and behavior*, vol. 2. Elsevier Science, Amsterdam, pp. 587–647.

Wingfield, J. C., Silverin, B., 2009. Ecophysiological studies of hormone-behavior relations in birds. In: Pfaff, D. W., Arnold, A. P., Etgen, A. M., Fahrbach, S. E., Rubin, R. T. (Eds.), *Hormones, brain, and behavior*, vol. 2. Academic Press, New York, pp. 817–854.

Wobber, V., Hare, B., Maboto, J., Lipson, S., Wrangham, R., Ellison, P. T., 2010. Differential changes in steroid hormones before competition in bonobos and chimpanzees. *Proc Natl Acad Sci USA* 107, 12457–12462.

Yirmiya, R., Avitsur, R., Donchin, O., Cohen, E., 1995. Interleukin-1 inhibits sexual behavior in female but not in male rats. *Brain Behav Immun* 9, 220–233.

Ylonen, H., Eccard, J. A., Jokinen, I., Sundell, J., 2006. Is the antipredatory response in behaviour reflected in stress measured in faecal corticosteroids in a small rodent? *Behav Ecol Sociobiol* 60, 350–358.

Zavjalov, E. L., Gerlinskaya, L. A., Moshkin, M. P., 2012. Factors of stress in a local population of water vole. *Zhurnal Obshchei Biologii* 73, 59–69 (in Russian, abstract in English).

Zuk, M., 1996. Disease, endocrine-immune interactions, and sexual selection. *Ecology* 77, 1037–1042.

Zuk, M., Johnsen, T. S., 1998. Seasonal changes in the relationship between ornamentation and immune response in red jungle fowl. *Proc R Soc Lond B* 265, 1631–1635.

Zuk, M., Stoehr, A. M., 2002. Immune defense and host life history. *Am Nat* 160, S9-S22.

Zwarts, L., Hulscher, J. B., Koopman, K., Zegers, P. M., 1996. Short-term variation in the body weight of oystercatchers *Haematopus ostralegus*: Effect of available feeding time by day and night, temperature and wind force. *Ardea* 84A, 357–372.

10

Modulation of the Adrenocortical Response to Stress

I. INTRODUCTION

One feature of corticosteroid responses to stress that ought to be obvious by this point is that corticosteroid release in response to labile perturbation factors is not a simple on/off response, but varies tremendously. Using the "stress series" (Chapters 3 and 6) where basal, maximum, and rates of corticosteroid increase can be compared among individuals as well as across populations and time, it quickly becomes clear that an individual's "normal" corticosteroid response can be modulated to fit the needs of the moment. Given that thus far we have emphasized how vital the adrenocortical response to acute perturbations is, why would animals modulate this response, especially down-regulation? Early work began by documenting that adrenocortical responses to stress varied daily, seasonally, and in relation to gender and social status (e.g., Sapolsky 1987; Wingfield 1994; Wingfield et al. 1995b), hinting at possible ecological bases. Since then, many investigations, in laboratory and field, have revealed that the adrenocortical response to stress is modulated consistently under many different environmental conditions and in relation to possible benefits to fitness (Wingfield et al. 1995b; Silverin 1998a; Sapolsky et al. 2000; Wingfield and Romero 2001; Romero 2002). Why does stress response modulation happen and how is it achieved?

A. Why Modulate the Response to Stress?

Growing evidence of variation in the magnitude of adrenocortical responses to stress, both seasonal and across populations, in breeding birds triggered a number of questions focused on understanding the ultimate causation that gave rise to the evolution of modulation of adrenocortical responses to stress. This then paved the way to determine why the stress response is modulated and the physiological mechanisms underlying those modulations (Sapolsky 1987; Wingfield et al. 1995b). Early hypotheses suggested that modulation of the baseline corticosteroid levels in blood and the adrenocortical responses to acute stress as a whole were functions of body size. Larger species have relatively greater reserves of fat and protein to withstand acute stresses (robustness) such as inclement weather. Bigger animals should therefore have an adrenocortical axis that is resistant to acute stress. Conversely, smaller species have relatively limited reserves of fat and protein and are vulnerable to starvation during perturbations. As a result, smaller species should retain a greater adrenocortical responsiveness. However, field studies in several arctic breeding birds failed to support this hypothesis (Wingfield et al. 1995b).

A second early hypothesis stated that variation in the magnitude of the adrenocortical response to stress is related to longevity. This fits well with life-history theory predicting that species with a limited life span, say one or two breeding seasons, are more resistant to acute stress, at least when breeding, to maximize reproductive success. The trade-off here is likely reduced post-breeding survival of adults. Conversely, species that have 5–10 or more potential breeding seasons should retain maximum sensitivity to acute perturbations and reduce their breeding efforts accordingly in favor of survival and later successful breeding (Wingfield et al. 1995b). This hypothesis, as well as life-history theory associated with aging, have been more extensively studied and will be discussed in this chapter (see also Chapter 9). Early ideas included a third hypothesis that gender differences in the adrenocortical responses to perturbations in arctic breeding birds (Figure 10.1; Wingfield et al. 1995b) may be associated with the degree of parental care provided (Figure 10.2; O'Reilly and Wingfield 2001). Those individuals providing more parental care are more resistant to identical acute perturbations than those that show less parental care, thus increasing fitness through extra effort made to raise young to independence. The trade-off again would be reduced over-winter survival (Wingfield et al. 1995b).

Arctic-breeding shorebirds are ideal tests of this hypothesis because in some, females provide parental care and males none (e.g., the pectoral sandpiper). In red phalaropes, males provide all parental care and females none, whereas in semi-palmated sandpipers, females and males share parental care equally. In western sandpipers, females show some parental care but males show more. The magnitudes of the adrenocortical responses to acute stress of capture, handling, and restraint in these species are consistent with this parental care hypothesis (Figure 10.2; O'Reilly and Wingfield 2001), a remarkable result at the time. Since then, many ecological and evolutionary bases of modulation of adrenocortical responses to acute perturbations of the environment have been put forward and will be

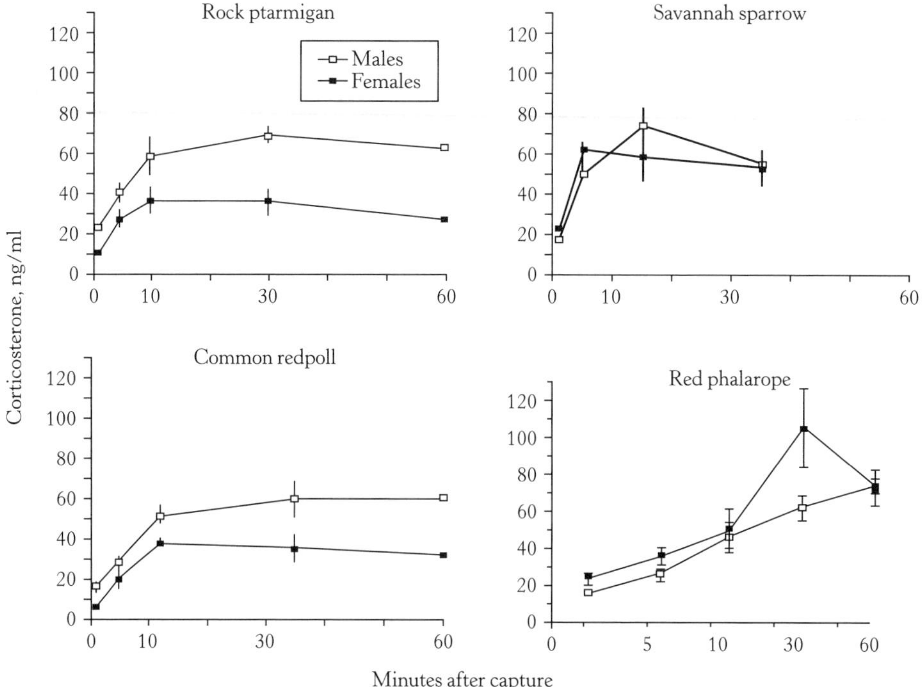

FIGURE 10.1: Plasma levels of corticosterone following capture, handling, and restraint in species of arctic birds sampled during the breeding season, including rock ptarmigans, savannah sparrows, redpolls, and red phalaropes.

From Wingfield et al. (1995b), courtesy of Allen Press.

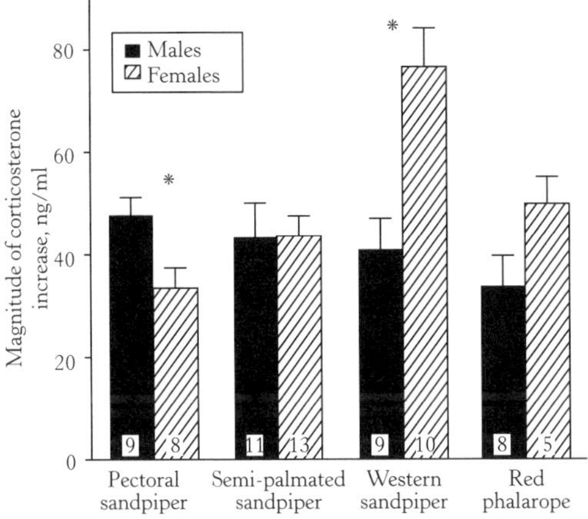

FIGURE 10.2: The increase in corticosterone in response to capture and handling as calculated by maximum (30-min) less baseline (3-min) concentrations. Asterisks indicate a significant difference between sexes within a species. In semi-palmated sandpipers, both sexes show equal parental care. In the pectoral sandpiper, females provide all care, whereas in the red phalarope, males provide all care. The western sandpiper is unusual because females provide parental care first (incubation) then males (escorting young). Three of the four species' results support the parental care hypothesis.

From O'Reilly and Wingfield (2001), courtesy of Elsevier.

summarized in this chapter. The discussion represents a classic example of integration of biology across several fields, from behavioral ecology and theory to cell and molecular mechanisms.

B. Types of Stress Modulation

There are now many ways known by which the adrenocortical responses to acute stress can be modulated, and we suspect even more await discovery. Wingfield and Sapolsky (2003) summarized some more recent examples in relation to the question of why some animals modulate the stress response while breeding (Table 10.1) and how that might occur (Table 10.2). It is useful to summarize the types of modulation of the stress responses both known from the literature and those predicted but not yet tested:

1. The first category encompasses changes due to developmental processes, including aging. Variations in prenatal and neonatal environment can result in different corticosteroid response, some of which can become permanent (see Chapters 5 and 11).
2. The second category includes daily changes typified by a circadian rhythm. Corticosteroid responses

TABLE 10.1: EVOLUTIONARY LOGIC BEHIND INSTANCES OF MAINTAINING REPRODUCTION DURING STRESS

Logic	Examples
A. Aged individuals, with minimal future reproductive success.	Leach's petrels
B. Seasonal breeder when environmental conditions are severe and/or time for actual reproduction is so short there is only one breeding event.	Arctic ground squirrels, many avian species, sea turtles, garter snakes
C. When both members of a breeding pair provide parental care, if the male is lost the remaining individual must work "double time" to raise young successfully.	Pied flycatcher
D. "Semelparous" species in which there is only a single round of breeding followed by programmed death.	Pacific salmon, lamprey, eels, Australian marsupial insectivores
E. Species where because of the transience of dominance, individuals may have only a short window of opportunity for mating.	Males of numerous tournament species
F. Alternate male reproductive morphs modulate effects of glucocorticosteroids on behavior according to dominance.	Tree lizards

Dickhoff (1989); Gregory et al. (1996); Knapp and Moore (1997); Silverin (1998b); Silverin and Wingfield (1998); O'Reilly et al. (1999); Valverde et al. (1999); Baker and O'Reilly (2000); Jessop et al. (2000); Wingfield and Romero (2001); Moore et al. (2001); Moore and Mason (2001); Oakwood et al. (2001); Sapolsky (2001). From Wingfield and Sapolsky (2003), courtesy of John Wiley and Sons.

TABLE 10.2: POTENTIAL MECHANISMS UNDERLYING RESISTANCE OF THE HYPOTHALAMO-PITUITARY-GONADAL AXIS TO STRESS

Mechanism	Examples
A. Blockade at the CNS level: stressors are not perceived as stressful.	Lekking species, breeding snow bunting
B. Blockade at the level of the HPA: failure to secrete glucocorticosteroids.	Many avian species, e.g., breeding Lapland longspurs, redpolls, garter snakes
C. Blockade at the level of the HPG: resistance of the gonadal axis to glucocorticosteroid actions.	Male olive baboons, arctic song birds
D. Compensatory stimulatory inputs to the gonad axis to counteract inhibitory glucocorticosteroid actions.	Male olive baboons, male arctic ground squirrels, dark-eyed junco
E. Protection from the actions of glucocorticosteroids by, for example, steroid-binding proteins.	Tree lizards

Deviche et al. (2001); Romero et al. (1998b; 1998c; 1998a; 1998); Jennings et al. (2000); Moore and Mason (2001); Sapolsky (2001). From Wingfield and Sapolsky (2003), courtesy of John Wiley and Sons.

are modulated around a daily cycle such that responses at some times of the day are quite different from those at other times (see Chapter 1). There is some evidence that tidal rhythms exist as well.

3. Seasonal changes related to life history stages such as reproduction, migrations, molts, winter strategies, and so forth.
4. This category reflects modulation of corticosteroid responses to match specific perturbations. In effect, corticosteroid responses are "titrated" to cope with major events such as inclement weather. Furthermore, stronger stressors elicit more corticosteroid release, and weaker stressors elicit less corticosteroid release (see Chapter 3).
5. As environmental variation and seasonality increase with latitude and altitude, then adrenocortical responses to similar stresses vary accordingly.
6. Similar variations in adrenocortical responses can occur along other environmental gradients such as rainfall, vegetation, and so on.
7. Population and social effects probably interact, especially in relation to the density of individuals and frequency of interactions, to modulate stress responses.
8. Predators and the risk of predation can have dramatic effects on stress responses, including susceptibility to other stresses.
9. Individual and gender differences in baseline as well as corticosteroid responses (rate of increase and maximum levels; see Chapter 9) vary in relation to personality as well as different allostatic states to produce variation in corticosteroid responses within the range of predictive and reactive homeostasis.

Although there remains much work to be done to assess the modulation of stress responses in all of the categories listed here, there is now a large body of evidence relating such modulation to ecological factors, allostatic load, and the underlying mechanisms by which modulation occurs (Table 10.2).

C. Some Theoretical Considerations

A theoretical approach to modulation of the stress response is needed to provide a framework for further integration of ecology, evolution, and mechanisms. Jacobs (1996) made an early attempt to do this by pointing out that if the value of expressing an emergency life-history stage (ELHS, Chapter 3) as a function of time of year and predictability (stability) of environmental conditions declines, then that value will reach a point at which it is no longer worth expressing. At this point, the adrenocortical response to stress that controls expression of the ELHS should be non-responsive (Figure 10.3). In other words, the adaptive value of the ELHS reflects the extent to which the adrenocortical response to stress should be expressed. As the adaptive value of expressing the ELHS decreases, it reaches a critical adaptive value when there is zero benefit (Figure 10.3), and the adrenocortical response to stress would be completely absent (Jacobs 1996). In general, it may always be adaptive to express the ELHS over a wide range of environmental predictability. It is possible that in environments with very low

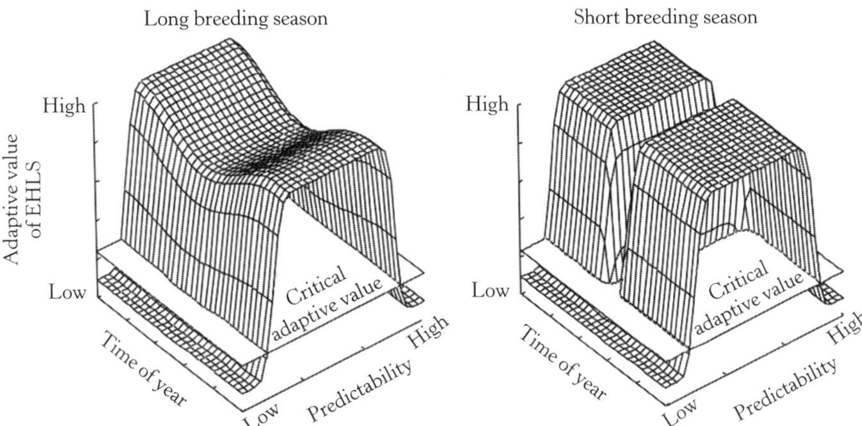

FIGURE 10.3: Three-dimensional figure showing the value of expressing an emergency life-history stage (ELHS) as a function of time of year and predictability (stability) of environmental conditions. The vertical axes are the adaptive value of the ELHS that also reflects the extent to which the adrenocortical response to stress should be expressed.

From Jacobs (1996), with permission.

predictability (chaotic) or very high predictability (constant) the ELHS would not confer any fitness advantage (i.e., below the critical adaptive value) and the stress response would be absent.

There are times during the life cycle when the ELHS may also have lower adaptive value. An example (right-hand panel of Figure 10.3) is a short breeding season when there is a trade-off of individual survival and reproductive success in the face of severe environmental conditions. Here the adaptive value of an ELHS falls below the critical level, and the stress response should be totally suppressed. In the left-hand panel (Figure 10.3), the trade-off of reproductive success and resistance to perturbations is weaker when the breeding season is longer, allowing several potential nesting events. In this case, the adaptive value of expressing an ELHS remains above the critical value and modulation of the stress response would be slight (Figure 10.3; from Jacobs 1996; Wingfield et al. 2011).

The degree to which an individual can be insensitive to a perturbation of the environment can be termed robustness (i.e., perception of an environmental perturbation can be altered, thus determining whether the individual responds or not). However, as the adaptive value of expressing an ELHS decreases, then if an adrenocortical response to the perturbation is triggered, the degree to which an individual responds can be termed "resistance." The resistance potential (suppressed adrenocortical response to stress) increases as the adaptive value of the ELHS decreases (Figure 10.4). This might be a linear response (solid line of Figure 10.4) or non-linear (dashed line of Figure 10.4), or somewhere between those lines (Wingfield et al. 2011). The resistance potential of a labile perturbation factor (LPF, often a stressor) varies with condition (Figure 10.5; Wingfield et al. 2011). Resistance potential is decreased with low body condition but increases as body condition improves (left-hand panel of Figure 10.5). Individuals in the best condition will be more robust and will show greater resistance to LPFs, resulting in the capacity to blunt adrenocortical responses to stress. Resistance potential will be less when LPFs are severe (dashed line of Figure 10.5) versus milder LPFs (solid line) and increases as the basic energetic costs of daily and seasonal routines (Ee + Ei) decrease. If the costs of daily/seasonal routines are low, extra resources can be dedicated to resisting the effects of LPFs. Resistance potential to LPFs decreases as another function of body condition: degree of infection and disease (right-hand panel). The slopes will be greater for severe LPFs and shallower for mild LPFS. Additionally, beginning resistance potential will be higher in individuals with lower costs of daily/seasonal routines (Figure 10.5; Wingfield et al. 2011). The mechanisms by which resistance potential is transduced into neural, endocrine and cell processes underlying HPA function remains to be determined.

Referring to Figure 10.5 again, we can explore how changes in LPF resistance potential can be affected by costs of daily and seasonal routines

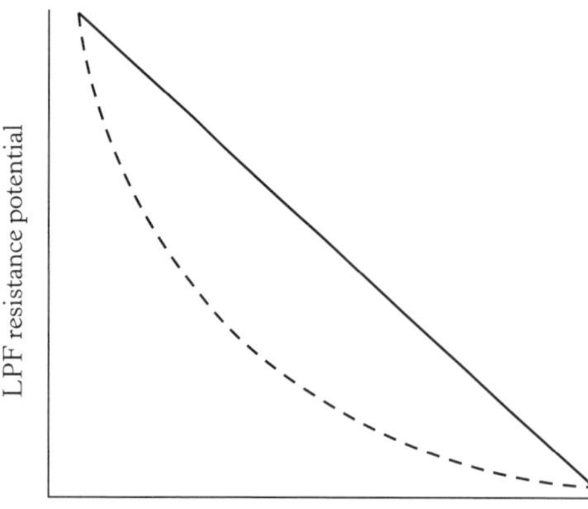

FIGURE 10.4: As the adaptive value of expressing an emergency life-history stage (ELHS) decreases, then the resistance potential (suppressed adrenocortical response to stress) increases. This might be a linear response (solid line) or non-linear (dashed line), or somewhere between those lines.

From Wingfield et al. (2011), courtesy of Springer-Verlag.

(Ee + Ei) and resource availability (Eg). If resistance potential is decreased by disease, human disturbance, invasive species, and so on, then Ee + Ei increases (top left panel of Figure 10.6). Any perturbation represented by Eo, and starting at the same time, triggers allostatic overload type 1 earlier (Wingfield et al. 2011). Higher Ee + Ei is similar to allostatic overload type 2 and shows how it could interact with overload type 1 (Figure 10.6, top panels). This effect can be exacerbated if Eg decreases and Ee + Ei increases (top right panel of Figure 10.6). In this case, type 1 allostatic overload will trigger an ELHS almost immediately (Wingfield et al. 2011). Conversely, a lower Ee + Ei will increase resistance potential, and any perturbation will take longer to result in allostatic overload type 1 and trigger an ELHS (lower left panel of Figure 10.6). If Eg also increases as Ee + Ei is lowered, then resistance potential becomes even greater (lower right panel of Figure 10.6; Wingfield et al. 2011).

An additional way of modeling LPF resistance potential is to consider the nature of Eo. The slope of Eo can be influenced by such factors as body condition (Figure 10.7; Wingfield et al. 2011). For example, the presence of larger fat depots, meaning more endogenous energy reserves, will result in progressively shallower Eo lines, with the steepest representing resistance potential with no fat reserves and the shallowest revealing resistance potential with more fat reserves (Figure 10.7). Thus an ELHS (resulting from allostatic overload type 1) will be triggered progressively later (greater resistance potential) in relation to the greater fat reserve that individual has. LPF resistance potential is thus increased with fat score in relation to the same Eo. The same curves can be generated for social status, with the steep curve for a subordinate and the shallowest for a dominant (Figure 10.7; Wingfield et al. 2011). Note that these curves are different from those generated earlier (Goymann and Wingfield 2004; Wingfield 2004).

It is important to point out that robustness, the ability to stave off triggering an adrenocortical response to acute perturbations, is different from resistance. They also may have completely separate control mechanisms—the varying degrees

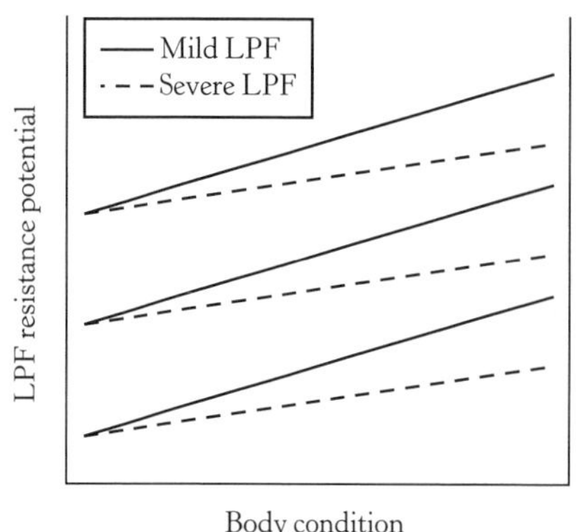

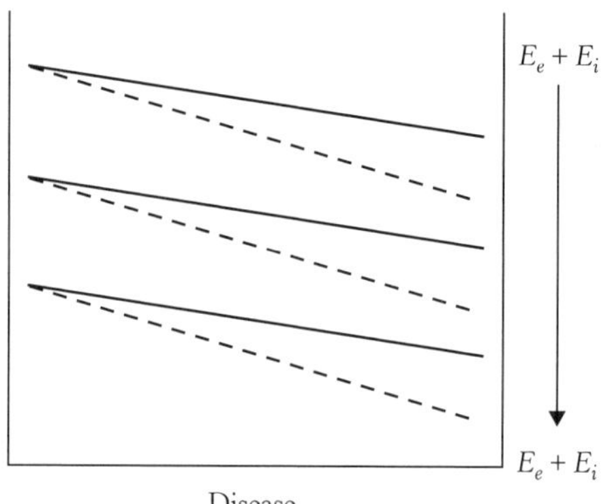

FIGURE 10.5: Labile perturbation factor (LPF) resistance potential varies with body condition and/or disease. Severe LPFs are indicated by dashed line, milder LPFs by solid line. Resistance potential also increases as basic energetic costs of daily and seasonal routines (Ee + Ei) decrease.

From Wingfield et al. (2011), courtesy of Springer Verlag.

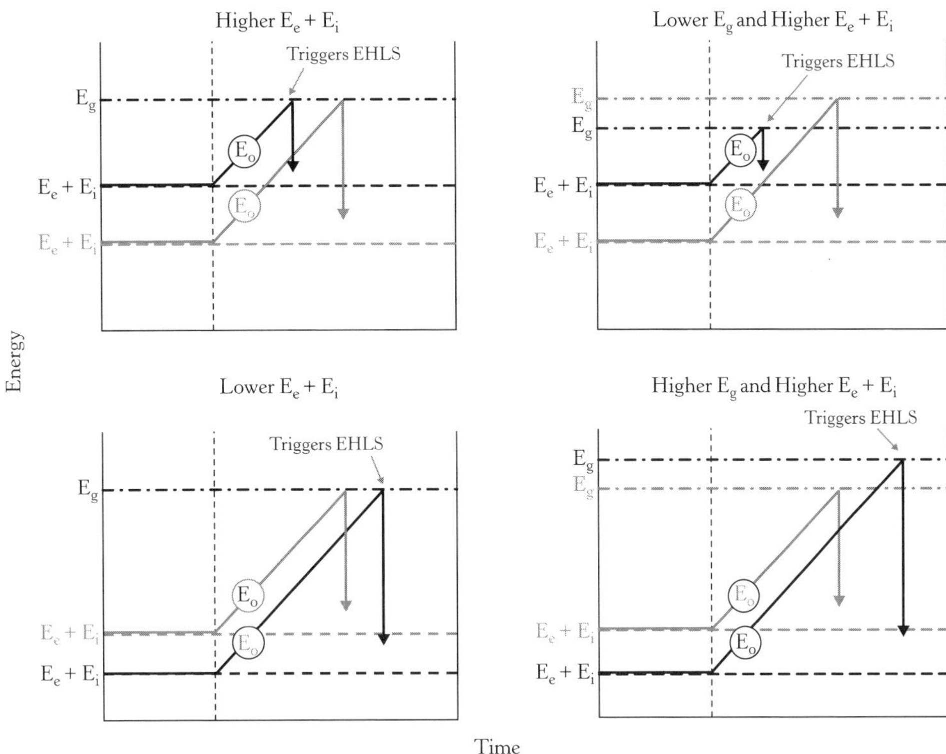

FIGURE 10.6: Building on Figure 10.5, this figure shows how changes in labile perturbation factor (LPF) resistance potential can be affected by costs of daily and seasonal routines (Ee + Ei) and resources available (Eg). Top left panel models an increase in Ee + Ei, and top right panel models an increase in Ee + Ei accompanied by a decrease in Eg. Conversely, lower left panel models a lower Ee + Ei, and lower right panel models an increase in Eg as well as a decrease in Ee + Ei.

From Wingfield et al. (2011), courtesy of Springer-Verlag.

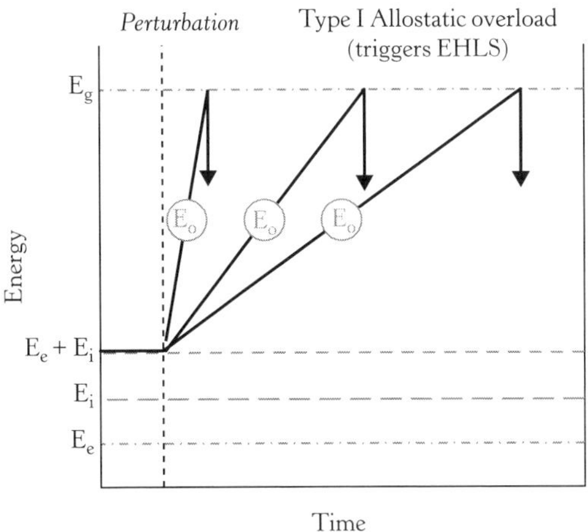

FIGURE 10.7: An additional way of modeling labile perturbation factor (LPF) resistance potential. Eo lines represent differences in fat depots, with the steepest representing no fat and the shallowest representing more fat.

From Wingfield et al. (2011), courtesy of Springer-Verlag.

to which the magnitude of the stress response is expressed once it has been triggered. Resistance can also include modulation of the responsiveness of target tissues through enzymatic degradation of glucocorticoids and changes in hormone receptors densities, and so on (Wingfield 2013a). "Resilience" in this sense refers to the ability to recover from the adrenocortical response to stress and the ELHS after the perturbation has passed. This will be especially true if body condition (e.g., fat stores) has been run down while coping with a perturbation. Resilience can also refer to the whole process and the ability of an individual to combat a perturbation, but here we prefer to focus it on the recovery from a perturbation—a process that remains largely unknown still.

II. DEVELOPMENTAL CHANGES

Offspring development is influenced in part by genetic effects determining the phenotype.

Environmental factors can have considerable influence on this process, especially maternal effects that are indirectly a consequence of environmental influences (e.g., Groothuis et al. 2005). Adrenocortical responses to acute stressors can change markedly during development, not only when the HPA axis first becomes active (see Chapter 5), but later in development as genetic, environmental, and maternal (in some cases also paternal) effects wax and wane. Aging effects also fit into this category. The phenotype that results may have developed a pattern of vulnerability to acute stressors (robustness), resistance of the HPA axis (as described earlier) once a perturbation is encountered, and resilience (i.e., the ability to recover following an acute stressor). This topic has been very well investigated in mammals, and studies of many non-mammal studies are appearing as well. These will be reviewed specifically in Chapter 11 and will not be treated separately here.

III. CHANGES IN DAILY AND SEASONAL ROUTINES

With few exceptions, organisms show daily and seasonal changes in morphology, physiology, and behavior in order to match routines of day and night and to match life history stages with season. Adrenocortical responses to stress are susceptible to major changes in the magnitude of the response as well (Sapolsky 1987; Wingfield 1994; Silverin 1998a; Wingfield and Romero 2001; Romero 2002). Examples of annual variation of corticosteroids are now widespread, but some important points can be made first.

A. Daily Changes of Corticosteroids

Overall, daily and seasonal changes in baseline plasma levels of corticosteroids are thought to regulate homeostatic processes such as energy balance in response to life cycle routines and in coping with unpredictable perturbations of the environment (e.g., Romero 2002). Although daily rhythms of corticosteroid levels in blood, saliva, urine, and feces reveal marked diel changes, some of which may be endogenous (circadian) rhythms, similar changes in maximum corticosteroid levels generated by acute stress are much less well known. It is an interesting question of whether the adrenocortical response to acute perturbations should be regulated from day to night, or whether the adaptive value of responding with facultative physiology and behavior would be selected for, regardless of time of day. In laboratory animals it is well known that HPA axis activity varies with time of day (e.g., Kant et al. 1986; Buckley and Schatzberg 2005), and may also have ultradian rhythms (Windle et al. 1998). More recently, studies of both captive and free-living animals have provided more insight (e.g., Breuner et al. 1999). How organisms in their natural habitat balance daily and seasonal routines with perturbations of the environment raises important questions about mechanisms by which they might achieve such adaptive responses.

In captive populations of Gambel's white-crowned sparrows, baseline plasma levels of corticosterone peaked toward the end of the dark period (inactive) and reached a nadir soon after onset of the light period (active). This pattern was similar in birds held on both long days and short days (Figure 10.8; Breuner et al. 1999). There were also daily changes in adrenocortical responses to acute stress (capture, handling, and restraint), as measured by maximum corticosterone levels in blood. Interestingly, maximum

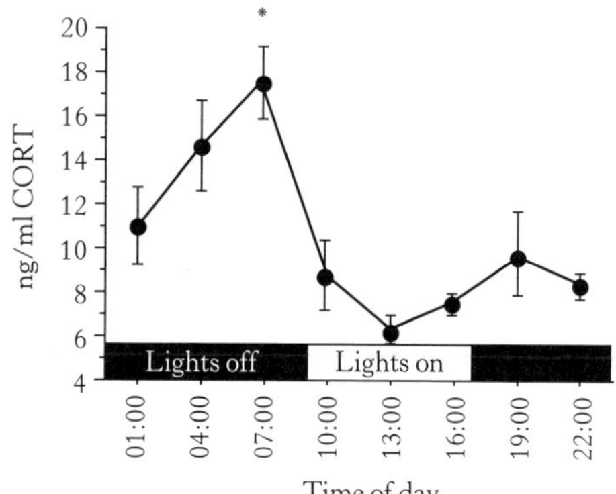

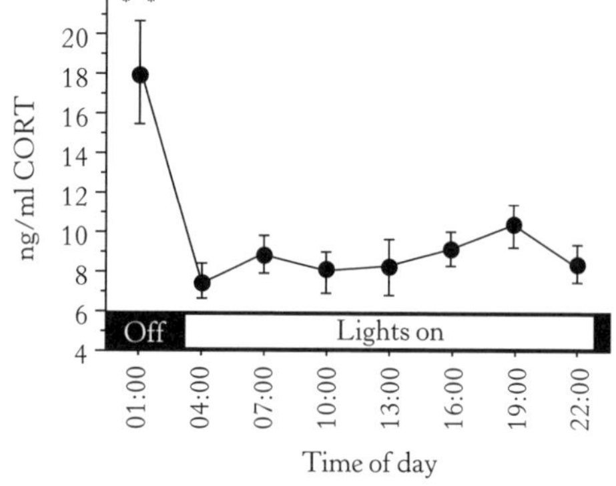

FIGURE 10.8: Basal corticosterone (CORT) levels in captive white-crowned sparrows held on short or long day photoperiods.

From Breuner et al. (1999), courtesy of Wiley-Liss.

corticosterone levels were found at the beginning of the active period (when baseline levels were lowest) and the patterns were similar to those found in mammals. As with baseline corticosterone, maximum levels generated by acute stress were similar on both long and short days (Figure 10.9; Breuner et al. 1999). In contrast, in captive and outdoor aviary-housed white-crowned and white-throated sparrows, Marra et al. (1995) found no significant differences in plasma levels of corticosterone with time of day. How modulation of the adrenocortical

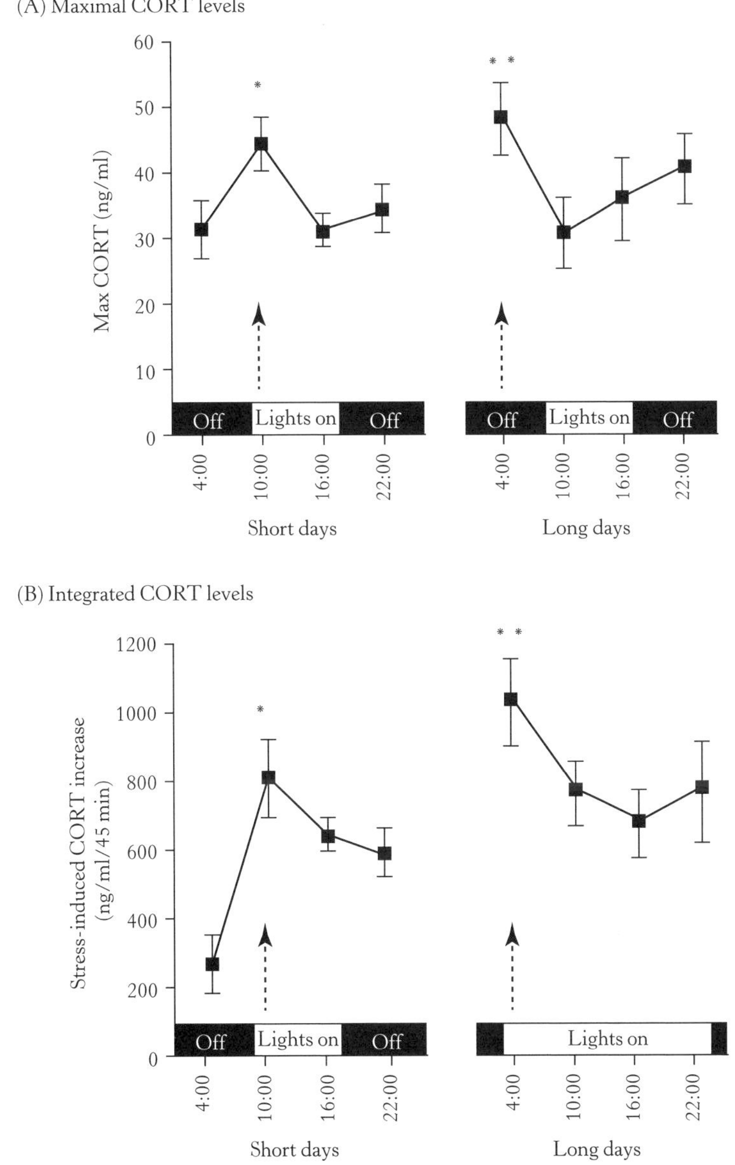

FIGURE 10.9: Stress-induced increase in corticosterone (CORT) in captive white-crowned sparrows under short- and long-day photoperiods. Arrows point to CORT levels just after lights on in both long and short days. (A) Maximal level of CORT experienced by each bird during 45 minutes of restraint (which may have occurred at 15, 30, or 45 min, depending on the individual). (B) An integrated measure of stress-induced CORT. To estimate the total CORT increase over the 45 minutes of restraint, we subtracted basal values (0 time point) from all four time points (0, 15, 30, and 45), and integrated the data (i.e., calculated the area under the resulting curve).

From Breuner et al. (1999), courtesy of Wiley-Liss.

response to perturbations of the environment in relation to time of day may be adaptive remains to be clarified.

In starlings, capture, handling, and restraint stress result in marked increases in plasma corticosterone levels at all times of day and night in all birds, both on short days and long days (Romero and Remage-Healey 2000). Baseline levels (i.e., within 3 minutes of capture) as well as maximum levels generated during the stress series varied with time of day and, in general, more corticosterone was released at night than during the day. As found in many free-living birds, both baseline and maximum stress levels of corticosterone were lowest during the pre-basic molt (Romero and Remage-Healey 2000). In a parallel study, Remage-Healey and Romero (2000) showed that plasma levels of glucose in captive starlings peaked during the midday (middle of the light period) and were lowest in the middle of the night. Furthermore, birds on long days had the highest levels of glucose and birds on short days the lowest. Starlings sampled while molting had intermediate circulating levels of glucose. Stress-induced levels of glucose showed no daily rhythm (Remage-Healey and Romero 2000).

In captive house sparrows housed on short and long day photoperiods, basal plasma levels of corticosterone were highest at night and lower during the day. The same pattern remained whether on long or short days or in pre-basic molt (Rich and Romero 2001). Although all birds on all treatments showed a marked increase in plasma corticosterone following acute stress (capture, handling, and restraint), only birds held on short days showed a change in daily rhythm, with blunted responses during the day-time hours (Rich and Romero 2001). This is different from the responses of white-crowned sparrows held on short and long days (Breuner et al. 1999). Why this variation is found across species remains unknown.

Great tits selected for different coping strategies, reactive versus proactive, showed marked changes in fecal levels of corticosteroid metabolites (Carere et al. 2003) with peaks early in the day (perhaps reflective of high circulating levels late in the night) and a nadir late in the day (perhaps because of lower plasma levels during the active period). Effects of time of day and response to social challenge tended to be higher in the reactive personality group (Carere et al. 2003).

As in the diurnally active white-crowned sparrow, plasma levels of corticosterone were significantly higher during the inactive period than during the active period in young western screech owls. However, this was opposite to white-crowned sparrows because the owls are nocturnal with the inactive period during the day (Dufty and Belthoff 1997). This is consistent with an effect of daily routine and activity, rather than time of day per se. There were no differences between sexes in the daily changes. Young screech owls showed a marked increase in corticosterone levels in response to handling and restraint, but it was not determined whether this changes with time of day.

Diel rhythms have been assessed in at least two free-living species. Since most free-living animals go into hiding during their inactive phase, thereby making sample collection very difficult, it might not be surprising that both species are island reptiles. Plasma levels of corticosterone showed no significant change from dusk, through the night, or during the day in males and females of a nocturnal reptile, the tuatara, sampled in the field in New Zealand (Tyrrell and Cree 1998). Baseline levels of corticosterone showed marked seasonal changes that were highest in gravid females just prior to egg-laying. Plasma levels of stress-induced corticosterone were generally positively correlated with body temperature and when active. In the Galápagos, marine iguanas captured every three hours show a marked diel rhythm (Figure 10.10; Woodley et al. 2003). Corticosterone levels were lower during the night and increased during the day. Interestingly, corticosterone levels dipped after the daily low tide when iguanas are foraging in the intertidal. When the two daily rhythms are adjusted so that the low tides coincide, a tidal rhythm is evident along with the diel rhythm (Figure 10.10). In captive American toads, baseline plasma corticosterone levels were highest in spring and autumn, with a daily high in the evening just prior to onset of activity (Pancak and Taylor 1983). Whether corticosterone responses to acute stress change seasonally and diurnally remains to be determined.

B. Annual Variation of Glucocorticoids along Environmental Gradients

Many free-living species modulate corticosteroid release seasonally (Romero 2002). Figure 10.11 provides a typical example from an avian species and shows that the magnitudes of both basal and stress-induced corticosteroid concentrations vary throughout the year. It appears that this variation results from changes in the secretory capacity of the adrenal/interrenal tissue since tissue volumes often correlate with plasma corticosteroid

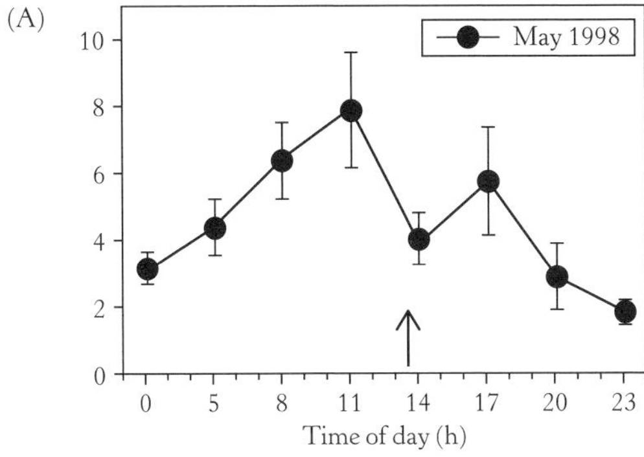

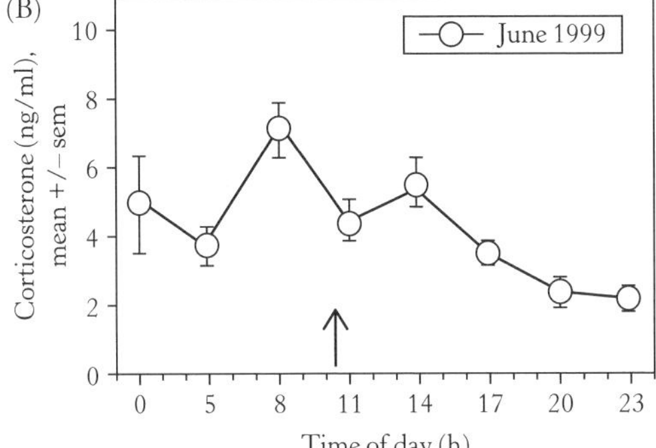

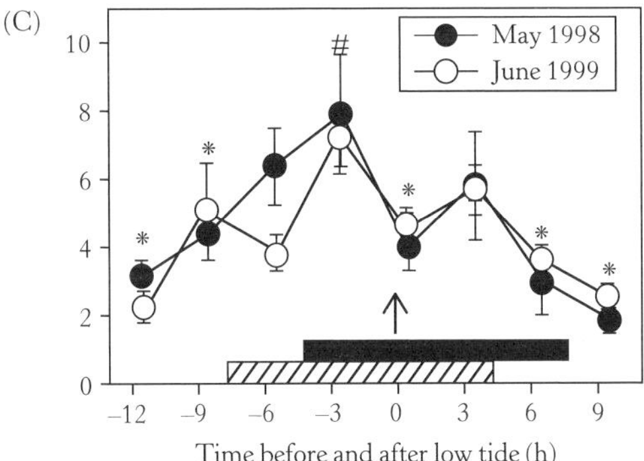

FIGURE 10.10: Plasma levels of baseline corticosterone in Galapagos marine iguanas. Arrows indicate time of low tide. (A) Profile from May 1998. (B) Profile from June 1999. (C) Profiles from May 1998 and June 1999 normalized according to the timing of low tide. Bars indicate the time span from 6 to 18 hours (day light) for each corticosterone profile (stippled bar, 1999; black bar, 1998).

Reprinted from (Woodley et al. 2003), with permission. Courtesy of Elesevier.

titers (reviewed for reptiles in Guillette et al. 1995). Furthermore, at least some of the modulation demonstrated in free-living individuals can be duplicated in captivity (for example, in both white-crowned sparrows [Marra et al. 1995; Romero et al. 1997] and house sparrows [Rich and Romero 2001; Romero et al. 2006]). Although not universally present in all species, the available evidence indicates that seasonal modulation of corticosteroid responses is common. Note also in Figure 10.11 that individuals held in captive conditions do not show the same annual variation in baseline and maximum corticosterone levels, indicating that environmental factors have a major role in modulating the adrenocortical response to perturbations (Romero et al. 1997; Romero and Wingfield 1999).

There is now considerable evidence that corticosteroid stress responses are modulated at the population level along environmental gradients such as latitude, altitude, rainfall, seasons, and so on. Next we will provide some examples, mostly from birds, to illustrate that patterns of modulation do occur and are in many ways consistent. Free-living song sparrows, sampled in western Washington State, show dramatic changes in the profile of plasma corticosterone responses to acute stress of capture, handling, and restraint (stress series, Figure 10.12; Wingfield et al. 1995b; J. C. Wingfield unpublished). Both baseline corticosterone levels and the maximum levels in the breeding season were much higher than in the non-breeding (winter) season and during the pre-basic (post-breeding) molt (Figure 10.12). A closer comparison of baseline and maximum corticosterone levels measured in the stress series of song sparrows emphasize how dramatic these changes with life-history stage and season are (Figure 10.13). If we examine only the breeding season, thereby holding season constant, and then compare across the environmental gradients of latitude and altitude, free-living male song sparrows show dramatic differences in the stress response at the subspecies and population level (Figure 10.14). Additionally, plotting the data in Figure 10.14 with just baseline and maximum corticosterone levels emphasizes the magnitude of the subspecies and population differences (Figure 10.15). The lowland, western Washington State, *M.m. morphna* data are from Figure 10.12. Additionally, a population of mountain *morphna* was sampled during the breeding season in Cascade Mountains between 1000 and 2000 meters elevation (Figures 10.14–10.15; J. C. Wingfield unpublished).

Mountain birds showed similar baseline corticosterone levels but greater maximum levels. Similar results have been obtained for an elevation gradient in dark-eyed juncos sampled in the mountains of British Columbia, Canada (Bears et al. 2003). Along a latitudinal gradient,

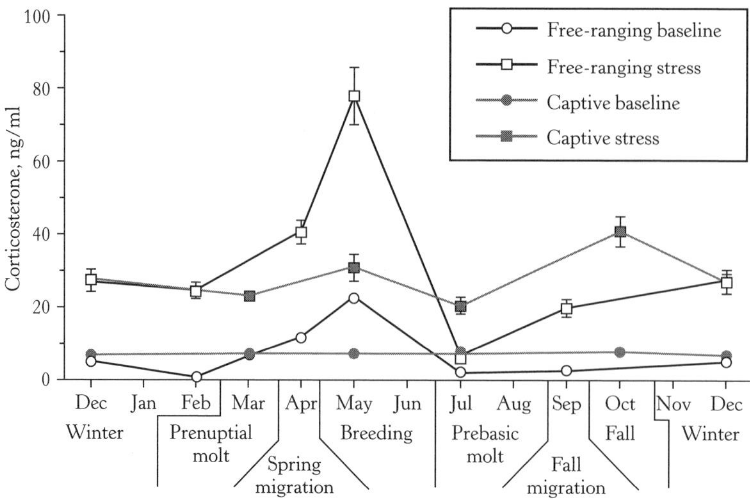

FIGURE 10.11: An example of seasonal corticosteroid modulation for free-living white-crowned sparrows. Both baseline and stress-induced corticosterone (GCs) vary over the course of the annual cycle. Of particular note is that patterns of baseline and maximum corticosterone in captive birds (grey lines) are much less variable over the year than in free-ranging animals. These data suggest considerable modulation of the adrenocortical response to stress by environmental factors not present in artificial laboratory conditions.

Reprinted with permission from (Romero 2002). Courtesy of Elsevier.

song sparrows sampled during the breeding season in coastal Sonoma County, California (Bodega Bay), *M.m. gouldi*, had the lowest baseline and profile of plasma corticosterone during a stress series (Figure 10.14), much lower than a population of *M.m. kenaiensis* sampled near the northern limit of their range at Cordova and the Copper River Delta, Alaska. The northernmost population had the highest baselines and the greatest stress response at the same stage

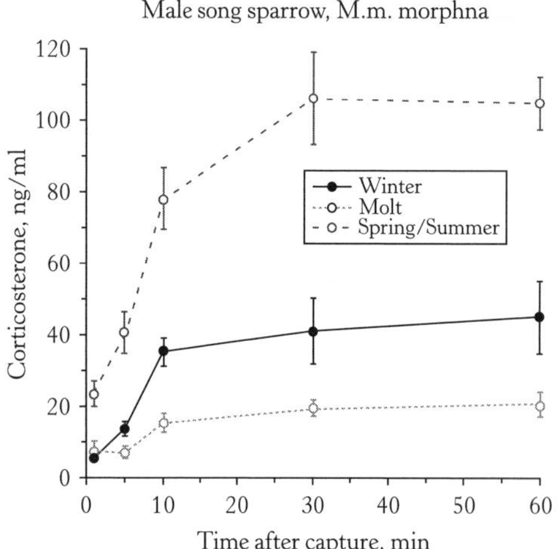

FIGURE 10.12: Adrenocortical responses to acute stress (capture, handling, and restraint) in free-living male song sparrows, *Melospiza melodia morphna*, sampled at different seasons in western Washington State. Lowest response was during pre-basic molt and greatest response in the breeding season.

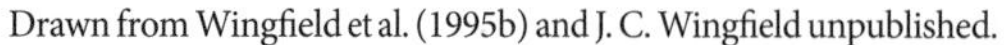
Drawn from Wingfield et al. (1995b) and J. C. Wingfield unpublished.

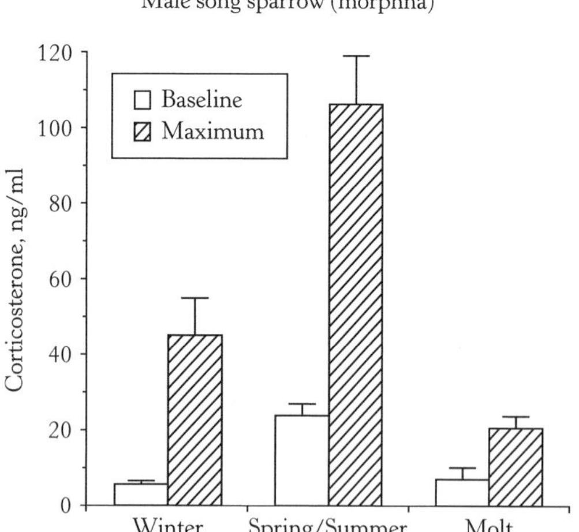

FIGURE 10.13: Comparisons of baseline (< 3 min post-capture) and maximum (30–60 min post-capture) plasma levels of corticosterone at different seasons in free-living male song sparrows in western Washington State.

Redrawn from Figure 10.12.

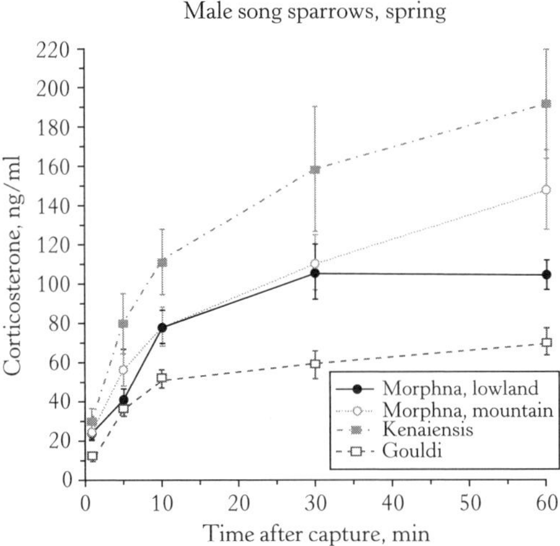

FIGURE 10.14: Plasma levels of corticosterone following capture, handling, and restraint in males of four taxa of song sparrows sampled during the breeding season. The northern population is *kenaiensis* and the southern population *morphna* from two localities, one on the lowlands of western Washington State, the other in the Cascade mountains of Washington State from 1500 to 2000 meters elevation. The *gouldi* population was sampled at Bodega Bay, Sonoma County, California. Drawn from Wingfield et al. (1995b) and J. C. Wingfield unpublished.

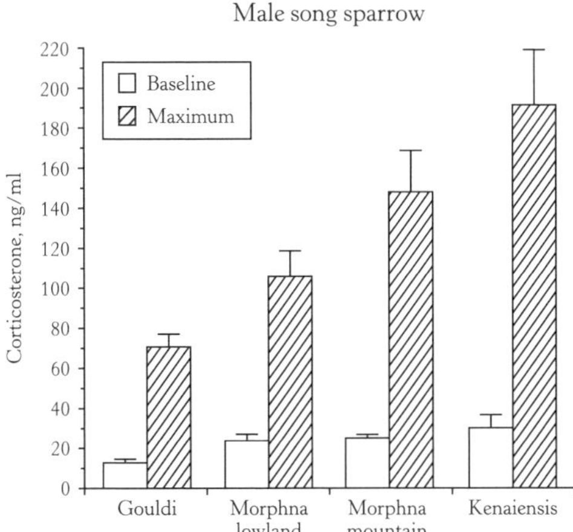

FIGURE 10.15: Comparison of baseline (i.e., < 3 min post-capture) and maximum (30–60 min post-capture) plasma levels of corticosterone in four taxa of free-living male song sparrows, *Melospiza melodia*. Drawn from Figure 10.14. Increasing maximum levels of corticosterone in relation to high altitude (mountain *morphna*) and latitude (*gouldi* southern, *kenaiensis* northern).

of breeding (Figure 10.14). Similar modulations of stress responses along latitudinal gradients have been measured in stress responses from free-living male bush warblers in Japan (Wingfield et al. 1995a), pied flycatchers, willow warblers, chaffinch, and bramblings sampled in southern and northern Sweden (Silverin et al. 1997; Silverin and Wingfield 1998; Silverin and Wingfield 2001).

Further detailed studies on seasonal and environmental gradient correlates of stress modulation reaffirm these trends. For example, seasonal modulation of the corticosteroid stress response occurs in the migratory Gambel's white-crowned sparrow sampled on its wintering and breeding grounds, but does not occur in the non-migratory Nuttall's subspecies sampled at the same times of year in coastal California (Bodega Bay, Sonoma County, Figure 10.16; Romero et al. 1997; Wingfield et al. 2004). These data suggest that not only can stress responses be modulated seasonally, but there is also a latitudinal gradient interaction as well. Free-living male *gambelii* sampled from winter through arrival on the breeding grounds after spring migration show a marked increase in baseline corticosterone as well as the magnitude of the stress response (Figure 10.17). Then the baseline plasma level of corticosterone and the maximum level during a stress series decline as the parental phase of breeding begins and continues through molt and the autumn migration back to the wintering grounds in California (Figures 10.17 and 10.18). These data are remarkable because they were collected from birds in the field undergoing seasonal changes along latitudinal gradients. Interestingly, female *gambelii* show similar changes in the seasonal and latitudinal stress responses but not as marked as in males (Figures 10.19 and 10.20). These data suggest that in addition to interactions of seasonal and latitudinal gradients, there are gender differences as well. These fascinating data allow a very comprehensive and detailed analysis of modulation of the stress response in free-living animals.

Field investigations of stress responses of free-living male white-crowned sparrows sampled at the beginning of the breeding season also show dramatic differences in baseline levels of corticosterone, stress profiles (Figure 10.21), and maximum levels after the stress series (Figure 10.22). Latitudinal differences in baselines and maximum levels are clear when comparing non-migratory and short distance migrants (*nutallii* and *pugetensis*, Figures 10.21 and 10.22) at lower latitudes versus *gambelii* sampled at

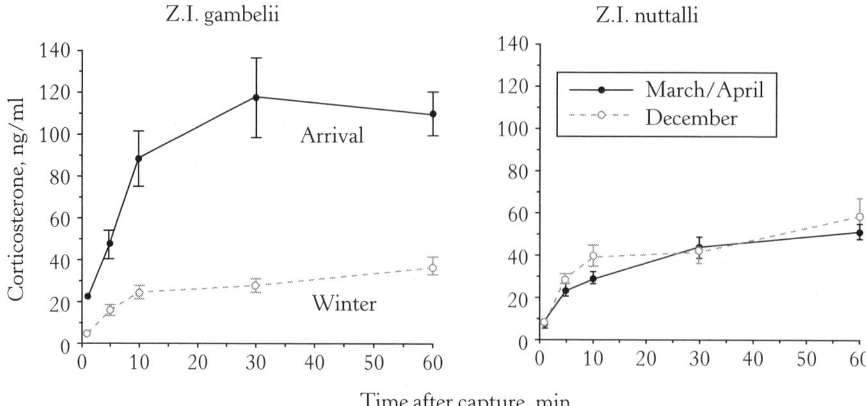

FIGURE 10.16: Seasonal modulation of the adrencocortical response to acute stress (capture, handling, and restraint) in free-living migratory white-crowned sparrows, *Zonotrichia leucophrys gambelii*, sampled in winter and on arrival on the breeding grounds (left-hand panel). Note that in the non-migratory subspecies, *Z.l. nuttallii*, sampled in the early breeding season and the non-breeding season, there is no modulation of the adrenocortical stress response (right-hand panel).

Redrawn from Romero et al. (1997) and Wingfield et al. (2004), courtesy of Academica Sinica.

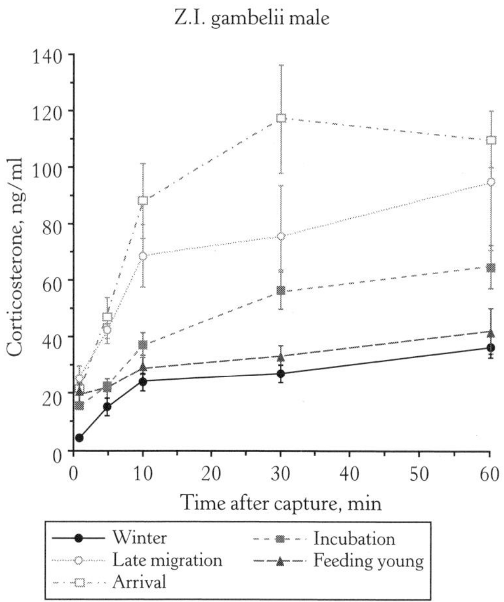

FIGURE 10.17: Seasonal changes in the plasma corticosterone stress response in free-living male Gambel's white-crowned sparrows. Birds were sampled on their breeding grounds in central and northern Alaska, during migration in Washington State and California, and on wintering grounds in California.

Redrawn from Romero et al. (1997), Holberton and Wingfield (2003), Meddle et al. (2002), and J. C. Wingfield unpublished.

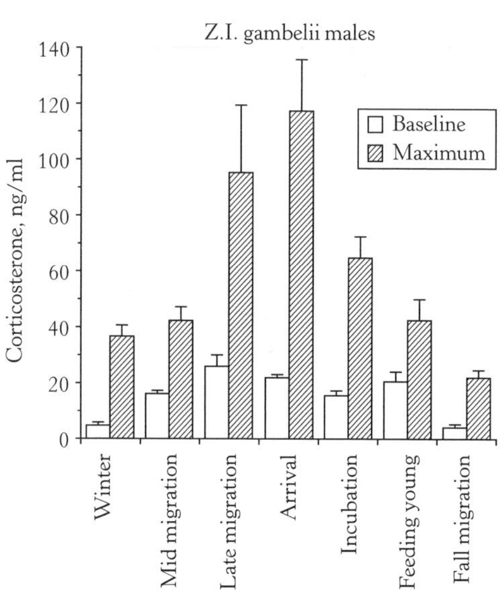

FIGURE 10.18: Seasonal changes in the baseline (< 3 min post-capture) and maximum (30–60 min post-capture) plasma corticosterone stress response in free-living male Gambel's white-crowned sparrows.

Drawn from data in Figure 10.17.

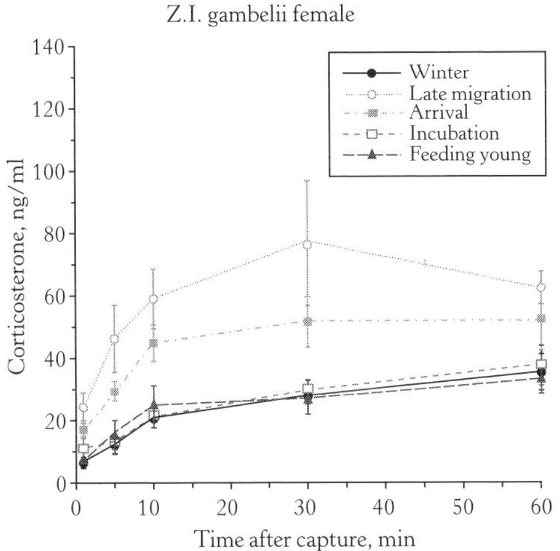

FIGURE 10.19: Seasonal changes in the plasma corticosterone stress response in free-living female Gambel's white-crowned sparrows. Samples were collected at sites as described in Figure 10.17.

Redrawn from Romero et al. (1997), Holberton and Wingfield (2003), and J. C.Wingfield unpublished.

the northern edge of the breeding range (from Romero et al. 1997; Romero and Wingfield 1999; Holberton and Wingfield 2003, J. C. Wingfield unpublished; Wingfield et al. 2004). Altitudinal gradients are also marked when comparing

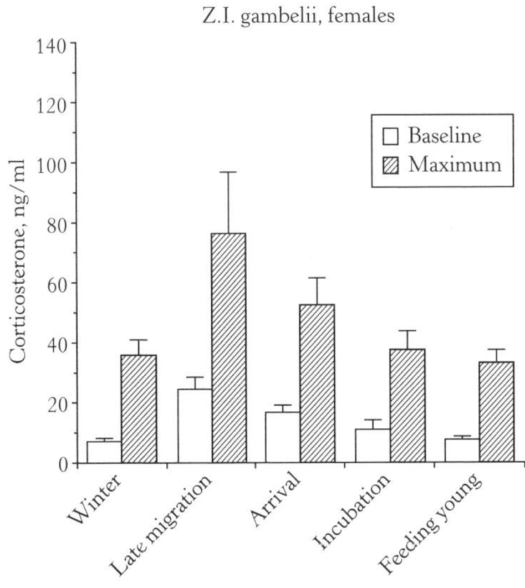

FIGURE 10.20: Seasonal changes in the baseline (< 3 min post-capture) and maximum (30–60 min post-capture) plasma corticosterone stress response in free-living female Gambel's white-crowned sparrows.

Drawn from data in the Figure 10.19.

nuttallii and *pugetensis* with *oriantha* sampled at 2500–3000 meters at Tioga Pass in the Sierra Nevada of California, and *gambelii* sampled at the southern limit of their breeding range, but at high altitude (Hart's Pass, 2500 meters) in the North Cascade Mountains of Washington State (Figures 10.21 and 10.22; J. C. Wingfield and M. C. Morton unpublished). Once again, a gender difference is apparent comparing the modulation of stress responses in females of the same subspecies and populations sampled at the beginning of the breeding season (Figure 10.23). The bottom line is that within closely related populations and subspecies the adrenocortical responses to acute stress (as measured by the profile of plasma levels of corticosterone) show variation with season, latitude, altitude, and gender.

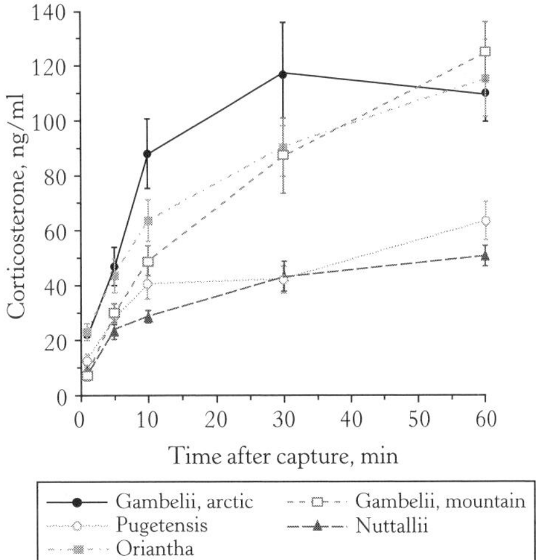

FIGURE 10.21: Increasing amplitude of the plasma corticosterone stress response with increasing latitude and altitude in five taxa of free-living male white-crowned sparrows, *Zonotrichia leucophrys*, sampled in the early breeding season. *Gambelii* were sampled at the northern limit of their range on the North Slope of Alaska, as well as near the southern limit of their breeding range at a high elevation site (2000 m) in the North Cascade Mountains (Hart's Pass), Washington State. *Z.l. pugetensis*, a short-distance migrant, were sampled in western Washington State, and *oriantha* were sampled at Tioga Pass (2500–3000 m) in the Sierra Nevada of California. *Nuttallii*, a non-migratory subspecies, were sampled at Bodega Bay on the coast of Sonoma County, California.

Redrawn from Romero et al. (1997), Holberton and Wingfield (2003), Wingfield et al., (2004), and J. C. Wingfield and M. C. Morton unpublished.

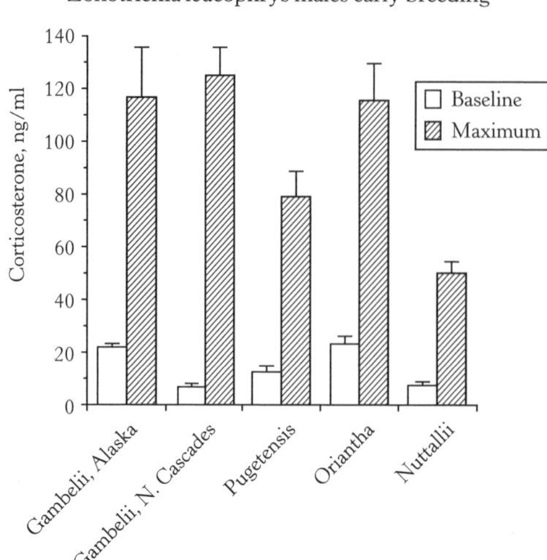

FIGURE 10.22: Increasing amplitude of the baseline (< 3 min post-capture) and maximum (30–60 min post-capture) plasma corticosterone stress response with increasing latitude and altitude in five taxa of free-living male white-crowned sparrows sampled in the early breeding season.

Redrawn from Figure 10.21.

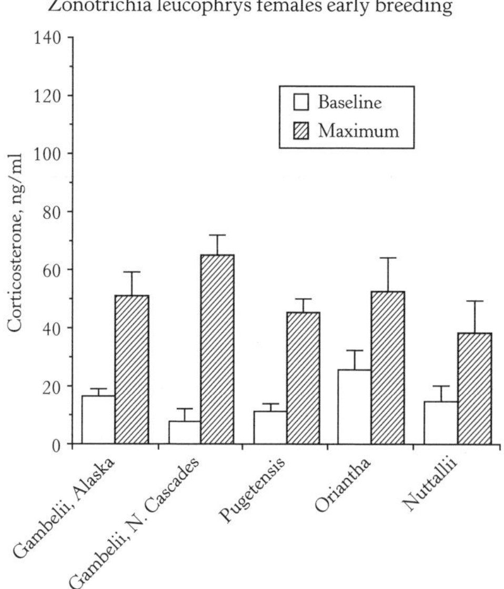

FIGURE 10.23: Increasing amplitude of the baseline (< 3 min post-capture) and maximum (30–60 min post-capture) plasma corticosterone stress response with increasing latitude and altitude in five taxa of free-living female white-crowned sparrows sampled in the early breeding season. Locations of sampling sites for each subspecies and population given in the caption to Figure 10.21.

Redrawn from Romero et al. (1997), Holberton and Wingfield (2003), and J. C. Wingfield and M. C. Morton unpublished.

Although the data reviewed thus far show consistent effects of latitude and altitude within closely related populations, not all similar studies on other species have been consistent. For example, semi-palmated sandpipers sampled while breeding in Alaska show lower stress responses at higher latitudes (Barrow) compared with lower latitudes (Nome in western Alaska, Figure 10.24; O'Reilly and Wingfield 2001). The reasons for this remain unclear, but O'Reilly and Wingfield (2001) were sampling populations within Alaska, that is, all were at high latitude and all were sampled during the parental phase (incubation) and not at the beginning of the breeding season as shown in earlier figures. The data in Figures 10.17–10.20 show that baseline corticosterone levels in Gambel's white-crowned sparrows decline during the parental phase. O'Reilly and Wingfield (2001) hypothesized that once the parental phase is underway, populations in more severe environments, such as at higher latitudes, would blunt the adrenocortical response to acute stressors, thereby ensuring successful breeding in the face of difficult environmental conditions (the high latitude hypothesis in breeding birds). The data in Figure 10.24 are consistent with this hypothesis. Note that male and female semi-palmated sandpipers show similar degrees of parental care (Figure 10.2) and thus gender differences do not confound the results

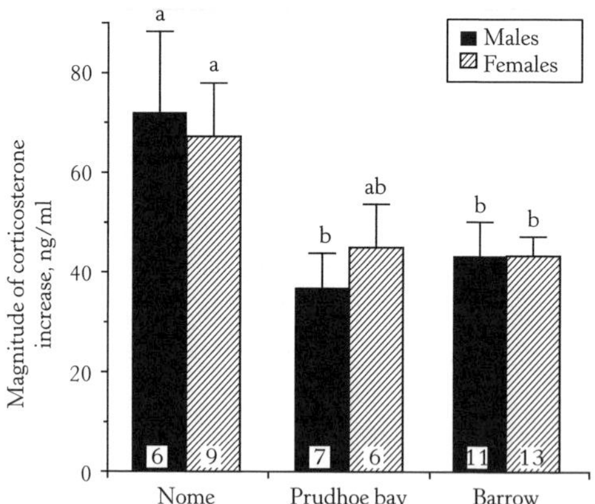

FIGURE 10.24: The increase in corticosterone in response to capture and handling in semi-palmated sandpipers as calculated by maximum (30 min) less baseline (3 min) concentrations. Comparisons were made within each gender, with different letters indicating significant differences between locations. The stress response is higher in Nome individuals than in Barrow individuals, supporting the High Latitude Hypothesis.

From O'Reilly and Wingfield (2001), courtesy of Elsevier.

(O'Reilly and Wingfield 2001). Differences among populations may also result from other, currently unknown, environmental gradients.

Many environmental gradients clearly interact to modulate the adrenocortical responses to acute perturbations. Changes in baseline corticosterone levels have been revealed along other types of gradients, such as aridity and distribution, in song wrens of Panama (Busch et al. 2011), and aridity with season in birds of the Sonoran desert (Chapter 8 of this volume; Wingfield et al. 1992). The aridity gradient data are also consistent with the high latitude hypothesis insofar as baseline and stress-induced plasma levels of corticosterone tend to be higher in more arid parts of the distribution (Busch et al. 2011) or during the hottest period of the year (Chapter 8; Wingfield et al. 1992). There are undoubtedly many more examples that await discovery along complex environmental and seasonal gradients worldwide, and in other vertebrate taxa.

There is accumulating evidence that severe perturbations of the environment, such as weather events, can also modulate the magnitude of the stress response. This was first noted in white-crowned sparrow (Puget Sound) males when a period of severe storm in 1980 increased the baseline levels of corticosterone to a degree greater than that found after another type of acute perturbation, the stress series, in the same population sampled at similar times in the breeding season (Figure 10.25; see also Chapter 8). Similar results were obtained when Lapland longspurs abandoned their nests during a severe snowstorm on the North Slope of Alaska (Astheimer et al. 1995). Other examples are given in Chapter 8.

Data on the modulation of the HPA axis have been summarized by Romero (2002) for vertebrates as a whole, providing new insight into changes in baseline levels of glucocorticoids as well as stress responses (e.g., Wingfield and Romero 2001; Wingfield and Sapolsky 2003; Landys et al. 2006). Clearly, modulation of stress responses to acute perturbations is a complex but well-orchestrated phenomenon, although the ecological, evolutionary, and mechanistic bases of these modulations are just beginning to be unraveled. Analysis of the reasons why and how modulation occurs will be the focus next.

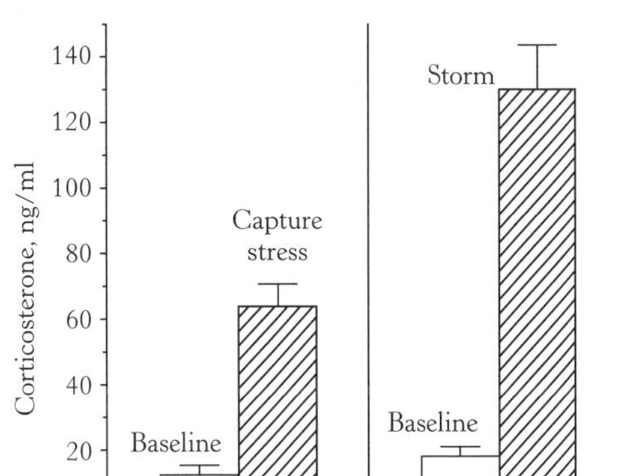

FIGURE 10.25: Effects of two different stresses, capture, handling, and restraint in the left panel and a severe storm in the right panel, on baseline (< 3 min post-capture) and maximum (30–60 min post-capture) plasma levels of corticosterone in free-living male white-crowned sparrows, (*pugetensis*) sampled during the breeding season in western Washington State.

Drawn from Wingfield et al. (1983), Addis et al. (2011), and J. C. Wingfield unpublished.

IV. HOW IS THE RESPONSE TO STRESS MODULATED?

Because of tremendous variation in technical details (e.g., plasma vs. fecal measurements of corticosteroids), it is often difficult to compare absolute corticosteroid concentrations. Consequently, the initial review of this phenomenon (Romero 2002) avoided direct comparisons and ranked whether corticosteroid concentrations were high, medium, or low during each part of the annual cycle (pre-breeding, breeding, or post-breeding seasons) relative to concentrations at other measured seasons from the same sex and same species. The review covered four major vertebrate taxa, including reptiles, amphibians, birds, and mammals. Unfortunately, there continue to be insufficient studies of free-living fish species to evaluate whether they also seasonally modulate corticosteroid responses. It appears that similar responses may occur in at least one fish species (e.g., Lu et al. 2007).

A. Mechanisms of Seasonal Change

It is clear that a majority of vertebrate species may seasonally modulate corticosteroid concentrations. Approximately 75% of all species studied show evidence of seasonal variation in corticosteroid responses in the initial review, and further recent studies have confirmed this approximate distribution. Furthermore, in some of the taxa, there are common patterns among species such that corticosteroid concentrations are higher or lower at similar times during the annual cycle. The percentages of pair-wise comparisons, where one specific season was found to have higher HPA activity than another season, are presented in Figure 10.26.

Perhaps the clearest seasonal rhythm in corticosteroid concentrations is seen in amphibians (Figure 10.26). Breeding corticosteroid titers in blood are higher than nearly all pre- and post-breeding conditions. A similar pattern is seen in reptile species, although it is not as robust. Most reptile species that are seasonal have peak corticosterone titers during the breeding period, but there are more exceptions than in amphibians. Furthermore, the evidence for an annual corticosteroid rhythm is much stronger for baseline concentrations because fewer studies have examined stress corticosteroid concentrations in free-living reptiles.

Avian species are the best studied of these four taxonomic groups (as reviewed earlier in this chapter). Baseline corticosteroid concentrations showed a strong seasonal peak during the early breeding season and an even stronger seasonal nadir during molt (Figure 10.26), but there are a number of interesting exceptions. In general, species with different molt dynamics (e.g., Romero and Wingfield 2001) or those that live in unique habitats such as the desert (e.g., Wingfield et al. 1992) do not show the same pattern of corticosteroid release. Understanding why certain species are exceptions to the general pattern is an area of ongoing research.

Strikingly, a nadir during molt is the only consistent seasonal difference in stress-induced corticosteroid concentrations in birds (Figure 10.26). Many species seasonally modulate stress-induced corticosteroid release, but an approximately equivalent number of species show high or low

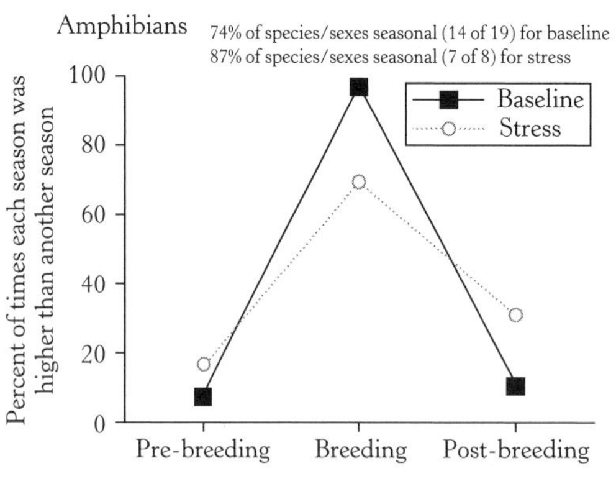

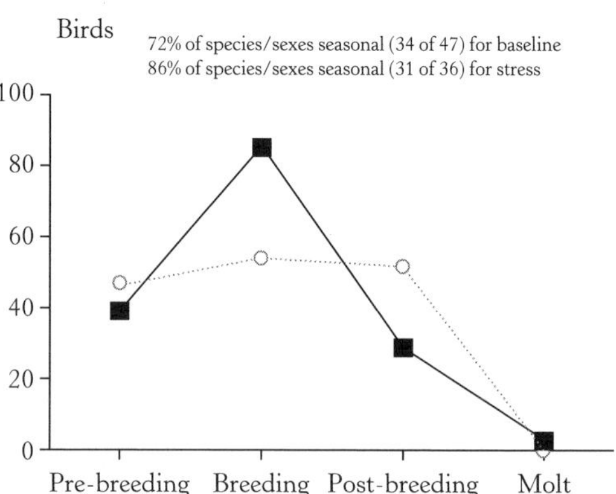

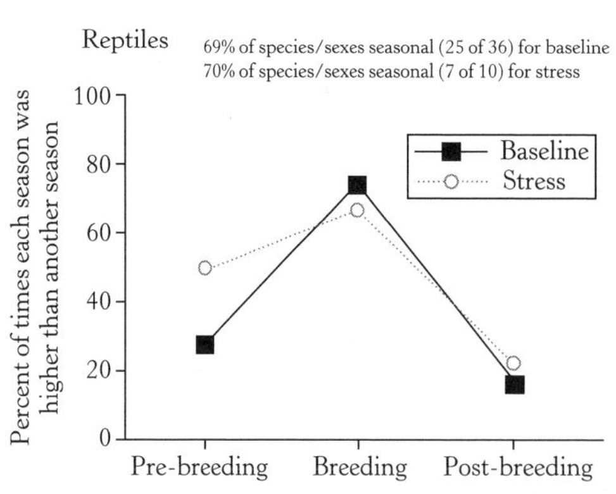

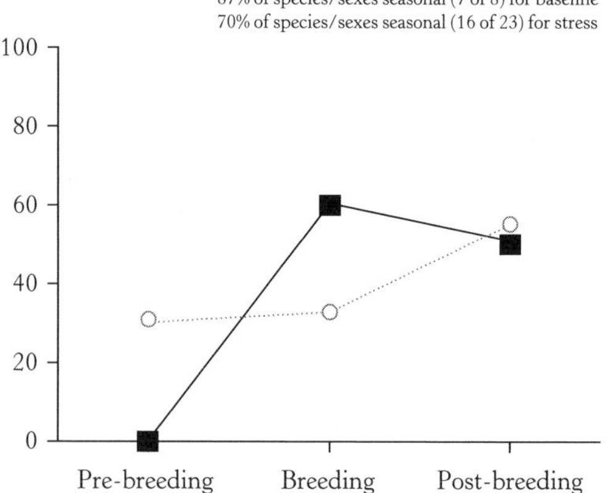

FIGURE 10.26: The percentage of species and sexes within those species that show the highest cortiosteroid concentrations during that phase of the annual cycle. Above each graph is an indication of the percentage of species of that taxon showing seasonal modulation of corticosteroid concentrations.

Reprinted with permission from Romero (2002). Courtesy of Elesevier.

corticosteroid concentrations in each season. Consequently, a seasonal peak in baseline corticosteroid titers does not necessarily coincide with a peak in HPA axis responsiveness.

Except for fish, free-living mammal species are the least studied vertebrate taxon. Most studies of mammals have found seasonal variation in both baseline and stress-induced corticosteroids, but there is no consensus on which season is higher (Figure 10.26). There are no consistent seasonal peaks or nadirs across species, suggesting that there is no consistent pattern of seasonal rhythmicity for this taxonomic group.

Annual variation of other components of the stress response, such as binding proteins and tissue sensitivity, must also be considered when determining mechanisms of stress modulation. Of course, from a physiological perspective, the fluctuation in corticosteroid titers is less important than the impact of those changes. The overall impact is essentially the integration of corticosteroid titers, transport, and tissue receptors and other cellular mechanisms such as hormone metabolizing enzymes (Wingfield 2013b). A number of studies have also found seasonal modulation in the capacity of CBG. As a general rule, CBG capacity increases when corticosteroid titers increase, although there are many exceptions (Malisch and Breuner 2010). However, CBG capacities and corticosteroid titers do not always change in parallel, and even when they do, CBG capacity does not always completely compensate for the change in titers. Consequently, when free steroid concentrations are estimated from CBG capacity and compared to total plasma corticosteroid titers, the seasonal rhythm occasionally changes, or disappears entirely (e.g., Monamy 1995; Boonstra et al. 2001; Breuner and Orchinik 2001; Romero et al. 2006; Wada et al. 2006). The physiological relevance of CBG changes is not yet entirely clear (see Chapter 2), but seasonal regulation of CBG capacity is another level at which corticosteroid's behavioral and physiological effects may be mediated (Lynn et al. 2003).

Of equal importance is the sensitivity of target tissues once corticosteroids arrive. Annual changes in corticosteroid concentrations could be accompanied by either compensatory or augmenting changes in corticosteroid receptors at target tissues. Work on this possibility is just beginning. Corticosteroid receptor numbers are known to change in laboratory studies and to alter corticosteroid's physiological effects (Munck and Náray-Fejes-Tóth 1992). Early evidence indicates that similar changes occur in the wild. Figure 10.27 shows that both type I (MR) and type II (GR) corticosteroid receptors vary seasonally in house sparrows that had been captive for only a few days. Interestingly, these receptor changes do not match the seasonal changes in corticosteroid titers in this species (Breuner and Orchinik 2001; Romero et al. 2006). However, type II receptor numbers do not change seasonally in one amphibian species, even though corticosteroid titers are highest during breeding (Denari and Ceballos 2006). Consequently, how receptor changes influence the physiological impact of seasonal variation of corticosteroid concentrations is not yet clear.

Other changes could also alter the physiological effects of corticosteroids. Examples include shifts in the relative amounts of 11ß-hydroxysteroid dehydrogenase enzymes that can activate and deactivate corticosteroids at the tissue level, or seasonal variation in corticosteroid clearance rates. Unfortunately, data examining potential changes in these parameters

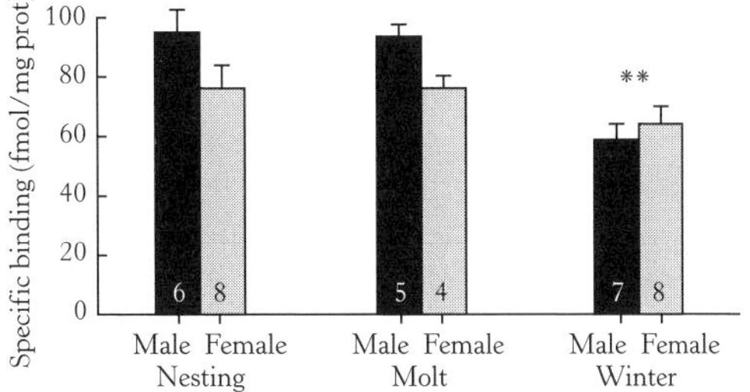

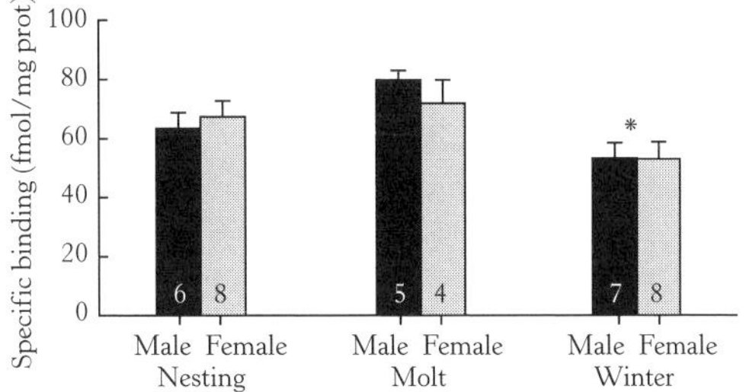

FIGURE 10.27: Yearly variability of (A) high-affinity (Type I) and (B) low-affinity (Type II) cytosolic corticosteroid receptors from house sparrow brains. In both receptors, capacity is lower during winter than during nesting or molting.

Reprinted with permission from Breuner and Orchinik (2001). Courtesy of Wiley.

in wild animals do not exist yet, but are vital to understanding any physiological consequences to annual corticosteroid rhythms.

What induces seasonal variation in corticosteroid concentrations, be it photoperiod, temperature, food availability, energetic demands, and so on, is currently unknown, although there is some evidence that implicates environmental modulation of the pineal (Sudhakumari et al. 2001). More is known about how seasonal changes in HPA function can regulate corticosteroid release. Although changes in adrenal mass are often positively correlated with corticosteroid release (e.g., Sheppard 1968; Amirat et al. 1980), simple variation in adrenal mass is not the entire story. Intriguingly, it appears that species differ in how they regulate modulation of the HPA axis. Some species regulate release directly at the adrenal, whereas in other species the primary regulatory point is at the pituitary or at the hypothalamus (Romero 2001).

i. Altered Adrenal Activity

There are several levels in the HPA axis that might change seasonally, each of which could ultimately lead to regulation of corticosteroid titers. The first level is at the adrenal cortex, where the adrenal tissue either can be exposed to a lower ACTH signal coming from the pituitary or can lose sensitivity to that ACTH signal.

ii. Altered Pituitary Activity

The second level is at the pituitary, where the corticotrophs that release ACTH either can be exposed to a lower secretagog signal coming from the hypothalamus, or can lose their sensitivity to the secretagog signal.

iii. Altered Hypothalamic Activity

The third level is at the hypothalamus, where there are at least three possibilities for a regulatory mechanism: fewer secretagogs could be released; the primary secretagog that is released could be shifted from a more potent secretagog (e.g., CRF in mammals) to a less potent secretagog (e.g., AVP in mammals); or secretagog-releasing cells could be less sensitive to inputs from higher brain centers.

iv. Changes in Negative Feedback of Glucocorticoids

Seasonal changes in corticosteroid negative feedback could regulate corticosteroid titers. Experiments intended to distinguish between these regulatory points generally follow the procedure detailed in Figure 10.28. Exogenous hormones are injected during the period when corticosteroid release is lowest in order to stimulate release of the downstream hormones. If exogenous secretagog injections successfully stimulate

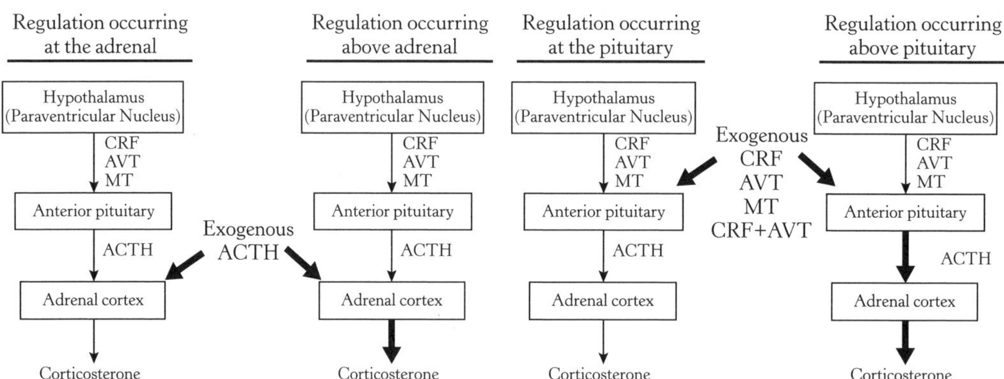

FIGURE 10.28: Procedure used to determine which level of the HPA axis is the regulatory point for modulating corticosteroid release. Exogenous releasing hormones (secretagogs) are injected at that point where corticosteroid titers are lowest. There are two possible outcomes for injection of each exogenous secretagog. The secretagog can be effective at stimulating endogenous release of its target hormone, thereby indicating that the target level would have responded further if a larger endogenous secretagog signal had been received. This would indicate that insufficient endogenous secretagog is reaching the target tissue to fully stimulate target hormone release, thus indicating that the primary regulatory site is above that target level of the HPA axis. Alternatively, the exogenous secretagog could be ineffective at stimulating endogenous release of its target hormone, thereby indicating that the target level would not respond, even if a larger endogenous secretagog signal had been received. This would then indicate that this target level of the HPA axis is the primary regulator of the lower corticosteroid release.

release of their target hormones, then the primary regulatory site in the HPA axis must lie above this point. The rationale is that the targeted level of the HPA axis would have produced a larger response were it exposed to higher concentrations of its secretagog. Since it does not respond maximally (i.e., there is a greater response to the exogenous signal), then the target site must be exposed to a lower endogenous signal coming from higher up in the axis. The inverse response, that the target tissue does not respond to the exogenous signal, indicates that this level of the HPA axis is the primary regulatory site. It would make no difference if this level received a larger endogenous signal from higher up in the axis—it has saturated its ability to respond.

A number of studies have used the protocol in Figure 10.28 to examine the site of HPA axis regulation during seasonal modulation of corticosteroid release. In all cases to date, there is a change in adrenal/interrenal sensitivity to ACTH. Even though exogenous ACTH is effective at eliciting corticosteroid release, its impact during seasons where corticosteroid titers are low is blunted vis-à-vis seasons where titers are higher (Astheimer et al. 1994; Romero et al. 1998b; Romero et al. 1998c; Romero et al. 1998a; Romero and Wingfield 1998; Carsia and John-Alder 2003; Romero 2006; Cartledge and Jones 2007). However, the adrenal is the primary site of regulation for only one species (Romero and Wingfield 1998), whereas two species regulate the change above the adrenal (but the experiments did not explore higher; Meddle et al. 2003; Cartledge and Jones 2007); two species primarily regulate the change in corticosteroid release at the pituitary (Romero et al. 1998a; Romero 2006), and two others at the hypothalamus (Romero et al. 1998b; Romero et al. 1998c). Other techniques, such as seasonal changes in CRF mRNA (Lu et al. 2007), also support a role for the hypothalamus. Figure 10.29 shows an example of these types of studies in house sparrows. Note in this study that regulation of the HPA axis changes seasonally.

It is not clear why the common phenomenon of seasonal modulation of corticosteroid titers should be regulated differently across species. Presumably, the importance for modulating the response is so great that the exact physiological mechanism used to accomplish this is relatively unimportant. In other words, there may be more than one way to accomplish the end result (different corticosteroid titers), and evolution favored whichever random mechanism changed first in each species (Wingfield 2013b, 2013a). On the other hand, we recently proposed an alternative hypothesis (Romero et al. 2000). Three of the species studied are arctic-breeding birds that are subject to highly fluctuating weather conditions. None of the three species showed any effects of weather on baseline corticosteroid titers during the breeding season, and only one showed a mild correlation between weather conditions and stress-induced titers. In all three species, however, corticosteroid titers were much lower during molt. Furthermore, they became highly sensitive to ambient weather conditions. In fact, in two of the species weather conditions explained 35%–88% of the individual variation in corticosteroid titers at the time of capture, depending upon the sex, the weather variable, and baseline versus stress-induced titers (Table 8.1). Interestingly, these two species regulated modulation of the HPA axis at the level of the hypothalamus. In contrast, the third species was less sensitive to weather conditions than the other two species, with only 20%–30% of the individual variation explained by ambient weather conditions. This species regulated its HPA axis at the level of the pituitary. These data led us to suggest that the higher the level of the HPA axis regulating corticosterone release, the more flexibility is retained to respond to changing environmental conditions (Romero et al. 2000), with implications for coping with unpredictable environments.

There has been little work examining the potential role of corticosterone negative feedback on seasonally regulated corticosteroid titers. Some data suggest that species can modulate the efficacy of negative feedback both daily (Romero and Wikelski 2006) and seasonally (Astheimer et al. 1994; Pyter et al. 2007; Lattin et al. 2012). Injections of a synthetic glucocorticoid, dexamethasone, provides a potent negative feedback signal to suppress ACTH release and thus plasma corticosterone levels. This method works because dexamethasone is hyperstimulating natural negative feedback. The very high levels of corticosteroids (dexamethasone + native corticosteroids) bind to receptors and shut down endogenous release. However, the antibodies used in most corticosteroid assays detect corticosterone or cortisol, but not dexamethasone. Consequently, the assays will reflect the decrease in the native corticosteroid, not the total amount of corticosteroids, and thus provides a measure of negative feedback. Note, however, that this method cannot be used to reduce the biological activity of corticosteroids—it does decrease secretion of the native corticosteroid, but only by making

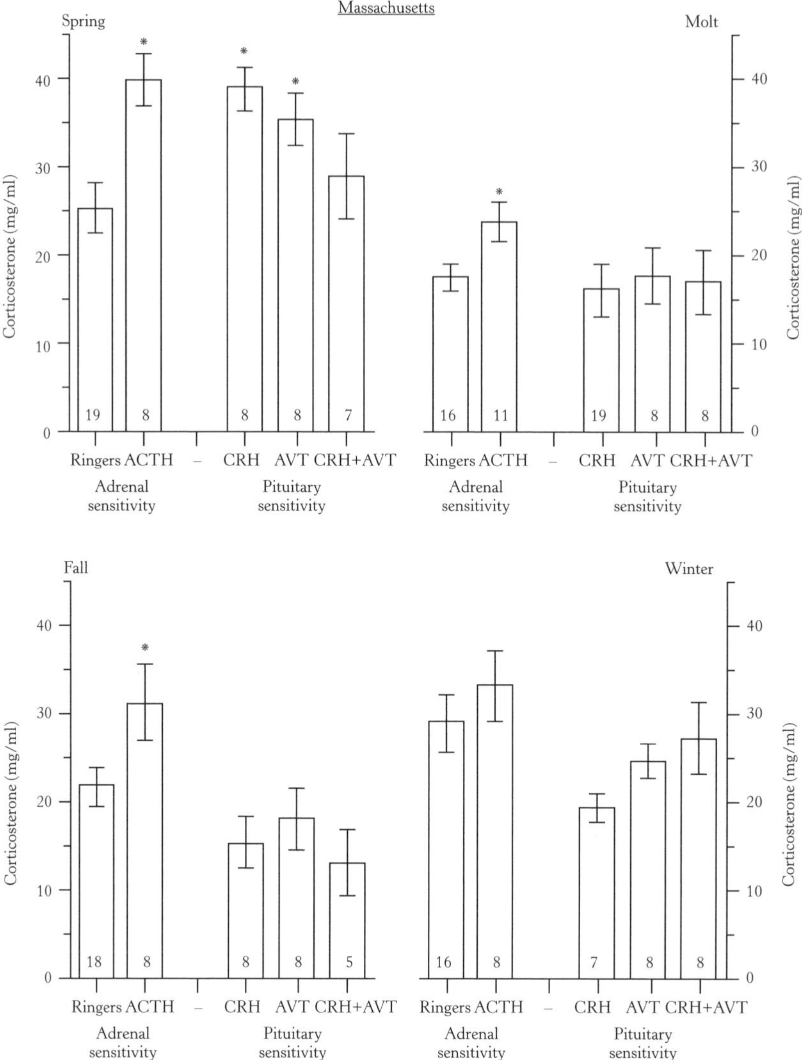

FIGURE 10.29: Seasonal differences in adrenal and pituitary sensitivities to exogenous administration of their respective releasing hormones in house sparrows captured in Massachusetts. Asterisks indicate significant differences compared to Ringers' injection for that season. Note that ACTH increased corticosterone levels in spring, molt, and fall, indicating that regulation was occurring above the level of the adrenal, whereas ACTH as not effective in winter, indicating that regulation was occurring at the adrenal in this season (see Figure 10.28). Conversely, CRH and AVT were effective in the spring indicating that in spring regulation was occurring above the level of the pituitary. CRH and AVT were ineffective the rest of the year, indicating that the pituitary was the site of regulation.

Reprinted from Romero (2006), with permission. Courtesy of Elsevier.

increases in native corticosteroid irrelevant by flooding the system with bioactive corticosteroids. An example of these types of data from Gambel's white-crowned sparrows is presented in Figure 10.30 (Astheimer et al. 1994). This is a widespread method in the biomedical literature to assess sensitivity to negative feedback (Carroll et al. 1981; Sapolsky and Altmann 1991; Sapolsky et al. 2000).

Injections of adrenocorticotrophic hormone (ACTH) into dexamethasone-treated male and female Gambel's white-crowned sparrows further showed how negative feedback can change seasonally. In non-breeding birds of both sexes, dexamethasone induced a suppression of corticosterone release and ACTH, but not saline, induced a rapid increase in plasma corticosterone levels (Figure 10.31). In contrast,

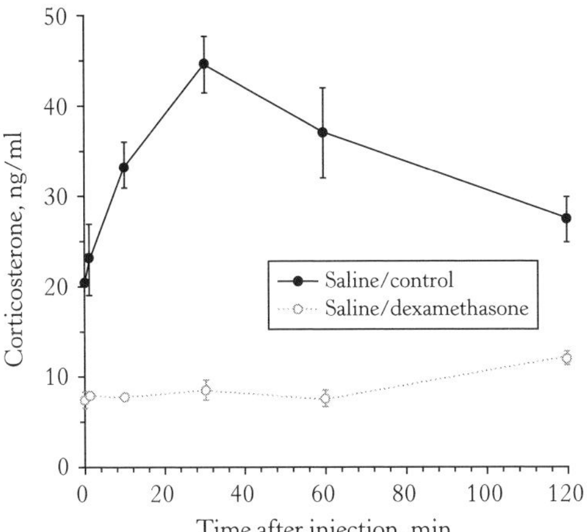

FIGURE 10.30: Injections of a synthetic glucocorticoid, dexamethasone, provides a potent negative feedback signal to suppress ACTH release and thus plasma corticosterone levels (in this case in Gambel's white-crowned sparrows). This is a widespread method in the biomedical literature to assess sensitivity to negative feedback.

From Astheimer et al. (1994), courtesy of Elsevier.

the same manipulations suggest that breeding male Gambel's white-crowned sparrows show decreased sensitivity to negative feedback, whereas females do not (Figure 10.32; Astheimer et al. 1994). Failure to respond to ACTH injection in dexamethasone-treated animals is an indication of changed sensitivity to feedback signals (i.e., dexamethasone fails to suppress ACTH and glucocorticoid release). This may explain gender differences in adrenocortical responses to acute stress in free-living Gambel's white-crowned sparrows at arrival on the breeding grounds (see also Figures 10.17–10.20).

Detailed studies exploring other aspects of seasonal regulation of HPA axis function (including secretagog receptor densities, levels of secretagog synthesis, and secretagog binding protein concentrations, for example) would be invaluable to understanding how animals seasonally regulate plasma corticosteroid concentrations. For example, exogenous testosterone can elevate corticosteroids in free-living birds (e.g., Ketterson et al. 1991; Schoech et al. 1999), suggesting a complex interaction between the gonadal and adrenal systems. The opposite, however, appears to occur in some lizards, where testosterone decreases sensitivity to ACTH in vitro (Carsia et al. 2008). Gonadal androgens could potentially be an important physiological regulator of seasonal changes in corticosteroid concentrations.

B. CBG and the Buffer Hypothesis

Circulating glucocorticoids are bound to corticosteroid-binding globulin (CBG), and while bound to this protein, it is believed that they are unable to enter cells and interact with

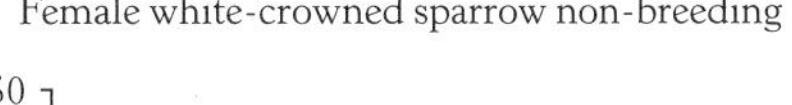

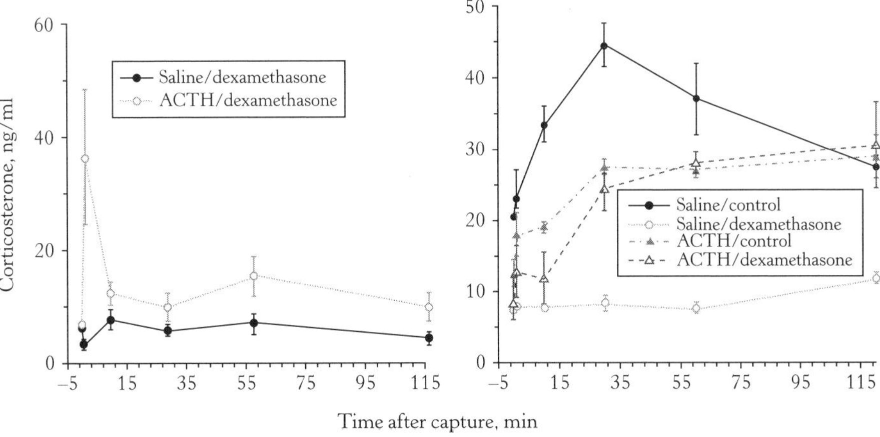

FIGURE 10.31: Injections of adrenocorticotrophic hormone (ACTH) into dexamethasone-treated male and female Gambel's white-crowned sparrows. In non-breeding males, ACTH but not saline induced a rapid increase in plasma corticosterone levels (left panel). In females, dexamethasone also decreases plasma corticosterone levels (right panel) compared to controls. ACTH also elicited an increase in plasma corticosterone in dexamethasone-treated females to levels similar to ACTH-injected controls (i.e., non-dexamethasone treated).

From Astheimer et al. (1994), courtesy of Elsevier.

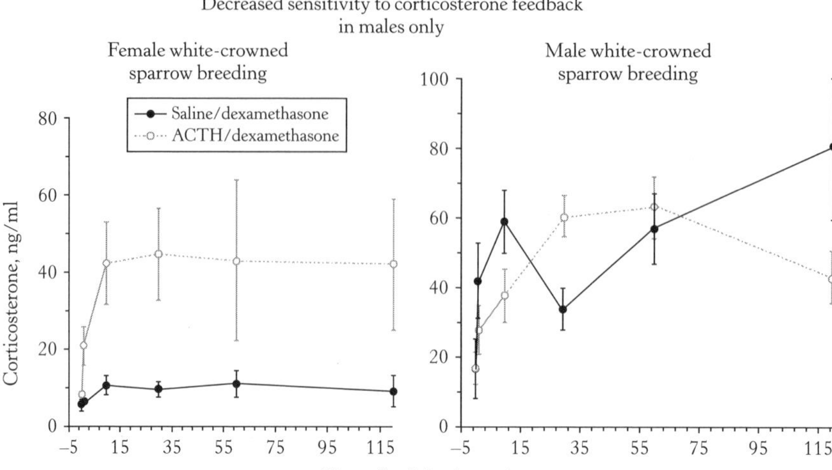

FIGURE 10.32: Failure to respond to ACTH injection in dexamethasone-treated animals is an indication of changed sensitivity to feedback signals (i.e., dexamethasone fails to suppress ACTH and glucocorticoid release). In this case, such manipulations suggest that breeding male Gambel's white-crowned sparrows show decreased sensitivity to negative feedback, whereas females do not. This may explain gender differences in adrenocortical responses to acute stress in free-living *gambelii* at arrival on the breeding grounds (see also Figures 10.17–10.20).

From Astheimer et al. (1994), courtesy of Elsevier.

receptors that mediate biological actions (see Chapter 2 of this volume; Breuner and Orchinik 2001; Breuner and Orchinik 2002). If this is the case, then it is possible that CBG levels are modulated to buffer increases in responsiveness to stress (CBG buffer hypothesis). The enhanced adrenocortical response to acute stress at arrival in male white-crowned sparrows in the Arctic (*Z.l. gambelii*) was accompanied by an increase in CBG levels compared with the high altitude population (*Z.l. oriantha*) in the Sierra Nevada of California and a lowland, mid-latitude breeding subspecies (*Z.l. pugetensis*) consistent with the buffer hypothesis (see Figures 10.17–10.20, 10.33; Romero and Wingfield 1999; Breuner et al. 2003). *Pugetensis* does not increase responsiveness to stress in early spring (but *gambelii* and *oriantha* do; Figures 10.17–10.20) and has a lower binding capacity of CBG, resulting in higher free levels of corticosterone 30 minutes post-capture than in *gambelii* and *oriantha* (Figure 10.33; Breuner et al. 2003). These data are consistent with the high latitude hypothesis (O'Reilly and Wingfield 2001) that the adrenocortical response to stress is actually reduced, even though total levels of corticosterone (bound and unbound to CBG) were high! Furthermore, there is growing evidence that the rise in CBG in early spring is regulated by rising testosterone levels in blood (Owen-Ashley 2004).

At least in *gambelii*, the increase in total corticosterone levels at arrival on the breeding grounds in Alaska is accompanied by reduced sensitivity to glucocorticoid feedback (Figure 10.32; Astheimer et al. 1994). However, although the CBG increase may buffer the effects of high glucocorticoids in response to acute stress (thus avoiding interruption of the breeding season in an environment when the time window for nesting is very short), a longer term stressor might result in triggering an emergency life-history stage and abandonment of a breeding attempt (Astheimer et al. 1995). It is possible that regulation of CBG expression could determine whether free levels of plasma corticosterone increase or decrease. In an experiment on captive male *gambelii* held on long days (mimicking summer), a 23-hour fast (typical of what may happen during a storm in northern Alaska) resulted in a decrease in plasma CBG (Figure 10.34), and despite no difference in total corticosterone levels, free levels increased significantly (Figure 10.34; Lynn et al. 2003). These data suggest that CBG levels can indeed be regulated, and can have potentially profound implications for free corticosterone and interaction with corticosteroid type II receptors and mineralocorticoid type

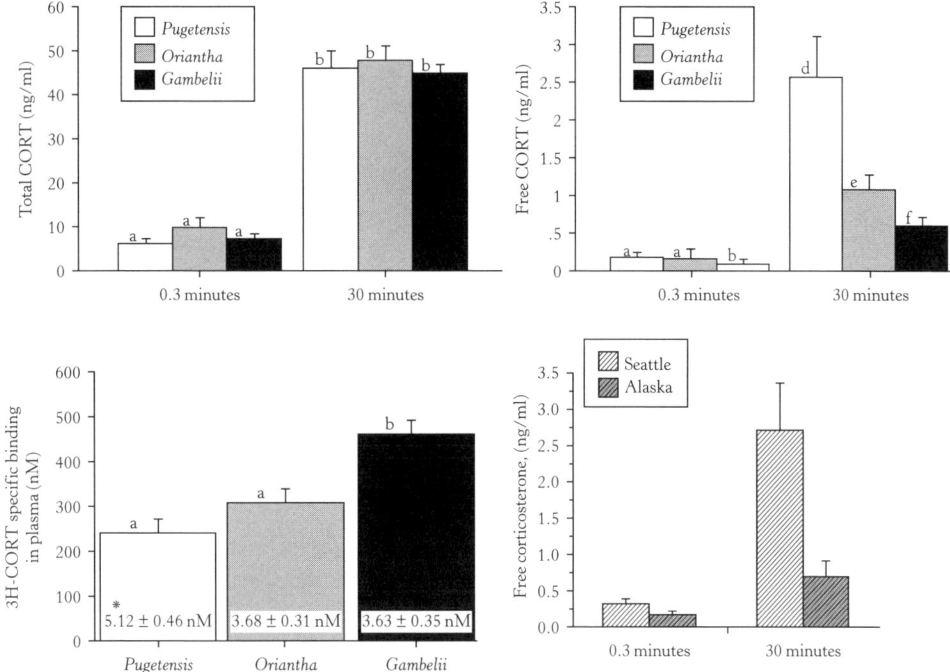

FIGURE 10.33: Corticosteroid-binding globulin potentially buffers high plasma levels of corticosterone in white-crowned sparrows. Top left: total corticosteroids (CORT) measured within 3 minutes of capture and after 30 minutes of capture and handling stress. There is no subspecies difference in either baseline or stress-induced CORT. Top right: calculated free CORT levels at capture and after 30 minutes of handling. Stress-induced free CORT levels are significantly different in each population. Consecutive letters denote significant differences. Bottom left: corticosteroid-binding globulin (CBG) capacity (bars) and affinity (inset) for *pugetensis, oriantha*, and *gambelii*. Bottom right: free levels of baseline corticosterone in Seattle birds versus Alaska birds and at 30 minutes of acute handling stress.

From Breuner et al. (2003), courtesy of the American Physiological Society.

I receptors. How CBG may be regulated remains unknown.

Corticosteroid interactions with tissues also appear to change. Genomic type I and type II receptor binding capacities in the brain and liver of white-crowned sparrows breeding near Seattle (*pugetensis*) and in Alaska (*gambelii*) are presented in Table 10.3 and Figure 10.35 (Breuner et al. 2003). There were no differences in binding capacity of Type I or II receptors with population in either liver or brain. However, Alaska birds tended to have lower binding capacity for both receptors in the brain (Figure 10.35; significant for type I but trend for type II). A measure of the number of type II receptors occupied (nM) at 30-minute free-corticosterone plasma levels in *pugetensis* and *gambelii* are presented in the top panel of Figure 10.36. Because the type II receptor has lower affinity for corticosteroids, it has been called the "stress receptor," as higher circulating levels are needed to saturate type II and increase gene expression (see Chapter 2). Remarkably, *gambelii* males breeding in Alaska appear to have less bound type II than *pugetensis* in both liver and brain (Figure 10.36). These data suggest that although male *gambelii* arrive on the breeding grounds with high levels of corticosterone, coincident high CBG buffers this and lowers free corticosterone and thus bound type II receptors (Figure 10.36; Breuner et al. 2003). Furthermore, estimations of type II receptor fractional occupancy after 30 minutes of capture and handling stress in both liver (bottom left of Figure 10.36) and brain (bottom right of Figure 10.36) show how CBG buffering can alter binding in *gambelii* and *pugetensis*. *Oriantha* that breed at altitude appear to have an intermediate response (Breuner et al. 2003).

It is important to recognize, however, that the buffer hypothesis for CBG function has not been conclusively established. There are alternate hypotheses for CBG function (see Chapter 2). Further research is needed to be able

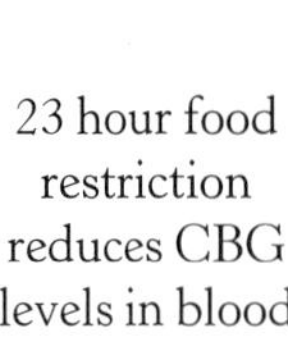

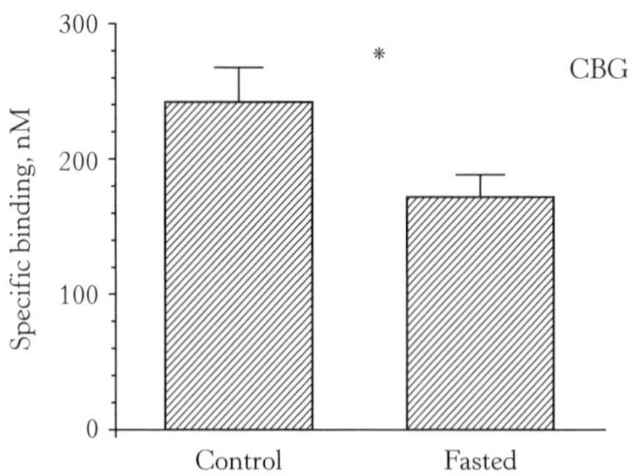

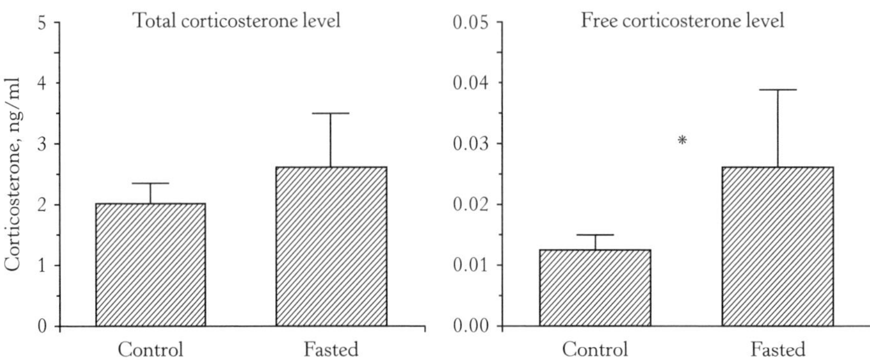

FIGURE 10.34: Total and free corticosterone (CORT) levels in captive male white-crowned sparrows after 23-hour fasted and control conditions. Lower left panel: birds held under fasted conditions showed no differences in total CORT levels. Upper right panel: specific binding of CORT by CBG decreased relative to control conditions. Lower right panel: calculated free CORT levels were higher in fasted birds.

Data adapted from Lynn et al. (2003), courtesy of Elsevier.

to distinguish the impact of CBG on corticosteroid function. Although the above data would require reinterpretation if CBG functioned differently than a buffer, the buffer hypothesis provides an attractive explanation for seasonal, latitudinal, and altitudinal differences in white-crowned sparrows. CBG modulation is potentially an important regulatory point in the variation in stress responses.

In conclusion, the highly integrative studies on white-crowned sparrows discussed throughout this chapter build on possible ecological bases of modulation of the adrenocortical responses to acute stress and explore the

TABLE 10.3: INTRACELLULAR RECEPTOR CAPACITY IN EACH WHITE-CROWNED SPARROW POPULATION

	Liver				Brain			
	High affinity		Low affinity		High affinity		Low affinity	
pugetensis	14.5	1.3	14.1	2.2	60.8	8.9	81.1	14.1
oriantha	15.2	1.3	20.0	2.0*	54.7	5.4	115.9	4.9*
gambelii	14.0	1.7	9.7	0.7	31.3	4.0*	50.3	12.1
ANOVA	$F = 0.2; P > 0.8$		$F = 8.8; P < 0.002$		$F = 5.9; P < 0.01$		$F = 8.8; P < 0.002$	

Values are means ± SE (in nM). *Population is significantly different from other populations within receptor type.
From Breuner et al. (2003), courtesy of the American Society of Physiologists.

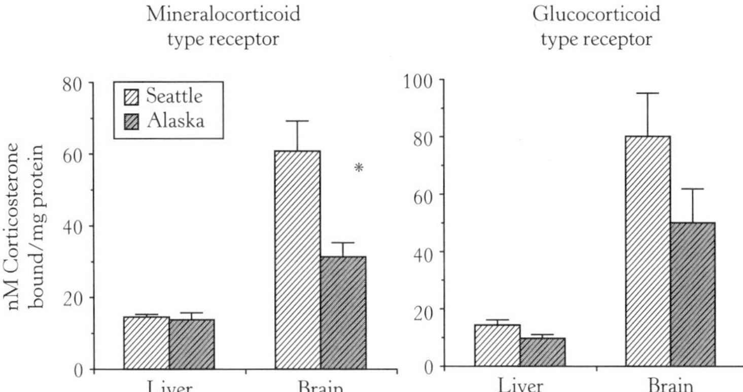

FIGURE 10.35: Genomic mineralocorticoid (type I; MR) and glucocorticoid (type II, GR) receptor binding in the brain and liver of white-crowned sparrows breeding near Seattle (*pugetensis*) and in Alaska (*gambelii*). Binding capacity data expressed as nM of tritiated corticosterone bound per mg of protein in the tissue sample. There were no differences in binding capacity of GR or MR with population in either liver or brain. However, Alaska birds tended to have lower binding capacity for GR and MR in the brain (significant for MR but trend for GR).

From Breuner et al. (2003), courtesy of the American Society of Physiology.

mechanisms underlying that modulation. This requires assessing three components of the HPA axis: first, control of the hormonal cascade leading to corticosteroid release; second, regulation of transport such as CBG activity; and third, regulation of responsiveness of the target tissue. These three foci of action, and thus regulation, may be widespread (Wingfield 2012, 2013a,

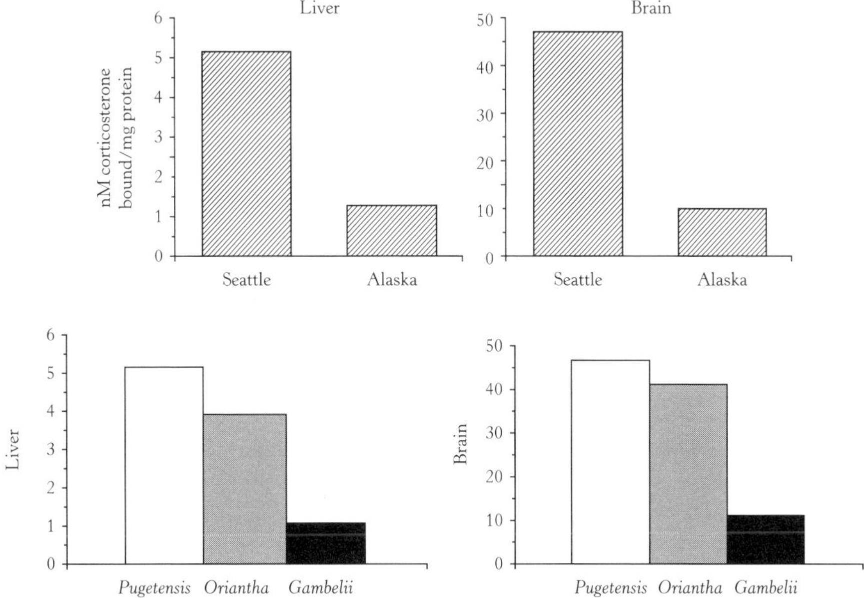

FIGURE 10.36: Top panels: glucocorticoid (type II, GR) receptors occupied (nM) at 30-minute free-corticosterone levels in Seattle (*pugetensis*) and Alaska (*gambelii*) white-crowned sparrows. Bottom panels: estimation of low-affinity GR fractional occupancy after 30 minutes of capture and handling stress in both liver and brain tissue.

From Breuner et al. (2003), courtesy of the American Physiological Society.

2013b), and investigations of other free-living organisms are needed.

C. Summary of Seasonal Changes in Four Vertebrate Taxa

Why does annual corticosteroid variation exist? Most wild species studied under natural conditions vary corticosteroids seasonally and, with the exception of mammalian species, the annual rhythm tends to peak during the breeding season (although in those studies that have looked at the breeding season in finer detail, high levels tend to occur just prior to breeding and then decrease once breeding commences). Which species will show an annual rhythm, however, is still not possible to predict. The modulation of corticosteroid release presents us with two interesting paradoxes. First, why should the highest corticosteroid concentrations tend to occur concurrent to breeding? What occurs during the breeding season that seems to require both elevated baseline titers as well as more robust responses to stressors? Second, if corticosteroid release is so important for survival (e.g., Darlington et al. 1990), then how do animals survive stressors at certain times of the year when they essentially fail to release corticosteroids? (Notice in Figure 10.11 that white-crowned sparrows undergoing a prebasic molt essentially fail to have a corticosteroid response to capture and handling; Romero 2002). The lack of response poses serious problems for the dogma that corticosteroids are essential for surviving stressors.

There are currently four potential explanations for why species seasonally modulate corticosteroid responses (Romero 2002). Each focuses on a different aspect of corticosteroid physiology and have different strengths and weaknesses.

i. The Energy Mobilization Hypothesis

The Energy Mobilization Hypothesis posits that corticosteroid concentrations will be highest during energetically costly times of the year. Because corticosteroids play an important role in energy mobilization, especially during stress (see Chapter 5), the highest corticosteroid titers should occur during those times of the year with the highest energetic demands (e.g., Anava et al. 2002). Consequently, this hypothesis predicts high corticosteroid concentrations during breeding because the reproductive process often requires substantial energy expenditure. This could certainly be true for females, who in most species bear the majority of the energy costs for raising the next generation. It might also be true for males in many species since breeding often entails increased energy costs associated with testosterone (Ketterson and Nolan 1999), attracting mates (Leary et al. 2008), feeding young (Kern et al. 2007), and territorial defense (Wingfield et al., 2001). Species that are exceptions to having peaks during breeding could also be explained with this hypothesis if other periods in the annual cycle are more energetically costly than breeding. In other words, the Energy Mobilization Hypothesis posits that elevated corticosteroid titers should coincide with those times of the annual cycle with the highest allostatic load.

Seasonal variation in corticosteroid responses in migratory passerine birds provides a test of the Energy Mobilization Hypothesis. Migratory passerines have four life-history stages that involve considerable energy expenditure: an often lengthy spring migration to the breeding grounds; breeding; a post-breeding molt where they replace all their body feathers; and a fall migration to the wintering grounds. It is not intuitively obvious which of these activities requires the most energy, and any distinctions would likely be subtle (such as rate of energy expenditure vs. total energy expenditure). Because all of these activities are energetically stressful (i.e., incur allostatic load), the Energy Mobilization Hypothesis would predict that corticosteroid concentrations would be highest during each of these activities, with little difference between them. However, the available evidence indicates that this is not the case. Figure 10.11 provides a good example. Molt is an almost universal period with the lowest corticosteroid concentrations in passerines (Romero 2002), even though molt is clearly a period of high allostatic load for these species. Similarly, allostatic load during migration is also high, yet corticosteroid concentrations do not correlate with this load. As an example, corticosteroid concentrations during the spring and fall migrations often differ, even though the migratory routes are identical (O'Reilly 1995).

The solution to the lack of correlation between seasonal corticosterone titers and allostatic load, however, may be that we simply are not assigning allostatic load properly. Perhaps allostatic load varies between these life-history stages more than we fully appreciate. As an example, desert birds shift the high corticosteroid periods from the breeding period to the post-breeding period (Wingfield et al. 1992). Although we might presume that breeding has a higher allostatic load, and should thus have higher corticosteroid titers, extreme heat and the lack of freely available water might make the post-breeding period more energetically costly (Chapter 8). Better estimates of allostatic load might better support the Energy Mobilization Hypothesis.

An analysis of corticosteroid titers in mammalian hibernators also fails to support the Energy Mobilization Hypothesis. Laboratory data indicate that corticosteroids synergize with insulin to regulate glucose and lipid trafficking to promote pre-hibernation hyperphagia (i.e., extensive fat accumulation). This led Dallman et al. (1993) to propose that corticosteroid concentrations would be higher in the fall in hibernators that require dramatically increased fat stores to survive the winter. Their proposal is consistent with the Energy Mobilization Hypothesis because the energy needed to support pre-hibernation hyperphagia must create a substantial allostatic load. Unfortunately, the available evidence is not supportive. Baseline corticosteroid concentrations have only been measured in two mammalian hibernators. Golden-mantled ground squirrels have the lowest corticosteroid titers as they deposit huge amounts of fat (Romero et al. 2008), opposite of Dallman et al.'s (1993) prediction. In contrast, yellow-pine chipmunks rely upon food caching rather than pre-hibernation hyperphagia to provide the energy to survive the winter, and yet they show the highest baseline corticosteroid concentrations just prior to entering their hibernaculae (Kenagy and Place 2000; Place and Kenagy 2000; Romero et al. 2008).

A similar lack of support for the Energy Mobilization Hypothesis comes from studies of stress-induced corticosteroid concentrations in hibernators, although these data should be interpreted with caution since the normal metabolic changes that allow fattening are proposed to be mediated by basal and not stress-induced concentrations of corticosteroids (Dallman et al. 1993; Sapolsky et al. 2000). Although the yellow-bellied marmot has stress-induced corticosteroid concentrations highest prior to hibernation (Armitage 1991), the golden-mantled ground squirrel has the lowest concentrations at this time (Boswell et al. 1994; Romero et al. 2008), and the arctic ground squirrel does not show a seasonal rhythm (Boonstra et al. 2001). Furthermore, yellow-pine chipmunks, who again do not undergo pre-hibernation fattening, show the highest stress-induced titers prior to hibernation (Romero et al. 2008).

The three examples discussed in this section, mammalian hibernation and avian migration and molt, highlight the insufficiency of the Energy Mobilization Hypothesis in providing a universal explanation for seasonal corticosteroid regulation. This does not mean, however, that the Energy Mobilization Hypothesis cannot be a powerful explanatory mechanism for certain species during at least some times of the year. Furthermore, energy utilization may modulate corticosteroid release, even if it does not drive the annual variation. Subtle differences in life-history strategies between species might make species-specific comparisons far more effective than simply treating each season as being equivalent for all species. For example, some species can prepare for energetically costly periods by storing energy as fat, thereby ensuring that energy is not in short supply at critical points. The Energy Mobilization Hypothesis would predict that the corticosteroid rhythm of such a species might be very different than in a sympatric species that does not accumulate fat. Similarly, bird migration should be interpreted in relation to both energy utilization and availability, information that studies rarely attempt to correlate with corticosteroid concentrations. Such studies would provide a much stronger connection to allostatic load.

On the other hand, approximately 70% of species seasonally regulate corticosteroid concentrations, and approximately 80% of those species show a peak just prior to and at the onset of breeding. If energy mobilization were the primary mechanism driving seasonal corticosteroid variation, future research should show breeding as the most energetically costly period for the majority of species. Consequently, although the Energy Mobilization Hypothesis does not have much current support, this may simply reflect our failure to accurately measure allostatic load. There is clearly enormous variation in how species gather, store, and utilize energy, which we are just beginning to be able to incorporate into models of allostatic load. Once we have better measures of allostatic load, it would be worth revisiting the Energy Mobilization Hypothesis to determine how well it explains corticosteroid variability during different life history stages.

ii. The Behavioral Hypothesis

The Behavioral Hypothesis proposes that annual variation in corticosteroid concentrations results from animals having specific requirements during each life-history stage for expressing (or not expressing) corticosteroid-mediated behaviors. For example, stress-induced corticosteroids can induce an animal to flee an area and relocate during adverse environmental conditions (see Chapter 9). While this might be an excellent strategy for most of the year, it could be catastrophic for an individual's overall fitness when relocation requires abandoning a nest or a breeding territory (Wingfield 1994). Abandoning a nest or breeding territory would be even worse for species with short breeding seasons and thus little ability to recover. The Behavior Hypothesis focuses specifically on the need to seasonally regulate the expression of these behaviors.

The foundation of the Behavioral Hypothesis stems from the theory of the emergency life-history stage (see Chapter 1). With this theory, when an animal is faced with an unpredictable stressor, it leaves its current life-history stage (e.g., breeding, migrating, etc.) and enters an all-purpose emergency life-history stage that allows the animal to cope with this unpredictable stressor (Wingfield 2003). The emergency life-history stage is characterized by (1) deactivation of territorial behavior; (2) activation of facultative behavior such as fleeing and/or seeking refuge; (3) changes in physiology such as energy mobilization; (4) continued movement until suitable habitat is discovered; and (5) settlement in an alternate habitat (Wingfield and Romero 2001). Notice that four of the five characteristics involve behavior. Also notice that the desirability of some of these behaviors, such as deactivating territorial behavior, will depend upon the initial life-history stage because deactivating territorial behavior will have different consequences at different times of the year.

There are some indications that behavioral responses to stress change seasonally. A good example from the laboratory is shown in Figure 10.37. The behavioral effects on white-crowned sparrow activity depend upon photoperiod (Breuner and Wingfield 2000), which is presumed to mimic seasonal differences found in the wild. Interestingly, at least with this system, corticosteroid effects on activity appear to be regulated by the non-genomic receptor (Breuner et al. 1998). Photoperiod also changes the fight-or-flight response to crowding in captive European starlings (Dickens et al. 2006). Although the laboratory provides a controlled setting to explore the interaction between corticosteroids and behavior, similar effects have been shown in the field.

Support for the Behavioral Hypothesis falls in two main categories. The first is evidence that corticosteroids alter behavior in free-living animals. Experimentally elevated corticosteroids reduce territorial aggression and home range size

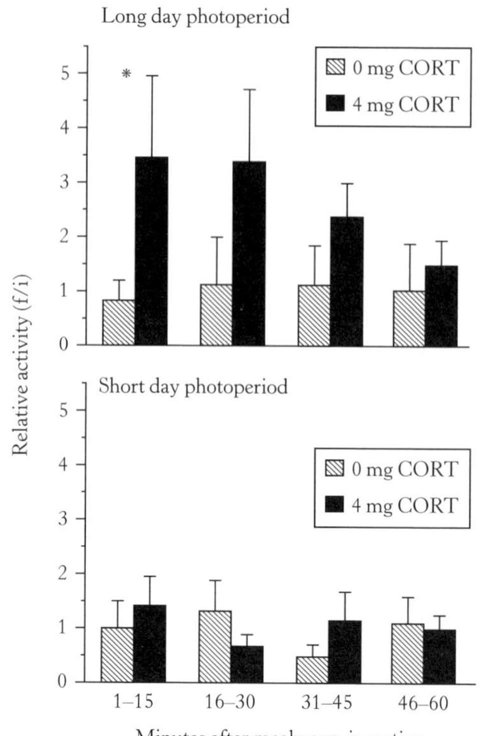

FIGURE 10.37: Changes in activity in response to administration of corticosterone in white-crowned sparrows. Corticosterone was provided in a mealworm that was then consumed. Note that corticosterone induced an increase in activity when birds were held on long days, but not when held on short days.

Reprinted with permission from Breuner and Wingfield (2000). Courtesy of Elsevier.

in many species (e.g., Wingfield and Silverin 1986; DeNardo and Sinervo 1994), although these studies have mostly used corticosteroid implants. High corticosteroid concentrations also suppress sexual behavior (e.g., Deviche et al. 1979; Moore and Miller 1984; Leary et al. 2006a) and parental behavior. Implants in breeding pied flycatchers can lead to less frequent feeding of young, inhibited nestling weight gain, and poor fledging of chicks (Silverin 1986), and corticosterone implants in free-living male song sparrows reduced territorial aggression compared to control implanted birds (Wingfield and Silverin 1986). Higher corticosteroid concentrations can even induce complete nest abandonment in pied flycatchers (Silverin 1986) and European starlings (Love et al. 2004), but this is not true in all species (Criscuolo et al. 2005). Decreased parental behavior, however, might be secondary to corticosteroid-induced reductions in prolactin titers (Angelier et al. 2009a). Although corticosteroids have well-established effects on food intake under laboratory conditions in both mammalian (Dallman et al. 2004) and avian (e.g., Gray et al. 1990; Astheimer et al. 1992) species, it is less clear whether corticosteroids alter foraging behavior in free-living animals. What little evidence exists suggests that corticosteroids can also stimulate foraging effort (e.g., Angelier et al. 2008). Finally, there is substantial and building evidence that corticosteroids are involved in escape behavior (reviewed in Wingfield and Romero 2001). However, whether escape behavior occurs can depend upon the nutritional status of the animal—when food is plentiful, the animal will likely seek refuge from the stressor, whereas when food is scarce the animal will likely emigrate from the area (termed irruptive movement; see Chapter 9).

The second category of support for the Behavioral Hypothesis is that seasonal changes in corticosteroid concentrations tend to correlate with seasonal changes in stress-induced behaviors. For example, desert birds (with variable breeding seasons under harsh conditions) have lower corticosteroid concentrations during the breeding season (Wingfield et al. 1992). This is consistent with avoiding the abandonment of nests during breeding. Perhaps the best examples, however, are from studies conducted entirely during the breeding life-history stage. When corticosteroid concentrations are measured throughout the breeding period in birds, corticosteroids tend to be lowest when the birds have the most to lose when abandoning the nest. In other words, titers are generally highest early during nest establishment and then gradually decrease as parental investment increases. This leads to the lowest concentrations occurring when parents are feeding young and just about to reap the benefits of successfully raising their young and increasing reproductive success (e.g., Reneerkens et al. 2002; Meddle et al. 2003; Li et al. 2008; Williams et al. 2008). The decrease over the breeding period has been proposed as the "parental care hypothesis" or "brood value hypothesis" (Wingfield et al. 1995b; Bokony et al. 2009). However, there is some evidence that the pattern changes when CBG changes are taken into account and a free corticosteroid titer is computed. In this case, the highest corticosteroid titers occur at the end of the breeding sequence (Love et al. 2004). Furthermore, for several species of arctic-breeding birds (Figure 10.2), the sex providing the most parental care (and thus with perhaps the most to lose from nest abandonment) had the lowest corticosteroid concentrations during the breeding season (e.g., O'Reilly and Wingfield 2001; Holberton and Wingfield 2003). There are counter examples, however. For example, in male meerkats who are parental helpers, increased feeding rates are correlated with increased corticosteroid concentrations (Carlson et al. 2006).

A further corollary to the Behavioral Hypothesis is that animals should be behaviorally resistant to the effects of exogenous corticosteroids during those periods when corticosteroids are low. Although the data are limited, there is evidence that corticosteroid insensitivity does occur. For example, corticosteroid implants have no impact on territorial defense in some (Astheimer et al. 2000; Meddle et al. 2003), but not all species (e.g., Meddle et al. 2002). Experimentally increasing clutch size, thereby producing more of an investment in chicks, also resulted in reduced sensitivity to stressors that increased as breeding progressed (Lendvai et al. 2007). Furthermore, in some environmental contexts where behavioral changes should not be favored, such as food shortages, behavior can become insensitive to corticosteroids (e.g., Cote et al. 2010). The sensitivity to stressors may also change. For example, some arctic-breeding birds are insensitive to ambient weather conditions when breeding, but are highly sensitive to weather conditions after breeding, even though those weather conditions are more benign (Romero et al. 2000).

Although the above evidence indicates that the Behavior Hypothesis is a very powerful explanation of why corticosteroid concentrations are modulated during the breeding season, the Behavior Hypothesis does not provide a good explanation for annual variation in corticosteroid concentrations outside the breeding season. The overall trend for most species (other than mammals) is that corticosteroid concentrations are highest just prior to and at the onset of the breeding season (Figure 10.11). If regulating corticosteroid concentrations seasonally were primarily to regulate the behavioral consequences of corticosteroid release, then the prediction would be that corticosteroid concentrations would be lowest during the breeding season. Consequently, the Behavior Hypothesis is likely to be useful in explaining the modulation of corticosteroid concentrations within a single season, but not very useful in explaining modulation across seasons.

Although not part of the original Behavior Hypothesis, behavior may play a different role in driving seasonal variation. Females of many species prefer males with low corticosteroid titers during mate selection (reviewed in Husak and Moore 2008). The mechanism seems to be an indirect effect in that high corticosteroids are correlated with poor male sexual signaling. For example, high corticosteroids decrease song quality in both avian (e.g., Spencer et al. 2003; Wada et al. 2008) and amphibian (e.g., Leary et al. 2006a; Leary et al. 2006b) species. Females then choose those males with the better signal. However, as with the Behavioral Hypothesis, female mate choice may explain individual differences but is unlikely to provide much explanatory power for understanding seasonal variation. Because mate choice occurs early in the breeding season, if mate choice were indeed driving seasonal corticosteroid variation, then corticosteroid titers should be lowest early in the breeding season. This is exactly opposite the pattern in most species. Moreover, lower corticosteroid titers favored during mate choice does not explain why most species have their highest titers of the year at this time.

iii. The Preparative Hypothesis

The Preparative Hypothesis proposes that annual variation in corticosteroid concentrations serves to modulate the priming of non-corticosteroid stress pathways during periods with different potential exposure to adverse conditions. Two important classes of physiological effects of corticosteroids are permissive effects that prime other physiological systems (e.g., epinephrine action) to work better under stress and preparative effects that help prepare the organism for subsequent stress responses (see Chapter 4). Corticosteroids have a priming effect on numerous physiological systems, many of which are necessary for survival under adverse conditions. Perhaps seasonal peaks in corticosteroid concentrations provide better priming effects during those times of year. This would then provide enhanced preparation for periods when adverse conditions are more common.

For many species, breeding can be a period when stress is more common. Many different stimuli are known to cause stress in wild animals, including severe storms (e.g., Smith et al. 1994), predation (e.g., Mason 1998), disease (e.g., Dunlap and Schall 1995), and social interactions (e.g. Sapolsky 2005). Many species, based on their life histories, may be able to predict that exposure to many of these stimuli is likely to increase during the breeding season. There are many potential examples. Predation may increase for amphibians that must congregate at a breeding pond, as well as for birds that are both much more active during mate choice and then tied to a nest for several weeks (e.g., Scheuerlein et al. 2001). For many species, competition for mates only occurs at the beginning of the breeding season and, especially for males, can include highly stressful social interactions and fights that can lead to death. Disease also may become more prevalent when individuals congregate for the breeding season, especially for diseases that do not go through a vector before infecting the next host. Energetic risk may also be predictable, especially if breeding reliably produces an increase in allostatic load. Furthermore, many physiological effects of corticosteroids help prepare the individual for a subsequent stressor, especially since one stressor (e.g., infection or a failed predator attack) can predispose that individual for a second stressor (e.g., further attacks on a weakened immune system or a second predatory attack on an exhausted or injured animal). The potential for being exposed to a stressor thus increases exponentially.

The Preparative Hypothesis predicts that increases in the frequency of stressors would result in higher corticosteroid concentrations. In other words, corticosteroid concentrations vary with different life-history stages in order to mediate changes in the preparedness of the non-corticosteroid pathways of the stress response. However, the Preparative Hypothesis does not require that each individual animal be subjected to more stressors, only that the chance of being subjected to a stressor is more likely. As a result, individuals that are fortunate enough to never be subjected to a stressor during that season still will show higher corticosteroid concentrations. In other words, corticosteroid titers respond to increased risk, not to increased exposure. This implies that changes in the risk of stressor exposure must be predictable over evolutionary time in order to result in repeatable annual variations in corticosteroid concentrations.

Seasonal changes in risk might explain why some species do not seasonally vary corticosteroid concentrations. If risk of stress exposure does not vary seasonally, neither will corticosteroid concentrations. In addition, because annual variation will coincide with variable risk, the annual peak does not have to coincide with breeding for every species. Because life-history traits will determine risk, breeding may not be the riskiest time of the year for every species. Note, however, that the emphasis on risk of stress exposure makes the hypothesis distinct from a hypothesis based upon allostatic load. Allostatic load and stressor risk may or may not coincide. This further distinguishes the Preparative Hypothesis from the Energetic Hypothesis.

Evidence for the Preparative Hypothesis is building. A few studies have now demonstrated a link between corticosteroid concentrations and the risk of adverse environmental conditions. A good example is in female brown lemmings (Romero et al. 2008), a small rodent that lives on the tundra plains in Alaska. They were captured by hand during two times of the year—in early June and in late July. Figure 10.38 shows that female lemmings show huge differences in their

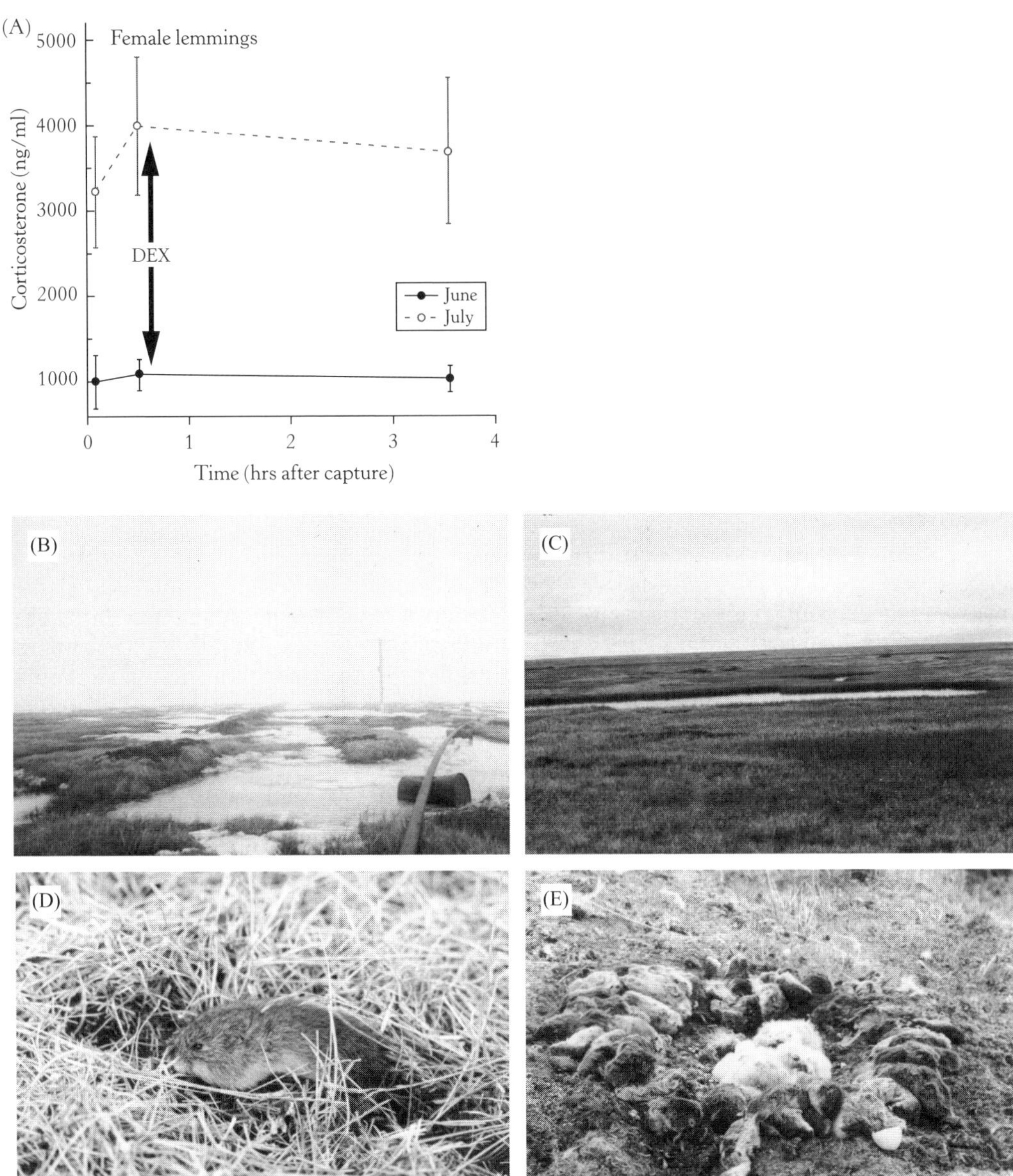

FIGURE 10.38: (A) Corticosterone concentrations from female brown lemmings trapped in June and July. The arrow marks when dexamethasone (DEX) was administered to the animals. Pictures of the tundra in early June (B) with plentiful snow cover for lemmings to hide from aerial predators and in late July (C) without any snow cover. When there is no snow cover, lemmings rely upon grass runways (D) to help escape from aerial predators. This is often unsuccessful, however, and snowy owls, among other predators, consume huge numbers of lemmings to feed growing chicks. (E) Snowy owl nest with 10 growing chicks and plentiful dead lemmings around the nest for the chicks to eat.

Data reprinted with permission from Romero et al. (2008). Courtesy of American Physiological Society. Photos by L. Michael Romero.

corticosteroid titers during these two periods. Although animals were trapped only six weeks apart, the changes in the habitat during this period are profound. Figure 10.38 shows pictures of the tundra in June when snow cover was greater than 50% and in July when there was no snow cover. The amount of snow cover can create very different predation pressures from aerial predators (an important predator in this habitat is the snowy owl). Snow cover protects the lemmings from avian predators, but when the snow is gone, defensive behaviors are limited. Permafrost prevents lemmings from digging burrows, so their primary defense is covered grass runways that help them hide and run from aerial predators (Figure 10.38.D). The predation pressure on lemmings can be intense (Figure 10.38.E). The loss of snow cover occurs at the same time the growing chicks from the aerial predators require more food. Lemmings provide the bulk of that food.

Corticosteroid concentrations were dramatically higher in July after the snow had melted and the high corticosteroid titers appear to be resistant to negative feedback. Injection of a synthetic corticosteroid, dexamethasone (see Chapter 6 and Figures 10.30–10.32) failed to reduce corticosterone concentrations. There is no evidence that females in July are facing chronic stress, however. In fact, juveniles are plentiful during both periods, which indicates reproductive success and suggests that animals were healthy. Furthermore, male lemmings do not show the same corticosteroid differences between June and July (Romero et al. 2008). Anecdotal evidence from counting the sex of lemming carcasses in snowy owl nests suggests that the sex ratio is roughly equivalent in June when there is extensive snow cover, but becomes heavily female biased in July when the snow cover is gone. Consequently, corticosteroid titers appear to track greater predation risk.

iv. The Brood Value Hypothesis

There are many trade-offs of hormone release in relation to life history traits. In species with higher annual adult survival, the adrenocortical responses to stress should be higher (Hau et al. 2010), probably resulting in loss or abandonment of the nest in favor of survival. A multi-species analysis showed that baseline plasma levels of corticosterone were inversely related to length of the breeding season and body size (Hau et al. 2010). As predicted, maximum plasma levels of corticosterone generated by stress series (Chapter 6) were higher in relation to adult survival and were lower in birds with lower body size. Risk-taking by parents in the presence of predators is predicted to increase as the age of the offspring increases or for young born earliest in the breeding season (i.e., with increasing value of the brood). Male collared flycatchers tended to return to feeding more quickly after experimental exposure to an avian predator when young were older or had hatched earlier (Michl et al. 2000). However, females took less risk by taking longer to return to feeding offspring after exposure to a predator, consistent with the "harm to offspring" hypothesis (i.e., that in the face of risk, individuals should be very cautious in exposing offspring to potential harm of predation). Brood value may increase if the brood size is reduced by predation, resulting in more parental effort (e.g., Poysa et al. 1997).

Bókony et al. (2009) conducted a meta-analysis of 64 avian species to assess the evidence for the Brood Value Hypothesis—specifically, when the value in terms of fitness of the current brood is high, then individuals should show greater resistance potential to acute stressors and the adrenocortical response is mitigated. If the value of the current brood is low, then susceptibility to acute perturbations should remain high (lower resistance potential) with a high likelihood of an adrenocortical response resulting in reduced reproductive success. Results of the analysis revealed that species with high value of the current brood showed generally blunted adrenocortical responses to acute stressors (Figure 10.39; Bókony et al. 2009). Furthermore, species with female-biased parental care showed lower adrenocortical responses to the same stressors than males (Figure 10.40; Bókony et al. 2009). Field investigations of Alaska breeding shorebirds showing different degrees of sex-biased parental care fit well with the Brood Value Hypothesis (Figure 10.2, O'Reilly and Wingfield 2001). In species with female-biased parental care, males show greater adrenocortical responses to acute stress, whereas in male-biased parental care the opposite trend was found. Species with no sex-biased parental care showed identical responses in males and females to acute stress (O'Reilly and Wingfield 2001).

Another alternative to the Brood Value Hypothesis is the Workload Hypothesis. Whereas large broods have the potential for increased reproductive success, the increased workload may have fitness consequences for the parents, resulting from increased workload. In free-living house sparrows, Lendvai and Chastel (2008) removed males in a pair during

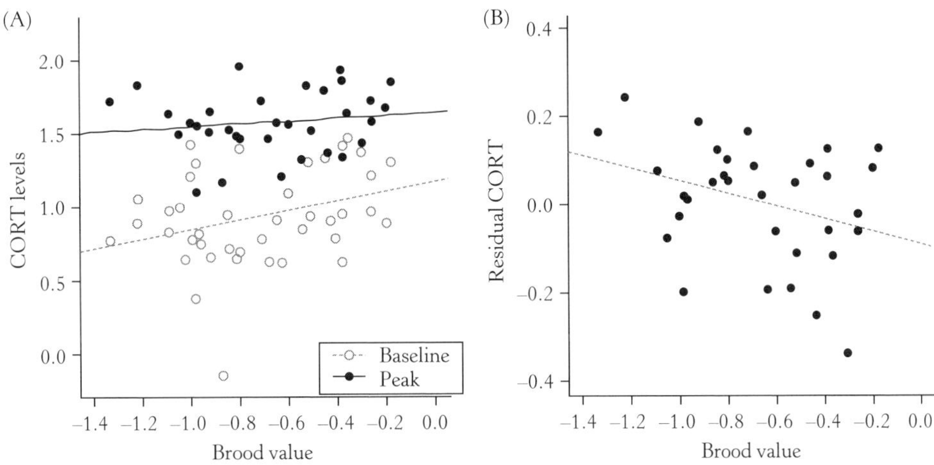

FIGURE 10.39: (A) Baseline and peak corticosterone (CORT) levels (ng mL1; log10 transformed) in relation to brood value. (B) Stress response, that is, peak CORT level controlled for baseline CORT level and breeding latitude (absolute distance from the equator), in relation to brood value. Brood value expresses the putative importance of current reproduction as $\log_{10}$ (clutch size/[clutch size xbroods per year x average reproductive life span]).

From Bókony et al. (2009), courtesy of University of Chicago Press.

the nestling feeding substage of breeding (both males and females feed young). Females temporarily without mates fed young more often but could not compensate fully, and thus nestlings declined in body condition. Females also showed increased adrenocortical responses to acute stress compared with controls, consistent with the brood value hypothesis (Lendvai and Chastel 2008). Note also that Hegner and Wingfield (1987b) showed that in breeding house sparrows, implants of testosterone into males decreased parental care, for which the female could not fully compensate, and reproductive success decreased significantly compared to pairs with a male given a control implant. In a second field experiment, brood size of house sparrows was manipulated. Increased brood size reduced the amount of time that males invested in nest site defense and mate-guarding, and females took longer to initiate a subsequent clutch of eggs and laid fewer eggs (Hegner and Wingfield 1987a). However, overwinter survival was not different between pairs with enlarged broods and reduced broods, and plasma levels of corticosterone were not affected by brood manipulation (Hegner and Wingfield 1987a). It is possible that this level of brood manipulation was not particularly stressful, or that food levels (Eg) in the environment were high enough to compensate for increased Eo. Lendvai et al. (2007) also manipulated brood size in house sparrows and found that parents feeding enlarged broods had a blunted adrenocortical response to acute stress compared with those attending reduced clutches. The latter data are consistent with the Brood Value Hypothesis, but the results differ from those of Hegner and Wingfield (Hegner and Wingfield 1987a). The contrast may result from difference in food available (Eg) to feed young.

In birds, environmental stress results in an increase in corticosterone release to promote survival and a decrease in prolactin release that has the potential to decrease parental effort in feeding young (Angelier and Chastel 2009). Thus it can be predicted that as brood value increases then corticosterone release would be reduced (modulated down) in the face of acute stress, whereas prolactin secretion would remain stable to promote parental behavior (Angelier and Chastel 2009). In the Antarctic breeding snow petrel, incubating birds had higher plasma levels of prolactin than failed breeders who had lost their nest. On the other hand, adrenocortical responses to acute stress were more related to body condition than reproductive status (Angelier et al. 2009b). Injection of ACTH into snow petrels showed that reduced corticosterone levels could be increased markedly compared with control-injected birds. Prolactin was not affected, suggesting that the HPA axis is not directly affecting release of prolactin (Angelier et al. 2009b). This independence of control of the HPA axis and prolactin may allow great plasticity in balancing brood value and individual survival.

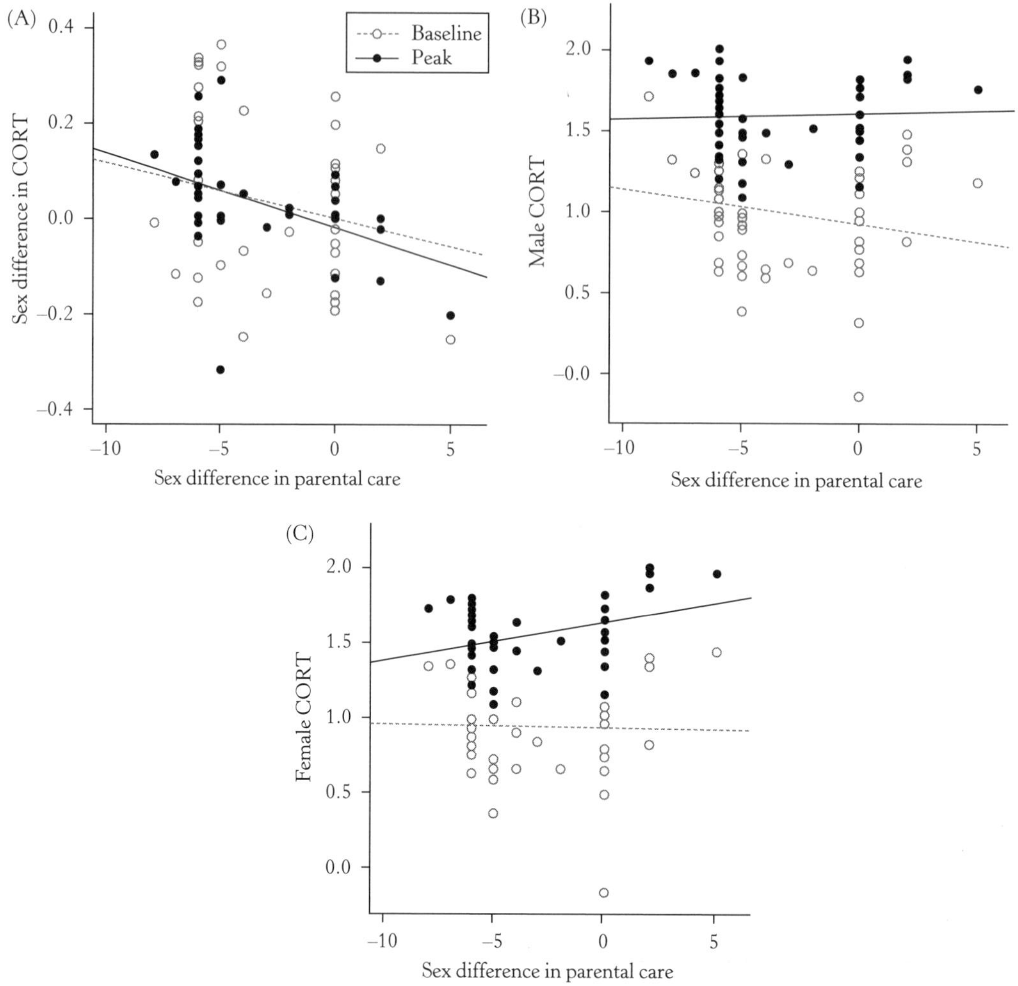

FIGURE 10.40: Sex differences in parental care (greater values indicate more male-biased care) in relation to sex differences in corticosterone (CORT) levels ($\log_{10}$ [male CORT/female CORT]; A), to male CORT level (B), and to female CORT level (ng/mL; $\log_{10}$ transformed; C).

From Bókony et al. (2009), courtesy of University of Chicago Press.

v. Conclusions of Seasonal Regulation

The Energy Mobilization, Behavioral, and Preparative hypotheses are derived from different aspects of corticosteroid physiology. For the Energy Mobilization Hypothesis, the increase in allostatic load is presumed to be the key driver of annual corticosteroid variability. The Behavior Hypothesis, however, suggests that the nature of the stressor is immaterial. Instead, the desired acute behavioral effects of corticosteroids, and specifically the need to attenuate typical corticosteroid-induced behavioral responses, drive the annual corticosteroid variability. Finally, the Preparative Hypothesis proposes that neither the nature of stressors nor corticosteroid's acute effects are relevant, but rather annual corticosteroid variability is an evolutionary consequence of seasonal differences in the risks of being exposed to stressors. The Energy Mobilization Hypothesis currently provides little explanatory power at the broad taxonomic level, but this primarily results from insufficient knowledge of how to compute allostatic load. Once a measure of allostatic load is developed that is independent of corticosteroid concentrations, the Energetic Hypothesis might prove the superior explanation. The Behavior Hypothesis, on the other hand, will likely prove most useful when comparing corticosteroid concentrations within a life-history stage, rather than comparisons across different life-history stages. Evidence for the Preparative Hypothesis is building. It has strong support from laboratory studies and is supported by recent field studies. It is likely, however, that all three mechanisms, as well as the brood value hypothesis, contribute to corticosteroid seasonal variability and that their relative contributions will differ by species. In the end, resolving why corticosteroids vary seasonally will further help us understand how corticosteroids contribute to free-living animals coping with and surviving adverse conditions.

V. INDIVIDUAL VARIATION

Differences between individuals, especially in coping style, can also modulate adrenocortical output. For example, great tits selected for different coping strategies showed overall increases in fecal corticosteroid metabolites in response to a social challenge (exposure to a dominant great tit). However, birds selected for reactive type (slow explorers, more cautious, and less aggressive) showed a strong fecal corticosteroid metabolite response to social stress, whereas those selected for more proactive personality (fast explorers, bolder, and more aggressive) showed very little response (Carere et al. 2003). Individual variation in baseline plasma levels of corticosterone as well as the adrenocortical response to stress varies markedly among individuals. In some cases, this variation can be so broad that means of HPA activity have doubtful value and the ecological basis for such variation becomes a more interesting question (see Williams 2008). A number of studies have commented on individual differences in not only plasma and/or fecal levels of corticosteroids and their metabolites, but also how they can change with development in different ways (e.g., Benhaiem et al. 2012). Behavioral interactions also have dramatic effects either directly or through maternal care, as shown in female mice that show increased fecal corticosteroid metabolites when exposed to soiled bedding of unfamiliar males. This in turn has important influences on maternal effects for offspring (Heiming et al. 2011) as another source of individual variation. High levels of social interactions during adolescence in mammals leads to decreased stress responsiveness as an adult (Lurzel et al. 2011). Indeed, social instability in general can result in changed responsiveness to stress in adults (Sachser et al. 2011), contributing to individual variation in HPA activity (Scheiber et al. 2005). This topic is reviewed in more depth in the next chapter and will not be dealt with further here.

VI. SEMELPARITY

Most vertebrates are iteroparous, meaning that once they reach adulthood they reproduce multiple times. Some are semelparous, compressing their lifetime reproductive output into a single breeding effort, followed by programmed death. Because there is only one breeding attempt, we can predict that the potentially inhibitory effects of environmental stress should be avoided and the typical adrenocortical responses to perturbations should be blunted. It would also be maladaptive for an environmental perturbation to interrupt reproductive function when there is a single opportunity to breed. Semelparity has been discovered in agnathan vertebrates such as lampreys (*Petromyzon* and *Lampetra* sp.), teleost fish, eels (*Anguilla* Sp.), and Pacific salmon (*Oncorhynchus* sp.; Figure 10.41; Dickhoff 1989) and a group of insectivorous dasyurid marsupials (Braithwaite and Lee 1979). Semelparity may occur in other species that are short-lived, but true semelparity is usually accompanied by evidence of programmed death. Typically, semelparous organisms progress through their first reproductive development despite deteriorating body condition and symptoms of severe stress, such as disease, muscle wasting, and cessation of feeding for weeks or months before breeding, all while development of the reproductive system occurs at the expense of body tissues (Larsen 1985).

There has been much speculation on why such a life-history strategy should evolve. Dickhoff (1989) summarizes the literature for Pacific salmon, suggesting that semelparity results because the upstream migration from the ocean, where they spend most of their lives and grow to adult size, is so energetically demanding. The salmon migrate long distances (in some cases, thousands of kilometers) and need to overcome substantial barriers such as waterfalls and rapids. Throughout this arduous migration, the reproductive system is maturing and may eventually comprise more than 30% of body weight. It is plausible then, that by the time they reach their spawning grounds, body condition has deteriorated to an extent that there are no reserves left for a migration back to the ocean. Programmed death may thus have evolved (Dickhoff 1989).

The behavioral and physiological correlates of semelparous salmonids are well investigated. As Pacific salmon mature, they enter rivers, frequently stop feeding, and the gastrointestinal tract

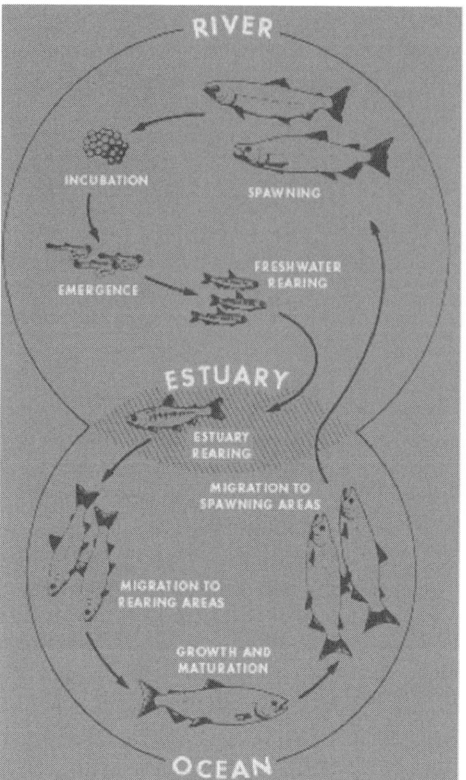

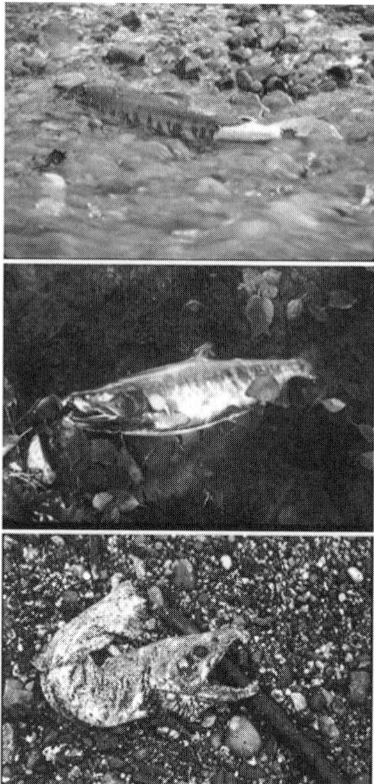

FIGURE 10.41: Schematic diagram of the life cycle of semelparous salmonids. The whole life cycle is ontogenetic with each life-history stage expressed only once. The fish spawn in fresh-water streams and the hatchlings eventually migrate downstream and metamorphose into a sea-going form (smoltification). After varying periods of feeding and growing in the ocean, they return to their natal streams, mate, lay eggs, and then die. Carcasses of the adults may be eaten by other animals or decompose, providing nutrients for the lotic system (right-hand panels). Diagram on the left from www.fish.washington.edu/hatchery/education.html.

Photos by John C. Wingfield.

atrophies as they begin the upstream migration to spawning grounds. Once at the spawning site, usually very close to where the individual hatched, male salmon fight to establish territories and attract mates. Females join in courtship with territorial males and dig nests (redds) in the gravel of streams. These metabolically demanding behaviors occur simultaneously with development of large gonads and mostly without feeding (Larsen 1985; Dickhoff 1989). The initial prediction was that under such conditions, semelparous salmon should reduce sensitivity to acute stressors and avoid interrupting the single upstream migration and spawning event (Table 10.1). Surprisingly, circulating levels of corticosteroids (cortisol) were elevated during the period of reproductive development and upstream migration (Donaldson and Fagerlund 1968). Adrenocortical cells of the interrenal tissue hypertrophied as cortisol titers increased (Fagerlund and McBride 1969) with the possibility of suppressing immune responses, exhausting metabolizable energy stores, especially muscle, leading to overwhelming infection by fungus and bacteria, which eventually leads to their demise (Dickhoff 1989). These data suggest that increasing allostatic load as migration and reproductive development progressed, coupled with zero Eg (they are aphagic), could easily explain hyperadrencortical activity leading to symptoms of chronic stress. Moreover, force feeding of maturing and spawned sockeye salmon in captivity reversed depletion of body condition and infection, resulting in prolonged life for up to 10 weeks (Dickhoff 1989). However, there is evidence that seemingly healthy post-spawned fish die eventually and never initiate a second attempt at breeding. Even the force-fed fish eventually die, suggesting than an endogenous program, or other factors, underlie the semelparous life-history strategy. Landlocked forms of sockeye, the kokanee salmon, which show a very short spawning migration in the upper Colorado River, have plasma levels of cortisol that are also elevated during the spawning migration (Carruth et al. 2000a). This suggests that rising cortisol during the upstream migration of semelparous salmon is not primarily a direct result of increased adrenocortical activity induced by a long-distance migration and salinity change. Some endogenous programmed death may be in operation—but why is there no suppression of the adrenocortical response to stress?

Despite increasing titers of blood cortisol, achieving levels which would result in suppressed reproductive development in most vertebrates, both sexes of Pacific salmon reach full maturity and shed gametes. This is accompanied by high circulating levels of gonadotropins and sex steroids, such as estradiol and 11-ketotestosterone, which peak for several weeks during the migration and before spawning (Sower and Schreck 1982; Dickhoff 1989). This high level of reproductive function occurs despite elevated corticosteroid levels and may actually potentiate hyperadrenocortical secretion. Experiments with captive salmon show that gonadectomy reduces hypersecretion of cortisol (Donaldson and Fagerlund 1970), and injections of androgens into gonadectomized males elevate the secretion of cortisol compared to controls (Fagerlund and Donaldson 1969).

Although the cellular mechanisms by which semelparous salmon are able to breed despite hyperadrenocortical function remain unknown, a possibility is that corticosteroid receptors in the brain and hypothalamo-pituitary-gonad axis could be down-regulated so that migration and reproductive function are not suppressed. Metabolic effects of high corticosteroid levels would be enabled, but without inhibiting breeding. Evidence to date shows that there is a corticosteroid receptor in cytosolic extracts from the brains of chinook salmon showing high affinity, low capacity, and different pharmacology of binding (Knoebl et al. 1996). This might be analogous to type I (MR) or type II (GR) receptors in tetrapod vertebrates. An assessment of corticosteroid receptor distribution measured the number of neurons staining positively for GRir in the brains of kokanee salmon that were sexually immature as well as in mature spawning individuals. The study showed a wide distribution of type II receptors in the brain, similar to what is found in mammals (Carruth et al. 2000b). Interestingly, the pattern of type II receptor expression in brains from spawning fish was similar to those of immature fish, contrary to predictions in Table 10.2. Moreover, olfactory regions revealed greater numbers of GRir neurons with nuclear locations in spawning fish. In contrast, staining for GRir in olfactory regions in immature fish appeared to be largely cytoplasmic (Carruth et al. 2000b). The significance of this difference is unclear.

Another intriguing story of semelparity involves small, shrew-like, marsupials, *Antechinus* sp. and *Phasogale calura*, from Australia. These animals develop to full maturity, then have a short mating period, followed by the death of all males (Figure 10.42; Wood 1970). Females then give birth to young and suckle them (Figure 10.42). After the offspring have weaned, most females die, although a few may breed in a second season (Woolley 1966). The complete mortality of the male population is a true case of semelparity. Removing males may reduce competition for food (Eg) when females are lactating—a period of high allostatic load. Mass death of males may also enable bigger litter size compared to closely related species that are iteroparous. This could be interpreted as a group selection argument, but more ecological studies may shed light on this.

As in Pacific salmon, circulating cortisol levels increase dramatically during reproductive development leading to mating (Figure 10.43; Barnett

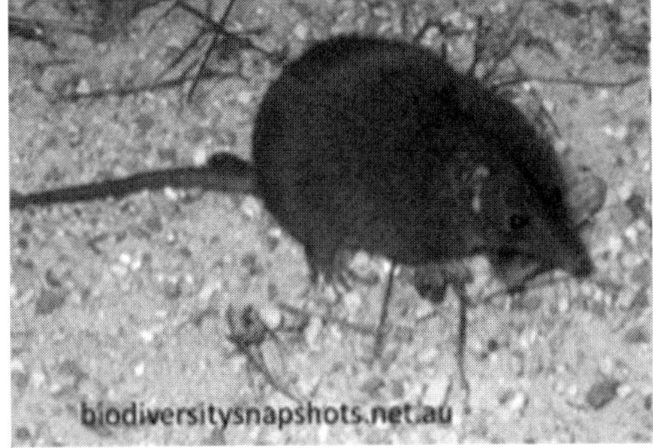

FIGURE 10.42: Life cycle of a semelparous marsupial insectivore, *Antechinus swaisoni*, from eastern Australia. In this species males die after their first mating season while females give birth and suckle young. Once the young are weaned adult females then die (almost all the population). Thus, in this species all males and virtually all females grow, become adult, breed once and then die. Courtesy of the Museum Victoria in Melbourne.

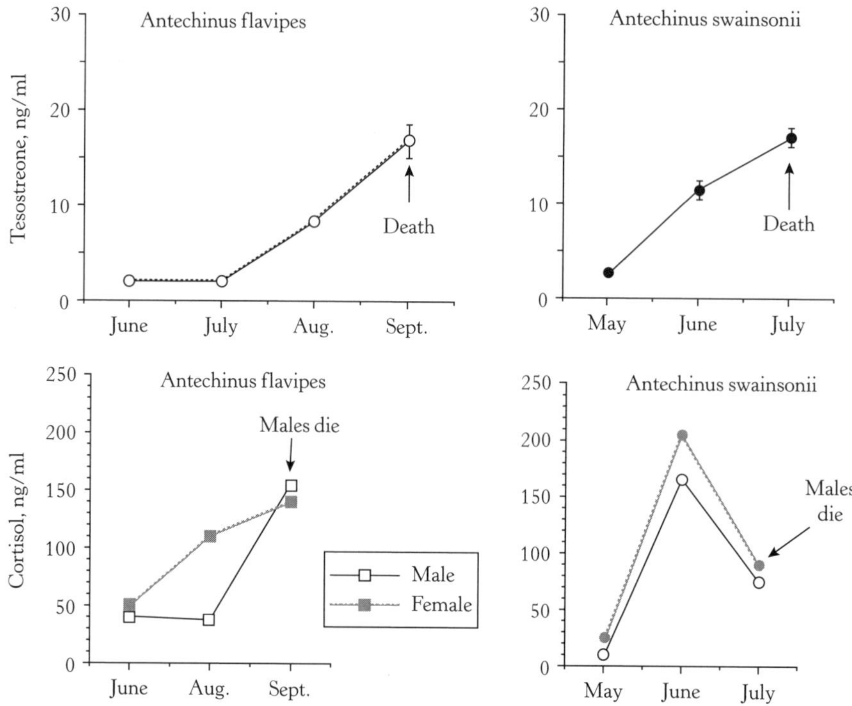

FIGURE 10.43: Patterns of testosterone and cortisol levels in the plasma from two species of semelparous marsupial insectivores, *Antechinus flavipes* and *A. swainsonii*. As testosterone levels peak during the breeding season, all males then die. In *A. flavipes*, females actually have higher cortisol levels than males leading up to breeding, but cortisol titers are identical in males and females when males die. Patterns of cortisol are identical in male and female *A. swainsonii* and even decrease prior to death.

From Barnett (1973), with permission and courtesy of the Zoological Society of Australia.

1973). The size of the adrenal gland also increased in male *A. stuarti* at mating (Barnett 1973). As testosterone levels peak during the breeding season, all males then die. In *A. flavipes*, females actually have higher cortisol levels than males leading up to breeding, but cortisol titers are identical in males and females when males die. Patterns of cortisol are identical in male and female *A. swainsonii* and even decrease prior to death (Barnett 1973). CBG binding capacity in plasma of male and female *Antechnus* sp. also changes during reproductive maturation (Figure 10.44). In August, when testosterone levels are high and males begin to die (Figure 10.43), CBG binding capacity is significantly less than in females, indicating that a large increase in free cortisol accompanies death (Figure 10.44; Bradley et al. 1976; Bradley et al. 1980; McDonald et al. 1981). In combination with the increased cortisol levels, there was a dramatic rise of free, biologically active cortisol. In contrast, in female *Antechinus*, which do not die until after the young have been weaned several weeks later, circulating levels of cortisol are as high as in males, but CBG binding capacity remained high, buffering circulating levels of cortisol (Figure 10.44; Bradley et al. 1976; Bradley et al. 1980).

It is possible that high plasma cortisol levels were a result of heightened aggressiveness of males during this breeding period as they competed for mates. Other changes in adrenocortical function have also been shown. Dexamethasone suppression tests revealed inhibition of plasma cortisol levels two months prior to the mating period, but not during the mating period (i.e., decreased sensitivity to cortisol negative feedback; McDonald et al. 1986). On the other hand, intramuscular injection of ACTH significantly increased circulating cortisol levels in males at both stages of reproductive function, suggesting that responsiveness of the adrenal cortex did not change. High ACTH concentrations also can result in decreased CBG levels (Bradley et al. 1980).

Does corticosteroid hypersecretion in *Antechinus* result in programmed death, as in Pacific salmonids? As mating begins, male *Antechnius* develop classic symptoms of chronic

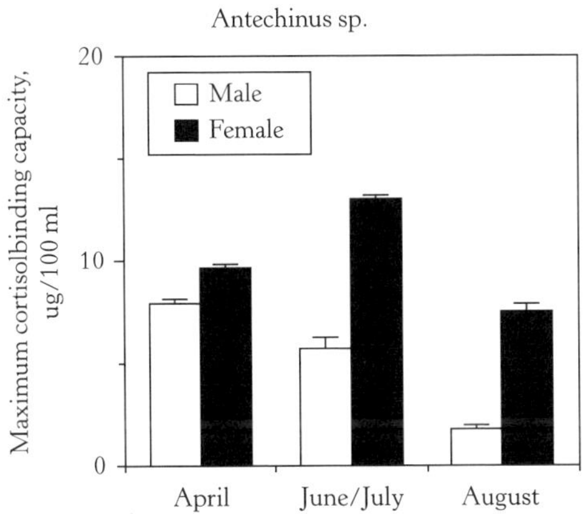

FIGURE 10.44: Corticosteroid-binding globulin binding capacity in plasma of male and female *Antechnus* sp. Note that in August when testosterone levels are high and males begin to die, CBG-binding capacity is significantly less than in females, indicating that a large increase in free cortisol accompanies death.

From Bradley et al. (1976), with permission and courtesy of the Endocrine Society, UK.

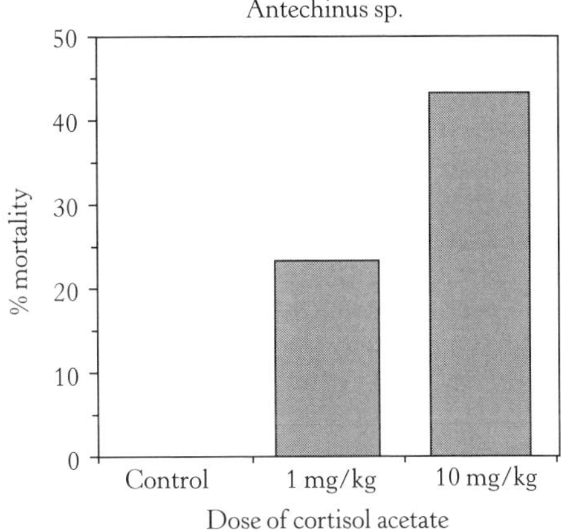

FIGURE 10.45: Effects of injections of cortisol acetate on the mortality of male *Antechinus* sp. Cortisol induces mortality in a dose-dependent manner.

From Bradley et al. (1975), with permission and courtesy of the Endocrine Society, UK.

stress (Figure 10.42), including moderate anemia, elevated parasite load, hepatic necrosis and abscesses, ulcers, hemorrhaging gastrointestinal tracts, and involuted splenic follicles (Barker et al. 1978; Bradley et al. 1980). Immunocompetence in male *Antechinus* was greater than in females prior to breeding, but as mating began, immunocompetence increased in females but declined precipitously in males. For example, serum immunoglobulin titers were lower in males than females, and an increase in endoparasite infection in males was accompanied by the pathologies cited previously (Barker et al. 1978; Bradley et al. 1980). As death approaches, males lose fur and body mass, become lethargic and show signs of being moribund (Figure 10.42; Woollard 1971), nitrogen balance malfunctions, and death ensues (Barnett 1973). Furthermore, intramuscular injections of cortisol acetate into males prior to the mating period resulted in increased mortality in a dose-dependent manner compared with controls, providing evidence that cortisol excess actually plays a role in programmed death in semelparous marsupials (Figure 10.45; Bradley et al. 1975).

As in Pacific salmon, and despite the increased adrenocortical response profile, reproductive function progresses with plasma levels of androgens rising in males to a maximum in August coincident with mating. Sex steroid levels then decline during rapid senescence (Bradley et al. 1980; McDonald et al. 1981; Bradley 1987). This is contra our original prediction that the adrenocortical function should be suppressed (Table 10.1). As also revealed in salmonids, activation of the gonadal axis appears to enable hyperadrenocorticism and subsequent pathologies. When male *Antechinus* are experimentally prevented from mating, they survive longer (Bradley 1985), and furthermore, if males have been castrated they too survive longer than intact males (Bradley et al. 1980). Interestingly, CBG binding capacity in blood remained high in castrated males compared with intact males, and injection of testosterone into castrates decreased CBG binding capacity (McDonald et al. 1981). In addition, males that survive the breeding season in captivity fail to show the increase in cortisol found in free-living males (Schmidt et al. 2006). There are remarkable parallels in the mechanisms underlying semelparity in Pacific salmon and Australian insectivorous marsupials. As discussed earlier, regulation can occur at three levels—control of the endocrine cascade leading to cortisol release, transport by CBG, and target tissue sensitivity.

Many small marsupials in Australia are iteroparous, and males survive beyond a single season. There is no increase in circulating cortisol as in semelparous species, remaining below the maximum binding capacity of CBG (McDonald et al. 1981). Curiously, in a dasyurid that is larger than *Antechinus*, the quoll (which thus presumably can store relatively more fat than the much smaller insectivorous marsupials), all males die after mating and show similar symptoms of senescence to *Antechinus*. Remarkably, there was apparently no increase in plasma cortisol in males—titers were similar to those in females, and CBG levels remained unchanged (Schmitt et al. 1989; Oakwood et al. 2001). Quolls also have a specialized fat storage organ in the tail and thus may be able to endure the mating season by drawing on these stores, preventing protein breakdown. But what triggers death in male quolls? Oakwood et al. (2001) and Schmitt et al. (1989) suggest that programmed senescence may be the cause. Hyper-secretion of corticosteroids in semelparous *Antechinus* may be a consequence of programmed senescence and not its cause.

VII. CONCLUSIONS

In many ways, this chapter was the most interesting for us to write. Modulation of corticosteroid release in response to different environmental conditions, other than circadian variation, is not a phenomenon that has attracted much attention from biomedical scientists. After all, if your research subjects are captive (and usually domesticated) animals held in constant laboratory conditions, there is little reason to suspect the diverse ways in which corticosteroid function varies that are discussed in this chapter. Consequently, these modulatory pathways are relatively new and primarily discovered in free-living animals. However, it is precisely the exploration of how and why corticosteroid function is modulated that we believe will help us understand the physiological role of corticosteroids. Furthermore, many studies to date have been truly integrative, spanning molecular and cellular mechanisms to field studies and ecology. Much of this work is just beginning, and there are many questions that still need to be addressed.

REFERENCES

Addis, E. A., Davis, J. E., Miner, B. E., Wingfield, J. C., 2011. Variation in circulating corticosterone levels is associated with altitudinal range expansion in a passerine bird. *Oecologia* 167, 369–378.

Amirat, Z., Khammar, F., Brudieux, R., 1980. Seasonal changes in plasma and adrenal concentrations of cortisol, corticosterone, aldosterone, and electrolytes in the adult male sand rat (*Psammomys obesus*). *Gen Comp Endocrinol* 40, 36–43.

Anava, A., Kam, M., Shkolnik, A., Degen, A. A., 2002. Seasonal daily, daytime and night-time field metabolic rates in Arabian babblers (*Turdoides squamiceps*). *J Exp Biol* 205, 3571–3575.

Angelier, F., Bost, C. A., Giraudeau, M., Bouteloup, G., Dano, S., Chastel, O., 2008. Corticosterone and foraging behavior in a diving seabird: The Adelie penguin, *Pygoscelis adeliae*. *Gen Comp Endocrinol* 156, 134–144.

Angelier, F., Chastel, O., 2009. Stress, prolactin and parental investment in birds: A review. *Gen Comp Endocrinol* 163, 142–148.

Angelier, F., Clement-Chastel, C., Welcker, J., Gabrielsen, G. W., Chastel, O., 2009a. How does corticosterone affect parental behaviour and reproductive success? A study of prolactin in black-legged kittiwakes. *Func Ecol* 23, 784–793.

Angelier, F., Moe, B., Blanc, S., Chastel, O., 2009b. What factors drive prolactin and corticosterone responses to stress in a long-lived bird species (snow petrel *Pagodroma nivea*)? *Physiol Biochem Zool* 82, 590–602.

Armitage, K. B., 1991. Factors affecting corticosteroid concentrations in yellow-bellied marmots. *Comp Biochem Physiol* 98A, 47–54.

Astheimer, L. B., Buttemer, W. A., Wingfield, J. C., 1992. Interactions of corticosterone with feeding, activity and metabolism in passerine birds. *Ornis Scan* 23, 355–365.

Astheimer, L. B., Buttemer, W. A., Wingfield, J. C., 1995. Seasonal and acute changes in adrenocortical responsiveness in an arctic-breeding bird. *Horm Behav* 29, 442–457.

Astheimer, L. B., Buttemer, W. A., Wingfield, J. C., 2000. Corticosterone treatment has no effect on reproductive hormones or aggressive behavior in free-living male tree sparrows, *Spizella arborea*. *Horm Behav* 37, 31–39.

Astheimer, L. B., Buttemer, W. A., Wingield, J. C., 1994. Gender and seasonal differences in the adrenocortical response to ACTH challenge in an Arctic passerine, *Zonotrichia leucophrys gambelii*. *Gen Comp Endocrinol* 94, 33–43.

Baker, J. G., O'Reilly, K. M., 2000. The effects of age, environmental conditions, and mass on the stress response of Leach's storm petrels. *Pacific Seabirds* 27, 31.

Barker, I. K., Beveridge, I., Bradley, A. J., Lee, A. K., 1978. Observations on spontaneous stress-related mortality among males of the dasyurid marsupial *Antechinus stuartii* MacLeay. *Aust J Zool* 26, 435–447.

Barnett, J. L., 1973. A stress response in *Antechinus stuartii* (MacLeay). *Aust J Zool* 21, 501–513.

Bears, H., Smith, J. N. M., Wingfield, J. C., 2003. Adrenocortical sensitivity to stress in Dark-eyed Juncos (*Junco hyemalis oregonus*) breeding in low and high elevation habitat. *Ecoscience* 10, 127–133.

Benhaiem, S., Dehnhard, M., Bonanni, R., Hofer, H., Goymann, W., Eulenberger, K., East, M. L., 2012. Validation of an enzyme immunoassay for the measurement of faecal glucocorticoid metabolites in spotted hyenas (*Crocuta crocuta*). *Gen Comp Endocrinol* 178, 265–271.

Bókony, V., Lendvai, A. Z., Liker, A., Angelier, F., Wingfield, J. C., Chastel, O., 2009. Stress response and the value of reproduction: are birds prudent parents? *Am Nat* 173, 589–598.

Boonstra, R., Hubbs, A. H., Lacey, E. A., McColl, C. J., 2001. Seasonal changes in glucocorticoid and testosterone concentrations in free-living arctic ground squirrels from the boreal forest of the Yukon. *Can J Zool* 79, 49–58.

Boswell, T., Woods, S. C., Kenagy, G. J., 1994. Seasonal changes in body mass, insulin, and glucocorticoids of free-living golden-mantled ground squirrels. *Gen Comp Endocrinol* 96, 339–346.

Bradley, A. J., 1985. Steroid binding proteins and life history in marsupials. In: Lofts, B., Holmes, W. N. (Eds.), *Current trends in comparative endocrinology.* Hong Kong University Press, Hong Kong, pp. 269–270.

Bradley, A. J., 1987. Stress and mortality in the red-tailed phasogale, *Phasogale calura* (Marsupalia: Dasyuridae). *Gen Comp Endocrinol* 67, 85–100.

Bradley, A. J., McDonald, I. R., Lee, A. K., 1975. Effect of exogenous cortisol on mortality of a dasyurid marsupial. *J Endocrinol* 66, 281–282.

Bradley, A. J., McDonald, I. R., Lee, A. K., 1976. Corticosteroid-binding globulin and mortality in a dasyurid marsupial. *J Endocrinol* 70, 323–324.

Bradley, A. J., McDonald, I. R., Lee, A. K., 1980. Stress and mortality in a small marsupial (*Antechinus stuartii*, Macleay). *Gen Comp Endocrinol* 40, 188–200.

Braithwaite, R. W., Lee, A. K., 1979. Mammalian example of semelparity. *Am Nat* 113, 151–155.

Breuner, C. W., Greenberg, A. L., Wingfield, J. C., 1998. Noninvasive corticosterone treatment rapidly increases activity in Gambel's white-crowned sparrows (*Zonotrichia leucophrys gambelii*). *Gen Comp Endocrinol* 111, 386–394.

Breuner, C. W., Orchinik, M., 2001. Seasonal regulation of membrane and intracellular corticosteroid receptors in the house sparrow brain. *J Neuroendocrinol* 13, 412–420.

Breuner, C. W., Orchinik, M., 2002. Beyond carrier proteins: Plasma binding proteins as mediators of corticosteroid action in vertebrates. *J Endocrinol* 175, 99–112.

Breuner, C. W., Orchinik, M., Hahn, T. P., Meddle, S. L., Moore, I. T., Owen-Ashley, N. T., Sperry, T. S., Wingfield, J. C., 2003. Differential mechanisms for regulation of the stress response across latitudinal gradients. *Am J Physiol* 285, R594–R600.

Breuner, C. W., Wingfield, J. C., 2000. Rapid behavioral response to corticosterone varies with photoperiod and dose. *Horm Behav* 37, 23.

Breuner, C. W., Wingfield, J. C., Romero, L. M., 1999. Diel rhythms of basal and stress-induced corticosterone in a wild, seasonal vertebrate, Gambel's white-crowned sparrow. *J Exp Zool* 284, 334–342.

Buckley, T. M., Schatzberg, A. F., 2005. Review: On the interactions of the hypothalamic-pituitary-adrenal (HPA) axis and sleep: Normal HPA axis activity and circadian rhythm, exemplary sleep disorders. *J Clin Endocrinol Metab* 90, 3106–3114.

Busch, D. S., Robinson, W. D., Robinson, T. R., Wingfield, J. C., 2011. Influence of proximity to a geographical range limit on the physiology of a tropical bird. *J Anim Ecol* 80, 640–649.

Carere, C., Groothuis, T. G. G., Moestl, E., Daan, S., Koolhaas, J. M., 2003. Fecal corticosteroids in a territorial bird selected for different personalities: Daily rhythm and the response to social stress. *Horm Behav* 43, 540–548.

Carlson, A. A., Manser, M. B., Young, A. J., Russell, A. F., Jordan, N. R., McNeilly, A. S., Clutton-Brock, T., 2006. Cortisol levels are positively associated with pup-feeding rates in male meerkats. *Proc R Soc Lond B* 273, 571–577.

Carroll, B., Feinberg, M., Greden, J., 1981. A specific laboratory test for the diagnosis of melancholia. *Arch Gen Psychiatry* 38, 15–23.

Carruth, L. L., Dores, R. M., Maldonado, T. A., Norris, D. O., Ruth, T., Jones, R. E., 2000a. Elevation of plasma cortisol during the spawning migration of landlocked kokanee salmon (*Oncorhynchus nerka kennerlyi*). *Comp Biochem Physiol C* 127, 123–131.

Carruth, L. L., Jones, R. E., Norris, D. O., 2000b. Cell density and intracellular translocation of glucocorticoid receptor-immunoreactive neurons in the kokanee salmon (*Oncorhynchus nerka kennerlyi*) brain, with an emphasis on the olfactory system. *Gen Comp Endocrinol* 117, 66–76.

Carsia, R. V., John-Alder, H., 2003. Seasonal alterations in adrenocortical cell function associated with stress-responsiveness and sex in the eastern fence lizard (*Sceloporus undulatus*). *Horm Behav* 43, 408–420.

Carsia, R. V., McIlroy, P. J., Cox, R. M., Barrett, M., John-Aldere, H. B., 2008. Gonadal modulation of in vitro steroidogenic properties of dispersed adrenocortical cells from Sceloporus lizards. *Gen Comp Endocrinol* 158, 202–210.

Cartledge, V. A., Jones, S. M., 2007. Does adrenal responsiveness vary with sex and reproductive status in *Egernia whitii*, a viviparous skink? *Gen Comp Endocrinol* 150, 132–139.

Cote, J., Clobert, J., Poloni, L. M., Haussy, C., Meylan, S., 2010. Food deprivation modifies corticosterone-dependent behavioural shifts in the common lizard. *Gen Comp Endocrinol* 166, 142–151.

Criscuolo, F., Chastel, O., Bertile, F., Gabrielsen, G. W., Le Maho, Y., Raclot, T., 2005. Corticosterone alone does not trigger a short term behavioural shift in incubating female common eiders *Somateria mollissima*, but does modify long term reproductive success. *J Avian Biol* 36, 306–312.

Dallman, M. F., la Fleur, S. E., Pecoraro, N. C., Gomez, F., Houshyar, H., Akana, S. F., 2004. Minireview: Glucocorticoids—food intake, abdominal obesity, and wealthy nations in 2004. *Endocrinology* 145, 2633–2638.

Dallman, M. F., Strack, A. M., Akana, S. F., Bradbury, M. J., Hanson, E. S., Scribner, K. A., Smith, M., 1993. Feast and famine: Critical role of glucocorticoids with insulin in daily energy flow. *Front Neuroendocrinol* 14, 303–347.

Darlington, D. N., Chew, G., Ha, T., Keil, L. C., Dallman, M. F., 1990. Corticosterone, but not glucose, treatment enables fasted adrenalectomized rats to survive moderate hemorrhage. *Endocrinology* 127, 766–772.

DeNardo, D. F., Sinervo, B., 1994. Effects of corticosterone on activity and home-range size of free-ranging male lizards. *Horm Behav* 28, 53–65.

Denari, D., Ceballos, N. R., 2006. Cytosolic glucocorticoid receptor in the testis of *Bufo arenarum*: Seasonal changes in its binding parameters. *Gen Comp Endocrinol* 147, 247–254.

Deviche, P., Breuner, C., Orchinik, M., 2001. Testosterone, corticosterone, and photoperiod interact to regulate plasma levels of binding globulin and free steroid hormone in Dark-eyed Juncos, Junco hyemalis. *GenCompar Endocrinol* 122, 67–77.

Deviche, P., Heyns, W., Balthazart, J., Hendrick, J. C., 1979. Inhibition of LH plasma-levels by corticosterone administration in the male duckling (Anas platyrhynchos). *IRCS Medical Sci Biochem* 7, 622–622.

Dickens, M. J., Nephew, B. C., Romero, L. M., 2006. Captive European starlings (*Sturnus vulgaris*) in breeding condition show an increased cardiovascular stress response to intruders. *Physiol Biochem Zool* 79, 937–943.

Dickhoff, W. W., 1989. Salmonids and annual fishes: death after sex. In: *Development, maturation, and senescence of neuroendocrine systems: A comparative approach*. Academic Press, New York, pp. 253–266.

Donaldson, E. M., Fagerlund, U. H. M., 1968. Changes in cortisol dynamics of sockeye salmon (*Oncorhynchus nerka*) resulting from sexual maturation. *Gen Comp Endocrinol* 11, 552–561.

Donaldson, E. M., Fagerlund, U. H. M., 1970. Effects of sexual maturation and gonadectomy at sexual maturity on cortisol secretion rate in sockeye salmon (*Oncorhynchus nerka*). *J Fish Res Bd Can* 27, 2287–2296.

Dufty, A. M. Jr, Belthoff, J. R., 1997. Corticosterone and the stress response in young western screech-owls: Effects of captivity, gender, and activity period. *Physiol Zool* 70, 143–149.

Dunlap, K. D., Schall, J. J., 1995. Hormonal alterations and reproductive inhibition in male fence lizards (*Sceloporus occidentalis*) infected with the malarial parasite *Plasmodium mexicanum*. *Physiol Zool* 68, 608–621.

Fagerlund, U. H. M., Donaldson, E. M., 1969. Effect of androgens on distribution and secretion of cortisol in gonadectomized male sockeye salmon (*Oncorhynchus nerka*). *Gen Comp Endocrinol* 12, 438–448.

Fagerlund, U. H. M., McBride, J. R., 1969. Suppression by dexamethasone of interrenal activity in adult sockeye salmon (*Oncorhynchus nerka*). *Gen Comp Endocrinol* 12, 651–657.

Goymann, W., Wingfield, J. C., 2004. Allostatic load, social status and stress hormones: the costs of social status matter. *Anim Behav* 67, 591–602.

Gray, J. M., Yarian, D., Ramenofsky, M., 1990. Corticosterone, foraging behavior, and metabolism in dark-eyed juncos, *Junco hyemalis*. *Gen Comp Endocrinol* 79, 375–384.

Gregory, L. F., Gross, T. S., Bolten, A. B., Bjorndal, K. A., Guillette, L. J., Jr., 1996. Plasma corticosterone concentrations associated with acute captivity stress in wild loggerhead sea turtles (*Caretta caretta*). *Gen Comp Endocrinol* 104, 312–320.

Groothuis, T. G. G., Muller, W., von Engelhardt, N., Carere, C., Eising, C., 2005. Maternal hormones as a tool to adjust offspring phenotype in avian species. *Neurosci Biobehav Rev* 29, 329–352.

Guillette, L. J., Cree, A., Rooney, A. A., 1995. Biology of stress: interactions with reproduction, immunology and intermediary metabolism. In: Warwick, C., Frye, F. L., Murphy, J. B. (Eds.), *Health and welfare of captive reptiles*. Chapman & Hall, London, pp. 32–81.

Hau, M., Ricklefs, R. E., Wikelski, M., Lee, K. A., Brawn, J. D., 2010. Corticosterone, testosterone and life-history strategies of birds. *Proc R Soc Lond B* 277, 3203–3212.

Hegner, R. E., Wingfield, J. C., 1987a. Effects of brood-size manipulations on parental investment, breeding success, and reproductive endocrinology of house sparrows. *Auk* 104, 470–480.

Hegner, R. E., Wingfield, J. C., 1987b. Effects of experimental manipulation of testosterone levels on parental investment and breeding success in male house sparrows. *Auk* 104, 462–469.

Heiming, R. S., Bodden, C., Jansen, F., Lewejohann, L., Kaiser, S., Lesch, K. P., Palme, R., Sachser, N., 2011. Living in a dangerous world decreases maternal care: A study in serotonin transporter knockout mice. *Horm Behav* 60, 397–407.

Holberton, R. L., Wingfield, J. C., 2003. Modulating the corticosterone stress response: a mechanism for balancing individual risk and reproductive success in Arctic-breeding sparrows? *Auk* 120, 1140–1150.

Husak, J. F., Moore, I. T., 2008. Stress hormones and mate choice. *Trends Ecol Evol* 23, 532–534.

Jacobs, J., 1996. *Regulation of life history stages within individuals in unpredictable environments.* PhD Dissertation, University of Washington, Seattle,

Jennings, D. H., Moore, M. C., Knapp, R., Matthews, L., Orchinik, M., 2000. Plasma steroid-binding globulin mediation of differences in stress reactivity in alternative male phenotypes in tree lizards, *Urosaurus ornatus*. *Gen Comp Endocrinol* 120, 289–299.

Jessop, T. S., Hamann, M., Read, M. A., Limpus, C. J., 2000. Evidence for a hormonal tactic maximizing green turtle reproduction in response to a pervasive ecological stressor. *Gen Comp Endocrinol* 118, 407–417.

Kant, G. J., Mougey, E. H., Meyerhoff, J. L., 1986. Diurnal variation in neuroendocrine response to stress in rats: Plasma ACTH, beta-endorphin, beta-LPH, corticosterone, prolactin and pituitary cyclic-AMP responses. *Neuroendocrinol* 43, 383–390.

Kenagy, G. J., Place, N. J., 2000. Seasonal changes in plasma glucocorticosteroids of free-living female yellow-pine chipmunks: Effects of reproduction and capture and handling. *Gen Comp Endocrinol* 117, 189–199.

Kern, M. D., Bacon, W., Long, D., Cowie, R. J., 2007. Blood metabolite levels in normal and handicapped pied flycatchers rearing broods of different sizes. *Comp Biochem Physiol A* 147, 70–76.

Ketterson, E. D., Nolan, V., Jr. 1999. Adaptation, exaptation, and constraint: a hormonal perspective. *Am Nat* 154, S4-S25.

Ketterson, E. D., Nolan, V., Jr., Wolf, L., Ziegenfus, C., Dufty, A. M., Jr., Ball, G. F., Johnsen, T., 1991. Testosterone and avian life histories: the effect of experimentally elevated testosterone on corticosterone and body mass in dark-eyed juncos. *Horm Behav* 25, 489–503.

Knapp, R., Moore, M. C., 1997. Male morphs in tree lizards have different testosterone responses to elevated levels of corticosterone. *Gen Comp Endocrinol* 107, 273–279.

Knoebl, I., Fitzpatrick, M. S., Schreck, C. B., 1996. Characterization of a glucocorticoid receptor in the brains of chinook salmon, *Oncorhynchus tshawytscha*. *Gen Comp Endocrinol* 101, 195–204.

Landys, M. M., Ramenofsky, M., Wingfield, J. C., 2006. Actions of glucocorticoids at a seasonal baseline as compared to stress-related levels in the regulation of periodic life processes. *Gen Comp Endocrinol* 148, 132–149.

Larsen, L. O., 1985. The role of hormones in reproduction and death in lampreys and other species which reproduce once and die. In: Lofts, B., Holmes, W. N. (Eds.), *Current trends in comparative endocrinology.* Academic Press, New York, pp. 613–616.

Lattin, C. R., Bauer, C. M., de Bruijn, R., Romero, L. M., 2012. Hypothalamus-pituitary-adrenal axis activity and the subsequent response to chronic stress differ depending upon life history stage. *Gen Comp Endocrinol* 178, 494–501.

Leary, C. J., Garcia, A. M., Knapp, R., 2006a. Elevated corticosterone levels elicit non-calling mating tactics in male toads independently of changes in circulating androgens. *Horm Behav* 49, 425–432.

Leary, C. J., Garcia, A. M., Knapp, R., 2006b. Stress hormone is implicated in satellite-caller associations and sexual selection in the Great Plains toad. *Am Nat* 168, 431–440.

Leary, C. J., Garcia, A. M., Knapp, R., Hawkins, D. L., 2008. Relationships among steroid hormone levels, vocal effort and body condition in an explosive-breeding toad. *Anim Behav* 76, 175–185.

Lendvai, A. Z., Chastel, O., 2008. Experimental mate-removal increases the stress response of female house sparrows: The effects of offspring value? *Horm Behav* 53, 395–401.

Lendvai, A. Z., Giraudeau, M., Chastel, O., 2007. Reproduction and modulation of the stress response: An experimental test in the house sparrow. *Proc R Soc Lond B* 274, 391–397.

Li, D. M., Wang, G., Wingfield, J. C., Zhang, Z., Ding, C. Q., Lei, F. M., 2008. Seasonal changes in adrenocortical responses to acute stress in Eurasian tree sparrow (Passer montanus) on the Tibetan Plateau: Comparison with house sparrow (P. domesticus) in North America and with the migratory P. domesticus in Qinghai Province. *Gen Comp Endocrinol* 158, 47–53.

Love, O. P., Breuner, C. W., Vézina, F., Williams, T. D., 2004. Mediation of a corticosterone-induced reproductive conflict. *Horm Behav* 46, 59–65.

Lu, W., Worthington, J., Riccardi, D., Balment, R. J., McCrohan, C. R., 2007. Seasonal changes in peptide, receptor and ion channel mRNA expression in the caudal neurosecretory system of the European flounder (*Platichthys flesus*). *Gen Comp Endocrinol* 153, 262–272.

Lurzel, S., Kaiser, S., Sachser, N., 2011. Social interaction decreases stress responsiveness during adolescence. *Psychoneuroendocrinology* 36, 1370–1377.

Lynn, S. E., Breuner, C.W., Wingfield, J. C., 2003. Short-term fasting affects locomotor activity, corticosterone, and corticosterone binding globulin in a migratory songbird. *Horm Behav* 43, 150–157.

Malisch, J. L., Breuner, C. W., 2010. Steroid-binding proteins and free steroids in birds. *Mol Cell Endocrinol* 316, 42–52.

Marra, P. P., Lampe, K. T., Tedford, B. L., 1995. Plasma corticosterone levels in two species of *Zonotrichia* sparrows under captive and free-living conditions. *Wilson Bull* 107, 296–305.

Mason, G., 1998. The physiology of the hunted deer. *Nature* 391, 22.

McDonald, I. R., Lee, A. K., Bradley, A. J., Than, K. A., 1981. Endocrine changes in dasyurid marsupials with differing mortality patterns. *Gen Comp Endocrinol* 44, 292–301.

McDonald, I. R., Lee, A. K., Than, K. A., Martin, R. W., 1986. Failure of glucocorticoid feedback in males of a population of small marsupials (*Antechinus swainsonii*) during the period of mating. *J Endocrinol* 108, 63–68.

Meddle, S. L., Owen-Ashley, N. T., Richardson, M. I., Wingfield, J. C., 2003. Modulation of the hypothalamic-pituitary-adrenal axis of an Arctic-breeding polygynandrous songbird, the Smith's longspur, *Calcarius pictus*. *Proc R Soc Lond B* 270, 1849–1856.

Meddle, S. L., Romero, L. M., Astheimer, L. B., Buttemer, W. A., Moore, I. T., Wingfield, J. C., 2002. Steroid hormone interrelationships with territorial aggression in an arctic-breeding songbird, Gambel's white-crowned sparrow, *Zonotrichia leucophrys gambelii*. *Horm Behav* 42, 212–221.

Michl, G., Torok, J., Garamszegi, L. Z., Toth, L., 2000. Sex-dependent risk taking in the collared flycatcher, *Ficedula albicollis*, when exposed to a predator at the nestling stage. *Anim Behav* 59, 623–628.

Monamy, V., 1995. Ecophysiology of a wild-living population of the velvet-furred rat, *Rattus lutreolus velutinus* (Rodentia: Muridae), in Tasmania. *Aust J Zool* 43, 583–600.

Moore, F. L., Miller, L. J., 1984. Stress induced inhibition of sexual behavior: Corticosterone inhibits courtship behaviors of a male amphibian. *Horm Behav* 18, 400–410.

Moore, I. T., Greene, M. J., Mason, R. T., 2001. Environmental and seasonal adaptations of the adrenocortical and gonadal responses to capture stress in two populations of the male garter snake, *Thamnophis sirtalis*. *J Exp Zool* 289, 99–108.

Moore, I. T., Mason, R. T., 2001. Behavioral and hormonal responses to corticosterone in the male red-sided garter snake, *Thamnophis sirtalis parietalis*. *Physiol Behav* 72, 669–674.

Munck, A., Náray-Fejes-Tóth, A., 1992. The ups and downs of glucocorticoid physiology: Permissive and supressive effects revisited. *Mol Cell Endocrinol* 90, C1–C4.

O'Reilly, K. M., Kurkinen, J. A., Savage, A. R., 1999. The effect of age and gender on the adrenocortical response to stress in Leach's storm-petrels. *Pacific Seabirds* 26, 42.

O'Reilly, K. M., Wingfield, J. C., 2001. Ecological factors underlying the adrenocortical response to capture stress in arctic-breeding shorebirds. *Gen Comp Endocrinol* 124, 1–11.

O'Reilly, M., 1995. *Ecological basis of endocrine phenomena: Field studies of Scolopacidae as model systems*. Thesis, Department of Zoology, University of Washington, Seattle.

Oakwood, M., Bradley, A.J., Cockburn, A., 2001. Semelparity in a large marsupial. *Proc R Soc Lond B* 268, 407–411.

Owen-Ashley, N. T., 2004. *Environmental regulation of immune-endocrine phenomena in songbirds*. Department of Zoology, University of Washington, Seattle.

Pancak, M. K., Taylor, D. H., 1983. Seasonal and daily plasma corticosterone rhythms in american toads, *Bufo americanus*. *Gen Comp Endocrinol* 50, 490–497.

Place, N. J., Kenagy, G. J., 2000. Seasonal changes in plasma testosterone and glucocorticosteroids in free-living male yellow-pine chipmunks and the response to capture and handling. *J Comp Physiol B* 170, 245–251.

Poysa, H., Virtanen, J., Milonoff, M., 1997. Common goldeneyes adjust maternal effort in relation to prior brood success and not current brood size. *Behav Ecol Sociobiol* 40, 101–106.

Pyter, L. M., Adelson, J. D., Nelson, R. J., 2007. Short days increase hypothalamic-pituitary-adrenal axis responsiveness. *Endocrinology* 148, 3402–3409.

Remage-Healey, L., Romero, L. M., 2000. Daily and seasonal variation in response to stress in captive starlings (*Sturnus vulgaris*): Glucose. *Gen Comp Endocrinol* 119, 60–68.

Reneerkens, J., Morrison, R. I. G., Ramenofsky, M., Piersma, T., Wingfield, J. C., 2002. Baseline and stress induced levels of corticosterone during different life cycle substages in a shorebird on the high arctic breeding grounds. *Physiol Biochem Zool* 75, 200–208.

Rich, E. L., Romero, L. M., 2001. Daily and photoperiod variations of basal and stress-induced corticosterone concentrations in house sparrows (*Passer domesticus*). *J Comp Physiol B* 171, 543–547.

Romero, L. M., 2001. Mechanisms underlying seasonal differences in the avian stress response. In: Dawson, A., Chaturvedi, C. M. (Eds.), *Avian endocrinology*. Narosa Publishing House, New Delhi, pp. 373–384.

Romero, L. M., 2002. Seasonal changes in plasma glucocorticoid concentrations in free-living vertebrates. *Gen Comp Endocrinol* 128, 1–24.

Romero, L. M., 2006. Seasonal changes in hypothalamic-pituitary-adrenal axis sensitivity in free-living house sparrows (*Passer domesticus*). *Gen Comp Endocrinol* 149, 66–71.

Romero, L. M., Cyr, N. E., Romero, R. C., 2006. Corticosterone responses change seasonally in free-living house sparrows (*Passer domesticus*). *Gen Comp Endocrinol* 149, 58–65.

Romero, L. M., Meister, C. J., Cyr, N. E., Kenagy, G. J., Wingfield, J. C., 2008. Seasonal glucocorticoid responses to capture in wild free-living mammals. *Am J Physiol* 294, R614–R622.

Romero, L. M., Ramenofsky, M., Wingfield, J. C., 1997. Season and migration alters the corticosterone response to capture and handling in an arctic migrant, the white-crowned sparrow (*Zonotrichia leucophrys gambelii*). *Comp Biochem Physiol* 116C, 171–177.

Romero, L. M., Reed, J. M., Wingfield, J. C., 2000. Effects of weather on corticosterone responses in wild free-living passerine birds. *Gen Comp Endocrinol* 118, 113–122.

Romero, L. M., Remage-Healey, L., 2000. Daily and seasonal variation in response to stress in captive starlings (*Sturnus vulgaris*): Corticosterone. *Gen Comp Endocrinol* 119, 52–59.

Romero, L. M., Soma, K. K., Wingfield, J. C., 1998a. Changes in pituitary and adrenal sensitivities allow the snow bunting (*Plectrophenax nivalis*), an Arctic-breeding song bird, to modulate corticosterone release seasonally. *J Comp Physiol B* 168, 353–358.

Romero, L. M., Soma, K. K., Wingfield, J. C., 1998b. Hypothalamic-pituitary-adrenal axis changes allow seasonal modulation of corticosterone in a bird. *Am J Physiol* 274, R1338-R1344.

Romero, L. M., Soma, K. K., Wingfield, J. C., 1998c. The hypothalamus and adrenal regulate modulation of corticosterone release in redpolls (*Carduelis flammea*—an arctic-breeding song bird). *Gen Comp Endocrinol* 109, 347–355.

Romero, L. M., Wikelski, M., 2006. Diurnal and nocturnal differences in hypothalamic-pituitary-adrenal axis function in Galapagos marine iguanas. *Gen Comp Endocrinol* 145, 177–181.

Romero, L. M., Wingfield, J. C., 1998. Seasonal changes in adrenal sensitivity alter corticosterone levels in Gambel's white-crowned sparrows (*Zonotrichia leucophyrys gambelii*). *Comp Biochem Physiol* 119C, 31–36.

Romero, L. M., Wingfield, J. C., 1999. Alterations in hypothalamic-pituitary-adrenal function associated with captivity in Gambel's white-crowned sparrows (*Zonotrichia leucophrys gambelii*). *Comp Biochem Physiol* 122B, 13–20.

Romero, L. M., Wingfield, J. C., 2001. Regulation of the hypothalamic-pituitary-adrenal axis in free-living pigeons. *J Comp Physiol B* 171, 231–235.

Sachser, N., Hennessy, M. B., Kaiser, S., 2011. Adaptive modulation of behavioural profiles by social stress during early phases of life and adolescence. *Neurosci Biobehav Rev* 35, 1518–1533.

Sapolsky, R. M., 1987. Stress, social status, and reproductive physiology in free-living baboons. In: Crews, D. (Ed.) *Psychobiology of reproductive behavior: An evolutionary perspective.* Prentice-Hall, Englewood Cliffs, NJ, pp. 291–322.

Sapolsky, R. M., 2001. Physiological and pathophysiological implications of social stress in mammals. In: McEwen, B. S., Goodman, H. M. (Eds.), *Handbook of physiology*; Section 7: *The endocrine system*; Vol. IV: *Coping with the environment: Neural and endocrine mechanisms.* Oxford University Press, New York, pp. 517–532.

Sapolsky, R. M., 2005. The influence of social hierarchy on primate health. *Science* 308, 648–652.

Sapolsky, R. M., Altmann, J., 1991. Incidence of hypercortisolism and dexamethasone resistance increases with age among wild baboons. *Biol Psych* 30, 1008–1016.

Sapolsky, R. M., Romero, L. M., Munck, A. U., 2000. How do glucocorticoids influence stress-responses? Integrating permissive, suppressive, stimulatory, and preparative actions. *Endocr Rev* 21, 55–89.

Scheiber, I. B. R., Kralj, S., Kotrschal, K., 2005. Sampling effort/frequency necessary to infer individual acute stress responses from fecal analysis in greylag geese (*Anser anser*). *Ann NY Acad Sci*, 1046, 154–167.

Scheuerlein, A., Van't Hof, T. J., Gwinner, E., 2001. Predators as stressors? Physiological and reproductive consequences of predation risk in tropical stonechats (Saxicola torquata axillaris). *Proc R Soc Lond B* 268, 1575.

Schmidt, A. L., Taggart, D. A., Holz, P., Temple-Smith, P. D., Bradley, A. J., 2006. Plasma steroids and steroid-binding capacity in male semelparous dasyurid marsupials (*Phascogale tapoatafa*) that survive beyond the breeding season in captivity. *Gen Comp Endocrinol* 149, 236–243.

Schmitt, L. H., Bradley, A. J., Kemper, C. M., Kitchener, D. J., Humphreys, W. F., How, R. A., 1989. Ecology and physiology of the Northern Quoll, *Dasyurus hallucatus* (Marsupalia, Dasyuridae), at Mitchell Plateau, Kimberly, Western Australia. *J Zool* 217, 539–558.

Schoech, S. J., Ketterson, E. D., Nolan, V., 1999. Exogenous testosterone and the adrenocortical response in dark-eyed juncos. *Auk* 116, 64–72.

Sheppard, D. H., 1968. Seasonal changes in body and adrenal weights of chipmunks (*Eutamias*). *J Mammal* 49, 463–474.

Silverin, B., 1986. Corticosterone-binding proteins and behavioral effects of high plasma levels of corticosterone during the breeding period in the pied flycatcher. *Gen Comp Endocrinol* 64, 67–74.

Silverin, B., 1998a. Stress responses in birds. *Avian Poultry Biol Rev* 9, 153.

Silverin, B., 1998b. Territorial behavioural and hormones of pied flycatchers in optimal and suboptimal habitats. *Anim Behav* 56, 811.

Silverin, B., Arvidsson, B., Wingfield, J., 1997. The adrenocortical responses to stress in breeding Willow Warblers *Phylloscopus trochilus* in Sweden: Effects of latitude and gender. *Func Ecol* 11, 376–384.

Silverin, B., Wingfield, J., 2001. The adrenocortical responses to stress in breeding male chaffinches *Fringilla coelebs* and bramblings *F. montifringill*, in Sweden. *Ornis Svecica* 11, 223–234.

Silverin, B., Wingfield, J. C., 1998. Adrenocortical responses to stress in breeding pied flycatchers *Ficedula hypoleuca*: Relation to latitude, sex and mating status. *J Avian Biol* 29, 228.

Smith, G. T., Wingfield, J. C., Veit, R. R., 1994. Adrenocortical response to stress in the common diving petrel, *Pelecanoides urinatrix*. *Physiol Zool* 67, 526–537.

Sower, S. A., Schreck, C. B., 1982. Steroid and thyroid hormones during sexual maturation of coho salmon (*Oncorhynchus kisutch*) in seawater or fresh water. *Gen Comp Endocrinol* 47, 42–53.

Spencer, K. A., Buchanan, K. L., Goldsmith, A. R., Catchpole, C. K., 2003. Song as an honest signal of developmental stress in the zebra finch (*Taeniopygia guttata*). *Horm Behav* 44, 132–139.

Sudhakumari, C. C., Haldar, C., Senthilkumaran, B., 2001. Seasonal changes in adrenal and gonadal activity in the quail, *Perdicula asiatica*: Involvement of the pineal gland. *Comp Biochem Physiol B* 128, 793–804.

Tyrrell, C. L., Cree, A., 1998. Relationships between corticosterone concentration and season, time of day and confinement in a wild reptile (tuatara, *Sphenodon punctatus*). *Gen Comp Endocrinol* 110, 97–108.

Valverde, R. A., Owens, D. W., Mackenzie, D. S., Amoss, M. S., 1999. Basal and stress-induced corticosterone levels in olive ridley sea turtles (*Lepidochelys olivacea*) in relation to their mass nesting behavior. *J Exp Zool 284*, 652–662.

Wada, H., Moore, I. T., Breuner, C. W., Wingfield, J. C., 2006. Stress responses in tropical sparrows: Comparing tropical and temperate Zonotrichia. *Physiol Biochem Zool* 79, 784–792.

Wada, H., Salvante, K. G., Stables, C., Wagner, E., Williams, T. D., Breuner, C. W., 2008. Adrenocortical responses in zebra finches (*Taeniopygia guttata*): Individual variation, repeatability, and relationship to phenotypic quality. *Horm Behav* 53, 472–480.

Williams, C. T., Kitaysky, A. S., Kettle, A. B., Buck, C. L., 2008. Corticosterone levels of tufted puffins vary with breeding stage, body condition index, and reproductive performance. *Gen Comp Endocrinol* 158, 29–35.

Williams, T. D., 2008. Individual variation in endocrine systems: moving beyond the "tyranny of the Golden Mean." *Phil Trans R Soc B* 363, 1687–1698.

Windle, R. J., Wood, S. A., Shanks, N., Lightman, S. L., Ingram, C. D., 1998. Ultradian rhythm of basal corticosterone release in the female rat: Dynamic interaction with the response to acute stress. *Endocrinology* 139, 443–450.

Wingfield, J. C., 1994. Modulation of the adrenocortical response to stress in birds. In: Davey, K. G., Peter, R. E., Tobe, S. S. (Eds.), *Perspectives in comparative endocrinology*. National Research Council of Canada, Ottawa, pp. 520–528.

Wingfield, J. C., 2003. Control of behavioural strategies for capricious environments. *Anim Behav* 66, 807–815.

Wingfield, J. C. (2004). Allostatic load and life cycles: implications for neuroendocrine mechanisms. In: Schulkin, J. (Ed.), *Allostasis, homeostasis and the costs of physiological adaptation*, Cambridge University Press, Cambridge, pp. 302–342.

Wingfield, J. C., 2012. Regulatory mechanisms that underlie phenology, behavior, and coping with environmental perturbations: An alternative look at biodiversity. *Auk* 129, 1–7.

Wingfield, J. C., 2013a. The comparative biology of environmental stress: behavioural endocrinology and variation in ability to cope with novel, changing environments. *Anim Behav* 85, 1127–1133.

Wingfield, J. C., 2013b. Ecological processes and the ecology of stress: The impacts of abiotic environmental factors. *Func Ecol* 27, 37–44.

Wingfield, J. C., Kelley, J. P., Angelier, F., 2011. What are extreme environmental conditions and how do organisms cope with them? *Curr Zool* 57, 363–374.

Wingfield, J. C., Kubokawa, K., Ishida, K., Ishii, S., Wada, M., 1995a. The adrenocortical response to stress in male bush warblers, *Cettia diphone*: A comparison of breeding populations in Honshu and Hokkaido, Japan. *Zool Sci* 12, 615–621.

Wingfield, J. C., Moore, M. C., Farner, D. S., 1983. Endocrine responses to inclement weather in naturally breeding populations of white-crowned sparrows (*Zonotrichia leucophrys pugetensis*). *Auk* 100, 56–62.

Wingfield, J. C., O'Reilly, K. M., Astheimer, L. B., 1995b. Modulation of the adrenocortical responses to acute stress in Arctic birds: A possible ecological basis. *Am Zool* 35, 285–294.

Wingfield, J. C., Owen-Ashley, N., Benowitz-Fredericks, Z. M., Lynn, S., Hahn, T. P., Wada, H., Breuner, C., Meddle, S., Romero, L. M., 2004. Arctic spring: the arrival biology of migrant birds. *Acta Zool Sinica* 50, 948–960.

Wingfield, J. C., Romero, L. M., 2001. Adrenocortical responses to stress and their modulation in free-living vertebrates. In: McEwen, B. S., Goodman, H. M. (Eds.), *Handbook of physiology*; Section 7: *The endocrine system*; Vol. IV: *Coping with the environment: Neural and endocrine mechanisms*. Oxford University Press, New York, pp. 211–234.

Wingfield, J. C., Sapolsky, R. M., 2003. Reproduction and resistance to stress: When and how. *J Neuroendocrinol* 15, 711.

Wingfield, J. C., Silverin, B., 1986. Effects of corticosterone on territorial behavior of free-living male song sparrows *Melospiza melodia*. *Horm Behav* 20, 405–417.

Wingfield, J. C., Lynn, S. E., Soma, K. K. (2001). Avoiding the "costs" of testosterone: ecological bases of hormone-behavior interactions. *Brain Behav. Evol.* 57, 239–251.

Wingfield, J. C., Vleck, C. M., Moore, M. C., 1992. Seasonal changes of the adrenocortical response to stress in birds of the Sonoran Desert. *J Exp Zool* 264, 419–428.

Wood, D. H., 1970. An ecological study of *Antechinus stuartii* (Marsupalia) in a southeast Queensland rain forest. *Aust J Zool* 18, 185–207.

Woodley, S. K., Painter, D. L., Moore, M. C., Wikelski, M., Romero, L. M., 2003. Effect of tidal cycle and food intake on the baseline plasma corticosterone rhythm in intertidally foraging marine iguanas. *Gen Comp Endocrinol* 132, 216–222.

Woollard, P., 1971. Differential mortality of *Antechinus stuartii* (MacLeay): Nitrogen balance and somatic changes. *Aust J Zool* 19, 347–353.

Woolley, P., 1966. Reproduction in Antechinus spp. and other dasyurid marsupials. *Symp Zool Soc Lond* 15, 281–294.

11

Development, Environmental, and Maternal Effects

I. INTRODUCTION

Virtually all organisms, including plants, fungi, and even some bacteria (e.g., Hoch 1998; Li and Piggot 2001) undergo some form of development from a single zygote to a functioning phenotype in a changing environment. This ontogenetic path of development is different from morphological, physiological, and behavioral changes that occur repeatedly from one season to another (Chapter 1). Ontogenetic development is not reversible as the organism goes through specific developmental stages until an adult form is reached. Although there are variations on this theme in semelparous versus iteroparous organisms (Chapter 1), such developmental paths are not fixed but are strongly influenced by environmental effects, including maternal and social influences (e.g., Gilbert 2005; Monaghan 2008). It is generally accepted that environmental inputs to developmental trajectories can have profound influences on fitness by "engineering" a phenotype that is adapted to the conditions under which it developed (West-Eberhard 2003; Pigliucci 2005). However, there are limits to how physical and social environmental conditions and maternal effects can influence development and fitness (Figure 11.1; Monaghan 2008). In many cases, there is plasticity in the phenotypes that develop from a single genome in relation to a given range of environmental conditions (reaction norm, Figure 11.1). As environmental conditions range outside the reaction norm and when parental responses to those environmental conditions also influence development (Monaghan 2008), then there are potential detriments to the fitness of the offspring that develop and eventually may lead to pathologies (Figure 11.1; Monaghan 2008).

In an insightful review, Monaghan (2008) presents some models intended to guide a more mechanistic approach to determining the endocrine mechanisms underlying environmental and maternal effects on development, as well as the fitness benefits (Figure 11.2). We present these ideas here because they have the potential to provide heuristic guidance as to how we may be able to integrate mechanisms with ecology. Figure 11.2a represents the environmental matching hypothesis that predicts expected fitness benefits under various combinations of environmental conditions early and in adult life (Monaghan 2008).

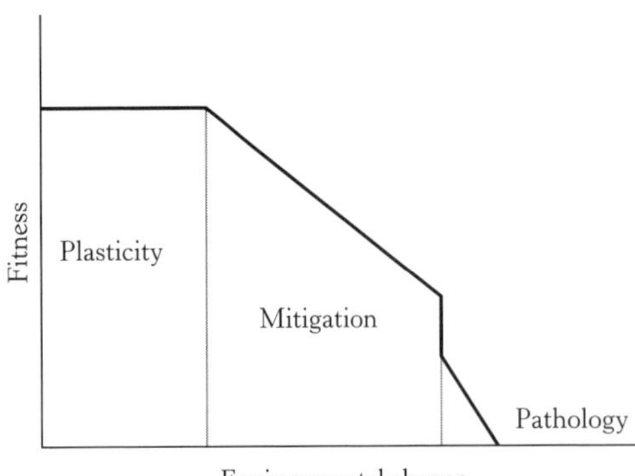

FIGURE 11.1: The effect of environmental change on fitness within the species reaction norm. As the environment during development changes (*x* axis), phenotypic changes will be triggered. Within a certain range of environmental change, no negative fitness consequences result from the development of an alternative phenotype; out of this range, fitness declines as the development of an optimal phenotype is constrained. The fitness decline is initially slow, since the phenotypic adjustments may mitigate the negative effects on fitness, and trade-offs between traits or across life-history stages may occur. Outside this "mitigation zone," pathologies develop and fitness drops dramatically.

From Monaghan (2008), with permission and courtesy of the Royal Society.

An example of an environmental condition, and one most likely to occur broadly, is food supply. Temperature, predators, rainfall, and other factors could also apply. Monaghan (2008) posits four important predictions as follows:

1. For those born in good conditions, fitness is highest under good adult conditions and progressively decreases as the adult environment deteriorates.
2. In good adult conditions, those individuals that developed under good conditions have higher fitness than those that developed under poor conditions.
3. For those born in poor conditions, fitness is highest when the environment matches that of development (i.e., poor), and progressively decreases as the adult environment departs from this (i.e., as the conditions in the adult environment improve).
4. In poor adult conditions, those individuals that developed under poor conditions have higher fitness than those that developed under good conditions. In effect, we have alternative phenotypes; to maintain fitness (i.e., to remain in the zone of tolerance shown in Figure 11.1), the developmental and the adult environments must match.

It is generally acknowledged that offspring that develop under good environmental conditions have a distinct fitness advantage over those that develop under poor conditions (Figure 11.2b; the silver spoon hypothesis; Pigliucci 2005; Monaghan 2008). In this scenario, those raised in good conditions match the environmental conditions as in Figure 11.2a, but those raised under poor conditions have a permanent disadvantage. Monaghan (2008) then posits four more predictions that can be tested:

1. For those born in good conditions, fitness is highest under good adult conditions and progressively decreases as the adult environment deteriorates.
2. In good adult conditions, those individuals that developed under good conditions have higher fitness than those that developed under poor conditions.
3. For those born in poor conditions, fitness is highest under good adult conditions and progressively decreases as the quality of the adult environment deteriorates.
4. Whatever the adult environment, those born in good conditions have a higher fitness than those born in poor conditions.

Under poor conditions, individuals will likely be developing in the "mitigation" zone of Figure 11.1, resulting in lower fitness. Monaghan (2008) goes on to suggest two more scenarios, such as in Figure 11.2c, in which good environmental conditions for the adult will likely result in greater fitness for offspring no matter what the developmental conditions were. On the other hand, a prediction here is that offspring born under poor conditions will have greater fitness than those raised under good conditions when they reach adulthood and begin breeding themselves. This example may be widespread (Monaghan 2008). In Figure 11.2d, a combination of 11.2a and 11.2b predicts that offspring raised in good conditions always fare well as adults, but this advantage deceases as adult environmental conditions become poorer. In contrast, those raised under poor conditions may do relatively better under poor conditions as an adult (Figure 11.2d;

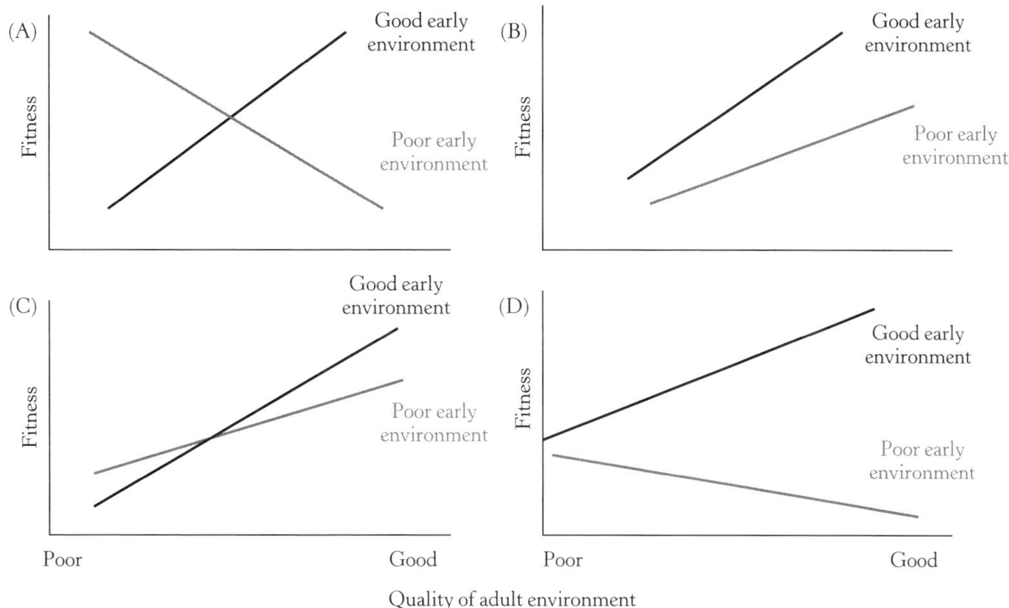

FIGURE 11.2: (A) Environmental matching. Here the adult environment changes in relation to levels of a particular parameter (e.g., resource low to resource high, stress low to stress high). Lines are shown for individuals developing at the low and high ends of the environmental spectrum. For those developing in both good and poor environments, fitness is the highest when the adult and developmental environments match. (B) Silver spoon effects. Here there is no environmental matching. Fitness always improves with improvement in the adult environment, and those born in poor conditions always have lower fitness than those born in good conditions. (C) Fitness always increases with resources in the adult environment, but when these are low, those born in such an environment have a fitness advantage over those not born in such conditions. (D) A combination of the silver spoon and environmental matching. For both those born in the good environment, fitness improves as the quality of the adult environment improves; for those born in the poor environment, fitness declines as the resources in the adult environment increase; however, whatever the adult environment, those born in the good environment always have higher fitness.

From Monaghan (2008), with permission and courtesy of the Royal Society.

Monaghan 2008). This framework may prove very useful for experimental tests of how maternal effects and environmental conditions interact to influence development and fitness.

Given the scope of this book, we now move on to address what mechanisms are involved in environmental and maternal effects on the ability of offspring to cope with environmental perturbations. Specifically, much of this chapter is devoted to how corticosteroids can alter developmental trajectories and can help mediate transitions between different life-history stages. Corticosteroids thus alter the ultimate phenotype of the individual, presumably by serving as the direct intermediary of how the environment interacts with the genome. Corticosteroids, therefore, are major players in phenotypic engineering, or the process of adjusting phenotypes to match the environment (Ketterson et al. 1996; Ketterson and Nolan 1999; Dufty et al. 2002).

II. CORTICOSTEROIDS IN PLACENTA AND YOLK

Hormonal manipulation of the embryo by corticosteroids has been known for many years in mammals (see Chapter 5). Could similar processes occur in non-mammalian species? It is clear that the sex steroids, and especially testosterone, can be differentially deposited in avian eggs (Schwabl 1993) and that the amount of testosterone can have profound phenotypic effects on the resultant offspring (Groothuis et al. 2005). Because the testosterone is of maternal origin (at least before the embryo begins synthesizing its own steroids), yolk steroids are thought to mediate maternal effects whereby the mother manipulates her offspring's developmental trajectories to specific phenotypes based upon environmental conditions (Groothuis and Schwabl 2008; Uller 2008). Perhaps the clearest example is of the mother depositing extra testosterone into some of the eggs of her clutch. The extra testosterone increases the aggressiveness of these chicks, thereby enhancing competition for scarce food during sibling rivalry (Schwabl et al. 1997). In effect, the mother is providing a non-genetic inheritance to her offspring.

It is important to remember that not all non-genomic hormonal modulations of phenotypes in embryos are evidence of maternal effects. In mammals that raise litters, there can be substantial "leakage" of hormones from one embryo to its sibling neighbor in the uterus (Ryan and Vandenbergh 2002). The result can be the masculinization (from androgens leaking from a neighboring brother) or feminization (from estrogens leaking from a neighboring sister) of the offspring. The mother presumably does not have any control over this process, even though the resulting phenotypes can alter fitness (Zielinski et al. 1992; Clark and Galef 1995; Drickamer 1996). On the other hand, maternal corticosteroids are presumed to be much higher than embryonic corticosteroids, and thus more likely to alter the phenotypes of siblings, although this has not yet been tested.

A. Avian Models

Given the central role of the stress response in mediating physiological changes in response to environmental stressors, it would make sense if avian mothers also exerted maternal effects through this system. Although there is some evidence that epinephrine is deposited in eggs in response to stressors (Moudgal et al. 1990), it is not yet known whether deposited epinephrine can alter the offspring's behavior. The majority of work has focused on whether mothers manipulate the deposition of corticosteroids into egg yolks.

To show that avian mothers can exert maternal effects through corticosteroids, two steps have to be shown. First, the increase in maternal corticosteroids must be deposited in the egg. The exact mechanisms for how this occurs are still being debated, but corticosteroid deposition may vary throughout the ovulation cycle (Okuliarová et al. 2010). Second, the extra corticosteroids must have an organizing effect on the growing embryo such that there is a change in phenotype. Avian species are excellent models for these studies because bird eggs are easy to access and manipulate, and birds generally produce only one egg per day. The later feature means that short-term stressors can have an impact on only one individual in the clutch. Evidence is currently building that both steps do, in fact, occur in birds.

Experimental increases in maternal corticosteroids have been accomplished in two ways: both by adding exogenous corticosteroids and by experimentally exposing the mothers to stressors. Both techniques have increased corticosteroid transfer to the yolks of eggs. Examples of exogenous corticosteroids resulting in elevated yolk corticosteroids include Japanese quail (Hayward and Wingfield 2004) and European starlings (Love et al. 2005; Love and Williams 2008a). Figure 11.3 shows an example of increased yolk corticosteroid after exposing barn swallows

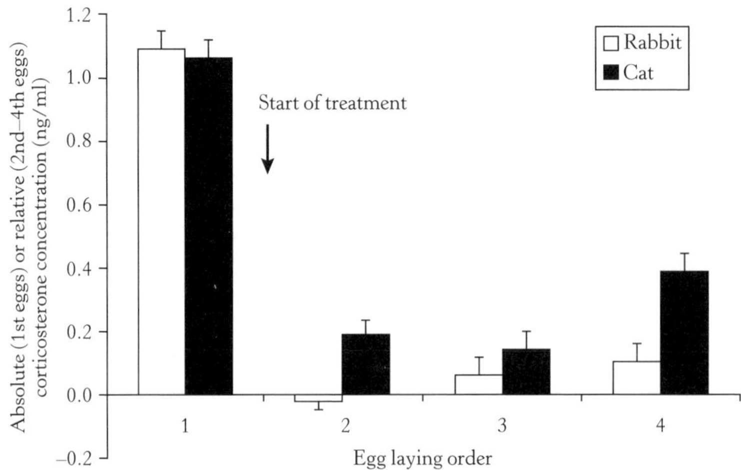

FIGURE 11.3: Effect of exposure to a predator (cat) or an herbivore (rabbit) on corticosterone concentrations in barn swallow eggs.

Reprinted with permission from Saino et al. (2005).

to a predator (Saino et al. 2005). A further example includes southern rockhopper penguins exposed to disturbance (Poisbleau et al. 2009b), but not all experiments that stress the mother result in corticosteroids deposited in the eggs (e.g., Janczak et al. 2007b; Poisbleau et al. 2009a). Furthermore, in quail selected for high and low corticosteroid responses, the quail with higher responses laid eggs with higher corticosteroid concentrations, although a response to a stressor was not additive (Hayward et al. 2005). On the other hand, a number of studies have failed to find a connection between stressors applied to the mother and subsequent increased deposition of corticosteroids in the egg (e.g., Cook et al. 2009).

Once the corticosteroids are deposited in the egg yolk, the assumption is that the embryo will take them up. However, it appears that the embryo has some control over how much of the maternally deposited steroid is actually used (von Engelhardt et al. 2009; Paitz et al. 2010). This fits models of an evolutionary conflict between what is best for the mother and what is best for the individual offspring. For example, using hormones to put some chicks at a disadvantage in sibling competition, and therefore aid in brood reduction, might increase the mother's fitness during periods of food scarcity, but it drastically decreases the chicks' survival probabilities. Consequently, it might not be a good assumption that what is in the egg necessarily will impact the growing embryo. It should also be borne in mind that as far as we are aware, there has been no demonstration of corticosteroid receptors in embryos very early in development and before the production of endogenous corticosterone by the embryo swamps concentrations found in yolk.

A growing number of studies in an ever widening spectrum of avian species indicate that increased corticosteroids in avian eggs, either indirectly via the mother or directly via exogenous administration, have long-term impacts on the chicks. The effects can be diverse, including changes in behavior (Rubolini et al. 2005; Freire et al. 2006; Janczak et al. 2006; Nordgreen et al. 2006), decreases in growth rates and survival (Eriksen et al. 2003; Hayward and Wingfield 2004; Love et al. 2005; Rubolini et al. 2005; Saino et al. 2005; Janczak et al. 2006), and changes in immune function (Love et al. 2005; Rubolini et al. 2005). Furthermore, effects on HPA reactivity are very similar to those seen in prenatally stressed mammals. Figure 11.4 indicates that increased corticosteroids in the egg result in increased HPA responses once those chicks reach adulthood

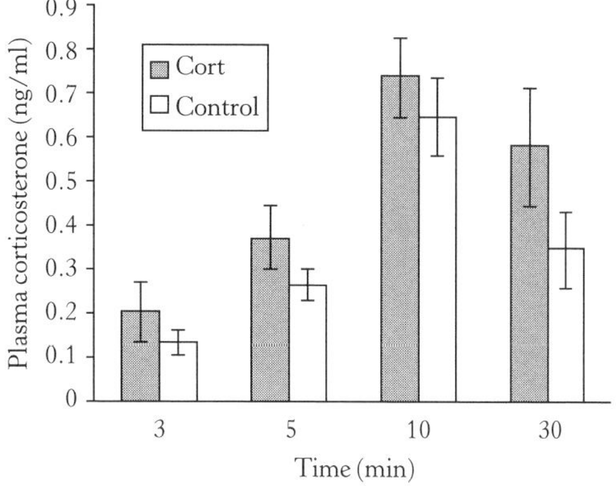

FIGURE 11.4: Corticosterone (CORT) responses to restraint are elevated in adult quail who were exposed to elevated corticosterone in the egg via mothers who were implanted with corticosterone implants during egg laying.

Reprinted with permission from Hayward and Wingfield (2004). Courtesy of Elsevier.

(Hayward and Wingfield 2004). However, the increased reactivity is not a feature of all species, or even with all manipulations. Figure 11.4 shows the effects of increasing the mother's corticosteroids, with the subsequent transfer to the eggs. However, directly injecting exogenous corticosteroids into the eggs had an opposite effect in females and no effect in males (Hayward et al. 2006). Similarly, exogenous corticosteroids placed in the egg yolk resulted in decreased HPA reactivity in European starlings, but applying stressors to these birds after hatch showed the predicted increase in reactivity (Love and Williams 2008b).

There are two potential reasons for detecting differences among species in responses to changes in yolk corticosteroids. First, it may relate to species' differences in life-history strategies. It might not make sense for all species to manipulate offspring phenotypes through maternal corticosteroids. For example, precocial species might not benefit from altering offspring quality, whereas altricial species could potentially use corticosteroids to mediate brood reduction during adverse environmental conditions (Love et al. 2008). Second, it might relate to environmental conditions post-hatch. Potential changes in phenotypes might be expressed under certain conditions, but not others (Janczak et al. 2007a).

Although the preceding data strongly suggest that corticosteroids can serve to mediate maternal effects in birds, recent data question whether the effects are truly a result of corticosteroids.

Corticosteroids are present in low concentrations in the yolk. Furthermore, the corticosteroids that are measured may not, in fact, be corticosteroids. Most studies have used radioimmunoassay or enzyme immunoassays to measure corticosteroid concentrations, but have not verified that the immunoreactivity actually reflects corticosteroid binding. A recent study using HPLC (high performance liquid chromatography) to separate various steroids suggests that the very low corticosteroid concentrations present in yolk are not measured by the antibodies used in the immunoassays (Rettenbacher et al. 2009). Instead, Figure 11.5 indicates that the antibodies are primarily cross-reacting with a number of different progestins. Earlier work had also implicated increases in progesterone in the egg yolk when the mother was exposed to stressors (Bertin et al. 2008). However, if earlier immunoassays truly are only measuring progestins, this raises intriguing questions on why increasing corticosteroids in the mother's plasma result in progestin increases in the egg. Furthermore, it will be difficult to determine what the corticosteroid manipulative experiments are truly telling us. A number of studies have indicated that increasing non-corticoid steroids (e.g., testosterone and progestins) to eggs can also induce changes to HPA function in a manner similar to the administration of exogenous corticosteroids (e.g., Daisley et al. 2005; Bertin et al. 2008). If corticosteroid concentrations in the egg do not change and are not really present, phenotypic changes resulting from the administration of exogenous corticosteroids to the eggs may tell us little about natural physiological and phenotypic changes. Clearly, substantial work is still required to verify that egg corticosteroids do indeed have physiological effects.

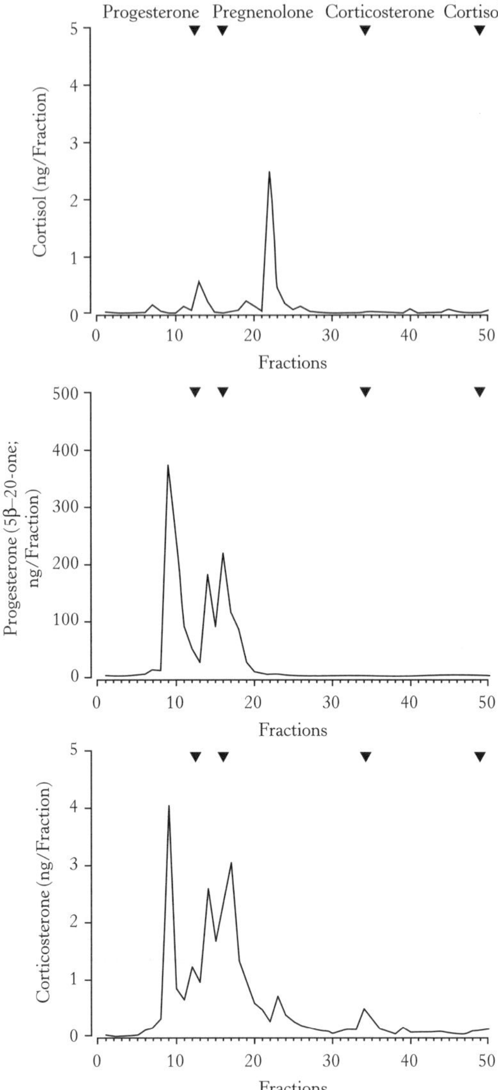

FIGURE 11.5: High-performance liquid chromatographic separations of a homogenized yolk extract. Immunoreactivity was measured with a cortisol, a progesterone, and a corticosterone enzyme immunoassay. Upside-down triangles mark the approximate elution positions of respective standards.

Reprinted with permission from Rettenbacher et al. (2009). Courtesy of Elsevier.

B. Reptilian Models

Unlike both birds and mammals, reptiles include egg-laying and live-bearing species. Both types have been the focus of studies on the role of corticosteroids prior to hatch/birth. In oviparous reptiles, the available evidence suggests that effects of corticosteroids in the egg yolk closely match those discussed in the preceding section in birds. Elevated corticosteroid concentrations in the female can be transferred to the eggs (Uller et al. 2009) and, once in the eggs, can alter embryonic growth (Uller et al. 2009) and anti-predator behavior (Uller and Olsson 2006).

More work has been done on viviparous species, primarily because their reproductive tactic is more similar to mammals in that embryonic exposure to corticosteroids is not limited to the time of yolk deposition. Embryos of viviparous lizards, however, seem to be more resistant to elevated maternal corticosteroid concentrations than are mammalian embryos. Increasing corticosteroid concentrations in the mother, either via natural stressors or artificial implants, can result in altered dispersal behavior (Meylan et al. 2002; Vercken et al. 2007), activity (Belliure et al. 2004; Meylan and Clobert 2004), and decreased growth and survival of embryos in some species (Cree et al. 2003; Meylan and Clobert 2005) but not others (Preest et al. 2005). Corticosteroids applied to the mother also increased juvenile survival rates in one lizard species (Meylan and Clobert 2005), but dramatically increased stillbirths in garter snakes (Robert et al. 2009). However, most of these studies indicate how little is actually changed in the offspring, with the documented changes subtle and overwhelmed by traits that do not change. Evidence suggests that the relatively simple placentas in these species are fully capable of buffering the growing embryos from the mother's steroids (Painter et al. 2002; Painter and Moore 2005), making it unclear how much of the maternal corticosteroids actually cross the placental barrier. If anything, the placentas of these viviparous lizards may be more capable steroid barriers than mammalian placentas. Perhaps as a consequence, the decease in sensitivity to environmental stressors that occurs in pregnant mammals does not occur in those species that have been examined (Cree et al. 2003; Preest et al. 2005), although behavioral mechanisms may allow females to avoid many stressors (Langkilde et al. 2005).

Similar to mammals, there is some evidence that corticosteroids help mediate hatching in oviparous lizards. Injection of corticosteroids into the egg significantly reduced the time to hatching, an effect that was blocked with a corticosteroid receptor antagonist (Weiss et al. 2007). Because lizard adrenal tissue is capable of producing corticosteroids at this period (Jennings et al. 2004), the endogenous corticosteroids that mediate hatching are presumably of embryonic origin. Any corticosteroids deposited by the mother are likely to have long since been metabolized. In contrast and even more similar to mammals, corticosteroids may regulate parturition in live-bearing reptiles as well. The source of these corticosteroids is likely to be embryonic (Girling and Jones 2006).

C. Fish Models

Similar mechanisms whereby corticosteroids are transferred to yolk (or embryos in viviparous species) may play a role in fish (Barry et al. 1995). Damselfish, for example, decrease the quality of eggs, and thus presumably the quality of offspring, when mothers are subjected to stressors of social crowding or increased heterospecific competition (McCormick 2006, 2009a). Once again, the decrease in quality appears to be mediated by corticosteroids. However, the relationship between stress and quality may be complex. Experimentally increased corticosteroids in the eggs alters endogenous rhythms (McCormick and Nechaev 2002) and decreases apparent offspring quality in several fish species (e.g., Eriksen et al. 2006), but the young survived longer in some species (Gagliano and McCormick 2009), and there appears to be little effect on quality in others (Stratholt et al. 1997). However, much like the long-term effects of prenatal stress in mammals and birds, increasing corticosteroid concentrations in eggs can alter stress responses later in life (Auperin and Geslin 2008).

D. Summary

Evidence is building that exposure to corticosteroids during development can have long-term and profound effects on the physiology and behavior of neonates of many species. Increasingly, these changes are being connected to changes in fitness later in life, and furthermore, they appear to result from the corticosteroid stress responses in the mother and thus are good examples of maternal effects. However, there remain some serious questions (for review, see Henriksen et al. 2011). First, it is not yet established how robust maternal transfer of corticosteroids is to the offspring, and at least for birds, whether the primary steroid is even a corticosteroid. Second, not all studies are showing phenotypic changes in the offspring from corticosteroid exposure, and it remains to be determined what the differences are between these species (e.g., Henriksen et al. 2011). Are there life-history differences or species-specific physiological differences that can predict whether corticosteroids can mediate maternal effects? Finally, we still lack a solid theoretical understanding of why a mother might want to phenotypically engineer her offspring. The assumption usually is that maternal corticosteroids can prepare offspring to cope with the environmental stressors facing the mother. This might make sense shortly after birth/hatch. For example, if the mother faces a stressor such as high predator densities, phenotypically altering her offspring with corticosteroids to cope with these predators would presumably provide a survival benefit. The benefit is less clear, however, if the environmental stressor is ephemeral or unlikely to affect the offspring throughout life. For long-lived species, for instance, predator density at birth/hatch is unlikely to predict predator densities throughout life, making the value of the phenotypic adjustments in utero or in the egg less apparent. Fortunately, both the theoretical and the empirical answers to these questions are currently the subject of intense study, and their solutions will have a profound impact on how we interpret the consequences of prenatal stressors in wildlife.

III. STRESS-INDUCED CHANGE IN SEX RATIOS

One interesting potential effect of maternal stress is an apparent skew in the sex ratios of offspring. Mothers faced with changing environmental conditions can alter the percentages of male and female offspring (e.g., Komdeur et al. 2002) (but see Ewen et al. 2004) and even the laying order of each sex (Badyaev et al. 2006). Because male and female offspring have the potential to provide different fitness advantages in different environments or under different conditions, skewing the sex ratio is predicted by life-history theory. For example, a son can mate with multiple females and thus has the potential to produce more grandchildren than a daughter, but only when males are not overrepresented in the population.

There are a number of potential physiological mechanisms that could underlie sex ratio skew (Krackow 1995; Pike and Petrie 2003), and maternal stress is gaining some support. For instance, increased cortisol in human mothers can result in pregnancy loss in the first few weeks after fertilization (Nepomnaschy et al. 2006), and manipulating maternal condition in birds can differentially alter the survival of sons and daughters (Nager et al. 1999). In fact, much of this work has been done on avian species. Because females are the heterogametic sex in birds, female birds could potentially manipulate chromosomal assortment during meiosis in order to skew the sex ratio to one sex or the other. There is a growing body of literature correlating maternal corticosterone concentrations during ovulation with skewed sex ratios. Data come from a number of different species, including Japanese quail (Pike and Petrie 2006), peahens (Pike and Petrie 2005a), pigeons (Pike 2005), European starlings (Love et al. 2005; Love and Williams 2008a). For example, experimental implants of corticosterone within baseline ranges resulted in a skew toward female offspring in white-crowned sparrows (Bonier et al. 2007). In addition, studies on zebra finches (Arnold et al. 2003), treecreepers (Suorsa et al. 2003), yellow-legged gulls (Alonso-Alvarez and Velando 2003), blue-footed boobies (Velando 2002), bell miners (e.g., Ewen et al. 2003), and jackdaws (Salomons et al. 2008) have shown skewed sex ratios after manipulations, such as lower food quality or body condition, that could potentially have resulted in stress. A few studies have also correlated yolk corticosterone with changing sex ratios (e.g., Pike and Petrie 2005b), with the yolk concentrations presumably reflecting the maternal corticosterone concentrations at the time of ovulation. As you can see, the taxonomic breadth of these studies is starting to build. Most of these studies support a pre-ovulatory mechanism for altering sex ratios, with one study suggesting that corticosteroids influence the segregation of sex chromosomes during meiosis (Gam et al. 2011). Although data come from studies using both natural stressors and experimental increases in corticosterone (i.e., implants), most of the data collected so far suggest that increased maternal corticosterone shifts the sex ratio toward females.

What a potential mechanism might be for corticosterone to influence primary sex ratio is not currently known. Increases in corticosterone concentrations may not even be causal, but instead only correlated with other unknown factors. However, corticosteroids are an attractive candidate for forming a functional link between environmental conditions and skewed sex ratio. Tantalizing evidence that corticosterone might be causative comes from species where sex ratios are environmentally determined. In one species (Warner et al. 2009), but not another (Warner et al. 2008), injecting corticosterone into the eggs skewed the sex ratio toward females. Finding a general corticosteroid mechanism for altering sex ratios would be an exciting advance in physiological ecology.

IV. STRESS HYPO-RESPONSIVE PERIOD AND THE ALTRICIAL VERSUS PRECOCIAL CONTINUUM

In many, if not most, species, the brain does not achieve adult function directly at birth, but continues to develop postnatally. The degree of brain development at birth depends greatly on the phenotype of the species. Some species are born relatively immature and must rely on their parents for a period of further development. This developmental strategy is known as altricial. Perhaps the most extreme example of altricial young is in marsupials, where the offspring, known as a joey, is born as little more than a fetus and requires an extensive developmental period in the pouch. Other species are born more somatically mature and rapidly become independent from their parents. This developmental strategy is known as precocial. An extreme example would be a sea turtle that immediately after hatch must dig its way out of the sand and rush for the water, all with no help from a parent. Clearly, a baby sea turtle's brain must be well developed at hatch. Most species are not so extreme, of course, and both birds and mammals show the full spectrum of developmental strategies from altricial to precocial.

A further concept in categorizing the spectrum from altricial to precocial is the difference between nidifugous, meaning that they leave the nest shortly after birth/hatching, and nidicolous, meaning that they stay at the nest. Precocial species are categorized as such based upon birth/hatching with open eyes and the capability of independent locomotion—both of which require a well-developed nervous system (Starck and Ricklefs 1998). Most precocial birds are thus nidifugous. Some precocial species are nidicolous, however, even though they are capable of independent locomotion. The interplay between neuronal development, mobility, and parental care produces the spectrum of altricial-precocial developmental strategies (Table 11.1).

Altricial species especially, however, may potentially have a problem. Their HPA axis is fully developed (because corticosteroids are necessary for birth/hatch) and can respond to a stressor, yet corticosteroids can be detrimental to growing neurons. These two features set up the paradox whereby a robust corticosteroid response during the altricial stage, a response presumably

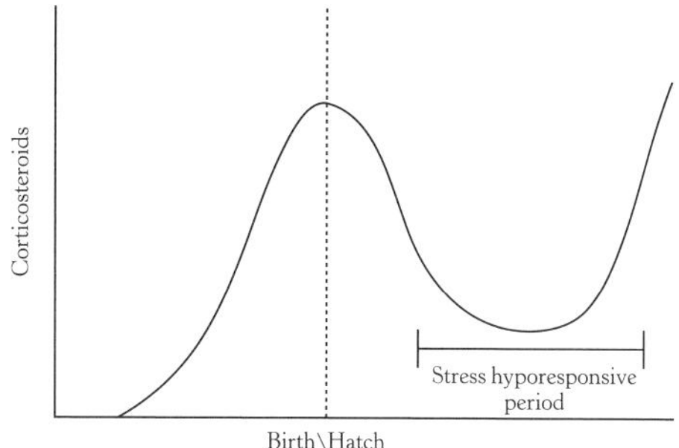

FIGURE 11.6: Schematic of the stress hyporesponsive period (SHRP). Corticosteroids are elevated to facility birth/hatch and then decrease to allow neuronal growth to progress (see also Chapter 5).

mounted to aid in survival of a stressor, could end up decreasing survival by compromising vital neuronal development. In many altricial mammals, the solution to this paradox is the stress hypo-responsive period (SHRP; see Chapter 5 and Figure 11.6). The neonates become hypo-responsive to stressors during the altricial period, thereby relying upon parental aid for survival while maximizing neuronal development. In effect, parental behavior serves as the stress response for altricial offspring.

The logic of having an SHRP in altricial neonates has generated the Developmental Hypothesis (reviewed by Wada 2008). Instead of the all-or-none response of an SHRP, the Developmental Hypothesis posits that an HPA response to a stressor will be stronger and occur sooner after birth/hatch as the developmental strategy moves from altricial to precocial. The Developmental Hypothesis is also an indirect test of the adaptive role of the SHRP. If the SHRP

TABLE 11.1: CHARACTERISTICS OF NESTLINGS

Type of Development	Down Present?	Eyes Open?	Mobile?	Feed Selves?	Parents Absent?
Precocial 1	Yes	Yes	Yes	Yes	Yes
Precocial 2	Yes	Yes	Yes	Yes*	No
Precocial 3	Yes	Yes	Yes	Yes^	No
Precocial 4	Yes	Yes	Yes	Yes/No	No
Semi-precocial	Yes	Yes	Yes/No	No	No
Semi-altricial 1	Yes	Yes	No	No	No
Semi-altricial 2	Yes	No	No	No	No
Altricial	No	No	No	No	No

* = Precocial 2 follow parents but find own food.
^ = Precocial 3 are shown food.
Characteristics of the developmental spectrum from altricial to precocial, specifically as it applies to avian species. Modified and reprinted with permission from Ehrlich et al. (1988).

is truly present to prevent damage to developing neurons, then the SHRP should be absent or attenuated in precocial species, perhaps even with a variable strength of the SHRP throughout the full spectrum of altricial to precocial developmental strategies. The evidence for an SHRP is extensive in laboratory rodents, is compelling in a few other biomedically and agriculturally important species, and is circumstantial in humans (Gunnar and Donzella 2002). Does an SHRP exist in other species, play a similar role in free-living conditions, and does its strength vary along the altricial-precocial continuum?

A. Free-Living Mammals

Since the laboratory data derive primarily from mammals, it would make sense to look first for an SHRP in other free-living mammalian species. Very little work has been done on this problem, but what does exist suggests that an SHRP is not universally present. For example, both Northern (Ortiz et al. 2003) and Southern (Engelhard et al. 2002) elephant seals have lower corticosteroid levels early during nursing than near the end of nursing. Furthermore, the response to restraint is lower shortly after birth, although the pups still mount a fairly robust response (Engelhard et al. 2002). Two studies, however, do not show an SHRP. Laboratory-bred degus, even though they are semi-precocial, have lower corticosteroid concentrations in the days after birth, although similar to other laboratory rodents, they mount a robust response to maternal separation (Gruss et al. 2006). Similarly, free-living baboon infants show high corticosteroid concentrations in the feces, which then decline during the juvenile years (Gesquiere et al. 2005). Clearly, however, these studies are insufficient, both in design and in species breadth, to conclude much about the presence of a SHRP in wild mammals.

B. Birds

The evidence is strong that an SHRP exists in several avian species. In domestic chickens, temperature stressors do not elicit corticosteroid release until about two days after hatch (Freeman and Flack 1980; Freeman 1982; Freeman and Manning 1984), even though the chicks are capable of mounting a response immediately at hatch (Mashaly 1991). There is also substantial circumstantial evidence in a number of free-living passerines (e.g., Romero et al. 1998; Schwabl 1999; Sims and Holberton 2000; Wada et al. 2007; Wada et al. 2009; Muller et al. 2010; Rensel et al. 2010a; Rensel et al. 2010b). An example is shown in Figure 11.7. HPA reactivity is lowest in the youngest chicks, and stressors sometimes fail to elicit any corticosteroid release, but these studies have not fully examined HPA function in embryos or chicks immediately after hatch, although based upon age-dependent corticosteroid receptor changes in the brain, there do not appear to be any changes in negative feedback (Wada and Breuner 2010). Without more data on HPA function, it is difficult to distinguish between an SHRP and developmental maturation of the HPA. Given the data from the laboratory, however, the later explanation seems unlikely. Furthermore, the role of corticosteroids in stimulating lung surfactant to aid in breathing in neonates appears to be conserved (Sullivan et al. 2003), suggesting that the HPA axis will be functional in later-term embryos and that corticosteroids are likely to increase just prior to hatch.

Although the evidence is reasonably strong for an SHRP in passerines, it is more mixed in other avian taxa with altricial and semi-altricial young. White storks (Blas et al. 2005; Blas et al. 2006), Magellanic penguins (Walker et al. 2005), thin-billed prions (Quillfeldt et al. 2009), black-legged kittiwakes (Fridinger et al. 2007), and American kestrels (Sockman and Schwabl 2001; Love et al. 2003b; Love et al. 2003a), for example, show a pattern similar to the passerines, but snowy owls (Romero et al. 2006) and Nazca boobies (Tarlow et al. 2001) do not.

There are very few data available for precocial birds. Most of the data come from chickens,

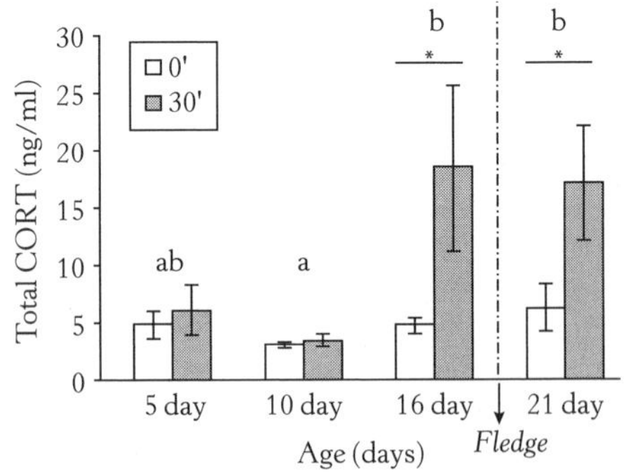

FIGURE 11.7: Changes in total corticosterone (CORT) secretion in response to handling stress, by age, in zebra finch nestlings. An asterisk denotes a significant adrenocortical response within the age group. Different letters indicate an overall age difference in adrenocortical responses.

Reprinted with permission from Wada et al. (2009). Courtesy of University of Chicago Press.

as described earlier. One study on mallard ducks indicated that HPA reactivity fit predictions—an adult-like response was present shortly after hatch (Holmes et al. 1989). The different responses between chickens and ducks appear to relate to steroidogenic capacity in the adrenal gland (Holmes et al. 1992). However, contrary to predictions from the Developmental Hypothesis, fecal concentrations of corticosteroid metabolites decreased after hatch in greylag geese (Frigerio et al. 2001), a precocial species. Interestingly, semi-precocial birds also seem to lack an SHRP (e.g., Adams et al. 2008). Many of these species are seabirds that are restricted to the nest and dependent upon parental feeding. However, these parents are foraging in the ocean and consequently must be absent from the nest for extended periods (often several days). This requires the chicks to be able to thermoregulate as quickly as possible. It appears that rapid maturation of thermoregulatory ability supports the absence of an SHRP, presumably because much of the neuron growth has already occurred.

One other feature of stress during early development also appears to be present in avian species. Individual variation in HPA reactivity of laboratory rodent pups depends a great deal on the degree of parental care (see Chapter 5). Likewise, the time spent away from the nest by female Florida scrub-jays correlated with nestling corticosteroid levels (Rensel et al. 2010b). The more time the female was absent, the higher the nestlings' corticosteroid levels (Figure 11.8).

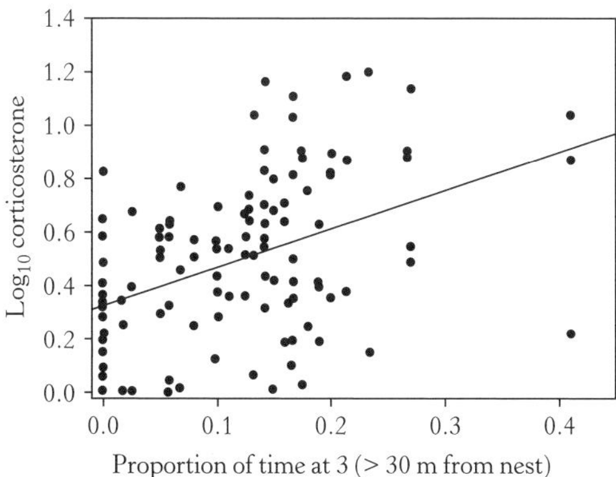

FIGURE 11.8: Nestling corticosterone regressed against the proportion of time that female breeders were away from the nest area in Florida scrub-jays. Category 3 refers to female breeders who have traveled at least 30 meters and out of sight of the observer.

Reprinted with permission from Rensel et al. (2010b). Courtesy of Elsevier.

Similarly, manipulating clutch size in nestlings can lead to different levels of testosterone deposited in the eggs when those nestlings become adults (Gil et al. 2004).

It is not yet clear whether the effects of stress in neonatal birds are long lasting, as occurs in rodents. It does appear that birds can modify HPA reactivity in their adult offspring by varying parental investment (Rensel et al. 2010b), and food restriction during development can alter HPA responses in adults in a number of species (e.g., Kitaysky et al. 2003; Pravosudov and Kitaysky 2006). However, other evidence suggests that HPA changes may be more ephemeral. A study of house sparrows indicated that manipulation of brood size changed HPA reactivity, with chicks from enlarged broods showing higher corticosteroid responses than chicks from small broods (Lendvai et al. 2009). However, this change disappeared a year later when these chicks became adults. It thus appears that we cannot assume that laboratory rodent models of neonatal stress will always apply to field conditions.

C. Reptiles

Few studies have explored whether there is an SHRP in reptiles. Corticosteroid concentrations do increase in the embryo prior to hatch in American alligators (Medler and Lance 1998), which has been linked to lung surfactant production (Sullivan et al. 2003). What is not known is whether this embryonic response continues or is attenuated after hatch (or birth in live-bearing species). In two closely related species of mountain spiny lizard, one viviparous and one oviparous, corticosteroid concentrations were elevated in the first few days postnatal compared to adults (Painter et al. 2002). In green sea turtles the evidence suggests that this species does appear to follow the Developmental Hypothesis. Corticosteroids spike as the hatchlings dig out of the sand and remain elevated for at least the first few hours of swimming out to sea (Hamann et al. 2007). There is thus no evidence for an SHRP in this species. Furthermore, data suggest that corticosteroids remain elevated throughout the juvenile period and only decline as the turtles reach breeding age (Jessop and Hamann 2005).

D. Amphibians

In contrast to reptiles, birds, and mammals, amphibians have a larval stage that is usually highly precocial. There are some exceptions where adults may carry larvae on the back (e.g.,

Wells 1977; Weygoldt 1987) or, in one exceptional case, carry eggs and larvae in the stomach, eventually regurgitating (analogous to giving birth) metamorphosed young (Corben et al. 1974). Corticosteroids have similar detrimental effects in growing larval amphibians by inhibiting growth (Glennemeier and Denver 2002a, 2002b). Consequently, it would make sense for amphibians to inhibit corticosteroid release prior to metamorphosis in a way that would be akin to an SHRP. This does occur in some species (e.g., Glennemeier and Denver 2001) but not in others (e.g., Glennemeier and Denver 2001). In the Pacific treefrog, tadpoles exposed to confinement stress in the field showed increases in whole-body corticosterone concentrations (Figure 11.9; Belden et al. 2005). Furthermore, treatment of tadpoles with corticosterone in water slowed growth (Figure 11.10; Belden et al. 2005), although the authors were careful to point out that corticosterone concentrations in treated tadpoles were higher than those induced by confinement stress in free-living tadpoles. The results, and those of other studies in which tadpoles were treated with corticosterone, should be interpreted with caution. Nonetheless, the presence of an SHRP is likely present in many species.

The developmental trajectory is sufficiently different and variable in amphibians that it is not clear whether comparing corticosteroid concentrations before and during metamorphosis is truly good evidence for an SHRP. The increase in corticosteroids is clearly part of metamorphosis and is also a result of the central role that CRF plays in regulating the metamorphic climax (Denver 2009). A similar burst of corticosteroids occurs during mammalian parturition (see later discussion in this chapter). If the developmental stage most closely analogous to mammalian birth is the metamorphic transition, rather than hatching, then the time to look for the presence of an SHRP is shortly after the metamorphic climax. This period does not appear to have been examined for differences in corticosteroid responses. Furthermore, it is not clear how much neuronal remodeling takes place after metamorphosis, so that an SHRP might not even be expected.

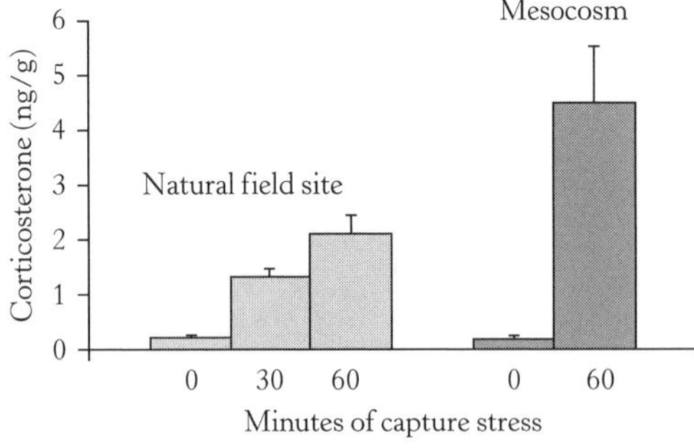

FIGURE 11.9: Mean whole-body corticosterone levels (ng/g) of Pacific treefrog tadpoles in response to confinement stress in a natural pond and outdoor mesocosms (a semi-natural enclosure).

From Belden et al. (2005), courtesy of the American Society of Ichthyologists and Herpetologists.

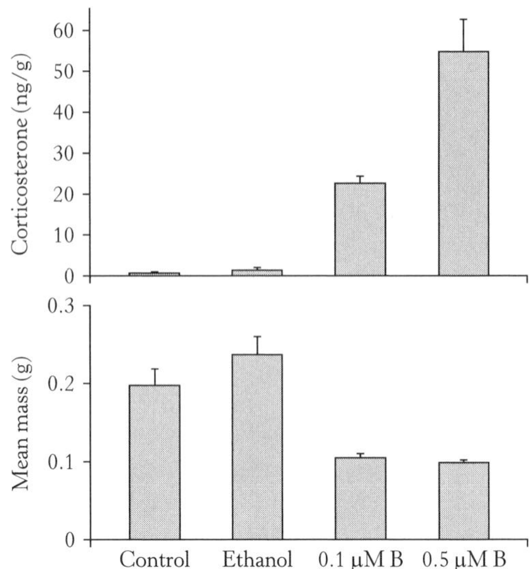

FIGURE 11.10: Mean whole-body corticosterone levels (ng/g) and mean mass (g) of Pacific treefrog tadpoles treated with exogenous corticosterone in the laboratory for 50 days.

From Belden et al. (2005), courtesy of the American Society of Ichthyologists and Herpetologists.

E. Fish

There is good evidence of an SHRP in many fish species (e.g., Barry et al. 1995; Carey and McCormick 1998; Pèrez-DomÌnguez and Holt 2006; Auperin and Geslin 2008; Alderman and Bernier 2009; Alsop and Vijayan 2009; Applebaum et al. 2010), but not all (e.g., Flik et al. 2002; Pepels and Balm 2004). An example is shown in Figure 11.11. Furthermore, in those species that do show an SHRP, its duration appears to vary widely between species, and there may also be a connection between corticosteroid concentrations and receptor densities (Deane and Woo 2003). Much of the difference

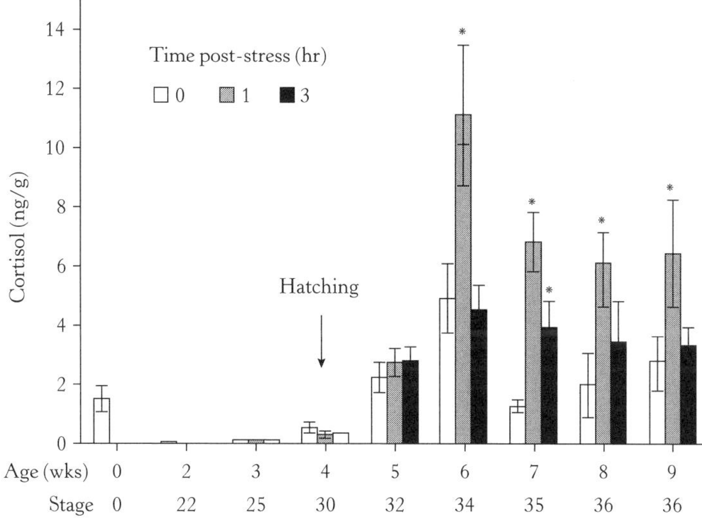

FIGURE 11.11: Changes in whole-body cortisol levels in rainbow trout in response to acute stress (30-sec handling followed immediately by a 30-sec 0°C cold shock) as a function of early developmental stage. Within each stage, asterisks indicate cortisol levels that are significantly different from pre-stress levels (i.e., 0 hr post-stress). Note the increase in cortisol at hatching and beyond, but a lack of a response to stress at 5 weeks.

Reprinted with permission from Barry et al. (1995). Courtesy of Elsevier.

between species may reside in the difference in egg size. Those species that produce small eggs often have an SHRP, whereas those with large eggs, and thus more maternal investment, often do not (Wada 2008). The difference between small and large egg fish species may be akin to the precocial-altricial spectrum in mammals and birds (Wada 2008).

The evidence for the Developmental Hypothesis continues to build. Although there are many exceptions, the available data indicate that there is a continuum in corticosteroid sensitivity to stress along the altricial-precocial gradient. However, substantial work, especially in increasing the taxonomic breadth, is required before concluding that the degree of neuronal development at birth/hatch is the primary variable explaining neonatal stress responses. Furthermore, work is just beginning to determine whether stressors during early life alter adult stress responses, as occurs in laboratory rodents.

V. BEGGING BEHAVIOR IN BIRDS

Many bird species are entirely dependent upon their parents for food shortly after hatch. Nature programs are full of examples on how these chicks signal to their parents that they are hungry—they beg. And the hungrier they are, the more frequently they beg. The evidence is growing that corticosteroids are a prime physiological regulator of this increase in begging rate. Perhaps the best example of this effect is in seabirds. Many seabirds nest at a distance from their feeding grounds and must make frequent foraging trips to satisfy their chicks. Both the amount and the quality of food available in the ocean, however, varies over time. Consequently, chicks can be well fed or poorly fed. When calories are sparse, chicks respond to a food shortage by increasing corticosteroid titers, both at baseline and in response to restraint stress (Kitaysky et al. 1999a; Kitaysky et al. 2001a). This in turn stimulates the chicks to signal their hunger by increasing their begging rates (Figure 11.12; also see Chapter 5). Although the role of corticosteroids in increasing begging has been shown experimentally using implants in captive animals (Kitaysky et al. 2001b; Kitaysky et al. 2003), it occurs in the field as well (Kitaysky et al. 2003; Quillfeldt et al. 2006; Villasenor and Drummond 2007), although perhaps not in all chicks in a brood (Vallarino et al. 2006). Figure 11.13 shows that the increase in begging rate then induces the parents to increase the amount of food delivered to the chicks (Kitaysky et al. 2001b; Quillfeldt et al. 2006).

An important test of the link between corticosteroids and begging is what happens when

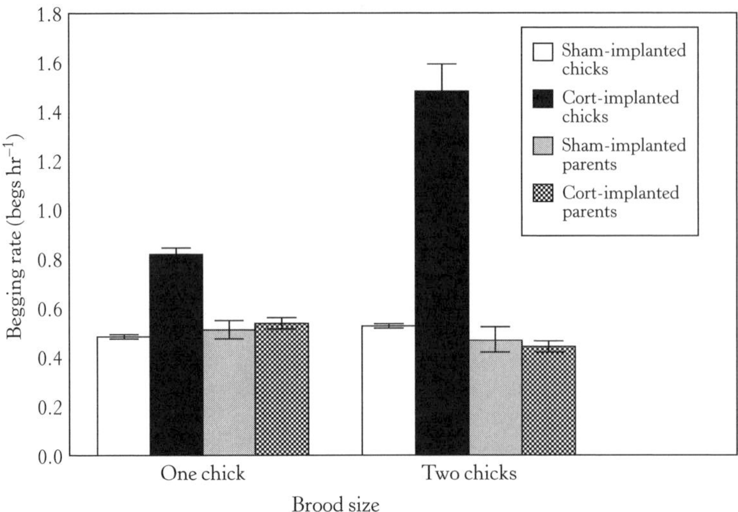

FIGURE 11.12: Behavioral responses of black-legged kittiwake chicks to experimentally increased circulating levels of corticosterone.

Reprinted with permission from Kitaysky et al. (2001b). Courtesy of Oxford University Press.

the parents do not respond to the chicks by increasing food delivery. One such species is the tufted puffin. In these species, chicks faced with a food shortage do not increase corticosteroid titers (Kitaysky et al. 2005), although they do appear to increase begging behavior (Williams et al. 2008a). In fact, tufted puffin chicks decrease corticosteroid titers, both baseline and stress-induced (Kitaysky et al. 2005), presumably as a way to preserve resources while maintaining as much growth as possible.

If conditions get really bad, parent puffins will stop feeding their chicks. As a result, many seabird species practice brood reduction, that is, they produce more eggs and chicks than they can normally feed. In some species, there is obligate

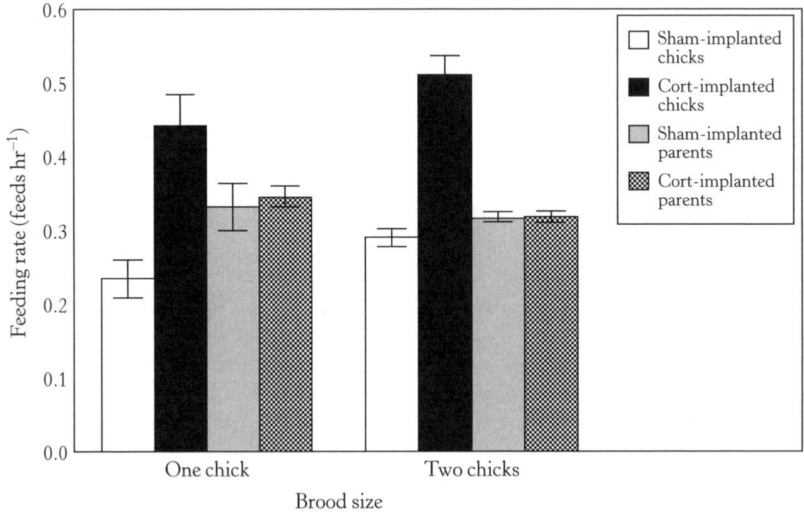

FIGURE 11.13: Behavioral responses of parent black-legged kittiwakes to experimentally increased circulating levels of corticosterone in their chicks.

Reprinted with permission from Kitaysky et al. (2001b). Courtesy of Oxford University Press.

brood reduction in which multiple eggs result in multiple chicks, but either the youngest chicks are never fed or the oldest chick kills its younger siblings. Corticosteroids appear to help facilitate the siblicide (delaMora et al. 1996; Tarlow et al. 2001; Vallarino et al. 2006). Other species have facultative brood reduction. In this case, multiple chicks can be successfully raised during bountiful years, but in other years the youngest chicks are not fed and are allowed to die. Once again, corticosteroids are thought to mediate abandonment of the youngest chicks (Wingfield et al. 1999; Angelier et al. 2007a).

One interesting result from these studies is the very strong correlation between chick corticosterone titers and the productivity surrounding the breeding colonies. Where ocean productivity is known to be low, the chicks from those colonies always have higher corticosteroid titers (Kitaysky et al. 1999b; Kitaysky et al. 2007; Williams et al. 2008b). In fact, the correlation between food availability and quality and chick corticosteroid titers is so strong that several researchers have proposed that chick corticosteroid titers can be used as an index for that years' productivity of the fishery (e.g., Buck et al. 2007; Benowitz-Fredericks et al. 2008; Brewer et al. 2008).

Although there has only been one study to date, it appears that the corticosteroid-induced elevation of begging rate is not restricted to seabirds. Experimental increases in corticosteroids resulted in a rapid increase in begging rate in white-crowned sparrow chicks as well (Wada and Breuner 2008). This suggests that corticosteroids are likely to affect begging rates in any species where parental feeding rates are sensitive to begging from the chicks.

One of the really fascinating features of corticosteroids and begging rates is that it has an effect on the parents. Parents will respond to their chicks by increasing foraging trips (Kitaysky et al. 2001b), probably resulting in an increase in their metabolic rate (Kitaysky et al. 2000). Remarkably, there often is no parallel change in corticosteroid titers in the parents. Corticosteroid-implanted adults do not increase chick feeding (Figure 11.12), although they do spend more time away from the nest (Kitaysky et al. 2001b). In fact, in other species, corticosteroid implants decrease feeding rates (e.g., Almasi et al. 2008; Horton and Holberton 2009). On the other hand, parents forced to increase foraging effort during chick feeding by clipping their wings do show an increase in corticosteroid titers (Harding et al. 2009). This suggests that an increase in allostatic load in the parents, but not the offspring, is what is inducing elevated corticosteroids.

The corticosteroid-induced increase in begging does have costs, however. It is undeniable that when food resources are limited, an increase in begging will increase the chances for survival, either through inducing greater parental feeding effort or through greater competitive advantage vis-à-vis siblings. So why don't chicks always increase corticosteroids and increase begging, even during good times? One answer appears to be a trade-off between getting more food and harming cognitive abilities. In kittiwake chicks provided exogenous corticosteroids, cognitive ability was greatly diminished (see Chapter 5). A second reason is that excessive begging may also bring unwanted attention to the chick. Begging sounds could alert predators to the location of the chicks or induce conspecific aggression (Müller et al. 2011). A third reason is to ensure the sending of an honest signal to the parent. The manipulation of parental behavior by chicks may be an interesting example of parent-offspring conflict, where the interests of the parent do not match the interests of the chicks (Muller et al. 2007). The chick may want to increase its food intake (by begging), but the parent may wish to ignore that signal. Excessive begging by the chick, therefore, may result in the begging becoming ineffective.

VI. CORTICOSTEROIDS IN FLEDGING, WEANING, AND PUBERTY

A number of important developmental events occur during the juvenile stage: altricial species leave the nest; young mammals are weaned; birds fledge (learn to fly); and many species undergo puberty. All of these events are associated with increases in corticosteroids.

A. Leaving the Nest (Fledging)

Behavioral changes that occur at fledging in birds are profound and are critical to survival. Young birds are still developing (growing) but must start to find food, avoid predators, locate good roost sites, and so on. Much of the data on this developmental transition have been collected from avian species. Furthermore, many of the studied species are altricial and fledge and leave the nest concurrently. This has made it difficult to distinguish between leaving the nest and fledging, although interpretations have usually focused more on the fledging behavior. Increased corticosteroid titers are associated with nest departure and fledging in American kestrels (Heath 1997; Sockman and Schwabl 2001), canaries (Schwabl 1999), thin-billed prions (Quillfeldt et al. 2007), and pied flycatchers (Kern et al. 2001). For example, in a study of white storks, Corbel and Groscolas (2008) found a four-fold increase in baseline plasma corticosterone levels of nestlings coincident with an increase in wing flapping. The timing and amplitude of this corticosterone increase were dependent upon hatching sequence, being less dramatic in later hatched chicks. In a second example, nestling American kestrels elevated plasma levels of corticosterone significantly as they prepared to depart the nest (Figure 11.14; Heath 1997).

It is important to note that many studies fail to find a correlation between increased corticosteroid titers and either leaving the nest or fledging. Examples include king penguins (Corbel et al. 2008; Corbel et al. 2009), American kestrels (Love et al. 2003a), and grey-faced petrels (Adams et al. 2008). For example, snowy owls nest on the ground, and all chicks disperse from the nest between ages 18–20 days, even though eggs hatch asynchronously. Because siblings can be of very different ages yet disperse at the same time, it suggests that chick dispersal from the nest is a developmentally regulated event. However, corticosterone titers do not increase at the time of dispersal (Figure 11.15; Romero et al. 2006). This study points out a major difference in studies: corticosteroid titers are often correlated with fledging in cavity-nesting birds but not ground-nesting birds. The difference may result from cavity nesters fledging and leaving the nest concurrently.

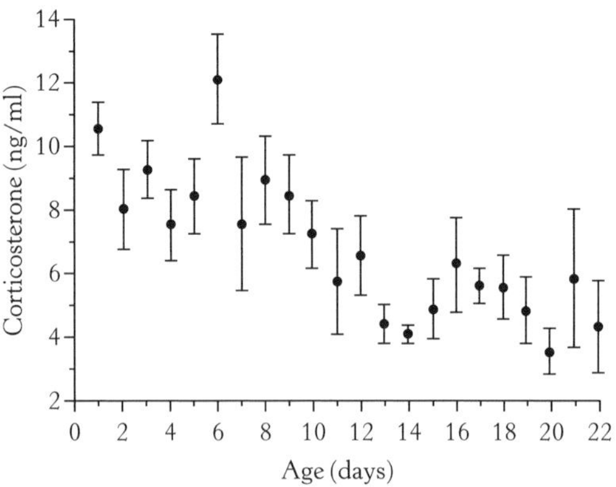

FIGURE 11.15: Corticosterone concentrations in snowy owl chicks as they age. Chicks disperse from their ground nests between ages 18 and 20 days, where there is no increase in corticosterone titers.

Reprinted with permission from Romero et al. (2006). Courtesy of Elsevier.

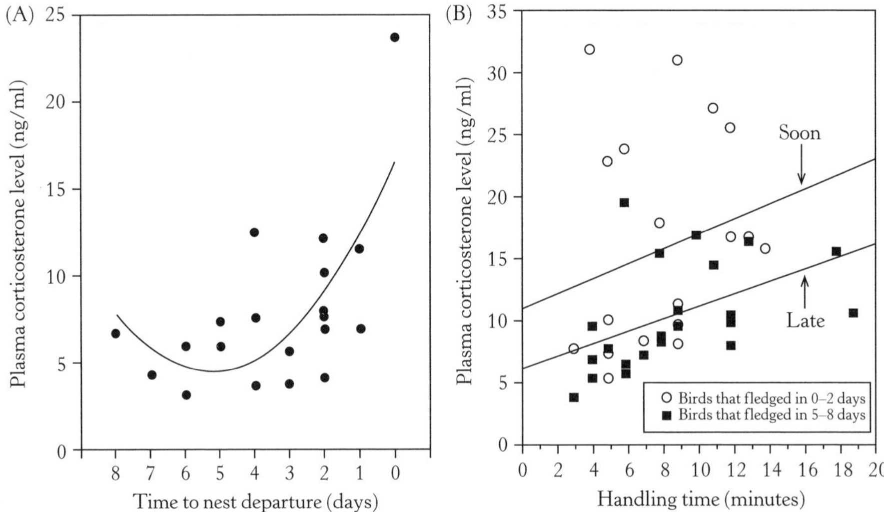

FIGURE 11.14: (A) The relationship between plasma corticosterone levels and time to nest departure ($r = 0.48$, $P < 0.005$) for American kestrels in southwestern Idaho. Solid circles represent individual nests. (B) The relationship among plasma corticosterone levels, time to nest departure, and handling time for American kestrels. There was no significant difference in rate of corticosterone increase between birds that left soon (0–2 days) and birds that left later (5–8 days, $P > 0.9$).

From Heath (1997), with permission and courtesy of the Cooper Onithological Society.

An additive effect of these two potentially stressful events may increase corticosteroids, whereas either event alone does not. Note also that in Gambel's white-crowned sparrows, plasma levels of corticosterone (baseline) remained low post-fledging and through the post-juvenile molt (Wingfield et al. 1980).

The question is, what factor would cause elevated corticosterone levels in fledging birds? A number of potential mechanisms have been proposed. The first possibility is a developmental effect. Under this hypothesis, corticosteroids help prime the individual for the greater activity associated with walking or flying. Elevated corticosteroids could be related to elevated metabolic activity associated with active flight away from the nest site. This is the presumed mechanism for species that fledge at the same time that they leave the nest (Heath 1997). Furthermore, Belthoff and Dufty (1998) suggest, based on a study on Western screech owls, that young birds in good body condition have high corticosterone levels. This situation could stimulate locomotor activity and thereby dispersal behavior. Lean birds should maintain low corticosterone levels, to keep gluconeogenesis low, and delay dispersal until their energy stores have improved. Once a set body condition is reached, corticosterone levels increase and induce dispersal. Further evidence comes from a mammalian species. Many rodents spend the first few weeks of life inside a protected burrow, from which they emerge several weeks after birth. A spike in corticosteroid levels accompanies burrow emergence in Belding's ground squirrels (Mateo 2006). Interestingly, captive individuals show a similar spike in corticosteroids at approximately the same time (Mateo 2006), suggesting that the spike is developmentally rather than environmentally driven.

A second potential mechanism is that corticosteroids increase as a result of increased predation pressure. As chicks get older, more vocal, and require more frequent parental feeding visits, the HPA axis could be responding to increased probability of being targeted by predators. This hypothesis fits with the proposed preparative actions of corticosteroids (see Chapter 4). Many corticosteroid-dependent behaviors are consistent with an attempt to escape from the stressor (Astheimer et al. 1992; Breuner et al. 1998). The association of corticosteroids with escape behaviors, concurrent with the release of corticosteroids during stressful conditions, led to the hypothesis that corticosteroids are the direct trigger for these escape movements (Wingfield and Ramenofsky 1997). However, there is little evidence to date of this mechanism underlying fledging or leaving the nest. In many species, the age of fledging is very synchronous (e.g., Romero et al. 2006) and, to our knowledge, corticosteroids have not been demonstrated to induce early fledging as a result of increased predation pressure.

A third potential mechanism is that hunger drives the increase in corticosteroids. If the growing chicks require more food than the parents can provide, the lack of food possibly induces fledging. This appears to be the proximal mechanism in white storks (Corbel and Groscolas 2008). In this case, the asynchronous hatching of white stork chicks indicated that the corticosteroid increase was not due to an endogenous signal, but rather to food restriction ameliorated by body condition.

Finally, the growing chicks could increase either crowding or sibling rivalry, both of which could initiate a stress response. Brood size and hatch order could potentially have a strong effect on chick corticosterone concentrations. Large brood sizes can lead to brood reduction in a number of species (e.g., Roulin et al. 1999; Ramos-Fernandez et al. 2000), with preferential mortality of the youngest chicks. The youngest chicks seem to be most vulnerable because parents fail to adequately provision these younger chicks when food is scarce. This creates a hierarchy whereby the parent can partition the available food to the greatest number of chicks by sacrificing the chicks it cannot feed. Better to feed a few chicks fully and let the others starve to death than to insufficiently feed all the chicks and risk losing the entire brood. This hierarchy, however, can produce intense inter-sibling rivalry for food. Food restriction can increase corticosteroid concentrations (e.g., Kitaysky et al. 1999a; Strochlic and Romero 2008), suggesting that inter-sibling rivalry could result in elevated corticosteroids in the youngest chicks of a nest. Although this is an attractive hypothesis, there is currently mixed evidence for it. Brood size was correlated with corticosteroid concentrations in pied flycatchers (Kern et al. 2001), but increased crowding, either through natural (Romero et al. 2006) or manipulated (Gil et al. 2008) changes in the number of chicks at a nest, had little effect on corticosteroid responses. Similarly in house sparrows, brood manipulations (smaller versus larger broods) had no effect on plasma corticosterone levels in either males or females. However, the inter-brood interval was longer in pairs that had raised larger broods (Hegner and Wingfield 1987).

B. Weaning

Weaning may also be a stressful period. Pups of Southern elephant seals had significantly higher cortisol concentrations shortly after weaning than did juveniles or adults (Ferreira et al. 2005), but there were no corticosteroid changes in the transition at the end of nursing in Northern elephant seals (Ortiz et al. 2003) or fur seals (Atkinson et al. 2011).

C. Puberty

A related developmental transition modulated by stress is puberty. The HPA axis appears to be greatly modified in many species during puberty (Romeo 2010). For example, laboratory rats have a different corticosteroid response prior to puberty than after, a change that is dependent upon neuronal development at puberty (Romeo and McEwen 2006). In free-living baboons, there is a marginally significant increase in corticosteroids in males and a significant decrease in corticosteroids in females concurrent to gonadal growth (Gesquiere et al. 2005). It is thus unclear whether corticosteroids are driving puberty. However, at least some aspects of puberty are regulated by corticosteroids in at least some species. For example, corticosteroids regulate a shift from play aggression to adult attacks during puberty in golden hamsters (Wommack and Delville 2007) and, in humans, stressful environmental conditions, such as poor parent-child relationships, can result in early puberty (Cameron et al. 2005).

VII. FACULTATIVE METAMORPHOSIS

Developmental transitions appear to be much more flexible in amphibians than in other vertebrate taxa. For example, many amphibians can alter the timing of hatching depending upon environmental conditions (Warkentin 2011), although this flexibility has not yet been linked to corticosteroids. On the other hand, similar to corticosteroid increases associated with hatching, birth, weaning, and fledging in other taxa, corticosteroids are critical in amphibian metamorphosis. Metamorphosis in amphibians is a complex re-engineering of nearly the entire body. Changes must occur in numerous physiological systems. Examples include the respiratory tract shifting from gills to lungs, the integument changing to prevent desiccation, locomotion changing from swimming to walking, and the excretory system changing how it regulates ion balances (Norris 2007). A number of hormones cooperate in regulating these changes; thyroid hormones, as well as hormones of the HPI (hypothalamic-pituitary-interrenal) axis, play a major role. One of the prime regulators is CRF, and in amphibians CRF plays a dual role—it not only stimulates ACTH release, but also is the primary TSH (thyroid stimulating hormone) releasing factor (Norris 2007). Consequently, CRF helps orchestrate the timing of metamorphosis (Denver 2009). Downstream from CRF release, corticosteroids and thyroid hormones synergize to initiate and sustain metamorphosis, with thyroid hormones playing the major role.

Although corticosteroids are important regulators of metamorphosis under normal circumstances, they also serve as a conduit for translating environmental information. They can modulate both the speed and the timing of metamorphosis. In other words, corticosteroids serve as the developmental signal to provide flexibility to the genetically determined phenotype in order to match current environmental conditions. In a recent review, Denver (2009) beautifully illustrates the many ways that environmental signals alter corticosteroid titers, which in turn alter metamorphosis. The following is one classic example.

Many amphibians use ephemeral pools or vernal ponds for their aquatic larval stage. These ponds are subject to drying, depending upon the extent of rainfall that year. Although ephemeral pools have the advantage of excluding fish predators, the larvae face the danger that the water will evaporate prior to completing metamorphosis. If this occurs, mass mortality ensues and breeding fails (Newman 1992). It would thus make sense for species that breed in these types of ponds to accelerate metamorphosis in dry years, and as long as they have achieved a minimum body size (Semlitsch et al. 1988), this is what they do. However, a reduced growth period prior to metamorphosis also results in smaller adults who are less likely to survive (Altwegg and Reyer 2003). Consequently, larvae attempt to time metamorphosis to derive the greatest amount of growth before running out of pond (Newman 1992). The regulators of this trade-off are the corticosteroids. When extra corticosteroids are administered to pre-metamorphic tadpoles, metamorphosis is accelerated (Galton 1990; Denver 2009).

There seem to be three potential triggers for increasing corticosterone titers. One is the extent of pond desiccation. For example, in the Western spade-foot toad, decreasing the water level in the laboratory results in an increase in corticosteroids (Denver 1998). A second potential trigger is increased tadpole densities. This makes sense because as the pond dries, bigger tadpoles are packed into a small space. Subjecting leopard frog tadpoles to increased conspecific density resulted in elevated corticosteroid titers (Glennemeier and Denver 2002a); similar results were found for tadpoles of Pacific treefrogs (Belden et al. 2005). The third potential trigger is decreases in food availability. Once again, bigger and hungrier tadpoles will quickly strip a pond of resources, especially as the pond dries. Consistent with this idea, leopard frog tadpoles increase corticosteroid titers when food is restricted (Crespi and Denver 2005). All three of these triggers elicit corticosteroid release and trigger accelerated metamorphosis.

Metamorphic changes are often regulated by corticosteroids in other species as well. Two major metamorphic changes in fish are known to be partially regulated by corticosteroids (Wada 2008). First, flatfish such as flounder undergo a number of morphometric changes as they shift from a classic bilateral body plan to one with both eyes on one side of the head. As in amphibians, this process is mostly regulated by thyroid hormones, but corticosteroids can accelerate the process (Dejesus et al. 1993; Wada et al. 2009). Second, young anadromous fish (ocean fish such as salmon that breed in fresh water) require extensive physiological remodeling as they transition from ion-poor fresh water to ion-rich seawater. This process is called smoltification. Corticosteroids are a major hormonal regulator of this transition, although in this case they synergize with growth hormone (Wada 2008; McCormick 2009b). Because corticosteroids appear to be the primary regulator of smoltification, increased corticosteroids do not so much accelerate the process as initiate the process in the first place.

VIII. AGING

For many years it did not seem to make much sense to look for changes in HPA function in aged wild animals. Although changes are known to occur in humans and captive animals (Pardon 2007; Pardon and Rattray 2008), how many wild animals manage to become old? After all, life expectancies of zoo animals are considerably longer than their wild counterparts. Furthermore, even if some individuals succeeded in navigating the gauntlets of disease, predation, and inclement habitat conditions, would they be so rare as to be of little consequence when trying to understand the biology of the majority of animals of that species?

A. Evidence for Corticosteroids and Senescence

It does appear, however, that individuals of at least some species survive to old age and experience senescence, as defined by age-dependent increases in mortality or decreases in fertility or immune function (Vleck et al. 2007). Much of the focus has been on long-lived seabirds, where multiyear field projects have produced large numbers of older individuals of known age. A number of studies have now attempted to determine if the oldest individuals in these populations show any indication of senescence in their HPA axes.

The data coming from these studies are intriguing. In common terns (Heidinger et al. 2006) and wandering albatrosses (Angelier et al. 2006), the ability of the oldest individuals to respond to capture and handling is attenuated compared to younger birds. At least part of this attenuation is due to a decrease in sensitivity of adrenal tissue to ACTH signals (Heidinger et al. 2008). These data support the idea that older individuals would inhibit stress responses in order to prevent corticosteroids from interfering with a limited number of remaining breeding attempts (Wingfield and Sapolsky 2003). However, this result does not apply to all species. In contrast to the common terns and wandering albatrosses, snow petrels showed no age-related changes in HPA function (Angelier et al. 2007b) or basal metabolic rate (Moe et al. 2007), and the oldest black-browed albatrosses had elevated corticosteroid titers (Angelier et al. 2007c). Furthermore, in a different study on wandering albatrosses, older males (but not females) failed to fully recover corticosteroid titers after a foraging trip, although there were no age-related differences in baseline titers (Lecomte et al. 2010). Interestingly, in several species prolactin may be a better indicator of breeding senescence than corticosteroids (Angelier and Chastel 2009).

It is currently unclear whether non-seabird species show corticosteroid changes with aging. Few studies have looked, but one found no indication that corticosteroids change (Brockman et al. 2009), and another showed that corticosteroid responses decreased in older, but not the oldest, individuals (Wilcoxen et al. 2011). However, senescence has been shown to occur in immune function in free-living animals (e.g., Hayward et al. 2009). Corticosteroid titers seem to be correlated with aging, but often it is not stress-induced titers that are the best predictors. In laboratory rats, behavioral traits, especially neophobia, are stronger predictors of longevity than corticosteroids, although increased baseline corticosterone titers had an additive effect (Cavigelli et al. 2009). In other words, the personality of individual rats is also correlated with corticosteroid titers (see later discussion in this chapter), and is a strong predictor of longevity. Whether similar processes are occurring in free-living animals has not yet been tested.

B. Telomere Length

One new and promising way of determining age in free-living populations is by measuring the length of telomeres. Telomeres are the short sequences of DNA that "cap" a chromosome. Without telomeres, each chromosome replication would lose a small part of the ends of the chromosome until eventually a key section would be lost. The cell would then either stop replicating or die. The cell delays this from occurring by providing a buffer of DNA—the telomere. Although telomerase, an enzyme that can repair telomeres, exists in many cells, the relative length of telomeres is a good index, at least in laboratory species, of the age of a cell, and by extension, the organism. Shortening of telomeres has also been correlated with aging in a number of free-living species of different taxa (e.g., Vleck et al. 2003; Hatase et al. 2008; Bize et al. 2009; Hartmann et al. 2009; Hayward et al. 2009). Furthermore, telomere shortening has been correlated with stressful events. For example, wild mice exposed to captive breeding conditions show significantly shorter telomeres (Kotrschal et al. 2007), chicken embryos exposed to extra corticosterone have shorter telomeres after hatching (Haussmann et al. 2012), and telomere shortening is correlated with adverse environmental conditions in free-living jackdaws (Salomons et al. 2009). In addition, telomere shortening seems to occur faster early in life (Monaghan and Haussmann 2006; Salomons et al. 2009), suggesting a further link between early developmental stressors and survival. Consequently, shorter telomeres appear to reflect greater exposure of the individual to environmental stressors and are correlated with shorter life spans, making telomere length another potential measure of the cumulative allostatic load experienced by the animal (see Chapter 6).

IX. INDIVIDUAL VARIATION AND HERITABILITY

Much of the discussion of this chapter leads up to a key idea: individuals vary in their responses to stressors. Some of this variation is undoubtedly genetic, but some is also developmentally regulated. How much is genetic and how much is environmental via development is still an open question, but it is becoming clear that developmentally induced differences can play an important role in the variation in individual differences in responses to stressors (reviewed by Schoech et al. 2011; Schoech et al. 2012).

One of the first questions to ask, however, is this: How much variation is there in individual responses? The biomedical literature, usually on laboratory rodents, clearly shows that individual animals have different reactions to stress, even when faced with the same stressors. Perhaps the best example is in the visible burrow system shown in Figure 11.16. In this model, four or five male rats are housed with two females. The entire group is housed in an apparatus with a central area that contains all the food and water. Leading out of this central area are passageways that connect to a number of burrows. The entire apparatus, including the central area, the burrows, and all passageways, are open at the top and thus visible to researchers (or more precisely, the researchers' cameras). When the rats are initially placed into the visible burrow system, the males quickly initiate fights and establish a dominance hierarchy (Blanchard and Blanchard 1989). The presence of the females enhances the male aggressiveness.

Once the male dominance hierarchy becomes established, the dominant male starts to monopolize the food and water source. He spends the most time in the central area, and the rest of the males spend their time waiting for the dominant male to leave the central area or braving attacks by cohabiting the central area with the dominant male (Blanchard and Blanchard 2003). As you can image, the subordinates perceive the dominant as a potent stressor and show significant symptoms of chronic stress (e.g., Blanchard et al. 1995). However, the physiological responses of the subordinates show great individual variability. Their responses generally fall into two broad categories—about 60% show extremely high corticosteroid levels and robust responses to other stressors such as restraint; and about 40% show a reduced or absent corticosteroid response to restraint (Blanchard et al. 1995). Subordinates are

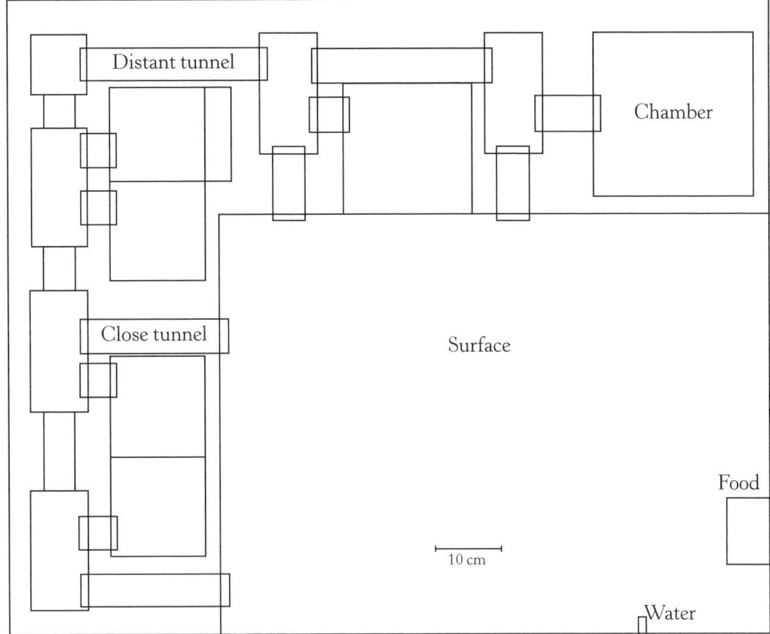

FIGURE 11.16: The visible burrow system. Six to seven rats live in the apparatus and form a stable dominance hierarchy. The subordinates, however, show many symptoms of chronic stress.

Reprinted with permission from Blanchard and Blanchard (1989). Courtesy of American Psychological Association.

indistinguishable on other measures, however, with both types of subordinates showing altered behavior, adrenal weights, and so on, compared to the dominant or controls. It is not yet clear why some subordinates show a robust response to restraint whereas others do not, but it is clear that these semi-natural laboratory studies can expose substantial individual differences.

Are these individual differences from laboratory studies evidence for individual differences in stress responses in wild animals? In some ways this question has an obvious answer since every field study documents some individual variation in responses. However, the question of whether this is meaningful variation reflecting underlying physiological differences, much like the differences between subtypes of subordinates in the visible burrow system, or whether the variability simply reflects the inevitable noise associated with field conditions, is still not fully resolved. Furthermore, this question is just now starting to be addressed. In many ways, the recent attention to individual differences reflects the maturation of field endocrinology in general, and of stress ecology in particular. Before one can start asking whether individuals vary in their responses, one has to determine what they are varying from. In other words, before testing the effects of individual variation, there has to be an idea of the mean response. Much of field endocrinology to date has been concerned with delineating and understanding the mean response. Now it is possible to ask what the variation is around those mean responses.

In an influential paper, Tony Williams lamented the lack of focus on individual variation in endocrine studies and called for a rejection of the "tyranny of the golden mean," as originally termed by Bennett (Williams 2008). He pointed out that few field endocrinology studies to date have estimated inter-individual variation and instead publish only the mean response. Williams introduced an important point, but part of the focus on means vis-à-vis variation has its root in disciplinary training. Those researchers who were trained as ecologists tend to focus on the individual variation, the grist of natural selection, whereas those researchers trained as physiologists tend to focus on mean responses to answer the question of how animals react. One of us (LMR) has the predilection of controlling the underlying variability in order to uncover the "normal" response, whereas the other (JCW) has the predilection of examining precisely the variation in order to explore how responses might have evolved. Both approaches are important and complementary.

Stress physiology, however, presents some difficult challenges for studying variation. One is actually identifying true variability. Field endocrinologists typically only have access to an animal once. It is very difficult, and often impossible, to retrap an animal. However, if we are to assess the role of inter-individual variation, these point samples, collected at a single moment of time, must accurately reflect the animal's "normal" or "usual" hormone titers and responses. In other words, point samples must reflect the "endocrine phenotype" of the individual so that individual differences found on one sampling occasion would be found consistently across many sampling occasions.

How likely are point samples to reflect the endocrine phenotype? Because responses of corticosteroids, not to mention the catecholamines, are so labile, this is a difficult question to answer. For example, suppose that 30 minutes prior to trapping, an animal was chased by a predator, unbeknownst to the researcher. The animal may very well have an elevated corticosteroid titer, but this reflects a physiological response to the predator, not a difference in the endocrine phenotype. The traditional response to this problem was to assume that there were no systematic biases among treatment groups in prior exposure to stressors. Calculation of means and subjecting the data to statistical analysis would then minimize this problem. However, if the focus is on the individual response rather than the mean, this approach is no longer possible. An alternative approach is to determine how well point samples reflect the endocrine phenotype in those few instances where multiple samples can be taken from the same individuals.

Given the difficulty of this task, it is not surprising that there have been few studies. A further complication is that many environmental factors, such as season, habitat, physiological condition, and so on, are known to alter corticosteroid titers and responses, so repeated captures must also control for these factors as well. It is encouraging that many studies to date indicate that single point samples reflect the endocrine phenotype of the individual. A classic example from great tits is shown in Figure 6.9. Field studies have generally shown a high repeatability of corticosteroid titers within an individual over multiple captures (e.g., Kralj-Fiser et al. 2007; Cockrem et al. 2009). However, even these studies can be difficult to interpret. Recent data suggest that wild animals alter their corticosteroid responses after multiple captures. Even though the mean responses to capture stress in two cohorts of birds captured several weeks apart were identical, birds sampled both times had a significantly lower corticosteroid response during the second capture (Lynn et al. 2010). Furthermore, repeatability might not be the important metric. Corticosteroid titers might not be repeatable, but if the same animal consistently has the highest (or lowest) titers, then a single point sample would represent the relative endocrine phenotype. The reverse can also be true—simply because an animal's response is repeatable does not necessarily indicate that it consistently has the highest or lowest endocrine phenotype of its cohort.

Data from captive and/or hand-reared wild animals are more equivocal than the field data. Several studies indicate a high level of repeatability across different samples (Cockrem and Silverin 2002; Love et al. 2003c; Schjolden et al. 2005) and substantial heritability (Tanck et al. 2001), but others do not (Romero and Reed 2008). In the latter study, each bird's baseline corticosteroid concentrations were ranked compared to its captive cohort to determine whether, despite intra-individual variation, the concentrations for each bird were consistently high or low. Not only were point samples from individual birds occasionally not consistent in rank between samples, an individual bird's rank was often not consistent between samples collected during the day and night (Romero and Reed 2008). Figure 11.17 shows the inter-sample variability from multiple bleeds of the same animal and how the relative rank in the cohort changes from day to night. In another study on zebra finches, there was a significant correlation between corticosteroid responses when sampled as chicks and later as adults in females, but not in males (Wada et al. 2008). This suggests that there might be sex differences in the stability of an endocrine phenotype for individual animals. Further variation can occur with laying order in birds, with first- and last-hatched chicks often differing in their corticosteroid responses (e.g., Schwabl 1999). Similar to field studies, there also appear to be differences in corticosteroid responses in captive animals bled for the first time and those subject to earlier sampling (Piersma and Ramenofsky 1998; Love et al. 2003c).

On the other hand, selection studies provide powerful evidence that individual variation does reflect the underlying endocrine phenotype. A number of species from diverse taxa have now been subjected to selective breeding experiments, based either upon the individual's baseline

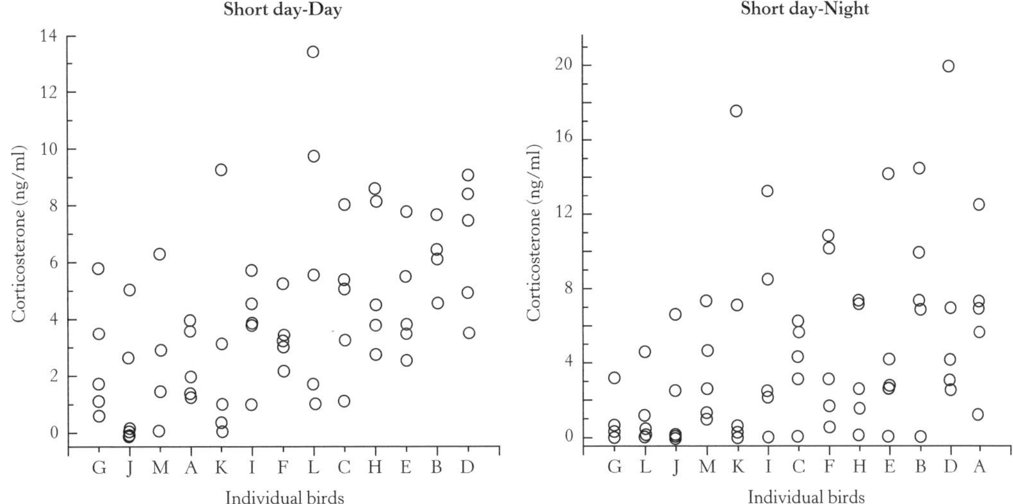

FIGURE 11.17: Corticosterone concentrations in captive house sparrows held on a short-day photoperiod. Points indicate individual corticosterone values from five different bleeds for each individual bird sampled during the day (left panel) and night (right panel). Individual birds are placed on the *x* axis in order of increasing mean corticosterone concentrations from the five bleeds. Note variability between bleeds of the same individual and that rankings are different during the day and night.

Reprinted with permission from Romero and Reed (2008). Courtesy of Elsevier.

corticosteroid titers or their response to a standardized stressor. Examples include Japanese quail (Satterlee and Johnson 1988; Jones et al. 1994; Satterlee and Jones 1997), chickens (Gross and Siegel 1985), turkeys (Brown and Nestor 1973), zebra finches (Evans et al. 2006), and rainbow trout (Øverli et al. 2002; Schjolden and Winberg 2007). These studies have successfully separated high and low corticosteroid lineages and have maintained these lines for several generations. Furthermore, selection for corticosteroids can have profound concurrent effects on behavioral responses (e.g., Øverli et al. 2005; Hodgson et al. 2007), and these behavioral changes may be mediated by changes in corticosteroid receptors (Hodgson et al. 2007). Conversely, corticosteroid concentrations co-vary with selection on other traits (e.g., Rodenburg et al. 2009). Mice selected for high voluntary wheel running, for example, show elevated baseline but not restraint-induced corticosteroid concentrations (Malisch et al. 2007; Malisch et al. 2008). Perhaps the best example, however, is in farmed silver foxes. Foxes selected for tameness not only decreased their aggressive behavior, but morphological and physiological traits changed in tandem, including a change in the function of the HPA axis (Krass et al. 1979; Oskina and Tinnikov 1992). How this occurs is not presently known. The evidence from selection studies suggests, therefore, that the individual variation in corticosteroid titers often found in free-living animals indicates true inter-individual variation and is not an artifact of random selection of a sample within a wide range of intra-individual variation.

In conclusion, even though the foundation of many field studies is the assumption that individual point samples will reflect the true endocrine phenotype of the animal at the time of capture, this fact has not yet been fully established. The data are far clearer for laboratory studies, with perhaps the best evidence being that single assessments of corticosteroid titers and/or responses can be used to select lines of high- and/or low-responding animals. But even in these cases, some data suggest substantial variation between different point samples. The problem is magnified in the field, where external factors, such as weather, predator presence, social interactions, and so on, can dramatically and rapidly adjust HPA function. This is certainly an area that requires more research, and given the vagaries of field conditions, it may never be satisfactorily resolved. Perhaps the best we can hope for is an acknowledgement that we can never be completely certain that a single point sample will represent a true endocrine phenotype for any individual. Consequently, studies that attempt to analyze individual differences should be interpreted cautiously. Studies of animals in the field under real challenges of everyday life will be instrumental in determining why and how animals adapt and will allow us to understand individual variation.

A. Personality as a Source of Variation

Although the selection studies detailed earlier clearly argue that a portion of the inter-individual variation is genetic in origin, the data from the rest of the chapter argue that at least some of the variation is derived during development. A further source of inter-individual variation that has attracted recent attention is in individual differences in how an animal responds to environmental stimuli. Animals show different coping styles, with some animals showing more fear or less aggression in novel situations and others showing enhanced exploration and more aggression in those same novel settings (see also Chapter 9). These differences have been termed "reactive and proactive coping styles," or "reactive and proactive personalities" (Koolhaas et al. 2007).

Studies in a number of species indicate that an individual's personality is consistent across time. This means that personalities can be heritable (Reale et al. 2007) and thus subject to selection. The genetic linkage is not absolute, however, since experience is known to shift the magnitude of responses in at least some species (Frost et al. 2007). If personalities are subject to selection, then why is more than one personality maintained? The answer appears to be that different personalities can have selective advantages depending upon environmental conditions (Dingemanse and Reale 2005; Koolhaas et al. 2007; Reale et al. 2007). Perhaps the best example of this comes from work on inter-uterine position (Ryan and Vandenbergh 2002). In many rodents and a few other species, hormones from one embryo can influence its sibling neighbor in the uterus. Since the horns of the uterus in these species can only accommodate single embryos in a line, each embryo has the potential of zero, one, or two brother or sister neighbors. The result is offspring that are either relatively masculinized (from androgens leaking from increasing numbers of neighboring brothers) or feminized (from estrogens leaking from increasing numbers of neighboring sisters). This creates a continuum of offspring from highly masculinized (two brother neighbors) to highly feminized (two sister neighbors) with concomitant differences in behavior. Furthermore, each of these behavioral phenotypes can provide a selective advantage depending upon environmental conditions (Clark and Galef 1995; Drickamer 1996; Ryan and Vandenbergh 2002). Although this example is from mammals, similar mechanisms appear to occur in other species bearing live young (Uller et al. 2005) or using testosterone deposited in yolks (e.g., Groothuis and Carere 2005; Tobler and Sandell 2007). There is also some evidence that corticosteroids can masculinize behavior as well (Knapp et al. 2011).

In contrast to the uterine horn example, which is clearly not regulated by genetics (whether the uterine neighbor is a brother or a sister is likely random), in wild birds and domesticated species consistent personalities (i.e., coping styles) have been experimentally demonstrated and shown to be heritable (see also Cockrem and Silverin 2002; Cockrem 2006; Evans et al. 2006). These differences persist in populations artificially selected for coping style and are thus useful for determining hormonal mechanisms (Evans et al. 2006). Using two zebra finch lines selected for a low or high corticosterone response to manual restraint, increasing corticosterone levels were correlated with elevated exploratory and risk-taking behaviors in the low corticosterone line but not in the high corticosterone line. The latter birds generally showed consistently greater risk-taking behaviors that were less sensitive to changing corticosterone titers. The authors conclude that, in general, higher corticosterone, at least following mild stress, may regulate exploratory behavior and risk-taking behavior, and that differences in corticosterone effects may be heritable.

Other types of studies also suggest potential ways in which environment could influence interpretation of personalities. Many factors could contribute to coping styles and their persistence within individuals regardless of possible genetic mechanisms. For example, first-hatched chicks of collared doves are bigger, and have lower baseline corticosterone and higher cell-mediated immune responses than second-hatched chicks (Eraud et al. 2008). These results could indicate possible bases of personalities/coping styles. Controlling for body size in collared dove chicks revealed that corticosterone levels were not directly related to cell-mediated immunity, but both were similar across sexes (Eraud et al. 2008). In a further experiment, they removed the first-laid egg (that would hatch the first chick) to eliminate the effects of egg quality and competition. Chicks in the second-laid egg were bigger and had lower levels of corticosterone and greater cell-mediated immunity than second chicks raised in two-chick broods. This suggests that body size effects, cell-mediated immunity, and corticosterone deficits are modulated by competition stress and probably not by genetics alone (Eraud et al. 2008).

There is growing evidence that personalities are also correlated with different responses to stress (Fucikova et al. 2009). In general, those individuals that have relatively active behavioral responses (a proactive personality) have lower corticosteroid responses than individuals with relatively passive behavioral responses (a reactive personality; e.g. Anestis et al. 2006; Cockrem 2007). In great tits, different fecal levels of corticosteroids were measured when confronted with an aggressive conspecific. Birds selected for slow responses tended to have a higher corticosteroid response, but this was lower the next day. High responders showed no corticosteroid response to an aggressor (Carere et al. 2003). These authors state that their results are evidence for coping styles in a wild bird, but inconsistencies across taxa indicate that much more work is needed to understand the behavioral ecology and control mechanisms for personalities and coping with perturbations of the environment. The personality differences can even extend to different morphological groups in a population. White-throated sparrow males have a white and a tan plumage morph (as do females, and these birds mate disassortively) that not only differ in behavior during mating, but also differ in their corticosteroid responses to restraint (Schwabl 1995). However, the correlations between corticosteroid and behavioral responses appear to be stronger in some species than others (Schjolden et al. 2005).

B. Impact of Development in Creating Variation in Stress Responses

Much of the work examining the long-term impact of corticosteroids during development has been done on laboratory rodents. Recent work has started to indicate that similar processes are occurring in both free-living (e.g., Landys et al. 2011) and captive wild animals. Early exposure to corticosteroids can profoundly alter an individual's phenotype in ways that can greatly change how that animal interacts with its environment.

One of the primary changes in phenotype that has been examined is change of the HPA response. In general, corticosteroid titers and responses to stress increase after early exposure to corticosteroids. For example, increases in corticosteroids in bird egg yolk result in higher activity of the HPA when those chicks become adults (Hayward and Wingfield 2004). Exposing growing western scrub-jays to a nutritional stressor also results in adults with stronger HPA activation (Pravosudov and Kitaysky 2006), which might be resultant of underlying changes to the hippocampus (Pravosudov et al. 2005). In contrast, either corticosteroids injected into egg yolks or exposure to a stressor after hatch resulted in attenuated corticosteroid responses to stressors five to six months later in rainbow trout (Auperin and Geslin 2008), and exposing mammalian mothers to stressors has had equivocal effects, with some studies showing increases (e.g., Boonstra and Singleton 1993) and others showing decreases (e.g., Osadchuk et al. 2003) in corticosteroid titers when offspring became adults. The difference in the mammalian studies may relate to the severity of the stressor applied to the mother. Given the robust effect on the HPA axis shown in laboratory rodents, most researchers assume that similar effects will be seen in free-living populations as well.

Early exposure to corticosteroids has been shown to alter subsequent immune function (see also Chapters 6 and 9). Both Japanese quail and zebra finches selected for high corticosteroid responses had greater humoral (antibody), but not cell-mediated, responses to a challenge than quail or zebra finches selected for low corticosteroid responses (Roberts et al. 2007c; Roberts et al. 2009). In contrast, male European starlings exposed to corticosteroids in the egg showed reduced cell-mediated immunity (Love et al. 2005). Clearly, more work is needed in this area. Furthermore, although numerous studies have examined corticosteroid effects on metabolic rates, whether early exposure results in long-term changes to metabolic rates has been infrequently studied, with some of the only available evidence suggesting no major effects (Spencer and Verhulst 2008).

A number of studies have also demonstrated that corticosteroid exposure during development can alter sexual signaling and mate choice (reviewed by Husak and Moore 2008). Much of this work has been done with birds. There are two major types of sexual signaling in birds—plumage and song. The quality of a male's song appears to be highly dependent upon developmental corticosteroid exposure. In general, exposing growing males to stressors during the period when they are learning their songs results in poorer quality songs (reviewed by MacDougall-Shackleton 2009;

Spencer and MacDougall-Shackleton 2011). This effect is likely regulated by corticosteroids because growing male zebra finches develop poorer songs when exposed to corticosteroids (Spencer et al. 2003; Spencer et al. 2005), an effect that appears to be mediated through decreases in the size of brain areas that regulate song learning (Buchanan et al. 2004; MacDonald et al. 2006) and corticosteroid receptor expression in song-control areas of the brain (Suzuki et al. 2011). Song quality also appears to be related to individual variation. Higher responses to capture and restraint correlate with lower quality songs in song sparrows (MacDougall-Shackleton et al. 2009). In sum, the evidence strongly supports the conclusion that male songbirds exposed to elevated corticosteroids during development have retarded growth of brain regions that regulate song learning, leading to lower quality songs and ultimately poorer success in attracting mates. The end result is lower reproductive fitness.

There is currently no consensus on whether corticosteroids exert developmental effects on sexually relevant plumage characteristics. In barn owls, implanted corticosteroids in nestlings significantly reduced melanin deposition into feathers, especially those feathers implicated in sexual selection (Roulin et al. 2008). Corticosteroids are also known to reduce feather quality (DesRochers et al. 2009), although this may not occur in young birds growing their first set of feathers (Butler et al. 2010). In crested auklets, the size of the showy feather ornament is inversely correlated with corticosteroids in males (Douglas et al. 2009). On the other hand, selection for divergent lines of zebra finches on the basis of corticosteroid responses failed to find any correlation with male sexual signal quality, although females did tend to prefer males from the line selected for lower responses (Roberts et al. 2007b). Individual variation in corticosteroid responses also seems to influence mate choice, with zebra finch males showing lower corticosteroid titers being favored by females (Roberts et al. 2007a). However, any effect on plumage may reflect a more general response. Corticosteroids also alter skin color in lizards (Fitze et al. 2009), suggesting that corticosteroids can alter areas of the integument important in sexual selection. In addition, much of this effect could potentially relate to the synthetic apparatus for corticosteroids being present in the skin (Slominski et al. 2007). The possibility that corticosteroids can directly alter the sexual signaling of many species by altering coloration of the integument remains an intriguing hypothesis.

Corticosteroid exposure during development also has profound and long-lasting effects on behavior. In general, corticosteroid exposure increases fear and decreases exploratory behavior—in other words, induces a more reactive personality. The results of this change can be manifested in a number of ways, all of which can have large impacts on the ultimate fitness of the animal.

Perhaps the best-studied behavioral change is that individuals with a more reactive personality are less likely to be aggressive or attain high rank and are thus at a competitive disadvantage compared to their peers. This has been shown in a number of taxa, including fish (e.g., Øverli et al. 2004; Schjolden and Winberg 2007) and some (Janczak et al. 2006; Spencer and Verhulst 2007) but not all (Roberts et al. 2007b) birds. The decrease in competitive advantage could clearly result in lower rank, reduced access to resources, and fewer opportunities to mate.

The corticosteroid-induced shift to a more reactive personality can have further downstream effects on locomotion. Trout selected for high corticosteroid responses showed increased locomotion when faced with a smaller competitor, but no increase in aggression (Øverli et al. 2002), which may be interpreted as an increase in flight behavior. The duration of corticosteroid exposure can also serve as a trigger for changes in locomotor behavior. For example, corticosteroid-exposed lizards show changes in overall activity (Belliure et al. 2004) and in juvenile dispersal (De Fraipont et al. 2000). Whether the juveniles stay or disperse (see Chapter 9), however, appears to depend upon a number of factors. The duration of corticosteroid exposure is important, with short exposures inducing dispersal and long durations inhibiting dispersal (Vercken et al. 2007), as is the timing of exposure, with prenatal exposure from older mothers being more potent than postnatal exposure (Meylan et al. 2002; Meylan et al. 2004). This response is reminiscent of the laboratory rodent studies that show small amounts of prenatal/neonatal exposure to corticosteroids to be beneficial, whereas larger exposures are detrimental.

A general role for corticosteroids in dispersal is unclear, however, because corticosteroids seem to have a general role in triggering dispersal in some (Silverin et al. 1989; Silverin 1997; Mateo 2006; Hamann et al. 2007) but not all (e.g., Strier and Ziegler 2000; Cease et al. 2007; Van Belle et al.

2009) species. However, there is a strong relationship between the quality of the natal environment and ultimate dispersal rates (reviewed by Benard and McCauley 2008). This suggests strongly that corticosteroids are connected to the decision to disperse, but the nature of this connection is not yet well defined.

Prenatal exposure to corticosteroids can also alter anti-predator behaviors. For example, young garter snakes exposed to maternal corticosteroids decreased tail lashing and reversal movements, both of which are effective anti-predator behaviors (Robert et al. 2009). Similarly, young lizards exposed to corticosteroids in the egg were slower to emerge from a shelter after being exposed to a simulated predator than non-exposed animals (Uller and Olsson 2006), suggesting greater fearfulness. Clearly, any changes in anti-predator behavior can have profound effects on ultimate survival.

C. Corticosteroids and Survival

The current evidence for the role of early corticosteroid exposure and survival of individuals is mixed. There is some evidence that early exposure to corticosteroids can be beneficial. Lizards exposed to corticosteroids in utero showed decreased body weight at hatch, but survived better when released to a natural environment (Meylan and Clobert 2005). Similar responses were seen with lizards treated as adults (Cote et al. 2006). In contrast, a number of other studies suggest that early exposure to corticosteroids will decrease survival. This seems especially true from three studies in birds. Barn swallows exposed to corticosteroids in the egg hatched at lower weight, which in this species is correlated with long-term survival (Saino et al. 2005). The stress response in nestling white storks was inversely correlated with survival—those nestlings with the greatest corticosteroid responses to capture and handling had the lowest recruitment, presumed to reflect survival, into the breeding population (Blas et al. 2007). Hoatzin chicks hatching in tourist areas, whose parents were thus presumably exposed to the stress of human visitation, showed lower survival to fledging (Mullner et al. 2004). A similar decrease in survival with early exposure to corticosteroids seems to occur in an example from mammals. Snowshoe hare females in the middle of a predator-induced population crash have elevated corticosteroid levels (Sheriff et al. 2009), which they presumably pass to their offspring through the placenta, and offspring of these females have significantly lower survival rates (Boonstra et al. 1998). Taken together, the available evidence suggests that early corticosteroid exposure can have a profound impact on survival, but what that impact might be is highly species-specific. Note also, however, that few studies have directly tested the link between survival and early exposure to corticosteroids. They instead have relied upon indirect correlations to the stressor.

X. CONCLUSIONS

Is there any way to make ultimate sense of the ecological role of early exposure to corticosteroids? There is an intriguing hypothesis that links maternal care, changes in HPA reactivity, and phenotypic adjustment to the current environment (Caldji et al. 2001; Cameron et al. 2005). Recall from Chapter 5 that poor maternal care can initiate a cascade in the offspring, in which an increase in DNA methylation leads to a decrease in corticosteroid receptor production, reduced efficacy of negative feedback, and ultimately elevated HPA reactivity. This elevated HPA reactivity in the daughters will result in poor maternal care provided to the next generation. Conversely, good maternal care leads to offspring with reduced DNA methylation, an increase in corticosteroid receptor production, more robust negative feedback, and reduced HPA reactivity. The reduced HPA reactivity then also propagates to the next generation. Consequently, under this scenario, poor mothering begets poor mothering and good mothering begets good mothering.

But perhaps these differences make ecological sense (Cameron et al. 2005). If resources are plentiful, then there may be a high likelihood of offspring survival. This would make it advantageous for the mother to invest in maternal care. The resultant "programming" of her offspring's HPA would further help the offspring survive in a benign environment. If the habitat were relatively benign, it might make sense to limit a stress response. On the other hand, a poor-resource environment would lead to a low likelihood of offspring survival. This would make it advantageous for the mother to invest her reproductive effort in many offspring with less individual attention rather than in fewer offspring with greater individual attention. This could be advantageous for the mother, giving her a greater chance to raise at least a few offspring, but might also be advantageous for the offspring. If the habitat is relatively poor, a robust stress response might greatly aid in survival. In a sense, the mother could use an epigenetic mechanism to "program" her offspring's defensive responses to maximize her offspring's ability to reproduce.

The evidence for this hypothesis is currently equivocal. However, there have been a number of critiques from theoretical grounds. First, the alterations in offspring phenotype may represent a physiological constraint (Rickard and Lummaa 2007). The HPA changes may or may not provide advantages or disadvantages, but selection cannot work on them—they are simply necessary byproducts that allow as normal a development as possible given the current conditions. Second, if the mother's environment is at all predictive of what her offspring will encounter, it is likely to be true only of the period soon after birth/hatch. In effect, the mother is making a "weather forecast" of future conditions (Wells 2007). It seems implausible, given the great variability in environmental conditions (see Chapter 1) that any predictive value would extend more than a few months. Especially for long-lived species, the environment during development may have little correlation with conditions the individual must cope with as an adult. Consequently, it may be in the offsprings' best interest to allow the mother to buffer the short-term environmental fluctuations as much as possible (Figures 11.1 and 11.2; see also Monaghan 2008). Under this scenario, the HPA changes reflect past, not future, conditions (Wells 2007).

On the other hand, maternal effects may facilitate the assimilation of these responses into the genome (Badyaev 2005). Although this may seem like Lamarkian evolution, whereby acquired characteristics are passed on to the next generation, there is a theoretical basis for the evolution of maternal effects (Badyaev and Uller 2009). In a horrible overgeneralization, the maternal effects can be incorporated in genetic heritability when random genetic mutations coincide with the maternal effects that are favored. Although there is some empirical support for this mechanism (Badyaev 2009), whether changes in the HPA axis provide an example is unknown.

The conclusion from this discussion is that it is not yet clear whether maternal effects on the HPA axis represent an adaptive response or pathology. Distinguishing between these two is an exciting avenue of ongoing research.

REFERENCES

Adams, N. J., Cockrem, J. F., Candy, E. J., Taylor, G. A., 2008. Non-precocial grey-faced petrel chicks (*Pterodroma macroptera gouldi*) show no age-related variation in corticosterone responses to capture and handling. *Gen Comp Endocrinol* 157, 86–90.

Alderman, S. L., Bernier, N. J., 2009. Ontogeny of the corticotropin-releasing factor system in zebrafish. *Gen Comp Endocrinol* 164, 61–69.

Almasi, B., Roulin, A., Jenni-Eiermann, S., Jenni, L., 2008. Parental investment and its sensitivity to corticosterone is linked to melanin-based coloration in barn owls. *Horm Behav* 54, 217–223.

Alonso-Alvarez, C., Velando, A., 2003. Female body condition and brood sex ratio in yellow-legged gulls *Larus cachinnans*. *Ibis* 145, 220–226.

Alsop, D., Vijayan, M. M., 2009. Molecular programming of the corticosteroid stress axis during zebrafish development. *Comp Biochem Physiol A* 153, 49–54.

Altwegg, R., Reyer, H. U., 2003. Patterns of natural selection on size at metamorphosis in water frogs. *Evolution* 57, 872–882.

Anestis, S. F., Bribiescas, R. G., Hasselschwert, D. L., 2006. Age, rank, and personality effects on the cortisol sedation stress response in young chimpanzees. *Physiol Behav* 89, 287–294.

Angelier, F., Chastel, O., 2009. Stress, prolactin and parental investment in birds: A review. *Gen Comp Endocrinol* 163, 142–148.

Angelier, F., Clement-Chastel, C., Gabrielsen, G. W., Chastel, O., 2007a. Corticosterone and time-activity black-legged budget: An experiment with kittiwakes. *Horm Behav* 52, 482–491.

Angelier, F., Moe, B., Weimerskirch, H., Chastel, O., 2007b. Age-specific reproductive success in a long-lived bird: Do older parents resist stress better? *J Anim Ecol* 76, 1181–1191.

Angelier, F., Shaffer, S. A., Weimerskirch, H., Chastel, O., 2006. Effect of age, breeding experience and senescence on corticosterone and prolactin levels in a long-lived seabird: The wandering albatross. *Gen Comp Endocrinol* 149, 1–9.

Angelier, F., Weimerskirch, H., Dano, S., Chastel, O., 2007c. Age, experience and reproductive performance in a long-lived bird: A hormonal perspective. *Behav Ecol Sociobiol* 61, 611–621.

Applebaum, S. L., Wilson, C. A., Holt, G. J., Nunez, B. S., 2010. The onset of cortisol synthesis and the stress response is independent of changes in CYP11B or CYP21 mRNA levels in larval red drum (*Sciaenops ocellatus*). *Gen Comp Endocrinol* 165, 269–276.

Arnold, K. E., Griffiths, R., Stevens, D. J., Orr, K. J., Adam, A., Houston, D. C., 2003. Subtle manipulation of egg sex ratio in birds. *Proc R Soc Lond B* 270, S216–S219.

Astheimer, L. B., Buttemer, W. A., Wingfield, J. C., 1992. Interactions of corticosterone with feeding, activity and metabolism in passerine birds. *Ornis Scan* 23, 355–365.

Atkinson, S., Arnould, J. P. Y., Mashburn, K. L., 2011. Plasma cortisol and thyroid hormone concentrations in pre-weaning Australian fur seal pups. *Gen Comp Endocrinol* 172, 277–281.

Auperin, B., Geslin, M., 2008. Plasma cortisol response to stress in juvenile rainbow trout is influenced by their life history during early development and by egg cortisol content. *Gen Comp Endocrinol* 158, 234–239.

Badyaev, A. V., 2005. Stress-induced variation in evolution: from behavioural plasticity to genetic assimilation. *Proc R Soc Lond B* 272, 877–886.

Badyaev, A. V., 2009. Evolutionary significance of phenotypic accommodation in novel environments: an empirical test of the Baldwin effect. *Phil Trans R Soc B* 364, 1125–1141.

Badyaev, A. V., Hamstra, T. L., Oh, K. P., Seaman, D. A. A., 2006. Sex-biased maternal effects reduce ectoparasite-induced mortality in a passerine bird. *Proc Natl Acad Sci USA* 103, 14406–14411.

Badyaev, A. V., Uller, T., 2009. Parental effects in ecology and evolution: mechanisms, processes and implications. *Phil Trans R Soc B* 364, 1169–1177.

Barry, T. P., Malison, J. A., Held, J. A., Parrish, J. J., 1995. Ontogeny of the cortisol stress-response in larval rainbow-trout. *Gen Comp Endocrinol* 97, 57–65.

Belden, L. K., Moore, I. T., Wingfield, J. C., Blaustein, A. R., 2005. Corticosterone and growth in Pacific Treefrog (*Hyla regilla*) tadpoles. *Copeia* 424–430.

Belliure, J., Meylan, S., Clobert, J., 2004. Prenatal and postnatal effects of corticosterone on Behavior in juveniles of the common lizard, *Lacerta vivipara*. *J Exp Zool A: Comp Exp Biol* 301A, 401–410.

Belthoff, J. R., Dufty, A. M., Jr. 1998. Corticosterone, body condition and locomotor activity: a model for dispersal in screech-owls. *Anim Behav* 55, 405–415.

Benard, M. F., McCauley, S. J., 2008. Integrating across life-history stages: Consequences of natal habitat effects on dispersal. *Am Nat* 171, 553–567.

Benowitz-Fredericks, Z. M., Shultz, M. T., Kitaysky, A. S., 2008. Stress hormones suggest opposite trends of food availability for planktivorous and piscivorous seabirds in 2 years. *Deep-Sea Res Part II Top Stud Oceanogr* 55, 1868–1876.

Bertin, A., Richard-Yris, M. A., Houdelier, C., Lumineau, S., Mostl, E., Kuchar, A., Hirschenhauser, K., Kotrschal, K., 2008. Habituation to humans affects yolk steroid levels and offspring phenotype in quail. *Horm Behav* 54, 396–402.

Bize, P., Criscuolo, F., Metcalfe, N. B., Nasir, L., Monaghan, P., 2009. Telomere dynamics rather than age predict life expectancy in the wild. *Proc R Soc Lond B* 276, 1679–1683.

Blanchard, D. C., Spencer, R. L., Weiss, S. M., Blanchard, R. J., McEwen, B., Sakai, R. R., 1995. Visible burrow system as a model of chronic social stress: Behavioral and neuroendocrine correlates. *Psychoneuroendocrinology* 20, 117–134.

Blanchard, R. J., Blanchard, D. C., 1989. Antipredator defensive behaviors in a visible burrow system. *J Comp Psychol* 103, 70–82.

Blanchard, R. J., Blanchard, D. C., 2003. Bringing natural behaviors into the laboratory: A tribute to Paul MacLean. *Physiol Behav* 79, 515–524.

Blas, J., Baos, R., Bortolotti, G. R., Marchant, T., Hiraldo, F., 2005. A multi-tier approach to identifying environmental stress in altricial nestling birds. *Func Ecol* 19, 315–322.

Blas, J., Baos, R., Bortolotti, G. R., Marchant, T. A., Hiraldo, F., 2006. Age-related variation in the adrenocortical response to stress in nestling white storks (*Ciconia ciconia*) supports the developmental hypothesis. *Gen Comp Endocrin*ol 148, 172–180.

Blas, J., Bortolotti, G. R., Tella, J. L., Baos, R., Marchant, T. A., 2007. Stress response during development predicts fitness in a wild, long lived vertebrate. *Proc Natl Acad Sci USA* 104, 8880–8884.

Bonier, F., Martin, P. R., Wingfield, J. C., 2007. Maternal corticosteroids influence primary offspring sex ratio in a free-ranging passerine bird. *Behav Ecol* 18, 1045–1050.

Boonstra, R., Hik, D., Singleton, G. P., Tinnikov, A., 1998. The impact of predator-induced stress on the snowshore hare cycle. *Ecol Monogr* 68, 371–394.

Boonstra, R., Singleton, G. R., 1993. Population declines in the snowshoe hare and the role of stress. *Gen Comp Endocrinol* 91, 126–143.

Breuner, C. W., Greenberg, A. L., Wingfield, J. C., 1998. Noninvasive corticosterone treatment rapidly increases activity in Gambel's white-crowned sparrows (*Zonotrichia leucophrys gambelii*). *Gen Comp Endocrinol* 111, 386–394.

Brewer, J. H., O'Reilly, K. M., Kildaw, S. D., Buck, C. L., 2008. Interannual variation in the adrenal responsiveness of black-legged kittiwake chicks (*Rissa tridactyla*). *Gen Comp Endocrinol* 156, 361–368.

Brockman, D. K., Cobden, A. K., Whitten, P. L., 2009. Birth season glucocorticoids are related to the presence of infants in sifaka (*Propithecus verreauxi*). *Proc R Soc Lond B* 276, 1855–1863.

Brown, K. I., Nestor, K. E., 1973. Some physiological responses of turkeys selected for high and low adrenal response to cold stress. *Poult Sci* 52, 1948–1954.

Buchanan, K. L., Leitner, S., Spencer, K. A., Goldsmith, A. R., Catchpole, C. K., 2004. Developmental stress selectively affects the song control nucleus HVC in the zebra finch. *Proc R Soc Lond B* 271, 2381–2386.

Buck, C. L., O'Reilly, K. A., Kildaw, S. D., 2007. Interannual variability of black-legged kittiwake productivity is reflected in baseline plasma corticosterone. *Gen Comp Endocrinol* 150, 430–436.

Butler, M. W., Leppert, L. L., Dufty, A. M., 2010. Effects of small increases in corticosterone levels on morphology, immune function, and feather development. *Physiol Biochem Zool* 83, 78–86.

Caldji, C., Liu, D., Sharma, S., Diorio, J., Francis, D., Meaney, M. J., Plotsky, P. M., 2001. Development of individual differences in behavioral and endocrine responses to stress: role of the postnatal environment. In: McEwen, B. S., Goodman, H. M. (Eds.), Handbook of physiology; Section 7: The endocrine system; Volume IV: Coping with the environment: Neural and endocrine mechanisms., Oxford University Press, New York, pp. 271–292.

Cameron, N. M., Champagne, F. A., Parent, C., Fish, E. W., Ozaki-Kuroda, K., Meaney, M. J., 2005. The programming of individual differences in defensive responses and reproductive strategies in the rat through variations in maternal care. *NeurosciBiobehav Rev* 29, 843–865.

Carere, C., Groothuis, T. G. G., Moestl, E., Daan, S., Koolhaas, J. M., 2003. Fecal corticosteroids in a territorial bird selected for different personalities: Daily rhythm and the response to social stress. *Horm Behav* 43, 540–548.

Carey, J. B., McCormick, S. D., 1998. Atlantic salmon smolts are more responsive to an acute handling and confinement stress than parr. *Aquaculture* 168, 237–253.

Cavigelli, S. A., Ragan, C. M., Michael, K. C., Kovacsics, C. E., Brliscke, A. P., 2009. Stable behavioral inhibition and glucocorticoid production as predictors of longevity. *Physiol Behav* 98, 205–214.

Cease, A. J., Lutterschmidt, D. I., Mason, R. T., 2007. Corticosterone and the transition from courtship behavior to dispersal in male red-sided garter snakes (Thamnophis sirtalis parietalis). *Gen Comp Endocrinol* 150, 124–131.

Clark, M. M., Galef, B. G., 1995. Prenatal influences on reproductive life-history strategies. *Trends Ecol Evolut* 10, 151–153.

Cockrem, J., 2006. Corticosterone stress responses and avian personalities. *J Ornithol* 147, 6–16.

Cockrem, J. F., 2007. Stress, corticosterone responses and avian personalities. *J Ornithol* 148, S169–S178.

Cockrem, J. F., Barrett, D. P., Candy, E. J., Potter, M. A., 2009. Corticosterone responses in birds: Individual variation and repeatability in Adelie penguins (*Pygoscelis adeliae*) and other species, and the use of power analysis to determine sample sizes. *Gen Comp Endocrinol* 163, 158–168.

Cockrem, J. F., Silverin, B., 2002. Variation within and between birds in corticosterone responses of great tits (*Parus major*). *Gen Comp Endocrinol* 125, 197–206.

Cook, N. J., Renema, R., Wilkinson, C., Schaefer, A. L., 2009. Comparisons among serum, egg albumin and yolk concentrations of corticosterone as biomarkers of basal and stimulated adrenocortical activity of laying hens. *Brit Poultry Sci* 50, 620–633.

Corbel, H., Geiger, S., Groscolas, R., 2010. Preparing to fledge: the adrenocortical and metabolic responses to stress in king penguin chicks. *Func Ecol.* 24, 82–92.

Corbel, H., Groscolas, R., 2008. A role for corticosterone and food restriction in the fledging of nestling white storks. *Horm Behav* 53, 557–566.

Corbel, H., Morlon, F., Groscolas, R., 2008. Is fledging in king penguin chicks related to changes in metabolic or endocrinal status? *Gen Comp Endocrinol* 155, 804–813.

Corben, C. J., Ingram, G. J., Tyler, M. J., 1974. Gastric brooding: Unique form of parental care in an Australian frog. *Science* 186, 946–947.

Cote, J., Clobert, J., Meylan, S., Fitze, P. S., 2006. Experimental enhancement of corticosterone levels positively affects subsequent male survival. *Horm Behav* 49, 320–327.

Cree, A., Tyrrell, C. L., Preest, M. R., Thorburn, D., Guillette, L. J., 2003. Protecting embryos from stress: corticosterone effects and the corticosterone response to capture and confinement during pregnancy in a live-bearing lizard (*Hoplodactylus maculatus*). *Gen Comp Endocrinol* 134, 316–329.

Crespi, E. J., Denver, R. J., 2005. Roles of stress hormones in food intake regulation in anuran amphibians throughout the life cycle. *Comp Biochem Physiol A* 141, 381–390.

Daisley, J. N., Bromundt, V., Mostl, E., Kotrschal, K., 2005. Enhanced yolk testosterone influences behavioral phenotype independent of sex in Japanese quail chicks *Coturnix japonica*. *Horm Behav* 47, 185–194.

De Fraipont, M., Clobert, J., John, H., Alder, S., 2000. Increased pre-natal maternal corticosterone promotes philopatry of offspring in common lizards *Lacerta vivipara*. *J Anim Ecol* 69, 404–413.

Deane, E. E., Woo, N. Y. S., 2003. Ontogeny of thyroid hormones, cortisol, hsp70 and hsp90 during silver sea bream larval development. *Life Sciences* 72, 805–818.

Dejesus, E. G., Hirano, T., Inui, Y., 1993. Flounder metamorphosis—its regulation by various hormones. *Fish Physiol Biochem* 11, 323–328.

delaMora, A. N., Drummond, H., Wingfield, J. C., 1996. Hormonal correlates of dominance and starvation-induced aggression in chicks of the blue-footed booby. *Ethology* 102, 748–761.

Denver, R. J., 1998. Hormonal correlates of environmentally induced metamorphosis in the Western spadefoot toad, *Scaphiopus hammondii*. *Gen Comp Endocrinol* 110, 326–336.

Denver, R. J., 2009. Stress hormones mediate environment-genotype interactions during amphibian development. *Gen Comp Endocrinol* 164, 20–31.

DesRochers, D. W., Reed, J. M., Awerman, J., Kluge, J., Wilkinson, J., van Griethuijsen, L. I., Aman, J., Romero, L. M., 2009. Exogenous and endogenous corticosterone alter feather quality. *Comp Biochem Physiol Part A: Mol Integr Physiol* 152, 46–52.

Dingemanse, N. J., Reale, D., 2005. Natural selection and animal personality. *Behaviour* 142, 1159–1184.

Douglas, H. D., Kitaysky, A. S., Kitaiskaia, E. V., Maccormick, A., Kelly, A., 2009. Size of ornament is negatively correlated with baseline corticosterone in males of a socially monogamous colonial seabird. *J Comp Physiol B* 179, 297–304.

Drickamer, L. C., 1996. Intra-uterine position and anogenital distance in house mice: Consequences under field conditions. *Anim Behav* 51, 925–934.

Dufty, A. M., Clobert, J., Moller, A. P., 2002. Hormones, developmental plasticity and adaptation. *Trends Ecol Evolut* 17, 190–196.

Ehrlich, P. R., Dobkin, D. S., Wheye, D., 1988. *The birder's handbook: A field guide to the natural history of North American birds.* Simon and Schuster, New York.

Engelhard, G. H., Brasseur, S., Hall, A. J., Burton, H. R., Reijnders, P. J. H., 2002. Adrenocortical responsiveness in southern elephant seal mothers and pups during lactation and the effect of scientific handling. *J Comp Physiol B* 172, 315–328.

Eraud, C., Trouve, C., Dano, S., Chastel, O., Faivre, B., 2008. Competition for resources modulates cell-mediated immunity and stress hormone level in nestling collared doves (*Streptopelia decaocto*). *Gen Comp Endocrinol* 155, 542–551.

Eriksen, M. S., Bakken, M., Espmark, A., Braastad, B. O., Salte, R., 2006. Prespawning stress in farmed Atlantic salmon Salmo salar: Maternal cortisol exposure and hyperthermia during embryonic development affect offspring survival, growth and incidence of malformations. *J Fish Biol* 69, 114–129.

Eriksen, M. S., Haug, A., Torjesen, P. A., Bakken, M., 2003. Prenatal exposure to corticosterone impairs embryonic development and increases fluctuating asymmetry in chickens (*Gallus gallus domesticus*). *Brit Poultry Sci* 44, 690–697.

Evans, M. R., Roberts, M. L., Buchanan, K. L., Goldsmith, A. R., 2006. Heritability of corticosterone response and changes in life history traits during selection in the zebra finch. *J Evolut Biol* 19, 343–352.

Ewen, J. G., Cassey, P., Moller, A. P., 2004. Facultative primary a lack of evidence sex ratio variation: A lack of evidence in birds? *Proc R Soc Lond B* 271, 1277–1282.

Ewen, J. G., Crozier, R. H., Cassey, P., Ward-Smith, T., Painter, J. N., Robertson, R. J., Jones, D. A., Clarke, M. F., 2003. Facultative control of offspring sex in the cooperatively breeding bell miner, *Manorina melanophrys. Behav Ecol* 14, 157–164.

Ferreira, A. P. S., Martinez, P. E., Colares, E. P., Robaldo, R. B., Berne, M. E. A., Filho, K. C. M., Bianchini, A., 2005. Serum immunoglobulin G concentration in Southern elephant seal, *Mirounga leonina* (Linnaeus, 1758), from Elephant Island (Antarctica): Sexual and adrenal steroid hormones effects. *Vet Immunol Immunopathol* 106, 239–245.

Fitze, P. S., Cote, J., San-Jose, L. M., Meylan, S., Isaksson, C., Andersson, S., Rossi, J. M., Clobert, J., 2009. Carotenoid-based colours reflect the stress response in the common lizard. *Plos One* 4, e5111.

Flik, G., Stouthart, X. J. H. X., Spanings, F. A. T., Lock, R. A. C., Fenwick, J. C., Wendelaar Bonga, S. E., 2002. Stress response to waterborne Cu during early life stages of carp, *Cyprinus carpio. Aquatic Toxicol* 56, 167–176.

Freeman, B. M., 1982. Stress non-responsiveness in the newly-hatched fowl. *Comp Biochem Physiol A* 72, 251–253.

Freeman, B. M., Flack, I. H., 1980. Effects of handling on plasma corticosterone concentrations in the immature domestic fowl. *Comp Biochem Physiol* 66A, 77–81.

Freeman, B. M., Manning, A. C. C., 1984. Re-establishment of the stress response in *Gallus domesticus* after hatching. *Comp Biochem Physiol* 78A, 267–270.

Freire, R., van Dort, S., Rogers, L. J., 2006. Pre- and post-hatching effects of corticosterone treatment on behavior of the domestic chick. *Horm Behav* 49, 157–165.

Fridinger, R. W., O'Reilly, K. M., Kildaw, S. D., Buck, C. L., 2007. Removal of a nest-mate elicits an age-dependent increase in plasma corticosterone of nestling black-legged kittiwakes. *J Field Ornith* 78, 93–99.

Frigerio, D., Moestl, E., Kotrschal, K., 2001. Excreted metabolites of gonadal steroid hormones and corticosterone in greylag geese (*Anser anser*) from hatching to fledging. *Gen Comp Endocrinol* 124, 246–255.

Frost, A. J., Winrow-Giffen, A., Ashley, P. J., Sneddon, L. U., 2007. Plasticity in animal personality traits: does prior experience alter the degree of boldness? *Proc R Soc Lond B* 274, 333–339.

Fucikova, E., Drent, P. J., Smits, N., van Oers, K., 2009. Handling stress as a measurement of personality in great tit nestlings (*Parus major*). *Ethology* 115, 366–374.

Gagliano, M., McCormick, M. I., 2009. Hormonally mediated maternal effects shape offspring survival potential in stressful environments. *Oecologia* 160, 657–665.

Galton, V. A., 1990. Mechanisms underlying the acceleration of thyroid hormone-induced tadpole metamorphosis by corticosterone. *Endocrinology* 127, 2997–3002.

Gam, A. E., Mendonca, M. T., Navara, K. J., 2011. Acute corticosterone treatment prior to ovulation biases offspring sex ratios towards males in zebra finches *Taeniopygia guttata. J Avian Biol* 42, 253–258.

Gesquiere, L. R., Altmann, J., Khan, M. Z., Couret, J., Yu, J. C., Endres, C. S., Lynch, J. W., Ogola, P., Fox, E. A., Alberts, S. C., Wango, E. O., 2005. Coming of age: Steroid hormones of wild immature baboons (*Papio cynocephalus*). *Am J Primatol* 67, 83–100.

Gil, D., Bulmer, E., Celis, P., Puerta, M., 2008. Increased sibling competition does not increase testosterone or corticosterone levels in nestlings of the spotless starling (*Sturnus unicolor*). *Horm Behav* 54, 238–243.

Gil, D., Heim, C., Bulmer, E., Rocha, M., Puerta, M., Naguib, M., 2004. Negative effects of early developmental stress on yolk testosterone levels in a passerine bird. *J Exp Biol* 207, 2215–2220.

Gilbert, S. F., 2005. Mechanisms for the environmental regulation of gene expression: Ecological aspects of animal development. *J Biosci* 30, 65–74.

Girling, J. E., Jones, S. A., 2006. In vitro steroid production by adrenals and kidney-gonads from embryonic southern snow skinks (*Niveoscincus microlepidotus*): Implications for the control of the timing of parturition? *Gen Comp Endocrinol* 145, 169–176.

Glennemeier, K. A., Denver, R. J., 2001. Developmental changes in interrenal responsiveness in anuran amphibians. In: *Annual meeting of the Society for Integrative and Comparative Biology*, Chicago, pp. 565–573.

Glennemeier, K. A., Denver, R. J., 2002a. Role for corticoids in mediating the response of Rana pipiens tadpoles to intraspecific competition. *J Exp Zool* 292, 32–40.

Glennemeier, K. A., Denver, R. J., 2002b. Small changes in whole-body corticosterone content affect larval *Rana pipiens* fitness components. *Gen Comp Endocrinol* 127, 16–25.

Groothuis, T. G. G., Carere, C., 2005. Avian personalities: Characterization and epigenesis. *Neurosci Biobehav Rev* 29, 137.

Groothuis, T. G. G., Muller, W., von Engelhardt, N., Carere, C., Eising, C., 2005. Maternal hormones as a tool to adjust offspring phenotype in avian species. *Neurosci Biobehav Rev* 29, 329–352.

Groothuis, T. G. G., Schwabl, H., 2008. Hormone-mediated maternal effects in birds: mechanisms matter but what do we know of them? *Phil Trans R Soc B* 363, 1647–1661.

Gross, W. B., Siegel, P. B., 1985. Selective breeding of chickens for corticosterone response to social stress. *Poult Sci* 64, 2230–2233.

Gruss, M., Westphal, S., Luley, C., Braun, K., 2006. Endocrine and behavioural plasticity in response to juvenile stress in the semi-precocial rodent *Octodon degus. Psychoneuroendocrinology* 31, 361–372.

Gunnar, M. R., Donzella, B., 2002. Social regulation of the cortisol levels in early human development. *Psychoneuroendocrinology* 27, 199–220.

Hamann, M., Jessop, T. S., Schauble, C. S., 2007. Fuel use and corticosterone dynamics in hatchling green sea turtles (*Chelonia mydas*) during natal dispersal. *J Exper Marine Biol Ecol* 353, 13–21.

Harding, A. M. A., Kitaysky, A. S., Hall, M. E., Welcker, J., Karnovsky, N. J., Talbot, S. L., Hamer, K. C., Gremillet, D., 2009. Flexibility in the parental effort of an Arctic-breeding seabird. *Func Ecol* 23, 348–358.

Hartmann, N., Reichwald, K., Lechel, A., Graf, M., Kirschner, J., Dorn, A., Terzibasi, E., Wellner, J., Platzer, M., Rudolph, K. L., Cellerino, A., Englert, C., 2009. Telomeres shorten while Tert expression increases during ageing of the short-lived fish *Nothobranchius furzeri*. Mech. *Ageing Dev* 130, 290–296.

Hatase, H., Sudo, R., Watanabe, K. K., Kasugai, T., Saito, T., Okamoto, H., Uchida, I., Tsukamoto, K., 2008. Shorter telomere length with age in the loggerhead turtle: a new hope for live sea turtle age estimation. *Genes Genet Syst* 83, 423–426.

Haussmann, M. F., Longenecker, A. S., Marchetto, N. M., Juliano, S. A., Bowden, R. M., 2012. Embryonic exposure to corticosterone modifies the juvenile stress response, oxidative stress and telomere length. *Proc R Soc Lond B* 279, 1447–1456.

Hayward, A. D., Wilson, A. J., Pilkington, J. G., Pemberton, J. M., Kruuk, L. E. B., 2009. Ageing in a variable habitat: Environmental stress affects senescence in parasite resistance in St Kilda Soay sheep. *Proc R Soc Lond B* 276, 3477–3485.

Hayward, L. S., Richardson, J. B., Grogan, M. N., Wingfield, J. C., 2006. Sex differences in the organizational effects of corticosterone in the egg yolk of quail. *Gen Comp Endocrinol* 146, 144–148.

Hayward, L. S., Satterlee, D. G., Wingfield, J. C., 2005. Japanese quail selected for high plasma corticosterone response deposit high levels of corticosterone in their eggs. *Physiol Biochem Zool* 78, 1026–1031.

Hayward, L. S., Wingfield, J. C., 2004. Maternal corticosterone is transferred to avian yolk and may alter offspring growth and adult phenotype. *Gen Comp Endocrinol* 135, 365–371.

Heath, J., 1997. Corticosterone levels during nest departure of juvenile American kestrels. *Condor* 99, 806–811.

Hegner, R. E., Wingfield, J. C., 1987. Effects of brood-size manipulations on parental investment, breeding success, and reproductive endocrinology of house sparrows. *Auk* 104, 470–480.

Heidinger, B. J., Nisbet, I. C. T., Ketterson, E. D., 2006. Older parents are less responsive to a stressor in a long-lived seabird: A mechanism for increased reproductive performance with age? *Proc R Soc Lond B* 273, 2227–2231.

Heidinger, B. J., Nisbet, I. C. T., Ketterson, E. D., 2008. Changes in adrenal capacity contribute to a decline in the stress response with age in a long-lived seabird. *Gen Comp Endocrinol* 156, 564–568.

Henriksen, R., Rettenbacher, S., Groothuis, T. G. G., 2011. Prenatal stress in birds: Pathways, effects, function and perspectives. *Neurosci Biobehav Rev* 35, 1484–1501.

Hoch, J. A., 1998. Initiation of bacterial development. *Curr Opin Microbiol* 1, 170–174.

Hodgson, Z. G., Meddle, S. L., Roberts, M. L., Buchanan, K. L., Evans, M. R., Metzdorf, R., Gahr, M., Healy, S. D., 2007. Spatial ability is impaired and hippocampal mineralocorticoid receptor mRNA expression reduced in zebra finches (*Taeniopygia guttata*) selected for acute high corticosterone response to stress. *Proc R Soc Lond B* 274, 239–245.

Holmes, W. N., Cronshaw, J., Collie, M. A., Rohde, K. E., 1992. Cellular aspects of the stress response in precocial neonates *Ornis Scan* 23, 388–397.

Holmes, W. N., Redondo, J. L., Cronshaw, J., 1989. Changes in the adrenal steroidogenic responsiveness of the mallard duck (*Anas-platyrhynchos*) during early post-natal development. *Comp Biochem Physiol A* 92, 403–408.

Horton, B. M., Holberton, R. L., 2009. Corticosterone manipulations alter morph-specific nestling provisioning behavior in male white-throated sparrows, *Zonotrichia albicollis*. *Horm Behav* 56, 510–518.

Husak, J. F., Moore, I. T., 2008. Stress hormones and mate choice. *Trends Ecol Evolut* 23, 532–534.

Janczak, A. M., Braastad, B. O., Bakken, M., 2006. Behavioural effects of embryonic exposure to corticosterone in chickens. *Appl Anim Behav Sci* 96, 69–82.

Janczak, A. M., Heikkilae, M., Valros, A., Torjesen, P., Andersen, I. L., Bakken, M., 2007a. Effects of embryonic corticosterone exposure and post-hatch handling on tonic immobility and willingness to compete in chicks. *Appl Anim Behav Sci* 107, 275–286.

Janczak, A. M., Torjesen, P., Palme, R., Bakken, M., 2007b. Effects of stress in hens on the behaviour of their offspring. *Appl Anim Behav Sci* 107, 66–77.

Jennings, D. H., Painter, D. L., Moore, M. C., 2004. Role of the adrenal gland in early post-hatching differentiation of alternative male phenotypes in the tree lezard (*Urosaurus ornatus*). *Gen Comp Endocrinol* 135, 81–89.

Jessop, T. S., Hamann, M., 2005. Interplay between age class, sex and stress response in green turtles (*Chelonia mydas*). *Aust J Zool* 53, 131–136.

Jones, R. B., Satterlee, D. G., Ryder, F. H., 1994. Fear of humans in Japanese quail selected for low or high adrenocortical response. *Physiol Behav* 56, 379–383.

Kern, M., Bacon, W., Long, D., Cowie, R. J., 2001. Possible roles for corticosterone and critical size in the fledging of nestling pied flycatchers. *Physiol Biochem Zool* 74, 651.

Ketterson, E.D., Nolan, V., Jr. 1999. Adaptation, exaptation, and constraint: A hormonal perspective. *Am Nat* 154, S4–S25.

Ketterson, E. D., Nolan, V., Cawthorn, M. J., Parker, P. G., Ziegenfus, C., 1996. Phenotypic engineering: Using hormones to explore the mechanistic and functional bases of phenotypic variation in nature. *Ibis* 138, 70–86.

Kitaysky, A. S., Hunt G. L., Jr., Flint, E. N., Rubega, M. A., Decker, M. B., 2000. Resource allocation in breeding seabirds: Responses to fluctuations in their food supply. *Mar Ecol Progr Ser* 206, 283.

Kitaysky, A. S., Kitaiskaia, E. V., Piatt, J. F., Wingfield, J. C., 2003. Benefits and costs of increased levels of corticosterone in seabird chicks. *Horm Behav* 43, 140–149.

Kitaysky, A. S., Kitaiskaia, E. V., Wingfield, J. C., Piatt, J. F., 2001a. Dietary restriction causes chronic elevation of corticosterone and enhances stress response in red-legged kittiwake chicks. *J Comp Physiol B* 171, 701.

Kitaysky, A. S., Piatt, J. F., Wingfield, J. C., 2007. Stress hormones link food availability and population processes in seabirds. *Mar Ecol Prog Ser* 352, 245–258.

Kitaysky, A. S., Piatt, J. F., Wingfield, J. C., Romano, M., 1999a. The adrenocortical stress-response of black-legged kittiwake chicks in relation to dietary restrictions. *J Comp Physiol B* 169, 303–310.

Kitaysky, A. S., Romano, M. D., Piatt, J. F., Wingfield, J. C., Kikuchi, M., 2005. The adrenocortical response of tufted puffin chicks to nutritional deficits. *Horm Behav* 47, 606–619.

Kitaysky, A. S., Wingfield, J. C., Piatt, J. F., 1999b. Dynamics of food availability, body condition and physiological stress response in breeding black-legged kittiwakes. *Func Ecol* 13, 577–584.

Kitaysky, A. S., Wingfield, J. C., Piatt, J. F., 2001b. Corticosterone facilitates begging and affects resource allocation in the black-legged kittiwake. *Behav Ecol* 12, 619.

Knapp, R., Marsh-Matthews, E., Vo, L., Rosencrans, S., 2011. Stress hormone masculinizes female morphology and behaviour. *Biol Lett* 7, 150–152.

Komdeur, J., Magrath, M. J. L., Krackow, S., 2002. Pre-ovulation control of hatchling sex ratio in the Seychelles warbler. *Proc R Soc Lond B* 269, 1067–1072.

Koolhaas, J. M., de Boer, S. F., Buwalda, B., van Reenen, K., 2007. Individual variation in coping with stress: A multidimensional approach of ultimate and proximate mechanisms. *Brain Behav Evol* 70, 218–226.

Kotrschal, A., Ilmonen, P., Penn, D. J., 2007. Stress impacts telomere dynamics. *Biol Lett* 3, 128–130.

Krackow, S., 1995. Potential mechanisms for sex-ratio adjustment in mammals and birds *Biol Rev Cambridge Phil Soc* 70, 225–241.

Kralj-Fiser, S., Scheiber, I. B. R., Blejec, A., Moestl, E., Kotrschal, K., 2007. Individualities in a flock of free-roaming greylag geese: Behavioral and physiological consistency over time and across situations. *Horm Behav* 51, 239–248.

Krass, P. M., Bazhan, N. M., Reshetnikov, S. S., Trut, L. N., 1979. Adrenal reactivity to ACTH age changes in silver foxes inheriting different defensive behaviors. *Biol Bull Acad Sci USSR* 6, 306–310.

Landys, M. M., Goymann, W., Slagsyold, T., 2011. Rearing conditions have long-term consequences for stress responsiveness in free-living great tits. *Gen Comp Endocrinol* 174, 219–224.

Langkilde, T., Lance, V. A., Shine, R., 2005. Ecological consequences of agonistic interactions in lizards. *Ecology* 86, 1650–1659.

Lecomte, V. J., Sorci, G., Cornet, S., Jaeger, A., Faivre, B., Arnoux, E., Gaillard, M., Trouve, C., Besson, D., Chastel, O., Weimerskirch, H., 2010. Patterns of aging in the long-lived wandering albatross. *Proc Natl Acad Sci USA* 107, 6370–6375.

Lendvai, D. M. Z., Loiseau, C., Sorci, G., Chastel, O., 2009. Early developmental conditions affect stress response in juvenile but not in adult house sparrows (*Passer domesticus*). *Gen Comp Endocrinol* 160, 30–35.

Li, Z. H., Piggot, P. J., 2001. Development of a two-part transcription probe to determine the completeness of temporal and spatial compartmentalization of gene expression during bacterial development. *Proc Natl Acad Sci USA* 98, 12538–12543.

Love, O. P., Bird, D. M., Shutt, L. J., 2003a. Corticosterone levels during post-natal development in captive American kestrels (*Falco sparverius*). *Gen Comp Endocrinol* 130, 135–141.

Love, O. P., Bird, D. M., Shutt, L. J., 2003b. Plasma corticosterone in American kestrel siblings: Effects of age, hatching order, and hatching asynchrony. *Horm Behav* 43, 480.

Love, O. P., Chin, E. H., Wynne-Edwards, K. E., Williams, T. D., 2005. Stress hormones: A link between maternal condition and sex-biased reproductive investment. *Am Nat* 166, 751–766.

Love, O. P., Gilchrist, H. G., Bety, J., Wynne-Edwards, K. E., Berzins, L., Williams, T. D., 2008. Using life-histories to predict and interpret variability in yolk hormones. In: *9th International Symposium on Avian Endocrinology*. Academic Press, Elsevier Science, Leuven, Belgium, pp. 169–174.

Love, O. P., Shutt, L. J., Silfies, J. S., Bird, D. M., 2003c. Repeated restraint and sampling results in reduced corticosterone levels in developing and adult captive American kestrels (*Falco sparverius*). *Physiol Biochem Zool* 76, 753–761.

Love, O. P., Williams, T. D., 2008a. The adaptive value of stress-induced phenotypes: Effects of maternally derived corticosterone on sex-biased investment, cost of reproduction, and maternal fitness. *Am Nat* 172, E135–E149.

Love, O. P., Williams, T. D., 2008b. Plasticity in the adrenocortical response of a free-living vertebrate: The role of pre- and post-natal developmental stress. *Horm Behav* 54, 496–505.

Lynn, S. E., Prince, L. E., Phillips, M. M., 2010. A single exposure to an acute stressor has lasting consequences for the hypothalamo-pituitary-adrenal response to stress in free-living birds. *Gen Comp Endocrinol* 165, 337–344.

MacDonald, I. F., Kempster, B., Zanette, L., MacDougall-Shackleton, S. A., 2006. Early nutritional stress impairs development of a song-control brain region in both male and female juvenile song sparrows (*Melospiza melodia*) at the onset of song learning. *Proc R Soc Lond B* 273, 2559–2564.

MacDougall-Shackleton, S. A., 2009. The importance of development: what songbirds can teach us. *Can J Exper Psychol* 63, 74–79.

MacDougall-Shackleton, S. A., Dindia, L., Newman, A. E. M., Potvin, D. A., Stewart, K. A., MacDougall-Shackleton, E. A., 2009. Stress, song and survival in sparrows. *Biol Lett* 5, 746–748.

Malisch, J. L., Breuner, C. W., Gomes, F. R., Chappell, M. A., Garland, T., 2008. Circadian pattern of total and free corticosterone concentrations, corticosteroid-binding globulin, and physical activity in mice selectively bred for high voluntary wheelrunning behaviour. *Gen Comp Endocrinol* 156, 210–217.

Malisch, J. L., Saltzman, W., Gomes, F. R., Rezende, E. L., Jeske, D. R., Garland, T., 2007. Baseline and stress-induced plasma corticosterone concentrations of mice selectively bred for high voluntary wheel running. *Physiol Biochem Zool* 80, 146–156.

Mashaly, M. M., 1991. Effect of exogenous corticosterone on chicken embryonic development. *Poult Sci* 70, 371–374.

Mateo, J. M., 2006. Developmental and geographic variation in stress hormones in wild Belding's ground squirrels (*Spermophilus beldingi*). *Horm Behav* 50, 718–725.

McCormick, M. I., 2006. Mothers matter: Crowding leads to stressed mothers and smaller offspring in marine fish. *Ecology* 87, 1104–1109.

McCormick, M. I., 2009a. Indirect effects of heterospecific interactions on progeny size through maternal stress. *Oikos* 118, 744–752.

McCormick, M. I., Nechaev, I. V., 2002. Influence of cortisol on developmental rhythms during embryogenesis in a tropical damselfish. *J Exp Zool* 293, 456–466.

McCormick, S. D., 2009b. Evolution of the hormonal control of animal performance: Insights from the seaward migration of salmon. *Integ Comp Biol* 49, 408–422.

Medler, K. F., Lance, V. A., 1998. Sex differences in plasma corticosterone levels in alligator (*Alligator mississippiensis*) embryos. *J Exp Zool* 280, 238–244.

Meylan, S., Belliure, J., Clobert, J., de Fraipont, M., 2002. Stress and body condition as prenatal and postnatal determinants of dispersal in the common lizard (*Lacerta vivipara*). *Horm Behav* 42, 319–326.

Meylan, S., Clobert, J., 2004. Maternal effects on offspring locomotion: Influence of density and corticosterone elevation in the lizard *Lacerta vivipara*. *Physiol Biochem Zool* 77, 450–458.

Meylan, S., Clobert, J., 2005. Is corticosterone-mediated phenotype development adaptive? Maternal corticosterone treatment enhances survival in male lizards. *Horm Behav* 48, 44–52.

Meylan, S., De Fraipont, M., Clobert, J., 2004. Maternal size and stress and offspring philopatry: An experimental study in the common lizard (*Lacerta vivipara*). *Ecoscience* 11, 123–129.

Moe, B., Angelier, F., Bech, C., Chastel, O., 2007. Is basal metabolic rate influenced by age in a long-lived seabird, the snow petrel? *J Exp Biol* 210, 3407–3414.

Monaghan, P., 2008. Early growth conditions, phenotypic development and environmental change. *Phil Trans R Soc B* 363, 1635–1645.

Monaghan, P., Haussmann, M. F., 2006. Do telomere dynamics link lifestyle and lifespan? *Trends Ecol Evolut* 21, 47–53.

Moudgal, R. P., Jagmohan, Panda, J. N., 1990. Epinephrine in egg yolk and abnormal eggshell calcification as the indicator of stress. *Indian J Animal Sci* 60, 53–54.

Muller, C., Jenni-Eiermann, S., Jenni, L., 2010. Development of the adrenocortical response to stress in Eurasian kestrel nestlings: Defence ability, age, brood hierarchy and condition. *Gen Comp Endocrinol* 168, 474–483.

Müller, M. S., Porter, E. T., Grace, J. K., Awkerman, J. A., Birchler, K. T., Gunderson, A. R., Schneider, E. G., Westbrock, M. A., Anderson, D. J., 2011. Maltreated nestlings exhibit correlated maltreatment as adults: Evidence of a "cycle of violence" in Nazca boobies (*Sula granti*). *Auk* 128, 615–619.

Muller, W., Lessells, C. M., Korsten, P., von Engelhardt, N., 2007. Manipulative signals in family conflict? On the function of maternal yolk hormones in birds. *Am Nat* 169, E84–E96.

Mullner, A., Linsenmair, K.E., Wikelski, M., 2004. Exposure to ecotourism reduces survival and affects stress response in hoatzin chicks (*Opisthocomus hoazin*). Biol Conserv 118, 549–558.

Nager, R. G., Monaghan, P., Griffiths, R., Houston, D. C., Dawson, R., 1999. Experimental demonstration that offspring sex ratio varies with maternal condition. *Proc Natl Acad Sci USA* 96, 570–573.

Nepomnaschy, P. A., Welch, K. B., McConnell, D. S., Low, B. S., Strassmann, B. I., England, B. G., 2006. Cortisol levels and very early pregnancy loss in humans. *Proc Natl Acad Sci USA* 103, 3938-3942.

Newman, R. A., 1992. Adaptive plasticity in amphibian metamorphosis. *Bioscience* 42, 671–678.

Nordgreen, J., Janczak, A. M., Bakken, M., 2006. Effects of prenatal exposure to corticosterone on filial imprinting in the domestic chick, Gallus gallus domesticus. *Anim Behav* 72, 1217–1228.

Norris, D. O., 2007. *Vertebrate endocrinology*. Academic Press, Boston.

Okuliarová, M., Šárniková, B., Rettenbacher, S., Škrobánek, P., Zeman, M., 2010. Yolk testosterone and corticosterone in hierarchical follicles and laid eggs of Japanese quail exposed to long-term restraint stress. *Gen Comp Endocrinol* 165, 91–96.

Ortiz, R. M., Houser, D. S., Wade, C. E., Ortiz, C. L., 2003. Hormonal changes associated with the transition between nursing and natural fasting in northern elephant seals (*Mirounga angustirostris*). *Gen Comp Endocrinol* 130, 78–83.

Osadchuk, L. V., Braastad, B. O., Hovland, A. L., Bakken, M., 2003. Reproductive and pituitary-adrenal axis parameters in normal and prenatally stressed prepubertal blue foxes (*Alopex lagopus*). *Anim Sci* 76, 413–420.

Oskina, I. N., Tinnikov, A. A., 1992. Interaction between cortisol and cortisol-binding protein in silver foxes (*Vulpes fulvus*). *Comp Biochem Physiol* 101A, 665–668.

Øverli, Ø., Korzan, W. J., Hoglund, E., Winberg, S., Bollig, H., Watt, M., Forster, G. L., Barton, B. A., Øverli, E., Renner, K. J., Summers, C. H., 2004. Stress coping style predicts aggression and social dominance in rainbow trout. *Horm Behav* 45, 235.

Øverli, Ø., Pottinger, T. G., Carrick, T. R., Øverli, E., Winberg, S., 2002. Differences in behaviour between rainbow trout selected for high- and low-stress responsiveness. *J Exp Biol* 205, 391–395.

Øverli, Ø., Winberg, S., Pottinger, T. G., 2005. Behavioral and neuroendocrine correlates of selection for stress responsiveness in rainbow trout: A review. *Integ Comp Biol* 45, 463–474.

Painter, D., Jennings, D. H., Moore, M. C., 2002. Placental buffering of maternal steroid hormone effects on fetal and yolk hormone levels: A comparative study of a viviparous lizard, *Sceloporus jarrovi*, and an oviparous lizard, *Sceloporus graciosus*. *Gen Comp Endocrinol* 127, 105–116.

Painter, D. L., Moore, M. C., 2005. Steroid hormone metabolism by the chorioallantoic placenta of the mountain spiny lizard *Sceloporus jarrovi* as a possible mechanism for buffering maternal-fetal hormone exchange. *Physiol Biochem Zool* 78, 364–372.

Paitz, R. T., Bowden, R. M., Casto, J. M., 2010. Embryonic modulation of maternal steroids in European starlings (*Sturnus vulgaris*). *Proc R Soc Lond B*. 278, 99–106.

Pardon, M. C., 2007. Stress and ageing interactions: A paradox in the context of shared etiological and physiopathological processes. *Brain Res Rev* 54, 251–273.

Pardon, M. C., Rattray, I., 2008. What do we know about the long-term consequences of stress on ageing and the progression of age-related neurodegenerative disorders? *Neurosci Biobehav Rev* 32, 1103–1120.

Pepels, P. P. L. M., Balm, P. H. M., 2004. Ontogeny of corticotropin-releasing factor and of hypothalamic-pituitary-interrenal axis responsiveness to stress in tilapia (*Oreochromis mossambicus*; Teleostei). *Gen Comp Endocrinol* 139, 251–265.

Pèrez-DomÌnguez, R., Holt, G. J., 2006. Interrenal and thyroid development in red drum (*Sciaenops ocellatus*): Effects of nursery environment on larval growth and cortisol concentration during settlement. *Gen Comp Endocrinol* 146, 108–118.

Piersma, T., Ramenofsky, M., 1998. Long-term decreases of corticosterone in captive migrant shorebirds that maintain seasonal mass and moult cycles. *J Avian Biol* 29, 97–104.

Pigliucci, M., 2005. Evolution of phenotypic plasticity: Where are we going now? *Trends Ecol Evolut* 20, 481–486.

Pike, T. W., 2005. Sex ratio manipulation in response to maternal condition in pigeons: evidence for pre-ovulatory follicle selection. *Behav Ecol Sociobiol* 58, 407–413.

Pike, T. W., Petrie, M., 2003. Potential mechanisms of avian sex manipulation. *Biol Rev* 78, 553–574.

Pike, T. W., Petrie, M., 2005a. Maternal body condition and plasma hormones affect offspring sex ratio in peafowl. *Anim Behav* 70, 745–751.

Pike, T. W., Petrie, M., 2005b. Offspring sex ratio is related to paternal train elaboration and yolk corticosterone in peafowl. *Biol Lett* 1, 204–207.

Pike, T. W., Petrie, M., 2006. Experimental evidence that corticosterone affects offspring sex ratios in quail. *Proc R Soc Lond B* 273, 1093–1098.

Poisbleau, M., Demongin, L., Angelier, F., Dano, S., Lacroix, A., Quillfeldt, P., 2009a. What ecological factors can affect albumen corticosterone levels in the clutches of seabirds? Timing of breeding, disturbance and laying order in rockhopper penguins (*Eudyptes chrysocome chrysocome*). *Gen Comp Endocrinol* 162, 139–145.

Poisbleau, M., Demongin, L., Trouve, C., Quillfeldt, P., 2009b. Maternal deposition of yolk corticosterone in clutches of southern rockhopper penguins (*Eudyptes chrysocome chrysocome*). *Horm Behav* 55, 500–506.

Pravosudov, V. V., Kitaysky, A. S., 2006. Effects of nutritional restrictions during post-hatching development on adrenocortical function in western scrub-jays (*Aphelocoma californica*). *Gen Comp Endocrinol* 145, 25–31.

Pravosudov, V. V., Lavenex, P., Omanska, A., 2005. Nutritional deficits during early development affect hippocampal structure and spatial memory later in life. *Behav Neurosci* 119, 1368–1374.

Preest, M. R., Cree, A., Tyrrell, C. L., 2005. ACTH-induced stress response during pregnancy in a viviparous gecko: No observed effect on offspring quality. *J Exp Zool A: Comp Exp Biol* 303A, 823–835.

Quillfeldt, P., Masello, J. F., Strange, I. J., Buchanan, K. L., 2006. Begging and provisioning of thin-billed prions, *Pachyptila belcheri*, are related to testosterone and corticosterone. *Anim Behav* 71, 1359.

Quillfeldt, P., Poisbleau, M., Chastel, O., Masello, J. F., 2007. Corticosterone in thin-billed prion Pachyptila belcheri chicks: Diel rhythm, timing of fledging and nutritional stress. *Naturwissenschaften* 94, 919–925.

Quillfeldt, P., Poisbleau, M., Chastel, O., Masello, J. F., 2009. Acute stress hyporesponsive period in nestling thin-billed prions *Pachyptila belcheri. J Comp Physiol A* 195, 91–98.

Ramos-Fernandez, G., Nunez-de la Mora, A., Wingfield, J. C., Drummond, H., 2000. Endocrine correlates of dominance in chicks of the blue-footed booby (*Sula nebouxii*): Testing the Challenge Hypothesis. *Ethol Ecol Evolution* 12, 27–34.

Reale, D., Reader, S. M., Sol, D., McDougall, P. T., Dingemanse, N. J., 2007. Integrating animal temperament within ecology and evolution. *Biol Rev* 82, 291–318.

Rensel, M. A., Boughton, R. K., Schoech, S. J., 2010a. Development of the adrenal stress response in the Florida scrub-jay (*Aphelocoma coerulescens*). *Gen Comp Endocrinol* 165, 255–261.

Rensel, M. A., Wilcoxen, T. E., Schoech, S. J., 2010b. The influence of nest attendance and provisioning on nestling stress physiology in the Florida scrub-jay. *Horm Behav* 57, 162–168.

Rettenbacher, S., Mostl, E., Groothuis, T. G. G., 2009. Gestagens and glucocorticoids in chicken eggs. *Gen Comp Endocrinol* 164, 125–129.

Rickard, I. J., Lummaa, V., 2007. The predictive adaptive response and metabolic syndrome: Challenges for the hypothesis. *Trends Endocrinol Metab* 18, 94–99.

Robert, K. A., Vleck, C., Bronikowski, A. M., 2009. The effects of maternal corticosterone levels on offspring behavior in fast- and slow-growth garter snakes (*Thamnophis elegans*). *Horm Behav* 55, 24–32.

Roberts, M. L., Buchanan, K. L., Bennett, A. T. D., Evans, M. R., 2007a. Mate choice in zebra finches: Does corticosterone play a role? *Anim Behav* 74, 921–929.

Roberts, M. L., Buchanan, K. L., Evans, M. R., Marin, R. H., Satterlee, D. G., 2009. The effects of testosterone on immune function in quail selected for divergent plasma corticosterone response. *J Exp Biol* 212, 3125–3131.

Roberts, M. L., Buchanan, K. L., Hasselquist, D., Bennett, A. T. D., Evans, M. R., 2007b. Physiological, morphological and behavioural effects of selecting zebra finches for divergent levels of corticosterone. *J Exp Biol* 210, 4368–4378.

Roberts, M. L., Buchanan, K. L., Hasselquist, D., Evans, M. R., 2007c. Effects of testosterone and corticosterone on immunocompetence in the zebra finch. *Horm Behav* 51, 126–134.

Rodenburg, T. B., Bolhuis, J. E., Koopmanschap, R. E., Ellen, E. D., Decuypere, E., 2009. Maternal care and selection for low mortality affect post-stress corticosterone and peripheral serotonin in laying hens. *Physiol Behav* 98, 519–523.

Romeo, R. D., 2010. Pubertal maturation and programming of hypothalamic-pituitary-adrenal reactivity. *Front Neuroendocrinol* 31, 232–240.

Romeo, R. D., McEwen, B. S., 2006. Stress and the adolescent brain. *Ann NY Acad Sci*, 1094, 202–214.

Romero, L. M., Holt, D. W., Maples, M., Wingfield, J. C., 2006. Corticosterone is not correlated with nest departure in snowy owl chicks (*Nyctea scandiaca*). *Gen Comp Endocrinol* 149, 119–123.

Romero, L. M., Reed, J. M., 2008. Repeatability of baseline corticosterone concentrations. *Gen Comp Endocrinol* 156, 27–33.

Romero, L. M., Soma, K. K., Wingfield, J. C., 1998. The hypothalamus and adrenal regulate modulation of corticosterone release in redpolls (*Carduelis flammea*—an arctic-breeding song bird). *Gen Comp Endocrinol* 109, 347–355.

Roulin, A., Almasi, B., Rossi-Pedruzzi, A., Ducrest, A. L., Wakamatsu, K., Miksik, I., Blount, J. D., Jenni-Eiermann, S., Jenni, L., 2008. Corticosterone mediates the condition-dependent component of melanin-based coloration. *Anim Behav* 75, 1351–1358.

Roulin, A., Ducrest, A.-L., Dijkstra, C., 1999. Effect of brood size manipulations on parents and offspring in the barn owl *Tyto alba*. *Ardea* 87, 91–100.

Rubolini, D., Romano, M., Boncoraglio, G., Ferrari, R. P., Martinelli, R., Galeotti, P., Fasola, M., Saino, N., 2005. Effects of elevated egg corticosterone levels on behavior, growth, and immunity of yellow-legged gull (*Larus michahellis*) chicks. *Horm Behav* 47, 592–605.

Ryan, B. C., Vandenbergh, J. G., 2002. Intrauterine position effects. *Neurosci Biobehav Rev* 26, 665–678.

Saino, N., Romano, M., Ferrari, R. P., Martinelli, R., Moller, A. P., 2005. Stressed mothers lay eggs with high corticosterone levels which produce low-quality offspring. *J Exp Zool* 303A, 998–1006.

Salomons, H. M., Dijkstra, C., Verhulst, S., 2008. Strong but variable associations between social dominance and clutch sex ratio in a colonial corvid. *Behav Ecol* 19, 417–424.

Salomons, H. M., Mulder, G. A., van de Zande, L., Haussmann, M. F., Linskens, M. H. K., Verhulst, S., 2009. Telomere shortening and survival in free-living corvids. *Proc R Soc Lond B* 276, 3157–3165.

Satterlee, D. G., Johnson, W. A., 1988. Selection of Japanese quail for contrasting blood corticosterone response to immobilization. *Poult Sci* 67, 25–32.

Satterlee, D. G., Jones, R. B., 1997. Ease of capture in Japanese quail of two lines divergently selected for adrenocortical response to immobilization. *Poult Sci* 76, 469–471.

Schjolden, J., Stoskhus, A., Winberg, S., 2005. Does individual variation in stress responses and agonistic behavior reflect divergent stress coping strategies in juvenile rainbow trout? *Physiol Biochem Zool* 78, 715–723.

Schjolden, J., Winberg, S., 2007. Genetically determined variation in stress responsiveness in rainbow trout: Behavior and neurobiology. *Brain Behav Evol* 70, 227–238.

Schoech, S. J., Rensel, M. A., Heiss, R. S., 2011. Short- and long-term effects of developmental corticosterone exposure on avian physiology, behavioral phenotype, cognition, and fitness: A review. *Curr Zool* 57, 514–530.

Schoech, S. J., Rensel, M. A., Wilcoxen, T. E., 2012. Here today, not gone tomorrow: Long-term effects of corticosterone. *J Ornithol* 153, S217–S226.

Schwabl, H., 1993. Yolk is a source of maternal testosterone for developing birds. *Proc Natl Acad Sci USA* 90, 11446–11450.

Schwabl, H., 1995. Individual variation of the acute adrenocortical response to stress in the white-throated sparrow. *Zoology* 99, 113–120.

Schwabl, H., 1999. Developmental changes and among-sibling variation of corticosterone levels in an altricial avian species. *Gen Comp Endocrinol* 116, 403–408.

Schwabl, H., Mock, D. W., Gieg, J. A., 1997. A hormonal mechanism for parental favouritism. *Nature* 386, 231–231.

Semlitsch, R. D., Scott, D. E., Pechmann, J. H. K., 1988. Time and size at metamorphosis related to adult fitness in *Ambystoma talpoideum*. *Ecology* 69, 184–192.

Sheriff, M. J., Krebs, C. J., Boonstra, R., 2009. The sensitive hare: sublethal effects of predator stress on reproduction in snowshoe hares. *J Anim Ecol* 78, 1249–1258.

Silverin, B., 1997. The stress response and autumn dispersal behaviour in willow tits. *Anim Behav* 53, 451–459.

Silverin, B., Viebke, P. A., Westin, J., 1989. Hormonal correlates of migration and territorial behavior in juvenile willow tits during autumn. *Gen Comp Endocrinol* 75, 148.

Sims, C. G., Holberton, R. L., 2000. Development of the corticosterone stress response in young northern mockingbirds (*Mimus polyglottos*). *Gen Comp Endocrinol* 119, 193–201.

Slominski, A., Wortsman, J., Tuckey, R. C., Paus, R., 2007. Differential expression of HPA axis homolog in the skin. *Mol Cell Endocrinol* 265, 143–149.

Sockman, K. W., Schwabl, H., 2001. Plasma corticosterone in nestling american kestrels: Effects of age, handling stress, yolk androgens, and body condition. *Gen Comp Endocrinol* 122, 205–212.

Spencer, K. A., Buchanan, K. L., Goldsmith, A. R., Catchpole, C. K., 2003. Song as an honest signal of developmental stress in the zebra finch (*Taeniopygia guttata*). *Horm Behav* 44, 132–139.

Spencer, K. A., MacDougall-Shackleton, S. A., 2011. Indicators of development as sexually selected traits: the developmental stress hypothesis in context. *Behav Ecol* 22, 1–9.

Spencer, K. A., Verhulst, S., 2007. Delayed behavioral effects of postnatal exposure to corticosterone in the zebra finch (*Taeniopygia guttata*). *Horm Behav* 51, 273–280.

Spencer, K. A., Verhulst, S., 2008. Post-natal exposure to corticosterone affects standard metabolic rate in the zebra finch (*Taeniopygia guttata*). *Gen Comp Endocrinol* 159, 250–256.

Spencer, K. A., Wimpenny, J. H., Buchanan, K. L., Lovell, P. G., Goldsmith, A. R., Catchpole, C. K., 2005. Developmental stress affects the attractiveness of male song and female choice in the zebra finch (*Taeniopygia guttata*). *Behav Ecol Sociobiol* 58, 423–428.

Starck, J. M., Ricklefs, R. E., 1998. Patterns of development: The altricial-precocial spectrum. In: Starck, J. M., Ricklefs, R. E. (Eds.), *Avian growth and development: Evolution within the altricial-precocial spectrum*. Oxford University Press, New York, pp. 3–30.

Stratholt, M. L., Donaldson, E. M., Liley, N. R., 1997. Stress induced elevation of plasma cortisol in adult female coho salmon (*Oncorhynchus kisutch*) is reflected in egg cortisol content, but does not appear to affect early development. *Aquaculture* 158, 141–153.

Strier, K. B., Ziegler, T. E., 2000. Lack of pubertal influences on female dispersal in muriqui monkeys, *Brachyteles arachnoides*. *Anim Behav* 59, 849–860.

Strochlic, D. E., Romero, L. M., 2008. The effects of chronic psychological and physical stress on feather replacement in European starlings (*Sturnus vulgaris*). *Comp Biochem Physiol Part A: Mol Integr Physiol* 149, 68–79.

Sullivan, L. C., Orgeig, S., Daniels, C. B., 2003. The role of extrinsic and intrinsic factors in the evolution of the control of pulmonary surfactant maturation during development in the amniotes. *Physiol Biochem Zool* 76, 281–295.

Suorsa, P., Helle, H., Huhta, E., Jantti, A., Nikula, A., Hakkarainen, H., 2003. Forest fragmentation is associated with primary brood sex ratio in the treecreeper (*Certhia familiaris*). *Proc R Soc Lond B* 270, 2215–2222.

Suzuki, K., Matsunaga, E., Kobayashi, T., Okanoya, K., 2011. Expression patterns of mineralocorticoid and glucocorticoid receptors in Bengalese finch (*Lonchura striata var. domestica*) brain suggest a relationship between stress hormones and song-system development. *Neuroscience* 194, 72–83.

Tanck, M. W. T., Vermeulen, K. J., Bovenhuis, H., Komen, H., 2001. Heredity of stress-related cortisol response in androgenetic common carp (*Cyprinus carpio L.*). *Aquaculture* 199, 283–294.

Tarlow, E. M., Wikelski, M., Anderson, D. J., 2001. Hormonal correlates of siblicide in Galapagos Nazca boobies. *Horm Behav* 40, 14–20.

Tobler, M., Sandell, M. I., 2007. Yolk testosterone modulates persistence of neophobic responses in adult zebra finches, *Taeniopygia guttata*. *Horm Behav* 52, 640–645.

Uller, T., 2008. Developmental plasticity and the evolution of parental effects. *Trends Ecol Evolut* 23, 432–438.

Uller, T., Hollander, J., Astheimer, L., Olsson, M., 2009. Sex-specific developmental plasticity in response to yolk corticosterone in an oviparous lizard. *J Exp Biol* 212, 1087–1091.

Uller, T., Meylan, S., De Fraipont, M., Clobert, J., 2005. Is sexual dimorphism affected by the combined action of prenatal stress and sex ratio? *J Exp Zool A: Comp Exp Biol* 303A, 1110–1114.

Uller, T., Olsson, M., 2006. Direct exposure to corticosterone during embryonic development influences behaviour in an ovoviviparous lizard. *Ethology* 112, 390–397.

Vallarino, A., Wingfield, J. C., Drummond, H., 2006. Does extra corticosterone elicit increased begging and submissiveness in subordinate booby (*Sula nebouxii*) chicks? *Gen Comp Endocrinol* 147, 297.

Van Belle, S., Estrada, A., Ziegler, T. E., Strier, K.B., 2009. Social and hormonal mechanisms underlying male reproductive strategies in black howler monkeys (*Alouatta pigra*). *Horm Behav* 56, 355–363.

Velando, A., 2002. Experimental manipulation of maternal effort produces differential effects in sons and daughters: Implications for adaptive sex ratios in the blue-footed booby. *Behav Ecol* 13, 443–449.

Vercken, E., de Fraipont, M., Dufty, A.M., Jr., Clobert, J., 2007. Mother's timing and duration of corticosterone exposure modulate offspring size and natal dispersal in the common lizard (*Lacerta vivipara*). *Horm Behav* 51, 379–386.

Villasenor, E., Drummond, H., 2007. Honest begging in the blue-footed booby: Signaling food deprivation and body condition. *Behav Ecol Sociobiol* 61, 1133–1142.

Vleck, C. M., Haussmann, M. F., Vleck, D., 2003. The natural history of telomeres: tools for aging animals and exploring the aging process. *Exper Gerontol* 38, 791–795.

Vleck, C. M., Haussmann, M. F., Vleck, D., 2007. Avian senescence: Underlying mechanisms. *J Ornithol* 148, S611–S624.

von Engelhardt, N., Henriksen, R., Groothuis, T. G. G., 2009. Steroids in chicken egg yolk: Metabolism and uptake during early embryonic development. *Gen Comp Endocrinol* 163, 175–183.

Wada, H., 2008. Glucocorticoids: Mediators of vertebrate ontogenetic transitions. *Gen Comp Endocrinol* 156, 441–453.

Wada, H., Breuner, C.W., 2008. Transient elevation of corticosterone alters begging behavior and growth of white-crowned sparrow nestlings. *J Exp Biol* 211, 1696–1703.

Wada, H., Breuner, C. W., 2010. Developmental changes in neural corticosteroid receptor binding capacity in altricial nestlings. *Devel Neurobiol* 70, 853–861.

Wada, H., Hahn, T. P., Breuner, C. W., 2007. Development of stress reactivity in white-crowned sparrow nestlings: Total corticosterone response increases with age, while free corticosterone response remains low. *Gen Comp Endocrinol* 150, 405–413.

Wada, H., Salvante, K. G., Stables, C., Wagner, E., Williams, T. D., Breuner, C.W., 2008. Adrenocortical responses in zebra finches (*Taeniopygia guttata*): Individual variation, repeatability, and relationship to phenotypic quality. *Horm Behav* 53, 472–480.

Wada, H., Salvante, K. G., Wagner, E., Williams, T. D., Breuner, C. W., 2009. Ontogeny and individual variation in the adrenocortical response of zebra finch (*Taeniopygia guttata*) nestlings. *Physiol Biochem Zool* 82, 325–331.

Walker, B. G., Wingfield, J. C., Boersma, P. D., 2005. Age and food deprivation affects expression of the glucocorticosteroid stress response in Magellanic penguin (*Spheniscus magellanicus*) chicks. *Physiol Biochem Zool* 78, 78–89.

Warkentin, K. M., 2011. Plasticity of hatching in amphibians: Evolution, trade-offs, cues and mechanisms. *Integ Comp Biol* 51, 111–127.

Warner, D. A., Lovern, M. B., Shine, R., 2008. Maternal influences on offspring phenotypes and sex ratios in a multi-clutching lizard with environmental sex determination. *Biol J Linnean Soc* 95, 256–266.

Warner, D. A., Radder, R. S., Shine, R., 2009. Corticosterone exposure during embryonic development affects offspring growth and sex ratios in opposing directions in two lizard species with environmental sex determination. *Physiol Biochem Zool* 82, 363–371.

Weiss, S. L., Johnston, G., Moore, M. C., 2007. Corticosterone stimulates hatching of late-term tree lizard embryos. *Comp Biochem Physiol A* 146, 360–365.

Wells, J. C. K., 2007. Flaws in the theory of predictive adaptive responses. *Trends Endocrinol Metab* 18, 331–337.

Wells, K. D., 1977. The social behaviour of anuran amphibians. *Anim Behav* 25, 666–693.

West-Eberhard, M., 2003. *Developmental plasticity and evolution*. Oxford University Press, Oxford.

Weygoldt, P., 1987. Evolution of parental care in dart poison frogs (Amphibia, Anura, Dendrobatidae). *Zeit Zool Syst Evolut* 25, 51–67.

Wilcoxen, T. E., Boughton, R. K., Bridge, E. S., Rensel, M. A., Schoech, S. J., 2011. Age-related differences in baseline and stress-induced corticosterone in Florida scrub-jays. *Gen Comp Endocrinol* 173, 461–466.

Williams, C. T., Kitaysky, A. S., Buck, C. L., 2008a. Food restricted tufted puffin (*Fratercula cirrhata*) nestlings increase vocal activity during handling without modulating total or free corticosterone. *J Ornithol* 149, 277–283.

Williams, C. T., Kitaysky, A. S., Kettle, A. B., Buck, C. L., 2008b. Corticosterone levels of tufted puffins vary with breeding stage, body condition index, and reproductive performance. *Gen Comp Endocrinol* 158, 29–35.

Williams, T. D., 2008. Individual variation in endocrine systems: Moving beyond the "tyranny of the Golden Mean." *Phil Trans R Soc B* 363, 1687–1698.

Wingfield, J. C., Ramenofsky, M., 1997. Corticosterone and facultative dispersal in response to unpredictable events. *Ardea* 85, 155–166.

Wingfield, J. C., Ramos-Fernandez, G., Nunez-de la Mora, A., Drummond, H., 1999. The effects of an "El Nino" southern oscillation event on reproduction in male and female blue-footed boobies, *Sula nebouxii*. *Gen Comp Endocrinol* 114, 163–172.

Wingfield, J. C., Sapolsky, R. M., 2003. Reproduction and resistance to stress: When and how. *J Neuroendocrinol* 15, 711.

Wingfield, J. C., Smith, J. P., Farner, D. S., 1980. Changes in plasma levels of luteinizing hormone, steroid, and thyroid hormones during the post-fledging development of white-crowned sparrows, *Zonotrichia leucophrys*. *Gen Comp Endocrinol* 41, 372–377.

Wommack, J. C., Delville, Y., 2007. Stress, aggression, and puberty: Neuroendocrine correlates of the development of agonistic behavior in golden hamsters. *Brain Behav Evol* 70, 267–273.

Zielinski, W. J., Vomsaal, F. S., Vandenbergh, J. G., 1992. The effect of intrauterine position on the survival, reproduction and home range size of female house mice (*Mus-musculus*). *Behav Ecol Sociobiol* 30, 185–191.

12

Global Change

Consequences of Human Disturbance

I. INTRODUCTION

Welcome to the Anthropocene! It is increasingly recognized that the era of the Holocene has changed dramatically in the past 100 years and that this human-dominated world has entered a new era, the "Anthropocene" (Crutzen and Stoemer 2000). Although this term is by no means fully accepted by all, it is a timely concept that captures the global changes that have already taken place and are happening right now. There is debate over when the Anthropocene began, some arguing that it started with the dawn of agriculture thousands of years ago, and others that it began with the industrial revolution of the mid-nineteenth century (Zalasiewicz et al. 2008; Zalasiewicz et al. 2010). At present, urbanization is spreading all over the world (Figure 12.1), covering hundreds of square kilometers and increasing. Now over 50% of the Earth's land surface has been modified by human activity such as agriculture, deforestation, and desertification (Hooke et al. 2012; Zalasiewicz et al. 2010). The full impact of the Anthropocene and what the future portends are major issues of our time. The combination of human disturbance and changing climate has altered our planet for the foreseeable future. How we will cope with this remains to be seen.

Our recent experience in the United States in 2014 brought it firmly home to us that we live in a world of increasing intensity, duration, and frequency of extreme events (see also Field et al. 2012): heat, cold, drought, floods, tornado swarms, hurricanes, and of course El Niño Southern Oscillation events. Add non-climatic events such as earthquakes, tsunamis, and volcanic eruptions, and it becomes clear that we face an unprecedented era of hazards and disasters. In Chapter 1 we discussed how Earth has always been a stressful planet and that there has been selection for coping mechanisms in all organisms, probably throughout the history of life. Nonetheless, the current trend of extreme events will likely have detrimental effects on organisms worldwide.

A whole new suite of environmental changes has relatively recently begun to have an impact on wild animals in addition to global climate change. The explosion of the human population and the resultant pressure on natural resources has created some unique changes to environments. These include the degradation, fragmentation, and modification of natural habitats, disturbances due to recreational activities, novel chemical challenges from pollution, and even the creation of novel habitats (cities; Figure 12.1). Each of these changes is unique to the evolutionary history of the affected species and has been collectively termed "human-induced rapid environmental change" (HIREC; Sih et al. 2011).

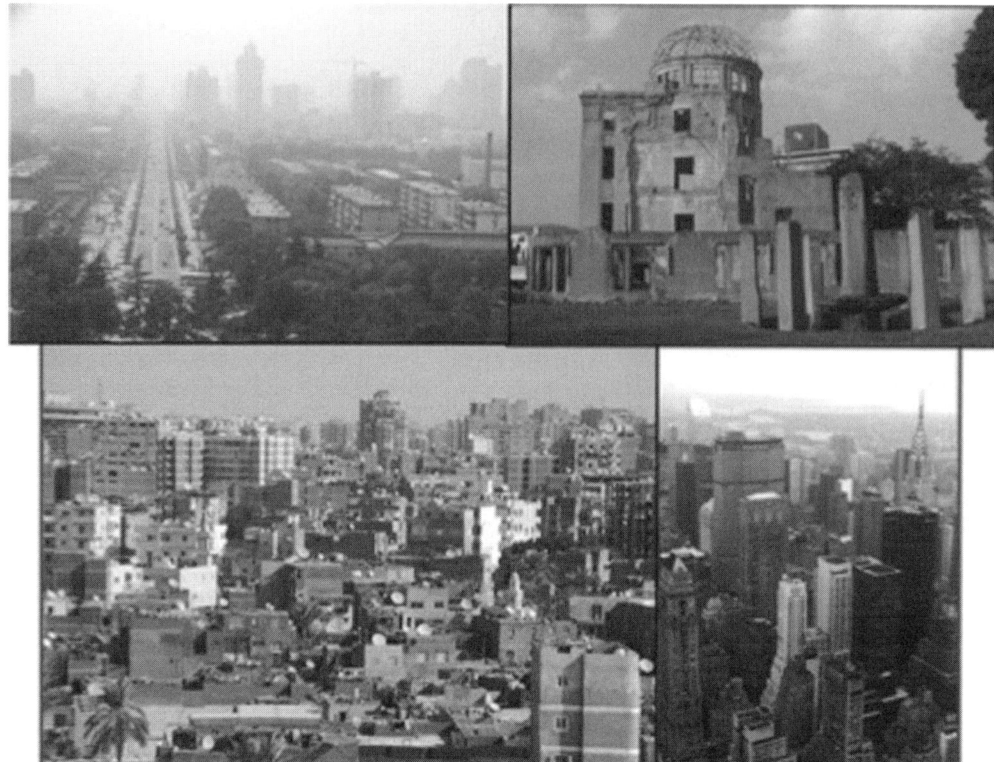

FIGURE 12.1: Types of urbanization across the globe. Some population centers cover hundreds of square kilometers and many are still growing. Upper left, Urbanization and smog in Xian, China. Upper right, ground zero at Hiroshima, site of atomic bomb explosion. Lower left, urbanization in Cairo, Egypt. Lower right, urbanization in New York City.

All photos by J. C. Wingfield.

A. What Is Global Climate Change?

All of us have seen graphs showing how the average temperature of the planet has increased steadily over the past 100 years. We also see how extreme events are increasing in frequency and intensity, resulting in dramatic swings from one extreme to another, heat then cold, drought then floods. So, the gradual warming trend is punctuated with these extreme swings, leaving us confused as to what is really happening. It is also probably challenging for plants and animals to cope with these changes as well. There have been dramatic impacts on the patterns of migrations, breeding seasons, and other aspects of the life cycles of organisms (e.g., Berthold 1993; Both and Visser 2001; Pulido et al. 2001; Thomas and Lennon 1999). For example, departure and arrival times of migrants, the timing of onset of breeding in some birds and other animals, the emergence of arthropods, and the flowering of many plants and trees are occurring earlier (e.g., Barrett 2002; Lehikoinen et al. 2006; Sparks and Menzel 2002). The timing of events in the autumn is much less well understood but also complex (Lehikoinen et al. 2006). Some populations remain unchanged as far as timing life-history stages, some terminate breeding later, and yet others earlier (Sparks and Menzel 2002). The implications for coping mechanisms remain unclear, but is possible that at a mechanistic level, hormonal cascades, regular timing of life-history stages, and the adrenocortical responses to acute perturbations may become mismatched with environmental phenology. Indeed, biological trends worldwide, including polar regions, are matching climate change predictions from mathematical models (Parmesan and Yohe 2003). Furthermore, behavioral patterns of individuals that change with season and social status may also be profoundly affected by changing environments, although exactly why and how remains unclear.

As reviewed in Chapter 1, changes in the physical environment can be grouped into two major types. The first group includes predictable changes such as seasons that determine the timing of stages in the predictable life cycle such as migration, reproduction, and molt. These are regulated by predictive cues such as annual photoperiod, rainfall, snow cover, temperature, and food availability (Wingfield et al. 1999a; Wingfield et al. 1999b; Wingfield 2006). Climate change is resulting in temporal shifts in many of these cues, but not in photoperiod. Thus the possibility exists for those species that rely on photoperiod changes to time events in the life cycle to become asynchronous (mismatched) with environmental conditions conducive for those life-history stages (Visser et al. 2006). Many species are more flexible in the timing of life-history stages, and local cues such as temperature can modulate the responses to photoperiod (e.g., Wingfield et al. 2003). These species should be able to adjust to climate changes, or may even shift the timing of life-history events too much (Both and Visser 2001; Both et al. 2005; Visser and Both 2005). The second type of environmental change involves unpredictable perturbations, such as storms, which are increasing in frequency and intensity. How the mechanisms underlying responses to both the predictable and unpredictable types of environment changes may contribute to phenotypic flexibility (i.e., the ability to adjust to global change) or inflexibility (i.e., vulnerability to global change) are key questions for the future (Wingfield 2005; Wingfield 2008b).

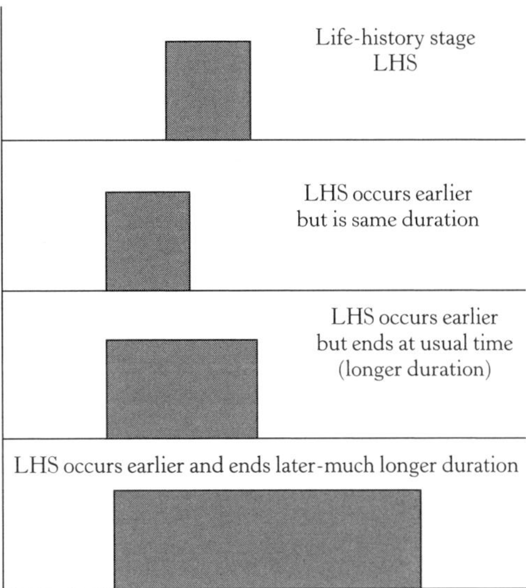

FIGURE 12.2: Global climate change, predictable variation: spring earlier, autumn later. Possible outcomes of early breeding accompanying global warming effects in north temperate regions.

From Wingfield (2008a), courtesy of Elsevier Press.

The annual cycle of many migratory songbirds, for example, consists of a fixed series of life-history changes whose timing and duration are regulated by combinations of environmental predictive cues (Figure 12.2; Wingfield 2008b). Any life-history stage, such as breeding, occurs at a specific time (e.g., spring). In a global warming scenario, the breeding season could be of the same duration but start earlier and end earlier. Another scenario could be that the life-history stage starts earlier but ends at the usual time, resulting in a net increase in duration. The fourth scenario could be that the life-history stage starts earlier, but because autumn also occurs later, then the life-history stage terminates later, resulting in an even greater increase in duration of that life-history stage (Figure 12.2; Wingfield 2008b). Any of these scenarios are possible, but what the underlying mechanisms might be and the scenario-specific consequences for responding to perturbations remain largely unknown.

This becomes even more complex and vexing if one considers that many animals, such as migratory songbirds, have many life-history stages, all of which could change in timing and duration (Figures 12.3 and 12.4; Wingfield 2008b). In Figure 12.3 there is an example of a migrant with five life-history stages—winter, vernal migration, breeding, molt, autumnal migration, and back to winter—that overlap very little. These occur in a fixed sequence and usually with specific durations (Figure 12.3). If spring occurs earlier and autumn later, then if just one life-history stage changes timing (i.e., occurs earlier; e.g., breeding; Figure 12.3), then other life-history stages are also affected and must shift their timing, and in the case of winter, duration. However, if the one life-history stage, breeding, starts earlier (top panel of Figure 12.4) or also ends later (middle panel of Figure 12.4), then other life-history stages shift more and more, in timing as well as duration. In the most complex situation, all life-history stages change timing and duration, and then there is an inevitable "pile up" of life-history stages with increasing overlap—the only way to accommodate changed phenology (lower panel of Figure 12.4). Clearly such changes could have serious consequences for regulatory mechanisms, and the energetic costs of overlapping life-history stages could reduce fitness markedly (Wingfield 2008b). Add to this the occurrence of extreme events resulting from global climate change, and the potentials for massive reproductive failure and high mortality in migration are high. Superimpose on these

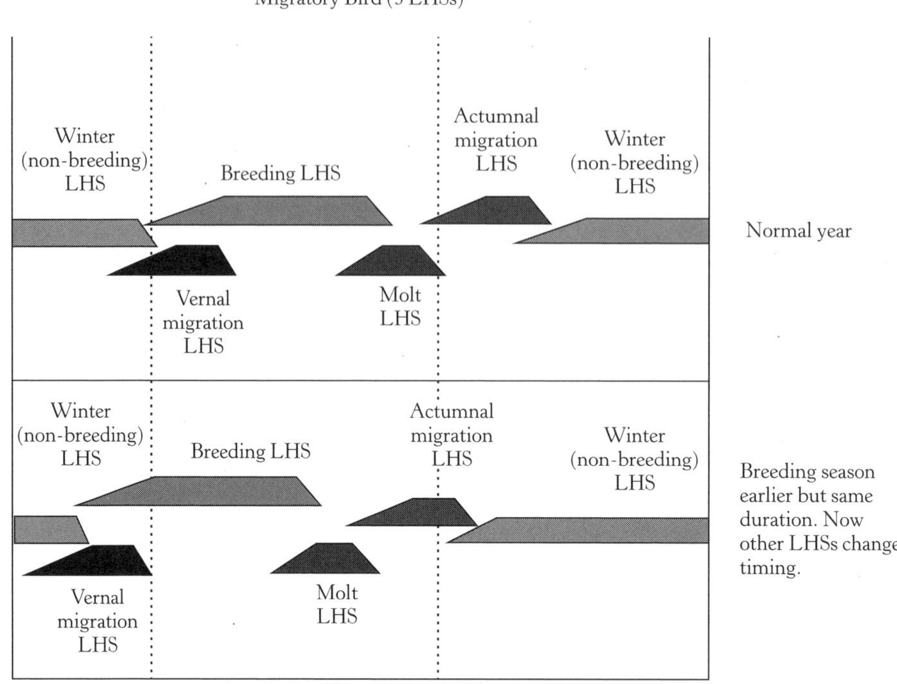

FIGURE 12.3: Global climate change, predictable variation: spring earlier, autumn later. Consequences of changed duration and timing of life history stages in a migratory bird in relation to global warming in north temperate regions. From Wingfield (2008a, 2008b), courtesy of Elsevier Press.

scenarios the increasing frequency of extreme events, and it becomes clear that many organisms face daunting environmental conditions.

B. What Are Extreme Environmental Conditions?

Extreme events brings to mind severe conditions such as in arctic-alpine habitats, deserts, and so on. However, we should be cautious when using the term "extreme conditions" because many plants and animals are well adapted for day-to-day survival in these environments. They probably are not "stressed" per se, even though such environments appear uninhabitable to us (e.g., Bartholomew 1958; Bartholomew 1964; Bartholomew 1966; Martin and Wiebe 2004). For example, fish adapted to the hyperbaric conditions of the ocean abyss always die when brought to the surface—which is to us a more hospitable environment. Nonetheless, although organisms living in what to us are extreme environments are well adapted, the additional energetic costs of breeding or molting can result in great demands of stored resources so that the potential for decreased fitness is great (e.g., Bartholomew 1964). Moreover, the severity in extreme environments (such as polar and alpine regions) to which an individual is adapted are predictable, allowing the organism to prepare for future life-history events such as breeding. Additional unpredictable extreme events such as storms may temporarily reduce food supply, providing further demands, and the combination of these two types of environmental pressures can be particularly taxing, leading to heightened allostatic load and even death. Many other local environmental factors, such as presence of predators, social status, infection, and injury, can be cumulative, resulting in "extreme conditions" even in mesic environments. Combinations of factors, both predictable and unpredictable, local and climatic, will determine how extreme an environment may be. Additionally, such cumulative conditions will also determine vulnerability to future perturbations (Wingfield 2008a). This is also known as a "carry-over effect." The dual concept of extreme environment versus extreme events suggests a framework to determine physiological and behavioral mechanisms.

Understanding how organisms respond to the increasing frequency and intensity of extreme

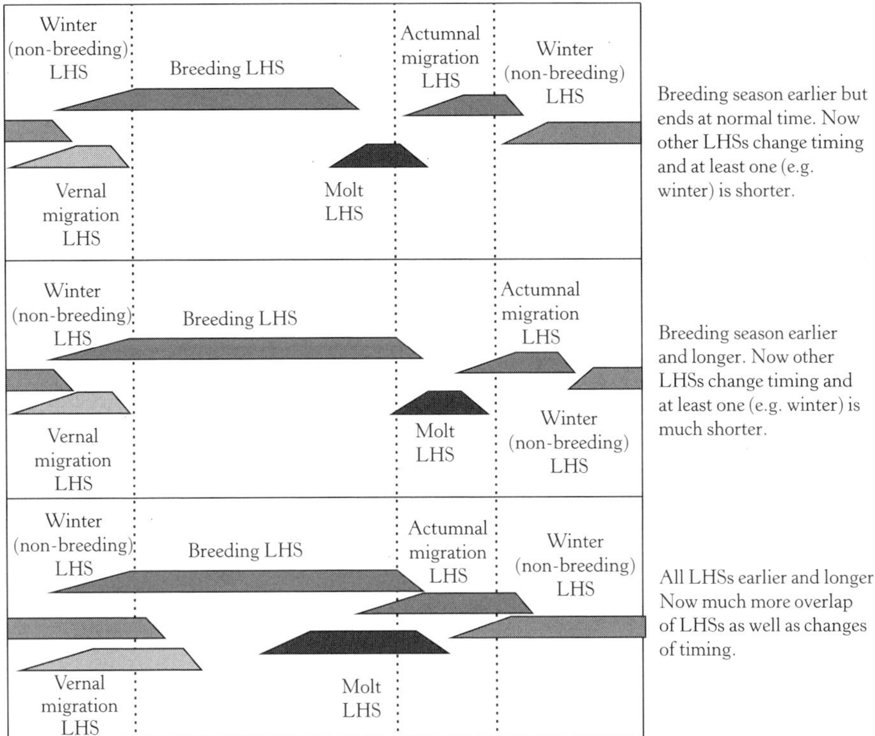

FIGURE 12.4: Global climate change, predictable variation: spring earlier, autumn later. Consequences of changed duration and timing of life history stages in a migratory bird in relation to global warming in north temperate regions. From Wingfield (2008a, 2008b), courtesy of Elsevier Press.

events will explain why some populations thrive and increase in such conditions, whereas others do not change, and yet others decline (e.g., Pörtner and Farrell 2008; Wingfield 2008a). Potentially catastrophic weather events, such as floods, droughts, storms, heat waves, and cold spells, have risen in frequency almost 10-fold in the past 50 years (Easterling et al. 2000; Beniston and Stephenson 2004). As a result, extinctions of plants and animals are increasing, and changes in distribution and phenology are shifting (Easterling et al. 2000; Meehl 2000). This ultimately leads to regulation of physiology, morphology, and behavior patterns as individuals adjust to climate change (Parmesan et al. 2000; Root 1988a, 1988b, 1994).

There are examples of severe events that can result in catastrophic reproductive failure and population decline. For example, a king penguin breeding colony on the Crozet Archipelago in the Southern Ocean was subjected to two sets of tsunami-generated waves, about two months apart, that inundated up to 44% of the colony, killing chicks and eggs (Viera et al. 2006). Similarly, the increase in the frequency of El Niño weather conditions has had a negative impact on Galápagos penguin populations (Vargas et al. 2006). How populations cope with and rebound from these events probably involves a degree of plasticity in coping with the dual effects of climate change and unpredictable extreme events.

How do we define extreme conditions? Answering this seemingly simple question is essential in order to understand how organisms might cope. Beniston and Stephenson (2004) suggest three criteria for evaluating extreme events and their occurrence:

1. How rare are these events? This requires some way to document their frequency.
2. How intense are they, and what is the threshold for this?
3. What impacts do they exert on environments and organisms in them (and what are the economic costs of damage)?

Extreme weather is generally considered as an event outside the normal range of weather conditions (measured over decades) and tends to be infrequent. Nonetheless, as mentioned above, such events appear to be increasing in recent decades (Francis and Hengeveld 1998). Taking a theoretical approach, if we consider a frequency distribution of weather phenomena such as temperature (Figure 12.5) as normally distributed, then most events will occur within the bell curve. The black shaded areas of Figure 12.5 represent extreme events, such as unusual heat at the right-hand end of the curve and intense cold at the left-hand end (Meehl 2000). Note that the boundaries of extreme events can be arbitrarily set at 95% confidence intervals, and where this boundary lies is an important question to be resolved (Beniston and Stephenson 2004). In this scenario, extreme events are rare and at the tails of the normal distribution, but if global warming results in a shift to the right of the normal distribution of weather events, an increase in extreme heat events will result (Figure 12.5). A shift in the mean to the left would result in more extreme cold events. Both are likely scenarios in global climate change (Meehl 2000). Changes in variance of weather/climate events, represented by a decreased frequency of the mean and an expanded bell curve, result in more extreme temperature events beyond the 95% confidence intervals (Figure 12.6). Moreover, the effect of a combination of decreased variance and a shift to the right of the mean (as in Figure 12.5), representing an increase in temperature due to global warming, is an even greater likelihood of extreme heat events (Figure 12.6). A shift to the left would result in more extreme cold events. Clearly, even slight changes in climate could mean more dramatic changes in frequency of extreme events.

Examples of such trends come from weather data in England showing that small elevations in

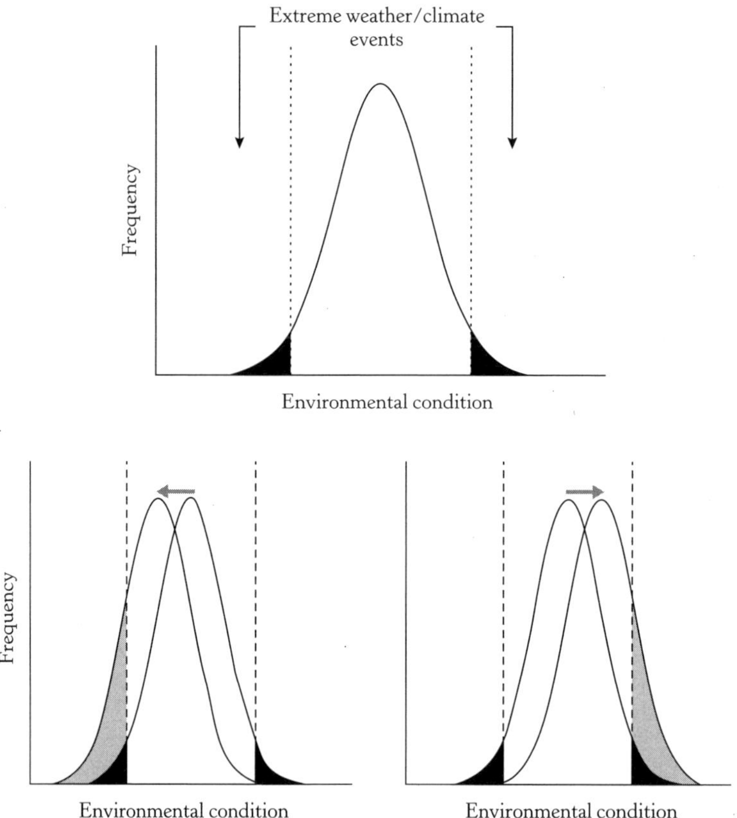

FIGURE 12.5: Weather or climatic variables such as temperature, assuming a normal distribution. The black shaded areas represent extreme events, such as extreme heat at the right end of the curve and extreme cold at the left end. The lower left-hand panel shows a shift in the mean frequency to the left, resulting in greater likelihood of more extreme cold events (gray shaded area). A shift in mean to the right (lower right-hand panel) results in greater likelihood of extreme heat events.

Modified and expanded from Meehl et al. (2000). With permission of the author and the American Meteorological Society.

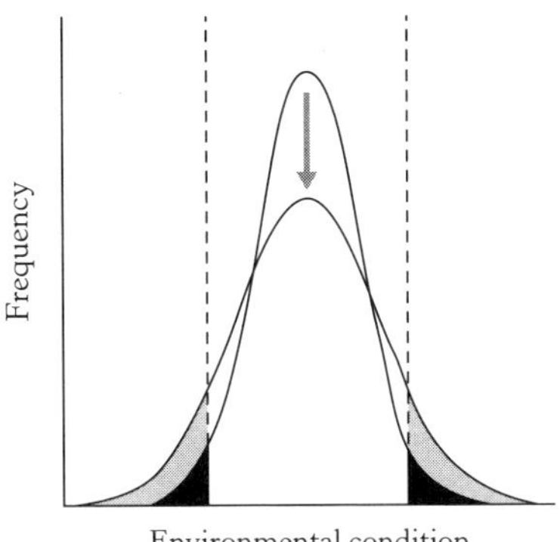

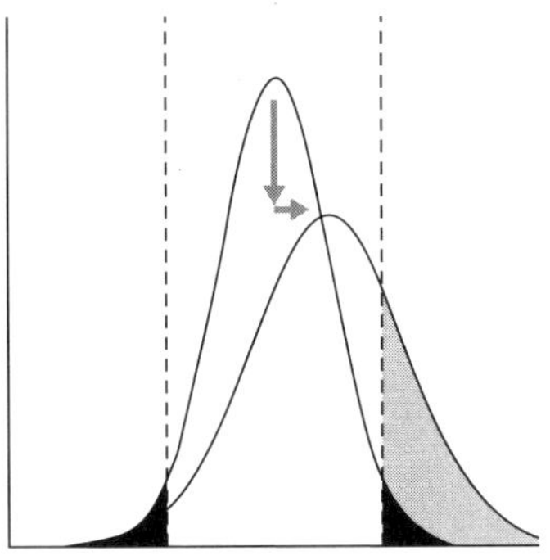

FIGURE 12.6: Weather or climatic variables such as temperature, assuming a normal distribution as shown in Figure 12.5. The black shaded areas represent extreme events, such as extreme heat at the right end of the curve and extreme cold at the left end. Left panel shows effects of a change in variance of weather events with the frequency of the mean decreasing and the curve expanding, resulting in more extreme temperature events (gray shading). Right panel shows the effects of a combination of decreased variance and a shift to the right with the mean. An even greater likelihood of extreme heat events results (gray shaded area). If the shift were to the left, then an increase in the likelihood of extreme cold events would occur.

Modified and expanded from Meehl et al. (2000), with permission of the author and the American Meteorological Society.

average temperature (e.g., 1–2°C) are accompanied by higher frequency of extreme summer heat from once every 75 years to once every 3 years (1.3%–33%; Francis and Hengeveld 1998; Munich Rev 2002). Another example, in France, shows a trend for reduced overnight temperatures over many years that is accompanied by greater frequency of hail storms and severe thunderstorms (Dessens 1995; Francis and Hengeveld 1998). In the United States warmer temperatures appear to be bringing heavier precipitation in many areas (Francis and Hengeveld 1998; Gordon et al. 1992). In fact, all types of extreme weather have increased in frequency and intensity, but in contrast, non-climatic events such as earthquakes have not (Francis and Hengeveld 1998). Note, however, that not all climate models agree as to how extreme weather events may be increasing (Meehl et al. 2000).

Changes in the frequency of extreme events in one locality are relatively easy to document over time, but we should be cautious when comparing extreme conditions in one area to another (Beniston and Stephenson 2004; Francis and Hengeveld 1998). For example, high winds on the ocean may not have as severe an impact on pelagic organisms as the same conditions would in a tropical forest. A modest 20-centimeter snow in Washington, D.C., to us represents an extreme condition, whereas the same amount would merely be an inconvenience in Montreal (Francis and Hengeveld 1998). Other important considerations include that it is inappropriate to assume that each individual in a population experiences extreme conditions in the same way. For example, an individual with a high-quality territory with shelter and food will be less affected by severe weather than a neighboring individual with a poor-quality territory containing less food and shelter. Habitat configuration is therefore an important consideration when comparing how individuals may cope with a changing world.

C. Habitat Configuration: Vulnerability of Local Habitat to Extreme Events

It is undoubtedly true to say that an individual experiences its habitat in a unique way, perhaps very differently from a neighbor just meters away. Internal differences such as parasite load, injuries, and social status are potentially important, as are external differences such as microhabitat, presence of predators, and so on. These also interact to give complex individual experiences of the environment, which in turn influence how organisms respond and regulate physiology, morphology, and behavior (Wingfield et al. 2011a; Wingfield et al. 2011b). The environmental conditions that an individual encounters can mean extremes for one but not necessarily another. The next question is, how is the habitat configured for a particular individual?

In a dictionary, "configuration" is defined as the way in which parts or elements of something are arranged to fit together. Configuration is also defined in the computational world as the manner in which software and internal and external hardware components of a computer system are arranged and interconnected so that the system functions correctly. For an organism, the integration of its internal state (parasites, energy reserves, injury, age) with external conditions in the habitat itself (territory/home range quality, weather and exposure, shelter, predators, population density), determines environmental conditions (Wingfield et al. 2011a; Wingfield et al. 2011b). Social status is also important and adds another dimension to habitat configuration.

It is critical for an individual to find a configuration of habitat that provides sufficient food for daily and annual routines, including internal components such as parasite load, injury, breeding (Ee + Ei + Eo—allostatic load), and that also provides shelter to cope with perturbations of the environment. Trophic resources (Eg from Chapter 3) available in that habitat must cover energetic costs. Unpredictable changes in habitat configuration from perturbations such as human disturbance can be an additional major threat with serious consequences for fitness (Wingfield et al. 2011a; Wingfield et al. 2011b). These complex interactions of external and internal factors are probably very extensive, and some examples are listed in Table 12.1 (Wingfield et al. 2011a). Prior experience of extreme events through learning is an important consideration that can provide skills for dealing with specific perturbations in the future. Making sense of such complex interactions requires a theoretical and biophysical approach that allows testable predictions about variation in biological processes under natural conditions, especially the interaction of abiotic and biotic factors. Porter et al. (2002) use models for ecological predictions concerning distribution, energetic requirements, and predator prey interactions that have direct relevance to identifying extreme conditions at the individual level. Their models include the following:

1. Porous insulation for fur/feathers;
2. Distributed heat generation and respiratory evaporation (lung models);
3. Coupled molar balance models of respiratory and digestive systems;
4. Animal posture, especially appendage effects, vital to estimates of field metabolism;
5. Steady state and transient capabilities;
6. Dynamic changes in local habitat selection by animals too hot or too cold out in the open (see Porter et al. 2002).

Pörtner and Farrell (2008) use models to predict how fishes adjust to changes in abiotic factors (e.g., temperature). Although these approaches to defining what constitutes extreme conditions should be tested widely, it is first pertinent to ask how these components of the external, internal, and social environments might combine to result in extreme conditions. Food and related resources are obvious potential factors (Table 12.2) and

TABLE 12.1: POTENTIAL COMPONENTS OF HABITAT CONFIGURATION

External	Internal
Territory/home range	Body condition
Location (central/peripheral)	Age
Food availability	Parasite load
Weather	Injury
Exposure to weather	Proactive/reactive coping style
Shelter	Social status
Population density	Pollutant load
Predator density/variety	Developmental experience
Human disturbance	Maternal (paternal) effects
Presence of mate (social status)	Ability to access food resources
Group size (social status)	
Heterospecific competition (non-predator)	
Invasive species	

From Wingfield et al. (2011a) with permission courtesy of Current Zoology.

TABLE 12.2: POTENTIAL FACTORS CONTRIBUTING TO AN "EXTREME ENVIRONMENT"

Food and related resources are obvious potential factors in the following scenarios:
Resources may be abundant for a limited but predictable period only.
Resources may be abundant for a limited but unpredictable period only.
Resources are never abundant; they are dispersed and difficult to obtain.
Resources are abundant (may be seasonally), but patchy (i.e., highly concentrated).

There are variable extremes of physical environment that can contribute to extreme conditions as follows:
Temperature extremes (well beyond the individual's thermo-neutral zone, predictable or unpredictable) may occur seasonally/daily.
Wind speed may vary in extremes seasonally/daily on a predictable schedule or is unpredictable.
Rainfall may show extreme variation seasonally/daily on a predictable schedule or is unpredictable.
Other factors that can contribute to an extreme environment include drought, fire, hypoxia, human disturbance (recreational, etc.; see Nisbet 2000; Walker et al. 2005a).

From Wingfield et al. (2011a) with permission courtesy of Current Zoology.

include resources being abundant for a limited but predictable period only; resources may be abundant for a limited but unpredictable period only; resources are never abundant, they are dispersed and difficult to obtain; resources are abundant, (e.g., seasonally), but patchy (i.e., highly concentrated; Wingfield et al. 2011a). In these cases, some individuals with poor territories or low social status have limited access to resources and are experiencing extreme conditions, whereas others with better territories and higher social status are not. Other variable extremes of the physical environment that contribute to extreme conditions include temperature (well beyond the individual's thermo-neutral zone), wind speed, and precipitation, which can all vary daily and seasonally in predictable or unpredictable ways (Table 12.2). Extremes of social environment, such as position in hierarchy, can determine access to critical resources, especially when rare and patchy (Wingfield et al. 2011a). Other examples are low partial pressure of oxygen, extremes of pH and osmotic pressure, trace element deficiency, high barometric pressure, and intense radiation. All of these contribute to what we would call an extreme environment (Table 12.2). Anthropogenic factors are important contributors to potentially extreme conditions, including environmental pollutants, human disturbance (direct and indirect), and habitat destruction/modification (Nisbet 2000; Walker et al. 2005a).

Organisms can acclimatize to any one of the above scenarios or use microhabitats in such extreme conditions or both. This applies to predictably extreme environments as well as unpredictable extremes. The question is, do problems arise as the individual or population encounters more than one set of extreme conditions outlined in the preceding paragraphs? This may be particularly harsh if two or more sets of conditions are out of phase with one another. For example, if three or four sets of conditions from Table 12.2 occurred in one habitat, simultaneously or sequentially, then these could result in extreme conditions (Wingfield et al. 2011a). Even in mesic habitats, extreme conditions could prevail if, for example, social extremes and human disturbance combined. Examples of how such factors may interact come from field studies of plants. In cold climates such as arctic and alpine zones, photoperiodic responses of plants regulate development at a time in spring when the likelihood of killing frosts is low (Keller and Körner 2003). In other words, an early warm spell could result in precocious development, followed by a return to sub-freezing conditions that would kill delicate spring growth (see also Heide et al. 1990). Plants become more responsive to local temperature as spring progresses. Prock and Körner (1996) showed that the transfer of arctic-alpine plants to different photoperiods resulted in marked changes in development. As global climate change results in earlier and earlier springs, plant development times have also advanced, but this may not be true for all arctic and alpine plants that are photoperiodic and resistant to temperature effects early in spring. These authors subjected 33 high alpine species of plants (from the east central Alps of Austria) to 12, 14.5, 15, and 16 hours of light per day and at two temperature regimes, 11/6°C and 18/8°C (day/night) temperature treatments. Shorter photoperiods tended to decrease flowering regardless of temperature treatment, whereas longer photoperiods resulted in flowering even at the colder temperatures. Overall there appeared to be three response types: species that are insensitive to temperatures to flower; species that flower only in warmer temperatures; and species flowering at cold temperatures only (Prock and Korner 1996).

Now that the nuances of global climate change have been discussed, we go on to present some examples of global change that indicate responses of the HPA axis. It should be noted that the direct effects of global climate change on adrenocortical responses to stress remain a potentially interesting but largely unknown entity.

II. URBANIZATION AND EXPLOITATION

The dramatic increase in the size of cities that has occurred with the growing human population has converted substantial areas from natural to urban and suburban habitats. This has resulted in two major changes: habitat loss and fragmentation; and the creation of novel habitats. Some species, especially those that tolerate large changes in environmental conditions (Bonier et al. 2007b) or are generally less fearful (Moller 2010), have been able to take advantage of the growing urban habitat and a few, such as pigeons (rock doves) and rats, have thrived in the center of cities. Films such as Pixar's *Ratatouille* have captured the foraging opportunities present in cities, but there is also a multitude of potential dangers. Are these dangers interpreted as stressors by the species that have adapted to live in cities, or in those that are in the process of making the transition to living in cities? Most current research suggests that they are.

One major aspect of urban areas is the noise. Noise can have a major impact on acoustic communication in a variety of species (e.g., Laiolo 2010; Warren et al. 2006). For example, birds can change the complexity (e.g., Hamao et al. 2011) and frequency range (e.g., Luther and Baptista 2010) of their songs when forced to make themselves heard over a city's background noise. Noise can also impact foraging behavior (Purser and Radford 2011). However, changes in behavior do not necessarily imply that there is a concomitant change in the physiological indices of stress.

Noise can directly elicit stress responses in laboratory rats (Baldwin 2007), but there has been little work on whether it can function as a stressor in free-living animals. In free-living sage grouse, lekking males had slightly higher fecal levels of corticosteroid metabolites when experimentally exposed to playback of human noise activity related to mining and road traffic (Figure 12.7; Blickley et al. 2012). Noise is assumed to cause stress in marine mammals (Nowacek et al. 2007; Wright et al. 2007), but there is little direct evidence. Low frequency acoustic disturbance from military sonars, energy development (seismic activity), construction, and so on, in oceans does reduce communication in whales, which is required to find mates, detect predators, and even navigate across vast expanse of ocean (Clark et al. 2009; Ellison et al. 2012; Hatch et al. 2012). A long-term study of North Atlantic right whales revealed a marked decrease in fecal levels of glucocorticoid metabolites when shipping and other noise-related events were decreased immediately after the events of September 11, 2001 (Rolland et al. 2012). Although this result was correlational with one event, it does raise the distinct possibility that noise may indeed be stressful for marine animals.

Other studies are equivocal. Ship sounds played back to free-living fish elicited a robust corticosteroid response (Wysocki et al. 2006), although another study suggests that a startle response, rather than the noise per se, is to blame (Smith et al. 2004). On the other hand, the sounds of jet aircraft did not elicit either a corticosteroid (Bartechi-Rozell and Romero, unpublished data) or a heart rate response (Ellis et al. 1991) and did not have an impact on nesting success in several bird species. Similarly, highly industrialized areas with more noise than suburban areas did not alter corticosteroid levels in house sparrows (Chavez-Zichinelli et al. 2010). The available data are thus mixed on whether noise is serving as a stressor for free-living animals. Although most studies suggest that noise does not elicit physiological responses, much more work is clearly needed.

An often under-appreciated consequence of urbanization, especially in wealthier countries, is a major increase in predator densities. House cats are often allowed to roam free and can have a devastating impact on local small bird and mammal populations (Beckerman et al. 2007; Forbush 1916; van Heezik et al. 2010). These are cats that are being fed by owners and so are not subject to normal predator-prey population dynamics (Churcher and Lawton 1987; Woods et al. 2003). (Humans are essentially subsidizing the predator

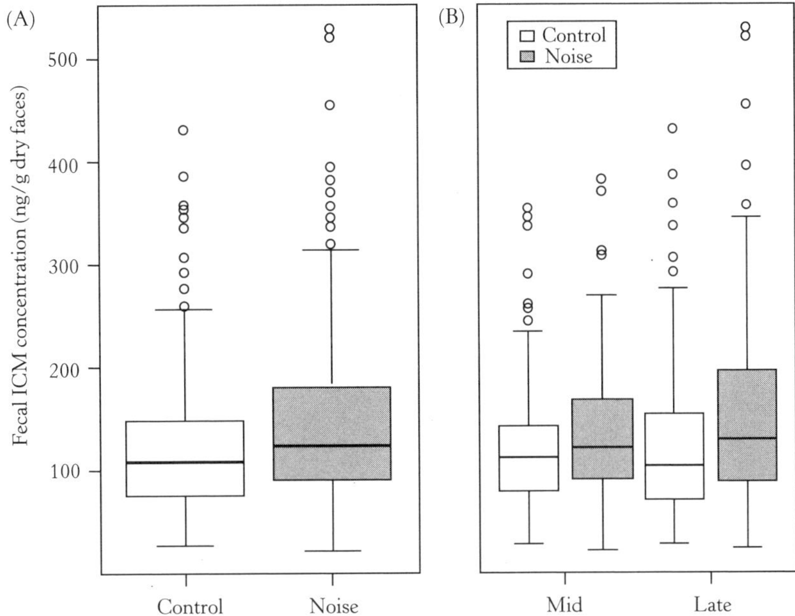

FIGURE 12.7: FCM (fecal corticosteroid metabolite) concentrations from control and noise-treated groups of free-living sage grouse. Data shown (A) pooled by season and (B) for mid- and late season samples. Horizontal line represents the median value, box ends represent upper and lower quartiles, whiskers represent maximum and minimum values and open circles represent outliers.

From Blickley et al. (2012) courtesy of *PLoS One*.

population.) The presence of predators is known to alter corticosteroid release (e.g., Scheuerlein et al. 2001), so the increased predator density is likely to be a major contributor to allostatic load.

Two pioneering series of studies have indicated that adapting to an urban environment can exert subtle changes to HPA axis function. One set of studies collected European blackbird chicks shortly after hatching from both urban and forest populations (Partecke et al. 2006b). These chicks were then hand-reared in equivalent captive conditions in a common garden experiment. Chicks born in an urban environment had a significantly lower corticosteroid response to handling, even though the basal concentrations were equivalent (Partecke et al. 2006b). The changes in HPA function were also accompanied by lower migratory behavior and earlier onset of gonadal regrowth in birds of urban origin (Partecke and Gwinner 2007). The differences likely originated from early rearing or maternal effects because there are no apparent genetic differences between the two populations (Partecke et al. 2006a), and the demographic evidence supports multiple colonizing events of urban centers rather than a single colonizing event and then radiation to new urban centers (Evans et al. 2009). Regardless of the ultimate underlying mechanism, the data suggest that the urban population has adjusted their HPA function to make them less sensitive to stressors. The decreased sensitivity, in turn, may provide the blackbirds a larger buffer to prevent entering an emergency life-history stage or avoiding homeostatic overload when breeding among plentiful urban stressors.

A second series of studies has focused on the colonization of urban areas in desert environments. Cities often provide attractive water sources for desert-adapted birds. Spillage from irrigation (i.e., watering grass lawns) can augment this precious resource, but managed plant assemblages from gardening can either increase or decrease the suitability of the urban habitat, depending upon which plants are cultivated (Fokidis 2011). In contrast to the decreased sensitivity to stressors detected in urban European blackbirds, several desert bird species had generally slightly augmented corticosteroid responses to capture and handling (Fokidis et al. 2009). In one of these species, birds occupying urban settings up-regulated pituitary sensitivity to arginine vasotocin and interrenal sensitivity to ACTH compared to birds in their natural desert habitat, suggesting that urban birds have a greater sensitivity to stressors

(Fokidis and Deviche 2011). However, the augmented corticosteroid responses were highly dependent upon life-history stage (Fokidis et al. 2009). In fact, the major effect of adjusting to the urban environment seems to have been a damping of the seasonal variation in corticosteroid responses. In extremely seasonal environments like the desert, urban areas may provide more predictable and benign conditions than the native habitat. In fact, an increase in defendable resources may underlie the observed increase in territoriality in urban settings, although this behavioral change was not accompanied by changes in corticosteroid responses (Fokidis et al. 2011). However, not all species successfully colonized the city (Fokidis et al. 2009), suggesting that not all species interpret the conditions as more predictable and benign. A common garden experiment, similar to the European blackbird studies, would help clarify whether these HPA changes truly reflected adjustment to urban living or were a consequence of differences in resource availability.

The European blackbird and desert bird studies highlight that we still have little understanding of how, or even whether, the HPA axis adjusts when adapting to urban habitats. The two sets of studies come to the opposite broad conclusions—European blackbirds damp corticosteroid responses, whereas the desert birds slightly augment responses. In neither case, however, was there a difference in baseline corticosteroid concentrations. A study on crow chicks supports this result (Heiss et al. 2009). In contrast, a number of other studies document changes in baseline concentrations. Male white-crowned sparrows in urban habitats have elevated baseline corticosterone compared to males in rural habitats, although females do not show this difference (Bonier et al. 2007a), and tree sparrows show progressively elevated baseline corticosterone as the degree of urbanization increases (Zhang et al. 2011). On the other hand, urban tree lizards have both lower baseline and stress-induced corticosterone compared to rural animals (French et al. 2008), and suburban Florida scrub jays have both lower baseline and elevated stress-induced corticosterone than rural scrub jays (Schoech et al. 2007). Other species show no change in corticosteroid concentrations (Chavez-Zichinelli et al. 2010). Clearly much more work is necessary to untangle the consequences of adjusting to an urban habitat, but the data to date suggest that there is no common strategy in how species balance the dangers of urban stressors with the benefits of urban resources.

III. HABITAT DEGRADATION AND FRAGMENTATION

One of the earliest attempts to link habitat degradation with stress responses was in a study on spotted owls. Wasser et al. (1997) compared fecal corticosterone metabolite concentrations in owls whose nests were near logging roads or recent timber harvests to those owls whose nests were in more pristine habitat. At least in males, nesting in proximity to these features of human activity resulted in elevated corticosterone metabolites (Figure 12.8), consistent with the presence of roads and habitat disruption being interpreted as a stressor.

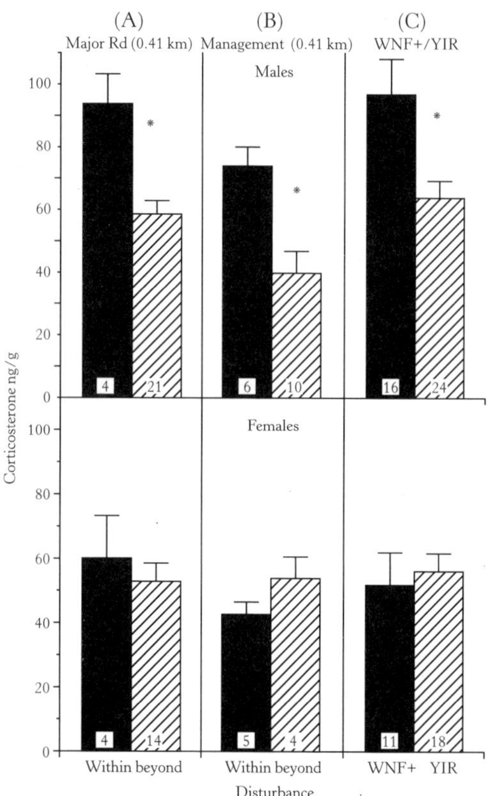

FIGURE 12.8: Mean fecal corticosterone levels in male and female spotted owls under three separate conditions: center of home range on the Yakama Indian Reservation (YIR) versus beyond a 0.41 km radius from a major logging road (A) or timber harvest activity (B), and YIR versus the more intensively harvested Wenatchee National Forest/ private industry lands checkerboard (WNF1), all on the eastern slope of the Cascade Mountains (C).

Asterisk is $p < 0.01$. Sample sizes shown in bars refer to number of individuals, with an average of three samples per individual. Reprinted with permission from Wasser et al. (1997) courtesy of Wiley Press.

What precisely induced the increase in corticosterone metabolites, however, is not entirely clear. Spotted owls generally prefer older and more mature forests (Buchanan et al. 1995; Williams et al. 2011), and areas around logging roads and recent timber harvests are better characterized as early successional habitats. Consequently, the owls likely interpret the presence of recent timber harvests as being less preferred habitat. Nesting in non-preferred habitat might serve as a stressor, but whether this assessment of habitat was what resulted in elevated corticosterone metabolites is not clear. There are a number of alternative hypotheses. First, females do not show a response (Figure 12.8), indicating that males and females may be interpreting the habitat changes differently. Wasser et al. (1997) suggested that the sex difference possibly reflected the predominant male role in territorial defense, but this has not yet been demonstrated. Second, the increase in corticosterone metabolites could reflect inferior or younger males establishing territories in suboptimal habitats. This would suggest that individual quality, not the habitat per se, may affect response to the stressor that was driving the changes in metabolites. Regardless of the underlying mechanism, however, human activities clearly had an impact on the corticosterone concentrations in the male owls—either directly by the males interpreting the habitat change as a stressor, or indirectly through lower quality males selecting territories in these habitats.

Determining whether habitat changes directly elicit a change in corticosteroid release or indirectly alter the quality of the animals present is a difficult problem. Natural differences in habitats are known to affect corticosteroid responses. For example, American redstarts overwinter in Jamaica in two different habitats that differ in overall quality, and this difference was reflected in corticosterone responses in the spring, just before the redstarts migrated north to their breeding sites (Marra and Holberton 1998). The redstarts in the poorer habitat had elevated baseline but attenuated stress-induced corticosterone concentrations. This highlights a major problem when interpreting the impact of habitat degradation—there is often little to distinguish human-degraded habitat from naturally poor habitat. For example, birds nesting on the edges of colonies (Herring and Ackerman 2011) or nesting in exposed areas (D'Alba et al. 2011) have elevated corticosteroid concentrations, but the reason appears to be poorer quality individuals occupying those nesting sites, rather than the habitat itself inducing allostatic load. This is a subtle point, but one with far-reaching consequences. Living in a poor neighborhood might elevate allostatic load, but suffering from a high allostatic load from other sources may also push individuals into living in that poor neighborhood, which could then add to allostatic load further. Distinguishing between these two possibilities can be very difficult.

Although the redstart data would suggest that natural and human-induced poor-quality habitat would result in similar corticosteroid changes, other data suggest that responses can be far more complicated. In some cases, habitat degradation could make the situation better—at least for some individuals. Figure 12.9 shows a vernal pond surrounded by urban development. Homan et al. (2003) studied corticosteroid responses from spotted salamanders breeding in two vernal pools—one where the surrounding habitat had recently been converted to a housing project, similar to Figure 12.9, and one that was relatively undeveloped. Not surprisingly, the salamander population plummeted in the developed pond (Homan et al. 2007), likely as a result of direct mortality from the construction. Adult spotted salamanders only use the ponds for breeding and spend most of the year hunting from burrows and from under logs in the surrounding upland habitat. Housing construction converts the upland habitat to buildings and lawns, with the bulldozers likely killing the adults. Those salamanders that survived and returned to the pond to breed had much lower baseline and stress-induced corticosterone concentrations compared to animals in the undeveloped pond. One interpretation of this result is that the surviving salamanders were less stressed than animals in the undeveloped pond. The large mortality event greatly decreased the density of breeding animals in the pond, so perhaps the attenuated corticosterone concentrations reflected a reduction in intra-specific competition and a perception that conditions had improved (at least for the surviving animals). One potential result of habitat destruction is an improvement in the conditions for the survivors. Because the animals that die are no longer available for study, habitat destruction could be interpreted as beneficial on the basis of corticosteroid responses, despite the fact that it killed lots of animals.

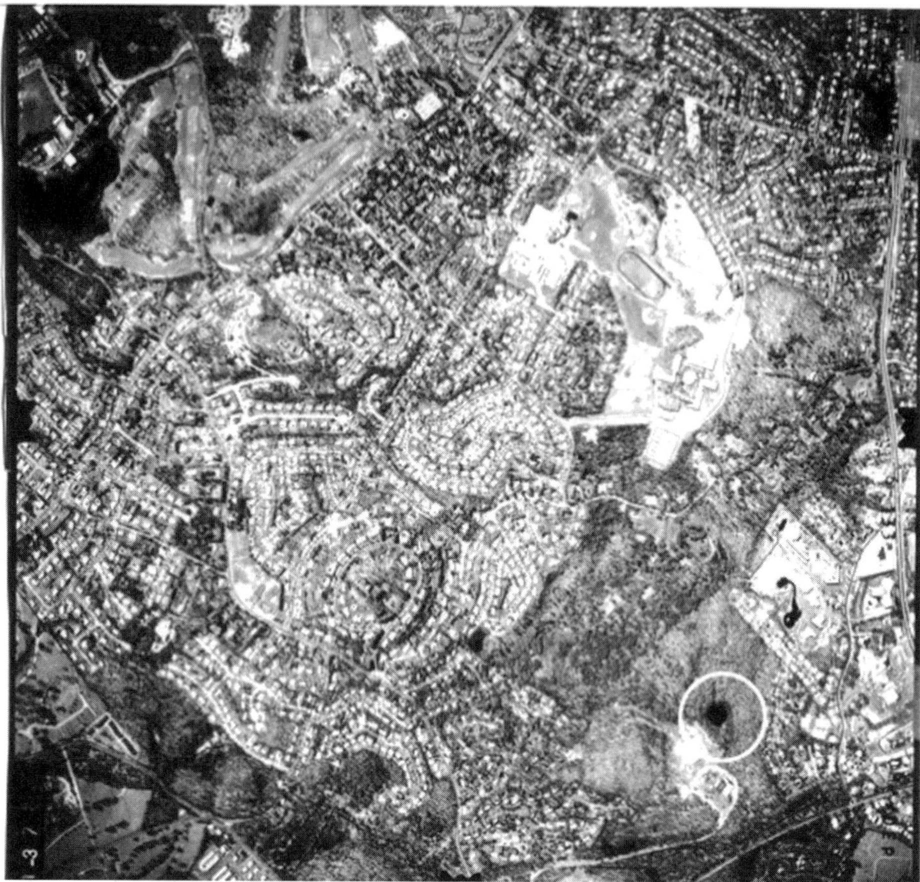

FIGURE 12.9: Example of a vernal pond surrounded by urban development.

A. Detecting Impacts of Potential Anthropogenic Stressors

You will notice from the preceding discussion, however, that the interpretations arising from the spotted owls and spotted salamanders are both contradictory and post hoc. A presumed stressor, habitat disturbance, elevated corticosterone in spotted owls but decreased corticosterone in spotted salamanders. The interpretations make sense, that the owls were stressed but the salamanders were not, but are they correct? What if the opposite result had been found in each study? If male owls near roads had lower corticosterone concentrations, couldn't we argue that the lower male density in suboptimal habitats reduced social stressors? And if the salamanders in the developed pond had higher corticosterone concentrations, couldn't we argue that development was stressful? In other words, logical explanations can be created to explain any result. What is needed is a way to test whether the explanations are correct. To do this, it would be important to know what the endocrine profile is for a chronically stressed wild animal. What do corticosteroid titers look like when a free-living wild animal has increased allostatic load, or enters allostatic overload?

Traditionally, researchers have attempted to address these questions by extrapolating from the biomedical literature. They assume that higher corticosteroid titers indicate increased allostatic load and/or overload. There are two problems with this assumption, however. First, substantial data suggest that corticosteroid responses in free-living animals can be quite different from responses described from highly inbred domesticated animals such as laboratory rats. Second, the biomedical literature itself is not entirely clear on the predicted corticosteroid response of a chronically stressed animal. Some of the key data come from a set of experiments utilizing what has been termed a "visible burrow system" (Blanchard and Blanchard 2003). The visible burrow system is a way of housing rats. Although there are a number of different designs (see Figure 11.16 in

Chapter 11), essentially each burrow system consists of a central open arena with multiple tunnels extending radially from the arena to a series of burrows. All of the water and food is placed in the center arena, thereby forcing all the animals to interact over the food and water. When multiple rats (especially males) are placed in the apparatus, one rat quickly becomes dominant and controls access to the food and water. The subordinates get access to food and water only when the dominant is absent or otherwise occupied.

It turns out that the visible burrow system is an ingenious apparatus for creating chronic stress. All of the subordinates suffer bite wounds, severe weight loss, behavioral changes consistent with depression, and elevated corticosterone concentrations (Blanchard et al. 1995). When exposed to a restraint stressor, however, 60% of the subordinates have normal increases in corticosterone, but 40% fail to increase corticosterone. Animals in the later group are classified as non-responders, whereas those that do respond to restraint are classified as responders. Although many other chronic stress protocols in the biomedical literature do not replicate this bimodal response, most of them utilize far more artificial conditions than the visible burrow system. By allowing animals to interact in an artificial colony rather than in small plastic cages, the visible burrow system is perhaps the closest representation of what a free-living animal might experience of all the paradigms used in biomedicine.

The implications of these studies can be profound for investigating responses to anthropogenic environmental changes. Think of the salamander study discussed earlier: Did the decreased corticosterone response in the salamanders in the developed pond result from a lower allostatic load because of the decrease in density? Or were they chronically stressed and reacting similarly to the non-responders in the visible burrow system? The traditional assumption is that all chronically stressed wild animals will have an endocrine profile similar to the responders, but that may not be the case. What is needed is an idea of what the endocrine profile looks like in a chronically stressed free-living animal. In other words, we need to try to recreate or simulate the dynamics of the visible burrow system with free-living animals. Studies thus need to ensure that animals are chronically stressed, but given the interpretation problems of whether common anthropogenic stressors such as habitat destruction are interpreted as stressors by the individual animals, it is insufficient to rely upon simple correlations with different environmental stimuli presumed to be stressors. A partial solution may be to establish chronic stressors in captive animals and then apply those stressors to free-living animals.

Unfortunately, the evidence to date indicates that there is no straightforward way to generate an endocrine profile for animals known to be chronically stressed. Laboratory evidence, however, suggests that captive wild animals may react more like the non-responders from the visible burrow system. In a series of studies of birds recently brought into captivity, animals were subjected to chronic stress by presenting a series of different acute stressors 4–5 times per day every day, on a rotating basis over a span of 3 weeks. Stressors included tapping cages, preventing perching, restraint, human voice, and so on. The syndrome that results is a dramatic loss of weight, lower baseline heart rates, attenuated heart rate responses to an acute stressor, and, as shown in Figure 12.10, lower baseline corticosterone and attenuated corticosterone responses to an acute stressor (Cyr et al. 2007; Cyr et al. 2009; Rich and Romero 2005). Using the first two weeks of captivity in freshly caught birds as another protocol for inducing chronic stress, Figure 12.11 indicates that there is a major attenuation in the ability to mount a fight-or-flight response (Dickens and Romero 2009). The endocrine profile for a chronically stressed wild animal held in captivity thus appears to be a *decrease* in corticosteroid and fight-or-flight responses. In other words, these captive studies indicate that the endocrine profile of wild birds exposed to chronic stress closely matches the non-responders from the visible burrow system.

When applied under field contexts, however, the picture is not as clear. Several studies have attempted to experimentally induce chronic stress and have obtained conflicting results. In one study, nesting European starling females were exposed to a similar chronic stress protocol as was used in the above laboratory studies. A series of different acute stressors was presented every day, four times per day, on a rotating basis over a span of 10 days. Stressors applied in the field included various predator models (Figure 12.12), human voice, human presence, and so on. Similar to results from the laboratory studies, females subjected to this protocol were exposed to elevated corticosterone concentrations but had a greatly attenuated response to capture, handling, and restraint (Cyr and Romero 2007, 2008). In other words, birds exposed to similar chronic

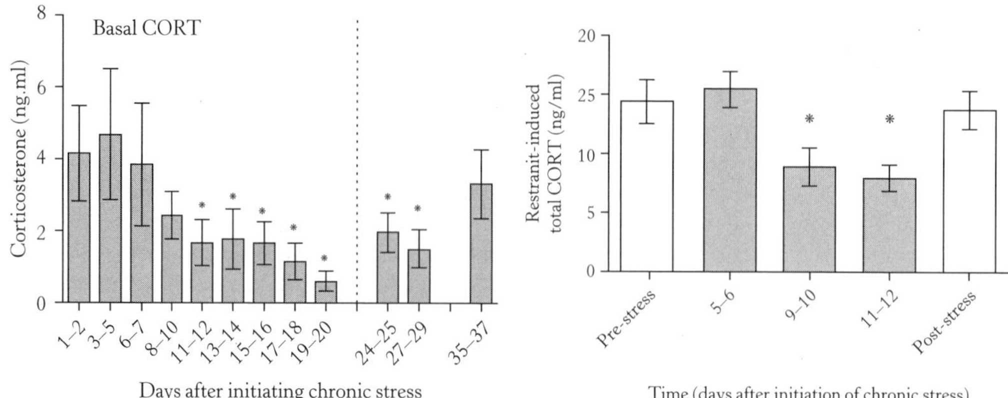

FIGURE 12.10: Change in baseline (left panel) and stress-induced (right panel) corticosterone concentrations in captive European starlings before, during, and after a period of chronic stress.

Reprinted with permission from Rich and Romero (2005) courtesy of American Physiological Society; Cyr et al. (2007) courtesy of Elsevier Press.

stress protocols under both field and laboratory conditions showed a similar endocrine response. Furthermore, that endocrine response was most similar to the non-responders from the visible burrow system.

On the other hand, another study repeated this experiment on two different species, white-eyed and black-capped vireos (Butler et al. 2009). In this case there were no changes in corticosterone responses. The birds clearly were disturbed by the stimuli because they increased alarm calls and distraction activities surrounding the nest, but corticosterone titers were equivalent to birds that were not exposed to rotating acute stressors. The differences in responses between the starlings and the two vireo species is intriguing and may be a consequence of different nesting strategies (Butler et al. 2009). Starlings are cavity nesters, and this strategy is typified by generally low nest mortality but, if the nest is depredated, high adult mortality results because of an inability to escape. Vireos, on the other hand, are open cup nesters.

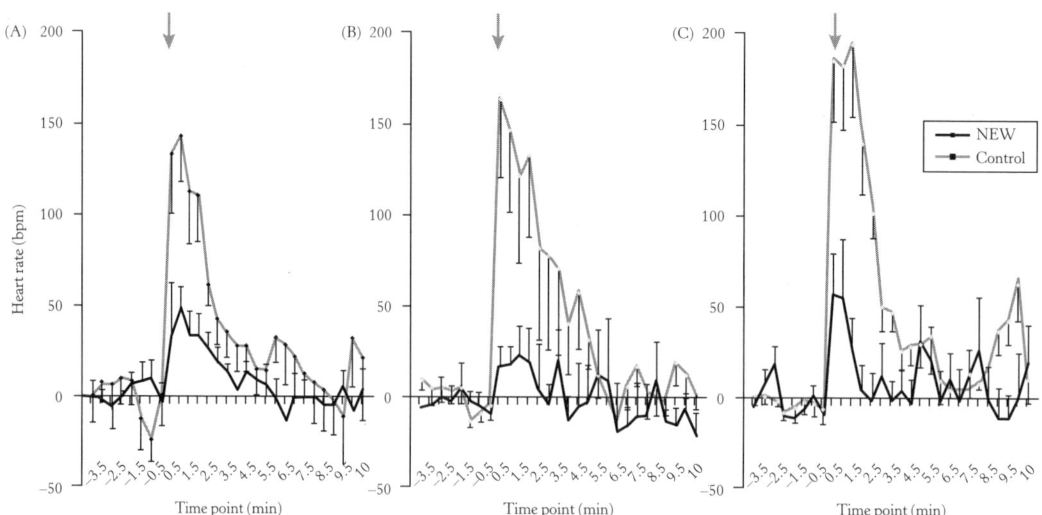

FIGURE 12.11: Heart rate responses to a startle stressor. Startle response for wild-caught, newly captive European starlings (new) and long-term captivity controls (controls) at (A) 36 h, (B) 88 h, or (C) 228 h after surgery. The arrow indicates the time period at which the startle was given.

Reprinted with permission from Dickens and Romero (2009) courtesy of University of Chicago Press.

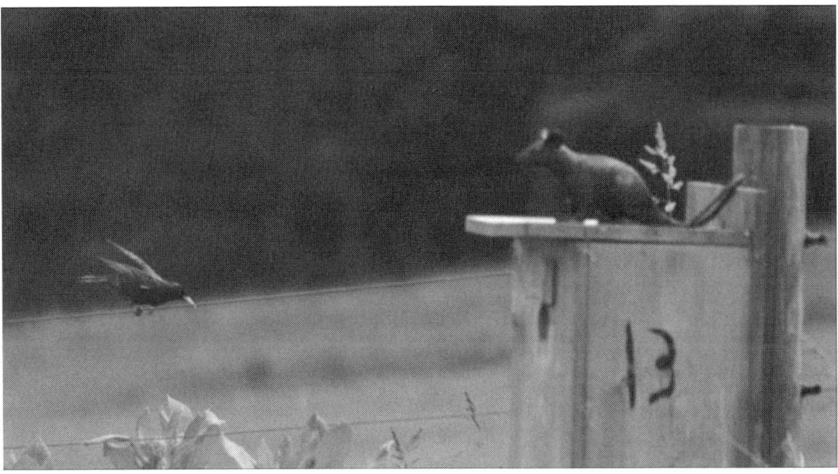

FIGURE 12.12: European starling female being exposed to a simulated predator (a fake rat) in order to induce chronic stress.

Photo courtesy of Jason Cyr.

The adults can easily see predators approaching and escape, so that nest predation rarely includes adult mortality. The key difference, therefore, may be whether the adult itself feels threatened by the stimuli used in the experiments. If the adult is threatened (i.e., starlings), then they mount acute responses that when summed 4 times per day for 3weeks becomes chronic stress. Conversely, when the adult is not threatened (i.e., vireos), a behavioral response but no endocrine stress response is mounted, even though the nest may be threatened. If this explanation is correct, only stimuli that threaten the individual itself, not stimuli that only threaten offspring (even if the threat is to the ultimate fitness of the individual), will elicit a stress response.

Regardless of the mechanism, the results from the starlings and vireos are rather disturbing. The data imply that it will be extremely difficult to predict a priori whether a given stimulus will elicit a stress response in free-living animals. In fact, a recent literature review of the impact of chronic stress on HPA axis function indicates that there is almost no consistency across studies, and studies are equally likely to report that chronic exposure to stressors results in increased, decreased, or no change in corticosteroid concentrations (Dickens and Romero 2013). Perhaps the best we can do is apply the lessons from the visible burrow system. Both the responders and non-responders altered their stress responses—just in opposite directions. Currently we have no way to predict whether a specific free-living individual or species will react like a responder or a non-responder, but deviations in either direction will indicate that the animal is likely suffering from chronic stress.

IV. RECREATIONAL DISTURBANCES

Perhaps some of the clearest examples of when anthropogenic disturbances are interpreted as stressors are following certain human recreational activities. Some of the early work on this topic studied the impact of snowmobiles on corticosteroid concentrations of wolves and elk (Creel et al. 2002). Snowmobile activity had a profound effect on fecal corticosteroid levels in both species, and the greater the snowmobile activity, the greater the corticosteroid levels. Elk were apparently unaffected when exposed to moderate numbers of snowmobiles (less than 300 entering their area of forest per day), but as the number of snowmobiles exceeded 300 and even 500 per day, corticosteroid levels increased. Interestingly, wheeled vehicles did not evoke the same type of response. Although this is a strong indication that snowmobiles were interpreted as stressors, there was no long-term impact on the demographics of either species. This suggests that even though snowmobile activity elicited acute stress responses, snowmobiles did not induce chronic stress.

The difference between the responses to snowmobiles and wheeled vehicles is intriguing. Wheeled vehicles are usually restricted to roads, so perhaps the difference is in the effects of roads. Roads can have complicated effects on animals that live near them. They can increase mortality and create barriers to movement (Taylor and

Goldingay 2010), but can also create habitat for species that prefer edges. Only a few studies have examined the impact of roads on corticosteroid responses. One on white-crowned sparrow nestlings found that corticosterone was elevated the closer the nest was to the road (Crino et al. 2011). Higher corticosterone was also correlated with increased body mass, suggesting a positive effect of the corticosterone, but this was offset by higher mortality through nest depredation. Although more work is needed to understand the impact of roads, it does appear that their proximity can alter HPA responses.

The situation is quite different with a number of grouse species in the European Alps exposed to alpine skiing. Black grouse build snow burrows for roosting during the winter, and these birds appear to be highly sensitive to human disturbance. As few as 2–11 ski or snowboard tracks within 500 meters of the burrow were sufficient to elevate fecal corticosteroid concentrations (Arlettaz et al. 2007). Furthermore, the levels attained in the feces were equivalent to levels after an intentional experimental flushing from the burrows. Although it is not clear whether the skiers actually flushed the birds, just a few transient, and presumably rapid, transits of a human near the burrow was sufficient to elicit a stress response. Similar results were obtained from capercaillie, another European grouse species. Capercaillie tended to avoid areas with high snow sport usage, but when they were in those areas their fecal corticosteroid concentrations were elevated compared to areas without snow sports (Thiel et al. 2008). Interestingly, the magnitude of the capercaillie response appears to depend upon the type of habitat (Thiel et al. 2011). Both of these species are currently declining in numbers, so in contrast to data from elk and wolves, human recreational activities could be contributing to the shrinking populations.

It will likely come as no surprise that hunting can also elicit a stress response in the hunted animal. However, how the hunting takes place can have a huge impact on the magnitude of the stress response. When red deer are run to ground before being killed, such as when hunted with dogs, their cortisol concentrations are over 70-fold higher than when cleanly shot from ambush (Bateson and Bradshaw 1997). The increase was especially pronounced when the pursuit exceeded 19 kilometers. Similar responses are likely from any hunting activity where the animal is exhausted prior to being killed (Mason 1998). For example, the time it takes to land a fish when angling has a clear impact on cortisol release—the longer it takes, the stronger the response (Cooke et al. 2002; Killen et al. 2003; Meka and McCormick 2005; Pottinger 1998; Suski et al. 2003). Furthermore, survival decreases the longer it takes to land the fish (i.e., the more exhausted the animal becomes; Cooke et al. 2002). Cougars are also hunted throughout much of their range in North America. Harlow et al. (1992) captured five animals and assessed plasma cortisol responses after ACTH injection in anesthetized animals. They then subjected the animals to chasing stress (i.e., simulated hunting) and tested with ACTH again. Plasma profiles of cortisol after ACTH were lower after having been chased than before the chase (Harlow et al. 1992). These data suggest that chasing resulted in a diminished capacity of the adrenal to respond to ACTH, although sample sizes were very small and, because chasing was performed after the initial test, the animals may have habituated to the captive situation. On the other hand, it does not appear that hunting pressure in and of itself elicits a stress response. Mourning doves in an area of active hunting lost weight, presumably due to reduced foraging time, but there was little effect on corticosteroid concentrations (Roy and Woolf 2001). In conclusion, responses of animals to hunting clearly vary markedly and may reflect the intensity of the chase and the perception of threat. Furthermore, hunting per se may not be stressful because a quick death prevents a stress response from occurring. But sport hunting that entails exhausting the animal can elicit extraordinarily strong responses.

V. ECOTOURISM

Although ecotourism is also a form of human recreation, it differs from the recreational activities discussed in the preceding section. As defined by Merriam-Webster, "ecotourism" is the practice of touring natural habitats in a manner meant to minimize ecological impact. In other words, the stated goal of ecotourism is to "take only photographs and leave only footprints," and definitely not to act as a major stressor to endemic wildlife. However, even taking photographs may affect some species (Huang et al. 2011). As a consequence, there has been great interest recently in determining whether ecotourism activities are major sources of stress to the observed wildlife.

Perhaps the best news for ecotourism is that the impact on stress response systems, if present at all, is quite subtle. Although tourists can clearly have an impact on behavior, they may not elicit a fight-or-flight response. Heart rate (and thus by extension the fight-or-flight response) has rarely been examined in ecotourism settings. When it has been measured, studies indicate that tourists do appear to elicit a heart rate response during their visit (Culik and Wilson 1995) and that human approach in general can elicit a heart rate response (e.g., Macarthur et al. 1982). On the other hand, many species also show a decrease in flight initiation distances (e.g., Mullner et al. 2004), the measure of how close an animal will allow the researcher to approach before moving, suggesting both habituation and the lack of a robust fight-or-flight response. Currently, however, there is no evidence of any long-term cardiac pathology (a hallmark of chronic stress or homeostatic overload) resulting from ecotourism, nor is there any indication of altered fight-or-flight responses to subsequent stressors. Consequently, the role of catecholamine release is likely to be transient.

In contrast, a number of studies have documented changes in HPA function in tourist-visited animals. One of the first attempts to measure tourist effects on the HPA responses to stress was in Magellanic penguins (Fowler 1999). Penguins visited by tourists had significantly lower baseline corticosterone concentrations. However, like the differences between salamanders and spotted owls discussed earlier in this chapter, it is not entirely clear whether the decrease represents habituation or is equivalent to non-responders to chronic stress. Tourist-visited penguins also failed to elevate corticosterone in response to 5 minutes of human presence at the nest. Considering that tourists rarely physically touch the birds, this lack of response likely represents habituation to the tourists' presence. Any habituation, however, appears to be only behavioral and not physiological. A subsequent study from the same population indicated that the reduced corticosterone response to capture and handling was partly due to a reduction in secretory capacity (Walker et al. 2006); tourist-visited birds were not capable of secreting the same amount of corticosterone. It is tempting to speculate that the intensity of tourist visitation was a major factor in the physiological changes. In the first study, penguins exposed to moderate human presence had normal HPA responses (Fowler 1999), suggesting that the more tourists, the greater the changes to the HPA axis. Furthermore, a study on a more recently established colony of Magellanic penguins that had far fewer annual or daily tourist visitations showed no HPA differences between naïve and tourist-visited animals (Villanueva et al. 2011). Unregulated tourism also altered corticosteroid responses in yellow-eyed penguins (Ellenberg et al. 2007), although in this case tourism evoked a sensitized response in which stress-induced corticosteroid titers were higher in visited animals.

Further evidence that tourist visitation is not benign comes from a study on Magellanic penguin chicks. Although the effects on adults appear to be quite subtle, the effects on chicks are more robust. Chicks appeared to be sensitized to stressors. Those chicks in the tourist-visited areas of the colony had accentuated corticosteroid responses to capture and handling (Walker et al. 2005b). This pattern is similar to the response in European starling chicks whose mothers were exposed to experimentally applied chronic stress (Cyr and Romero 2007). The accentuated response is transient, however, and disappears as the chicks get older. The underlying mechanism for this transient increase is not clear. In fact, the youngest chicks cannot thermoregulate and thus are still brooded by their parents, so how the information of human presence even gets conveyed to the chicks is a bit of a mystery. Walker et al. (2005b) suggest an intriguing hypothesis that an elevated heart rate from the brooding parents is the signal of danger to the chicks. If true, this would be a fascinating mechanism connecting the fight-or-flight response of the parents to changes in the HPA axis in the chicks.

Another good example of an enhanced HPA response in tourist-visited animals is in hoatzin chicks (Mullner et al. 2004). Hoatzins are large brightly colored birds of the equatorial Amazon and attractive targets for ecotourism. Tourist-exposed birds had much higher corticosteroid responses to capture and handling than non-exposed birds, and this was accompanied by a large decrease in offspring survival. Once again, the magnitude of the effect was correlated with the intensity of tourist visits, with chick survivorship decreasing as the number of visitors increased. However, in contrast to the HPA changes in penguin chicks, hoatzin chicks were most affected as juveniles, rather than nestlings. The corticosteroid responses to capture and handling in tourist-exposed and naïve nestlings were identical. It thus appears that ecotourism sensitized the juveniles to subsequent stressors. Consequently, although an accentuated corticosteroid response in tourist-visited chicks appears common, the sensitive ages appear to differ across species.

Changes in HPA function resulting from ecotourism are not restricted to birds. European pine martens excrete more corticosteroids in their feces as the average daily number of visitors increases (Barja et al. 2007), suggesting that corticosteroid release has been up-regulated. Two studies on marine iguanas from the Galápagos, however, indicate that how HPA function changes is not consistent even within a species. In one study, tourist-visited animals had a lower corticosteroid response than naïve animals (Romero and Wikelski 2002a), whereas the exact opposite was found in a subsequent study (French et al. 2010). In a further complication, the elevated corticosteroid response in the second study only occurred when the animals were not breeding—there were no differences between tourist-visited and naïve animals during the breeding season (French et al. 2010). Why these two studies should differ is not clear. The studies were performed on different islands, but that seems to be too simple an explanation. Unfortunately, there is no record of the relative intensities of tourist visitation, but tourism is high at most permitted sites in the Galápagos. Without further data, we currently have no way to predict whether different populations of marine iguanas will respond to tourism with an increase or a decrease in HPA function.

Interestingly, it appears that ecotourism has little effect on the baseline concentrations of corticosteroids. Only two studies, the earliest study in Magellanic penguins (Fowler 1999) and a study in yellow-eyed penguins (Ellenberg et al. 2007), documented an increase in baseline corticosteroid concentrations associated with tourism. In contrast, there were no differences in baseline concentrations from other studies in penguins (Walker et al. 2005b; Walker et al. 2006; Villanueva et al. 2011), from the work on hoatzins (Mullner et al. 2004), or from either study on marine iguanas (French et al. 2010; Romero and Wikelski 2002a). The weight of evidence thus suggests that ecotourism is not directly acting as a stressor to these animals. If it were, we would expect to find robust and persistent elevations of baseline corticosteroid concentrations across studies. Instead, ecotourism's major impact appears to be in altering the HPA axis sensitivity to additional stressors. This change may still alter a tourist-visited individual's ability to cope with additional stressors vis-à-vis unvisited animals, but if those additional stressors are mild or do not occur, the overall impact on the animal will be negligible.

In conclusion, ecotourism per se seems to have little impact on the stress responses of most animals. However, like many other stimuli, there can be substantial differences in sensitivity from animals in different age classes or in different life-history stages. Furthermore, the intensity of ecotourism can be a factor, with high-intensity activities eliciting changes in the HPA axis that are not apparent at lower intensities. What is not yet clear is whether any of the HPA axis changes have a long-term impact on the survival of these animals. Tourist activities can decrease reproductive success, but this may be unrelated to changes in stress physiology. Even if ecotourism does have an impact, conservation managers will have to decide whether the dangers to the individual animals, and often only a small proportion of the animals of a population, outweighs the benefits of the education and economic activity that help preserve these species and their habitats.

VI. POLLUTION

Pollution created by human activities has clearly had a major impact on wildlife. The physiological impacts can range from the devastating, such as the massive mortality accompanying oil spills, to the subtle, such as sub-lethal effects on the endocrine system that have been termed "endocrine disruption" (Colborn et al. 1996). The majority of work that has studied how pollution affects endocrine systems has focused on the various reproductive axes, especially effects on testosterone and estradiol. Much less work has focused on impacts to the corticosteroid system and, to our knowledge, there have not been any studies examining the effects of toxicants on catecholamine release. The emerging picture is quite different from the effects of other potential anthropogenic stressors discussed earlier in this chapter. The majority of studies indicate that toxicants generally inhibit HPA function.

One of the problems with any toxicant study is choosing the toxicant. Field studies are plagued by mixtures of toxicants, and even if investigators invest the time and expense to characterize the mixture, it is not clear which toxicants contributed to the overall endocrine effect. The problem is exacerbated by the realization that mixtures differ with sites and the growing reality that there is likely to be no remaining completely pristine environment left on earth. This last point is especially troubling because it becomes difficult to identify an appropriate control site. One partial solution to this problem has been to focus on various fish species living in polluted streams or rivers. The source of a toxicant can often be determined, and the upstream habitat can be used as a control for the downstream polluted habitat. Partly as a consequence, fish studies have provided the foundation for much of our understanding of toxicant effects on HPA function.

A number of toxicants have been assessed for their role in inducing altered corticosteroid release under natural conditions. Heavy metals seem to act as endocrine disruptors of the HPA axis in fish. Several, such as cadmium, mercury, and copper, inhibit cortisol production in vitro (Lacroix and Hontela 2004) and depress cortisol responses to stressors in both free-living fish (e.g., Gravel et al. 2005; Hontela et al. 1992; Hontela et al. 1995; Laflamme et al. 2000; Levesque et al. 2003) and under controlled laboratory conditions (e.g., Bleau et al. 1996; Kirubagaran and Joy 1991). In general, a decrease in the capacity to secrete cortisol appears to be common in fish species exposed to heavy metals (Hontela et al. 1997; Hontela 1998). The consequences can be subtle, but severe. Figure 12.13 shows data from brown trout captured upstream and downstream of a site of major heavy metal contamination. There is little apparent physical difference between the two populations, and both groups of fish appear healthy. However, when exposed to capture and a lengthy period of confinement, the fish from the contaminated site were unable to increase cortisol at the same rate as upstream fish (Figure 12.13), even though both groups reached similar maximum concentrations (Norris et al. 1999). Furthermore, the downstream fish were unable to maintain these elevated cortisol concentrations for the full 24 hours of the experiment. Although this is a subtle difference, the impact was devastating. All the contaminated fish died during the procedure, whereas none of the controls died (Norris 2000). Maintaining the cortisol response over the full 24 hours appears to be necessary to survive the 24 hours of confinement; the history of heavy metal exposure prevented a sustained response and doomed those animals.

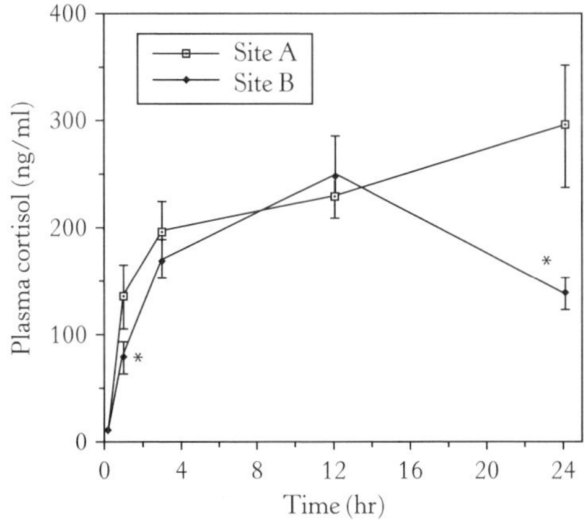

FIGURE 12.13: Plasma levels of cortisol following acute confinement of free-living brown trout. Site B is a downstream contaminated site and Site A is the upstream uncontaminated control site. Fish from Site B are unable to maintain cortisol levels after 24 hours of continuous confinement when compared to trout from Site A.

Reprinted with permission from Norris et al. (1999) courtesy of Elsevier Press.

The conclusion of toxicants generally depressing corticosteroid responses is not as clear in other taxa as it is in fish. A growing number of studies indicate an often similar, but not identical, dynamic effect occurring in various bird species. However, the responses to toxicants change, depending upon the developmental stage of the bird as well as the specific toxicant. A series of studies in a single species, tree swallows, illustrates these differences. PCB contamination in adults resulted in a lower stress response but no change in baseline concentrations (Franceschini et al. 2008), similar to the fish studies described in the preceding paragraph. On the other hand, nestling tree swallows had a higher stress response when exposed to PCBs, with again no effect on baseline concentrations (Franceschini et al. 2008). Dioxins, mercury, and chlorinated hydrocarbons had nearly the opposite effect on tree swallow nestlings, with lower baseline titers and no impact on stress-induced titers (Franceschini et al. 2008; Franceschini et al. 2009; Martinovic et al. 2003), whereas adults showed lower baseline corticosteroid titers as mercury levels increased (Figure 12.14) with no effect on stress-induced titers (Franceschini et al. 2009). These studies, conducted on the same species with animals living in similar habitats, highlight the difficulties of extrapolating results from one species to other species, from one toxicant to another, and even extrapolating results within a species across different life-history stages.

Other studies further emphasize the difficulty of extrapolating effects. Glaucous gulls contaminated with a variety of pollutants showed elevated baseline titers of corticosterone, but only males showed a reduced response to capture and restraint (Verboven et al. 2010). In mudpuppies, a mix of pollutants resulted in decreased corticosteroid release after capture, in females but not males and only at one site (Gendron et al. 1997). This decrease, however, correlated with a decrease in responsiveness to ACTH. In common

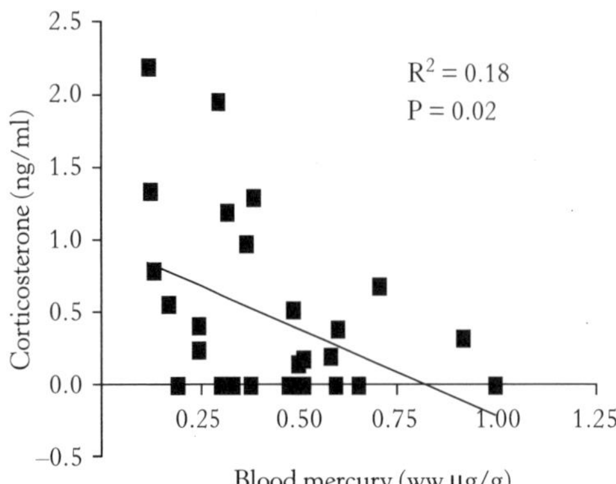

FIGURE 12.14: Correlation between mercury levels measured in the blood and baseline corticosterone concentrations in tree swallows.

Reprinted with permission from Franceschini et al. (2009) courtesy of Springer Press.

eiders, selenium decreased stress-induced corticosteroid concentrations, cadmium increased stress-induced corticosteroids but only in incubating females, and mercury had no effect (Wayland et al. 2002; Wayland et al. 2003). On the other hand, selenium exposure did not alter the corticosteroid response to capture and confinement in white suckers (Miller et al. 2009b), or two different trout species (Miller et al. 2009a), even though other indices of a stress response, such as glucose levels, did change and acute exposure to selenium increases corticosteroid titers (Miller et al. 2007). No relationship was found between corticosteroid and mercury in bald eagle nestlings (Bowerman et al. 2002) or adult white ibises (Heath and Frederick 2005), and mercury and cadmium had no effect on stress-induced corticosteroids in common eiders (Wayland et al. 2003). White suckers and mountain whitefish also did not alter corticosteroid release in response to a mixture of pesticides (Quinn et al. 2010).

These studies are only examples of the wide variety of species and toxicants that have been tested. The take-home message seems to be that, although most toxicants appear to decrease corticosteroid release in most species, the effect is not universal. Other toxicants seem to have minimal, if any, effects on HPA axis function. Perhaps this is not surprising considering the diversity of toxic chemicals.

On the other hand, only a minority of studies documented an increase in corticosteroid release. For example, heavily contaminated beluga whales (Beland et al. 1993) have adrenal hypertrophy consistent with augmented corticosteroid release (Deguise et al. 1995; Lair et al. 1997). One of the best examples, however, comes from two studies on the effects of coal combustion waste on southern toads. Figure 12.15A shows that baseline corticosteroid titers were greatly elevated at a polluted pond during both the middle and late portions of the breeding season (Hopkins et al. 1997). In contrast, coal waste only elevated testosterone titers during the late breeding season. This increase in corticosterone appears to be a result of constant stimulation of the adrenal tissue. Exogenous ACTH stimulated corticosterone release in toads from the control sites but not in

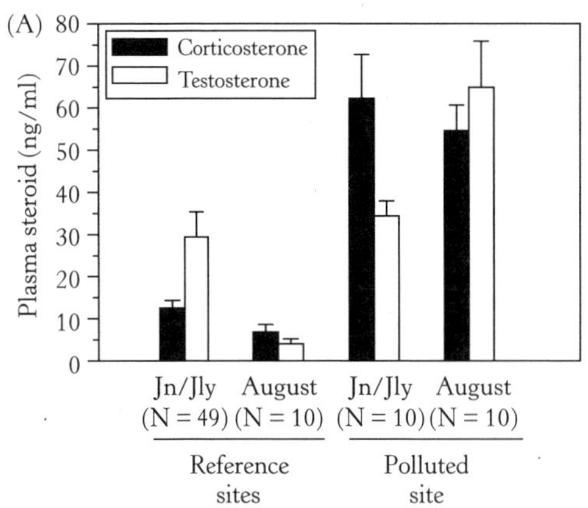

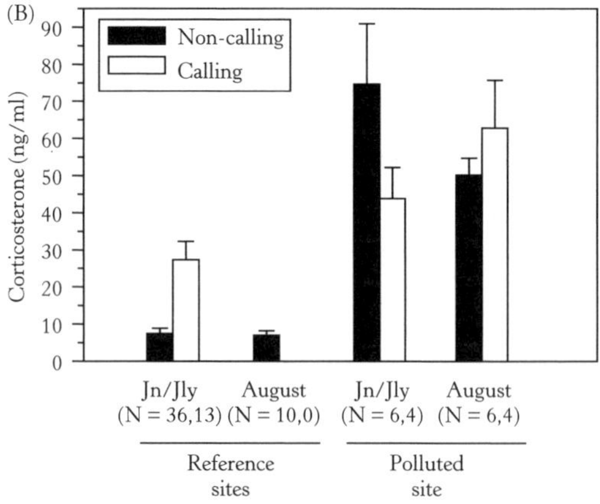

FIGURE 12.15: Circulating corticosterone and testosterone levels (A) and circulating corticosterone levels in calling and non-calling (B) male toads captured at a polluted site and at nearby reference sites. Toads were captured in June/July (Jn/Jly) and August at each site. No calling males were captured at the reference sites in August.

Reprinted with permission from Hopkins et al. (1997) courtesy of Elsevier Press.

the toads from the polluted site, suggesting that endogenous ACTH was greatly elevated and saturated the ability of the adrenal tissue to respond (Hopkins et al. 1999). In addition, Hopkins et al. (1999) also implicated impaired corticosteroid clearance from the liver in maintaining the high corticosterone concentrations.

The really interesting result, however, is shown in Figure 12.15B. Normally, toads that are calling, and thus actively attempting to attract mates, have elevated corticosterone titers. The large elevation in corticosterone in the toads from the polluted pond completely swamped this difference. Corticosterone was elevated regardless of month or behavior. This chronic elevation of corticosterone in non-calling toads from the polluted site may have profound consequences on the timing of reproductive behavior, and therefore overall fitness, because calling behavior continued much longer at the polluted site than at nearby reference sites (Hopkins et al. 1997). To date, this remains one of the few studies to link contaminant exposure effects on corticosteroid release with changes in behavior.

Oil spills are another example where toxicant-induced changes in corticosteroids have been implicated with ecologically important consequences. Oiling obviously can kill animals outright, but even small amounts of oil can affect an animal, potentially via changes in corticosteroid function. For example, lightly oiled Magellanic penguin females had elevated corticosterone titers and ended up with reduced nesting success (Fowler et al. 1995). One of the strongest connections between oiling, corticosteroids, and fitness, however, is from a series of studies on Galápagos marine iguanas.

The foundation for the oil spill studies on the marine iguanas was an earlier study on the corticosteroid effects during a previous El Niño. During 1997 and 1998 one of the longest and most severe El Niños on record struck the Galápagos Islands (Oberhuber et al. 1998), resulting in widespread starvation. Many animals were in extremely poor condition, and carcasses were abundant. We also sampled animals exactly one year after the El Niño event, during a "normal" year. Corticosterone levels were generally low during the 1999 La Niña feast period, but the 1998 El Niño famine resulted in both higher baseline and capture-stress induced corticosterone concentrations (Romero and Wikelski 2001). Corticosterone levels were higher during El Niño, even though absolute corticosterone levels differed between islands. Different ocean currents created different local conditions on each island, and when combined with variation in the average body mass of iguanas on each island, the result was that estimates of overall survival differed between islands. These survival estimates, however, were highly correlated with the mean stress-induced corticosterone levels for the respective island (Romero and Wikelski 2001). Stress-induced corticosterone levels, therefore, predicted overall population health.

This relationship between corticosteroids and health provided a template for assessing the impact of a small oil spill. On January 17, 2001, an oil tanker spilled roughly 3 million liters of diesel and bunker oil. Blood samples collected 3 days before and 7 days after the spill on the same population of marine iguanas showed a large increase in both baseline and stress-induced corticosterone titers in oiled individuals (Wikelski et al. 2001). Figure 12.16 shows that the corticosterone-to-survival relationship from the El Niño could be used to predict survival of the oiled iguanas. Normal corticosterone concentrations predicted an annual survival rate of more than 95%, typical of normal survival rates during good conditions (Laurie 1989; Wikelski et al. 1997). In contrast, corticosterone concentrations from oiled iguanas predicted mortality rates of about 40%. As shown in Figure 12.17, actual mortality determined approximately one year later was reasonably close at 62% (Wikelski et al. 2002).

Importantly, mortality did not occur immediately after the spill. Animals died over the ensuing few months, likely because the iguana's

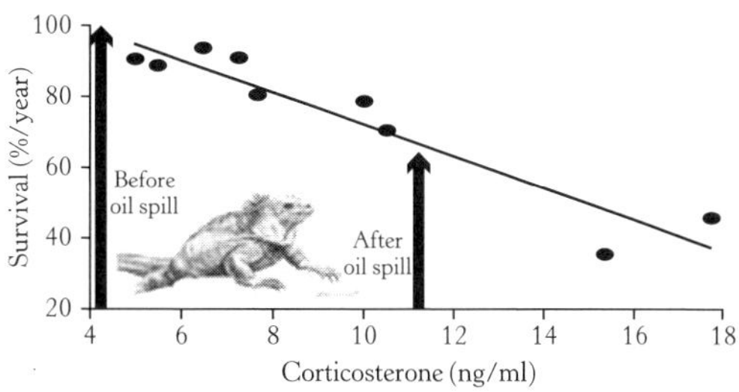

FIGURE 12.16: Correlation between yearly survival and corticosterone responses to capture and handling in Galápagos marine iguanas from six different islands during 1999 and during the El Niño of 1998. Each data point represents the mean ±SE for one island in one year. The linear regression line indicates the predicted survival rate based on population counts. The vertical arrows show the corticosterone levels of marine iguanas before and after an oil spill hit Santa Fe island.

Reprinted with permission from Romero and Wikelski (2002b) courtesy of Pergemon-Elsevier Science Press.

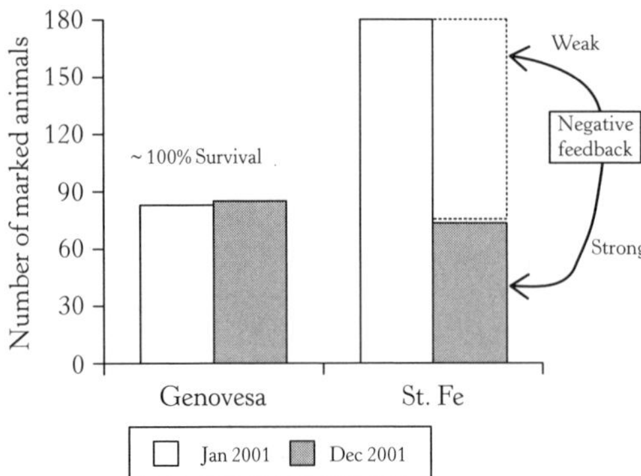

FIGURE 12.17: Population counts of Galápagos marine iguanas on Genovesa (control island) and Santa Fe (oil contaminated island) before (Jan. 2001) and about 1 year after (Dec. 2001) the oil spill. The estimated total Santa Fe iguana population declined dramatically, while the Genovesa control population was stable.

Adapted with permission from Romero and Wikelski (2002b) courtesy of Pergemon-Elsevier Science Press.

endosymbiotic hindgut bacteria were wiped out by consumed oil (Romero and Wikelski 2002b). The marine iguanas still foraged normally and appeared fine, but could not actually digest the food. The reason the survivorship relationship in Figure 12.16 was reasonably successful in predicting mortality, therefore, was that the oiled iguanas also died of starvation. A recent study also can provide a potential mechanism for which iguanas were likely to die from the oil spill. During an El Niño, iguanas that have the strongest negative feedback, in other words are best able to limit corticosteroid release after stressors, are the most likely to survive (Romero and Wikelski 2010). As shown in Figure 12.17, these data predict that the surviving iguanas from the oil spill were also likely to show stronger negative feedback.

All of us are aware of the catastrophic oil spills resulting in massive environmental damage and thousands to hundreds of thousands of animals dying, but less well appreciated are small, deliberate, oils spills occurring on oceans worldwide that also contribute to mortality and decreased reproductive success in many marine organisms (Boersma 2012). Studies now are beginning to show that even small quantities of oil on skin, fur, and feathers, or ingested in small amounts (e.g., from preening oiled feathers) can have serious effects on health and reproductive function (e.g., Holmes et al. 1978a; Holmes et al. 1978b). As Boersma (2012) points out, oil spills will never go away, but management of how ships clean out oil tanks, increased awareness of what spills do, and creation of marine-protected areas that exclude ships and the possibility of spills could go a long way to mitigate effects of partial oiling.

Finally, there are also a number of non-traditional forms of pollution that are starting to attract attention. For example, Cieslar et al. (2008) investigated the effects of static electric fields from nearby high-voltage DC lines in rats. The rats were exposed for 56 days, 8 hours per day, at intensities of 0, 16, 25 and 35 kV/m. Static electric fields increased insulin and thyroid hormones and decreased corticosterone plasma levels. Intensities above 16 kV/m were most effective. In another example, tadpoles of the Cascades frog show decreased survival if exposed to UV-B radiation in the field for 42 days compared with controls shielded from UV-B. Although these tadpoles show a confinement-induced increase in whole body corticosterone, indicating a typical adrenocortical response to stress, exposure to UV-B radiation did not affect corticosterone levels (Belden et al. 2003).

In conclusion, the impact of pollution on HPA function defies easy categorization. The majority of studies report a decrease in corticosteroid responses to stressors. A few studies link this decrease to desensitization of corticosteroidogenic tissue to ACTH, suggesting an effect directly on the steroid-producing cells. That chemicals prove to be toxic to corticosteroidogenic cells is probably not surprising. The result is an inability to properly initiate and sustain corticosteroid responses. Although this might not kill the animals outright, it can make them far more vulnerable to subsequent stressors, as occurs in fish bathed in water with elevated heavy metals (Figure 12.13; Norris et al. 1999). The toxicants have increased the affected animals' allostatic load and have greatly reduced their reactive scope. On the other hand, there are a number of toxicants that have the opposite effect—they stimulate excessive corticosteroid release. Rather than simply decreasing the individual's reactive scope, the elevated corticosteroid levels induce pathological behaviors, as seen in toads bathed in water with coal combustion waste (Hopkins et al. 1997), and corticosteroid-mediated starvation physiology follows, as seen with the oil spill and marine iguanas (Wikelski et al. 2002). These toxicant-induced symptoms are more typical of allostatic overload. Although we cannot yet predict whether a specific species will have a blunted or accentuated corticosteroid response when faced with a specific toxicant (or specific mixture of toxicants), it is clear that either result can have devastating consequences for the affected individuals. Of all the human-induced changes to our environment, pollution may be the worst in terms of affecting the HPA axis.

VII. ENDOCRINE DISRUPTION AND PERCEPTION AND TRANSDUCTION OF ENVIRONMENTAL CUES

There is no doubt that hundreds, indeed thousands, of chemicals comprise a major group of environmental factors that animals and plants must cope with (Crews et al. 2000; McLachlan 2001). In the preceding section we discussed how these chemicals disrupt endocrine systems, especially the HPA axis, but in this section we will consider how endocrine disrupting chemicals (EDCs) might interfere with pathways of transduction of environmental cues and thus alter how an organism might respond to global change, including labile perturbation factors (Figure 12.18).

We discussed in Chapter 1 how an animal in its natural environment responds to changes in that environment and the types of responses. In other words, pollutants may act as toxic chemicals reducing fitness, but there is emerging evidence that at sub-toxic levels some chemicals may disrupt endocrine systems by altering perception of the environment. An organism uses some sensory modality or modalities to perceive the environment as it changes and then must transduce that information into neural, neuroendocrine, and endocrine secretions. These pathways then orchestrate morphological, physiological, and behavioral responses as the individual acclimates. Different levels of feedback also regulate the extent of the responses, and these too could be disrupted by pollutants (Figure 12.18). This allows us to look at the bigger picture from environmental change to response and to consider mechanisms by which endocrine disruption could interfere.

A. Endocrine Disrupting Chemicals (EDCs) in the Context of Life Cycles

Of the hundreds, perhaps thousands, of papers published on EDCs and mixtures of those chemicals (more relevant for animals in their natural habitat), most demonstrate that EDCs have not only endocrine disrupting effects but are often carcinogenic and have additional toxic properties (Crews et al. 2000; National Research Council 1999). Laboratory experiments reveal that EDCs can interact with a hormone receptor, or disrupt

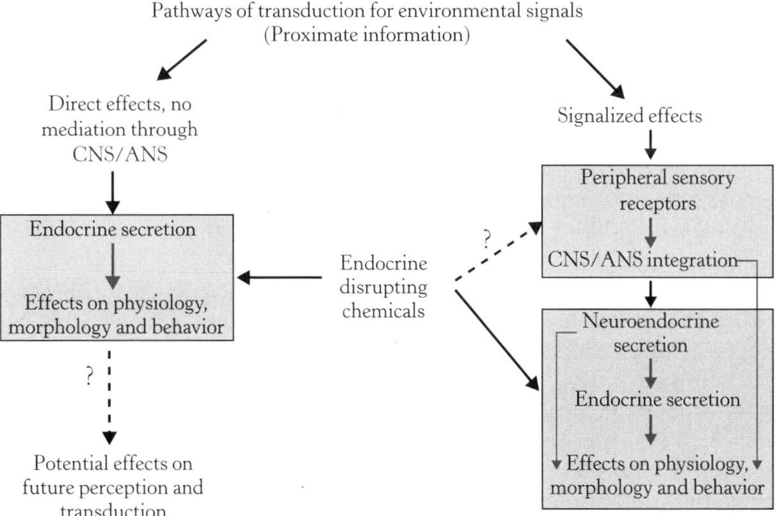

FIGURE 12.18: Potential pathways by which endocrine disrupting chemicals (EDCs) may influence environmental response pathways. Classically, many EDCs act directly on endocrine cells or their target tissues, but how these effects may influence the future ability of the individual to perceive and respond to environmental signals is much less well known. EDCs may also affect specific sensory modalities and transduction mechanisms through the nervous system, thus indirectly affecting neuroendocrine and endocrine secretions downstream. Disruption of sensory neural inputs could have major implications for how organisms respond to environmental signals.

From Wingfield and Mukai (2009), courtesy of Elsevier Press.

endocrine action in other ways, such as synthesis of the hormone, secretion, transport, and clearance from the blood (e.g., Crews et al. 2000; Kendall et al. 1998; National Research Council 1999; Norris and Carr 2006). This information is then used to assess risk and regulatory policy and could be useful for environmental mitigation and conservation. Classic model organisms, such as rats, mice, quail, chickens, or constructs of receptor/reporter genes in vitro, allow screening of large numbers of chemicals (e.g., National Research Council 1999). However, endocrine disrupting actions in populations of animals in their natural habitat are not easily extrapolated from the laboratory (Wingfield and Mukai 2009).

Natural populations of animals undoubtedly have greater genetic variation compared to highly inbred laboratory strains, which form the basis for much of our knowledge of the effects of EDCs. However, it also appears that wild populations of rats and mice that are not inbred apparently can survive the actions of EDCs more effectively. Although some individuals die from toxic effects and endocrine disruption, others continue to reproduce and the population can maintain numbers, or even increase (Wingfield and Mukai 2009). This raises a number of questions: Are some individuals in free-living populations more resistant to the effects of EDCs? Do some respond to their environment in different ways? Are some able to reduce exposure to EDCs? The answers are probably in the affirmative for all vertebrate species, especially invasive species that seem to be thriving across the globe. However, some species may be more vulnerable to many EDCs, such as those at high trophic levels, predators, that accrue high levels because of bioaccumulation and biomagnification (Wingfield and Mukai 2009).

Another question from the general literature is, why do some species survive and cope with EDCs better than others? There may be genetic differences in receptor forms and actions (Karchner et al. 2006; Lee et al. 2007), different metabolism of the hormone (Scheuhammer et al. 2008), and differences in other aspects of endocrine function such as transport. Nonetheless, it is also probable that variation in coping with EDCs includes how an organism responds to its environment (Wingfield and Mukai 2009).

B. Effects on Perception and Transduction of Environmental Cues

Because EDCs alter endocrine function by mimicking, blocking, and/or interfering with their endogenous ligands, and disrupt metabolism and degradation of the receptors, hormones, or their carrier proteins (Figure 12.18; Wingfield and Mukai 2009), it could be argued that EDCs have direct effects on endocrine cells independently of any signalized pathway of perception, transduction, and response (Figure 12.18; Wingfield and Mukai 2009). This could influence "downstream" events of how individuals transduce and respond to environmental signals in the future (left-hand part of Figure 12.18). The "upstream" components of responsiveness to labile perturbation factors is much less well known. Could EDCs alter perception of environment and transduction of that information (right-hand part of Figure 12.18; Wingfield and Mukai 2009)?

Wingfield and Mukai (2009) summarize many examples of how EDCs influence perception of the environment, transduction of the environmental signal, and the ensuing morphological, physiological, and behavioral responses in relation to photoperiodic effects, social interactions, and responses to local predictive cues. Effects of EDCs on unpredictable environmental perturbations are less well known, but there is growing evidence that EDCs can interfere with the coping mechanisms, including the emergency life-history stage (Norris 2000; Propper 2005). If EDCs are interfering with mechanisms by which neuroendocrine and endocrine secretions respond to labile perturbation factors, then major issues arise that go far beyond laboratory studies. Indeed, other impacts of HIREC (human-induced rapid environmental change), such as permanent perturbation factors, could be greatly exacerbated by EDCs. As discussed in the previous section, evidence suggests that environmental chemicals of anthropogenic origin, particularly as mixtures, are having detrimental effects on the adrenocortical responses to stress in animals in their natural environment (e.g., Propper 2005). (Refer again to Figure 12.13 as an example.) But EDC effects on coping with labile perturbation factors go beyond just interfering with HPA function. In mammals, corticosteroids influence memory consolidation (Melcangi and Panzica 2006), which could be important for how the animal reacts to the same perturbation in the future. Furthermore, the adrenocortical responses and cognitive-memory pathways could be impaired both directly and indirectly by EDCs, resulting in inappropriate responses to labile perturbation factors in the future.

EDCs can have effects on developing organisms influencing maternal physiology and behavior (e.g., Kendall et al. 1998; National Research

Council 1999; Norris and Carr 2006). In water birds breeding in the Great Lakes region of North America, exposures to organochlorines such as DDT caused embryo mortality, edema, and deformities including eggshell thinning (Gilbertson et al. 1991; Lundholm and Bartonek 1992). Additionally, behavioral disruption in adult birds resulted in abandonment of nests and eggs. Much less well known is whether EDCs change the perception of the environment by the mother (or father in the case of paternal effects), and what implications there may be for developmental effects downstream and even across generations (Wingfield and Mukai 2009). In a laboratory study, Hayward et al. (2006) exposed eggs of Japanese quail to corticosterone, resulting in altered development and behavioral phenotype of chicks. Stressors during egg formation and the transfer of corticosteroids to egg yolk or maternal licking/grooming in rodents can have profound effects on the behavioral phenotypes of offspring, including how they respond to stress, by altering corticosteroid receptor expression (Caldji et al. 1998). It is entirely possible that interference effects of EDCs on maternal/paternal behaviors could also affect the offsprings' ability to cope with perturbations later in life.

Although endocrine systems are influenced directly by environmental cues, they are also linked to sensory transduction pathways that are vulnerable to disruption. Global gene expression profiling and functional pathway analysis will be tools to explore novel genes involved in responses to the environment. How EDCs affect these relevant pathways should be a major focus of future work. Pathologies and death may not always occur, but fitness could be reduced. If fitness were reduced by 10%–20%, then over time there could be a marked population decline.

On a final note, predators are exposed to higher levels of EDCs by consuming large numbers of contaminated prey (i.e., bioaccumulation) and thus tend to be more susceptible. Not only does this create a problem for the predator species itself, but it could also have serious implications for other species at the ecosystem level. Changing abundance and distribution of predators can precipitate declines and/or population explosions of other species, particularly prey. Changes in herbivore populations could then further disrupt ecosystems, particularly vegetation patterns, with more far-reaching effects. Ecological effects following detrimental effects of EDCs on predators or keystone species could be catastrophic for biodiversity (Wingfield and Mukai 2009).

VIII. CONCLUSIONS

The question posed at the beginning of this chapter was whether human activities and human-induced changes to the environment are interpreted as stressors by wildlife. The answer is a resounding yes, but with many caveats. Some changes and activities, such as pollution and hunting, can be interpreted as incredibly strong stressors. These anthropogenic changes have profound impacts on individuals and populations. Other anthropogenic changes, however, such as ecotourism and urbanization, affect animals much more subtly. We can document changes in corticosteroid and catecholamine release, but the long-term impacts on the individuals are far less clear. The subtle endocrine changes may not ultimately alter an individual's fitness. How EDCs disrupt perception of the environment and transduction of this information, or interfere with patterns of behavior, will also be critical for us to understand. What is clear is that the stress response is an important physiological system for coping with anthropogenic changes, just as it is an important physiological system for coping with natural environmental changes. Humans continue to have varied and far-reaching impacts on the environment. What the studies of this chapter have shown is that sometimes the stress response is able to help animals cope, and other times it is insufficient to the task. The implications for conservation and reducing loss of biodiversity will be discussed in the next chapter.

REFERENCES

Arlettaz, R., Patthey, P., Baltic, M., Leu, T., Schaub, M., Palme, R., Jenni-Eiermann, S., 2007. Spreading free-riding snow sports represent a novel serious threat for wildlife. *Proc R Soc Lond B* 274, 1219–1224.

Baldwin, A. L., 2007. Effects of noise on rodent physiology. *Int J Comp Psychol* 20, 134–144.

Barja, I., Silvan, G., Rosellini, S., Pineiro, A., Gonzalez-Gil, A., Camacho, L., Illera, J. C., 2007. Stress physiological responses to tourist pressure in a wild population of European pine marten. *J Ster Biochem Mol Biol* 104, 136–142.

Barrett, R. T., 2002. The phenology of spring bird migration to north Norway. *Bird Study* 49, 270–277.

Bartholomew, G. A., 1958. The role of physiology in the distribution of terrestrial vertebrates. In: Hubbs, I. (Ed.), *Zoogeography*, Washington, D.C.: American Association for the Advancement of Science, pp. 81–95.

Bartholomew, G. A., 1964. The roles of physiology and behaviour in the maintenance of homeostasis in the desert environment. In: Hughes, G. M. (Ed.), *Homeostasis and Feedback Mechanisms*, Symp. Soc. Exp. Biol. Cambridge University Press, Cambridge, U.K. 18, 7–29.

Bartholomew, G. A., 1966. Interaction of physiology and behavior under natural conditions. In: Bowman, R. I. (Ed.), *The Galápagos: Proceedings of the Symposia of the Galápagos International Scientific Project*. University of California Press, Los Angeles, pp. 39–45.

Bateson, P., Bradshaw, E. L., 1997. Physiological effects of hunting red deer (*Cervus elaphus*). *Proc R Soc Lond B* 264, 1707–1714.

Beckerman, A. P., Boots, M., Gaston, K. J., 2007. Urban bird declines and the fear of cats. *Anim Conserv* 10, 320–325.

Beland, P., Deguise, S., Girard, C., Lagace, A., Martineau, D., Michaud, R., Muir, D. C. G., Norstrom, R. J., Pelletier, E., Ray, S., Shugart, L. R., 1993. Toxic compounds and health and reproductive effects in St. Lawrence beluga whales. *J Gt Lakes Res* 19, 766–775.

Belden, L. K., Moore, I. T., Mason, R. T., Wingfield, J. C., Blaustein, A. R., 2003. Survival, the hormonal stress response and UV-B avoidance in Cascades Frog tadpoles (*Rana cascadae*) exposed to UV-B radiation. *Func Ecol* 17, 409–416.

Beniston, M., Stephenson, D. B., 2004. Extreme climatic events and their evolution under changing climatic conditions. *Global Planet Change* 44, 1–9.

Berthold, P., 1993. *Bird migration: A general survey.* Oxford University Press, New York.

Blanchard, D. C., Spencer, R. L., Weiss, S. M., Blanchard, R. J., McEwen, B., Sakai, R. R., 1995. Visible burrow system as a model of chronic social stress: Behavioral and neuroendocrine correlates. *Psychoneuroendocrinology* 20, 117–134.

Blanchard, R. J., Blanchard, D. C., 2003. Bringing natural behaviors into the laboratory: A tribute to Paul MacLean. *Physiol Behav* 79, 515–524.

Bleau, H., Daniel, C., Chevalier, G., vanTra, H., Hontela, A., 1996. Effects of acute exposure to mercury chloride and methylmercury on plasma cortisol, T3, T4, glucose and liver glycogen in rainbow trout (*Oncorhynchus mykiss*). *Aquatic Toxicology* 34, 221–235.

Blickley, J. L., Word, K. R., Krakauer, A. H., Phillips, J. L., Sells, S. N., Taff, C. C., Wingfield, J. C., Patricelli, G. L., 2012. Experimental chronic noise is related to elevated fecal corticosteroid metabolites in lekking male greater sage-grouse (*Centrocercus urophasianus*). *Plos One* 7, e50462.

Boersma, P. D., 2012. Penguins and petroleum: lessons in conservation ecology. *Front Ecol Environ* 10, 218–219.

Bonier, F., Martin, P. R., Sheldon, K. S., Jensen, J. P., Foltz, S. L., Wingfield, J. C., 2007a. Sex-specific consequences of life in the city. *Behav Ecol* 18, 121–129.

Bonier, F., Martin, P. R., Wingfield, J. C., 2007b. Urban birds have broader environmental tolerance. *Biol Lett* 3, 670–673.

Both, C., Bijlsma, R. G., Visser, M. E., 2005. Climatic effects on timing of spring migration and breeding in a long-distance migrant, the pied flycatcher *Ficedula hypoleuca*. *J Avian Biol* 36, 368–373.

Both, C., Visser, M. E., 2001. Adjustment to climate change is constrained by arrival date in a long-distance migrant bird. *Nature* 411, 296–298.

Bowerman, W. W., Mehne, C. J., Best, D. A., Refsal, K. R., Lombardini, S., Bridges, W. C., 2002. Adrenal corticotropin hormone and nestling bald eagle corticosterone levels. *Bull Environ Contam Toxicol* 68, 355–360.

Buchanan, J. B., Irwin, L. L., McCutchen, E. L., 1995. Within-stand nest-site selection by spotted owls in the Eastern Washington Cascades. *J Wildlife Manage* 59, 301–310.

Butler, L. K., Bisson, I. A., Hayden, T. J., Wikelski, M., Romero, L. M., 2009. Adrenocortical responses to offspring-directed threats in two open-nesting birds. *Gen Comp Endocrinol* 162, 313–318.

Caldji, C., Tannenbaum, B., Sharma, S., Francis, D., Plotsky, P. M., Meaney, M. J., 1998. Maternal care during infancy regulates the development of neural systems mediating the expression of fearfulness in the rat. *Proc Natl Acad Sci USA* 95, 5335–5340.

Chavez-Zichinelli, C. A., MacGregor-Fors, I., Rohana, P.vT., Valdez, R., Romano, M.vC., Schondube, J.vE., 2010. Stress responses of the House Sparrow (*Passer domesticus*) to different urban land uses. *Landscape Urban Plan* 98, 183–189.

Churcher, P. B., Lawton, J. H., 1987. Predation by domestic cats in an English village. *J Zool* 212, 439–455.

Cieslar, G., Sowa, P., Kos-Kudla, B., Sieron, A., 2008. Influence of static electric field generated nearby high vltage direct current transmission lines on hormonal activity of experimental animals. In: Krawczyk, A., Kubacki, R. (Eds.), *Electromagnetic field, health and environment.* IOS Press, Amsterdam, pp. 72–78.

Clark, C. W., Ellison, W. T., Southall, B. L., Hatch, L., Van Parijs, S. M., Frankel, A., Ponirakis, D., 2009. Acoustic masking in marine ecosystems: intuitions, analysis, and implication. *Marine Ecol Progress Ser* 395, 201–222.

Colborn, T., Dumanoski, D., Meyers, J. P., 1996. *Our stolen future.* Dutton, New York.

Cooke, S. J., Schreer, J. F., Wahl, D. H., Philipp, D. P., 2002. Physiological impacts of catch-and-release angling practices on largemouth bass and smallmouth bass. In: Philipp, D. P., Ridgway, M. S. (Eds.), *Black bass: Ecology, conservation, and management.* American Fisheries Society, Bethesda, MD, vol. 31. pp. 489–512.

Creel, S., Fox, J. E., Hardy, A., Sands, J., Garrott, B., Peterson, R. O., 2002. Snowmobile activity and glucocorticoid stress responses in wolves and elk. *Conserv Biol* 16, 809–814.

Crews, D., Willingham, E., Skipper, J. K., 2000. Endocrine disruptors: Present issues, future directions. *Q Rev Biol* 75, 243–260.

Crino, O. L., Van Oorschot, B. K., Johnson, E. E., Malisch, J. L., Breuner, C. W., 2011. Proximity to a high traffic road: Glucocorticoid and life history consequences for nestling white-crowned sparrows. *Gen Comp Endocrinol* 173, 323–332.

Crutzen, P. J., Stoemer, E. F., 2000. The Anthropocene. *Global Change Newsletter* 41, 17–18.

Culik, B. M., Wilson, R. P., 1995. Penguins disturbed by tourists. *Nature* 376, 301–302.

Cyr, N. E., Dickens, M. J., Romero, L. M., 2009. Heart rate and heart rate variability responses to acute and chronic stress in a wild-caught passerine bird. *Physiol Biochem Zool* 82, 332–344.

Cyr, N. E., Earle, K., Tam, C., Romero, L. M., 2007. The effect of chronic psychological stress on corticosterone, plasma metabolites, and immune responsiveness in European starlings. *Gen Comp Endocrinol* 154, 59–66.

Cyr, N. E., Romero, L. M., 2007. Chronic stress in free-living European starlings reduces corticosterone concentrations and reproductive success. *Gen Comp Endocrinol* 151, 82–89.

Cyr, N. E., Romero, L. M., 2008. Fecal glucocorticoid metabolites of experimentally stressed captive and free-living starlings: Implications for conservation research. *Gen Comp Endocrinol* 158, 20–28.

D'Alba, L., Spencer, K. A., Nager, R. G., Monaghan, P., 2011. State dependent effects of elevated hormone: Nest site quality, corticosterone levels and reproductive performance in the common eider. *Gen Comp Endocrinol* 172, 218–224.

Deguise, S., Martineau, D., Beland, P., Fournier, M., 1995. Possible mechanisms of action of environmental contaminants on St Lawrence beluga whales (*Delphinapterus leucas*). *Environ Health Perspect* 103, 73–77.

Dessens, J., 1995. Severe convective weather in the context of a nighttime global warming. *Geophys Res Let* 22, 1241–1244.

Dickens, M. J., Romero, L. M., 2009. Wild European starlings (*Sturnus vulgaris*) adjust to captivity with sustained sympathetic nervous system drive and a reduced fight-or-flight response. *Physiol Biochem Zool* 82, 603–610.

Dickens, M. J., Romero, L. M., 2013. A consensus endocrine profile for a chronically stressed wild animal does not exist. *Gen Comp Endocrinol* 191, 177–189.

Easterling, D. R., Meehl, G. A., Parmesan, C., Changnon, S. A., Karl, T. R., Mearns, L. O., 2000. Climate extremes: Observations, modeling, and impacts. *Science* 289, 2068–2074.

Ellenberg, U., Setiawan, A. N., Cree, A., Houston, D. M., Seddon, P. J., 2007. Elevated hormonal stress response and reduced reproductive output in Yellow-eyed penguins exposed to unregulated tourism. *Gen Comp Endocrinol* 152, 54–63.

Ellis, D. H., Ellis, C. H., Mindell, D. P., 1991. Raptor responses to low-level jet aircraft and sonic-booms. *Environ Pollut* 74, 53–83.

Ellison, W. T., Southall, B. L., Clark, C. W., Frankel, A. S., 2012. A new context-based approach to assess marine mammal behavioral responses to anthropogenic sounds. *Conserv Biol* 26, 21–28.

Evans, K. L., Gaston, K. J., Frantz, A. C., Simeoni, M., Sharp, S. P., McGowan, A., Dawson, D. A., Walasz, K., Partecke, J., Burke, T., Hatchwell, B. J., 2009. Independent colonization of multiple urban centres by a formerly forest specialist bird species. *Proc R Soc Lond B* 276, 2403–2410.

Field, C. B., Barros, V., Stocker, T. F., Dahe, Q., Dokken, D. J., Ebi, K., Mastrandrea, M. D., Mach, K. J., Plattner, G.-K., Allen, S. K., Tignor, M., Midgley, P. M. (Eds.), 2012. Managing the risks of extreme events and disasters to advance climate change adaptation. Special Report of the IPCC. Cambridge University Press, Cambridge.

Fokidis, H. B., 2011. Homeowners associations: Friend or foe to native desert avifauna? Conservation concerns and opportunities for research. *J Arid Environ* 75, 394–396.

Fokidis, H. B., Orchinik, M., Deviche, P., 2009. Corticosterone and corticosteroid binding globulin in birds: Relation to urbanization in a desert city. *Gen Comp Endocrinol* 160, 259–270.

Fokidis, H. B., Orchinik, M., Deviche, P., 2011. Context-specific territorial behavior in urban birds: No evidence for involvement of testosterone or corticosterone. *Horm Behav* 59, 133–143.

Fokidis, H. B., Deviche, P., 2011. Plasma corticosterone of city and desert Curve-billed Thrashers, *Toxostoma curvirostre*, in response to stress-related peptide administration. *Comp Biochem Physiol A* 159, 32–38.

Forbush, E. H., 1916. The domestic cat: Bird killer, mouser, and destroyer of wild life; means of utilizing and controlling it. The Commonwealth of Massachusetts State Board of Agriculture, *Economic biology*—Bulletin No 2. Wright & Potter, Boston, p. 112.

Fowler, G. S., 1999. Behavioral and hormonal responses of Magellanic penguins (*Spheniscus magellanicus*) to tourism and nest site visitation. *Biol Conserv* 90, 143–149.

Fowler, G. S., Wingfield, J. C., Boersma, P. D., 1995. Hormonal and reproductive effects of low levels of petroleum fouling in megallanic penguins. *Auk* 111, 20–27.

Franceschini, M. D., Custer, C. M., Custer, T. W., Reed, J. M., Romero, L. M., 2008. Corticosterone stress response in tree swallows, *Tachycineta bicolor*, nesting near PCB and dioxin contaminated rivers. *Environ Toxicol Chem* 27, 2326–2331.

Franceschini, M. D., Lane, O. P., Evers, D. C., Reed, J. M., Hoskins, B., Romero, L. M., 2009. The corticosterone stress response and mercury contamination in tree swallows, *Tachycineta Bicolor. Ecotoxicology* 18, 514–521.

Francis, D., Hengeveld, H., 1998. Extreme weather and climate change. Minister of Supply and Services, Canada., Minister of the Environment, Ontario, p. 31.

French, S. S., DeNardo, D. F., Greives, T. J., Strand, C. R., Demas, G. E., 2010. Human disturbance alters endocrine and immune responses in the Galapagos marine iguana (Amblyrhynchus cristatus). *Horm Behav* 58, 792–799.

French, S. S., Fokidis, H. B., Moore, M. C., 2008. Variation in stress and innate immunity in the tree lizard (*Urosaurus ornatus*) across an urban-rural gradient. *J Comp Physiol B* 178, 997–1005.

Gendron, A. D., Bishop, C. A., Fortin, R., Hontela, A., 1997. In vivo testing of the functional integrity of the corticosterone-producing axis in mudpuppy (amphibia) exposed to chlorinated hydrocarbons in the wild. *Environ Toxicol Chem* 16, 1694–1706.

Gilbertson, M., Kubiak, T., Ludwig, J., Fox, G., 1991. Great Lakes embryo mortality, edema, and deformities syndrome (GLEMEDS) in colonial fish-eating birds: similarity to chick-edema disease. *J Toxicol Environ Health* 33, 455–520.

Gordon, H. B., Whetton, P. H., Pittock, A. B., Fowler, A. M., Haylock, M. R., 1992. Simulated changes in daily rainfall intensity due to the enhanced greenhouse effect: implications for extreme rainfall events. *Climate Dynamics* 8, 83–102.

Gravel, A., Campbell, P. G. C., Hontela, A., 2005. Disruption of the hypothalamo-pituitary-interrenal axis in 1+ yellow perch (*Perca flavescens*) chronically exposed to metals in the environment. *Can J Fish Aquat Sci* 62, 982–990.

Hamao, S., Watanabe, M., Mori, Y., 2011. Urban noise and male density affect songs in the great tit Parus major. *Ethol Ecol Evolution* 23, 111–119.

Harlow, H. J., Lindzey, F. G., Vansickle, W. D., Gern, W. A., 1992. Stress response of cougars to nonlethal pursuit by hunters. *Can J Zool* 70, 136–139.

Hatch, L. T., Clark, C. W., Van Parijs, S. M., Frankel, A. S., Ponirakis, D. W., 2012. Quantifying loss of acoustic communication space for right whales in and around a U.S. National Marine Sanctuary. *Conserv Biol* 26, 983–994.

Hayward, L. S., Richardson, J. B., Grogan, M. N., Wingfield, J. C., 2006. Sex differences in the organizational effects of corticosterone in the egg yolk of quail. *Gen Comp Endocrinol* 146, 144–148.

Heath, J. A., Frederick, P. C., 2005. Relationships among mercury concentrations, hormones, and nesting effort of White Ibises (*Eudocimus albus*) in the Florida Everglades. *Auk* 122, 255–267.

Heide, O. M., Pedersen, K., Dahl, E., 1990. Environmental control of flowering and morphology in the high-arctic *Cerastium regelii*, and the taxonomic status of C. jenisejense. *Nordic J Botany* 10, 141–147.

Heiss, R. S., Clark, A. B., McGowan, K. J., 2009. Growth and nutritional state of American Crow nestlings vary between urban and rural habitats. *Ecological Applic* 19, 829–839.

Herring, G., Ackerman, J. T., 2011. California gull chicks raised near colony edges have elevated stress levels. *Gen Comp Endocrinol* 173, 72–77.

Holmes, W. N., Cavanaugh, K. P., Cronshaw, J., 1978a. Effects of ingested petroleum on oviposition and some aspects of reproduction in experimental colonies of mallard ducks (Anas-platyrhynchos). *J Reprod Fertil* 54, 335.

Holmes, W. N., Cronshaw, J., Gorsline, J., 1978b. Some effects of ingested petroleum on seawater-adapted ducks (*Anas-platyrhynchos*). *Environ Res* 17, 177–190.

Homan, R. N., Regosin, J. V., Rodrigues, D. M., Reed, J. M., Windmiller, B. S., Romero, L. M., 2003. Impacts of varying habitat quality on the physiological stress of spotted salamanders (*Ambystoma maculatum*). *Anim Conserv* 6, 11–18.

Homan, R. N., Windmiller, B. S., Reed, J. M., 2007. Comparative life histories of two sympatric Ambystoma species at a breeding pond in Massachusetts. *J Herp* 41, 401–409.

Hontela, A., 1998. Interrenal dysfunction in fish from contaminated sites: In vivo and in vitro assessment. *Environ Toxicol Chem* 17, 44–48.

Hontela, A., Daniel, C., Rasmussen, J. B., 1997. Structural and functional impairment of the hypothalamo-pituitary-interrenal axis in fish exposed to bleached kraft mill effluent in the St Maurice River, Quebec. *Ecotoxicology* 6, 1–12.

Hontela, A., Dumont, P., Duclos, D., Fortin, R., 1995. Endocrine and metabolic dysfunction in yellow perch, *Perca flavescens*, exposed to organic contaminants and heavy metals in the St Lawrence River, *Environ Toxicol Chem* 14, 725–731.

Hontela, A., Rasmussen, J. B., Audet, C., Chevalier, G., 1992. Impaired cortisol stress response in fish from environments polluted by PAHs, PCBs, and mercury. *Arch Environ Contam Toxicol* 22, 278–283.

Hooke, R. L., Martin-Duque, J. F., Pedraza, J., 2012. Land transformation by humans: A review. *Geol Soc Amer Today* 22, 4–10.

Hopkins, W. A., Mendonça, M. T., Congdon, J. D., 1997. Increased circulating levels of testosterone and corticosterone in southern toads, *Bufo terrestris*, exposed to coal combustion waste. *Gen Comp Endocrinol* 108, 237–246.

Hopkins, W. A., Mendonça, M. T., Congdon, J. D., 1999. Responsiveness of the hypothalamo-pituitary-interrenal axis in an amphibian (*Bufo terrestris*) exposed to coal combustion wastes. *Comp Biochem Physiol* 122C, 191-196.

Huang, B., Lubarsky, K., Teng, T., Blumstein, D. T., 2011. Take only pictures, leave only . . . fear? The effects of photography on the West Indian anole Anolis cristatellus. *Curr Zoology* 57, 77–82.

Karchner, S. I., Franks, D. G., Kennedy, S. W., Hahn, M. E., 2006. The molecular basis for differential dioxin sensitivity in birds: Role of the aryl hydrocarbon receptor. *Proc Natl Acad Sci USA* 103, 6252–6257.

Keller, F., Körner, C., 2003. The role of photoperiodism in alpine plant development. *Arctic Antarctic Alpine Res* 35, 361–368.

Kendall, R., Dickerson, R., Giesy, J., Suk, W., 1998. Principles and processes for evaluating endocrine disruption in wildlife. SEATAC Press, Pensacola, FL.

Killen, S. S., Suski, C. D., Morrissey, M. B., Dyment, P., Furimsky, M., Tufts, B. L., 2003. Physiological responses of walleyes to live-release angling tournaments. *N Am J Fish Manage* 23, 1238–1246.

Kirubagaran, R., Joy, K. P., 1991. Changes in adrenocortical pituitary activity in the catfish, Clarias batrachus (L), after mercury treatment. *Ecotoxicol Environ Safety* 22, 36–44.

Lacroix, A., Hontela, A., 2004. A comparative assessment of the adrenotoxic effects of cadmium in two teleost species, rainbow trout, *Oncorhynchus mykiss*, and yellow perch, *Perca flavescens*. *Aquatic Toxicol* 67, 13–21.

Laflamme, J. S., Couillard, Y., Campbell, P. G. C., Hontela, A., 2000. Interrenal metallothionein and cortisol secretion in relation to Cd, Cu, and Zn exposure in yellow perch, *Perca flavescens*, from Abitibi lakes. *Can J Fish Aquat Sci* 57, 1692–1700.

Laiolo, P., 2010. The emerging significance of bioacoustics in animal species conservation. *Biol Conserv* 143, 1635–1645.

Lair, S., Beland, P., DeGuise, S., Martineau, D., 1997. Adrenal hyperplastic and degenerative changes in beluga whales. *J Wildlife Dis* 33, 430–437.

Laurie, W. A., 1989. Effects of the 1982–1983 El Nino-Southern Oscillation event on marine iguana (*Amblyrhynchus cristatus*, Bell, 1825) populations in the Galapagos islands. In: Glynn, P. (Ed.) *Global ecological consequences of the 1982–1983 El Nino-Southern Oscillation*. Elsevier, New York, pp. 121–141.

Lee, J. S., Kim, E. Y., Iwata, H., Tanabe, S., 2007. Molecular characterization and tissue distribution of aryl hydrocarbon receptor nuclear translocator isoforms, ARNT1 and ARNT2, and identification of novel splice variants in common cormorant (Phalacrocorax carbo). *Comp Biochem Physiol C* 145, 379–393.

Lehikoinen, E., Sparks, T. H., Zalakevicius, M., 2006. Arrival and departure dates. In: Møller, A. P., Fiedler, W., Berthold, P. (Eds.), *Birds and climate change*. Elsevier, Amsterdam, pp. 1-31.

Levesque, H. M., Dorval, J., Hontela, A., Van Der Kraak, G. J., Campbell, P. G. C., 2003. Hormonal, morphological, and physiological responses of yellow perch (*Perca flavescens*) to chronic environmental metal exposures. *J Toxicol Environ Health A* 66, 657–676.

Lundholm, C. E., Bartonek, M., 1992. Effects of p,p'-DDE and some other chlorinated hydrocarbons on the formation of prostaglandins by the avian eggshell gland mucosa. *Arch Toxicol* 66, 387-391.

Luther, D., Baptista, L., 2010. Urban noise and the cultural evolution of bird songs. *Proc R Soc Lond B* 277, 469–473.

Macarthur, R. A., Geist, V., Johnston, R. H., 1982. Cardiac and behavioral responses of mountain sheep to human disturbance. *J Wildlife Manage* 46, 351–358.

Marra, P. P., Holberton, R. L., 1998. Corticosterone levels as indicators of habitat quality: effects of habitat segregation in a migratory bird during the non-breeding season. *Oecologia* 116, 284–292.

Martin, K., Wiebe, K. L., 2004. Coping mechanisms of alpine and arctic breeding birds: Extreme weather and limitations to reproductive resilience. *Integ Comp Biol* 44, 177–185.

Martinovic, B., Lean, D., Bishop, C. A., Birmingham, E., Secord, A., Jock, K., 2003. Health of tree swallow (*Tachycineta bicolor*) nestlings exposed to chlorinated hydrocarbons in the St. Lawrence River basin. Part II. Basal and stress plasma corticosterone concentrations. *J Toxicol Environ Health A* 66, 2015–2029.

Mason, G., 1998. The physiology of the hunted deer. *Nature* 391, 22.

McLachlan, J. A., 2001. Environmental signaling: What embryos and evolution teach us about endocrine disrupting chemicals. *Endocr Rev* 22, 319–341.

Meehl, G. A., 2000. An introduction to trends in extreme weather and climate events: Observations, socioeconomic impacts, terrestrial ecological impacts, and model projections. *Bull Am Meteorol Soc* 81, 413–416.

Meehl, G. A., Zwiers, F., Evans, J., Knutson, T., Mearns, L., Whetton, P., 2000. Trends in extreme weather and climate events: Issues related to modeling extremes in projections of future climate change. *Bull Am Meteorol Soc* 81, 427–436.

Meka, J. M., McCormick, S. D., 2005. Physiological response of wild rainbow trout to angling: impact of angling duration, fish size, body condition, and temperature. *Fisheries Res (Amsterdam)* 72, 311–322.

Melcangi, R. C., Panzica, G. C., 2006. Neuroactive steroids: Old players in a new game. *Neuroscience* 138, 733–739.

Miller, L. L., Rasmussen, J. B., Palace, V. P., Hontela, A., 2009a. The physiological stress response and oxidative stress biomarkers in rainbow trout and brook trout from selenium-impacted streams in a coal mining region. *J Applied Toxicol* 29, 681–688.

Miller, L. L., Rasmussen, J. B., Palace, V. P., Hontela, A., 2009b. Physiological stress response in white suckers from agricultural drain waters containing pesticides and selenium. *Ecotoxicol Environ Safety* 72, 1249–1256.

Miller, L. L., Wang, F., Palace, V. P., Hontela, A., 2007. Effects of acute and subchronic exposures to waterborne selenite on the physiological stress response and oxidative stress indicators in juvenile rainbow trout. *Aquatic Toxicol* 83, 263–271.

Moller, A. P., 2010. Interspecific variation in fear responses predicts urbanization in birds. *Behav Ecol* 21, 365–371.

Mullner, A., Linsenmair, K. E., Wikelski, M., 2004. Exposure to ecotourism reduces survival and affects stress response in hoatzin chicks (*Opisthocomus hoazin*). *Biol Conserv* 118, 549–558.

Munich Rev, 2002. *Topics: An annual review of natural catastrophes.* Munich Reinsurance Company Publications, Munich.

National Research Council, 1999. *Hormonally active agents in the environment.* Report of the Committee on Hormonally Active Agents in the Environment, Commission on Life Sciences, National Research Council. National Academies Press, Washington, DC.

Nisbet, I. C. T., 2000. Disturbance, habituation, and management of waterbird colonies. *Waterbirds* 23, 312–332.

Norris, D. O., 2000. Endocrine disruptors of the stress axis in natural populations: How can we tell? *Am Zool* 40, 393–401.

Norris, D. O., Carr, J. A., 2006. Endocrine disruption. Oxford Univ. Press, New York.

Norris, D. O., Donahue, S., Dores, R. M., Lee, J. K., Maldonado, T. A., Ruth, T., Woodling, J. D., 1999. Impaired adrenocortical response to stress by brown trout, *Salmo trutta*, living in metal-contaminated waters of the Eagle River, Colorado. *Gen Comp Endocrinol* 113, 1–8.

Nowacek, D. P., Thorne, L. H., Johnston, D. W., Tyack, P. L., 2007. Responses of cetaceans to anthropogenic noise. *Mammal Review* 37, 81–115.

Oberhuber, J. M., Roeckner, E., Christoph, M., Esch, M., Latif, M., 1998. Predicting the 97 El-Nino event with a global climate model. *Geophys Res Let* 25, 2273–2276.

Parmesan, C., Root, T. L., Willig, M. R., 2000. Impacts of extreme weather and climate on terrestrial biota. *Bull Am Meteorol Soc* 81, 443–450.

Parmesan, C., Yohe, G., 2003. A globally coherent fingerprint of climate change impacts across natural systems. *Nature* 421, 37–42.

Partecke, J., Gwinner, E., 2007. Increased sedentariness in European blackbirds following urbanization: A consequence of local adaptation? *Ecology* 88, 882–890.

Partecke, J., Gwinner, E., Bensch, S., 2006a. Is urbanisation of European blackbirds (*Turdus merula*) associated with genetic differentiation? *J Ornithol* 147, 549–552.

Partecke, J., Schwabl, I., Gwinner, E., 2006b. Stress and the city: Urbanization and its effects on the stress physiology in European blackbirds. *Ecology* 87, 1945–1952.

Porter, W. P., Sabo, J. L., Tracy, C. R., Reichman, O. J., Ramankutty, N., 2002. Physiology on a landscape scale: Plant-animal interactions. *Integ Comp Biol* 42, 431–453.

Pörtner, H. O., Farrell, A. P., 2008. Ecology: Physiology and climate change. *Science* 322, 690–692.

Pottinger, T. G., 1998. Changes in blood cortisol, glucose and lactate in carp retained in anglers' keepnets. *J Fish Biol* 53, 728–742.

Prock, S., Korner, C., 1996. A cross-continental comparison of phenology, leaf dynamics and dry matter allocation in Arctic and temperate zone herbaceous plants from contrasting altitudes. *Ecol Bull* 45, 93–103.

Propper, C. R., 2005. The study of endocrine-disrupting compounds: Past approaches and new directions. *Integ Comp Biol* 45, 194–200.

Pulido, F., Berthold, P., Mohr, G., Querner, U., 2001. Heritability of the timing of autumn migration in a natural bird population. *Proc R Soc Lond B* 268, 953–959.

Purser, J., Radford, A. N., 2011. Acoustic noise induces attention shifts and reduces foraging performance in three-spined sticklebacks (*Gasterosteus aculeatus*). *Plos One* 6, e17478.

Quinn, A. L., Rasmussen, J. B., Hontela, A., 2010. Physiological stress response of Mountain Whitefish (Prosopium williamsoni) and White Sucker (Catostomus commersoni) sampled along a gradient of temperature and agrichemicals in the Oldman River, Alberta. *Environ Biol Fish* 88, 119–131.

Rich, E. L., Romero, L. M., 2005. Exposure to chronic stress downregulates corticosterone responses to acute stressors. *Am J Physiol* 288, R1628–R1636.

Rolland, R. M., Parks, S. E., Hunt, K. E., Castellote, M., Corkeron, P. J., Nowacek, D. P., Wasser, S. K., Kraus, S. D., 2012. Evidence that ship noise increases stress in right whales. *Proc R Soc Lond B* 279, 2363–2368.

Romero, L. M., Wikelski, M., 2001. Corticosterone levels predict survival probabilities of Galápagos marine iguanas during El Niño events. *Proc Natl Acad Sci USA* 98, 7366–7370.

Romero, L. M., Wikelski, M., 2002a. Exposure to tourism reduces stress-induced corticosterone levels in Galápagos marine iguanas. *Biol Conserv* 108, 371–374.

Romero, L. M., Wikelski, M., 2002b. Severe effects of low-level oil contamination on wildlife predicted by the corticosterone-stress response: Preliminary data and a research agenda. *Spill Sci Technol Bull* 7, 309–313.

Romero, L. M., Wikelski, M., 2010. Stress physiology as a predictor of survival in Galapagos marine iguanas. *Proc R Soc Lond B* 277, 3157–3162.

Root, T., 1988a. Energy constraints on avian distributions and abundances. *Ecology* 69, 330–339.

Root, T., 1988b. Environmental factors associated with avian distributional boundaries. *J Biog*eography 15, 489–505.

Root, T. L., 1994. Scientific/philosophical challenges of global change research: a case study of climatic changes on birds. *Proc Am Philos Soc* 138, 377–384.

Roy, C., Woolf, A., 2001. Effects of hunting and hunting-hour extension on mourning dove foraging and physiology. *J Wildlife Manage* 65, 808–815.

Scheuerlein, A., Van't Hof, T. J., Gwinner, E., 2001. Predators as stressors? Physiological and reproductive consequences of predation risk in tropical stonechats (*Saxicola torquata axillaris*). *Proc R Soc Lond B* 268, 1575.

Scheuhammer, A. M., Basu, N., Burgess, N. M., Elliott, J. E., Campbell, G. D., Wayland, M., Champoux, L., Rodrigue, J., 2008. Relationships among mercury, selenium, and neurochemical parameters in common loons (*Gavia immer*) and bald eagles (*Haliaeetus leucocephalus*). *Ecotoxicol (London)* 17, 93–101.

Schoech, S. J., Bowman, R., Bridge, E. S., Boughton, R. K., 2007. Baseline and acute levels of corticosterone in Florida Scrub-Jays (*Aphelocoma coerulescens*): Effects of food supplementation, suburban habitat, and year. *Gen Comp Endocrinol* 154, 150–160.

Sih, A., Ferrari, M. C. O., Harris, D. J., 2011. Evolution and behavioural responses to human-induced rapid environmental change. *Evolut Applic* 4, 367–387.

Smith, M. E., Kane, A. S., Popper, A. N., 2004. Noise-induced stress response and hearing loss in goldfish (*Carassius auratus*). *J Exp Biol* 207, 427–435.

Sparks, T. H., Menzel, A., 2002. Observed changes in seasons: An overview. *Int J Climatol* 22, 1715–1725.

Suski, C. D., Killen, S. S., Morrissey, M. B., Lund, S. G., Tufts, B. L., 2003. Physiological changes in largemouth bass caused by live-release angling tournaments in southeastern Ontario. *N Am J Fish Manage* 23, 760–769.

Taylor, B. D., Goldingay, R. L., 2010. Roads and wildlife: impacts, mitigation and implications for wildlife management in Australia. *Wildlife Res* 37, 320–331.

Thiel, D., Jenni-Eiermann, S., Braunisch, V., Palme, R., Jenni, L., 2008. Ski tourism affects habitat use and evokes a physiological stress response in capercaillie *Tetrao urogallus*: A new methodological approach. *J Applied Ecology*. 45, 845–853.

Thiel, D., Jenni-Eiermann, S., Palme, R., Jenni, L., 2011. Winter tourism increases stress hormone levels in the Capercaillie *Tetrao urogallus*. *Ibis* 153, 122–133.

Thomas, C. D., Lennon, J. J., 1999. Birds extend their ranges northwards. *Nature* 399, 213–213.

van Heezik, Y., Smyth, A., Adams, A., Gordon, J., 2010. Do domestic cats impose an unsustainable harvest on urban bird populations? *Biol Conserv* 143, 121–130.

Vargas, F. H., Harrison, S., Rea, S., Macdonald, D. W., 2006. Biological effects of El Nino on the Galapagos penguin. *Biol Conserv* 127, 107–114.

Verboven, N., Verreault, J., Letcher, R. J., Gabrielsen, G. W., Evans, N. P., 2010. Adrenocortical function of Arctic-breeding glaucous gulls in relation to persistent organic pollutants. *Gen Comp Endocrinol* 166, 25–32.

Viera, V. M., Le Bohec, C., Côté, S. D., Groscolas, R., 2006. Massive breeding failures following a tsunami in a colonial seabird. *Polar Biol* 29, 713–716.

Villanueva, C., Walker, B., Bertellotti, M., 2012. A matter of history: Effects of tourism on physiology, behaviour and breeding parameters in Magellanic Penguins (*Spheniscus magellanicus*) at two colonies in Argentina. *J Ornithol* 153, 219–228.

Visser, M. E., Both, C., 2005. Shifts in phenology due to global climate change: The need for a yardstick. *Proc R Soc Lond B* 272, 2561–2569.

Visser, M. E., Both, C., Lambrechts, M. M., 2006. Global climate change leads to mistimed avian reproduction. In: Møller, A. P., Fielder, W., Berthold, P. (Eds.), *Birds and global climate change*. Elsevier, Amsterdam, pp. 89–110.

Walker, B. G., Boersma, P. D., Wingfield, J. C., 2005a. Field endocrinology and conservation biology. *Integ Comp Biol* 45, 12–18.

Walker, B. G., Boersma, P. D., Wingfield, J. C., 2005b. Physiological and behavioral differences in Magellanic Penguin chicks in undisturbed and tourist-visited locations of a colony. *Conserv Biol* 19, 1571–1577.

Walker, B. G., Boersma, P. D., Wingfield, J. C., 2006. Habituation of adult magellanic penguins to human visitation as expressed through behavior and corticosterone secretion. *Conserv Biol* 20, 146–154.

Warren, P. S., Katti, M., Ermann, M., Brazel, A., 2006. Urban bioacoustics: It's not just noise. *Anim Behav* 71, 491–502.

Wasser, S. K., Bevis, K., King, G., Hanson, E., 1997. Noninvasive physiological measures of disturbance in the Northern Spotted Owl. *Conserv Biol* 11, 1019–1022.

Wayland, M., Gilchrist, H. G., Marchant, T., Keating, J., Smits, J. E., 2002. Immune function, stress response, and body condition in arctic-breeding common eiders in relation to cadmium, mercury, and selenium concentrations. *Environ Res* 90, 47–60.

Wayland, M., Smits, J. E. G., Gilchrist, H. G., Marchant, T., Keating, J., 2003. Biomarker responses in nesting, common eiders in the Canadian arctic in relation to tissue cadmium, mercury and selenium concentrations. *Ecotoxicology* 12, 225–237.

Wikelski, M., Carrillo, V., Trillmich, F., 1997. Energy limits to body size in a grazing reptile, the Galapagos marine iguana. *Ecology* 78, 2204–2217.

Wikelski, M., Romero, L. M., Snell, H. L., 2001. Marine iguanas oiled in the Galápagos. *Science* 292, 437–438.

Wikelski, M., Wong, V., Chevalier, B., Rattenborg, N., Snell, H. L., 2002. Marine iguanas die from trace oil pollution. *Nature* 417, 607–608.

Williams, P. J., Gutierrez, R. J., Whitmore, S. A., 2011. Home range and habitat selection of spotted owls in the Central Sierra Nevada. *J Wildlife Manage* 75, 333–343.

Wingfield, J. C., 2005. The concept of allostasis: Coping with a capricious environment. *J Mammal* 86, 248–254.

Wingfield, J. C., 2006. Communicative behaviors, hormone-behavior interactions, and reproduction in vertebrates. In: Neill, J.D. (Ed.), *Physiology of reproduction*. Academic Press, New York, pp. 1995–2040.

Wingfield, J. C., 2008a. Comparative endocrinology, environment and global change. *Gen Comp Endocrinol* 157, 207–216.

Wingfield, J. C., 2008b. Organization of vertebrate annual cycles: implications for control mechanisms. *Philos Trans Roy Soc B* 363, 425–441.

Wingfield, J. C., Hahn, T. P., Maney, D. L., Schoech, S. J., Wada, M., Morton, M. L., 2003. Effects of temperature on photoperiodically induced reproductive development, circulating plasma luteinizing hormone and thyroid hormones, body mass, fat deposition and molt in mountain white-crowned sparrows, Zonotrichia leucophrys oriantha. *Gen Comp Endocrinol* 131, 143–158.

Wingfield, J. C., Jacobs, J. D., Soma, K., Maney, D. L., Hunt, K., Wisti-Peterson, D., Meddle, S., Ramenofsky, M., Sullivan, K., 1999a. Testosterone, aggression and communication: Ecological bases of endocrine phenomena. In: Hauser, M., Konishi, M. (Eds.), *The design of animal communication*. MIT Press, Cambridge, MA, pp. 255–284.

Wingfield, J. C., Jacobs, J. D., Tramontin, A. D., Perfito, N., Meddle, S., Maney, D. L., Soma, K., 1999b. Toward an ecological basis of hormone-behavior interactions in reproduction of birds. In: Wallen, K., Schneider, J. (Eds.), *Reproduction in context*. MIT Press, Cambridge, MA, pp. 85–128.

Wingfield, J. C., Kelley, J. P., Angelier, F., 2011a. What are extreme environmental conditions and how do organisms cope with them? *Curr Zool* 57, 363–374.

Wingfield, J. C., Kelley, J. P., Angelier, F., Chastel, O., Lei, F. M., Lynn, S. E., Miner, B., Davis, J. E., Li, D. M., Wang, G., 2011b. Organism-environment interactions in a changing world: a mechanistic approach. *J Ornithol* 152, 279–288.

Wingfield, J. C., Mukai, M., 2009. Endocrine disruption in the context of life cycles: Perception and transduction of environmental cues. *Gen Comp Endocrinol* 163, 92–96.

Woods, M., McDonald, R. A., Harris, S., 2003. Predation of wildlife by domestic cats *Felis catus* in Great Britain. *Mammal Rev* 33, 174–188.

Wright, A. J., Aguilar Soto, N., Baldwin, A. L., Bateson, M., Beale, C. M., Clark, C., Deak, T., Edwards, E. F., Fernández, A., Godinho, A., Hatch, L., Kakuschke, A., Lusseau, D., Martineau, D., Romero, L. M., Weilgart, L., Wintle, B., Notarbartolo di Sciara, G., Martin, V., 2007. Do marine mammals experience stress related to anthropogenic noise? Int J Comp Psychol 20, 274–316.

Wysocki, L. E., Dittami, J. P., Ladich, F., 2006. Ship noise and cortisol secretion in European freshwater fishes. *Biol Conserv* 128, 501–508.

Zalasiewicz, J., Williams, M., Smith, A., Barry, T. L., Coe, A. L., Brown, P. R., Brenchly, P., Cantrill, D., Gale, A., Gibbard, P., Gregory, F. J., Hounslow, M. W., Kerr, A. C., Pearson, P., Knox, R., Powell, J., Waters, C., Marshal, J., Oates, M., Rawson, P., Stone, P., 2008. Are we now living in the Anthropocene? *Geo Soc Amer Today* 18, 4–8.

Zalasiewicz, J., Williams, M., Steffen, W., Crutzen, P., 2010. The new world of the Anthropocene. *Environ Sci Technol* 44, 2228-2231.

Zhang, S. P., Lei, F. M., Liu, S. L., Li, D. M., Chen, C., Wang, P. Z., 2011. Variation in baseline corticosterone levels of Tree Sparrow (*Passer montanus*) populations along an urban gradient in Beijing, China. *J Ornithol* 152, 801–806.

13

Global Change

Conservation Implications and the Role of Stress Physiology

I. INTRODUCTION

Human disturbance and global change are detrimental to biodiversity. Habitat degradation, pollution, invasive species, and so on, can have devastating effects on populations of all organisms. Conservation biology is the discipline dedicated to figuring out how to reverse those trends and restore habitats, eliminate invasive species, and rehabilitate and reintroduce native plants and animals. Conservation biology is one of the fastest growing fields in biology. For over 100 years there has been some attention paid to species conservation—at least at the level of recognizing that species are natural resources and that some were disappearing. Of course, Rachel Carson's *Silent Spring* (1962) drew the public's attention to species loss due to human activities, but people were concerned with conserving species much earlier than this. The field of conservation biology grew steadily from these roots and has now gained a foothold in the scientific community. There are now a number of journals that specialize on publishing papers that focus on the intersection between biology and the conservation of species.

Conservation biology is a bit unusual as a scientific discipline. The distinguishing feature of conservation biology, and what separates it as a distinct area of biology, is that it is goal oriented—the end result of any research in this area should be to aid in the preservation of species and their habitats. Conservation biologists use the scientific method to define and resolve problems, but the results all have an application, usually to help increase the likelihood of persistence of a species. As a result, conservation biology has enlisted the aid of other biological disciplines, such as behavioral ecology and population genetics.

There are historical roots of conservation-related biology in physiological ecology (Tracy et al. 2006) as well as field endocrinology (e.g., Busch and Hayward 2009). One of the newest emerging sub-disciplines in conservation biology is conservation physiology, and a major focus has been on the endocrinology of the stress response. In order to understand problems associated with population decline and how to conserve species, it is important to understand physiological changes associated with environmental change (Wikelski and Cooke 2006). A review of investigations measuring glucocorticoids in blood, feces, and so on, by Busch and Hayward (2009) is useful because it points out that there are inconsistencies in results: some studies show a relationship with fitness, some with human disturbance, pollution, and so on, whereas many do not. There may be methodological differences that explain these inconsistencies, but it is also highly likely that variation across species and habitat, time of year, social status, body condition, and so on, determine the "exposome" of each individual. In other words, a stressor at one time of year may not be as detrimental as at another time of year, dependent upon allostatic load (see Chapter 3). Endocrine studies of wildlife have specific roles in determining whether a threatened population is stressed by human disturbance or related perturbations, or whether some aspects of the habitat have changed, resulting in failed reproductive function (Wingfield et al. 1997; Berger et al. 1999).

Field and laboratory investigations of wild vertebrates are essential to assess conservation efforts and possible problems associated with saving threatened species. It is particularly important to consider individual differences within populations as well (Cockrem 2005). Using minimally invasive techniques (such as collection of blood samples) or non-invasive techniques (such as collection of fecal samples) can help determine processes which may be related to the decline of a population. Although the non-invasive nature of fecal glucocorticoid metabolite measurements are attractive and indeed are very useful for conservation biology and decision-making, care should be taken in interpreting results too broadly and without proper controls or reference samples (see Chapter 6; e.g., Millspaugh and Washburn 2004). The use of template species that are common and easily studied can allow closely related but critically endangered species to be characterized using spot samples on the template to reveal if plasma or fecal levels of steroids, for example, fall within normal breeding limits or are outside the normal range and suggest dysfunction (Wingfield et al. 2000). Research in animal welfare in captivity has been criticized for not utilizing a framework based on scientific thinking on a broad scale from mechanisms at physiological levels to behavioral ecology (Korte et al. 2007). The same criticism should be exercised in mechanistic approaches to conservation biology.

II. THEORY OF CONSERVATION ENDOCRINOLOGY

The gold standard in conservation is population numbers. If the number of individuals is stable or increasing, the population is considered to be in good health. If the number of individuals is decreasing, however, the population is generally considered to be in trouble, especially if there are few individuals remaining. One of the main goals of conservation biology, therefore, is to determine how human disturbances have an impact on population numbers.

There are, of course, major problems associated with this approach. Perhaps the most important is that, by the very nature of connecting disturbances with population numbers, much of this work is post hoc. Population declines are documented after the initiation of a human disturbance. This is great for conclusively showing that human disturbances have an effect, but it does not allow for predicting the impact of a specific disturbance so that population declines can potentially be avoided. Waiting to demonstrate a measurable decline in population numbers may be too late for many species. As a consequence, substantial work in conservation biology has also focused on determining methods and techniques that can predict population declines, and thus forestall their occurrence.

Although many conservation biologists have relied upon established principles of ecology, and especially the development of mathematical models, to predict the impacts of various human disturbances, others have focused on the organismal biology of the species themselves. Panel A of Figure 13.1 shows a schematic of the approach. The central question is whether human disturbances will result in changes in population numbers. A number of approaches have been tried using empirical data (as compared to mathematical models) to predict whether a specific human disturbance will result in population declines. One of these approaches is to use behavior. The idea is that changes in behavior induced by a specific disturbance can be used as a predictive index for decreased survival or reproductive success. For example, decreases in home range size could anticipate decreases in reproductive output, altered dispersal patterns could disrupt important migratory movements, and altered vocalization behavior, such as in birds or cetaceans, could make it more difficult to find a mate or food resources.

Although there is considerable promise in using behavioral ecology data to predict impacts on population numbers (e.g., Caro 1999; Anthony and Blumstein 2000), the results have not been particularly impressive (e.g., Caro 2007). Perhaps an example will illustrate why. What if we build a new road through a habitat? Many species do not like the open-habitat nature of a road or the accompanying noise, so they actively avoid it. Consequently, building that road will be predicted to elicit a measurable change in behavior (i.e., avoiding the road). However, simply avoiding an object like a road may have no impact on reproductive success, and thus no impact on

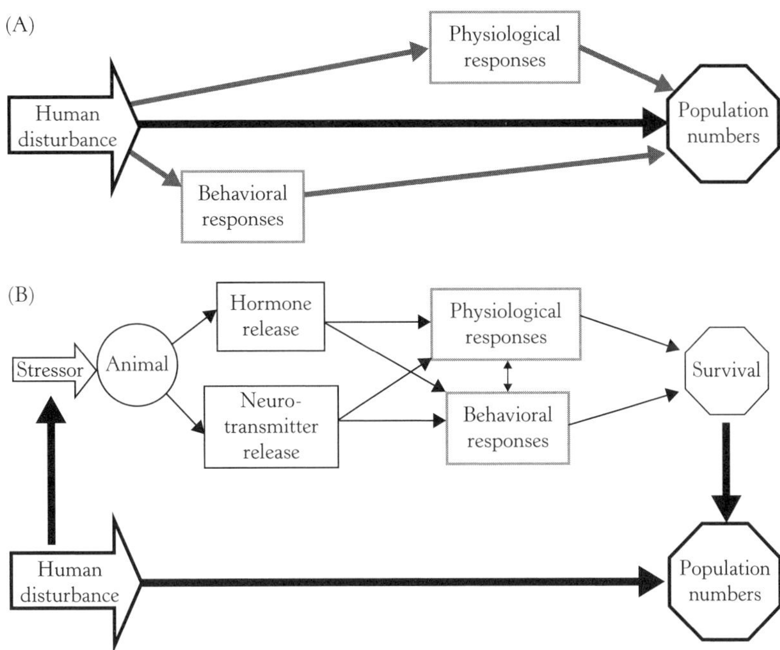

FIGURE 13.1: Schematic of the use of behavioral and physiological responses in predicting changes in population numbers (A) and specifically the use of the physiological responses to stress (B). Together, these schematics represent the theoretically underpinning of using stress in a conservation context.

actual population numbers. As a consequence, behavioral changes are often insufficient in and of themselves to create a strong predictor between human disturbances and population declines.

A second approach has been to use physiological responses as a predictor of population declines. A number of physiological systems have been studied, including reproduction (e.g., Berger et al. 1999; McNab 2006), migration (e.g., Wingfield 2008), immune responses (e.g., Foley et al. 2011; Ujvari and Belov 2011), energy regulation (e.g., Stevenson 2006; Tracy et al. 2006), thermal tolerances (e.g., Somero 2010; Somero 2011), body condition (e.g., Stevenson and Woods 2006), and so on. A number of authors have identified this growing body of work as a new sub-discipline termed "conservation physiology" (Wikelski and Cooke 2006), and when applied specifically to hormonal responses, "conservation endocrinology" (Wingfield et al. 1997; Cockrem and Ishii 1999; Cockrem 2005; Walker et al. 2005). This is a burgeoning field, attracting numerous young investigators, and is currently being applied to many traditional conservation concerns, including the monitoring of wild populations, captive breeding, and reintroductions.

One physiological system that is particularly attractive for conservation physiology is the adrenocortical response to stress (Hofer and East 1998). The reason should be obvious. The stress response systems are intimately connected with health, and high levels of stress mediators often anticipate bigger problems. This has been the major focus of this book, especially Chapter 3. If animals are in allostatic or homeostatic overload, they are likely to face lower survival and/or reproductive success. Finding an individual in allostatic overload is, therefore, a major predictor of the overall health of the animal. After all, this is essentially what human physicians do when they diagnose stress-related pathologies: they are connecting the stress response mediators with greater future risk of disease.

The rationale for using stress mediators in a conservation context is similar. The thinking goes something like this: If we can demonstrate allostatic or homeostatic overload in individual animals exposed to human disturbances, then this is likely to impact the overall health of the animal and result in decreased survival and/or reproductive success. If we then aggregate the health of the individuals in a population, it will give us an indication of the health of the population as a whole. In other words, overall population numbers are assumed to be a summation of the survival and reproduction of each individual within that population. So if a specific human disturbance elicits a stress response in an individual animal, its response will "scale up" to project an overall impact of that disturbance on the population as a whole. To state this in one further way, if population health is a summation of individual health, then decreases in individual health will signify a potential decrease in population health. As a consequence, the stress response of individual animals can be used as a predictor of the impact on population numbers. The predictive power of individual responses will be further heightened in those social species that learn from each other (Cornelius et al. 2010). Panel B of Figure 13.1 shows a schematic of this relationship.

Stress physiology has been used in a number of conservation contexts. The rest of this chapter will be devoted to discussing some of these applications.

III. THE NATURE OF HUMAN DISTURBANCES

Not all human disturbances have identical impacts on free-living animals. Nisbet (2000) created eight categories of disturbances, which are presented in Table 13.1. These types of disturbances vary in their projected impact on the individual animal. One interesting feature about Nisbet's categories is the distinction between researchers, visitors, managers, and "vandals." Although many of the impacts may be perceived as roughly equivalent

TABLE 13.1: TYPES OF HUMAN DISTURBANCES AND THEIR POTENTIAL EFFECTS ON WILDLIFE

Types of Disturbance	Types of Effects
1. "Research procedures" Activities by investigators that are applied to individuals.	1. Physiological effects (e.g., increases in heart rate) without overt changes in behavior. These effects should not be classified as "adverse" unless they decrease survival or reproductive success.
2. "Investigator intrusions" Activities by investigators that affect animals and/or species other than those individually targeted (e.g., the impact on nontargeted individuals on repeatedly entering a colony).	2. Moving away from a nest, territory, feeding site, etc., and then returning after the disturbance ends. Effects should not be regarded as "adverse" unless movement results in losses of nest, status, food resources, etc.
3. "Visitor intrusions" Activities by humans other than investigators that disturb animals deliberately (e.g., by taking photographs) or incidentally (e.g., during recreation).	3. Permanent movement away from a nest, territory, feeding site, or other resource (i.e., abandonment or desertion). May not be "adverse" if other areas are available.
4. "Visitor approaches" Approaches by humans that do not directly induce movements away from the intruder, but do induce changes in alarm and vigilance.	4. Abandonment of a colony or home range in colonial or group living species. May have adverse effects of alternative sites are unavailable or less favorable.
5. "Vehicle activities" Movements of motor vehicles, boats, or aircraft in or close to animal populations.	5. Direct reduction in reproductive effort or reproductive success (e.g., loss of young, failure to attract mate, failure to find suitable territory, etc.).
6. "Positive management" Activity by managers designed to benefit animals (e.g., erecting fences, controlling predators, etc.).	6. Increase in adult mortality in local, regional, or total populations
7. "Negative management" Activity by managers designed to reduce numbers or control activity of animals (e.g., hunting, modifying the habitat, etc.).	
8. "Persecution, harassment, vandalism" Activity by humans intended to harm animals (e.g., destroying nests, indiscriminate hunting, pursuing animals with animals or vehicles, etc.).	

Adapted from Nisbet (2000) and Walker et al. (2005).

by the animals in question (for example, animals likely perceive little difference between investigator and visitor intrusions), the distinctions can be important in terms of study design and certainly in terms of conservation priorities. Equivalent disturbances could be considered necessary from investigators, tolerated by visitors, and intolerable from vandals. Notice also that these categories highlight the distinction between classical physiology and conservation biology. The distinctions between these different classes of disturbances would be irrelevant to a classical physiologist, but if your goal is to preserve species, the origins and intentions of the disturbances are as important, and perhaps more important, than the disturbances themselves.

Regardless of the source of the human disturbance, Nisbet (2000) identified a number of types of effects on the affected animals. Table 13.1 presents six of these effects (although Nisbet originally distinguished between more types of effects, several can be combined [cf. Walker et al. 2005]). Notice that all of these effects refer to measurable changes in the behavior of the animals, yet Nisbet is careful to distinguish between those changes that have long-term adverse effects on survival and successful reproduction. For our purposes, Nisbet's insights can be rephrased to indicate that not all stress responses will have an impact on species' persistence. This categorization fits nicely with the concepts of allostasis and reactive scope. Only those responses that push the animal into allostatic or homeostatic overload will be important in a conservation context. The short-term responses in the predictive or reactive homeostatic ranges are important for immediately responding to the human disturbance, but will not affect the animals' long-term survival or reproductive success. Impacts that threaten species persistence are only ensured with categories 5 and 6 in Table 13.1, are likely with categories 3 and 4, but are probably rare with categories 1 and 2. It is important to keep these distinctions in mind while interpreting data related to stress physiology and conservation.

One additional feature that Nisbet (2000) identifies is how an animal adjusts its responses to human disturbance. Animals can both habituate to and tolerate disturbance. Habituation refers to the animal becoming accustomed to the disturbance, realizing that it is not actually a stressor, and resuming normal activity (see Chapter 3). Tolerating a disturbance, on the other hand, refers to a threshold under which an animal is disturbed but chooses not to respond. Distinguishing between habituation and tolerance is often ignored in conservation research, yet there are quite different consequences of the two responses on the biology of the animal (Bejder et al. 2009; Cyr and Romero 2009).

Physiological techniques, especially those that monitor the fight-or-flight response, can be invaluable in determining whether a reduction in a behavioral response is due to a higher tolerance or to habituation (e.g., Steen et al. 1988). Since the fight-or-flight response is highly sensitive to stressors, the lack of a response is excellent evidence of habituation, whereas the presence of a fight-or-flight response in the absence of overt behavioral changes should indicate tolerance. The only caveat is that care must be taken to distinguish between a true fight-or-flight response and a simple startle response.

A number of studies have used increases in heart rate as an indication of the fight-or-flight response in order to evaluate the impact of human disturbances. For example, several penguin species living in human-visited colonies show increased heart rates (Nimon et al. 1995; Nimon et al. 1996). However, the penguin studies and a recent set of studies on vireos highlight that what we think is human disturbance might not be interpreted that way by the animals themselves. And even if the animals do interpret the human disturbances as stressors, the animals may habituate quickly and show little long-term effects. For example, two species of vireos were equipped with specialized transmitters that allowed the heart rate to be monitored in free-living birds (Bisson et al. 2009; Bisson et al. 2011). These birds were then exposed to a variety of stressors, including human disturbance (chasing the birds around). Many of these presumed stressors failed to elicit any increase in heart rate, and even when there was an increase, it quickly returned to baseline. As a consequence, the increased heart rate had essentially zero impact on the daily energy expenditure of the bird. The birds presumably knew that the human disturbance had occurred and mounted the equivalent of a startle response, but quickly acclimated and failed to show any other signs of disruption to their daily routine (Bisson et al. 2009; Bisson et al. 2011).

Investigator disturbance also may not activate the HPA axis. Black-legged kittiwakes are seabirds that nest in large colonies along cliffs. Consequently, in order to study one bird, the entire colony must be disturbed. However, human disturbance does not appear to act as a stressor (Kitaysky et al. 2010). For example, one study on black-legged kittiwake chicks had three treatments: chicks that were previously handled; chicks that were exposed to a nearby investigator and thus were exposed to colony disturbance; and chicks that had never been previously exposed to any human disturbance. There were no differences in corticosteroid release between the groups (Brewer et al. 2008). Although a potential explanation for this result is that chicks from this species simply do not respond to disturbance, other studies indicate that they can mount a stress response (e.g., Kitaysky et al. 1999), indicating that black-legged kittiwake chicks simply do not interpret investigator presence as a stressor.

The penguin, vireo, and kittiwake studies illustrate Nisbet's ideas nicely. The type of disturbance, in this case investigator and/or tourist disturbances, can clearly elicit physiological and behavioral responses. However, in none of these studies did the physiological responses approach allostatic or homeostatic overload. Consequently, even though it makes intuitive sense to presume that human presence would be detrimental to the animals, the measurements of stress physiology provide strong evidence that the animals are not suffering any long-term detriments. When combined with conservation goals (i.e., knowledge gained through research, education gained through tourism), stress physiological measurements provide conservation managers with a predictive tool to assess whether certain activities are likely to affect population numbers for a species.

A. Marking and Tracking Techniques

Stress physiology has been used extensively to monitor the impact of various marking and tracking techniques. One of the earliest examples of this to appear in the conservation literature concerned the impact of handling in African wild dogs. In the 1970s and 1980s, wild dog numbers began a significant decline. As part of the monitoring program, a number of animals were given radio collars to track movement, assess the degree of human interactions, and so on. For reasons unknown, all the dog packs where radio collars were used died out shortly thereafter. In 1992, Burrows (1992) proposed that a stress-induced emergence of rabies could be the reason that all these dogs died. His reasoning was thus: many wild dogs have evidence of subclinical rabies infections; the handling required to dart, anesthetize, and affix radio collars would result in substantial corticosteroid release; corticosteroids are known to be immunosuppressive; ergo, handling-induced corticosteroid release allowed latent rabies infections to kill the handled animals. Before the animals died, they spread the rabies to their pack mates, leading to the death of the entire pack. Obviously, this hypothesis had profound implications for the conservation of wild dogs. Burrows (1992) was essentially claiming that researchers were inadvertently killing the very animals they were attempting to save.

There was substantial indirect evidence for this hypothesis, foremost being that only the packs where animals were handled died, an event extremely unlikely by chance alone (Burrows et al. 1994; Burrows et al. 1995). However, Burrows never directly tested whether radio collaring resulted in corticosteroid release. Certainly Burrows and colleagues were correct that darting and handling would result in corticosteroid release, but if we can put Burrows's hypothesis in a more modern context, his hypothesis really was assuming that the handling-induced corticosteroid release would result in allostatic or homeostatic overload. Transient increases in corticosteroids would be unlikely to inhibit the immune system sufficiently to induce the eruption of a latent infection.

Creel et al. (1997) attempted to address the question of whether wearing a radio collar results in chronic corticosteroid release. They measured fecal corticosteroids in animals both with and without collars. They found no correlation between fecal corticosteroids and collaring status over many months. Because fecal titers better reflect long-term elevations of corticosteroids, indicative of allostatic load, these data provided strong support that radio collaring did not result in animals entering allostatic or homeostatic overload. There is still the possibility that corticosteroids affect subclinical rabies infections differently, especially if rabies is preferentially attacked by the cellular arm of the immune system (East et al. 1997), and Creel et al. did not collect fecal samples from dogs in a population with high rabies infection rates. However, the weight of the evidence suggests that radio collaring does not result in substantial increase in allostatic load in wild dogs (Creel 1997).

So, in the end, was Burrows correct? Of course we will never know for certain. The critical data were the causes of death of the handled dogs, and those data were never collected. The available evidence suggests that death resulted from a complicated situation, with numerous environmental and anthropogenic factors certainly playing a role. However, the corticosteroid data clearly indicated that radio collaring did not result in chronic stress.

Perhaps the most lasting legacy of Burrows's hypothesis was the identification of stress as a potential impact of research that could result in negative consequences. As a result, many studies have subsequently examined the stress responses of animals carrying various transmitters in order to assess the impact. These studies have now spanned a number of taxa, from fish (e.g., Jepsen et al. 2001; Lower et al. 2005; DeLonay et al. 2007), reptiles (e.g., Rittenhouse et al. 2005; Sperry et al. 2009), birds (e.g., Wells et al. 2003; O'Hearn et al. 2005; Schulz et al. 2005; Davis et al. 2008; Pereira et al. 2009), and mammals (e.g., Schradin 2008; Moll et al. 2009). In general, these studies show that, unsurprisingly, the process of either implanting a transmitter or affixing a transmitter externally (such as a radio collar) elicits a large acute increase in corticosteroid release. All studies to date, however, indicate that transmitters do not result in chronic corticosteroid release, although different placement sites of the transmitters can affect mortality (Makiguchi and Ueda 2009). When corticosteroid titers do indicate a negative impact, it is often the handling itself, not the transmitter per se, that creates the problem. For example, plasma corticosteroids did not change four weeks after handling and other invasive procedures in gopher tortoises (Kahn et al. 2007), but handling had long-term impacts on corticosteroid responses in eastern bluebirds (Lynn et al. 2010). This clearly suggests that responses can be quite different among species. Part of the negative impact can also result from the extra attention paid to tagged animals (Sharpe et al. 2009). The sum of the data, however, indicates that transmitters are not creating a long-term negative impact on the individual animals (but for effects on behavior, see Barron et al. 2010), and therefore are not a major conservation concern. In fact, the lack of a stress response in giant pandas helped establish that radio collaring was not injurious to this species (Durnin et al. 2004).

In contrast, the conservation benefits can be huge. Tagging can provide information about ranges, habitat utilization, migratory routes, and so on, that are simply unobtainable through other methods (Cooke et al. 2004; Cooke et al. 2006; Bridge et al. 2011). The twin innovations of electronic miniaturization and novel tracking technologies have begun to open up some really exciting possibilities for future research. Radio collars are beginning to be replaced by geolocators, GPS transmitters, and other devices. For example, video collars can now provide not only location, but also video of the habitat from the perspective of the individual animal (Moll et al. 2009). Important conservation concerns can be addressed if these new devices do not cause harm to the animals, and stress physiology can continue to provide these data. Consequently, it was important to show that video collars also did not induce an increase in fecal corticosteroids (Moll et al. 2009).

Other marking techniques, such as toe clipping, are more controversial. Toe clipping has a long history for marking animals in ecological studies. It has been used especially in small amphibians and lizards where other marking techniques are impractical or impossible (Funk et al. 2005). Amputating a toe (or several toes) can seem an extreme technique for the sole purpose of later identification of an animal, and many people are uncomfortable with the practice. The technique itself has become a source of substantial controversy. But is it actually harmful to the animals? The evidence is mixed. Whereas some studies indicate that toe-clipped animals have lower survivorship compared to other marking techniques (Davis and Ovaska 2001; May 2004; McCarthy and Parris 2004), others show that there is little long-term impact (Funk et al. 2005; Grafe et al. 2011). Much of the difference between studies likely results from how different species react to the clipping. One potential solution to determine whether toe clipping is problematic to a specific species, without inflicting clipping on large numbers of animals to generate survival data (not to mention the investment of time), is to determine whether toe clipping results in allostatic or homeostatic overload on a small subset of animals. This is parallel to the goal of determining whether less invasive anthropogenic disturbances, such as habitat destruction, impact threatened species, as was presented at the beginning of this chapter.

Several studies have used corticosteroid measurements to address this question. Those that have addressed toe clipping in small lizards indicate that toe clipping does not result in long-term increases in corticosteroids. In fact, microchip implantation, a commonly suggested alternative to toe clipping, resulted in higher corticosteroid concentrations in one study (Langkilde and Shine 2006), and poorer locomotor performance in another (Le Galliard et al. 2011). Toe clipping in several neonatal mammal species similarly did not result in decreased apparent survival (Fisher and Blomberg 2009) or chronic corticosteroid release (Schaefer et al. 2010). It thus appears that toe clipping may not be as problematic as many people believe.

However, the impact of toe clipping appears to be species-specific. Amphibians might be more sensitive to the technique than other taxa. Cane toads maintain elevated corticosteroid concentrations 72 hours after toe clipping, which was a distinctly stronger stressor than handling (Narayan et al. 2011). However, this study did not examine corticosteroid release after 72 hours, so the long-term impact is not clear. On the other hand, epinephrine and norepinephine levels in two species of salamanders were similar in toe-clipped and control animals (Kinkead et al. 2006).

Our intent in the previous discussion is not to try to provide answers to the growing controversy of toe clipping. Like many impacts of specific techniques on wildlife, species appear to differ in their sensitivity. Perhaps most of the disparate data on toe clipping's impact on survival is as simple as how well the different species tolerate the clipping. If this is so, measurements of stress physiology are likely to provide a tool for determining which species are more likely to be at risk.

B. Rehabilitation and Reintroduction

One major activity in conservation is rehabilitation. Sick or injured wildlife often must be treated before being released to the wild. A number of studies have used corticosteroid physiology to assess different treatment techniques and regimens. Corticosteroid physiology has proven invaluable for pointing rehabilitators away from problematic techniques, or for reassuring them that certain techniques do not produce long-term harm. For example, injured and infected California sea lions subjected to restraint and corrective surgery did not show any long-term changes in fecal corticosteroid release (Petrauskas et al. 2008), suggesting that the sea lions tolerated the surgery. Similarly, captive river otters being prepared for reintroduction do not show increases in fecal corticosteroids (Rothschild et al. 2008).

However, not all rehabilitation techniques are found to be benign. A prime example of this is cleaning birds after an oil spill. Oil on the ocean surface can coat the external surface of many organisms such as Magellanic penguins, with fatal results unless the oil is cleaned (Figure 13.2; Fowler et al. 1995). Cleaning the oil from fouled birds as a way to mitigate the impact of an oil spill is a popular activity and creates terrific visuals for the evening news. Successful cleaning does increase survival and reproduction (Weston et al. 2008; Wolfaardt et al. 2009), and the rehabilitated birds often have lower reproductive success than un-oiled birds (e.g., Giese et al. 2000).

Studies on corticosteroids, however, have indicated that cleaning by itself can result in elevated corticosteroids (Briggs et al. 1997). Washing creates a strong corticosteroid response in several penguin species (Fowler et al. 1995; Lampen 2007), and although washing oiled penguins in a rehabilitation center resulted in only transient

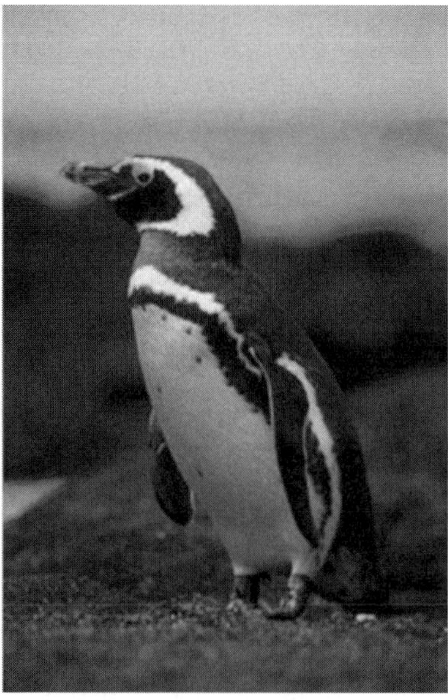

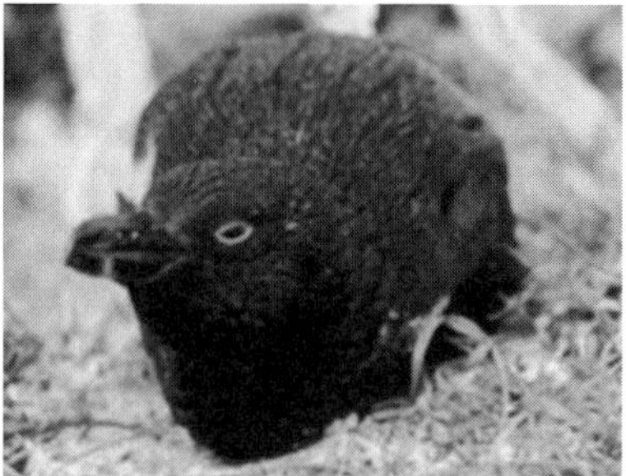

FIGURE 13.2: Magellanic penguin (left) and oiled (right).

Photos courtesy of P. D. Boersma.

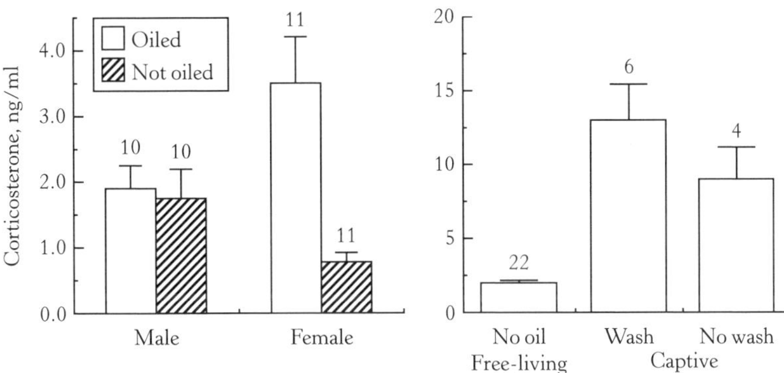

FIGURE 13.3: Effects of oiling and subsequent washing in captivity on plasma levels of corticosterone in Magellanic penguins. Females appear to be more affected by oiling than males although washing procedures were apparently very stressful.

From Fowler et al. (1995), courtesy of the American Ornithologists Union.

elevated fecal corticosteroids, the elevated corticosteroid levels were about the same magnitude as the original placement into captivity (Lampen 2007). Clearly, the washing is quite stressful to these birds, and waterproofing of their plumage must occur before release, which can take days to weeks. Furthermore, prior oiling can have detrimental effects on reproduction, at least in male Magellanic penguins (Figures 13.3 and 13.4; Fowler et al. 1995). Given these results, animals would benefit from modified cleaning techniques designed to minimize corticosteroid release.

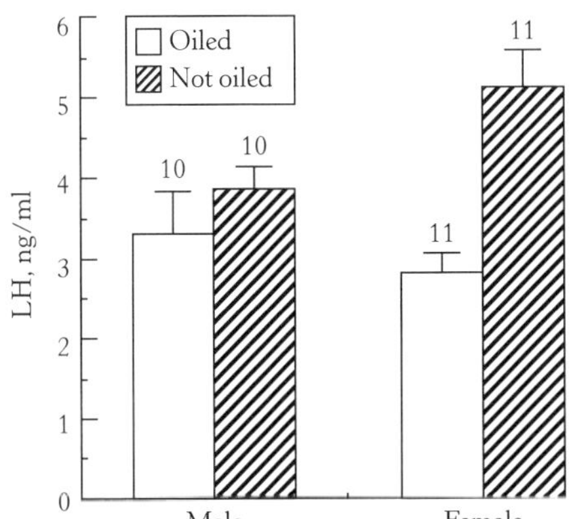

FIGURE 13.4: Plasma levels of luteinizing hormone were reduced in female, but not male Magellanic penguins following oiling.

From Fowler et al. (1995), courtesy of the American Ornithologists Union.

Rehabilitation is clearly a last-ditch conservation activity. Animals brought into rehabilitation facilities are usually desperately in need of veterinary care. This is unlikely to ever change. Measurements of stress physiology, however, can allow the optimization of rehabilitation techniques to give the animals the best chance to return to the wild.

Many of these techniques can also be applied more broadly than just in rehabilitation. The entire field of animal welfare science is dedicated to ensuring appropriate and non-stressful housing in zoos and conservation settings. Research in animal welfare in captivity has been criticized for not utilizing a framework based on scientific thinking on a broad scale from mechanisms at physiological levels to behavioral ecology (Korte et al. 2007). Assessing stress physiology is an important technique in the toolkit (e.g. Mason 2010). One major focus is how to determine the appropriateness of housing because different species, even closely related ones, can differ quite dramatically in how they react to different captive conditions (reviewed by Mason 2010). Measuring corticosteroid and catecholamine release is a powerful index of how well individual animals tolerate and/or thrive in their captive environments.

Work in this area has been progressing for a long time. For example, decreasing pen size, from housing in a yard to smaller pens, including restraint with a neck collar, resulted in elevated corticosteroid levels and increased responsiveness to ACTH injection in Holstein calves (Friend et al. 1985). This was accompanied by a gradation of stress responses over the treatments. However, different methods of housing chickens, including deep litter and larger enriched environment cages versus standard cages, did not necessarily have effects on plasma corticosteroid levels (Pavlik et al. 2008). These authors conclude that the type of housing was not particularly stressful. Similarly, duration of crating (10 per container) and transport of broiler chickens also did not influence plasma levels of corticosterone, epinephrine, or norepinephrine (Kannan et al. 1997). On the other hand, crating and confinement was found to elevate circulating corticosterone (e.g., Kannan and Mench 1996).

Shelter and body condition of dairy cows can combine to have important effects mitigating winter conditions. Cows held outside in fields during winter conditions had higher plasma T4, cortisol, and fecal corticosteroid levels than cows housed in sheds (Tucker et al. 2007). Cold-stressed sheep show marked increases in plasma cortisol compared with control sheep that were not exposed to cold and wet. Application of plastic "coats" allowed cold-stressed sheep to maintain core temperature, and plasma cortisol levels did not increase and remained similar to sheep that were not exposed to cold (Ellis et al. 1985).

Captive breeding of critically endangered species is a classic conservation strategy. Conservation biology has succeeded in many cases by taking critically endangered species into captivity and breeding them for reintroduction into the wild. The high-tech techniques used in these programs, including in vitro fertilization technology, modern genetics, and so on, are truly impressive. However, adrenocortical responses to stress during this period, particularly when individuals are reintroduced into the field, will be critical to assess how "stressed" such reintroduced individuals may be and thus how likely they will be to survive under natural conditions (see section later in this chapter on translocations). For example, fecal measures of corticosteroid metabolites in captive whooping cranes showed typical responses to many environmental stresses such as storms and physical stresses such as capture and restraint (Hartup et al. 2005). However, the reintroduction process, including migration "training" by guidance with ultra-light aircraft, did not affect fecal corticosteroids, suggesting that chronic stress may not be a problem in this species (Hartup et al. 2005).

C. Assessing Management Techniques: Buffers

As discussed earlier in this chapter, part of the essence of conservation biology is the making of decisions and policies that impact wild populations. These policies are intended to be beneficial for the species, but there are often competing priorities, such as human economic concerns, that can shape the ultimate policy that gets adopted. Given that many of these policies have to be put into place without the benefit of years of study, there is often a question as to whether the policy is scientifically appropriate. Eventually, each policy will be tested to determine its impact and then adjusted. The hope is that this iterative process will eventually produce a good workable policy.

There are many techniques that conservation biologists use to test the usefulness of different conservation policies. Stress physiology is providing another tool to assess the impact on animals. An excellent early example is the testing of corticosteroids in spotted owls (Wasser et al. 1997). Spotted owls are specialists of old-growth forests in the Northwest of the United States whose numbers are declining due to habitat destruction. The species' status has become highly contentious between conservationists trying to protect old-growth forests and the financial interests of loggers and the associated communities. In order to help protect spotted owls, the US Fish and Wildlife Service established 0.41 kilometer buffer zones around nests that limited human activities.

Wasser et al. (1997) tested whether the 0.41 kilometer buffer zone was biologically meaningful to the birds. They assayed fecal samples for corticosteroids from nests that were closer than 0.41 kilometers from a major logging road with those nests where the nearest logging road was outside this buffer zone. The result was increased fecal corticosteroids from males where the logging road was inside the buffer zone (see Figure 12.8 in Chapter 12). Interestingly, the increase was not seen in females. These data showed that the 0.41 kilometer buffer distance might not be ideal, but did successfully distinguish between animals that were and were not affected by the logging activity.

In a further study on a federally threatened population of northern spotted owls in California, it was suspected that proximity to roads and human disturbance from motorcycle and other off-road vehicle activity were having a detrimental effect on reproductive success. Experimental exposure of free-living pairs of owls to one hour of motorcycle activity (simulating a racing event called an enduro) resulted in an overall increase in fecal corticosteroid metabolite levels (Figure 13.5; Hayward et al. 2011). Males and juveniles showed the greatest response (Figure 13.6). Effects of motorcycle disturbance varied with gender, age,

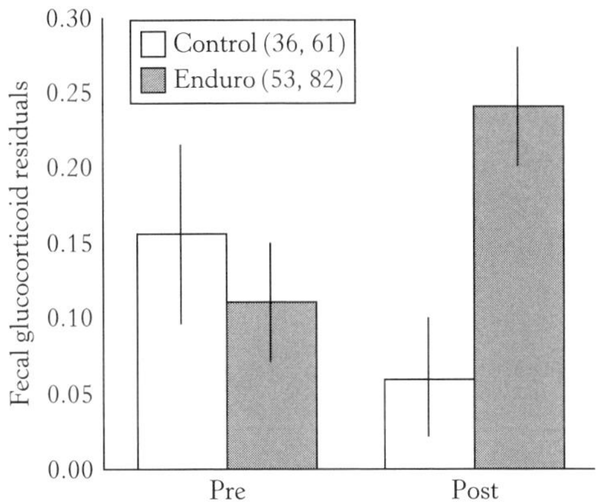

FIGURE 13.5: Spotted owl fecal GC residuals before (pre) and after (post) one hour of experimentally applied motorcycle exposure on treated (enduro) and control sites (no motorcycles). Standard error is shown. Average residuals were adjusted to make values positive for graphing. Samples sizes are shown in parentheses.

From Hayward et al. (2011), courtesy of the Ecological Society of America.

and month but were generally less in non-nesting birds and those that attempted nesting but failed (Hayward et al. 2011). Furthermore, spotted owl pairs nesting near heavily used roads tended to fledge fewer young, suggesting an impact of disturbance on reproductive success via potential stress responses (Hayward et al. 2011). However,

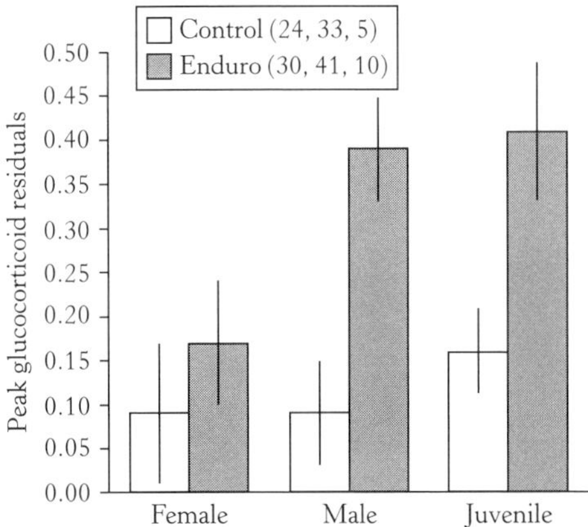

FIGURE 13.6: Peak fecal GC residuals post-treatment split by sex in spotted owls exposed (enduro) or not exposed (control) to motorcycles. Standard error is shown. Average residuals were adjusted to make values positive for graphing. Samples sizes are shown in parentheses.

From Hayward et al. (2011), courtesy of the Ecological Society of America.

similar studies on other populations of spotted owls obtained equivocal results in relation to disturbance (Tempel and Gutierrez 2003, 2004). This may be partially explained by differences in the collection and processing of samples.

The importance of maintaining a buffer distance between human recreation activity and wildlife is not restricted to birds. For example, caribou exposed to snowmobile and helicopter skiing activity in British Columbia had higher fecal corticosteroid metabolite concentrations than caribou sampled in areas where motorized recreation was not allowed (Freeman 1996). This effect was apparent up to 10 kilometers from snowmobile activity! Similarly, variation in fecal levels of corticosteroid metabolites in elk herds in South Dakota were related to vehicle use along primary roads in the Black Hills region and to the density of roads (Millspaugh et al. 2001). The authors also point out that more extensive studies of seasonal changes in fecal corticosteroid metabolites in undisturbed elk populations will be important to confirm these correlations.

There are also a number of studies on elephants that have documented corticosteroid responses to nearby human activities. For example, poaching can have long-term impacts on African elephant populations in Tanzania. Females from groups that did not have an old matriarch and had weaker social bonds had higher fecal corticosteroid metabolite levels than groups with a matriarch (Gobush et al. 2008). Elephants in areas with a higher risk of poaching also tended to have higher fecal corticosteroid metabolite levels than those from areas with lower poaching risk (Gobush et al. 2008). In addition, forest elephants in Gabon are more and more frequently exposed to human disturbance associated with the petroleum industry. However, fecal corticosteroid metabolite levels in forest elephants near human disturbance actually were lower than those from elephants not exposed to such activity (Munshi-South et al. 2008). The authors suggest that forest elephants may habituate well to human disturbance.

The importance of defining appropriate buffer zones might be most apparent in ecotourism settings, where tourists usually want to get as close to animals as possible. Ecotourism has the potential to increase stress (see Chapter 12), especially in breeding populations, and reintroduced animals could be particularly vulnerable. Breeding Magellanic penguins in coastal Argentina that were not accustomed to tourist visits showed increased head turns (a defensive behavior also

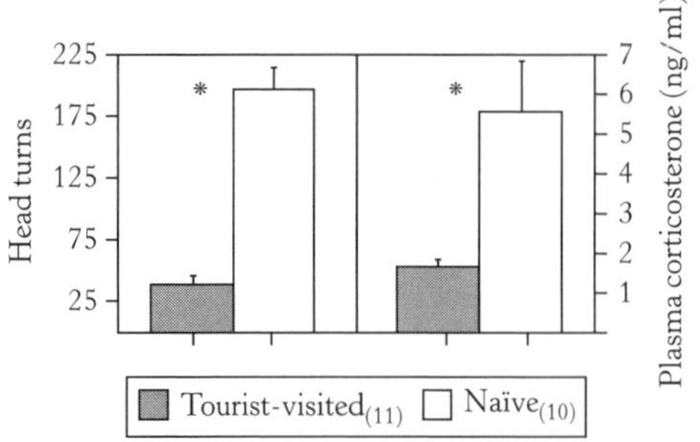

FIGURE 13.7: Defensive head turns (left) and plasma corticosterone levels (right) after 15 minutes of a standardized human visits in Magellanic penguin adults nesting in either tourist-visited (n = 11) or naïve (n = 10) areas of the Punta Tombo colony, Argentina. Modified from data presented in Figure 1 in Walker et al. (2006).

From Walker et al. (2008), courtesy of the Neotropical Ornithological Society.

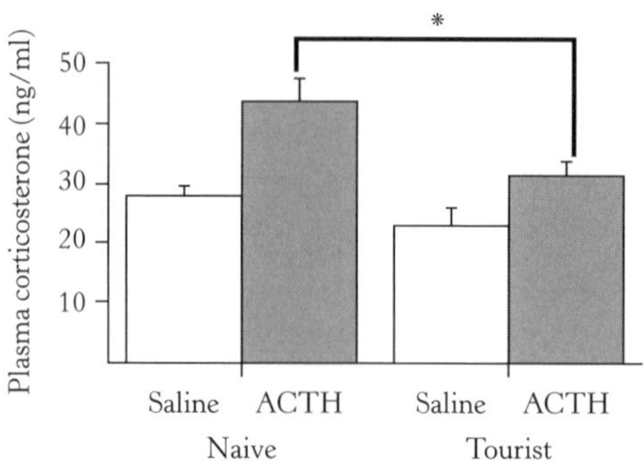

FIGURE 13.9: Plasma corticosterone levels at 45 minutes post-injection of either saline or ACTH for both tourist-visited and naïve adult Magellanic penguins. Data modified from Figure 3 in Walker et al. (2006).

From Walker et al. (2008), courtesy of the Neotropical Ornithological Society.

indicating alarm) accompanied by elevated plasma corticosterone levels when exposed to tourists (Figure 13.7 Walker et al. 2006; Walker et al. 2008). Walker et al. (2006) also showed that penguins exposed to long-term tourist visitation, and presumably habituated to tourists, had fewer head turns (Figure 13.7 tourist-visited animals) and blunted adrenocortical responses to capture stress than did naïve animals (Figure 13.8). Furthermore, penguins naïve to tourists showed greater responses to ACTH injection than penguins that were exposed to tourist visits (Figure 13.9; see also Walker et al. 2008)). However, perhaps even more troubling, newly hatched chicks in burrows with parents showed a greater adrenocortical responses to handling stress in areas where tourists visited versus areas of the breeding colony that were protected from tourists (Figure 13.10; Walker et al. 2005; Walker et al. 2008). These data suggest that although adults may appear to habituate to eco-tourism, chicks are somehow able to respond in the opposite manner. Implications for conservation, including reintroductions, are important, and these data should

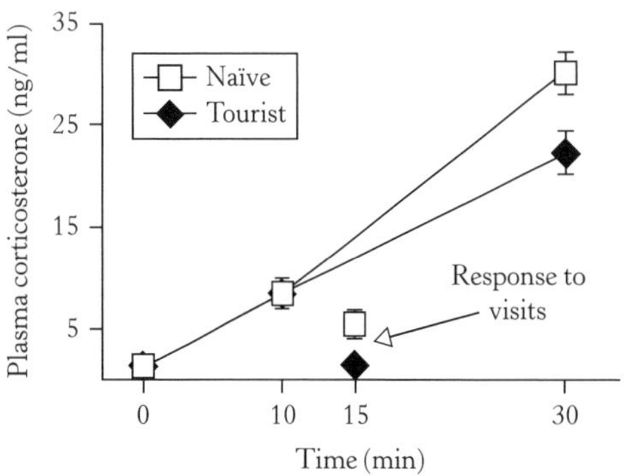

FIGURE 13.8: Corticosterone concentration increase in response to 30 minutes of capture and restraint in Magellanic penguins in tourist-visited (n = 10) or naïve (n = 10) areas of the colony as compared to levels of corticosterone in penguins in both groups (n = 11 and n = 10 for tourist-visited and naïve, respectively) subjected to 15 minutes of a standardized human visit. Original data from Figure 2 in Walker et al. (2006).

From Walker et al. (2008), courtesy of the Neotropical Ornithological Society.

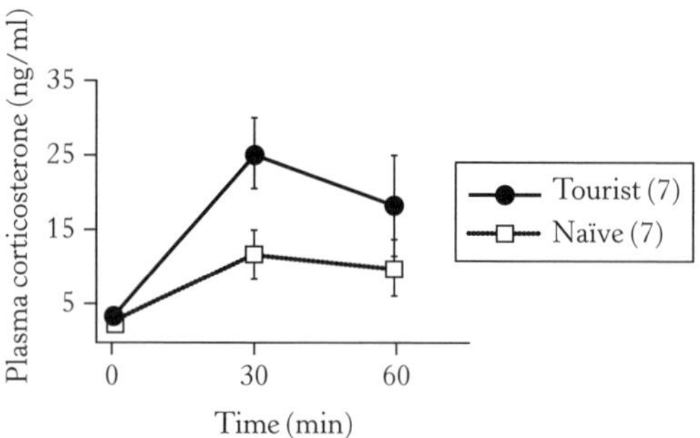

FIGURE 13.10: Pattern of corticosterone secretion in response to capture and restraint in newly—hatched (< 5 day) Magellanic penguin chicks in both naïve and tourist-visited areas of Punta Tombo, Argentina. Data taken from Figure 2 in Walker et al. (2005).

From Walker et al. (2008), courtesy of the Neotropical Ornithological Society.

help in deriving acceptable buffer distances between tourists and penguins.

In many areas, whales have become especially attractive for ecotourism activities. Endocrine profiles, particularly stress responses, are virtually unknown for cetaceans, particularly in their natural habitat. Hunt et al. (2006) were able to collect fecal samples from North Atlantic right whales at sea and analyzed these samples for corticosteroid metabolites. They found that levels were highest in pregnant females and mature males, lower in lactating females, and lowest in non-reproductive females and immature animals. In one case they were able to sample a right whale entangled in fishing nets that had an extremely high fecal corticosteroid metabolite level, suggesting that even collection of fecal samples at sea can provide meaningful data on endocrine responses of free-living cetaceans to environmental perturbations (Hunt et al. 2006). The value of measuring fecal corticosteroid metabolites in cetaceans became apparent during a "natural" experiment (see Chapter 12) (Rolland et al. 2012). These data suggest that shipping noise, including from whale-watching boats involved in the ecotourism industry, have the potential to elicit adrenocortical responses in cetaceans.

Free-living animals are exposed to local inhabitants as well as tourists. Increasing density of human populations and incursions into natural areas for pastoralist activity increased fecal glucocorticoid metabolites in adult male spotted hyenas in Kenya. Spotted hyenas from areas not exposed to pastoralist activity had lower levels. Interestingly, anthropogenic activity associated with tourism had no effects on fecal corticosteroid metabolites (Van Meter et al. 2009). The increase in corticosteroids could signal increased mortality risk. For example, high fecal corticosteroid metabolite levels in free-living ring-tailed lemurs in Madagascar were associated with higher mortality rates than animals with lower levels (Pride 2005). Curiously, in eastern wild turkey hens, plasma corticosterone was weakly negatively correlated with risk of mortality (Nicholson et al. 2000). Although more data are needed, the authors explain this seemingly paradoxical result by suggesting that high corticosterone may increase the likelihood of "freezing" behavior, thus avoiding risk of mortality by predation. In contrast, there were no effects of human presence or activity on fecal glucocorticoid metabolite levels in Alaska brown bears (von der Ohe et al. 2004).

In conclusion, one important function of conservation managers is to create an appropriate separation between human activities and wildlife. The implementation of an appropriate buffer distance is subjected to many competing biological and social goals. It is becoming increasingly clear from the studies presented here that a major complication in this process is that different species have very different responses to human activities, and thus require different size buffers. Stress physiology is a tool of increasing utility for helping conservation managers settle on appropriate buffer sizes.

D. Assessing Management Techniques: Habitat Quality

Another important task of the conservation community is prioritizing which habitats to protect in order to have the maximal positive impact on a species. Economic resources available for species protection are finite, so it is important to maintain the most important habitats for species preservation. A number of important tools have been developed to help make these choices, and stress physiology can provide some help (Homyack 2012). It is still not entirely clear, however, how useful corticosteroid concentrations will be in measuring changes in habitat quality. Do normal habitat differences result in different corticosteroid titers? Although few studies have explored this question directly, the evidence suggests that there is no clear-cut answer. Studies in various salamander species indicate that corticosteroid titers do not change, even when habitat is clearly degraded. Eastern hellbenders, a large salamander in the Eastern United States, had equivalent corticosteroid titers in forested and degraded habitat (Hopkins and DuRant 2011), and surviving spotted salamanders actually had lower corticosteroid titers in a pond that had recently undergone a major human-induced mortality event (Homan et al. 2003). Furthermore, spotted salamanders traversing poor and good microhabitats during their migration away from a breeding pond had equivalent corticosteroid titers (Homan et al. 2003). Similar lack of habitat differences have been seen in mammalian (e.g., Sauerwein et al. 2004; Mateo 2006), and avian (e.g., Owen et al. 2005) species.

In contrast, there are other examples where natural habitat differences and/or changes have been shown to stimulate corticosteroid release (e.g., Cash and Holberton 2005). For example, measures of fecal corticosteroid levels in Carolina chickadees from a human residential site, a recently logged forest site (disturbed), and an undisturbed forest site showed that levels were greatest in birds at the disturbed site than at the other two sites (Lucas et al. 2006). Chickadees from the disturbed site also had lower body weight than at the undisturbed site. Similarly, black howler monkeys in fragmented forest of Mexico had higher fecal corticosteroid metabolite levels than monkeys sampled in more contiguous forests (Martinez-Mota et al. 2007). Interestingly, the authors showed that monkeys from fragmented habitats also traveled at higher frequencies—consistent with greater corticosteroid levels. Potential effects of habitat fragmentation are further underscored by observations of Western fence lizards, sampled both within their geographic range and at the edge of their range or in isolated populations (Figure 13.11; Dunlap and Wingfield 1995). Lizards sampled in the central part of their range tended to have a reduced corticosterone response to capture and handing (especially in the breeding season, April; Figure 13.12) compared to animals sampled at sites peripheral to their normal range. This habitat difference was particularly marked in the non-breeding season in August (Figure 13.12; Dunlap and Wingfield 1995). Habitat fragmentation and a disproportionate number of individuals at the edge of their preferred habitat might exacerbate these differences in adrenocortical response to capture and handling.

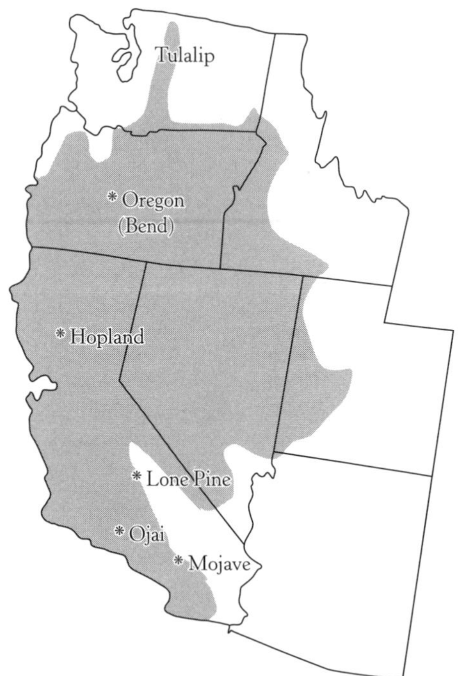

FIGURE 13.11: Geographical distribution (shaded area) of western fence lizards and the locations of six study sites (asterisks). Range is taken from Sites et al. (1992). Tulalip, Lone Pine, and Mojave are at the periphery, and Ojai, Hopland, and Oregon are in the central part of the species range.

From Dunlap and Wingfield (1995), courtesy of Wiley-Liss.

Even when corticosteroid titers do correlate with habitat quality, corticosteroids might not be a good metric to use in assessing habitat quality for conservation purposes. For example, wintering American redstarts occupy two different habitats that differ in prey availability. Not surprisingly, redstarts occupying the poorer habitat had elevated corticosteroid titers (Marra and Holberton 1998). Unfortunately, this information is useless for conservation purposes because redstarts partition these habitats—males are more likely to occupy the better habitat, and females are more likely to occupy the poorer habitat. If corticosteroid concentrations were used to prioritize habitat conservation, female numbers would suffer disproportionately.

The redstart data highlight a further theoretical reason for urging caution when using stress physiology to assess habitat quality. In order to be useful in making conservation decisions, any change in the stress response must be a consequence of living in the habitat in question. In other words, the individual animals living in that habitat must see the habitat itself as being stressful. The alternative is that poorer competitive individuals are pushed into a habitat. For example, if better habitat is occupied by older adults who push juveniles into more marginal habitat, animals in the marginal habitat might indeed have altered HPA responses. However, this would be a consequence of the stress of poorer competitive ability in the juveniles, not of the poor habitat. A similar case may occur with the redstarts: the elevated corticosteroids in the females may result from aggressive exclusion from the better habitat by males, not the fact of living in the poorer habitat per se. This is an important distinction. In these two examples, the habitats occupied by the juveniles or the females may be poorer and less desirable, but those habitats are still vital from a conservation perspective.

E. Assessing Management Techniques: Translocation

Perhaps the best example of how stress physiology can be used to assess a conservation tool is in translocation. Translocation is the process of moving rare or endangered animals from areas of local abundance to areas where they have

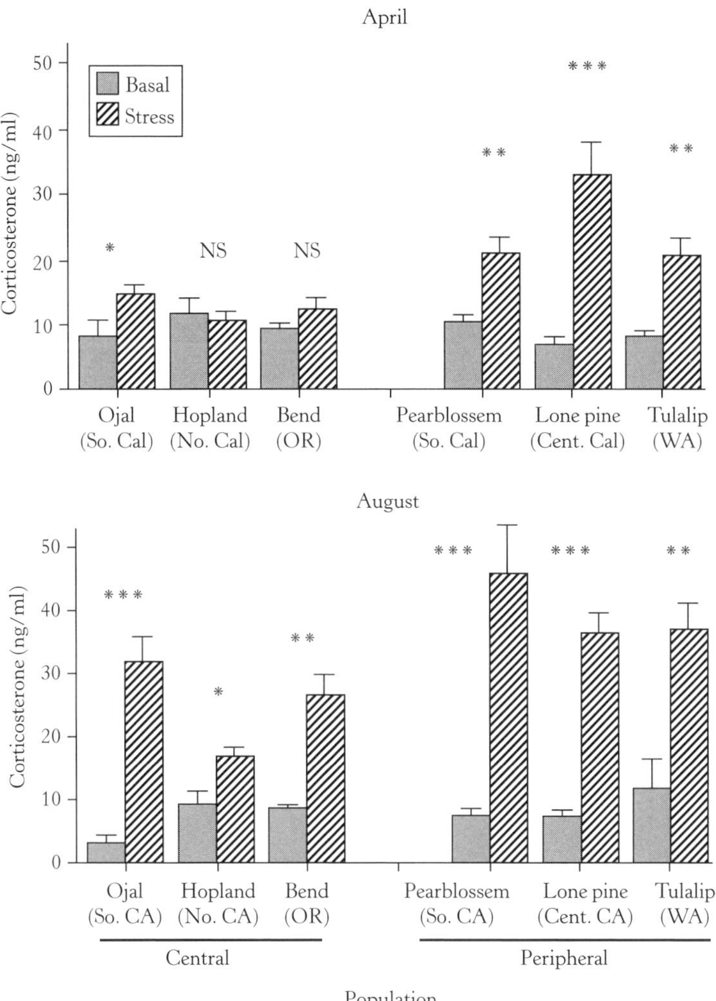

FIGURE 13.12: Plasma corticosterone concentration (mean ± SE; n = 9–25) in six populations of western fence lizards during April and August. Blood was collected immediately after capture (within 1 minute) for basal concentrations (filled bars) or 1 hour after capture for stress concentrations (hatched bars).

Asterisks indicate significant differences between basal and stress values: * $P < 0.05$; ** $P < 0.01$; *** $P < 0.001$; NS, not significant.

From Dunlap and Wingfield (1995), courtesy of Wiley-Liss.

been extirpated. Translocation is an increasingly important conservation tool. The goal is to "seed" the new area and re-establish viable populations. In fact, translocation, or "assisted migration/colonization," has been proposed as an excellent tactic to rescue species that have lost, or are about to lose, their native habitats due to global climate change (Hoegh-Guldberg et al. 2008).

Unfortunately, translocation traditionally has a low rate of success (Griffith et al. 1989). The underlying causes of translocation failure are often poorly understood, primarily because of difficulties in conducting adequate follow-up (Fischer and Lindenmayer 2000). We do know, however, that survival during the period immediately following the release of animals into a novel environment, the establishment phase, is critical to the creation of a self-sustaining population (Armstrong and Seddon 2008). But consider what those animals have just experienced prior to and during their release: they have been captured; held in captivity; prodded, poked, and handled, "donating" various body fluids for health assessments; loaded into cages; jostled in strange ways during transport; thrown together with new conspecifics; released into a completely novel place that may be quite different from anything they have previously experienced; and finally must survive after release with no idea where the food and water are, the location of refuges, the type, density, and location of predators, and so on. The preceding list reads like the ultimate recipe for creating chronic stress in an animal. Given all that we know about the impacts of chronic stress, it is little wonder that translocations have had such dismal success rates.

Nonetheless, the potential conservation rewards for successfully establishing a new population can be enormous. Translocation can represent an emergency conservation intervention, but when translocation uses small numbers of rare animals, the challenge of chronic stress is centrally important. Consequently, stress physiology may provide key data in the debate about whether or not translocation is a feasible tactic to rescue at-risk species (Ricciardi and Simberloff 2009a, 2009b).

There is substantial evidence that the translocation procedure does result in increased allostatic load, and potentially even allostatic/homeostatic overload. A recent review (Dickens et al. 2010) broke the translocation process into four component parts: (1) capture and handling, (2) captivity or some form of prolonged restraint, (3) transport, and (4) release into an unfamiliar location. Evidence (presented in the following text) suggests that each of these stressors elicit acute and/or persistent stress responses.

First, capture and handling clearly elicit strong and persistent stress responses. Chapter 6 presents much of the effects of different trapping techniques. In fact, capture and restraint are considered one of the best ways to elicit and study the maximal stress response in wild animals (Wingfield and Romero 2001). Furthermore, capture can result in overexertion and tearing of muscles, a phenomenon called capture myopathy. Capture myopathy can be a major source of mortality during capture of a wide range of mammalian (Kock et al. 1987; Beringer et al. 1996; Cattet et al. 2008) and avian (Hofle et al. 2004; Hanley et al. 2005; Marco et al. 2006) species and is exacerbated by the surge of epinephrine from the fight-or-flight response (Montane et al. 2002). Even after release to the wild, a single capture and handling incident can have lasting negative impacts on the future capacity for an animal to mount an acute stress response (Dickens et al. 2009b; Lynn et al. 2010), and capture myopathy can significantly decrease overall body condition (Cattet et al. 2008) and the ability to escape predation (Montane et al. 2002).

Second, translocation procedures usually require an extended period of captivity for disease screening or quarantine (Teixeira et al. 2007). There are a number of powerful stressors associated with recent captivity (reviewed by Morgan and Tromborg 2007), including lack of adequate stimulation in housing (Young 2003), crowding (Nephew and Romero 2003), and unnatural social environments (Rogovin et al. 2003). These stressors are all known to elicit powerful and persistent stress responses that can affect animals for weeks. For example, placement of previously wild birds into captivity results in profound dysregulation of the sympathetic nervous system consistent with long-lasting elevation in catecholamines (Dickens and Romero 2009). Such exposure has the potential to damage the cardiovascular system (Oneill et al. 1997). The evidence of incipient cardiovascular disease in translocated animals (Letty et al. 2003) could cause serious problems for individuals facing imminent release. In addition, animals new to captivity can experience a virtual elimination of the fight-or-flight response to mild startle stimuli lasting for at least 10 days (Dickens and Romero 2009). When released, the lack of a startle response might be catastrophic if a predator suddenly attacked.

Similar changes occur in the HPA response. Corticosteroid release is temporarily altered in many species newly brought into captivity (e.g., Coddington and Cree 1995; Davidson et al. 1997; Baker et al. 1998; Franceschini et al. 2008). A good example of the range of HPA changes associated with recent captivity is a series of studies on the chukar, a Eurasian partridge. Introduction to captivity resulted in substantial dysregulation of the corticosteroid response (Dickens et al. 2009c). First, chukars had elevated baseline corticosteroids during the first 5 days of captivity. Although these baseline concentrations seemed to recover by day 5, a strong attenuation of the normal corticosteroid response to experimental restraint continued until day 9 of captivity. This was accompanied by a complete failure of negative feedback. These changes in HPA function persisted for at least 31 days after release of the chukar to a new habitat (Dickens et al. 2009b). The inability to adequately initiate and terminate corticosteroid release is a potentially serious endocrinological outcome of translocation. The combined disruption of normal flight-or-flight and corticosteroid responses in newly released animals might make it very difficult to adequately cope with the novel conditions at the release site. This transition from reactive homeostasis to homeostatic overload may occur in as little as one day (although the timing may be different in different species), suggesting that the captivity portion of the translocation process is a critical stage in inducing allostatic overload in translocated animals.

Third, transport also exposes animals to a wide range of stressors (reviewed by Fazio and Ferlazzo 2003) that results in increased corticosteroid secretion (e.g., Davis and Parker 1986; Coddington and Cree 1995; Young et al. 2002; Millspaugh et al. 2007; Aoyama et al. 2008) and increased heart rate (e.g., Waas et al. 1997; Zapata et al. 2004). The distance, or time in transit, an animal is transported appears to have a large effect on the eventual response (Chacon et al. 2005). Some species appear relatively resistant to transportation effects (Congleton et al. 2000). For example, transport duration did not affect plasma corticosteroids in broiler chickens (Knowles et al. 1996) or in steers (Blecha et al. 1984), but long journeys resulted in slightly higher cortisol levels in rabbits undergoing transport compared with those subjected to shorter duration trips (Liste et al. 2006). However, in many species the impact on the HPA axis can be profound. For example, 14 hours of transport resulted in chukar being completely unable to mount a corticosteroid response to restraint upon arrival (Dickens et al. 2009c). It also appears that animals do not habituate to multiple transportation events, either in corticosteroids or in heart rate (Waas et al. 1999). This inability could dramatically affect an animal's ability to survive if it is released immediately after transport.

Fourth, exposure to a novel environment is a well-known and persistent psychological stressor. In fact, Chapter 3 discussed in detail how novelty is considered one of the defining features of a stressor in biomedical studies. It is difficult to image a more novel situation for a free-living animal than its abrupt release to a new habitat with unknown dangers. Although it has not been measured, the animals must experience a profound stress response. Considering that the novelty persists for some time, it would not be surprising if the new habitat by itself resulted in translocated animals entering allostatic overload.

When the translocation process is broken down into the above four components, the conclusion is that translocation must result in unavoidable allostatic overload (Dickens et al. 2010). How long overload lasts following translocation remains an open question. This is clearly an area of great importance in understanding the effects of translocation on stress physiology; however, very few studies have attempted to answer this question (but see Franceschini et al. 2008; Viljoen et al. 2008), and it is reasonable to expect that there will be substantial variation. Recovery time will likely depend on several factors, such as the sensitivity of the species, the intensity and duration of the stressors, and the number of stressors the animal encounters following release. In addition, release strategies may also play a role in the long-term effects.

The implications from the research to date are not encouraging for the health of translocated animals. The example of the changed stress response in chukar (Dickens et al. 2009b) is likely to be a common profile: altered baseline corticosteroids; attenuated corticosteroid responses to stressors; disrupted corticosteroid negative feedback; and an attenuated fight-or-flight response. The lack of sufficient acute fight-or-flight and corticosteroid responses might be immediately lethal, especially if trying to escape predators. But this is also combined with impaired corticosteroid negative feedback, resulting in long-term overexposure to corticosteroids. This overexposure is likely what is measured when determining fecal corticosteroids in translocated animals. Dickens et al. (2010) presented the schematic in Figure 13.13 to explain the overall endocrine responses of translocated animals. Translocated animals will have an elevated resting heart rate paired with an attenuated fight-or-flight response. This is paired with a reduced corticosteroid response with inadequate negative feedback, so that the HPA axis remains activated and the exposure to stress-induced corticosteroid concentrations is sustained. This physiological picture of a translocated animal describes an individual incapable of mounting an appropriate stress response.

The allostatic or homeostatic overload suggested by the translocation process should result in increased mortality consistent with symptoms of chronic stress. This appears to be what occurs. When translocations have been accompanied with extensive follow-up studies, an increase in mortality in the weeks to months following release is often noted (Mumme and Below 1999; Reinert and Rupert 1999; Pinter-Wollman et al. 2009a). Specifically, five major causes of translocation failure have been identified. Although several factors, such as increased encounters with roads (Chiarello et al. 2004; Sullivan et al. 2004) and cardiac pathology (Letty et al. 2000), can kill animals, the most common cause of direct mortality is predation (Moreno et al. 1996; Van Zant and Wooten 2003; Matson et al. 2004; Rominger

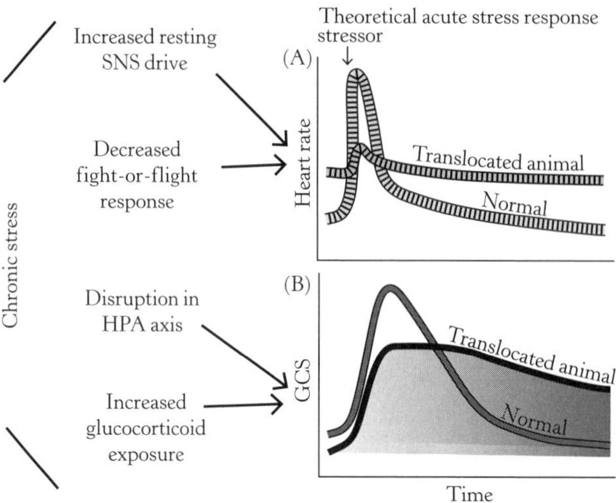

FIGURE 13.13: When translocated animals encounter a stressor in the wild (indicated by arrow), the acute stress response may be altered. First, as compared to a non-chronically stressed animal, the translocated animal will lack an adequate fight-or-flight response. In addition, the chronically stressed translocated animal may have an attenuated corticosteroid negative feedback response due to disruption of the HPA axis, and this attenuation will lead to a sustained release of the stress hormone, causing greater overall exposure (indicated by the filled in area beneath the curve) to potentially damaging stress-induced concentrations of corticosteroids.

Reprinted with permission from Dickens et al. (2010).

et al. 2004; Rouco et al. 2008; Moorhouse et al. 2009). This makes the lack of a quick reaction to a startle cue in chronically stressed animals (Dickens and Romero 2009) especially alarming. The fight-or-flight response is the primary physiological system for coping with immediate danger. When survival depends upon an immediate response, any delay in that response can be lethal. Consequently, the attenuation of the fight-or-flight response would make a prey animal less likely to escape a predator's attack. Similarly, for the translocated predator, losing the enhanced alertness and diversion of energy to the muscles that is promoted by the sympathetic nervous system response could result in missing an opportunity for a meal. Clearly, an increase in predation on a translocated population is primarily related to the presence of predators, especially if there are new or more predators at the release location, and this has no relation to whether or not the released animals are chronically stressed. If a predator never attacks, a fight-or-flight response will never be needed. However, the probability of translocation failure due to predation is amplified when the translocated population is composed of chronically stressed animals with impaired fight-or-flight responses and impaired physiological ability to recover following a stressor.

A second major source of mortality in translocated animals is starvation (Work et al. 1999; Islam et al. 2008). Pre-existing conditions of the release site are likely the primary reason for starvation. A release site with poor food availability or resource limitation directly contributes to starvation (Knapp 2001; Nolet et al. 2005; Moorhouse et al. 2009). Moreover, if the release site is marginally adequate and the chronically stressed animals have a greater requirement for energy and a decreased capacity to take in nutrients, the translocated population is more vulnerable to succumb to starvation.

Disease is the third major source of mortality in translocated animals (Nolet et al. 1997; Rosatte et al. 2002; Moreno et al. 2004). Pre-existing environmental conditions, such as the presence of pathogens (Nelson et al. 2002), clearly play a primary role in disease-related mortality, but additional pre-existing population conditions, such as susceptibility to these pathogens due to bottleneck effects in the population (Hale and Briskie 2007), may also play a role. After all, an animal cannot die of infectious disease unless it has been exposed to a pathogen. But, if a high pathogen risk exists at the release site and chronic stress down-regulates the ability of the translocated animals to fight disease, the translocated population will be more vulnerable to succumbing to disease-related mortality after release to the wild.

Of course, translocation failure does not result only from mortality. A decrease in reproductive capacity of the translocation population (Lloyd and Powlesland 1994; Wolf et al. 1998; Ortiz-Catedral and Brunton 2008) could also contribute to the failure to establish a new breeding population. Many factors can alter reproductive capacity in translocated populations, such as skewed sex ratios resulting from skewed dispersal or survival (Moehrenschlager and Macdonald 2003), lack of adequate nesting sites (Hooson and Jamieson 2004), or decreased offspring viability due to inbreeding effects (Briskie and Mackintosh 2004). None of these factors is linked to chronic stress which can make the impact of these environmental conditions more severe. In translocated populations, individuals will be more likely to suffer limited reproduction due to the effects of chronic stress. For example, impacts on reproduction will be exacerbated if chronic stress inhibits the functioning of the reproductive axis, or if it prevents animals from establishing territories or defending a nest site. Consequently, the combination of pre-existing environmental conditions and chronic stress will lead to reduced reproductive output in the overall population.

Dispersal of released animals away from the release site is a further source of translocation failure (Dickens et al. 2009a). Dispersal is a major concern for translocation efforts since it not only decreases the number of animals available to establish a population at the new location, but it also increases the potential for predation and starvation (Letty et al. 2007). Stress increases the likelihood of dispersal (Wingfield and Ramenofsky 1997). Understanding the propensity for translocated individuals to move as a stress avoidance behavior is an important consideration for translocation efforts. When the effect of chronic stress leads to movement away from the release site, it may leave the remaining population too small for adequate establishment.

Notice that one common theme of the major sources of translocation failure (reproductive failure, disease, starvation, and behavior such as irruptive movements) is that they are all made worse by the symptoms of homeostatic overload. Even though the direct causes for translocation failure are likely external factors, such as predators or pathogens, the vulnerability to these external factors is exacerbated among the translocated individuals by increased allostatic load and having stress mediators in overload. Dickens et al. (2010) proposed the schematic in Figure 13.14 to illustrate the connection between the five commonly cited causes of translocation failure (disease, decreased reproduction, predation, starvation, and movement away from the release site) as lines with independent start points leading to translocation failure. Stress is the common underlying physiological mechanism that can exacerbate the effects of each external factor and thus contribute to translocation failure. In other words, stress increases the vulnerability of the translocated population to succumbing to such external factors. This is an important point. The increase in allostatic load does not doom an animal to translocation failure; it makes the animals in a translocated population more vulnerable to the factors that directly contribute to translocation failure.

So translocated animals are chronically stressed. Does this preclude translocation as a conservation tool? The consensus seems to be that translocation is not condemned, but that we need procedures to accommodate the increased vulnerability of the translocated individuals to succumbing to pre-existing environmental conditions. Translocation success ultimately relies on four major factors (Griffith et al. 1989), all of which can be directly affected by stress. First is the number of founders (which depends on post-release survival and dispersal as well as the number released). Improving post-release survival and site fidelity by reducing the effects of chronic stress could reduce the number of animals required for successful establishment. Second is reproduction rate. Decreasing the magnitude and persistence of chronic stress can remove the brake on the reproductive system applied by stress mediators in homeostatic overload. Third is survival rate, and the removal of chronic stress can increase survival odds. Fourth is genetic variability. Decreasing the magnitude of stress may improve the genetic variability of the translocated population because different personalities could suffer selective mortality as a result of stress exposure that selects for individuals at one end of the coping strategy spectrum (Koolhaas et al. 1999). Although translocated animals will be chronically stressed to some degree, the above analysis suggests that decreasing the severity and the duration of chronic stress could enhance translocation success.

Dickens et al. (2010) suggest a number of strategies for decreasing the magnitude and/or

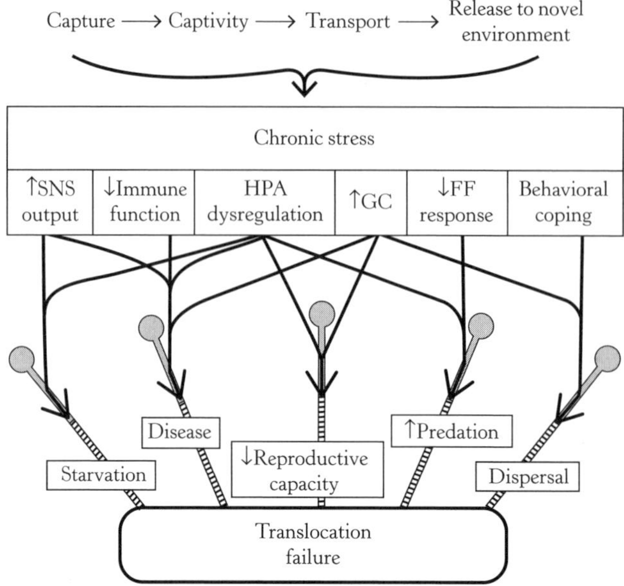

FIGURE 13.14: Schematic demonstrating the link between the translocation procedure, chronic stress, and translocation failure. Since the basic components of translocation induce simultaneous and sustained acute stress responses, they can push an animal into a state of allostatic or homeostatic overload, resulting in increased sympathetic nervous system (SNS) output, decreased immune function, increased glucocorticoid (GC) exposure, hypothalamic-pituitary-adrenal (HPA) axis dysregulation (e.g., disrupted GC negative feedback), decreased fight-or-flight (FF) responsiveness, and behavioral coping. These chronic stress effects then increase the *vulnerability* to factors linked to translocation failure, such as starvation, disease, decreased reproductive capacity, predation, and dispersal.

Reprinted with permission from Dickens et al. (2010).

duration of stress during the translocation process. The idea is to reduce the overall exposure to successive or persistent acute stressors during and following translocation in order to minimize the chance that translocation results in allostatic overload. One suggestion is to reduce the duration of handling during trapping. Trapping will inevitably cause stress in a wild animal, but reducing the subsequent handling will potentially minimize the impact. Dickens et al. (2010) also suggest using species-specific features of the captive environment, such as group housing in social species, to reduce stress during captivity. Key features are to decrease the total number of human visits, improve the predictability of the timing of visits (Bassett and Buchanan-Smith 2007), and restrict visits to the same person at the same time of day. A third suggestion is to decrease the stress of transport. Extensive research on farm animal transportation indicates that specific aspects of transport, such as vehicle design, stacking density, ventilation, and even the quality of the road and the standard of driving, highly impact the stress imposed on the transported animals (Fazio and Ferlazzo 2003). Finally, Dickens et al. (2010) gave some recommendations about reducing the novelty of the release site. Suggestions included releasing animals (1) inside their core range (Wolf et al. 1996) during the least stressful season, especially in terms of pathogen exposure (Nelson et al. 2002); (2) with familiar conspecifics in social species; (3) using a "soft-release" strategy (Armstrong and Seddon 2008) in which animals adjust to the area in a special designed enclosure before being released (Bright and Morris 1994); and ensuring (4) low predator density (Short et al. 1992), (5) minimal local competition (Linklater and Swaisgood 2008), (6) adequate access to refuges (Moreno et al. 1996; Cabezas and Moreno 2007), and (7) adequate food resources (Schoech et al. 2008; Pinter-Wollman et al. 2009b).

In conclusion, translocation is a conservation technique that has benefited greatly from the application of stress physiology. The poor success rate of translocations appears to be directly related to the physiological responses of the translocated animals. Understanding those physiological responses has allowed concrete recommendations to potentially improve translocation success. These recommendations are relatively new, so it is not yet known whether following these guidelines will improve actual success. However, these recommendations have the potential to rescue translocation as a viable conservation technique. Success was so dismal that many researchers have recommended abandoning the technique, or at least suggesting that it has very limited utility (e.g., Ricciardi and Simberloff 2009b). The application of stress physiology to a current conservation problem is what makes the work on translocation such a good example of conservation physiology.

F. Assessing Management Techniques: Invasive Species

A major form of human-induced rapid environmental change is the introduction of species to environments in which they are not native. This can be intentional, such as the "naturalization" of Australia and New Zealand by British colonizers that introduced familiar plants and animals from their native England. The results were generally detrimental to many indigenous and endemic species. Or, introduction of alien species can be accidental, being carried in containers on ships and so forth, or the result of human error, allowing invasive species to escape. However, not all alien species of plants and animals are successful. Many populations die out, and others seem to thrive and spread remarkably quickly. What determines whether a species will be successful or not in colonizing non-native habitat? Behavioral flexibility (i.e., the ability to adapt many suites of behaviors when presented with novel habitats) may be an important trait in successful invasive species. Flexibility may also arise through innovation in which an invasive species can "invent" new behaviors to fit novel situations (Wright et al. 2010). However, this flexibility might await suitable human disturbance to allow an established invasive species to become even more successful and spread rapidly into yet additional habitat (Freed and Cann 2012).

Corticosteroids might also be important in the colonization of new habitats. House sparrows are an incredibly successful invasive species and are now found in many places throughout the world. Evidence suggests that they recently were introduced to Mombasa, Kenya, and have been slowly expanding their range from this initial beachhead. Liebl and Martin (2012) used distance from Mombasa as an index of the time since introduction, with the birds farthest from Mombasa being assumed to be at the vanguard of the invasion. Corticosterone responses to capture and handling increased the farther the birds were from Mombasa, as did exploratory behavior (Liebl and Martin 2012). It is not yet clear whether these changes in corticosterone responses are helping to promote the invasion, but it is an intriguing hypothesis.

G. Assessing Management Techniques: Fisheries Maintenance

A technique related to translocation is the introduction of captive-bred animals back to the wild (Hartup et al. 2004; Hartup et al. 2005). Reintroduction shares two of the major stressors with translocation: transport and release to a novel environment. Because the animals are bred, captivity and capture are less of a problem. One of the big areas where reintroduction has been studied in relation to stress is in fisheries. Restocking of hatchery-raised fish is a common tool in fisheries management. There has been substantial work in using corticosteroid release as a marker to minimize the stress of the reintroduction process, and thus increase survival.

There are many physiological factors that can play into successful introduction of fishery-hatched fish, including rearing conditions (e.g., Clarke et al. 2010), transportation methods and densities (e.g., Congleton et al. 2000; Sulikowski et al. 2006), and release conditions. Physiological indices of stress, and specifically corticosteroid release, have been used to assess each of these factors (Pickering 1992). For example, because loading into transport containers was found to contribute most to corticosteroid release and the fish could not rapidly recover, transport by barge resulted in lower corticosteroid titers at release than transport by truck simply because the barges took longer and thus provided the fish with a longer time to recover (Maule et al. 1988). Determining HPA axis function has turned out to be an effective method for refining fish husbandry (Schreck 2010) and transportation techniques (Schreck et al. 1995). However, the usefulness for assessing reintroduction techniques is still unclear. Corticosteroids do not always correlate with survival and return rates in hatchery-raised salmon (Beckman et al. 1999).

HPA axis physiology has also been used to assess the efficacy of various methods to transport wild migrating fish around man-made obstructions such as dams. Fish ladders have been used for decades to aid fish migration, but fish do not always use them. Corticosteroid release has been used to assess fish ladder designs (Ferguson et al. 2007). In general, it seems that fish ladders do not induce corticosteroid release either in fish who succeed or do not succeed in circumnavigating the obstruction (Pon et al. 2009a; Pon et al. 2009b). The avoidance of corticosteroid release appears to be especially important in fish migrating around dams. A high allostatic load from the transit itself makes the animals highly vulnerable to predation (Mesa 1994) and oxidative stress (Welker and Congleton 2009), although the effect may be temporary (Olla et al. 1992). On the other hand, low corticosteroid release in transported juvenile fish (Specker and Schreck 1980; Maule et al. 1988) correlates with low predation risk (Schreck et al. 2006). In other words, when corticosteroids are high, predation is increased, but when transportation techniques minimize corticosteroid release, predation is diminished. This link between corticosteroid titers and predation risk is a major benefit for using corticosteroids to assess techniques to get migrating fish around obstructions such as hydroelectric dams.

IV. GLOBAL CLIMATE CHANGE

Perhaps no other anthropogenic change has the potential to affect wildlife as profoundly as global climate change. The impact of climate change on species distributions and survival is the focus of intense scientific interest. Climate change is predicted to affect numerous life-history stages, from migration (e.g., DeLeon et al. 2011) to reproduction (e.g., Visser et al. 2004). As we have seen throughout this book, many of these life-history events are regulated by the stress response. In Chapter 12 we discussed how climate change might impact animals. In this section, we will focus on how stress physiology is being used to address issues arising from climate change.

The considerable database on global climate change indicates that the predictable seasonal change in weather is shifting. This includes earlier springs, shorter winters, or changes in rainy and dry seasons. Organisms must shift their life cycles to match changing phenology, and those that are unable to adjust become "mismatched" with serious consequences for fitness (e.g., Visser et al. 2004). Superimpose on this the increased frequency and intensity of unpredictable weather events, and coping strategies such as the emergency life-history stage will be expressed more frequently and for longer periods of time (Wingfield et al. 2011). If these conditions are short-lived, then an individual can probably cope without significant loss of fitness (i.e., increase allostatic load but maintain stress mediators in the reactive homeostasis range). But, if such conditions persist for weeks and months, or occur frequently as predicted for severe weather events, then the individual may enter allostatic or homeostatic overload. However, Chapter 3 presented the idea that it is the unpredictable nature of events that can make them stressors. In other words, climate is not a stressor, but weather can be. This means that climate change per se is unlikely to elicit a stress response, but extreme weather events that are becoming more widespread and frequent may.

Corticosteroids may provide the physiological and behavioral coping mechanism that allows vertebrates to acclimatize in the short term and adapt in the longer term. Chapter 3 showed that allostasis and reactive scope link energetic demands and the wear and tear of everyday life with the added effects of environmental perturbations (McEwen 2000; McEwen and Wingfield 2003; McEwen and Wingfield 2010). We expect allostatic load to be high in organisms living in changing environments, especially when attempting to breed. When unpredictable perturbations of the environment are taken into account, allostatic load increases further (*Eo*). If the sum of *Ee*, *Ei*, and *Eo* exceeds available trophic resources (Eg), then negative energy balance results in allostatic overload type 1 (McEwen and Wingfield 2003; Romero et al. 2009; McEwen and Wingfield 2010). Hormonal mediators of allostasis such as corticosteroids then trigger the emergency life-history stage, shifting the individual into a coping mode that reduces allostatic load to manageable levels (McEwen and Wingfield 2003; Korte et al. 2005; Romero et al. 2009; McEwen and Wingfield 2010).

There is an urgent need for more investigations of hormone regulatory mechanisms for physiology and behavior in a changing climate. One model for how this work might progress is from birds breeding on the arctic tundra. For migrant birds arriving in the Arctic in spring, the potential for allostatic overload type 1 is very great. A variety of strategies, including micro-habitats, varied diets, and so on, are used, as well as hormone-behavior adaptations, to allow them to cope so that breeding can begin as soon as conditions are favorable (Wingfield and Hunt 2002; Wingfield et al. 2004). The hormone-behavior adaptations include the following:

1. Testosterone secretion is attenuated because territoriality and excess courtship may be too costly in arctic environments.

2. During breeding/molt events, sensitivity to acute stress is reduced, thereby enhancing reproductive success or development of a vital new integument to combat extreme conditions during the rest of the year. This reduced sensitivity could include (a) modulated response of the adrenocortical response to stress, (b) reduced sensitivity to high corticosteroid levels, or (c) a combination of a and b.
3. Increased corticosteroid binding protein (CBP) will buffer any acute responses to stress.
4. The enzyme 11-beta-hydroxysteroid dehydrogenase (HSD) can convert corticosteroids to an inactive form, thus providing a deactivation shunt. Conversely, another form of this enzyme potentiates the active form, ensuring activation corticosteroid and mineralocorticoid receptors. Future studies of these enzyme systems that determine access of corticosteroids to receptors within the cell will likely be pivotal.
5. There is changed sensitivity of the HPA axis, as well as altered feedback sensitivity of corticosteroids.

Much more work remains to be done to determine mechanisms by which these changes occur, how they are regulated, and how diverse these mechanisms may be across populations in different ecosystems and hemispheres. Are there constraints on the regulatory mechanisms with which vertebrates cope with extreme conditions, or have they evolved many different ways to endure? As pointed out by Martin and Wiebe (2004), organisms that live in extreme environments and/or are exposed to unpredictable perturbations that result in extreme events have evolved physiological and behavioral strategies to cope. The allostasis model allows a framework to explain individual as well as population changes in allostatic load (McEwen and Wingfield 2003). This includes resilience or the ability to resist environmental perturbations that would normally result in allostatic overload type 1.

We are just now starting to understand how these factors can affect the stress response. For example, captive birds will initiate both corticosteroid and heart rate responses to a transient rapid 3°C change in temperature (de Bruijn and Romero 2011), indicating that they are highly sensitive to small changes in air temperature. Free-ranging birds also show increased fecal corticosteroid metabolites with changes in barometric pressure (Frigerio et al. 2004), suggesting that they can detect impending storms. However, experimental evidence indicates that habitat configuration is very important in the response, since arctic birds are sensitive to inclement weather at some times of the year, but not others (Romero et al. 2000).

Storms can have a dramatic impact on food availability, leading some bird species to abandon territories and migrate to lower altitudes (Boyle et al. 2010). These kinds of irruptive migrations can be initiated by elevated corticosteroid titers (see Chapter 9), as they were in this study. In addition, corticosteroids appear to be involved in altitudinal range expansion (Addis et al. 2011), suggesting that the HPA axis may help determine which species, and which individuals, are best able to cope with an increase in storms. Furthermore, corticosteroids play a role in smoltification (the process of young fish, such as salmon, becoming physiologically ready to move from fresh to seawater), and the process is partially regulated by water temperature. Climate change could disrupt this process by increasing water temperatures, leading to inappropriate timing of smoltification (Bjornsson et al. 2011). Fish species differ in their sensitivity to changes in water temperature (Quinn et al. 2010), however, suggesting that climate change will impact species differently.

In summary, organisms are vulnerable to unpredictable perturbations that can tax an individual beyond the reaction norms for morphology, physiology, and behavior. Even for populations in benign environments, some individuals may have chronically elevated allostatic load because of low social status, poor territory quality, and injury or infection. Taken together, such high allostatic load represents extreme conditions compared with nearby neighbors that have a lower allostatic load. In addition, different species may be able to cope with high allostatic load better than others (Boonstra 2004). Understanding the physiological mechanisms by which organisms cope with climate change have advanced over the past decades, but the hormonal mechanisms by which physiological and behavioral responses to extreme events are regulated have lagged behind. The concepts of allostasis and reactive scope, and the related concepts of allostatic load and overload, have potential as a framework to determine if vertebrates in their environment are experiencing extreme conditions and to understand the hormonal control (reactive scope) mechanisms. Integrating hormonal, physiological, and behavioral studies will be key to understanding why some populations and individuals are able to cope with extremes and others are not.

V. CONCLUSIONS

Species conservation has become a major topic of discussion for the public throughout the world. Although various groups have been concerned with species survival for centuries, the attempt to apply concepts from physiology is relatively recent. The specific application of stress physiology is more recent still. In this chapter we have presented the theoretical basis for using stress physiology, have shown some of the problems where measurements of stress physiology have been applied, and have concluded with a discussion of global climate change, where applying stress physiology has just begun but is likely to prove fruitful.

There is an urgent need to understand the mechanisms by which organisms cope with a changing environment. Such mechanisms may shed considerable insight on why some individuals flourish and others succumb (Wingfield 2008). Comparative stress endocrinology has a major role to play here because neuroendocrine and endocrine control systems, in conjunction with direct neural regulation, are the major links between perception of environment and morphological, physiological, and behavioral responses. Understanding these links in the context of conservation concerns will be key to resolving variation in responsiveness to changing environments (Wingfield 2008).

The introduction of the allostasis and reactive scope models of stress are also opening up new avenues of research. For example, a recent mathematical model used concepts of allostasis, especially allostatic load, to generate theoretical predictions on how populations would react to increases in the average amount of stress experienced by individuals in that population (Fefferman and Romero 2013). The idea was to predict how much stress individuals could withstand before negative impacts on population size would be detectable. The model predicted several non-intuitive results, including (1) populations where the average individual was exposed to high levels of stress relied preferentially on the oldest and most physically fit individuals for reproduction and population persistence; and (2) this reliance on the most physically fit individuals led to the average physical condition being highest in the populations where the average individual experienced the most stress. These results generated two major testable predictions with important conservation implications: that the average physical condition of individuals in a population may be a poor measure of how much stress the population is experiencing; and that any disturbance which affects the oldest and most physically fit individuals could have a disproportionate effect on the population. Although these predictions remain to be empirically tested, the generation, and even the conception, of this type of model was difficult if not impossible using the traditional model of stress (see Chapter 3).

We predict that conservation will quickly become a major emphasis in comparative stress physiology, and it would not surprise us if it becomes the dominant topic for studies of stress in wild animals in the near future. Conservation is of growing concern to the next generation of comparative endocrinologists, and we anticipate that, just as cancer became the dominant justification for cell biology, conservation will become the dominant justification for understanding the stress physiology of wild animals. This is good, because much remains to be done, and there is an immediate need.

REFERENCES

Addis, E. A., Davis, J. E., Miner, B. E., Wingfield, J. C., 2011. Variation in circulating corticosterone levels is associated with altitudinal range expansion in a passerine bird. *Oecologia* 167, 369–378.

Anthony, L. L., Blumstein, D. T., 2000. Integrating behaviour into wildlife conservation: the multiple ways that behaviour can reduce N-e. *Biol Conserv* 95, 303–315.

Aoyama, M., Negishi, A., Abe, A., Maejima, Y., Sugita, S., 2008. Short-term transportation in a small vehicle affects the physiological state and subsequent water consumption in goats. *Anim Sci J* 79, 526–533.

Armstrong, D. P., Seddon, P. J., 2008. Directions in reintroduction biology. *Trends Ecol Evol* 23, 20–25.

Baker, M. L., Gemmell, E., Gemmell, R. T., 1998. Physiological changes in brushtail possums, *Trichosurus vulpecula*, transferred from the wild to captivity. *J Exp Zool* 280, 203–212.

Barron, D. G., Brawn, J. D., Weatherhead, P. J., 2010. Meta-analysis of transmitter effects on avian behaviour and ecology. *Methods Ecol Evol* 1, 180–187.

Bassett, L., Buchanan-Smith, H. M., 2007. Effects of predictability on the welfare of captive animals. *Appl Anim Behav Sci* 102, 223–245.

Beckman, B. R., Dickhoff, W. W., Zaugg, W. S., Sharpe, C., Hirtzel, S., Schrock, R., Larsen, D. A., Ewing, R. D., Palmisano, A., Schreck, C. B.,

Mahnken, C. V. W., 1999. Growth, smoltification, and smolt-to-adult return of spring chinook salmon from hatcheries on the Deschutes River, Oregon. *Trans Am Fish Soc* 128, 1125–1150.

Bejder, L., Samuels, A., Whitehead, H., Finn, H., Allen, S., 2009. Impact assessment research: Use and misuse of habituation, sensitisation and tolerance in describing wildlife responses to anthropogenic stimuli. *Mar Ecol-Prog Ser* 395, 177–185.

Berger, J., Testa, J. W., Roffe, T., Monfort, S. L., 1999. Conservation endocrinology: A noninvasive tool to understand relationships between carnivore colonization and ecological carrying capacity. *Conserv Biol* 13, 980–989.

Beringer, J., Hansen, L. P., Wilding, W., Fischer, J., Sheriff, S. L., 1996. Factors affecting capture myopathy in white-tailed deer. *J Wildlife Manage* 60, 373–380.

Bisson, I. A., Butler, L. K., Hayden, T. J., Kelley, P., Adelman, J. S., Romero, L. M., Wikelski, M. C., 2011. Energetic response to human disturbance in an endangered songbird. *Anim Conserv* 14, 484–491.

Bisson, I. A., Butler, L. K., Hayden, T. J., Romero, L. M., Wikelski, M. C., 2009. No energetic cost of anthropogenic disturbance in a songbird. *Proc R Soc Lond B* 276, 961–969.

Bjornsson, B. T., Stefansson, S. O., McCormick, S. D., 2011. Environmental endocrinology of salmon smoltification. *Gen Comp Endocrinol* 170, 290–298.

Blecha, F., Boyles, S. L., Riley, J. G., 1984. Shipping suppresses lymphocyte blastogenic responses in Angus and Brahman X Angus feeder calves. *J Anim Sci* 59, 576–583.

Boonstra, R., 2004. Coping with changing northern environments: The role of the stress axis in birds and mammals. *Integ Comp Biol* 44, 95–108.

Boyle, W. A., Norris, D. R., Guglielmo, C. G., 2010. Storms drive altitudinal migration in a tropical bird. *Proc R Soc Lond B* 277, 2511–2519.

Brewer, J. H., O'Reilly, K. M., Buck, C. L., 2008. Effect of investigator disturbance on corticosterone concentrations of Black-legged Kittiwake chicks. *J Field Ornith* 79, 391–398.

Bridge, E. S., Thorup, K., Bowlin, M. S., Chilson, P. B., Diehl, R. H., Fleron, R. W., Hartl, P., Kays, R., Kelly, J. F., Robinson, W. D., Wikelski, M., 2011. Technology on the move: Recent and forthcoming innovations for tracking migratory birds. *Bioscience* 61, 689–698.

Briggs, K. T., Gershwin, M. E., Anderson, D. W., 1997. Consequences of petrochemical ingestion and stress on the immune system of seabirds. *ICES J Mar Sci* 54, 718–725.

Bright, P. W., Morris, P. A., 1994. Animal translocation for conservation: Performance of dormice in relation to release methods, origin and season. *J Appled Ecology* 31, 699–708.

Briskie, J. V., Mackintosh, M., 2004. Hatching failure increases with severity of population bottlenecks in birds. *Proc Natl Acad Sci USA* 101, 558–561.

Burrows, R., 1992. Rabies in wild dogs. *Nature* 359, 277–277.

Burrows, R., Hofer, H., East, M. L., 1994. Demography, extinction and intervention in a small population—the case of the Serengeti wild dogs. *Proc R Soc Lond B* 256, 281–292.

Burrows, R., Hofer, H., East, M. L., 1995. Population-dynamics, intervention and survival in African wild dogs (Lycaon-pictus). *Proc R Soc Lond B* 262, 235–245.

Busch, D. S., Hayward, L. S., 2009. Stress in a conservation context: A discussion of glucocorticoid actions and how levels change with conservation-relevant variables. *Biol Conserv* 142, 2844–2853.

Cabezas, S., Moreno, S., 2007. An experimental study of translocation success and habitat improvement in wild rabbits. *Anim Conserv* 10, 340–348.

Caro, T., 1999. The behaviour-ìconservation interface. *Trends Ecol Evol* 14, 366–369.

Caro, T., 2007. Behavior and conservation: a bridge too far? *Trends Ecol Evol* 22, 394–400.

Carson, R., 1962. *Silent spring.* Houghton Mifflin, New York.

Cash, W. B., Holberton, R. L., 2005. Endocrine and behavioral response to a decline in habitat quality: Effects of pond drying on the slider turtle, Trachemys scripta. *J Exp Zool A: Comp Exp Biol* 303A, 872–879.

Cattet, M., Boulanger, J., Stenhouse, G., Powell, R. A., Reynolds-Hogland, M. L., 2008. An evaluation of long-term capture effects in ursids: Implications for wildlife welfare and research. *J Mammal* 89, 973–990.

Chacon, G., Garcia-Belenguer, S., Villarroel, M., Maria, G. A., 2005. Effect of transport stress on physiological responses of male bovines. *Dtsch Tierarztl Wochenschr* 112, 465–469.

Chiarello, A. G., Chivers, D. J., Bassi, C., Amelia, M., Maciel, F., Moreira, L. S., Bazzalo, M., 2004. A translocation experiment for the conservation of maned sloths, Bradypus torquatus (Xenarthra, Bradypodidae). *Biol Conserv* 118, 421–430.

Clarke, L. R., Flesher, M. W., Whitesel, T. A., Vonderohe, G. R., Carmichael, R. W., 2010. Postrelease performance of acclimated and directly released hatchery summer steelhead into Oregon tributaries of the Snake River. *N Am J Fish Manage* 30, 1098–1109.

Cockrem, J. F., 2005. Conservation and behavioral neuroendocrinology. *Horm Behav* 48, 492–501.

Cockrem, J. F., Ishii, S., 1999. Conservation endocrinology: A new field of comparative endocrinology. In: Kwon, H. B., Joss, J. M., Ishii, S. (Eds.), Recent progress in molecular and comparative endocrinology. Hormone Research Center, Kwangju, Korea, pp. 413–418.

Coddington, E. J., Cree, A., 1995. Effect of acute captivity stress on plasma concentrations of corticosterone and sex steroids in female whistling frogs *Litoria ewingi*. *Gen Comp Endocrinol* 100, 33–38.

Congleton, J. L., LaVoie, W. J., Schreck, C. B., Davis, L. E., 2000. Stress indices in migrating juvenile Chinook salmon and steelhead of wild and hatchery origin before and after barge transportation. *Trans Am Fish Soc* 129, 946–961.

Cooke, S. J., Hinch, S. G., Crossin, G. T., Patterson, D. A., English, K. K., Healey, M. C., Shrimpton, J. M., Van Der Kraak, G., Farrell, A. P., 2006. Mechanistic basis of individual mortality in pacific salmon during spawning migrations. *Ecology* 87, 1575–1586.

Cooke, S. J., Hinch, S. G., Wikelski, M., Andrews, R. D., Kuchel, L. J., Wolcott, T. G., Butler, P. J., 2004. Biotelemetry: A mechanistic approach to ecology. *Trends Ecol Evol* 19, 334–343.

Cornelius, J. M., Breuner, C. W., Hahn, T. P., 2010. Under a neighbour's influence: public information affects stress hormones and behaviour of a songbird. *Proc R Soc Lond B* 277, 2399–2404.

Creel, S., 1997. Handling of African wild dogs and chronic stress: Reply. *Conserv Biol* 11, 1454–1456.

Creel, S., Creel, N. M., Monfort, S. L., 1997. Radiocollaring and stress hormones in african wild dogs. *Conserv Biol* 11, 544–548.

Cyr, N. E., Romero, L. M., 2009. Identifying hormonal habituation in field studies of stress. *Gen Comp Endocrinol* 161, 295–303.

Davidson, G. W., Thorarensen, H. T., Lokman, M., Davie, P. S., 1997. Stress of capture and captivity in kahawai *Arripis trutta* (Bloch and Schneider) (*Perciformes: Arripidae*). *Comp Biochem Physiol A* 118, 1405–1410.

Davis, A. K., Diggs, N. E., Cooper, R. J., Marra, P. P., 2008. Hematological stress indices reveal no effect of radio-transmitters on wintering Hermit Thrushes. *J Field Ornith* 79, 293–297.

Davis, K. B., Parker, N. C., 1986. Plasma corticosteroid stress response of 14 species of warmwater fish to transportation. *Trans Am Fish Soc* 115, 495–499.

Davis, T. M., Ovaska, K., 2001. Individual recognition of amphibians: Effects of toe clipping and fluorescent tagging on the salamander *Plethodon vehiculum*. *J Herp* 35, 217–225.

de Bruijn, R., Romero, L. M., 2011. Behavioral and physiological responses of wild-caught European starlings (*Sturnus vulgaris*) to a minor, rapid change in ambient temperature. *Comp Biochem Physiol A* 160, 260–266.

DeLeon, R. L., DeLeon, E. E., Rising, G. R., 2011. Influence of climate change on avian migrants' first arrival dates. *Condor* 113, 915–923.

DeLonay, A. J., Papoulias, D. M., Wildhaber, M. L., Annis, M. L., Bryan, J. L., Griffith, S. A., Holan, S. H., Tillitt, D. E., 2007. Use of behavioral and physiological indicators to evaluate Scaphirhynchus sturgeon spawning success. *J Appl Ichthyol* 23, 428–435.

Dickens, M. J., Delehanty, D. J., Reed, J. M., Romero, L. M., 2009a. What happens to translocated game birds that "disappear"? *Anim Conserv* 12, 418–425.

Dickens, M. J., Delehanty, D. J., Romero, L. M., 2009b. Stress and translocation: alterations in the stress physiology of translocated birds. *Proc R Soc Lond B* 276, 2051–2056.

Dickens, M. J., Delehanty, D. J., Romero, L. M., 2010. Stress: An inevitable component of animal translocation. *Biol Conserv* 143, 1329–1341.

Dickens, M. J., Earle, K., Romero, L. M., 2009c. Initial transference of wild birds to captivity alters stress physiology. *Gen Comp Endocrinol* 160, 76–83.

Dickens, M. J., Romero, L. M., 2009. Wild European starlings (*Sturnus vulgaris*) adjust to captivity with sustained sympathetic nervous system drive and a reduced Fight-or-Flight response. *Physiol Biochem Zool* 82, 603–610.

Dunlap, K. D., Wingfield, J. C., 1995. External and internal influences on indices of physiological stress: I. Seasonal and population variation in adrenocortical secretion of free-living lizards, *Sceloporus occidentalis*. *J Exp Zool* 271, 36–46.

Durnin, M. E., Swaisgood, R. R., Czekala, N., Zhang, H. M., 2004. Effects of radiocollars on giant panda stress-related behavior and hormones. *J Wildlife Manage* 68, 987–992.

East, M. L., Hofer, H., Burrows, R., 1997. Stress hormones and radiocollaring of African wild dogs. *Conserv Biol.* 11, 1451–1453.

Ellis, T., Bradley, A., Watson, F., Elliott, K., Smith, G., Mcgrath, M., Dolling, M., 1985. Protection of recently shorn sheep against adverse weather using plastic coats. *Aust Vet J* 62, 213–218.

Fazio, E., Ferlazzo, A., 2003. Evaluation of stress during transport. *Vet Res Comm* 27, 519–524.

Fefferman, N. H., Romero, L. M., 2013. Can physiological stress alter population persistance? A model with conservation implications. *Conserv Physiol* 1, cot012.

Ferguson, J. W., Sandford, B. P., Reagan, R. E., Gilbreath, L. G., Meyer, E. B., Ledgerwood, R. D., Adams, N. S., 2007. Bypass system modification at Bonneville Dam on the Columbia River improved the survival of juvenile salmon. *Trans Ame Fish Soc* 136, 1487–1510.

Fischer, J., Lindenmayer, D. B., 2000. An assessment of the published results of animal relocations. *Biol Conserv* 96, 1–11.

Fisher, D. O., Blomberg, S. P., 2009. Toe-bud clipping of juvenile small marsupials for ecological field research: No detectable negative effects on growth or survival. *Austral Ecol* 34, 858–865.

Foley, J., Clifford, D., Castle, K., Cryan, P., Ostfeld, R. S., 2011. Investigating and managing the rapid emergence of white-nose syndrome, a novel, fatal, infectious disease of hibernating bats. *Conserv Biol* 25, 223–231.

Fowler, G. S., Wingfield, J. C., Boersma, P. D., 1995. Hormonal and reproductive effects of low levels of petroleum fouling in megallanic penguins. *Auk* 111, 20–27.

Franceschini, M. D., Rubenstein, D. I., Low, B., Romero, L. M., 2008. Fecal glucocorticoid metabolites as an indicator of stress during translocation and acclimation in an endangered large mammal, the Grevy's zebra. *Anim Conserv* 11, 263–269.

Freed, L. A., Cann, R. L., 2012. Increase of an introduced bird competitor in old-growth forest associated with restoration. *NeoBiota* 13, 43–60.

Freeman, N. L., 1996. *Motorized backcountry recreation and stress response in mountain caribou* (Rangifer tarandus caribou). MS Thesis, University of Calgary, p. 75.

Friend, T. H., Dellmeier, G. R., Gbur, E. E., 1985. Comparison of four methods of calf confinement. I. Physiology. *J Anim Sci* 60, 1095–1101.

Frigerio, D., Dittami, J., Mostl, E., Kotrschal, K., 2004. Excreted corticosterone metabolites co-vary with ambient temperature and air pressure in male Greylag geese (*Anser anser*). *Gen Comp Endocrinol* 137, 29–36.

Funk, W. C., Donnelly, M. A., Lips, K. R., 2005. Alternative views of amphibian toe-clipping. *Nature* 433, 193–193.

Giese, M., Goldsworthy, S. D., Gales, R., Brothers, N., Hamill, J., 2000. Effects of the Iron Baron oil spill on little penguins (*Eudyptula minor*). III. Breeding success of rehabilitated oiled birds. *Wildlife Res* 27, 583–591.

Gobush, K. S., Mutayoba, B. M., Wasser, S. K., 2008. Long-term impacts of poaching on relatedness, stress physiology, and reproductive output of adult female African elephants. *Conserv Biol* 22, 1590–1599.

Grafe, T. U., Stewart, M. M., Lampert, K. P., Rodel, M. O., 2011. Putting toe clipping into perspective: A viable method for marking anurans. *J Herp* 45, 28–35.

Griffith, B., Scott, J. M., Carpenter, J. W., Reed, C., 1989. Translocation as a species conservation tool: Status and strategy. *Science* 245, 477–480.

Hale, K. A., Briskie, J. V., 2007. Decreased immunocompetence in a severely bottlenecked population of an endemic New Zealand bird. *Anim Conserv* 10, 2–10.

Hanley, C. S., Thomas, N. J., Paul-Murphy, J., Hartup, B. K., 2005. Exertional myopathy in whooping cranes (Grus americana) with prognostic guidelines. *J Zoo Wildlife Med* 36, 489–497.

Hartup, B. K., Olsen, G. H., Czekala, N. M., 2005. Fecal corticoid monitoring in whooping cranes (*Grus americana*) undergoing reintroduction. *Zoo Biology* 24, 15–28.

Hartup, B. K., Olsen, G. H., Czekala, N. M., Paul-Murphy, J., Langenberg, J. A., 2004. Levels of fecal corticosterone in sandhill cranes during a human-led migration. *J Wildlife Dis* 40, 267–272.

Hayward, L. S., Bowles, A. E., Ha, J. C., Wasser, S. K., 2011. Impacts of acute and long-term vehicle exposure on physiology and reproductive success of the northern spotted owl. *Ecosphere* 2, 1–20.

Hoegh-Guldberg, O., Hughes, L., McIntyre, S., Lindenmayer, D. B., Parmesan, C., Possingham, H. P., Thomas, C. D., 2008. Assisted colonization and rapid climate change. *Science* 321, 345–346.

Hofer, H., East, M. L., 1998. Biological conservation and stress. In: Moller, A. P., Milinski, M., Slater, P. J. B. (Eds.), *Stress and behavior*, vol. 27. Elsevier Academic Press, San Diego, pp. 405–525.

Hofle, U., Millan, J., Gortazar, C., Buenestado, F. J., Marco, I., Villafuerte, R., 2004. Self-injury and capture myopathy in net-captured juvenile red-legged partridge with necklace radiotags. *Wildlife Soc Bull* 32, 344–350.

Homan, R. N., Regosin, J. V., Rodrigues, D. M., Reed, J. M., Windmiller, B. S., Romero, L. M., 2003. Impacts of varying habitat quality on the physiological stress of spotted salamanders (*Ambystoma maculatum*). *Anim Conserv* 6, 11–18.

Homyack, J. A., 2012. Evaluating habitat quality of vertebrates using conservation physiology tools. *Wildlife Res* 37, 332–342.

Hooson, S., Jamieson, I. G., 2004. Variation in breeding success among reintroduced island populations of South Island Saddlebacks Philesturnus carunculatus carunculatus. *Ibis* 146, 417–426.

Hopkins, W. A., DuRant, S. E., 2011. Innate immunity and stress physiology of eastern hellbenders (*Cryptobranchus alleganiensis*) from two stream reaches with differing habitat quality. *Gen Comp Endocrinol* 174, 107–115.

Hunt, K. E., Rolland, R. A., Kraus, S. D., Wasser, S. K., 2006. Analysis of fecal glucocorticoids in the North Atlantic right whale (*Eubalaena glacialis*). *Gen Comp Endocrinol* 148, 260–272.

Islam, M. Z. U., Ismail, K., Boug, A., 2008. Re-introduction of the Red-necked Ostrich, *Struthio camelus camelus*, in Mahazat as-Sayd Protected Area in central Saudi Arabia. *Zool Middle East* 44, 31–40.

Jepsen, N., Davis, L. E., Schreck, C. B., Siddens, B., 2001. The physiological response of chinook salmon smolts to two methods of radio-tagging. Trans Ame Fish Soc 130, 495–500.

Kahn, P. F., Guyer, C., Mendonca, M. T., 2007. Handling, blood sampling, and temporary captivity do not affect plasma corticosterone or movement patterns of Gopher Tortoises (*Gopherus polyphemus*). *Copeia* 614–621.

Kannan, G., Heath, J. L., Wabeck, C. J., Souza, M. C. P., Howe, J. C., Mench, J. A., 1997. Effects of crating and transport on stress and meat quality characteristics in broilers. *Poult Sci* 76, 523–529.

Kannan, G., Mench, J. A., 1996. Influence of different handling methods and crating periods on plasma corticosterone concentrations in broilers. *Brit Poultry Sci* 37, 21–31.

Kinkead, K. E., Lanham, J. D., Montanucci, M. R., 2006. Comparison of anesthesia and marking techniques on stress and behavioral responses in two Desmognathus salamanders. *J Herp* 40, 323–328.

Kitaysky, A. S., Piatt, J. F., Hatch, S. A., Kitaiskaia, E. V., Benowitz-Fredericks, Z. M., Shultz, M. T., Wingfield, J. C., 2010. Food availability and population processes: severity of nutritional stress during reproduction predicts survival of long-lived seabirds. *Func Ecol* 24, 625–637.

Kitaysky, A. S., Piatt, J. F., Wingfield, J. C., Romano, M., 1999. The adrenocortical stress-response of Black-legged Kittiwake chicks in relation to dietary restrictions. *J Comp Physiol B* 169, 303–310.

Knapp, C. R., 2001. Status of a translocated Cyclura iguana colony in the Bahamas. *J Herp* 35, 239–248.

Knowles, T. G., Ball, R. C., Warriss, P. D., Edwards, J. E., 1996. A survey to investigate potential dehydration in slaughtered broiler chickens. *Brit Vet J* 152, 307–314.

Kock, M. D., Clark, R. K., Franti, C. E., Jessup, D. A., Wehausen, J. D., 1987. Effects of capture on biological parameters in free-ranging bighorn sheep (*Ovis-canadensis*): Evaluation of normal, stressed and mortality outcomes and documentation of postcapture survival. *J Wildlife Dis* 23, 652–662.

Koolhaas, J. M., Korte, S. M., De Boer, S. F., Van Der Vegt, B. J., Van Reenen, C. G., Hopster, H., De Jong, I. C., Ruis, M. A. W., Blokhuis, H. J., 1999. Coping styles in animals: current status in behavior and stress-physiology. *Neurosci Biobehav Rev* 23, 925–935.

Korte, S. M., Koolhaas, J. M., Wingfield, J. C., McEwen, B. S., 2005. The Darwinian concept of stress: benefits of allostasis and costs of allostatic load and the trade-offs in health and disease. *Neurosci Biobehav Rev* 29, 3–38.

Korte, S. M., Olivier, B., Koolhaas, J. M., 2007. A new animal welfare concept based on allostasis. *Physiol Behav* 92, 422–428.

Lampen, F., 2007. Faecal corticosterone concentration as an indicator of stress in African penguins (*Spheniscus demersus*). In: Department of Production Animal Studies, MS, Univesity of Pretoria, Pretoria, p. 84.

Langkilde, T., Shine, R., 2006. How much stress do researchers inflict on their study animals? A case study using a scincid lizard, *Eulamprus heatwolei*. *J Exp Biol* 209, 1035–1043.

Le Galliard, J. F., Paquet, M., Pantelic, Z., Perret, S., 2011. Effects of miniature transponders on physiological stress, locomotor activity, growth and survival in small lizards. *Amphibia-Reptilia* 32, 177–183.

Letty, J., Aubineau, J., Marchandeau, S., Clobert, J., 2003. Effect of translocation on survival in wild rabbit (*Oryctolagus cuniculus*). *Mamm Biol* 68, 250–255.

Letty, J., Marchandeau, S., Aubineau, J., 2007. Problems encountered by individuals in animal translocations: Lessons from field studies. *Ecoscience* 14, 420–431.

Letty, J., Marchandeau, S., Clobert, J., Aubineau, J., 2000. Improving translocation success: an experimental study of anti-stress treatment and release method for wild rabbits. *Anim Conserv* 3, 211–219.

Liebl, A. L., Martin, L. B., 2012. Exploratory behaviour and stressor hyper-responsiveness facilitate range expansion of an introduced songbird. *Proc R Soc Lond B* 279, 4375–4381.

Linklater, W. L., Swaisgood, R. R., 2008. Reserve size, conspecific density, and translocation success for black rhinoceros. *J Wildlife Manage* 72, 1059–1068.

Liste, G., Maria, G. A., Buil, T., Garcia-Belenguer, S., Chacon, G., Olleta, J. L., Sanudo, C., Villarroel, M., 2006. Journey length and high temperatures: Effects on rabbit welfare and meat quality. *Dtsch Tierarztl Wochenschr* 113, 59–64.

Lloyd, B. D., Powlesland, R. G., 1994. The decline of kakapo *Strigops habroptilus* and attempts at conservation by translocation. *Biol Conserv* 69, 75–85.

Lower, N., Moore, A., Scott, A. P., Ellis, T., James, J. D., Russell, I. C., 2005. A non-invasive method to assess the impact of electronic tag insertion on stress levels in fishes. *J Fish Biology* 67, 1202–1212.

Lucas, J. R., Freeberg, T. M., Egbert, J., Schwabl, H., 2006. Fecal corticosterone, body mass, and caching rates of Carolina chickadees (Poecile carolinensis) from disturbed and undisturbed sites. *Horm Behav* 49, 634–643.

Lynn, S. E., Prince, L. E., Phillips, M. M., 2010. A single exposure to an acute stressor has lasting consequences for the hypothalamo-pituitary-adrenal response to stress in free-living birds. *Gen Comp Endocrinol* 165, 337–344.

Makiguchi, Y., Ueda, H., 2009. Effects of external and surgically implanted dummy radio transmitters on mortality, swimming performance and physiological status of juvenile masu salmon *Oncorhynchus masou*. *J Fish Biol* 74, 304–311.

Marco, I., Mentaberre, G., Ponjoan, A., Bota, G., Manosa, S., Lavin, S., 2006. Capture myopathy in little bustards after trapping and marking. *J Wildlife Dis* 42, 889–891.

Marra, P. P., Holberton, R. L., 1998. Corticosterone levels as indicators of habitat quality: Effects of habitat segregation in a migratory bird during the non-breeding season. *Oecologia* 116, 284–292.

Martin, K., Wiebe, K. L., 2004. Coping mechanisms of alpine and arctic breeding birds: Extreme weather and limitations to reproductive resilience. *Integ Comp Biol* 44, 177–185.

Martinez-Mota, R., Valdespino, C., Sanchez-Ramos, M. A., Serio-Silva, J. C., 2007. Effects of forest fragmentation on the physiological stress response of black howler monkeys. *Anim Conserv* 10, 374–379.

Mason, G. J., 2010. Species differences in responses to captivity: stress, welfare and the comparative method. *Trends Ecol Evol* 25, 713–721.

Mateo, J. M., 2006. Developmental and geographic variation in stress hormones in wild Belding's ground squirrels (Spermophilus beldingi). *Horm Behav* 50, 718–725.

Matson, T. K., Goldizen, A. W., Jarman, P. J., 2004. Factors affecting the success of translocations of the black-faced impala in Namibia. *Biol Conserv* 116, 359–365.

Maule, A. G., Schreck, C. B., Bradford, C. S., Barton, B. A., 1988. Physiological effects of collecting and transporting emigrating juvenile chinook salmon past dams on the Columbia River. *Trans Am Fish Soc* 117, 245–261.

May, R. M., 2004. Ecology: Ethics and amphibians. *Nature* 431, 403–403.

McCarthy, M. A., Parris, K. M., 2004. Clarifying the effect of toe clipping on frogs with Bayesian statistics. *J Appl Ecol* 41, 780–786.

McEwen, B. S., 2000. Allostasis and allostatic load: implications for neuropsychopharmacology. *Neuropsychopharmacology.* 22, 108–124.

McEwen, B. S., Wingfield, J. C., 2003. The concept of allostasis in biology and biomedicine. *Horm Behav* 43, 2–15.

McEwen, B. S., Wingfield, J. C., 2010. What is in a name? Integrating homeostasis, allostasis and stress. *Horm Behav* 57, 105–111.

McNab, B. K., 2006. The energetics of reproduction in endotherms and its implication for their conservation. *Integ Comp Biol* 46, 1159–1168.

Mesa, M. G., 1994. Effects of multiple acute stressors on the predator avoidance ability and physiology of juvenile chinook salmon. *Trans Am Fish Soc* 123, 786–793.

Millspaugh, J. J., Burke, T., Van Dyk, G., Slotow, R., Washburn, B. E., Woods, R. J., 2007. Stress response of working African elephants to transportation and safari adventures. *J Wildlife Manage* 71, 1257–1260.

Millspaugh, J. J., Washburn, B. E., 2004. Use of fecal glucocorticoid metabolite measures in conservation biology research: Considerations for application and interpretation. *Gen Comp Endocrinol* 138, 189.

Millspaugh, J. J., Woods, R. J., Hunt, K. E., Raedeke, K. J., Brundige, G. C., Washburn, B. E., Wasser, S. K., 2001. Fecal glucocorticoid assays and the physiological stress response in elk. *Wildlife Soc Bull* 29, 899–907.

Moehrenschlager, A., Macdonald, D. W., 2003. Movement and survival parameters of translocated and resident swift foxes *Vulpes velox*. *Anim Conserv* 6, 199–206.

Moll, R. J., Millspaugh, J. J., Beringer, J., Sartwell, J., Woods, R. J., Vercauteren, K. C., 2009. Physiological stress response of captive white-tailed deer to video collars. *J Wildlife Manage* 73, 609–614.

Montane, J., Marco, I., Manteca, X., Lopez, J., Lavin, S., 2002. Delayed acute capture myopathy in three roe deer. *J Vet Med A* 49, 93–98.

Moorhouse, T. P., Gelling, M., Macdonald, D. W., 2009. Effects of habitat quality upon reintroduction success in water voles: Evidence from a replicated experiment. *Biol Conserv* 142, 53–60.

Moreno, S., Villafuerte, R., Cabezas, S., Lombardi, L., 2004. Wild rabbit restocking for predator conservation in Spain. *Biol Conserv* 118, 183–193.

Moreno, S., Villafuerte, R., Delibes, M., 1996. Cover is safe during the day but dangerous at night: The use of vegetation by European wild rabbits. *Can J Zool* 74, 1656–1660.

Morgan, K. N., Tromborg, C. T., 2007. Sources of stress in captivity. *Appl Anim Behav Sci* 102, 262–302.

Mumme, R. L., Below, T. H., 1999. Evaluation of translocation for the threatened Florida scrub-jay. *J Wildlife Manage* 63, 833–842.

Munshi-South, J., Tchignoumba, L., Brown, J., Abbondanza, N., Maldonado, J. E., Henderson, A., Alonso, A., 2008. Physiological indicators of stress in African forest elephants (*Loxodonta africana cyclotis*) in relation to petroleum operations in Gabon, Central Africa. *Diver Distrib* 14, 995–1003.

Narayan, E. J., Molinia, F. C., Kindermann, C., Cockrem, J. F., Hero, J. M., 2011. Urinary corticosterone responses to capture and toe-clipping in the cane toad (*Rhinella marina*) indicate that toe-clipping is a stressor for amphibians. *Gen Comp Endocrinol* 174, 238–245.

Nelson, R. J., Demas, G. E., Klein, S. L., Kriegsfeld, L. J., 2002. *Seasonal patterns of stress, immune function, and disease.* Cambridge University Press, Cambridge.

Nephew, B. C., Romero, L. M., 2003. Behavioral, physiological, and endocrine responses of starlings to acute increases in density. *Horm Behav* 44, 222–232.

Nicholson, D. S., Lochmiller, R. L., Stewart, M. D., Masters, R. E., Leslie, D. M., 2000. Risk factors associated with capture-related death in eastern wild turkey hens. *J Wildlife Dis* 36, 308–315.

Nimon, A. J., Schroter, R. C., Oxenham, R. K. C., 1996. Artificial eggs: Measuring heart rate and effects of disturbance in nesting penguins. *Physiol Behav* 60, 1019–1022.

Nimon, A. J., Schroter, R. C., Stonehouse, B., 1995. Heart-rate of disturbed penguins *Nature* 374, 415–415.

Nisbet, I. C. T., 2000. Disturbance, habituation, and management of waterbird colonies—Commentary. *Waterbirds* 23, 312–332.

Nolet, B. A., Broekhuizen, S., Dorrestein, G. M., Rienks, K. M., 1997. Infectious diseases as main causes of mortality to beavers Castor fiber after translocation to the Netherlands. *J Zool* 241, 35–42.

Nolet, B.A., Broftova, L., Heitkonig, I. M. A., Vorel, A., Kostkan, V., 2005. Slow growth of a translocated beaver population partly due to a climatic shift in food quality. *Oikos* 111, 632–640.

O'Hearn, P. P., Romero, L. M., Carlson, R., Delehanty, D. J., 2005. Effective subcutaneous radiotransmitter implantation into the furcular cavity of chukars. *Wildlife Soc Bull* 33, 1033–1046.

Olla, B. L., Davis, M. W., Schreck, C. B., 1992. Comparison of predator avoidance capabilities with corticosteroid levels induced by stress in juvenile coho salmon *Trans Am Fish Soc* 121, 544–547.

O'Neill, M., Sears, C. E., Paterson, D. J., 1997. Interactive effects of K+, acid, norepinephrine, and ischemia on the heart: Implications for exercise. *J Appl Physiol* 82, 1046–1052.

Ortiz-Catedral, L., Brunton, D. H., 2008. Clutch parameters and reproductive success of a translocated population of red-crowned parakeet (*Cyanoramphus novaezelandiae*). *Aust J Zool* 56, 389–393.

Owen, J. C., Sogge, M. K., Kern, M. D., 2005. Habitat and sex differences in physiological condition of breeding Southwestern Willow Flycatchers (*Empidonax traillii extimus*). *Auk* 122, 1261–1270.

Pavlik, A., Jezova, D., Zapletal, D., Bakos, J., Jelinek, P., 2008. Impact of housing technology on blood plasma corticosterone levels in laying hens. *Acta Vet Hung* 56, 515–527.

Pereira, R. J. G., Granzinolli, M. A. M., De Barros, F. M., Duarte, J. M. B., 2009. Influence of radiotransmitters on fecal glucocorticoid levels of free-ranging male American kestrels. *J Wildlife Manage* 73, 772–778.

Petrauskas, L., Atkinson, S., Gulland, F., Mellish, J.-A., Horning, M., 2008. Monitoring glucocorticoid response to rehabilitation and research procedures in California and Steller sea lions. *J Exper Zool A*309A, 73–82.

Pickering, A. D., 1992. Rainbow trout husbandry: Management of the stress response. *Aquaculture* 100, 125–139.

Pinter-Wollman, N., Isbell, L. A., Hart, L. A., 2009a. Assessing translocation outcome: Comparing behavioral and physiological aspects of translocated and resident African elephants (Loxodonta africana). *Biol Conserv* 142, 1116–1124.

Pinter-Wollman, N., Isbell, L. A., Hart, L. A., 2009b. The relationship between social behaviour and habitat familiarity in African elephants (*Loxodonta africana*). *Proc R Soc Lond B* 276, 1009–1014.

Pon, L. B., Hinch, S. G., Cooke, S. J., Patterson, D. A., Farrell, A. P., 2009a. A comparison of the physiological condition, and fishway passage time and success of migrant adult sockeye salmon at Seton River Dam, British Columbia, under three operational water discharge rates. *N Am J Fish Manage* 29, 1195–1205.

Pon, L. B., Hinch, S. G., Cooke, S. J., Patterson, D. A., Farrell, A. P., 2009b. Physiological, energetic and behavioural correlates of successful fishway passage of adult sockeye salmon Oncorhynchus nerka in the Seton River, British Columbia. *J Fish Biol* 74, 1323–1336.

Pride, R. E., 2005. High faecal glucocorticoid levels predict mortality in ring-tailed lemurs (*Lemur catta*). *Biol Lett* 1, 60.

Quinn, A. L., Rasmussen, J. B., Hontela, A., 2010. Physiological stress response of Mountain Whitefish (*Prosopium williamsoni*) and White Sucker (*Catostomus commersoni*) sampled along a gradient of temperature and agrichemicals in the Oldman River, Alberta. *Environ Biol Fish* 88, 119–131.

Reinert, H. K., Rupert, R. R., 1999. Impacts of translocation on behavior and survival of timber rattlesnakes, *Crotalus horridus*. *J Herp* 33, 45–61.

Ricciardi, A., Simberloff, D., 2009a. Assisted colonization is not a viable conservation strategy. *Trends Ecol Evol* 24, 248–253.

Ricciardi, A., Simberloff, D., 2009b. Assisted colonization: good intentions and dubious risk assessment. *Trends Ecol Evol* 24, 476–477.

Rittenhouse, C. D., Millspaugh, J. J., Washburn, B. E., Hubbard, M. W., 2005. Effects of radiotransmitters on fecal glucocorticoid metabolite levels of three-toed box turtles in captivity. *Wildlife Soc Bull* 33, 706–713.

Rogovin, K., Randall, J. A., Kolosova, I., Moshkin, M., 2003. Social correlates of stress in adult males of the great gerbil, *Rhombomys opimus*, in years of high and low population densities. *Horm Behav* 43, 132–139.

Rolland, R. M., Parks, S. E., Hunt, K. E., Castellote, M., Corkeron, P. J., Nowacek, D. P., Wasser, S. K., Kraus, S. D., 2012. Evidence that ship noise increases stress in right whales. *Proc R Soc Lond B* 279, 2363–2368.

Romero, L. M., Dickens, M. J., Cyr, N. E., 2009. The reactive scope model—a new model integrating homeostasis, allostasis, and stress. *Horm Behav* 55, 375–389.

Romero, L. M., Reed, J. M., Wingfield, J. C., 2000. Effects of weather on corticosterone responses in wild free-living passerine birds. *Gen Comp Endocrinol* 118, 113–122.

Rominger, E. M., Whitlaw, H. A., Weybright, D. L., Dunn, W. C., Ballard, W. B., 2004. The influence of mountain lion predation on bighorn sheep translocations. *J Wildlife Manage* 68, 993–999.

Rosatte, R., Hamr, J., Ranta, B., Young, J., Cool, N., 2002. Elk restoration in Ontario, Canada: Infectious disease management strategy, 1998–2001. In: Gibbs, E. P. J., Bokma, B. H. (Eds.), *Domestic animal/wildlife interface: Issue for disease control, conservation, sustainable food production, and emerging diseases*, vol. 969. New York Acad Sciences, New York, pp. 358–365.

Rothschild, D. M., Serfass, T. L., Seddon, W. L., Hegde, L., Fritz, R. S., 2008. Using fecal glucocorticoids to assess stress levels in captive river otters. *J Wildlife Manage* 72, 138–142.

Rouco, C., Ferreras, P., Castro, F., Villafuerte, R., 2008. The effect of exclusion of terrestrial predators on short-term survival of translocated European wild rabbits. *Wildlife Res* 35, 625–632.

Sauerwein, H., Muller, U., Brussel, H., Lutz, W., Mostl, E., 2004. Establishing baseline values of parameters potentially indicative of chronic stress in red deer (*Cervus elaphus*) from different habitats in western Germany. *Eur J Wildlife Res* 50, 168–172.

Schaefer, D. C., Asner, I. N., Seifert, B., Burki, K., Cinelli, P., 2010. Analysis of physiological and behavioural parameters in mice after toe clipping as newborns. *Lab Anim* 44, 7–13.

Schoech, S. J., Bridge, E. S., Boughton, R. K., Reynolds, S. J., Atwell, J. W., Bowman, R., 2008. Food supplementation: A tool to increase reproductive output. A case study in the threatened Florida Scrub-Jay. *Biol Conserv* 141, 162–173.

Schradin, C., 2008. Seasonal changes in testosterone and corticosterone levels in four social classes of a desert dwelling sociable rodent. *Horm Behav* 53, 573–579.

Schreck, C. B., 2010. Stress and fish reproduction: The roles of allostasis and hormesis. *Gen Comp Endocrinol* 165, 549–556.

Schreck, C. B., Jonsson, L., Feist, G., Reno, P., 1995. Conditioning improves performance of juvenile Chinook salmon, *Oncorhynchus tshawytscha*, to transportation stress. *Aquaculture* 135, 99–110.

Schreck, C. B., Stahl, T. P., Davis, L. E., Roby, D. D., Clemens, B. J., 2006. Mortality estimates of juvenile spring-summer Chinook salmon in the Lower Columbia River and estuary, 190–1998: Evidence for delayed mortality? *Trans Am Fishe Soc* 135, 457–475.

Schulz, J. H., Millspaugh, J. J., Washburn, B. E., Bermudez, A. J., Tomlinson, J. L., Mong, T. W., He, Z., 2005. Physiological effects of radiotransmitters on mourning doves. *Wildlife Soc Bull* 33, 1092–1100.

Sharpe, F., Bolton, M., Sheldon, R., Ratcliffe, N., 2009. Effects of color banding, radio tagging, and repeated handling on the condition and survival of Lapwing chicks and consequences for estimates of breeding productivity. *J Field Ornith* 80, 101–110.

Short, J., Bradshaw, S. D., Giles, J., Prince, R. I. T., Wilson, G. R., 1992. Reintroduction of macropods (Marsupialia macropodoidea) in Australia: A review. *Biol Conserv* 62, 189–204.

Somero, G. N., 2010. The physiology of climate change: how potentials for acclimatization and genetic adaptation will determine "winners" and "losers." *J Exp Biol* 213, 912–920.

Somero, G. N., 2011. Comparative physiology: a "crystal ball" for predicting consequences of global change. *Am J Physiol* 301, R1–R14.

Specker, J. L., Schreck, C. B., 1980. Stress responses to transportation and fitness for marine survival in coho salmon (*Oncorhynchus kisutch*) smolts. *Can J Fish Aquat Sci* 37, 765–769.

Sperry, J. H., Butler, L. K., Romero, L. M., Weatherhead, P. J., 2009. Effects of parasitic infection and radio-transmitters on condition, hematological characteristics and corticosterone concentrations in Texas ratsnakes. *J Zool* 278, 100–107.

Steen, J. B., Gabrielsen, G. W., Kanwisher, J. W., 1988. Physiological aspects of freezing behavior in willow ptarmigan hens. *Acta Physiol Scand* 134, 299–304.

Stevenson, R. D., 2006. Ecophysiology and conservation: The contribution of energetics—introduction to the symposium. *Integ Comp Biol* 46, 1088–1092.

Stevenson, R. D., Woods, W. A., 2006. Condition indices for conservation: new uses for evolving tools. *Integ Comp Biol* 46, 1169–1190.

Sulikowski, J. A., Fairchild, E. A., Rennels, N., Howell, W. H., Tsang, P. C. W., 2006. The effects of transport density on cortisol levels in juvenile winter flounder, *Pseudopleuronectes americanus*. *J World Aqua Soc* 37, 107–112.

Sullivan, B. K., Kwiatkowski, M. A., Schuett, G. W., 2004. Translocation of urban Gila Monsters: A problematic conservation tool. *Biol Conserv* 117, 235–242.

Teixeira, C. P., De Azevedo, C. S., Mendl, M., Cipreste, C. F., Young, R. J., 2007. Revisiting translocation and reintroduction programmes: the importance of considering stress. *Anim Behav* 73, 1–13.

Tempel, D. J., Gutierrez, R. J., 2003. Fecal corticosterone levels in California spotted owls exposed to low-intensity chainsaw sound. *Wildlife Soc Bull* 31, 698–702.

Tempel, D. J., Gutierrez, R. J., 2004. Factors related to fecal corticosterone levels in California spotted owls: Implications for assessing chronic stress. *Conserv Biol* 18, 538–547.

Tracy, C. R., Nussear, K. E., Esque, T. C., Dean-Bradley, K., DeFalco, L. A., Castle, K. T., Zimmerman, L. C., Espinoza, R. E., Barber, A. M., 2006. The importance of physiological ecology in conservation biology. *Integ Comp Biol* 46, 1191–1205.

Tucker, C. B., Rogers, A. R., Verkerk, G. A., Kendall, P. E., Webster, J. R., Matthews, L. R., 2007. Effects of shelter and body condition on the behaviour and physiology of dairy cattle in winter. *Appl Anim Behav Sci* 105, 1–13.

Ujvari, B., Belov, K., 2011. Major histocompatibility complex (MHC) markers in conservation biology. *Int J Mol Sci* 12, 5168–5186.

Van Meter, P. E., French, J. A., Dloniak, S. M., Watts, H. E., Kolowski, J. M., Holekamp, K. E., 2009. Fecal glucocorticoids reflect socio-ecological and anthropogenic stressors in the lives of wild spotted hyenas. *Horm Behav* 55, 329–337.

Van Zant, J. L., Wooten, M. C., 2003. Translocation of Choctawhatchee beach mice (*Peromyscus polionotus allophrys*): Hard lessons learned. *Biol Conserv* 112, 405–413.

Viljoen, J. J., Ganswindt, A., du Toit, J. T., Langbauer, W. R., Jr 2008. Translocation stress and faecal glucocorticoid metabolite levels in free-ranging African savanna elephants. *S Afr J Wildlife Res* 38, 146–152.

Visser, M. E., Both, C., Lambrechts, M. M., 2004. Global climate change leads to mistimed avian reproduction. *Adv Ecol Res*35, 89–110.

von der Ohe, C. G., Wasser, S. K., Hunt, K. E., Servheen, C., 2004. Factors associated with fecal glucocorticoids in Alaskan Brown bears (*Ursus arctos horribilis*). *Physiol Biochem Zool* 77, 313–320.

Waas, J. R., Ingram, J. R., Matthews, L. R., 1997. Physiological responses of red deer (Cervus elaphus) to conditions experienced during road transport. *Physiol Behav* 61, 931–938.

Waas, J. R., Ingram, J. R., Matthews, L. R., 1999. Real-time physiological responses of red deer to translocations. *J Wildlife Manage* 63, 1152–1162.

Walker, B. G., Boersma, P. D., Wingfield, J. C., 2005. Field endocrinology and conservation biology. *Integ Comp Biol* 45, 12–18.

Walker, B. G., Boersma, P. D., Wingfield, J. C., 2006. Habituation of adult Magellanic penguins to human visitation as expressed through behavior and corticosterone secretion. *Conserv Biol* 20, 146–154.

Walker, B. G., Wingfield, J. C., Boersma, P. D., 2008. Tourism and Magellanic penguins (*Spheniscus magellanicus*): An example of applying field endocrinology to conservation problems. *Ornitologia Neotropical* 19S, 219–228.

Wasser, S. K., Bevis, K., King, G., Hanson, E., 1997. Noninvasive physiological measures of disturbance in the Northern Spotted Owl. *Conserv Biol* 11, 1019–1022.

Welker, T. L., Congleton, J. L., 2009. Preliminary examination of oxidative stress in juvenile spring Chinook salmon *Oncorhynchus tshawytscha* of wild origin sampled from transport barges. *J Fish Biol* 75, 1895–1905.

Wells, K. M. S., Washburn, B. E., Millspaugh, J. J., Ryan, M. R., Hubbard, M. W., 2003. Effects of radio-transmitters on fecal glucocorticoid levels in captive Dickcissels. *Condor* 105, 805–810.

Weston, M. A., Dann, P., Jessop, R., Fallaw, J., Dakin, R., Ball, D., 2008. Can oiled shorebirds and their nests and eggs be successfully rehabilitated? A case study involving the threatened Hooded Plover *Thinornis rubricollis* in south-eastern Australia. *Waterbirds* 31, 127–132.

Wikelski, M., Cooke, S. J., 2006. Conservation physiology. *Trends Ecol Evol* 21, 38–46.

Wingfield, J. C., 2008. Comparative endocrinology, environment and global change. *Gen Comp Endocrinol* 157, 207–216.

Wingfield, J. C., Hunt, K., Breuner, C., Dunlap, K., Fowler, G. S., Freed, L., Lepson, J., 1997. Environmental stress, field endocrinology, and conservation biology. In: Clemmons, J. R., Buchholz, R. (Eds.), *Behavioral approaches to conservation in the wild*. Cambridge University Press, Cambridge, U.K., pp. 95–131.

Wingfield, J. C., Hunt, K. E., 2002. Arctic spring: Hormone-behavior interactions in a severe environment. *Comp Biochem Physiol B* 132, 275–286.

Wingfield, J. C., Ishii, S., Kikuchi, M., Wakabayashi, S., Sakai, H., Yamaguchi, N., Wada, M., Chikatsuji, K., 2000. Biology of a critically endangered species, the Toki (Japanese Crested Ibis) *Nipponia nippon*. *Ibis* 142, 1–11.

Wingfield, J. C., Kelley, J. P., Angelier, F., 2011. What are extreme environmental conditions and how do organisms cope with them? *Curr Zool* 57, 363–374.

Wingfield, J. C., Owen-Ashley, N., Benowitz-Fredericks, Z. M., Lynn, S., Hahn, T. P., Wada, H., Breuner, C., Meddle, S., Romero, L. M., 2004. Arctic spring: The arrival biology of migrant birds. *Acta Zool Sinica* 50, 948–960.

Wingfield, J. C., Ramenofsky, M., 1997. Corticosterone and facultative dispersal in response to unpredictable events. *Ardea* 85, 155–166.

Wingfield, J. C., Romero, L. M., 2001. Adrenocortical responses to stress and their modulation in free-living vertebrates. In: McEwen, B. S., Goodman, H. M. (Eds.), *Handbook of physiology;* Section 7: *The endocrine system;* Vol. IV: *Coping with the environment: Neural and endocrine mechanisms*. Oxford University Press, New York, pp. 211–234.

Wolf, C. M., Garland, T., Griffith, B., 1998. Predictors of avian and mammalian translocation success: reanalysis with phylogenetically independent contrasts. *Biol Conserv* 86, 243–255.

Wolf, C. M., Griffith, B., Reed, C., Temple, S. A., 1996. Avian and mammalian translocations: Update and reanalysis of 1987 survey data. *Conserv Biol* 10, 1142–1154.

Wolfaardt, A. C., Williams, A. J., Underhill, L. G., Crawford, R. J. M., Whittington, P. A., 2009. Review of the rescue, rehabilitation and restoration of oiled seabirds in South Africa, especially African penguins *Spheniscus demersus* and Cape gannets *Morus capensis*, 1983–2005. *Afr J Marine Sci* 31, 31–54.

Work, T. M., Massey, J. G., Johnson, L., Dougill, S., Banko, P. C., 1999. Survival and physiologic response of common amakihi and Japanese white-eyes during simulated translocation. *Condor* 101, 21–27.

Wright, T. F., Eberhard, J. R., Hobson, E. A., Avery, M. L., Russello, M. A., 2010. Behavioral flexibility and species invasions: the adaptive flexibility hypothesis. *Ethol Ecol Evolution* 22, 393–404.

Young, F. A., Kajiura, S. M., Visser, G. J., Correia, J. P. S., Smith, M. F. L., 2002. Notes on the long-term transport of the scalloped hammerhead shark (*Sphyrna lewini*). *Zoo Biol* 21, 243–251.

Young, R. J., 2003. *Environmental enrichment for captive animals*. Blackwell Synergy, Oxford.

Zapata, B., Gimpel, J., Bonacic, C., Gonzalez, B., Riveros, J., Ramirez, A., Bas, F., Macdonald, D. W., 2004. The effect of transport on cortisol, glucose, heart rate, leukocytes and body weight in captive-reared guanacos (*Lama guanicoe*). *Anim Welfare* 13, 439–444.

14

Conclusions and the Future

A persistent message of this book has been that the mechanisms underlying responses to perturbations of the environment are common to all vertebrates despite the extremely diverse types, frequencies, durations, and intensities of perturbations. These responses have been the focus of biomedical, agricultural, and environmental research in relation to deleterious effects of chronic stress, but the highly adaptive behavioral and physiological responses that occur immediately following a perturbation have received much less focus. We hope this book will draw attention to the beneficial aspects of these coping strategies, especially in relation to the anti-stress concepts. It is surprising to us that at the time of writing, there is no center or focus on the comparative biology of stress responses. There are centers for biomedical aspects of stress, for example psychosocial aspects, but nothing that centers on the early components of the stress response in a broadly comparative sense. The interrelationships of cellular aspects of the stress response, including heat shock protein function, DNA repair, and mitigation of oxidative damage, remain to be explored in detail. We also hope this book will focus attention on stress biology as a concept worthy of its own emphasis at a time when the planet is changing in rapid and frequently disruptive ways. In this final chapter we summarize some big issues that will likely be the subject of future research. We also point out where developments of new technologies and cyber-infrastructure will enable the integration of molecular, cell, and physiological responses with behavior on a scale unimaginable just a few years ago.

I. BIOLOGICAL VERSUS BIOMEDICAL ISSUES: BIOLOGY OF STRESS IN NATURAL CONTEXTS

Chronic stress is a major biomedical issue and is also crucial in agriculture/aquaculture- and conservation-related concerns. The first part of this book made extensive use of the knowledge gained by countless laboratories around the world dedicated to trying to understand and ameliorate the diseases of chronic stress. However, chronic stress in free-living organisms is usually accompanied by widespread mortality, resulting in selection for coping mechanisms that allow some individuals to survive. Such selection has undoubtedly been in operation for hundreds of millions of years, even before the rise of vertebrates, yet we know much less about these fascinating aspects of stress biology. Since all of our long lines of ancestors managed to survive, at least long enough to have us, an understanding of these selection pressures should be the foundation for all the biomedical and agricultural research. It is truly amazing, for example, that we still cannot answer the basic question of whether the release of corticosteroids ultimately is good or bad for survival. Understanding the coping mechanisms of the initial stress responses could allow us to prepare for potentially stressful conditions (e.g., in humans, long-duration space flight) as well as provide us with new insights into how to treat chronic stress and adjust our societies and infrastructure accordingly.

There is a great need to build a cyber-infrastructure that will allow the synthetic analysis of existing data on environmental cycles, and their changes in recent years, as well as increased intensity and frequency of climatic events. This database could then be integrated with ecosystem data on biodiversity and genomics, proteomics, and metabolomics of individuals as they cope with the routine annual cycles as well as unpredictable perturbations of all kinds. Such massive integration of huge data sets will require an (as yet) absent cyber-infrastructure that includes repositories of diverse data sets with open access but also with standards for uploading new data. Such repositories must be inter-operable across diverse data sets (e.g., genomics, morphology, behavior, physiology, environmental, etc.) and must be curated as computational platforms develop and change. A tall order, but an era when such integration and data-enabled science are possible is just around the corner. The effects on comparative stress biology will be profound.

A key concept here is the "exposome"—the cumulative sum of all exposures to environmental conditions, physical, social, and internal, from conception to death (Wild 2005). The exposome evolves throughout the life of an individual and is completely unique. As a result, the exposome is a highly variable and dynamic entity (Wild, 2005). Good and bad components (exposures) can interact to determine the future physiological and behavioral responses to environmental events of all kinds. The external exposome includes the physical environment, abiotic and biotic, as well as human-induced rapid environmental change (HIREC; Sih 2013). The social exposome includes agonistic and affiliative behavioral interactions, with social status playing an important role. In contrast, the internal exposome includes homeostatic damage such as oxidative stress, pollutants, infection, and other pathologies. Such a concept is only just beginning to be applied to environmental biology and will be essential to understanding individual differences in morphology, physiology, and behavior, including responding to perturbations of the environment. A major question here is how to measure the exposome, or at least estimate it, so we can understand individual differences (Smith and Rappaport 2009).

Interesting questions deriving from the concept of the exposome include the following: Can cells retain information of the exposome early in life and transmit this "knowledge" to other cells throughout the life span of the individual? To what extent is it also possible that one individual can pass on exposome information to another, either by cultural transfer of information through learning, or through epigenetic factors, including maternal effects? We can expect dramatic developments in these areas in the future (Smith and Rappaport 2009).

II. GLOBAL WARMING: FINITE STATE MACHINE MODELS PREDICT PROBLEMS WITH LIFE CYCLES

In Chapter 12 we outlined how finite state diversity (i.e., the number of life-history stages adjusted for the duration of each stage) may have a huge impact on the extent to which individuals may be able to cope with global warming and changing phenology. In general, those organisms that inhabit environments with a wide range of environmental conditions (e.g., cold winters and warm summers, or migrants that cross many climatic zones) have greater finite state diversity than organisms inhabiting more constant environments (e.g., at lower latitudes or in marine-dominated habitats). The more life-history stages a species expresses, the more adjustments in duration and timing of each must be addressed. Although there is some evidence of "micro-evolution" of changed timing and duration of some life-history stages (e.g., Visser et al. 2006), how this translates to the entire annual cycle and what the mechanisms are remain almost completely unknown.

Questions that remain include the following: How do organisms adjust to changing phenology? Does this include flexibility within an individual, resulting in rapid shifts in the "perception-transduction-response" systems (Figure 14.1) to change morphology, physiology and behavior (Wingfield 2012)? Or, is there rapid micro-evolution resulting in selection for those individuals with the best "fit" to current environmental conditions (Visser et al. 2006)? There is evidence from European songbirds, for example, that within three generations one can select for non-migratory to migratory life-history stages and vice versa (e.g., Pulido and Berthold 2010), suggesting that such rapid evolution can indeed occur. Other populations show range expansions (or reductions) moving into habitat that now is most favored for breeding or wintering (e.g., Berthold 1995). How does this occur—that is, what makes a pioneer? Does this just involve

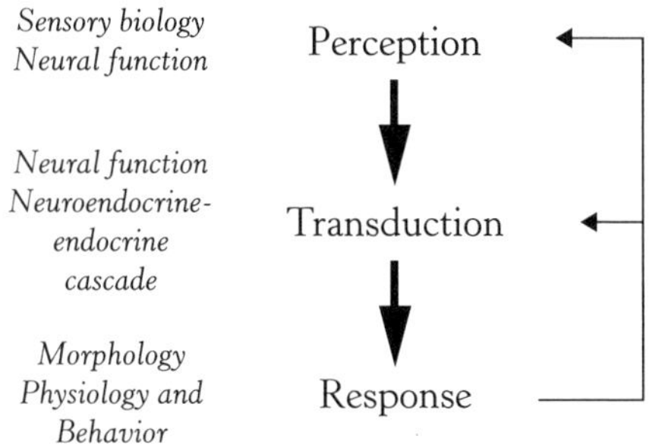

FIGURE 14.1: Perception-transduction-response. Vertebrates perceive their physical, social, and internal environments through sensory receptors that activate neural function. These signals are transduced within the brain and are converted to hormonal (neuroendocrine and endocrine) cascades that result in specific hormonal signals that elicit morphological, physiological, and behavioral responses relevant to the environmental change. Note that there are feedback systems (mostly negative) from the response to transduction and perhaps even to perception.

From Wingfield (2012), courtesy of University of California Press.

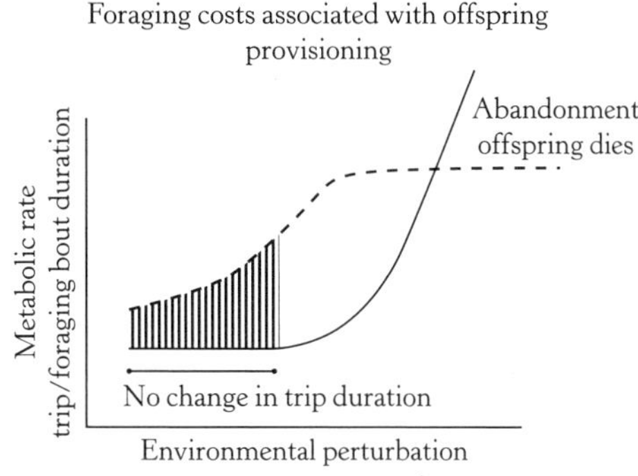

FIGURE 14.2: A conceptual model of how parents should respond to environmental perturbation that causes a reduction in prey availability. The dashed line represents FMR (functional metabolic rate) and the solid line is trip duration.

From Costa (2007), with permission and courtesy of Wiley Interscience.

some migratory overshoots that find themselves in suitable habitat and successfully breed or over winter in the best condition?

One major avenue for future research is to model the responses of individuals to perturbations of the environment in relation to Eg (the amount of energy available in terms of trophic resources and stored fat, etc.) that the animal can utilize and either survive the perturbation in the best condition possible or use it to move away from the source of the perturbation until environmental conditions improve (e.g., Wingfield et al. 1998; Wingfield and Ramenofsky 1999). In Chapter 7 it became very clear that perturbations of the environment may act indirectly on food availability (Eg) and both directly and indirectly on individuals. Machmer and Ydenberg (1990) model food availability and energy expended to obtain food in ospreys. Their results indicate a clear need to have some estimate in Eg in any model. This is further illustrated in modeling of the effects of food availability and perturbations of the environment in relation to the abandonment of offspring when the equivalent of allostatic overload type I occurs (Figure 14.2; Costa 2007, 2012). Furthermore, many aspects of the life cycle of marine pinnipeds may be influenced by food availability, energy expended in obtaining it, and the life cycle (Figure 14.3; Costa 2012). There are many parallels to the allostasis and reactive scope models discussed in Chapter 3. Modeling of these concepts could provide many new insights into how organisms in general cope with an unpredictable world and, most important, could provide new hypotheses and predictions to test possible mechanisms.

III. WHAT WE NEED TO KNOW TO MAKE ACCURATE PREDICTIONS ABOUT POPULATIONS AND MECHANISMS: THREE LEVELS OF HORMONE REGULATION

Throughout this book we have observed that there are diverse ways in which organisms respond to predictable internal and external environmental change such as time of day, seasons, and social interactions, as well as diverse ways of coping with perturbations in those internal and external conditions. In vertebrates the "perception-transduction-response" system (Figure 14.1; Wingfield 2012) is key to how organisms fare in relation to global change, including direct human disturbance. The first step is perception of the environment through sensory mechanisms, followed by rapid neural transduction within the central nervous system and then by neuroendocrine and endocrine cascades to regulate morphological and physiological responses of target tissues. There also appear to be diverse ways in which individuals

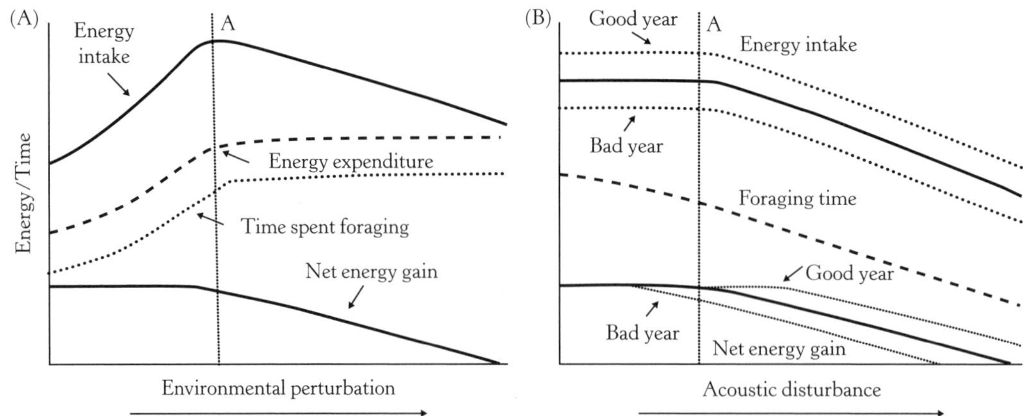

FIGURE 14.3: (A) Response of an animal to reductions in prey availability due to environmental perturbation such as an EI Niño Southern Oscillation (ENSO) event. (B) Response to acoustic disturbance. Vertical dotted line (A) is the point beyond which the animal can no longer adjust its behavior to accommodate the perturbation and goes into an energy deficit. In (B), in a bad year, animals have less ability to accommodate to acoustic disturbance, whereas in a better than average year (good year), animals have a greater capacity.

From Costa (2012), with permission and courtesy of Springer-Verlag.

can respond to the same environmental change, indicating multiple mechanisms (a response dimension of biodiversity) through which the perception-transduction-response complex can be regulated (Wingfield 2008; Wingfield and Mukai 2009).

Population, individual, and habitat differences all impinge upon specific temporal aspects of the life cycle, resulting in highly conserved molecular, cellular, and physiological mechanisms of the perception-transduction-response axis. Nonetheless, there are many potential variations on this conserved network, allowing selection to act on many different components of the network, yet resulting in similar morphological, physiological, or behavioral effects (Wingfield 2008; Wingfield et al. 2011a; Wingfield et al. 2011b; Wingfield 2012). For example, we often assume that the Southern Hemisphere is the mirror image of the Northern in terms of environmental gradients and so on, but even superficial observation of the globe reveals a Northern Hemisphere dominated by land masses surrounding a polar ocean, whereas in the Southern Hemisphere there is a polar landmass surrounded by oceans. These differences have profound influences on seasonality, habitats, and climates (e.g., Ghalambor et al. 2006). For these reasons, regulatory networks of adaptation/acclimation to environments at high latitudes and high altitudes, including the adrenocortical response to perturbations and so on, in the two hemispheres may appear to be very similar at the organism-environment interaction level, but show marked variations at mechanistic levels (Wingfield 2008, 2012). Moreover, specific cell mechanisms within these conserved networks can be adjusted to "customize" the responses of individuals and populations to specific environments, gender, age, and so on (Martin et al. 2011). Furthermore, there is more than one way in which individuals may respond to the same environmental challenge (i.e., alternate points of regulation within the network, all of which could affect fitness in similar ways; Williams 2008; Hau and Wingfield 2011; Martin et al. 2011; Wingfield et al. 2011a; Wingfield et al. 2011b; Wingfield 2012).

Evidence for diversity of mechanisms or regulation in seasonal changes of morphology, physiology, and behavior has been proposed. Examples include the physiology nexus of Ricklefs and Wikelski (2002) and phenotypic flexibility by Piersma and Gils (2011). It is also important to note that networks of physiological responses result from developmental experience and environmental influences, including maternal effects, and have been discussed by Martin et al. (2011) and Cohen et al. (2012). These include regulatory endocrine systems and neural circuits that underlie control mechanisms.

As discussed in Chapter 3, hormones, such as those in the HPA axis, serve as the signaling molecules following the perception-transduction-response system and circulate in the blood (endocrine actions) from their sites of synthesis and secretion to their targets

(Figure 14.4; Wingfield 2012, 2013). They can also act locally on other cell types (called paracrine actions) or provide short-loop feedback to the cell of origin (autocrine actions). In many cases a single hormone can have all three major types of action—distant, local, and self-feedback.

Once released into the blood stream, circulating hormones such as steroids, thyroid hormones, and some peptides are bound to carrier proteins—another point of potential regulation (Figure 14.4; Wingfield 2013). Corticosteroid-binding proteins are synthesized mainly in the liver, but the mechanisms of regulation remain poorly known. On reaching their target organs, hormones initiate cell responses by binding to specialized proteins called receptors. The hormone-receptor complex is what triggers responses of the cell that underlie morphological, physiological, and behavioral effects (Figure 14.4; Wingfield 2013). In the case of the HPA axis, these receptors would be primarily glucocorticoid receptor (GR) and mineralocorticoid receptor (MR) (see Chapter 3).

Looking at Figure 14.4 summarizing the functioning of the HPA axis, it is clear that there is more than one way of regulating perception-transduction-response axes in relation to acclimation to environmental change. These are from Wingfield (2012):

1. The regulation of hormone secretion from perception of the environmental stimulus and transduction by the brain, resulting in release of neuroendocrine signals from the hypothalamus. This then triggers release of tropic hormones from the anterior pituitary gland and, in turn, peripheral endocrine secretions that regulate morphological, physiological, and behavioral responses (Figure 14.4).
2. Once released into the peripheral blood, transport of hormones such as steroids, thyroid hormones, and some peptides involves binding to carrier proteins (Figure 14.4; e.g., Breuner and Orchinik 2002; Nelson 2011).
3. Once the hormone signal arrives at a target cell (e.g., in the brain or liver), there are multiple fates of that hormone that can have profound influences on the type of response (Figure 14.4; e.g., Wingfield 2006). For example, there are two isozymes of 11β-hydroxysteroid dehydrogenase (11β-HSD) that apparently play different roles in corticosteroid metabolism (Holmes et al. 2001). Type 1 can be bi-directional in tissue homogenates, but in vivo acts mostly as a reductase, regenerating active corticosteroids from circulating 11-ketosteroids. Type 2 acts to inactivate corticosteroids. 11β-HSD knockout mice show signs of hypertension arising from activation of MR receptor by corticosteroids in the absence of the protection from the type 2 enzyme (Holmes et al. 2001) and show subtler effects with reduced corticosteroid-induced processes such as gluconeogenesis when fasting, and lower glucose levels in response to obesity or stress (Holmes et al. 2001). Regulation of 11-βHSD activity involves two gene splices and may regulate local production of corticosteroids in neural tissue, immune system, and skin (i.e., extra-adrenal sources; Schmidt et al. 2008; Taves et al. 2011a; Taves et al. 2011b).

All components of the HPA perception-transduction-response axes, from the cascade of hormone secretion to hormone actions (Figure 14.4), are potential sites of regulation of how an individual may respond to daily metabolic needs as well as to perturbations of the environment. Different, yet similar, changes at multiple regulatory points can ultimately have the same phenotypic effect—the final morphological, physiological, or behavioral response can be accomplished via highly diverse mechanisms. This means that the ways in which an individual may respond to similar environmental cues will form a suite of phenotypes that may develop under specific environmental conditions. Several phenotypes may thus have a high degree of fitness in how they respond simultaneously to the same perturbation. It is not necessarily true that there are only limited ways by which organisms respond to environmental change (e.g., Hau and Wingfield 2011). Focusing more on the HPA axis and Figure 14.4, the diversity of these potential points of regulatory mechanisms becomes apparent.

IV. FITNESS CONSEQUENCES

The adrenocortical response to stress is generally thought to be adaptive in allowing organisms to cope with environmental perturbations in the best shape possible and then return to their normal life cycles (Wingfield et al. 1998; Sapolsky et al. 2000; Wingfield and Romero 2001). Much less attention has been given to showing the benefits of the stress response at the individual and

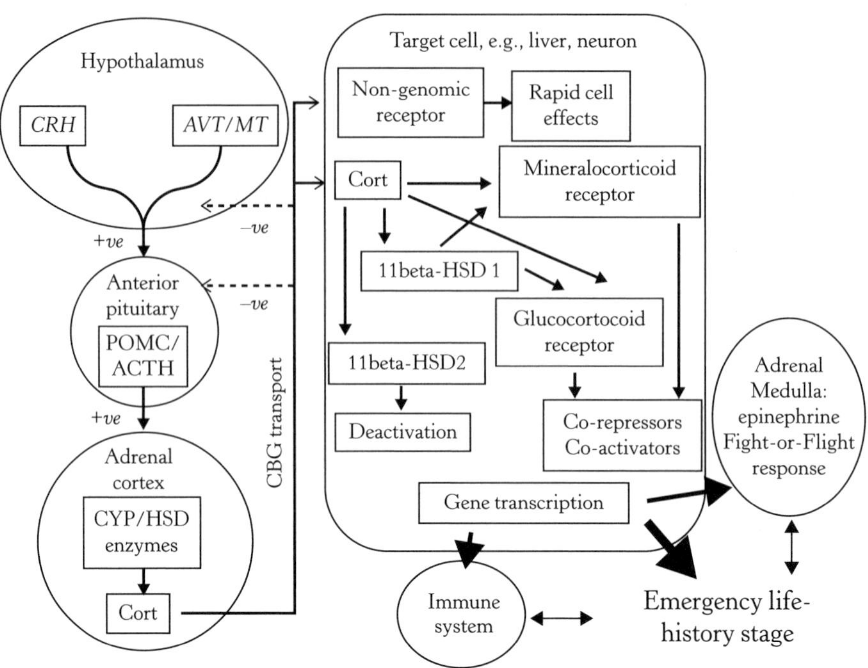

FIGURE 14.4: The three-part regulatory system of secretion control, transport, and hormone responses: the adrenocortical response to acute environmental perturbations that trigger an emergency life-history stage (ELHS). The left-hand part of the figure represents the hormone secretion cascade, in this case the hypothalamo-pituitary-adrenal cortex (HPA) axis. Perturbations of the environment are perceived by sensory modalities, and that information is transduced into neuropeptide secretions, such as corticotropin-releasing hormone (CRH), arginine vasotocin (AVT), and mesotocin (MT), which regulate expression of a precursor or pro-peptide hormone, pro-opiomelanocortin (POMC), in the anterior pituitary. POMC can be then cleaved to give several peptides, including adrenocorticotropin (ACTH). Release of ACTH from the pituitary gland into the blood is also regulated by CRH and AVT. ACTH acts on adrenocortical cells to activate CYP enzymes, including hydroxysteroid dehydrogenases that synthesize corticosteroids such as corticosterone (Cort). Release of Cort into the blood is a major endpoint of the cascade of events that are part of the adrenocortical response to stress. Once in the blood, Cort circulates bound to a carrier protein corticosteroid-binding globulin (CBG) which is part of the transport part of the system (lines). Cort provides negative feedback signals for ACTH release from the pituitary, as well as CRH release from the hypothalamus. More than 90% of Cort circulating in avian blood is bound by CBG. On reaching target cells, such as liver or neurons in the brain involved in the emergency life-history (coping) stage, it is thought that only Cort unbound to CBG can enter cells. Once inside the cell there are two types of genomic receptors that can bind Cort and become gene transcription factors. The mineralocorticoid type receptor (MR) binds with high affinity and so can be saturated at low levels of Cort. The glucocorticoid type receptor (GR) has a lower affinity for Cort and is saturated only at higher concentrations of Cort. Thus GR has been proposed as the "stress" receptor. Note also that there is strong evidence for a membrane receptor (non-genomic) that mediates rapid behavioral effects within minutes. The genomic receptors have effects through gene transcription (different genes affected by each receptor type) and thus require up to several hours for biological effects to be manifest. There are also steroidogenic enzymes expressed in target cells that can modulate how much Cort encounters at least genomic receptors (right-hand part of the Figure). 11beta-hydroxysteroid-dehydrogenase (11beta-HSD) has two major forms—1 and 2. 11beta-HSD 2 converts corticosterone to deoxycorticosterone, which cannot bind to any known Cort receptor and is a deactivation shunt. 11beta-HSD 1 tends to have the opposite effect, enhancing Cort and thus the likelihood of binding to MR or GR. Co-repressors and co-activators also are points of regulation for gene transcription and responses that control the emergency life-history stage and affect the immune system. The adrenal medulla of mammals (medullary cells in birds are called chromaffin) is a key component of the fight-or-flight response (far right-hand part of the figure) secreting epinephrine. This neuroendocrine system is also involved in the emergency life-history stage. This three-part system (hormone cascade, transport in blood, and response networks in the target cells) is also well conserved across vertebrates, but the diversity of ways by which specific components can be regulated to modulate responsiveness to stress is very great.

From Wingfield (2013), courtesy of Elsevier.

population levels in relation to fitness gained (Magee et al. 2006; Breuner et al. 2008; Lancaster et al. 2008; Bonier et al. 2009a). Breuner et al. (2008) point out that the majority of comparative studies on adrenocortical function in vertebrates fall within three general categories (Figure 14.5), as follows:

1. Regulation of secretion (and other components of action discussed earlier and in Figure 14.4): environmental, developmental, physiological, and social effects that alter the acute corticosteroid response, discussing the expected fitness benefit of the change in response.
2. Performance measures: corticosteroid activation or suppression of intermediate performance measures, and the expected fitness benefit of the change in performance.
3. Fitness effects: association of acute corticosteroid reactivity with direct measures of survival or reproductive output. However, much more work is needed in this area to fully assess whether a corticosteroid stress response does increase fitness.

It should be noted that it is not clear whether single studies showing a beneficial effect of corticosteroids to cope with one perturbation may have much relevance to the rest of the individual's life and thus overall fitness. This will require much longer term sampling, possibly not very tractable at present. Dufty et al. (2002) suggest that studying hormone dynamics throughout the developmental trajectory of individuals will likely reveal more pertinent information than just studying samples taken at one point in time.

Several ideas have been put forward to understand how corticosteroids may be related to fitness. For example, Bonier et al. (2007c) predicted that urban birds are more likely to be broadly tolerant of environmental conditions than rural congeners. Fitness of a bird with narrow tolerance (Figure 14.6) is reduced markedly with any changes in the environment. In contrast, a bird with broad tolerance (Figure 14.6) has maximum fitness across a wide range of environmental conditions. In animals with broad tolerance, fitness only declines at more extreme conditions. If an area where the two species coexist becomes urbanized, environmental conditions will shift, and are more likely to fall within the range of tolerance of a bird with broad environmental tolerance than that of a bird with narrow tolerance (Figure 14.6; Bonier et al. 2007c). These ideas of tolerance in urban birds led Bonier et al. (2009a) to formulate a theoretical foundation called the corticosteroid-fitness hypothesis. This hypothesis states:

a. Baseline corticosteroid levels are predicted to increase with environmental challenges (tenet 1, Figure 14.7).
b. Increasing environmental challenges are associated with decreasing fitness because resources must be reallocated toward coping with these challenges at the expense of reproduction or self-maintenance (tenet 2, Figure 14.7).
c. In combination, these two tenets lead to the central prediction of the

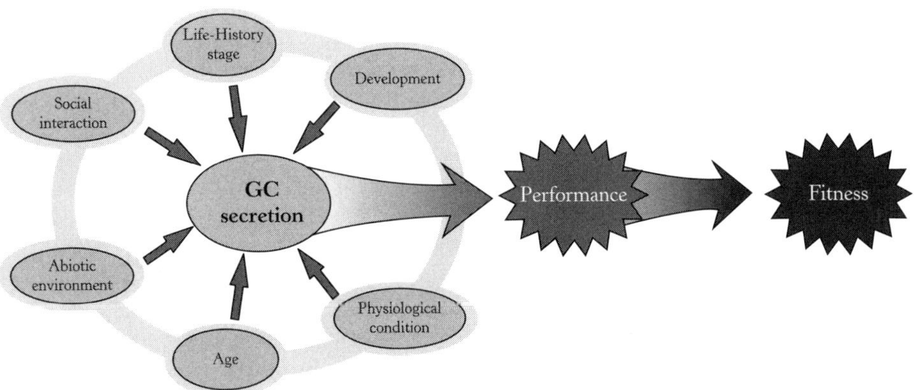

FIGURE 14.5: A framework illustrating the relationships between environment, GC secretion, intermediate performance measures, and fitness.

From Breuner et al. (2008), with permission and courtesy of Elsevier.

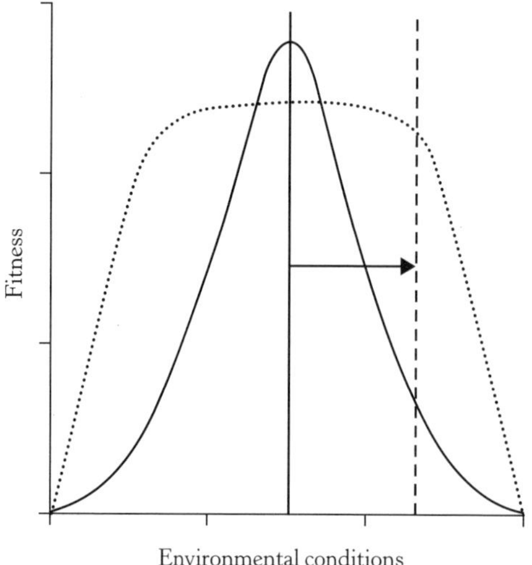

FIGURE 14.6: Illustration that urban birds are more likely to be broadly tolerant of environmental conditions than rural congeners. Solid curve indicates fitness of a bird with narrow tolerance. Dotted curve indicates fitness of a bird with broad tolerance. If an area where the two species coexist becomes urbanized (arrow), environmental conditions (vertical lines) will shift, and are more likely to fall within the range of tolerance of a bird with broad environmental tolerance than that of a bird with narrow tolerance.

From Bonier et al. (2007c), courtesy of the Royal Society, London.

> corticosteroid-fitness hypothesis: a negative relationship between baseline corticosteroids and fitness (Figure 14.7; Bonier et al. 2009a).

A further refinement of these ideas led to a recent conceptual model that outlines the potential relationship between baseline or fecal corticosteroids or corticosteroid responsiveness, and survival or reproductive success (Figure 14.8a; Busch and Hayward 2009). This model emphasizes that a middle level of corticosteroids provides the most fitness; fitness decreases when corticosteroids are both too low or too high. The proposal that mid-level corticosteroid concentrations provide the most fitness meshes nicely with both allostasis and reactive scope, where corticosteroid levels that are too high induce allostatic/homeostatic overload and corticosteroid levels that are too low induce homeostatic failure. Busch and Hayward (2009) then model predictions for baseline, fecal, and stress-induced corticosteroids, as well as fitness, as the duration and intensity of disturbance increase (Figure 14.8b).

An interesting test of these ideas is presented in Figures 14.9–14.11. Male white-crowned sparrows living in urban habitats along the Pacific Coast of the United States had higher baseline levels of corticosterone than males in rural habitats (Figure 14.9; Bonier et al. 2007a). In contrast, female white-crowned sparrows had similar baseline corticosterone in both types of habitat. A follow-up study then measured reproductive success in one urban population. Corticosterone levels had no relationship to male reproductive success, regardless of paternity (Figure 14.10; Bonier et al. 2007a), but females with higher baseline corticosterone fledged fewer offspring (Figure 14.11). In other words, the higher the female's corticosterone, the lower the fitness, consistent with the corticosteroid-fitness hypothesis. In addition, although parasitic infections also correlated with reproductive success in females, it did not in males, and there were no correlations of infections with plasma corticosterone in either sex (Bonier et al. 2007a).

The impact of corticosterone on fitness, however, can also be subtle. In another experiment,

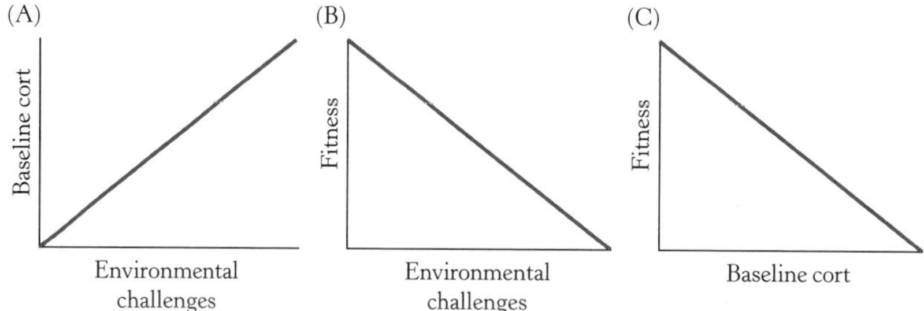

FIGURE 14.7: The theoretical foundation of the corticosteroid (cort)-fitness hypothesis. (A) Baseline corticosteroid levels increase with environmental challenges (tenet 1). (B) Increasing environmental challenges decrease fitness (tenet 2). (C) In combination, the result is a negative relationship between baseline corticosteroid and fitness.

From Bonier et al. (2009a), courtesy of Elsevier.

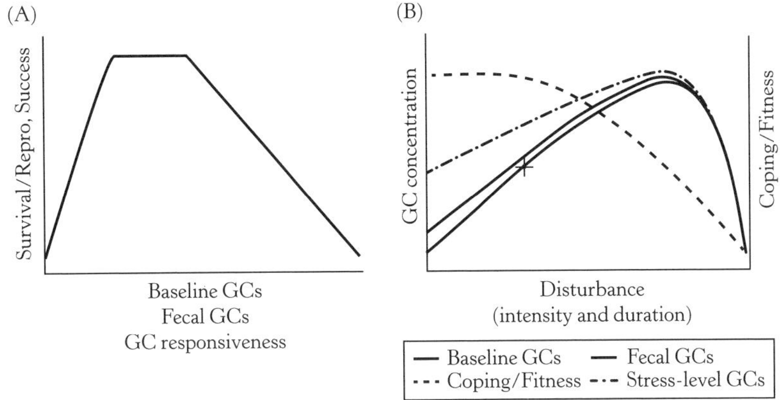

FIGURE 14.8: Conceptual models outlining the potential relationship: (A) between baseline or fecal corticosteroids (GCs) or GC responsiveness and survival or reproductive success and (B) among duration and intensity of disturbance, baseline GCs (solid line), fecal GCs (dotted line), stress-level GCs (dot-dashed line), and fitness/ability to cope with stressors (dashed line). The star indicates the point at which baseline GC titers reach chronic stress levels and condition begins declining.

From Busch and Hayward (2009), courtesy of Elsevier.

free-living female Puget Sound white-crowned sparrows were studied in an urban environment on the University of Washington campus, Seattle. Breeding females with elevated baseline levels of corticosterone produced more female offspring.

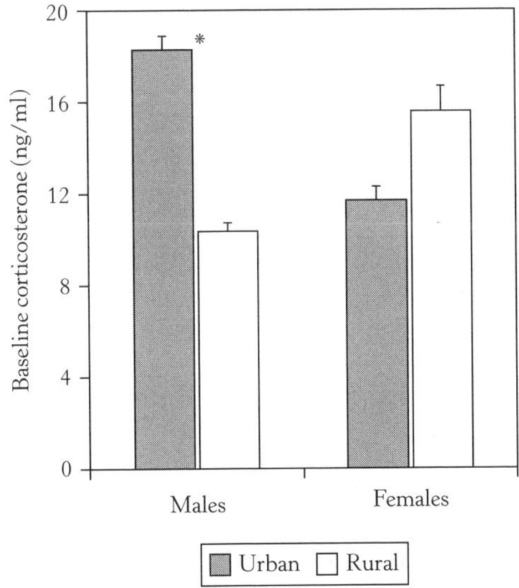

FIGURE 14.9: Comparison of baseline corticosterone levels in male and female white-crowned sparrows breeding in urban (black bars) and rural (white bars) habitat. Urban males had significantly higher baseline corticosterone levels than rural conspecifics. There were no differences between urban and rural female birds' hormone levels. Asterisk (*) denotes a significance at the $P = 0.05$ level.

From Bonier et al. (2007a), courtesy of Oxford University Press.

These correlational data were supported by a field experiment in which corticosterone was implanted subcutaneously to moderately elevate corticosterone (i.e., within the baseline range, A–B, Chapter 3). The elevated corticosterone also resulted in the production of more female embryos (sexed genetically) than males (Bonier et al. 2007b). The combination of the two experiments on white-crowned sparrows indicates that high baseline corticosterone had a profound impact. Not only did females show decreased reproductive success, but they shifted the sex ratio of their young toward females.

This example in white-crowned sparrows is only one example of recent tests of the corticosteroid-fitness hypothesis. There is an increasing volume of literature relating baseline, as well as stress-induced, blood levels of corticosteroids to body condition, parasite load, and survival, with ultimate inferences to fitness (Figures 14.5–14.8). A review of over 50 investigations of vertebrates by Bonier et al. (2009a) revealed that there is evidence for negative, positive, or no relationships of baseline corticosteroid levels in circulation with estimates of fitness. Much more investigation is needed to determine why such variation exists and why the relationship can shift within populations and with time in individuals (Bonier et al. 2009a).

There are a number of excellent empirical studies that support the corticosteroid-fitness hypothesis. For example, corticosteroid levels in some seabirds are linked to fish availability (e.g., Kitaysky et al. 1999). This can lead to differences

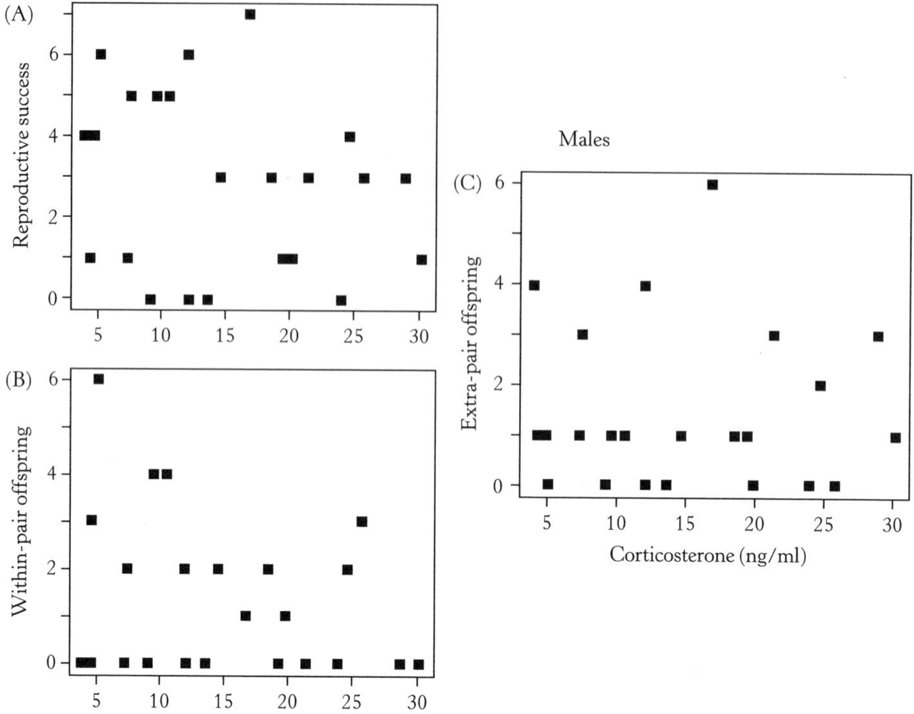

FIGURE 14.10: Poisson regression of cumulative seasonal reproductive success (number of offspring fledged during one breeding season) on male white-crowned sparrow baseline corticosterone levels. There was no relationship between male reproductive success and baseline corticosterone for total number of offspring fledged (A), number of within-pair offspring (B, those sired with the social mate), or number of extra-pair offspring (C, those sired with another female in the population).

From Bonier et al. (2007a), courtesy of Oxford University Press.

in reproductive success, with increasing baseline levels of circulating corticosterone correlated with decreasing productivity in terms of the number of chicks fledged (Buck et al. 2007). On the other hand, Lanctot et al. (2003) concluded that corticosterone levels were not a reliable indicator of food availability in an experiment in which black-legged kittiwakes were given supplemental food. Another example of corticosteroids altering reproductive success is that baseline corticosterone predicted fledging success in free-living house sparrows. Both sexes with low pre-breeding baseline corticosterone levels raised the most offspring (Ouyang et al. 2011). There were no relationships with circulating levels of prolactin. Furthermore, stress-induced plasma levels of corticosterone were negatively correlated with provisioning rates of young (Ouyang et al. 2011). High baseline corticosteroids can also impact survival. In male lizards, treatment with corticosterone increased energy expenditure, food intake, and activity during the day. In combination, these effects increased survival, suggesting an adaptive role for the adrenocortical response to stress (Cote et al. 2006). For another example, high fecal corticosteroid metabolite levels in free-living ring-tailed lemurs in Madagascar were associated with higher mortality rates than animals with lower levels (Pride 2005).

The support for the corticosteroid-fitness hypothesis, however, can also be context dependent. Figure 14.12 shows that experimentally elevated corticosterone had opposite impacts on survival and reproduction in two morphs of female side-blotched lizards with distinct reproductive strategies (Lancaster et al. 2008). Furthermore, it is not always clear what the impact of corticosteroids will be on the offspring (see Chapter 11). Do stressed females reduce or enhance survival in their offspring? In at least one experiment, the answer can be both. Corticosterone treatment of pregnant female lizards resulted in offspring with smaller body size and lower body condition. However, survival of male offspring from

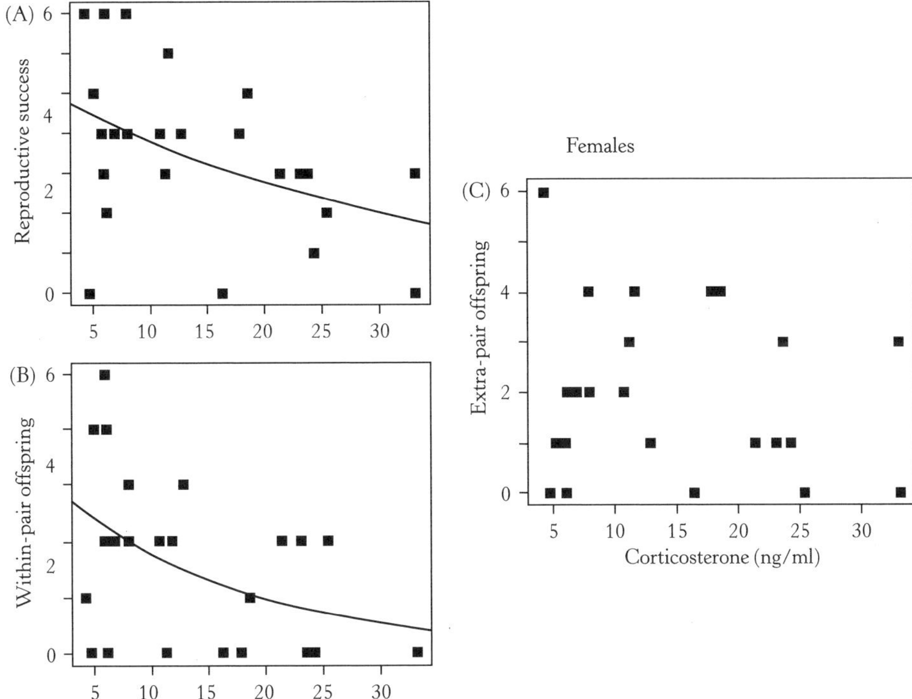

FIGURE 14.11: Poisson regression of cumulative seasonal reproductive success (number of offspring fledged during one breeding season) on female white-crowned sparrow baseline corticosterone levels. Females with high baseline corticosterone levels fledged fewer offspring (A) and had fewer within-pair offspring (B, those sired by the social mate) than females with low hormone levels. There was no relationship between a female's baseline corticosterone level and number of extra-pair offspring (C).

From Bonier et al. (2007a), courtesy of Oxford University Press.

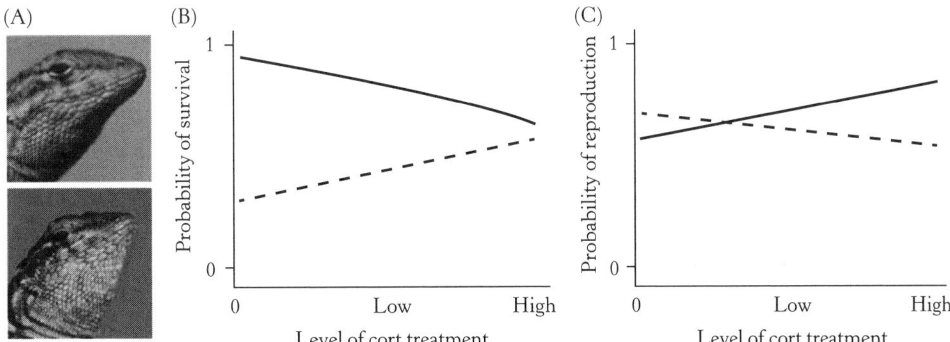

FIGURE 14.12: Variation in the corticosteroid (cort)-fitness relationship within female side-blotched lizards. (A) Experimentally increased corticosterone had opposite effects in two morphs with distinct reproductive strategies (orange, r-strategist; and yellow, K-strategist females). High corticosterone increased the probability of short-term survival (B) but decreased the probability of reproduction (C) in yellow females (dashed blue line), and increased reproduction but reduced survival in orange females (solid orange line).

(A) reproduced with permission from Barry Sinervo. (B) and (C) reproduced from Lancaster et al. (2008) and Bonier et al. (2009a), with permission.

corticosterone-treated females was increased (Meylan and Clobert 2005).

A modification of the corticosteroid-fitness hypothesis emphasizes the shifting of resources to reproduction. Using allostasis (Chapter 3), an increase in baseline corticosteroids could help support the continuance of reproduction despite the accompanying increase in allostatic load. This can be called the corticosteroid-adaptation hypothesis because the elevated corticosteroids are promoting the reallocation of resources to reproduction (Bonier et al. 2009a). There is some empirical support for the corticosteroid-adaptation hypothesis. In the breeding house sparrows discussed earlier, although birds with low pre-breeding baseline corticosterone raised the most offspring, this was accompanied by higher baseline corticosterone during breeding (Ouyang et al. 2011). It is possible that high reproductive effort may have resulted in higher secretion of corticosterone. Two further examples are shown in Figure 14.13. In Figure 14.13b, corticosteroid levels measured early in breeding were negatively correlated with reproductive success in male bluegill sunfish. Males with higher baseline corticosteroids were more likely to abandon their nests. Furthermore, males that abandoned earliest had the highest corticosteroid levels. In Figure 14.13c, an experimental reduction in brood size later in the breeding effort resulted in reduced baseline corticosteroid levels relative to fish with larger unmanipulated broods. This suggests that corticosteroids help mediate reproductive investment, with more offspring requiring higher corticosteroid concentrations. Figure 14.13e shows a similar pattern in breeding female tree swallows. There is again a negative relationship between baseline corticosteroids and reproductive investment (clutch mass) early in the breeding season. Furthermore, in Figure 14.13f higher corticosteroid levels were correlated with increased nestling growth later in the breeding season, another metric of reproductive investment (Magee et al. 2006).

In contrast to positive effects of corticosteroids on fitness, others have found deleterious effects, also called carryover effects, of high

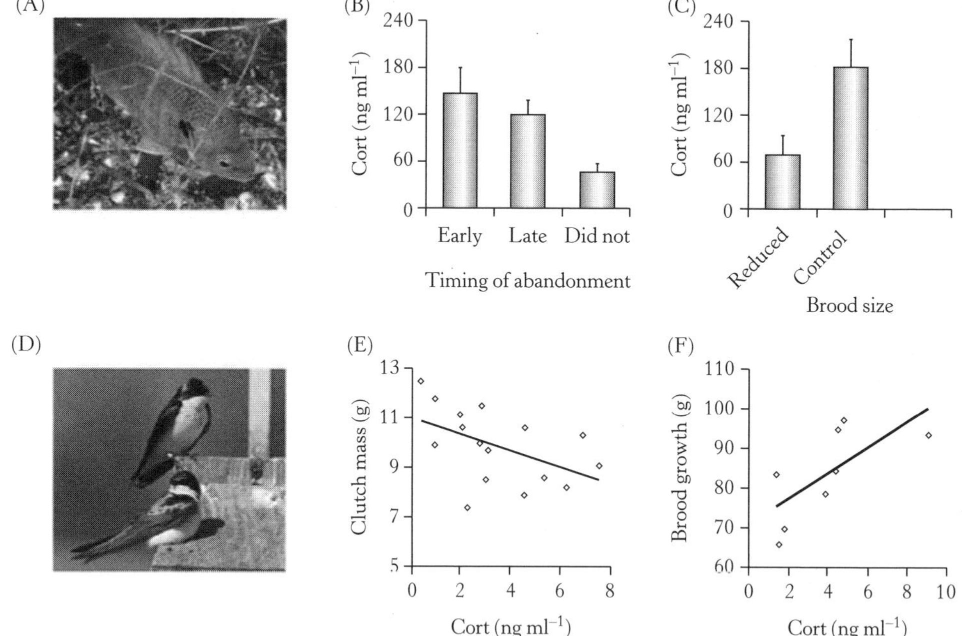

FIGURE 14.13: Empirical support for the corticosteroid-adaptation hypothesis. In male bluegill sunfish (A), baseline corticosteroid levels were negatively correlated with the timing of nest abandonment (B) and positively correlated with an experimental reduction in brood size (C). In breeding female tree swallows (D), baseline corticosteroids were negatively correlated with (clutch mass) early in the breeding season (E), and positively correlated with total growth of all nestlings in a brood over 8 days later in the breeding season (F).

(A) reproduced with permission from Bryan D. Neff, (B) and (C) adapted with permission from data provided in Magee et al. (2006), (D) reproduced with permission from P-G Bentz, and (E) and (F) adapted with permission from Bonier et al. (2009b). Fig. from Bonier et al. (2009a), with permission.

corticosteroids following a stressful episode. In wild largemouth bass, implants of cortisol were used to raise plasma levels for about 5 days. Immediately after cortisol treatment, fish showed increased activity compared with controls. After treatment ended, the effect on activity disappeared (O'Connor et al., 2010). However, in the following winter during severe conditions many fish in this population died, but previously cortisol-treated fish died sooner than controls and showed decreased activity levels before other fish. These data suggest carryover effects of adrenocortical surges associated with stress and ecological consequences on broader temporal scales (O'Connor et al. 2010).

In southern Sweden, pied flycatchers prefer to nest in deciduous forests rather than coniferous forests. As a result, density of breeding birds and reproductive success were highest in the deciduous forest. Simulated territorial intrusions to test aggression of breeding birds in the two habitats showed that flycatchers were generally more aggressive in response to territorial intrusions and had higher plasma levels of testosterone in the deciduous versus coniferous forest (Silverin 1998). However, circulating levels of corticosterone were also higher in the preferred habitat, deciduous forest, than in the suboptimal coniferous forest (Silverin 1998). This may have been because the density of birds was higher and there was more competition in the preferred habitat. These data are the opposite of what many others found and emphasize that many factors should be taken into consideration when determining adrenocortical responses to habitat quality (for further discussion, see Chapter 12).

A further complication to the corticosteroid-fitness hypothesis is that corticosteroid responses can be modulated (see Chapter 10). For example, the amount of reproductive potential remaining during an individual's life span, known as the brood-value hypothesis, can change how that individual will respond to stressors (Wingfield and Sapolsky 2003). Figure 14.14 shows data from a review that examined both baseline and peak corticosterone levels during breeding in relation to brood value in 64 bird species (Bókony et al. 2009). Baseline values were higher as brood value increased (Figure 14.14A), supporting the corticosteroid-adaptation hypothesis. However, peak corticosterone levels following capture stress, but controlled for baseline levels and breeding latitude, decreased in relation to brood value (Figure 14.14B). This indicates that the corticosteroid relationship to fitness can be quite complex. Furthermore, sex differences in parental care indicated that the sex that provided the most parental care tended to have lower baseline and peak corticosterone levels (Figure 14.15; Bókony et al. 2009).

Finally, Busch and Hayward (2009) presented a flow chart for using allostasis to help interpret results from field studies on baseline, fecal, and stress-level corticosteroid titers (Figure 14.16). In

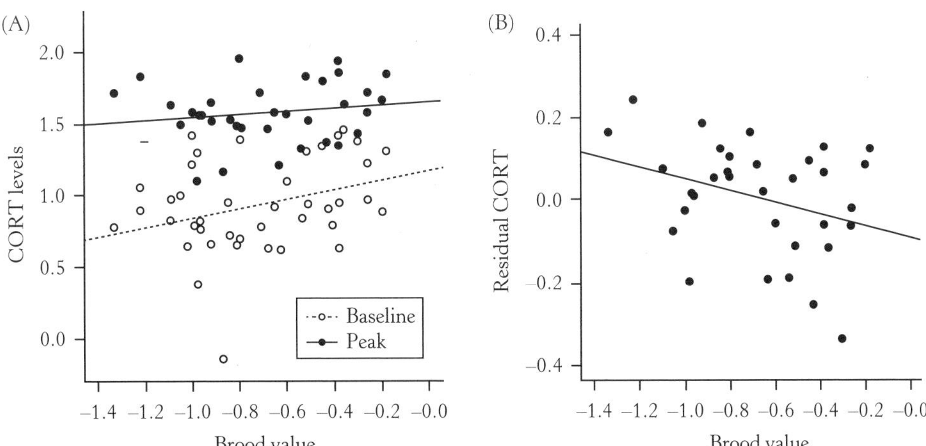

FIGURE 14.14: (A) Baseline and peak corticosterone (CORT) levels (ng mL1; log10 transformed) in relation to brood value. (B) Stress response (peak CORT level) controlled for baseline CORT level and breeding latitude (absolute distance from the equator), in relation to brood value. Brood value expresses the putative importance of current reproduction as log10 (clutch size/[clutch size × broods per year × average reproductive life span]).

From Bokony et al. (2009), courtesy of University of Chicago Press.

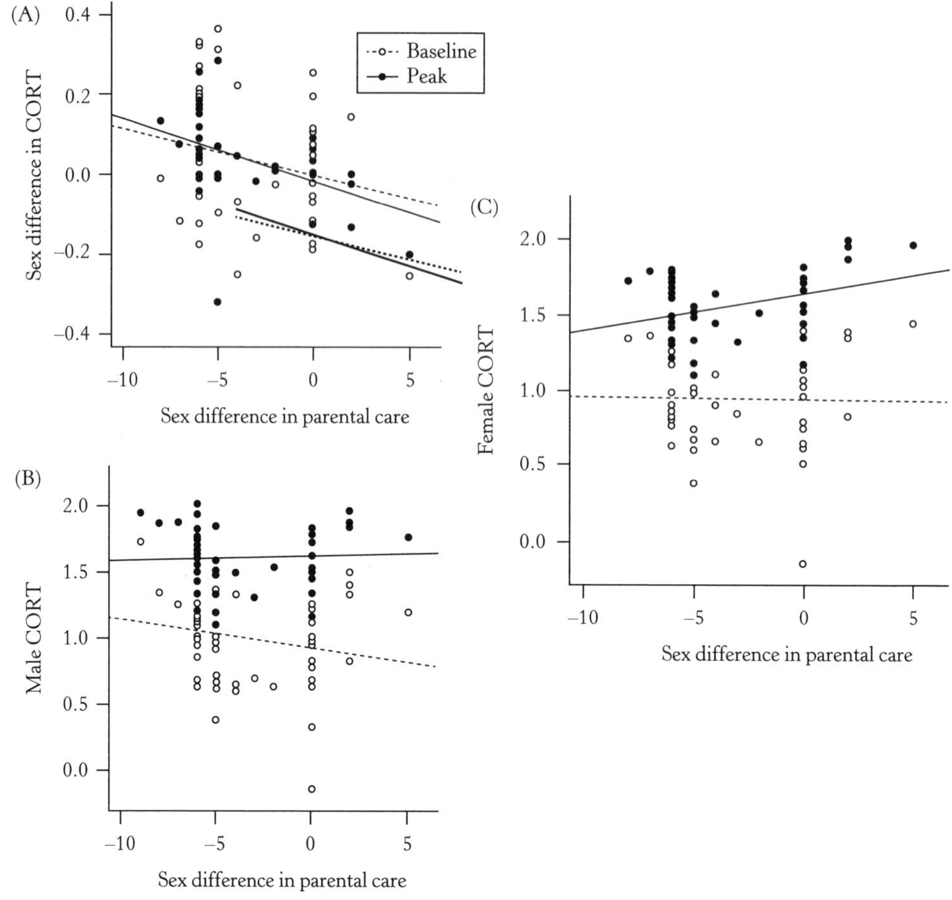

FIGURE 14.15: Sex differences in parental care (greater values indicate more male-biased care) in relation to sex differences in corticosterone (CORT) levels (log10 [male CORT/female CORT]; A), to male CORT level (B), and to female CORT level (ng mL1; log10 transformed; C).

From Bokony et al. (2009), courtesy of University of Chicago Press.

this flow chart, stress-level titers can be induced via a standardized protocol (e.g., capture and restraint) or chemical challenge (e.g., injection with the releaser hormone adrenocorticotropic hormone, ACTH). The key concept arising from this flow chart is that any difference in corticosteroid titers can reduce the animal's ability to cope.

V. RANGE EXPANSIONS

As climate change continues, or following introduction by humans, many species of plants and animals are changing their natural ranges as suitable habitat appears. For example, over the past 300 years the brown-headed cowbird has expanded its range from primarily the prairies of central North America throughout the eastern part of the continent as well as the West, including the Sierra Nevada. This range expansion appears to have been facilitated by human-disturbed areas, particularly agriculture, clearing forest for grazing and horse corrals (Rothstein et al. 1980). In western bluebirds, a combination of high aggression in some individuals and dispersal allowed them to move to the "invasion" front and displace the less aggressive mountain bluebirds, thus facilitating range expansion (Duckworth and Badyaev 2007). Maternal effects when resources are low may be important mechanisms by which female western bluebirds manipulate aggression and dispersion in male chicks (Duckworth 2009). After range expansion and isolation, rapid diversification of populations can occur (Mila et al. 2007), resulting in rapid evolution of traits such as migration (e.g., Able and Belthoff 1998).

A subspecies of dark-eyed junco breeds in the mountains of southern California and is a

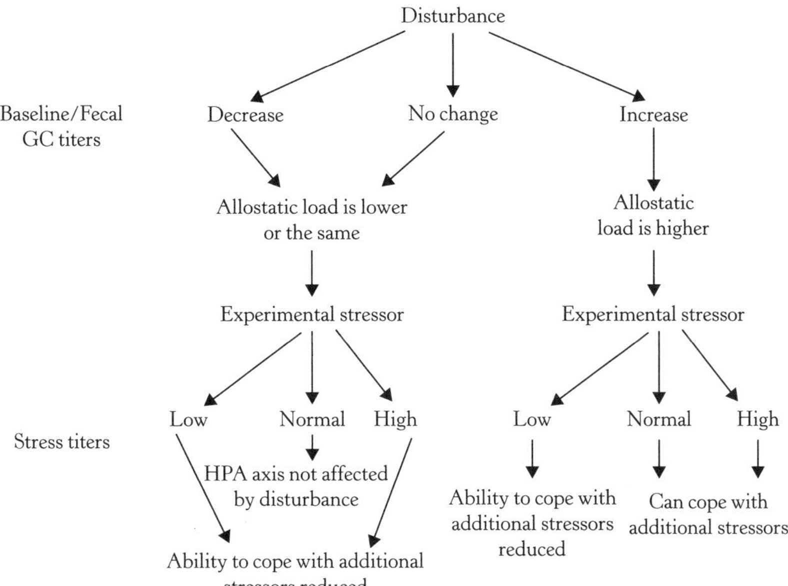

FIGURE 14.16: Flow chart indicating how results from field studies on baseline, fecal, and stress-level GC titers could be interpreted in relation to allostatic load and ability to cope with additional stressors.

From Busch and Hayward (2009), courtesy of Elsevier Press.

short-distance migrant wintering along the coast of southern California. About 30 years ago a small subpopulation remained on the wintering grounds and began breeding. This newly established breeding population now raises more broods per year than the ancestral mountain-breeding population (Yeh and Price 2004). Following the colonization of urban wintering habitat by breeding dark-eyed juncos, urban birds had consistently lower adrenocortical responses to capture stress (Figure 14.17; Atwell et al. 2012) and a negative covariation between maximum corticosterone and exploratory behavior. These population differences persisted in a common garden experiment of birds from ancestral habitat and the urban colonizers (Atwell et al. 2012).

In another type of range expansion, Puget Sound white-crowned sparrows had an original breeding distribution along the coast of Oregon and Washington states. In the past 60 years they have colonized inland urban sites, including human-disturbed areas such as farmland and forest clear-cuts, and more recently have extended their breeding range into the Cascade Mountains and beyond (Figure 14.18; Addis et al. 2011). The birds that colonized urban habitats and those invading human-disturbed areas in the mountains had higher baseline corticosterone levels than birds breeding in ancestral habitat and also greater than in a non-migratory subspecies in coastal California and a native high-elevation subspecies (Figure 14.19). Additionally, the range expanders into the mountains also had higher "integrated corticosterone" (i.e., a measure of the total amount of corticosterone secreted, Figure 14.20; Addis et al. 2011). When the profiles of individual patterns of corticosterone release following capture and handling were compared, the population that had expanded its range into the mountains showed tremendous individual variation, some showing no response and others exhibiting the highest levels of corticosterone ever measured in avian blood (Figure 14.21; Addis et al. 2011). This individual variation was far greater than in the birds still breeding in ancestral coastal habitat, the coastal California subspecies and the mountain subspecies that breeds in natural alpine meadows and less so in disturbed habitat (Figure 14.21; Addis et al. 2011). The significance of this finding remains to be clarified, but it does the raise the question of "what makes a pioneer?" Is it large variation of traits among individuals, such as the stress response, and then selection for those phenotypes best adapted to the new environment? Do corticosteroids play additional, heretofore unknown, roles in range expansion and adaptation?

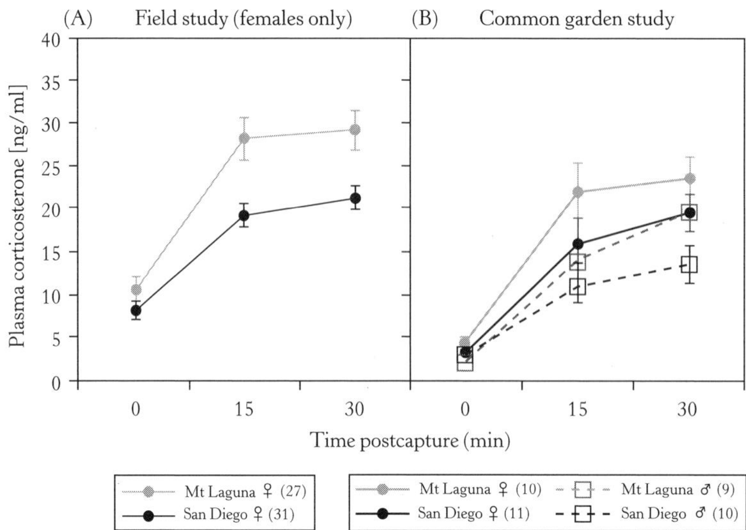

FIGURE 4.17: Initial (baseline) and stress-induced plasma corticosterone in colonist (San Diego) and ancestral range populations of dark-eyed juncos. Data are from (A) field study of free-living nesting females and (B) a captive common garden study of birds raised from early life under identical aviary conditions. Note the significant population differences in both maximum corticosterone and corticosterone responsiveness in both field and common garden studies, and also the sex differences in the common garden.

From Atwell et al. (2012), with permission and courtesy of Oxford University Press.

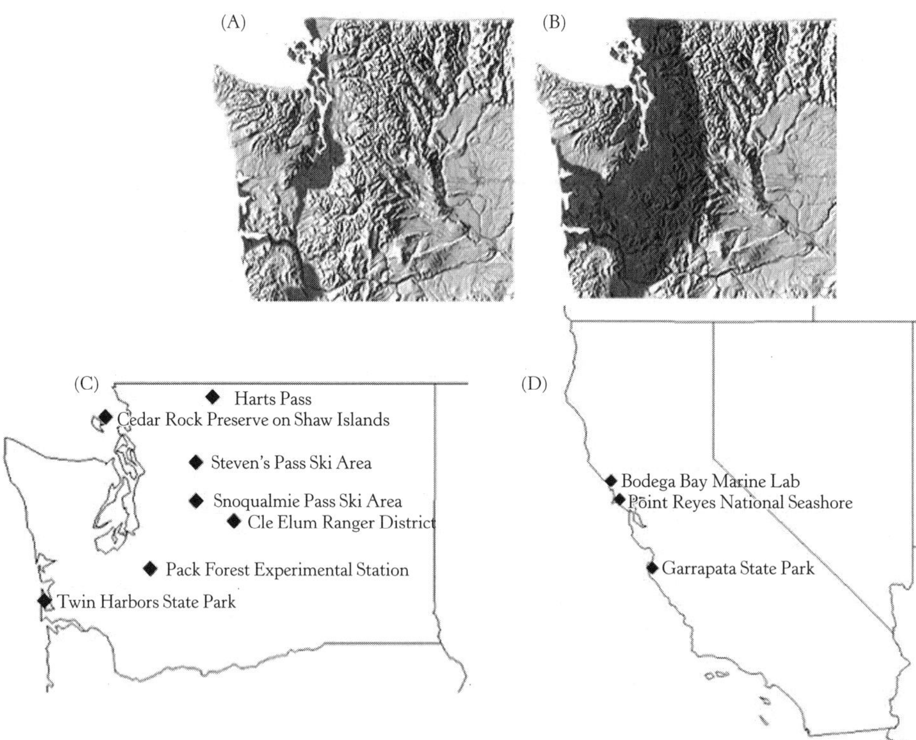

FIGURE 14.18: Distribution of Puget Sound white-crowned sparrows in Washington State shown in dark grey. (A) pre-1940 (Blanchard 1941); (B) present day (J. C. Wingfield, pers. obs.); (C) fields sites in Washington State; (D) field sites in California.

Base map from Thelin and Pike (1991). From Addis et al. (2011), courtesy of Elsevier.

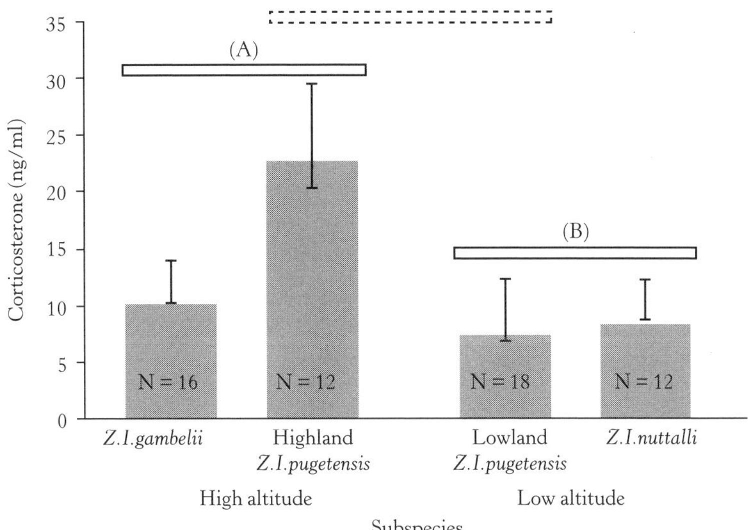

FIGURE 14.19: Mean baseline corticosterone levels differed among white-crowned sparrow populations. Using the AICc best fit model (Altitude) the two high-altitude populations (A) group separately from the two low-altitude populations (B), as shown by the solid horizontal brackets. By direct comparison, baseline corticosterone levels are different between highland and lowland *pugetensis*, as shown by the dashed horizontal bracket.

From Addis et al. (2011), courtesy of Elsevier.

VI. RELEVANCE TO HUMAN SOCIETY: HABITAT DEGRADATION AND HUMAN BEHAVIOR

Although this book has focused on vertebrates as experimental animals in their natural habitats and the laboratory as models for understanding the comparative biology of stress and HIREC (human-induced rapid environmental change), it is important here to consider what the implications may be for humans—that is, the role for the adaptive responses to stress, rather than just the clinical aspects of chronic stress.

A. Human Socioeconomic Status

Socioeconomic status (SES) is an important predictor of a range of health outcomes, but it is not entirely consistent with individuals simply

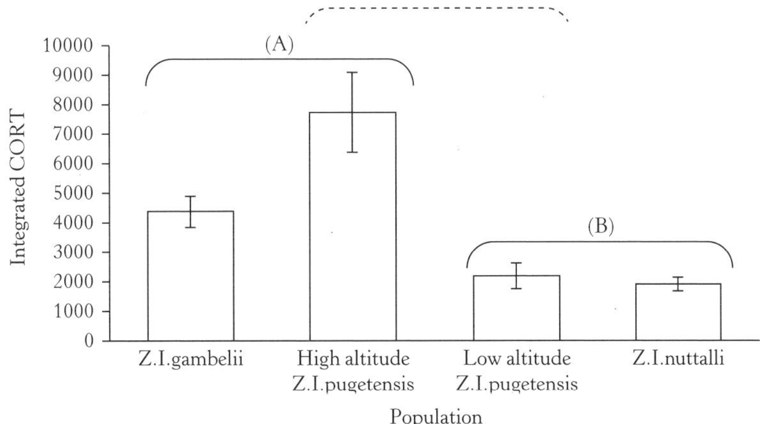

FIGURE 14.20: Integrated corticosterone responses across subspecies of white-crowned sparrows. Using the AICc best fit model (Altitude) the two high-altitude populations (A) group separately from the two low-altitude populations (B), as shown by the solid horizontal brackets. By direct comparison, integrated corticosterone levels are different between highland and lowland *pugetensis*, as shown by the dashed horizontal bracket.

From Addis et al. (2011), courtesy of Elsevier.

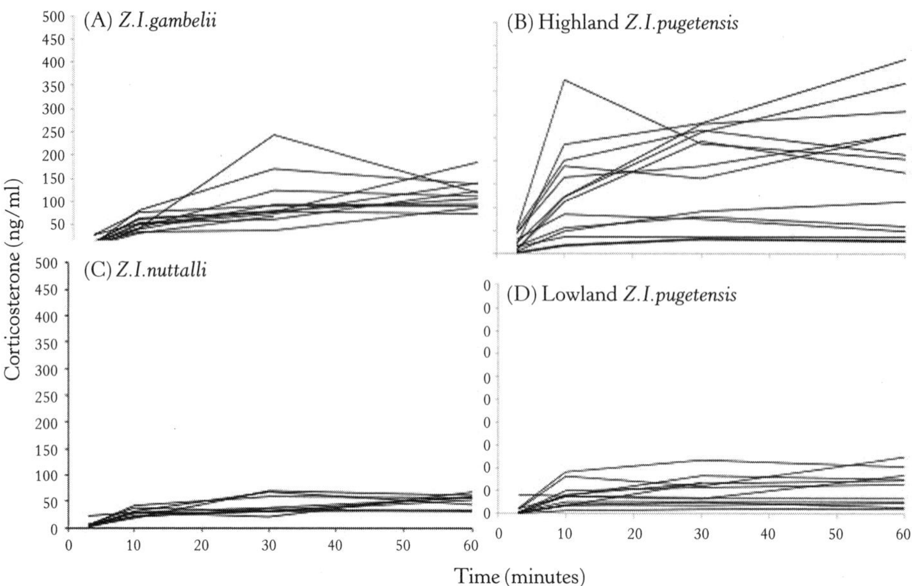

FIGURE 14.21: Individual integrated corticosterone responses for each population. Variance is different between populations. (A) *Z. l. gambelii*; (B) Highland *Z. l. pugetensis*; (C) *Z. l. nuttalli*; and (D) Lowland *Z. l. pugetensis*.

From Addis et al. (2011), courtesy of Elsevier.

suffering from chronic stress (Baum et al. 1999). There is a large body of evidence showing that low SES is accompanied by reduced mental and physical health (Figure 3.22; McEwen 2000; Lupien et al. 2001), possibly because of greater exposure to stressful life events. High SES people can also be susceptible, perhaps through work-related issues. This is a form of allostatic overload type II that could also result in high circulating levels of glucocorticoids such as cortisol (McEwen and Wingfield 2003). For example, in a study of over 300 children of three age cohorts from low, medium, and high SES neighborhoods, it was shown that salivary cortisol was lowest in the high SES group compared with medium and low SES and was evident as early as age six (Figure 14.22; Lupien et al. 2000). Furthermore, the child's cortisol levels were significantly correlated with the degree of depression of the mother.

In another example, Cohen et al. (2006b) found that lower SES was accompanied by higher cortisol levels in saliva later in the day (i.e., a flatter daily rhythm compared with those in higher SES). However, these differences were small, and it is not clear whether they are biologically significant. SES determined by assessing income plus education was associated with higher salivary cortisol levels (determined by area under the curve from multiple samples collected over three days) in low SES compered to medium or high SES (Figure 14.23; Cohen et al. 2006a). Furthermore, urinary levels of epinephrine and norepinephrine were similarly related to SES (Figure 14.23; Cohen et al. 2006a). There was no effect of age, gender, or race. In general, salivary cortisol levels tend to be higher in lower SES men than in high SES men, with the morning rise being blunted and higher levels late in the day in low SES people.

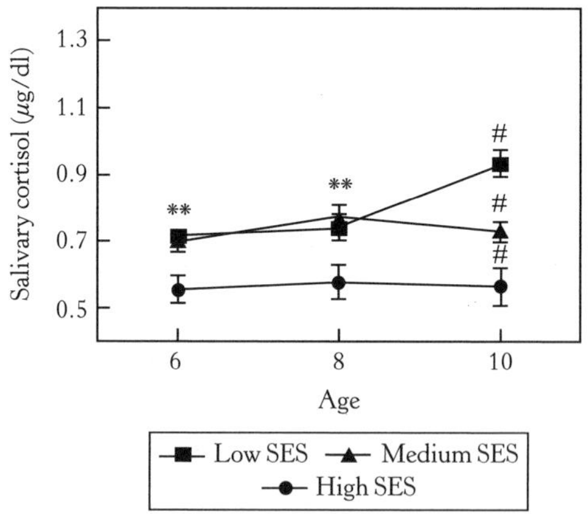

FIGURE 14.22: Morning basal cortisol levels in children aged 6, 8, and 10 years and with low, medium, and high socioeconomic status (SES).

**Significantly different from high SES. # All between-group differences significant.

From Lupien et al. (2000) with permission and courtesy of Cambridge University Press.

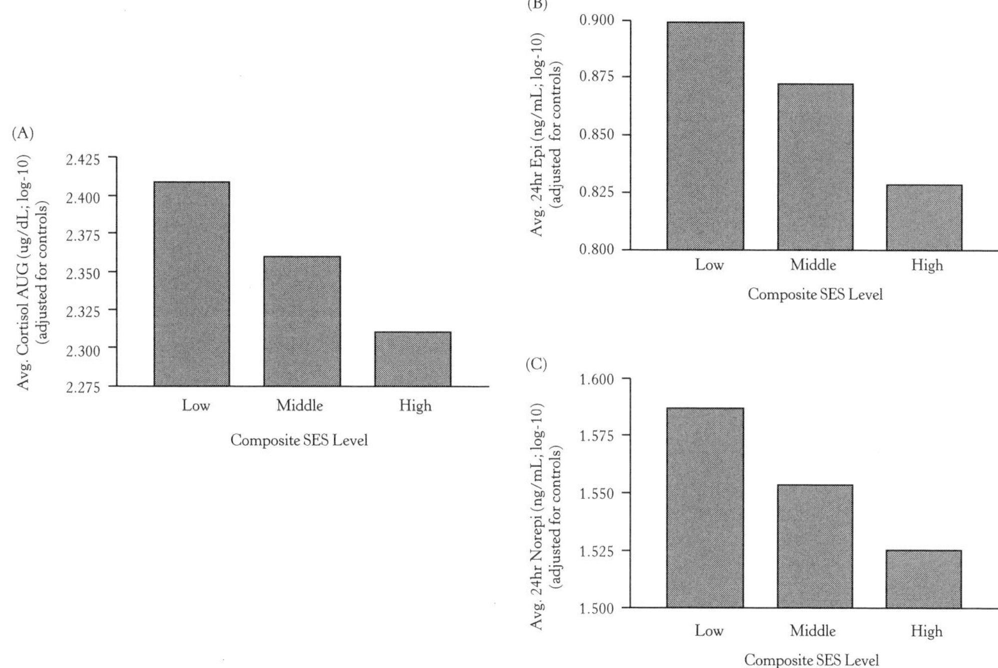

FIGURE 14.23: (A) Association between composite (income + education) SES and saliva cortisol (area under the curve) averaged across 3 days of sampling. The *y* axis range corresponds to the 25th and 75th percentiles. (B) Association between composite (income + education) SES and 24-hour urine epinephrine (B) and norepinephrine (C) averaged across 2 days of sampling. The y axis range corresponds to the 25th and 75th percentiles.

From Cohen et al. (2006a), with permission and courtesy of Lippincott, Williams and Wilkins Inc. and the American Psychosomatic Society.

In a third example, SES can alter the ways in which people interpret the environment. Job demands can have a dramatic effect to increase salivary cortisol at waking, particularly in low SES men and women (Figure 14.24; Kunz-Ebrecht et al. 2004). Curiously, low control over job demands resulted in higher saliva cortisol in high SES men over the day (Figure 14.24). Kunz-Ebrecht et al. (2004) conclude that while low SES tends to blunt the daily rhythm of cortisol, low control over job demands appear to have different effects.

What is striking about the data on SES in humans is how closely it matches much of the data presented in this book from free-living animals. Poor neighborhoods appear to induce increases in corticosteroids regardless of species. It is clear that what we see in free-living animals is not so different from what we see in humans, and visa versa. Much of what we learn about the impacts of human-induced rapid environmental change (HIRAC) in wild animals will likely be applicable to humans as well.

B. Refugees

The pictures of refugee exoduses in Rwanda and Bosnia (Figure 14.25) appear very similar to the movements of animals away from areas where severe perturbations of the environment have occurred. Are these phenomena analogous or even homologous? Are the mechanisms involved the same?

In refugees that had fled from East Germany to the West, plasma levels of cortisol overall tended to be lower than in controls, but this was not significant. However, blood cortisol levels were higher in a subgroup of refugees with major depressive disorder (Bauer et al. 1994). The authors concluded that the HPA axis may adapt during severe long-term stress. A group of refugees from Kosovo with post-traumatic stress disorder (PTSD) actually had lower salivary cortisol than refugees without, and compared to refugees in follow-up studies up to 1.5 years later (Roth et al. 2006). In recently settled refugees in Sweden, there was a high incidence of PTSD, and non-depressed individuals in this group had higher blood levels of

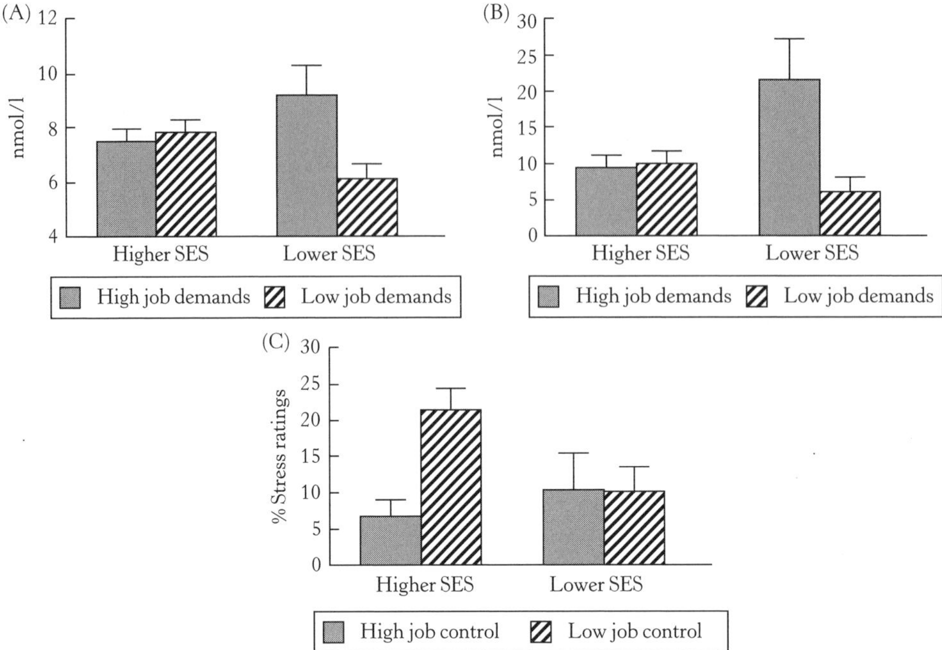

FIGURE 14.24: (A) Mean cortisol response to waking in relation to job demands in higher and lower SES participants. (B) Mean cortisol level over the working day in relation to job demands in higher and lower SES women. (C) Proportion of high stress ratings through the day in relation to job control in higher and lower SES participants. Error bars are s.e.m.

From Kunz-Ebrecht et al. (2004), with permission and courtesy of Pergamon Press.

dehydroepiandrosterone (DHEA) sulphate compared to non-depressed individuals without PTSD (Sondergaard et al. 2002). Plasma levels of cortisol tended to show the opposite trends, that is, higher in non-depressed PTSD refugees, and generally in people with distress compared to controls (Sondergaard and Theorell 2003).

Male genocide survivors from Rwanda, with and without PTSD, showed no differences in diurnal profiles of salivary cortisol (Eckart et al. 2009). There were no differences in plasma cortisol profiles in refugee children from Iraq who had been re-settled in Sweden (Söndergaard 2002). Displaced women in the Balkan region

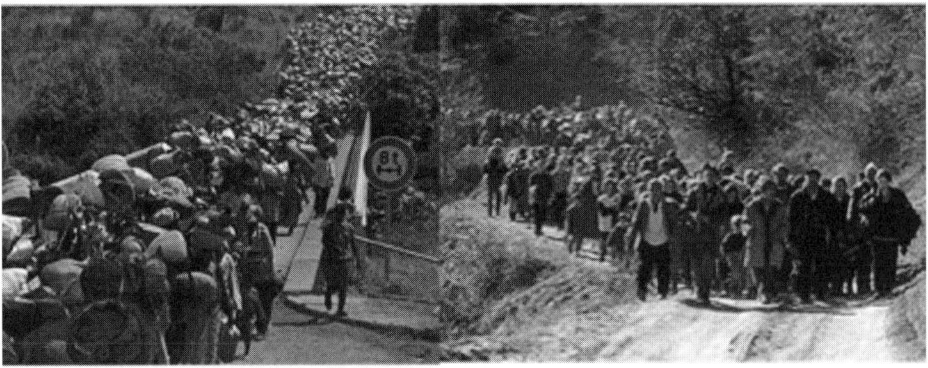

FIGURE 14.25: Refugees in Rwanda (left, courtesy of the British Broadcasting Corporation and the Balkans (right, courtesy of the Economist). Large numbers of people are forced by violence and/or climatic events to abandon their homes and villages, moving long distances to find shelter and safety. Are such movements similar to those seen in many animals in response to perturbations of the environment? Could control mechanisms also be similar?

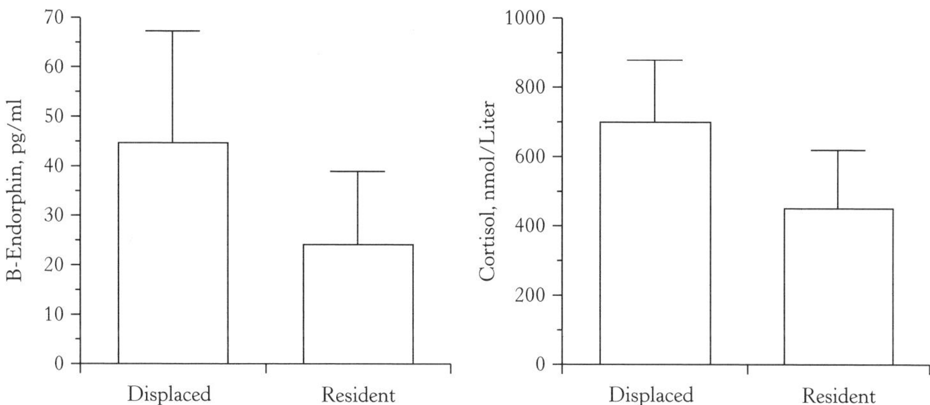

FIGURE 14.26: Plasma levels of beta-endorphins (left panel) and cortisol (right panel) in refugees (displaced column) from the Balkans compared with residents.

Drawn from data in Sabioncello et al. (2000), with permission and courtesy of the American Psychosomatic Society.

conflict showed higher serum cortisol, prolactin, and endorphin levels (Figure 14.26) than control women who were not displaced (Sabioncello et al. 2000). Refugees from Somalia who had taken residence in Canada and had experienced severe trauma were more susceptible to additional stressors of everyday life. The daily rise in salivary cortisol was exaggerated in trauma victims, but the HPA response to additional stressors was blunted, suggesting an impaired ability to respond to continuing day-to-day perturbations (Figure 14.27; Matheson et al. 2008). Child refugees from conflict areas such as the Balkans and Iraq often develop an apathetic or unconscious state, unable to communicate and even unable to eat. Plasma levels of cortisol at baseline generally were lower in these children compared to controls not exhibiting these behavioral symptoms (Söndergaard et al. 2012). This is consistent with chronic stress effects. Bosnian war refugees with PTSD had lower salivary corticosteroid levels and showed a reduced increase in corticosteroids post-waking that did control subjects not suffering from PTSD. This is also consistent with effects of chronic stress blunting the HPA axis responses to daily life and additional stressors (Figure 14.28;

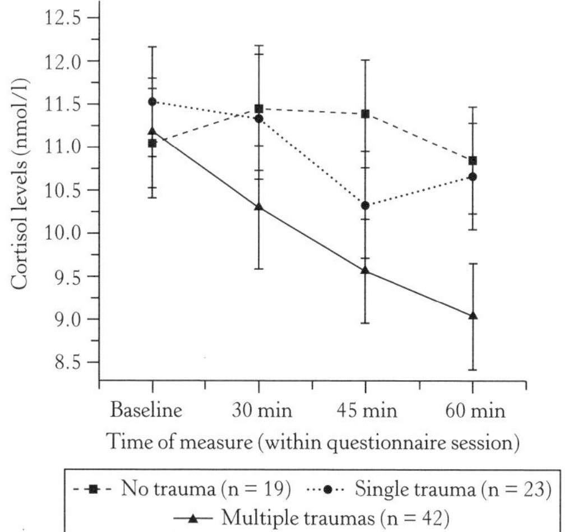

FIGURE 14.27: Absolute cortisol levels (nmol/l ±SE) over the course of the questionnaire session as a function of whether participants had not experienced a trauma, had experienced only one type of trauma, or had experienced multiple types of trauma. The questionaire addressed past traumatic experiences leading to their fleeing Somalia.

From Matheson et al. (2008), with permission and courtesy of Springer-Verlag.

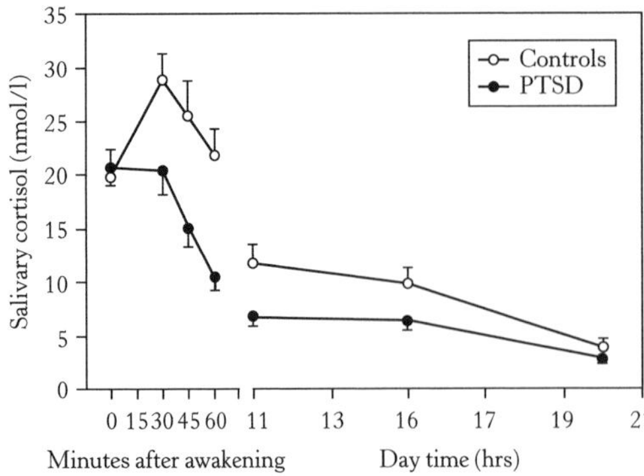

FIGURE 14.28: Cortisol response to awakening and short daytime cortisol levels in Bosnian war refugees with post-traumatic stress disorder (PTSD) and in control subjects.

From Rohleder et al. (2004), with permission and courtesy of Elsevier.

Rohleder et al. 2004). Cortisol levels in saliva of military personnel were generally lower in individuals that showed better military performance and fewer indications of PTSD (Morgan et al. 2004).

In a review and meta-analysis, Meewisse et al. (2007) found that while PTSD was generally accompanied by decreased responsiveness of the HPA axis to daily rhythms and stress, there are examples of increased cortisol or no change. Reasons for this could be many, but in general, studies on human refugees are always conducted after they have reached a haven, and data represent adapted or long-term situations. It is not surprising that correlations with cortisol and other stress hormones do not show consistent patterns. Samples would need to be collected during the traumatic events leading to the refugees actually leaving. This underscores how important it is to study free-living animal species under a variety of stressors (perturbations of the environment) to gain a true picture of how organisms actually respond during an unpredictable event. The basic biology of coping mechanisms remains to be explored in full depth.

VII. A FINAL WORD

As we discussed at the beginning of Chapter 1, stress has been an astonishingly successful concept in biology. It has revolutionized how many of us categorize our interactions with our physical and social environment. Stress has had a tremendous impact on clinical medicine, psychological health, social interactions, job satisfaction, and many other aspects of our lives. What we hope has become clear in this book is that stress is also an important organizing principle in understanding how wild animals cope in their natural environments.

When considering the scope of this book, it is amazing how much we already know about how wild animals respond physiologically, hormonally, and behaviorally to unanticipated changes in their environments. Each chapter in the second half of this book has explored these mechanisms in reference to stressors that animals routinely face. It is clear that there is considerable overlap in each of these systems, and in many ways the division of this book into these specific chapters is quite arbitrary. For example, an individual animal's developmental history (Chapter 11) will influence how it responds to inclement weather (Chapter 8), injury (Chapter 9), or human disturbance (Chapter 12). In turn, an individual's history with injury, sickness, and so on, can ultimately influence that individual's offspring's developmental trajectory. Unraveling this tangled web of causes, responses, impacts, accommodations, and modulations can be truly daunting. That we've made so much progress is very gratifying.

However, it is also clear that we have a tremendous amount still to learn. For example, refer again to Figure 14.4. In many ways this figure represents a central theme of this book. It shows, and in fact grossly simplifies, the incredible complexity of mechanisms involved in transducing an environmental signal into a coordinated response that allows an individual to enter an emergency life-history stage. Completely missing from Figure 14.4 are the higher brain functions that interpret whether a stimulus is indeed a stressor. We know that many of the steps enumerated in Figure 14.4 play vital roles in regulating stress responses. Other steps, however, are not so well studied. Much of the work over the next few decades should focus on some of these understudied steps. As more and better tools become available to field endocrinologists, progress on these problems should occur rapidly.

Next, we list what we consider the major unresolved challenges in stress physiology. Although the list is not exhaustive, we hope that it will help guide research in the future.

1. What is the source of individual variation?
    a. How heritable are stress responses?
    b. Do baselines and stress-induced increases vary independently?
    c. What is a stress phenotype?

   d. How plastic is that phenotype?
   e. Does the stress phenotype change predictably over the life span?
   f. Is there an individual benefit to this plasticity (i.e., fitness)?
2. What is the link between individual variation and vulnerability?
   a. How is this influenced by epigenetic mechanisms, developmental experience, maternal effects, and so on?
3. Scaling: How do you link subcellular/cellular responses to organism effects/responses?
   a. How do we incorporate variations in regulation of secretion, transport, and target cell responses?
4. Scaling: How do you link organism responses to population-level effects?
5. When does a beneficial short-term response become problematic chronic stress?
6. How do the three "arms" of the stress response—HPA, sympathetic, behavior—interact to form an integrated stress response?
   a. How does the immune system interact with these responses?
7. How do anthropogenic impacts alter stress physiology?
   a. Impacts of urbanization
   b. Impacts of global climate change
   c. Effects of invasive species
   d. Impacts of habitat degradation
   e. Integration of stress responses with biotic and abiotic environmental features
   f. Why do different populations respond differently? Is it phylogeny and/or adaptation?

Finally, we would like to leave the reader with a sense of why studying stress in wild animals is so important. We believe that there are two broad reasons. First, we anticipate a major benefit in gaining a fundamental understanding of how the stress response allows animals, including humans, to cope with adverse environmental stimuli. Ever since Selye (1946) proposed that the corticosteroids were primary mediators for the stress response, science has struggled to understand why these hormones were released. It has always struck us as odd that 70+ years later, we still really don't know something as fundamental as whether corticosteroid release during a stressor helps an animal survive or hastens that animal's demise. After all, once we discovered that diabetes was a disease related to insulin, we worked hard (and continue to work hard) to understand what insulin does under normal conditions. Why haven't we done the same for the corticosteroids? Chapter 3 presented a bit of the history of how science has swung back and forth in concluding whether corticosteroids are a net positive or negative in aiding survival. We know that corticosteroid excess can lead to disease, but why are corticosteroids released in the first place? Many recent biomedical studies have started to address this question, including showing that corticosteroids help alter behavior after trauma (Zohar et al. 2011), protect neurons during stress (Rao et al. 2012), help in learning (Liston et al. 2013), and help in regulating mitochondrial function (Du et al. 2009). However, when all is said and done, studies on modern Western humans, and the highly domesticated lab animal surrogates, are poorly positioned to answer this question. As we presented in Chapter 1, perhaps the four most important stressors for wild animals are inclement weather, attacks by predators, exposure to infectious disease, and famine. These stressors provided the selective pressure for the evolution of the stress response. Although these four stressors were undoubtedly major influences for our pre-modern ancestors as well, modern Western humans rarely face them. As a consequence, we are more likely to discover why corticosteroids are secreted during stress by studying wild animals still subjected to the selective pressures that selected for the vertebrate stress response.

The second major importance for continuing studies of stress in wild animals is that it will help us understand the impact of the Anthropocene. As discussed in Chapter 13, human-induced rapid environmental change (HIREC) is here. We cannot avoid it. The best we can do is understand how HIREC will affect different species and determine how we can ameliorate the impact. The stress physiology of wild species has an important role to play, but we are just beginning to understand the links between HIREC, stress responses, and population persistence. We anticipate that work on these problems will comprise a major, if not the majority, of effort in the field of endocrinology of stress in the foreseeable future. HIREC is shaping up to be the preeminent challenge for environmental scientists in the twenty-first century. An understanding of how the stress response helps affected individuals cope physiologically will form a major piece of the puzzle in deciding how humanity ought to respond.

REFERENCES

Able, K. P., Belthoff, J. R., 1998. Rapid 'evolution' of migratory behaviour in the introduced house finch of eastern North America. *Proc R Soc Lond B* 265, 2063–2071.

Addis, E. A., Davis, J. E., Miner, B. E., Wingfield, J. C., 2011. Variation in circulating corticosterone levels is associated with altitudinal range expansion in a passerine bird. *Oecologia* 167, 369–378.

Atwell, J. W., Cardoso, G. C., Whittaker, D. J., Campbell-Nelson, S., Robertson, K. W., Ketterson, E. D., 2012. Boldness behavior and stress physiology in a novel urban environment suggest rapid correlated evolutionary adaptation. *Behav Ecol* 23, 960–969.

Bauer, M., Priebe, S., Graf, K. J., Kurten, I., Baumgartner, A., 1994. Psychological and endocrine abnormalities in refugees from East Germany: Part II. Serum levels of cortisol, prolactin, luteinizing hormone, follicle stimulating hormone, and testosterone. *Psychiatry Res* 51, 75–85.

Baum, A., Garofalo, J. P., Yali, A.M., 1999. Socioeconomic status and chronic stress—Does stress account for SES effects on health? In: Adler, N. E., Marmot, M., McEwen, B., Stewart, J. (Eds.), *Socioeconomic status and health in industrial nations: Social, psychological, and biological pathways*, vol. 896. New York Acad Sciences, New York, pp. 131–144.

Berthold, P., 1995. Microevolution of migratory behavior illustrated by the blackcap Sylvia-atricapilla: 1993 Witherby-Lecture. *Bird Study* 42, 89–100.

Blanchard, B., 1941. The white-crowned sparrows (*Zonotrichia leucophrys*) of the Pacific seaboard: Environment and annual cycle. *Univ Calif Publ Zool* 46, 1–178.

Bókony, V., Lendvai, A. Z., Liker, A., Angelier, F., Wingfield, J. C., Chastel, O., 2009. Stress response and the value of reproduction: Are birds prudent parents? *Am Nat* 173, 589–598.

Bonier, F., Martin, P. R., Moore, I. T., Wingfield, J. C., 2009a. Do baseline glucocorticoids predict fitness? *Trends Ecol Evolu* 24, 634–642.

Bonier, F., Martin, P. R., Sheldon, K. S., Jensen, J. P., Foltz, S. L., Wingfield, J. C., 2007a. Sex-specific consequences of life in the city. *Behav Ecol* 18, 121–129.

Bonier, F., Martin, P. R., Wingfield, J. C., 2007b. Maternal corticosteroids influence primary offspring sex ratio in a free-ranging passerine bird. *Behav Ecol* 18, 1045–1050.

Bonier, F., Martin, P. R., Wingfield, J. C., 2007c. Urban birds have broader environmental tolerance. *Biol Lett* 3, 670–673.

Bonier, F., Moore, I. T., Martin, P. R., Robertson, R. J., 2009b. The relationship between fitness and baseline glucocorticoids in a passerine bird. *Gen Comp Endocrinol* 163, 208–213.

Breuner, C. W., Orchinik, M., 2002. Beyond carrier proteins: plasma binding proteins as mediators of corticosteroid action in vertebrates. *J Endocrinol* 175, 99–112.

Breuner, C. W., Patterson, S. H., Hahn, T. P., 2008. In search of relationships between the acute adrenocortical response and fitness. *Gen Comp Endocrinol* 157, 288–295.

Buck, C. L., O'Reilly, K. A., Kildaw, S. D., 2007. Interannual variability of Black-legged Kittiwake productivity is reflected in baseline plasma corticosterone. *Gen Comp Endocrinol* 150, 430–436.

Busch, D. S., Hayward, L. S., 2009. Stress in a conservation context: A discussion of glucocorticoid actions and how levels change with conservation-relevant variables. *Biol Conserv* 142, 2844–2853.

Cohen, A. A., Martin, L. B., Wingfield, J. C., McWilliams, S. R., Dunne, J. A., 2012. Physiological regulatory networks: Ecological roles and evolutionary constraints. *Trends Ecology Evol* 27, 428–435.

Cohen, S., Doyle, W. J., Baum, A., 2006a. Socioeconomic status is associated with stress hormones. *Psychosom Med* 68, 414–420.

Cohen, S., Schwartz, J. E., Epel, E., Kirschbaum, C., Sidney, S., Seeman, T., 2006b. Socioeconomic status, race, and diurnal cortisol decline in the Coronary Artery Risk Development in Young Adults (CARDIA) Study. *Psychosom Med* 68, 41–50.

Costa, D. P., 2007. A conceptual model of the variation in parental attendance in response to environmental fluctuation: foraging energetics of lactating sea lions and fur seals. Aquat Conserv 17, S44–S52.

Costa, D. P., 2012. A bioenergetics approach to developing a population consequences of acoustic disturbance model. In: Popper, A. N., Hawkins, A. (Eds.), *The effects of noise on aquatic life*, vol. 730, *Advances in experimental medicine and biology*. Springer, Berlin, pp. 423–426.

Cote, J., Clobert, J., Meylan, S., Fitze, P.S., 2006. Experimental enhancement of corticosterone levels positively affects subsequent male survival. *Horm Behav* 49, 320–327.

Du, J., Wang, Y., Hunter, R., Wei, Y. L., Blumenthal, R., Falke, C., Khairova, R., Zhou, R. L., Yuan, P. X., Machado-Vieira, R., McEwen, B. S., Manji, H. K., 2009. Dynamic regulation of mitochondrial function by glucocorticoids. *Proc Natl Acad Sci USA* 106, 3543–3548.

Duckworth, R. A., 2009. Maternal effects and range expansion: A key factor in a dynamic process? *Philos Trans R Soc B* 364, 1075–1086.

Duckworth, R. A., Badyaev, A. V., 2007. Coupling of dispersal and aggression facilitates the rapid range expansion of a passerine bird. *Proc Natl Acad Sci USA* 104, 15017-15022.

Dufty, A. M., Clobert, J., Moller, A. P., 2002. Hormones, developmental plasticity and adaptation. *Trends Ecol Evol* 17, 190–196.

Eckart, C., Engler, H., Riether, C., Kolassa, S., Elbert, T., Kolassa, I. T., 2009. No PTSD-related differences in diurnal cortisol profiles of genocide survivors. *Psychoneuroendocrinology* 34, 523–531.

Ghalambor, C. K., Huey, R. B., Martin, P. R., Tewksbury, J. J., Wang, G., 2006. Are mountain passes higher in the tropics? Janzen's hypothesis revisited. *Integ Comp Biol* 46, 5–17.

Hau, M., Wingfield, J. C., 2011. Hormonally-regulated trade-offs: evolutionary variability and phenotypic plasticity in testosterone signaling pathways. In: Flatt, T., Heyland, A. (Eds.), *Mechanisms of life history evolution: The genetics and physiology of life history traits and trade-offs*, Oxford University Press, Oxford, pp. 349–361.

Holmes, M.C., Kotelevtsev, Y., Mullins, J. J., Seckl, J.R., 2001. Phenotypic analysis of mice bearing targeted deletions of 11 beta-hydroxysteroid dehydrogenases 1 and 2 genes. *Mol Cell Endocrinol* 171, 15–20.

Kitaysky, A.S., Wingfield, J.C., Piatt, J.F., 1999. Dynamics of food availability, body condition and physiological stress response in breeding Black-legged Kittiwakes. Func Ecol 13, 577–584.

Kunz-Ebrecht, S. R., Kirschbaum, C., Steptoe, A., 2004. Work stress, socioeconomic status and neuroendocrine activation over the working day. *Soc Sci Med* 58, 1523–1530.

Lancaster, L. T., Hazard, L. C., Clobert, J., Sinervo, B. R., 2008. Corticosterone manipulation reveals differences in hierarchical organization of multidimensional reproductive trade-offs in r-strategist and K-strategist females. *J Evol Biol* 21, 556–565.

Lanctot, R. B., Hatch, S. A., Gill, V. A., Eens, M., 2003. Are corticosterone levels a good indicator of food availability and reproductive performance in a kittiwake colony? *Horm Behav* 43, 489–502.

Liston, C., Cichon, J. M., Jeanneteau, F., Jia, Z. P., Chao, M. V., Gan, W. B., 2013. Circadian glucocorticoid oscillations promote learning-dependent synapse formation and maintenance. *Nature Neurosci* 16, 698.

Lupien, S. J., King, S., Meaney, M. J., McEwen, B. S., 2000. Child's stress hormone levels correlate with mother's socioeconomic status and depressive state. *Biol Psych* 48, 976–980.

Lupien, S. J., King, S., Meaney, M. J., McEwen, B. S., 2001. Can poverty get under your skin? Basal cortisol levels and cognitive function in children from low and high socioeconomic status. *Devel Psychopathol* 13, 653–676.

Machmer, M. M., Ydenberg, R. C., 1990. Weather and osprey foraging energetics *Can J Zool* 68, 40–43.

Magee, S. E., Neff, B. D., Knapp, R., 2006. Plasma levels of androgens and cortisol in relation to breeding behavior in parental male bluegill sunfish, *Lepomis macrochirus*. *Horm Behav* 49, 598–609.

Martin, L. B., Liebl, A. L., Trotter, J. H., Richards, C. L., McCoy, K., McCoy, M. W., 2011. Integrator networks: Illuminating the black box linking genotype and phenotype. *Integ Comp Biol* 51, 514–527.

Matheson, K., Jorden, S., Anisman, H., 2008. Relations between trauma experiences and psychological, physical and neuroendocrine functioning among Somali refugees: Mediating role of coping with acculturation stressors. *J Immigrant Minority Health* 10, 291–304.

McEwen, B. S., 2000. Allostasis and allostatic load: Implications for neuropsychopharmacology. *Neuropsychopharmacology* 22, 108–124.

McEwen, B. S., Wingfield, J. C., 2003. The concept of allostasis in biology and biomedicine. *Horm Behav* 43, 2–15.

Meewisse, M. L., Reitsma, J. B., De Vries, G. J., Gersons, B. P. R., Olff, M., 2007. Cortisol and post-traumatic stress disorder in adults—Systematic review and meta-analysis. *Brit J Psychiatry* 191, 387–392.

Meylan,S.,Clobert,J.,2005.Iscorticosterone-mediated phenotype development adaptive? Maternal corticosterone treatment enhances survival in male lizards. *Horm Behav* 48, 44–52.

Mila, B., McCormack, J. E., Castaneda, G., Wayne, R. K., Smith, T. B., 2007. Recent postglacial range expansion drives the rapid diversification of a songbird lineage in the genus Junco. *Proc R Soc Lond B* 274, 2653–2660.

Morgan, C.A., Southwick, S., Hazlett, G., Rasmusson, A., Hoyt, G., Zimolo, Z., Charney, D., 2004. Relationships among plasma dehydroepiandrosterone sulfate and cortisol levels, symptoms of dissociation, and objective performance in humans exposed to acute stress. *Arch Gen Psychiatry* 61, 819–825.

Nelson, R. J., 2011. *An introduction to behavioral endocrinology*, 4th Edition. Sinauer Associates, Sunderland, MA.

O'Connor, C. M., Gilmour, K. M., Arlinghaus, R., Hasler, C. T., Philipp, D. P., Cooke, S. J., 2010. seasonal carryover effects following the administration of cortisol to a wild teleost fish. *Physiol Biochem Zool* 83, 950–957.

Ouyang, J. Q., Sharp, P. J., Dawson, A., Quetting, M., Hau, M., 2011. Hormone levels predict individual differences in reproductive success in a passerine bird. *Proc R Soc Lond B* 278, 2537–2545.

Piersma, T., van Gils, J.A., 2011. *The flexible phenotype: A body-centred integration of ecology, physiology, and behavior.* Oxford University Press, Oxford.

Pride, R. E., 2005. High faecal glucocorticoid levels predict mortality in ring-tailed lemurs (*Lemur catta*). *Biol Lett* 1, 60.

Pulido, F., Berthold, P., 2010. Current selection for lower migratory activity will drive the evolution of residency in a migratory bird population. *Proc Natl Acad Sci USA* 107, 7341-7346.

Rao, R. P., Anilkumar, S., McEwen, B. S., Chattarji, S., 2012. Glucocorticoids protect against the delayed behavioral and cellular effects of acute stress on the amygdala. *Biol Psych* 72, 466–475.

Ricklefs, R. E., Wikelski, M., 2002. The physiology/life-history nexus. *Trends Ecol Evol* 17, 462–468.

Rohleder, N., Joksimovic, L., Wolf, J. M., Kirschbaum, C., 2004. Hypocortisolism and increased glucocorticoid sensitivity of pro-inflammatory cytokine production in Bosnian war refugees with posttraumatic stress disorder. *Biol Psych* 55, 745–751.

Roth, G., Ekbad, S., Agren, H., 2006. A longitudinal study of PTSD in a sample of adult mass-evacuated Kosovars, some of whom returned to their home country. *Eur Psychiatry* 21, 152–159.

Rothstein, S. I., Verner, J., Stevens, E., 1980. Range expansion and diurnal changes in dispersion of the brown-headed cowbird in the Sierra Nevada. *Auk* 97, 253–267.

Sabioncello, A., Kocijan-Hercigonja, D., Rabatic, S., Tomasic, J., Jeren, T., Matijevic, L., Rijavec, M., Dekaris, D., 2000. Immune, endocrine, and psychological responses in civilians displaced by war. *Psychosom Med* 62, 502–508.

Sapolsky, R. M., Romero, L. M., Munck, A. U., 2000. How do glucocorticoids influence stress-responses? Integrating permissive, suppressive, stimulatory, and preparative actions. *Endocr Rev* 21, 55–89.

Schmidt, K. L., Pradhan, D. S., Shah, A. H., Charlier, T. D., Chin, E. H., Soma, K. K., 2008. Neurosteroids, immunosteroids, and the Balkanization of endocrinology. *Gen Comp Endocrinol* 157, 266–274.

Selye, H., 1946. The general adaptation syndrome and the diseases of adaptation. *J Clin Endocrinol* 6, 117–230.

Sih, A., 2013. Understanding variation in behavioural responses to human-induced rapid environmental change: a conceptual overview. *Anim Behav* 85, 1077–1088.

Silverin, B., 1998. Territorial behavioural and hormones of pied flycatchers in optimal and suboptimal habitats. *Anim Behav* 56, 811.

Smith, M. T., Rappaport, S. M., 2009. Building Exposure Biology Centers to Put the E into "G x E" Interaction Studies. *Environ Health Perspect* 117, A334–A335.

Söndergaard, H. P., 2002. *Post-traumatic stress disorder and life events among recently settled refugees.* Doctor of Medical Science Thesis, Karolinska Institute, Stockholm, Sweden.

Söndergaard, H. P., Hansson, L. O., Theorell, T., 2002. Elevated blood levels of dehydroepiandrosterone sulphate vary with symptom load in posttraumatic stress disorder: Findings from a longitudinal study of refugees in Sweden. *Psychother Psychosom* 71, 298–303.

Söndergaard, H. P., Kushnir, M. M., Aronsson, B., Sandstedt, P., Bergquist, J., 2012. Patterns of endogenous steroids in apathetic refugee children are compatible with long-term stress. *BMC Res Notes* 5, 186.

Söndergaard, H. P., Theorell, T., 2003. A longitudinal study of hormonal reactions accompanying life events in recently resettled refugees. *Psychother Psychosom* 72, 49–58.

Taves, M. D., Gomez-Sanchez, C. E., Soma, K. K., 2011a. Extra-adrenal glucocorticoids and mineralocorticoids: Evidence for local synthesis, regulation, and function. *Am J Physiol* 301, E11–E24.

Taves, M. D., Ma, C., Heimovics, S. A., Saldanha, C. J., Soma, K. K., 2011b. Measurement of steroid concentrations in brain tissue: methodological considerations. *Front Endocrin* 2, 1–13.

Thelin, G., Pike, R., 1991. Landforms of the conterminous United States: A digital scaled relief portrayal. Miscellaneous Investigation, USGS, Renton, VA.

Visser, M. E., Both, C., Lambrechts, M. M., 2006. Global climate change leads to mistimed avian reproduction. In: Møller, A. P., Fielder, W., Berthold, P. (Eds.), *Birds and global climate change*, Elsevier, Amsterdam, pp. 89–110.

Wild, C. P., 2005. Complementing the genome with an "exposome": The outstanding challenge of environmental exposure measurement in molecular epidemiology. *Cancer Epidem Biomar Prev* 14, 1847–1850.

Williams, T. D., 2008. Individual variation in endocrine systems: Moving beyond the "tyranny of the Golden Mean." *Phil Trans R Soc B* 363, 1687–1698.

Wingfield, J. C., 2006. Communicative behaviors, hormone-behavior interactions, and reproduction in vertebrates. In: Neill, J. D. (Ed.), *Physiology of reproduction*, Academic Press, New York, pp. 1995–2040.

Wingfield, J. C., 2008. Comparative endocrinology, environment and global change. *Gen Comp Endocrinol* 157, 207–216.

Wingfield, J. C., 2012. Regulatory mechanisms that underlie phenology, behavior, and coping with environmental perturbations: An alternative look at biodiversity. *Auk* 129, 1–7.

Wingfield, J. C., 2013. The comparative biology of environmental stress: Behavioural endocrinology and variation in ability to cope with novel, changing environments. *Anim Behav* 85, 1127–1133.

Wingfield, J. C., Kelley, J. P., Angelier, F., 2011a. What are extreme environmental conditions and how do organisms cope with them? *Curr Zool* 57, 363–374.

Wingfield, J. C., Kelley, J. P., Angelier, F., Chastel, O., Lei, F. M., Lynn, S. E., Miner, B., Davis, J. E., Li, D. M., Wang, G., 2011b. Organism-environment interactions in a changing world: a mechanistic approach. *J Ornithol* 152, 279–288.

Wingfield, J. C., Maney, D. L., Breuner, C. W., Jacobs, J. D., Lynn, S., Ramenofsky, M., Richardson, R. D., 1998. Ecological bases of hormone-behavior interactions: The "emergency life history stage." *Integ Comp Biol* 38, 191.

Wingfield, J. C., Mukai, M., 2009. Endocrine disruption in the context of life cycles: Perception and transduction of environmental cues. *Gen Comp Endocrinol* 163, 92–96.

Wingfield, J. C., Ramenofsky, M., 1999. Hormones and the behavioral ecology of stress. In: Balm, P. H. M. (Ed.), *Stress Physiology in Animals*, Sheffield Academic Press, Sheffield, U.K., pp. 1–51.

Wingfield, J. C., Romero, L. M., 2001. Adrenocortical responses to stress and their modulation in free-living vertebrates. In: McEwen, B. S., Goodman, H. M. (Eds.), *Handbook of physiology*; Section 7: *The endocrine system*; Vol. IV: *Coping with the environment: Neural and endocrine mechanisms*. Oxford University Press, New York, pp. 211–234.

Wingfield, J. C., Sapolsky, R. M., 2003. Reproduction and resistance to stress: When and how. *J Neuroendocrinol* 15, 711.

Yeh, P. J., Price, T. D., 2004. Adaptive phenotypic plasticity and the successful colonization of a novel environment. *Am Nat* 164, 531–542.

Zohar, J., Yahalom, H., Kozlovsky, N., Cwikel-Hamzany, S., Matar, M. A., Kaplan, Z., Yehuda, R., Cohen, H., 2011. High dose hydrocortisone immediately after trauma may alter the trajectory of PTSD: Interplay between clinical and animal studies. *Eur Neuropsychopharmacology* 21, 796–809.

GLOSSARY OF SPECIES NAMES

English Name	Latin Name
Abert's towhee	*Piplo aberti*
Adélie penguin	*Pygoscelis adeliei*
African elephant	*Loxodonta africana*
Alaska brown bear	*Ursus arctos*
albatross	*Diomedea* sp
alpine swift	*Apus melba*
American alligator	*Alligator mississippiensis*
American goldfinch	*Carduelis tristis*
American kestrel	*Falco sparverius*
American opossum	*Didelphis marsupialis*
American pipit	*Anthus spinoletta*
American redstart	*Setophaga ruticilla*
American toad	*Bufo americanus*
Arctic char	*Salvelinus alpinus*
Arctic fox	*Alopex lagopus*
Arctic ground squirrel	*Spermophilus parryii*
Asian elephant	*Elephas maximus*
Atlantic croaker	*Micropogonias undulatus*
Atlantic salmon	*Salmo salar*
Australian blue-tongued skink	*Tiliqua scincoides*
Australian sub-alpine skink	*Bassiana duperreyi*
baboon	*Papio cyanocephalus*
bald eagle	*Haliaeetus leucocephalus*
bank vole	*Clethrionomys glareolus*
barbell	*Barbus barbus*
barn swallow	*Hirundo rustica*
barn owl	*Tyto alba*
bar-tailed godwit	*Limosa lapponic*
beaver	*Castor canadensis*
Belding's ground squirrel	*Spermophilus beldingi*
bell miner	*Manorina melanophrys*
beluga whale	*Delphinapterus leucas*
black-bellied plover	*Pluvialis squatorola*
black-browed albatross	*Thallasarche melanophris*
black-capped chickadee	*Poecile atricapilla*
black-capped vireo	*Vireo atricapilla*
black duck	*Anas rubripes*

black grouse	*Tetrao tetrix*
black howler monkey	*Alouatta pigra*
black kite	*Milvus nigrans*
black-legged kittiwake	*Rissa tridactyla*
black-tailed deer	*Odocoileus hemionus*
black tailed gnatcatcher	*Polioptila melanura*
black-throated sparrow	*Amphispiza bilineata*
blind mole-rat	*Spalax ehrenbergi*
blue-footed boobies	*Sula nebouxi*
bluegill sunfish	*Lepomis macrochirus*
blue gourami	*Trichogaster trichopterus*
blue mao mao	*Scorpis violaceus*
blue monkey	*Cercopithecus mitis*
blue tit	*Parus caeruleus*
bobwhite quail	*Colinus virginianus*
bonobo	*Pan paniscus*
boreal chickadee	*Poecile hudsonica*
boreal toad	*Bufo boreas*
bottlenose dolphin	*Tursiops truncatus*
box turtle	*Terrapene ornata*
brambling	*Fringilla montifringilla*
Brandt's vole	*Lasiopodomys brandtii*
brook trout	*Salvelinus fontinalis*
brown-headed cowbird	*Molothrus ater*
brown lemming	*Lemmus trimucronatus*
brown tree snake	*Boiga irregularis*
brown trout	*Salmo trutta*
bullfrog	*Rana catesbeiana*
bushtit	*Psaltriparus minmus*
bush warbler	*Cettia diphone*
cactus wren	*Campylorhynchus brunneicapillus*
California sea lion	*Zalophus californianus*
camel	*Camelus dromadarius*
Canadian lynx	*Lynx canadensis*
canary	*Serinus canaria*
cane toad	*Rhinella marina*
capercaillie	*Tetrao urogallus*
caribou	*Rangifer tarandus*
Carolina chickadee	*Poecile carolinensis*
carp	*Cyprinus carpio*
Cascades frog	*Rana cascadae*
cattle egrets	*Bubulcus ibis*
chacma baboon	*Papio hamadryas*
chaffinch	*Fringilla coelebs*
channel catfish	*Ictalurus punctatus*
chestnut-backed chickadee	*Poecile rufescens*
chiffchaff	*Phylloscopus collybita*
chimpanzee	*Pan troglodytes*
chinook salmon	*Oneorhynchus tshawytscha*
chub	*Leuciscus cephalus*
chukar	*Alectoris chukar*
cliff swallow	*Petrochelidon pyrrhonota*
coal tit	*Parus ater*
coho salmon	*Oncorhynchus kisutch*

collared dove	*Streptopelia decaocto*
collared flycatcher	*Ficedula albicollis*
collared lizard	*Crotaphytus nebrius*
common blackbird	*Turdus merula*
common diving petrel	*Pelecanoides urinatrix*
common eider	*Somateria mollissima*
common hamster	*Cricetus cricetus*
common murre	*Uria aalge*
common nighthawk	Chordeiles minor
common tern	*Sterna hirundo*
Cory's shearwater	*Calonectris diomedea*
cougar	*Felis concolor*
coyote	*Canis latrans*
crested auklet	*Aethia cristatella*
crossbill	*Loxia spp*
crow	*Corvus brachyrhynchos*
curve-billed thrasher	*Toxostoma curvirostra*
cutthroat trout	*Onchorhynchus clarkii*
damselfish	*Pomacentrus amboinensis*
dark-eyed junco	*Junco hyemalis*
degu	*Octodon degu*
desert iguana	*Dipsosaurus dorsalis*
desert tortoises	*Gopherus agassizii*
dollyvarden	*Salvelinus malma*
downy woodpecker	*Picoides pubescens*
dusky flycatcher	*Empidonax oberholseri*
dwarf mongoose	*Helogale parvula*
eastern bluebird	*Sialia sialis*
eastern hellbender	*Cryptobranchus alleganiensis*
eastern fence lizard	*Sceloporus undulatus*
elk	*Cervus elephus*
emperor penguin	*Aptenodytes forsteri*
Eurasian tree creeper	*Certhia familiaris*
Eurasian water vole	*Arvicola amphibious*
European badger	*Meles meles*
European blackbird	*Turdus merula*
European carp	*Cyprinus carpio*
European hare	*Lepus europaeus*
European pine marten	*Martes martes*
European rabbit	*Oryctolagus cuniculus*
European sand lizard	*Lacerta agilis*
European sparrow hawk	*Accipiter nisus*
European starling	*Sturnus vulgaris*
European stonechat	*Saxicola torquata rubicola*
Fijian ground frog	*Platymantis vitiana*
fiscal shrike	*Lanius collaris*
flightless cormorant	*Phalacrocorax harrisi*
Florida manatee	*Trichechus manatus latirostris*
Florida scrub jay	*Aphelocoma coeruleus*
flounder	*Paralichthys olivaceus*
forest elephant	*Loxodonta africana cyclotis*
freckled nightjar	Caprimulgus tristigma
fur seal	*Arctocephalus tropicalis*

Galapagos dove	*Zenaida galapagoensis*
Galapagos finch	*Geospiza* sp.
Galapagos marine iguana	*Amblyrhynchus cristatus*
Galapagos mockingbird	*Nesomimus parvulus*
Galapagos penguin	*Spheniscus mediculus*
garden warbler	*Sylvia borin*
garter snake	*Thamnophis sirtalis*
gecko	*Hoplodactylus maculatus*
gelada baboon	*Theropithecus gelada*
gentoo penguin	*Pygoscelis papua*
giant kokopu	*Galaxias argenteus*
giant panda	*Ailuropoda melanoleuca*
gilthead sea bream	*Sparus aurata*
glass eel	*Anguilla anguilla*
glaucous gull	*Larus hyperboreus*
golden-crowned sparrow	*Zonotrichia atricapilla*
golden hamster	*Mesocricetus auratus*
golden-mantled ground squirrel	*Spermophilus saturatus*
gopher tortoise	*Gopherus polyphemus*
Gouldian finch	*Erythrura gouldiae*
great bustard	*Otis tarda*
great frigate bird	*Fregatta minor*
great gerbil	*Rhombomys opimus*
great knot	*Calidris tenuirostris*
great spotted woodpecker	*Dendrocopus major*
great tit	*Parus major*
green toad	*Bufo viridis*
green turtle	*Chelonia mydas*
grey-faced petrel	*Pterodroma macroptera gouldi*
greylag goose	*Anser anser*
grizzly bear	*Ursus arctos*
grouse	Aves, Tetraonidae
Gulf toadfish	*Opsanus beta*
Gunther's vole	*Microtus socialis*
hamadryas baboon	*Papio hamadryas*
harlequin duck	*Histrionicus histrionicus*
Harris' sparrows	*Zonotrichia querula*
hen harrier	*Circus cyaneus*
hermit thrush	*Catharus guttatus*
hoatzin	*Opisthocomus hoazin*
house mouse	*Mus musculus*
house sparrow	*Passer domesticus*
Humboldt penguin	*Spheniscus humboldti*
iguana	*Iguana iguana*
Inca dove	*Scardafella inca*
jackdaw	*Corvus monedula*
Japanese eel	*Anguilla japonica*
Japanese quail	*Coturnix coturnix japonica*
Kemp's ridley sea turtle	*Lepidochelys kempii*
king penguin	*Aptenodytes patagonicus*
kokanee salmon	*Oncorhynchus nerka kennerlyi*
lake trout	*Salmo trutta*
Lapland longspur	*Calcarius lapponicus*

largemouth bass	*Micropterus salmoides*
Laysan albatross	*Phoebastria immutabilis*
Leach's petrel	*Oceanodroma leucorhoa*
leopard frog	*Rana pipiens*
Lingcod	*Ophiodon elongatus*
little auk	*Alle alle*
little blue penguin	*Eudyptula minor*
lizard	*Lacerta vivipara*
loggerhead turtle	*Caretta caretta*
Magellanic penguin	*Spheniscus magellanicus*
mallard	*Anas platyrhynchos*
marmoset	*Callithrix jacchus*
marsh tit	*Parus palustris*
marten	*Martes martes*
meadow vole	*Microtus pensylvanicus*
meerkat	*Suricata suricatta*
mountain bluebird	*Sialia currucoides*
mountain chickadee	*Poecile gambeli*
mountain spiny lizard	*Sceloporus jarrovi and S. graciosus*
mountain whitefish	*Prosopium williamsoni*
mourning dove	*Zenaida macroura*
mudpuppy	*Necturus maculosus*
musk ox	*Ovibos moschatus*
Nazca boobie	*Sula granti*
New Zealand white rabbit	*Oryctolagus cuniculus*
North Atlantic right whale	*Eubalaena glacialis*
northern elephant seal	*Mirounga angustirostris*
northern giant petrel	*Macronectes halli*
Nutcracker	*Nucifraga caryocatactes*
olive baboon	*Papio anubis*
osprey	*Pandion haliatus*
owlet-nightjar	Aegotheles cristatus
oystercatcher	*Haematopus ostralegus*
Pacific treefrog	*Hyla regilla*
parrotfish	*Sparisoma* and *Scarus* sp.
peahen	*Pavo cristatus*
pectoral sandpiper	*Calidris melanotos*
pied flycatcher	*Ficedula hypoleuca*
pigeon	*Columba livia*
pine siskin	*Carduelis pinus*
pintail	*Anas acuta*
poorwill	Phalaenoptilus nuttalli
prairie vole	*Microtus ochrogaster*
pronghorn antelope	*Antilocapra americana*
Puerto Rican tody	*Todus mexicanus*
quoll	*Dasyurus hallucatus*
racoon dog	*Nyctereutes procyonoides*
raven	*Corvus corax*
rainbow trout	*Oncorhynchus mykiss*
red deer	*Cervus elaphus*
red-footed boobie	*Sula sula*
red fox	*Vulpes vulpes*
red knot	*Calidris canutus*

red-legged kittiwake	*Rissa brevirostris*
red-legged partridge	*Alectoris rufa*
red phalarope	*Phalaropus lobatus*
redpoll	*Carduelis flammea*
red porgy	*Pagrus pagrus*
redshank	*Tringa tetanus*
red-sided garter snake	*Thamnophis sirtalis parietalis*
reindeer	*Rangifer tarandus tarandus*
rhesus macaque	*Macaca mulatta*
rhinoceros auklet	*Cerorhinca monocerata*
ring dove	*Streptopelia risoria*
ring-tailed lemur	*Lemur catta*
river otter	*Luta lutra*
rockhopper penguin	*Eudyptes chrysocome*
rock ptarmigan	*Lagopus mutus*
roe deer	*Capreolus capreolus*
rough-skinned newt	*Taricha torosa*
royal penguin	*Eudyptes schlegeli*
rufous hummingbird	*Selasphorus rufus*
sage grouse	*Centrocercus urophasianus*
Sandwich tern	*Sterna sandvicensis*
savannah sparrow	*Passerculus sandvichensis*
semi-palmated sandpiper	*Calidris pusilla*
Siberian hamster	*Phodopus sungorus*
Siberian tit	*Parus cinctus*
side-blotched lizard	*Uta stansburiana*
sifaka	*Propithecus verreauxi*
silver fox	*Vulpes fulvus*
snow bunting	*Plectrophenax nivalis*
snow petrel	*Pagodroma nivea*
snowshoe hare	*Lepus americanus*
snowy owl	*Nyctea scandiaca*
sociable weaver	*Philetairus socius*
sockeye salmon	*Oncorhynchus nerka*
song sparrow	*Melospiza melodia*
song wren	*Cyphorhinus phaeocephalus*
southern elephant seal	*Mirounga leonine*
southern toad	*Bufo terrestris*
speckled dace	*Rhinichthys osculus*
sperm whale	*Physeter macrocephalus*
spiny mouse	*Acomys cahirinus*
spotted hyena	*Crocuta crocuta*
spotted owl	*Strix occidentalis*
spotted salamander	*Ambystoma maculatum*
spotfin chub	*Erimonax monachus*
Steller's sea lion	*Eumetopias jubatus*
stonechat	*Saxicola torquata axillaris*
sucker	*Catostomus* sp
striped bass	*Morone saxatalis*
sunshine bass	*Morone* sp.
superb starling	*Lamprotornis superbus*
tamar wallaby	*Macropus eugenii*
Tengmalm's owl	*Aegolius funereus*

tawny frogmouth	Podargus strigoides
tawny owl	*Strix aluco*
Texas toad	*Bufo speciosus*
thick-billed murre	*Uria lomvia*
thin-billed prion	*Pachyptila belcheri*
tiger shark	*Galeocerdo cuvier*
tilapia	*Oreochromis mossambicus*
toad	*Bufo arenarum* and *Bufo paracnemis*
treecreeper	*Certhia familiaris*
tree lizard	*Urosaurus ornatus*
tree sparrow	*Passer montanus*
tree swallow	*Tachycineta bicolor*
Trinidadian guppy	*Poecilia reticulata*
Tuatara	*Sphenodon punctatus*
tufted puffin	*Fratercula cirrhata*
turkey	*Melagris gallapavo*
verdin	*Auriparus flaviceps*
vole	*Microtus* sp.
walleye	*Stizostedion vitreum*
wandering albatross	*Diomedea exulans*
weasel	*Mustella nivalis*
western bluebird	*Sialia mexicana*
western fence lizard	*Sceloporus occidentalis*
western sandpiper	*Calidris mauri*
western screech-owl	*Otus asio* and *O. kennicottii*
western scrub-jay	*Aphelocoma californica*
western spadefoot toad	*Scaphiopus hammondi*
whip-poor-will	Chordeiles vociferous
white-breasted nuthatch	*Sitta carolinensis*
white-browed sparrow weaver	*Plocepasser mahali*
white-crowned sparrow	*Zonotrichia leucophrys*
white-crowned sparrow, Gambel's	*Zonotrichia leucophrys gambelii*
white-crowned sparrow, mountain	*Zonotrichia leucophrys oriantha*
white-crowned sparrow, Nuttall's	*Zonotrichia leucophrys nuttalli*
white-crowned sparrow, Puget Sound	*Zonotrichia leucophrys pugetensis*
white-eyed vireo	*Vireo griseus*
white-faced capuchin	*Cebus capuchinus*
white-tailed deer	*Odocoileus virginianus*
white ibis	*Eudocimus albus*
white stork	*Ciconia ciconia*
white sturgeon	*Accipenser transmontanus*
white sucker	*Catostomus commersonii*
white-tailed ptarmigan	*Lagopus leucurus*
whitetail shiners	*Cyprinella galatura*
white-throated sparrow	*Zonotrichia albicollis*
whooping crane	*Grus americana*
wild dog	*Lycaon pictus*
willow ptarmigan	*Lagopus lagopus*
willow tit	Parus montanus
willow warbler	*Phylloscopus trochilus*
Wilson's storm-petrel	*Oceanites oceanicus*
winter flounder	*Pseudopleuronectes americanus*
wolf	*Canis lupus*

woodchuck	*Marmota monax*
yellow-bellied marmot	*Marmota flaviventris*
yellow bunting	*Emberiza citrinella*
yellow-eyed penguin	*Megadyptes antipodes*
yellow-legged gull	*Larus cachinnans*
yellow-pine chipmunk	*Tamias amoenus*
zebra finch	*Taenopygia guttata*
zebra fish	*Danio danio*

INDEX